Healthy for Life

Wellness and the Art of Living

Brian K. Williams

Sharon M. Knight
East Carolina University

Brooks/Cole Publishing Company
Pacific Grove, California

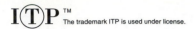 ™ The trademark ITP is used under license.

Brooks/Cole Publishing Company
A Division of Wadsworth, Inc.

Printed in the United States of America

10 9 8 7 6 5 4 3 2 1

Library of Congress Cataloging-in-Publication Data

Williams, Brian K., [date]
    Healthy for life : wellness and the art of living / Brian K. Williams. Sharon M. Knight.
        p. cm.
    Includes bibliographical references and index.
    ISBN 0-534-15498-0
    1. Health. I. Knight, Sharon M. II. Title.
RA776.W684   1993
613--dc20   93-32748
                                 CIP

Sponsoring Editor: Marianne Taflinger
Contracting Editor: Frank Ruggirello
Editorial Assistants: Virge Perelli-Minetti and Rhonda Gray Sands
Production Coordinator: Jerry Holloway
Production: Stacey C. Sawyer, Sawyer & Williams
Copy Editor: Anita Wagner
Cover Design: MaryEllen Podgorski and Vernon Boes
Interior Design: MaryEllen Podgorski
Cover Photograph: © Tom Bean, Allstock, Inc.
Interior Illustrations: GTS Graphics, Inc.
Dummy: Stacey C. Sawyer
Permissions: David Sweet
Photo Research: Linda L. Rill, LLR Research
Composition: GTS Graphics, Inc.
Color Separation: GTS Graphics, Inc.
Printing and Binding: Arcata Graphics/Hawkins
Cover Printing: Phoenix Color Corp.

Credits appear at the end of the book.

To Stacey, who performed a production miracle.

–B. K. W.

To my family and students, who continually enrich my life.

–S. M. K.

Contents in Brief

About the Organization:

16 units, 37 chapters: For ease of instruction and learning, the material has been arranged into 16 units, adaptable for 16-week semester or 10-week quarter classes. Each unit contains 2–4 chapters.

Small, self-contained chapters: All chapters are self-contained and may be read independently of each other. Thus, chapters may be assigned in any order or omitted, at the instructor's option.

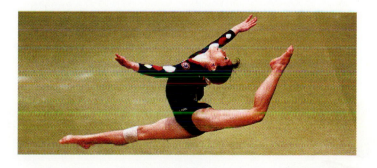

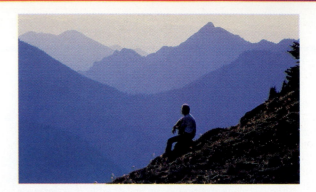

Preface to the Instructor

A college offers many important and interesting courses for students. But only one course is truly concerned with teaching them how to live: *yours.*

This idea may seem rather presumptuous. However, one can easily see that most college-level instruction has other priorities: to give students a well-rounded education, to teach them how to think, to prepare them for careers or graduate or professional training. Even introductory courses in psychology, ethics, and religion are mainly concerned with some of these other goals.

By contrast, an introductory course in health is specifically aimed at teaching or reinforcing skills in *how to live*—in providing students with the physical, intellectual, emotional, social, and spiritual platform from which they can pursue all their other college and life goals. For one to be successful in many other things in life, one must first be successful in health. Thus, more than any other course, in our opinion, a course in health offers students the knowledge and skills they can apply life-long, through ups and downs in careers and relationships and personal fortunes.

It is particularly unfortunate, therefore, that so many students treat the introductory health course as "just another course" to be checked off en route to the college degree. In this book, we try to do everything possible to alter this perception. We try to help students realize that they are here not just in pursuit of another grade but to analyze their lives and learn habits of body, mind, and spirit that will affect them in important ways in all the years ahead.

The Audience for and Goals of This Book

Intended readers are college students in a one-term introductory health course. The goals of the book are to show students how to respond flexibly in health matters and how to achieve high-level wellness and peak performance.

HEALTHY FOR LIFE: Wellness and the Art of Living is designed for use as a college textbook to accompany a one-semester or one-quarter introductory course in health science. More specifically, the book is intended to help readers learn the following:

- *"Response-ability"—flexibility in avoiding and coping with ill health:* We try to give students the tools for what has been called "re-sponse-ability"—the ability to respond flexibly and creatively to new events. In particular, we try to show readers how to avoid and cope with ill health in all five dimensions—physical, mental, emotional, social, and spiritual.

- *The art of living—achieving high-level wellness and peak performance:* Health, of course, is not merely the avoidance of illness. We try to show readers how they can go beyond mere good health to achieve high-level wellness—that is, to realize themselves to the fullest, to become peak performers.

Both themes are constantly reinforced throughout the text in the sections headed "Strategy for Living."

Why This Book Is Different

This book offers flexible organization, reinforces student learning with built-in mastery devices and personalized ways to help students "own" the material, provides art that instructs as well as entertains, and covers material both in breadth and in depth.

This textbook is, we think, quite distinctive in a number of ways. It offers:

1. Flexible organization to give the instructor many options.

2. Reinforcement for learning with built-in repetition.

3. Reinforcement for learning with ways to help students "own" the material.

4. Art that instructs and informs as well as entertains.

5. Coverage of material in depth and in breadth.

We elaborate on these features below.

1. Flexible Organization: Chapters May Be Taught Out of Order or Skipped
Because many instructors have difficulty tailoring their reading assignments to fit a 10-week or 16-week term, we have arranged the text material in two ways:

- *Into 16 units:* Material has been arranged into 16 major divisions, or units. For instructors who wish to proceed more or less chronologically through the book, this organization works out to a unit a week in a 16-week semester system or about 1½ units a week in a 10-week quarter system. Each unit contains 2–4 chapters.

- *Into 37 chapters:* The material has also been arranged into 37 generally small, self-contained chapters, which may be read independently of one another. *Chapters may be assigned in any order or eliminated entirely*, as the instructor chooses. To permit this smorgasbord of options, we have repeated the definition of key terms throughout the text. Small chapters also give readers the sense of satisfaction that comes with mastering material in easily digestible portions.

2. Reinforcement for Learning: Offering Built-In Repetition

How do people learn? One major way, of course, is by repetition. Accordingly, *we have built repetition into the book* to reinforce the same information over and over, as follows:

- *Unit table of contents:* Each unit opens with a table of contents listing the titles and headings of the 2–4 chapters within the unit.
- *Learning objectives:* Chapters begin with learning objectives setting forth the questions the student should try to answer in reading the material.
- *Section summaries:* Each section opens with a section summary or abstract—the material in blue type immediately following the section heading—that offers a preview of the material to come.
- *Material in "bite-size" portions, with headings:* Major ideas are presented in bite-size form, with generous use of advance organizers, headings, bulleted lists, and new paragraphing when a new idea is introduced.

In addition, for students whose study skills may be rusty, we have presented a crash course in study techniques at the end of Unit 1. This is the Life Skills essay entitled "Better Organization and Time Management."

3. Reinforcement for Learning: Helping Readers "Own" the Material

Another principle of learning is that students have to mentally "own" the material—personalize it, incorporate it into their own experience. We have tried to encourage this ownership through the following devices:

- *Interesting writing:* Studies have found that textbooks written in an imaginative style significantly improve students' ability to retain information. Thus, we have tried to employ a number of journalistic devices—such as the short biographical sketch, the colorful fact, the apt direct quote—to make the material as interesting as possible.
- *Real anecdotes and examples:* We believe that examples take on much more significance when they are true rather than fictionalized. Accordingly, we have scouted the general press for real episodes involving real people of both traditional and nontraditional student age in order to introduce or support concepts. In addition, to eliminate the usual barriers of remoteness between textbook writers and readers, we have drawn on a few life experiences of our own. We hope to suggest by all these examples the relevance of the health lessons to the reader's own life.
- *Self Discovery questionnaires:* Most people are curious about where they stand or how they are faring in matters of health. Although many health texts provide student inventories to make material relevant to the reader and provide feedback on health practices, we believe ours are unusual both in number and in scope. Some of our Self Discoveries cover somewhat unusual topics—for example, TV watching, the need for excitement, and "spendaholism."
- *800-HELP toll-free phone numbers:* At the end of most chapters, we present toll-free 800 numbers of helpful sources dealing with the matters we have just discussed. Readers thus have the *immediate* opportunity to follow through on the material on their own.
- *Life Skill essays:* We have chosen not to distract the student's reading of the text with a lot of boxes, notes in the margins, and similar bits of information. Instead, we have tried to concentrate topics for "student enrichment" purposes in a short student-involvement essay at the end of each unit.

This Life Skill essay—which may be assigned or not at the instructor's option and which may also be used as the basis for class discussion—begins with a few short questions that invite the student to examine his or her feelings or assumptions about the topic at hand. The essay then goes on to examine the living skills to be considered in relation to the topic.

Examples of Life Skill topics include *spirituality* (in "The Will to Believe: The Search for Guides, Not Gurus"), *assertiveness* (in "Developing Assertiveness: Speaking Out for Safe Sex"), *drugs* (in "Coming to Terms with 'the Drug Problem' "), and *intellectual health* (in "Intellectual Health: Critical Thinking and the Art of Living").

4. Art That Informs as Well as Entertains Many college textbooks often use art, particularly photos, simply to break up a gray page of words (on the assumption that readers raised on television don't handle such pages well). We believe, however, that art should be *didactic*—it should inform and instruct as well as entertain.

With only a few exceptions, most of the illustrations in this book are designed to reinforce concepts discussed in the text. Although we present some photographs that simply stand alone, for the most part we have tried to couple photos with additional information: an elaboration of the discussion in the text, some how-to advice, an interesting quotation, or a piece of line art.

In addition, we have tried to deal with the irritating matter of *page flipping* between text reference and illustration in two ways: (1) wherever possible, positioning illustrations on the same page spread where the reference occurs and (2) by using colored dots (●●●●) to help readers easily find their way back from the illustration to the place in the text where they left off reading.

5. Coverage That Is Both Deep and Broad A glance at the Notes section in the back of the book will, we hope, show the instructor that our research is both deep and broad. Our sources cover not only many scholarly journals and books but also articles from the general press and some popular books, which often provide the apt anecdote or quotation that scholarly sources do not.

In addition, some of our chapters and sections cover material not routinely treated in introductory texts in this area. These include:

- Non-drug dependency issues—gambling, spendaholism, workaholism, codependency
- Alternative health therapies and quackery
- Violence and sexual victimization
- Voluntarism in the cause of environmentalism
- Relationship issues
- Abusive parents

We also deal with the spiritual, intellectual, and social dimensions of health in ways that we have not found elsewhere.

Convenient, "Turn-Key" Teaching Package

The instructional package includes an Annotated Instructor's Edition, an Instructor's Manual, transparencies, test bank, and study guide.

We offer a great deal of assistance in teaching materials in hopes that an instructor can simply "turn the key" to launch an instructional program. Knowing the value of instructors' time, we have stressed convenience and effectiveness, offering teaching materials that eliminate time-wasting preparations. This allows instructors to do what they do best: engage the students in this exciting subject, develop their enthusiasm and interest in health, and tailor topics as appropriate for their particular classes.

Some features of this instructional package are as follows:

An Annotated Instructor's Edition We make two versions of the textbook available. The first is the text for the student. The second is the *Annotated Instructor's Edition*, the same text with marginal annotations for the instructor—anecdotes, statistics, quotations, observations, and suggested in-class discussion questions and activities.

A Separate Instructor's Manual The separate Instructor's Manual includes lecture notes, class activities, and instructional resources.

The Instructor's Manual also includes:

- *"How to teach health" tips:* Teaching health science is not the same as teaching other disciplines. Thus, we have included in the Instructor's Manual suggestions for most effectively presenting health concepts.
- *Informative, entertaining lectures:* The startling statistic, the poignant story, the amusing anecdote—we include these as "asides" in the lecture notes for instructors to use to enliven their classroom presentations.
- *Big-type lecture notes:* The lecture notes in the

instructor's manual are printed in big type, to make them easily readable at a rostrum.

Transparency Visuals Health science is a particularly visual subject. Many times, however, the transparencies developed by publishers are created as an afterthought. As part of our "turn-key" instructional package, we have paid special attention to the preparation of transparencies. Particularly important, they have been *upsized*, so that they can be easily seen even from the back of a large lecture hall.

Test Bank The test-bank was created by the well-respected health educator Herb Jones of Ball State University, who has had over 30 years of teaching experience. He has prepared meaningful questions linked to the learning objectives at the beginning of each chapter. The test bank offers over 1000 questions, broken down as follows for each chapter: 15 multiple-choice, 25 true-false, 10 short-answer, and 5 to 10 matching items.

Study Guide for Students A separate study guide is available to provide students with further learning reinforcement. It consists of learning objectives, matching terms and definitions, short answers, multiple-choice questions, and a few personal-insight questions that are linked to the Life Skills sections in the text. The study guide provides reminders of key terms, questions that require more than word definitions to answer, and multiple-choice questions that test general knowledge of specific important points. The guide was prepared by Anita Wagner and Richard Reser.

Acknowledgments

Two names are on the front of this book, but a great many others are powerful contributors to its development.

This book began under the administration of Frank Ruggirello, Steve Rutter, and Dick Greenberg of Wadsworth Publishing Company, to whom we are exceedingly grateful. Throughout we were fortunate to have as our steady contact Jerry Holloway, one of the warmest and most patient of men and a friend and colleague of Brian's for over 30 years. Jerry, you're the greatest. He was backed by other old colleagues and friends—Bill Ralph, Peggy Meehan, Pat Brewer, Stephen Rapley, and Kathy Head. Folks,

thanks for all your help. We also greatly appreciate the cheerfulness and efficiency of Rhonda Gray Sands in editorial and the number-juggling assistance of Diana Spence in manufacturing.

The book continued with the support of Wayne Oler, CEO of Wadsworth, Inc., a friend of long standing and publisher when Brian was coauthor of *Invitation to Health*. It was Wayne who felt our book would be more compatible with the list at Brooks/Cole Publishing Company and directed us there. Wayne, we're grateful for your support, but what is this karma that throws you and Brian together doing health books?

At Brooks/Cole, we were lucky to have as our sponsoring editor Marianne Taflinger, whose attention to detail, concerns about lining up all necessary support, and cheerful sense of humor gave us a powerful second wind. Marianne, thanks for the great job of taking up the baton; we're excitedly looking forward to working with you in the future. We are also grateful to editorial assistant Virge Perelli-Minetti, who went out of her way to assist us on many matters and was Marianne's able right hand.

Standing behind Marianne and Virge were some powerful supporters in Vicki Knight, managing editor; Craig Barth, vice president, editorial; and Bill Roberts, president. We much appreciate having you in our corner and look forward to many years of association.

The Brooks/Cole marketing staff has done everything authors could expect a publisher to do. Adrian Perenon, director of marketing, reappeared in Brian's life after many years, a sign we have to view as fortuitous. He was ably assisted by Susan Hays, our championship marketing manager; Leslie Mata, advertising product manager and scribbler first class; and Barbara Smallwood, our conscientious marketing assistant. Some enthusiastic salespeople also contributed to the marketing plans—Jack Fox, Stacey Steiner, Joanne Terhaar and Jeff Wilhelm—and we owe them heartfelt thanks.

Ellen Brownstein, production manager, held our hands as we went into the final stretch and oversaw the troubleshooting of some last-minute glitches, and we appreciate her responsible and caring interest. We also greatly appreciate the last-minute efforts of Vernon Boes on the cover. In addition, we are grateful to Bill Bokermann, who lent his moral support and stood ready to render aid when called upon.

Outside of Wadsworth and Brooks/Cole, we were ably assisted by a community of first-rate publishing professionals. Directing the production of the entire enterprise was Stacey Sawyer—Brooks/Cole alumna,

Brian's wife and life companion, and an author herself and hence able to understand authors' travails. Stacey, you probably used every trick you've ever learned in publishing in the course of putting together this complicated package against horrendous deadlines. Also, it was you who lined up the top-rate talent that we are lucky enough to be able to acknowledge below. In addition, you did a sensational job of dummying the book, indeed putting this task at the top of your list when prudence might have suggested otherwise. Moreover, you provided emotional support when the times were toughest. Thank you for everything. You could not have done more.

We consider it our huge good fortune that we were able to get the services of MaryEllen Podgorski, truly one of the finest book designers in the United States, if not the universe. MaryEllen is the very original force behind the stunning use of color, the pop-out quotation marks, and the creative play between visual and typographic elements. MaryEllen, you really know how to do it!

We don't know how she does it, but photo researcher Linda Rill seems to have a special gift for finding the right selection of photographs. Indeed, Linda's task was much like that of an illustrator, for she was asked to find the very best photograph to illustrate a particular quotation or concept. She also has a very wonderful eye for the offbeat.

The great permissions-seeking game was wonderfully executed by David Sweet. David is adept at all the detective work that that pursuit requires and has the greatest patience in pursuing loose ends.

Anita Wagner performed a careful copyediting of the manuscript, removing from the public eye probably a wheelbarrow-load of potential embarrassments. Her patience with the notes section alone deserves some sort of award. Anita was ably backstopped by proofreaders Linda McPhee and Beverly Zegarski, whose keen eyes have, we hoped, sanitized the book of the kind of typos, inconsistencies, and other nuisances that forever bedevil authors.

The work performed by GTS Graphics, led by Elliott Derman and Bennett Derman, and Sherrie Beyen, has been first cabin all the way. Many thanks to them and also to artists Danny Barillaro, Chris Burke, Michelle Gauthe, Mark Jaensch, and Mary Zelinski.

Both authors are grateful for the terrific assistance of Herb Jones for the superb job on the test bank and of Anita Wagner and Rick Reser for their excellent work on the study guide. We also want to express our deep appreciation to the authors of the instructor's manual for their conscientious contributions: Karen Vail-Smith, Lisa Jenkins, Jennifer Phillips, Kathy Brown, and Louise Evans.

Finally, there are always people who were not directly involved in the book but who must be acknowledged nevertheless. Brian wishes to express his high regard for Dianne Hales, with whom he was associated for several years and whose work he admires. As ever, he also wants to thank not only Stacey but also Gertrude, Sylvia, Kirk, Susan, and Michael for their continuing warmth and support.

Acknowledgment of Reviewers

We are grateful to the following people for their reviews on earlier drafts of all or part of the book: Nancy Baldwin, Edinboro State University; Danny Ballard, Texas A & M University; Rick Barnes, East Carolina University; Marsha Campos, Modesto City College; Rosemary Clark, City College of San Francisco; Bryan Cooke, University of North Colorado; Sandra Cross, California State University, San Bernardino; Paul Finnicum, Arkansas State University; Fred Fridinger, University of North Texas; Kathie Garbe, Youngstown University; Bernard Green, Valdosta State College, Leslie Hickcox, Linn Benton Community College; Norm Hoffman, Bakersfield College; William Hotchkiss, Slippery Rock University; Herb Jones, Ball State University; Henry Petraki, Palm Beach Community College; Frances Poe, Washoe Medical Center, Reno; Susan Radius, Towson State University; Kerry Redican, Virginia Polytechnic Institute and State University; Gayle Schmidt, Texas A & M University; Christine Hamilton Smith, California State University, Northridge; Sherm Sowby, California State University, Fresno; and Richard W. Wilson, Western Kentucky University.

Write to Us

We welcome your response to this book, for we are truly trying to make it as useful as possible. Write to us in care of Marianne Taflinger, Health Science Editor, Brooks/Cole Publishing Co., 511 Forest Lodge Road, Pacific Grove, CA 93950-9968.

Brian K. Williams, M.A.
Sharon M. Knight, Ph.D.

Detailed Contents

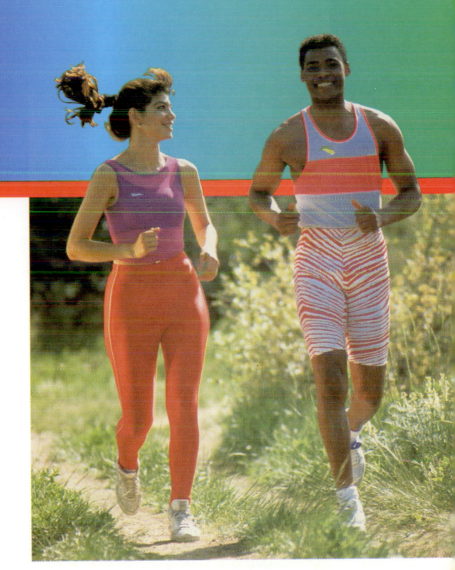

First, do no harm.

That's the most important advice medical schools teach future doctors about treating patients. And, if asked, that's the first advice doctors would give patients about treating themselves. It's also daily wisdom we can all use—for dealing both with ourselves and with others.

Not doing harm is the first lesson to be learned about health. But beyond that are the far more exciting lessons to be learned in what might be called *the art of living*—the art of using all the resources available to you to enhance your life.

The art of living, it has been said, is something that is not easily taught. Yet it is perhaps the most important subject that one can study. Living *is* an art, the art of discovering who you are, your personal boundaries and potential, the choices available to you, and your willingness to act in ways that will advance your and others' well-being.

The purpose of this book, then, is to show you how to do the following:

- *Discover ways of improving the quality of life:* The art of living is not about learning how to avoid or cope with the things that are wrong with one's life. It is about expanding one's knowledge as to the great possibilities life has to offer and then learning how to make the changes necessary to realize them.

- *Improve your ability to respond flexibly to new situations:* Life is a series of new situations, but some people respond inflexibly, as though every new event was the same as situations in the past. This kind of rigid behavior closes off options to new opportunities. Part of learning how to respond flexibly is to improve one's decision making—to learn how to ask the right ques-

tions—to sharpen critical thinking skills. This means learning how to think creatively, to define what your values are, to distinguish among different authorities.

- *Take responsibility and make desirable changes:* It is one thing to know the right course of action, another thing to do it. We all know that making certain changes can be difficult. Still, even *not* making a change is to take some sort of action. Whether you act or not in a given matter, the choice is your responsibility. In this book we try to suggest ways you can take responsibility and make desirable changes.

Learning the art of living is nothing less than learning to develop our "genius, power, and magic," to use Goethe's words. As the German poet wrote:

Whatever you can do, or dream you can begin, begin it. Boldness has genius, power, and magic in it.

1 Health and the Art of Living

▶ What is the meaning of *good health* and *bad health*?

▶ To what extent are we responsible for our own health?

If pain were for sale, would you buy it? Would you pay good money every day, knowing that in the end it would make you feel awful, perhaps cause you terrible agony?

For several years one of the authors actually did that: Beginning in high school, I levied a daily "tax" on myself, first only small change, but later dollar bills. As the "tax" increased, so did my nervousness, irritability, fatigue, and general discomfort. I also began coughing more, and one morning I was so overcome by a painful coughing attack that I could hardly get out of bed. At that point I realized I was probably killing myself.

What produced this? You've probably guessed: cigarettes. Of course, I didn't set out deliberately to buy pain and suffering. In fact, I thought I was doing the opposite. I took up smoking to ease pain of a psychological sort— that of feeling awkward in social situations. But although cigarettes might have partly alleviated my social unease, their addiction created new discomforts—physical, mental, and emotional. And breaking the habit was also definitely not a pleasurable experience.

A major aspect of the art of living is learning to clarify one's attitude toward pain and pleasure. We must learn what pains we are willing to endure in the short run, and what pleasures we will forego, in order to have far less pain and greater pleasure in the long run—to attain, in other words, optimum *well-being*. In fact, what this striving aims for is the very definition of health:

> **Health** *is the achievement of physical, mental, emotional, social, and spiritual well-being.*

Is this how you would define health? Perhaps not. You might wish to take a minute and consider what good health means to you before reading on.

What Is *Good Health*?

Do any of the following exclusively define good health: the absence of illness, living longer, or having vitality?

We hear the words *good health* used so often that we may think we know what they mean when in fact we may not. Let's consider the principal meanings people attach to the term.

Is Good Health the Absence of Illness?

Ask the average person what *good health* is, and the response is likely to be stated in terms of its opposite: the absence of disease, of pain, of disability. Ask what *poor health* is, and you're apt to hear words such as "disease" or "sickness" or "germs."

Is good health just the absence of disease-causing organisms? In many big-city hospitals, a great many health problems have nothing to do with germs, points out medical-ethics consultant Bruce Hilton. Surgeons regularly practice "battlefield medicine," attending to the multiple gunshot and knife wounds of the victims of violence. Or they sew up car-crash survivors, many of whom did not wear seatbelts, many of whose accidents were alcohol-caused. In the psychiatric wing, a high proportion of patients have cocaine or other drug-related problems. In the nursery, undersized crack-cocaine babies fight to survive. Other newborns won't live out the year because their mothers didn't have access to prenatal health care. Elsewhere cigarette smokers await their turn for radiation treatment of their lung cancer or respiratory therapy for their emphysema. Indeed, if you were to walk around the hospital you would turn up many other reasons for poor health, says Hilton: "skin cancer from too many days on the beach, or people whose disease was food—too much, not the right kind, or too little."[1]

Certainly we can agree that all these problems add up to ill health. But if they were removed, would people be truly healthy?

Is Good Health Living Longer? "Life's a dance," says Arizonan William Van Hooser. "Take it one step at a time and keep listening for the music."[2]

At age 102 Hooser may have reason to be so upbeat, for he has far surpassed the life span of most Americans. But he is also part of a rapidly increasing group. The U.S. Census Bureau estimates there are 25,000 **centenarians**—people age 100 or more—in the United States, 10 times the number of 30 years ago. Does this mean, then, that the true biological limit of human life is being pushed past the century mark?

From time to time, reports appear of 120- or 140-year-old Russians or of similarly long-lived people in South America or China. Invariably such accounts turn out to be unprovable. The world's *documented* oldest person, as listed in *The Guinness Book of World Records,* is Jeanne Calment of France, age 117.[3]

Some researchers have suggested that, with some exceptions, the body's natural degeneration limits human life to about 85 years.[4] Other authorities disagree. They point out that previous predictions of a biological limit on life span have turned out to be incorrect.

At present, the Japanese have the longest life expectancy among citizens of 33 industrialized nations. The average life expectancy at birth in Japan was 79.1 years in 1987, according to the federal Centers for Disease Control and Prevention in Atlanta.[5] Canada, where people can expect to live an average of 76.5 years, ranked sixth (along with Greece and the Netherlands). The United States, where average life expectancy is 75, is 13th—behind Australia, Israel, and most European countries. (*See* ● *Figure 1.1.**) Life expectancy for American men is 71, for American women 78.

But is defining health by death rates and life expectancy useful? By this definition, a long-lived person in a coma or with severe paralysis would be considered healthy.[6] Most people, then, would probably vote to define health by a "disability standard"—as freedom from disease and from being incapacitated. In other words, *quality* of life becomes more important than *length* of life.

*●●●●*What do the colored dots mean?* The dot in a figure reference is a reading aid to help the eye find the figure and then easily locate where you left off reading in the text.

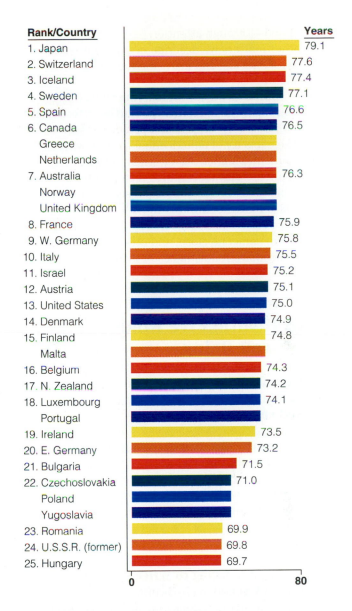

Rank/Country	Years
1. Japan	79.1
2. Switzerland	77.6
3. Iceland	77.4
4. Sweden	77.1
5. Spain	76.6
6. Canada	76.5
Greece	
Netherlands	
7. Australia	76.3
Norway	
United Kingdom	
8. France	75.9
9. W. Germany	75.8
10. Italy	75.5
11. Israel	75.2
12. Austria	75.1
13. United States	75.0
14. Denmark	74.9
15. Finland	74.8
Malta	
16. Belgium	74.3
17. N. Zealand	74.2
18. Luxembourg	74.1
Portugal	
19. Ireland	73.5
20. E. Germany	73.2
21. Bulgaria	71.5
22. Czechoslovakia	71.0
Poland	
Yugoslavia	
23. Romania	69.9
24. U.S.S.R. (former)	69.8
25. Hungary	69.7

0   80

● **Figure 1.1 Life expectancy in developed countries.** Lower life expectancies, as in the countries of Eastern Europe and the former Soviet Union, are probably caused by poor health habits, such as high rates of smoking and inadequate diets.

Is Good Health Having Vitality? One aspect of quality of life is how *vigorous* one is. Two medical researchers have suggested that the essence of health is **vitality,** defined as a person's ability to function with vigor.[7] Although it requires lifelong vigilance, vitality can be maintained—through attention to exercise, diet, and other matters we describe in this book—despite advancing age and many mental and physical limitations.

Another way of considering vitality is as health potential. **Health potential,** according to one writer, consists of a person's reserves— "the capacity of an individual to cope with environmental influences and thus keep in balance."[8] Having reserves means not only being able to resist harmful disease organisms. It also means being able to withstand the adverse effects of noise, ionizing radiation, the loss of someone close, and other negative or hazardous circumstances of living.

The Five Dimensions of Health: Five Kinds of Well-Being

Health is the achievement of physical, mental (intellectual), emotional, social, and spiritual well-being.

Being without illness, living long, and having vitality are all partial ways of thinking about good health. But we have said that health consists of attaining *well-being* in five areas: physical, mental, emotional, social, and spiritual.

Let us see how we arrived at this.

Health According to WHO: Physical, Mental, and Social Well-Being One of the most widely used definitions of health is that given by WHO, the Geneva-based World Health Organization, an arm of the United Nations. *Health,* they say, "is a state of complete physical, mental, and social well-being and not merely the absence of disease and infirmity." Note that true health doesn't involve just your body. It also involves your mind and how you interact with those around you.

Holistic Health: Adding Emotional and Spiritual Well-Being The idea of **holistic health** adds *emotional* and *spiritual* well-being to WHO's *physical, mental,* and *social* dimensions of health. The word *holism* refers to interacting wholes—the concern with com-

plete systems rather than isolated parts. In this view, a person's health is measured by his or her functioning in *all* areas of life. Thus, a person who may be incapacitated physically may still be healthy on the other four of the five dimensions. Moreover, that person need not be consistently *un*healthy on the physical dimension.

The Five Dimensions of Health Let us consider these five dimensions:

1. *Physical:* **Physical health** means not only the absence of disease or risk behaviors that might lead to disease, but also physical fitness, functioning body systems, and minimal exposure to such abuses as drugs, stress, and environmental hazards.

2. *Mental or intellectual:* **Mental health,** or **intellectual health,** may be described as having to do with intellect or thinking or cognition, as opposed to feeling. Thus, mental or intellectual health covers such activities as speaking, writing, analyzing, and judgment.

3. *Emotional:* **Emotional health** is concerned with matters of feeling, as opposed to thinking. It covers such areas as self-esteem, love, empathy, and expression of appropriate feelings.

4. *Social:* **Social health** has to do with one's well-being in interacting with others: the comfort level of being involved with others, the kinds of social skills, the care and concern for others, and ability to respect differences.

5. *Spiritual:* **Spiritual health** could be defined as the ability to love and be loved.[9] Spiritual health, says Richard Eberst of Adelphi University, "includes trust, integrity, principles and ethics, the purpose or drive in life, basic survival instincts, feelings of selflessness, degree of pleasure-seeking qualities, commitment to some higher process or being and the ability to believe in concepts that are not subject to 'state of the art' [or customary] explanation."[10]

All five health dimensions overlap and affect one another. Thus, when you make improvements in one area of well-being, they may affect several other areas. Exercise, for example, may improve your mood and give you energy that makes you work or study more efficiently, which in turn may lessen your work and study worries and improve your social interactions.

Toward High-Level Wellness and Peak Performance

Health may be considered as a hierarchy, with optimum health consisting of high-level wellness and peak performance.

Health, we said, is the attainment of physical, mental (intellectual), emotional, social, and spiritual well-being. All these together may be considered as a continuum or a hierarchy. (*See* ● *Figure 1.2.*) Note that at the bottom end is early and needless death, at the top end is *high-level wellness.* Most people, of course, are somewhere in between. In this book, we are concerned not merely with avoiding disabling illness but with helping you to achieve total wellness, to become a peak performer.

High-Level Wellness People who are holistically healthy are often said to have achieved a high level of **wellness.** *Wellness* and *illness* are opposites, of course. But wellness also suggests that people's health should not be measured just by the absence of disease but by how satisfactorily they achieve what is known as their *human potential*—their ability to realize themselves to the fullest.

Peak Performance The phenomenon of **peak performance** refers to repeated performance at the height of one's abilities in order to produce great accomplishments. Psychologist Charles Garfield spent years studying top achievers in various fields and concluded that the qualities they showed could be adopted by others to further their own development. "The differences between peak performers and ordinary performers do not stem primarily from the situations in which they operate," Garfield writes in his book *Peak Performers.* "The differences appear in the attitude and skills a peak performer brings to a situation."[11]

Some of the qualities that Garfield found characterize high-performing individuals as follows:

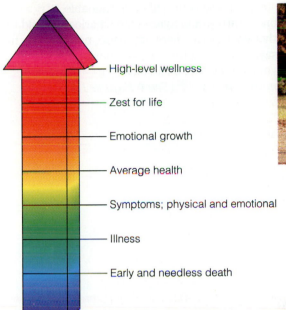

- High-level wellness
- Zest for life
- Emotional growth
- Average health
- Symptoms; physical and emotional
- Illness
- Early and needless death

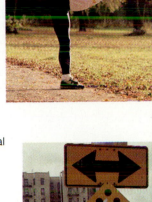

● **Figure 1.2 The hierarchy of health.** Health may be ranked from early and needless death up to high-level wellness.

- *Missions that motivate:* Peak performers have made an internal decision to excel; they have a sense of mission.

- *Results in real time:* They consistently reach their goals, in both short and long time frames.

- *Self-management through self-mastery:* They are self-confident, able to see both the big and little pictures, and able to mentally rehearse the achievements they wish to attain.

- *Team building/team playing:* They are team players, expanding their own potentialities by aligning themselves with others.

- *Course correction:* They are able to change course when they make mistakes.

- *Change management:* They are able to anticipate difficulties and opportunities, adapt to them, and act to preserve what is best.

Do these sound like unattainable attributes? We would agree with Charles Garfield that peak performers are made, not born. As he says, searching for the peak performer within yourself has one basic meaning—asking, *What more can I be?*[12] (See ● *Figure 1.3.*)

● **Figure 1.3 Peak performers are made, not born.**

“*You recognize yourself as a person who was born not as a peak performer but as a learner. With the capacity to grow, change, and reach for the highest possibilities of human nature, you regard yourself as a person in process. Not perfect, but a person who keeps asking:* What more can I be? . . . *And answering for yourself.*”

—Charles Garfield (1986). *Peak performers.* New York: Morrow, pp. 288–289.

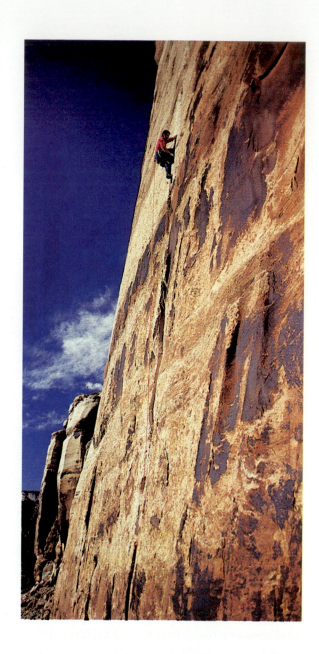

1.7

*Chapter 2
Health Status,
Personal
Responsibility,
and Mastering
Change*

2   Health Status, Personal Responsibility, and Mastering Change

▶ What is the present status of health in the United States?

▶ What kinds of general health goals should we try to realize?

▶ Why are lifestyle matters important in health?

Next time you are out on the highway, take a look at the cars around you. Then pretend your body is one of them. Could you let yourself become almost completely deteriorated, like the rustbucket pickup truck in the lane next to you, then have it lovingly restored, like that bright-chromed classic convertible over there?

Unfortunately, the analogy between people and cars does not hold up: you cannot simply replace all the parts in people the way you can in automobiles. Yet the American health care system—the most expensive in the world, costing $700 billion a year—spends a great deal of its resources trying to "restore" people to their previous health.

Is the system working? If not, what should we be doing instead?

American Health, Then and Now

During the past century, life expectancy has risen because of improvements in public health, drugs and medical technology, and better lifestyle. Still, a great many Americans are in ill health, and many suffer premature deaths—young people principally from injuries and violence, adults from cancer and heart disease—most of which are preventable by lifestyle changes. The lesson is: your habits matter.

More than a century ago, people were pretty much obliged to look after their own health, because the "health authorities" themselves were not much more knowledgeable. Then came the revolutions that have led to modern medicine.

From Public Health to Lifestyle Over the past 100 years or so, death rates have declined through three stages, according to Donald M. Vickery.[13] (*See ● Figure 2.1.*)

- *Age of Environment—Improved public health:* From about 1885 until the 1930s, public health policies and improvements in the environment dramatically lowered death rates, especially those for infant mortality. During this period, city health departments were established, city water supplies were cleaned up, milk became pasteurized, and public health campaigns were introduced.

- *Age of Medicine—Improved drugs and technology:* In the 1930s, sulfa drugs, penicillin, and other antibiotics were introduced, further accelerating the drop in death rates. However, in the early 1950s, life-expectancy rates stopped increasing, even though many high-tech innovations—open-heart surgery, polio vaccine, and so on—continued to be introduced.

- *Age of Lifestyle—Better living habits:* It was not until the 1970s that life-expectancy rates began to increase again. This coincided with attempts to deal with what are called **lifestyle disorders**—ill health brought about by individuals' behavior patterns, such as those involving eating, safety, and drug use.

Today we are still living in the Age of Lifestyle. Unfortunately, people find lifestyle a lot less fascinating than medical wizardry. "We're so in love with the chrome and glitter of high-tech medicine," says medical-ethics consultant Bruce Hilton, "we forget to ask how the patient got this way . . . . How many people remember that Barney Clark, the first artificial-heart patient, whose bravery we all admired, had been a lifelong chain smoker?"[14]

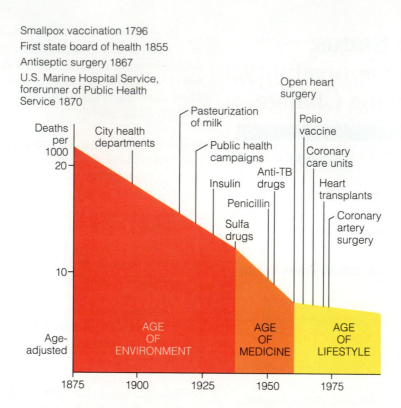

Smallpox vaccination 1796
First state board of health 1855
Antiseptic surgery 1867
U.S. Marine Hospital Service, forerunner of Public Health Service 1870

● **Figure 2.1 One hundred years of health advancement.**

Physician Donald Vickery describes three stages of health advancement in the United States that took place in the 100 years between 1885 and 1985:

- In stage 1, the *Age of Environment* (approximately 1875–1935), 70% of the decline in the death rate occurred *before* the introduction of wonder drugs and organ transplants—the result of improvements in the environment and public health policy.

- In stage 2, the *Age of Medicine* (approximately 1935–1955), there was further progress resulting from antibiotics and other drugs.

- In stage 3, the *Age of Lifestyle* (approximately 1955–present), for several years life-expectancy rates no longer improved, despite the introduction of many high-tech innovations such as open-heart surgery. Then, in the early 1970s, death rates began to decline again as the effects of lifestyle programs took hold, with their emphasis on less fat in the diet, more exercise, and reduction in tobacco use.

Is *Everyone* Sick? Where have these ages of health advancement brought us today? A researcher on the staff of former U.S. surgeon general C. Everett Koop added up the numbers of Americans suffering from various diseases. He found, according to Koop, "that the total

1.9

*Chapter 2
Health Status,
Personal
Responsibility,
and Mastering
Change*

exceeded by a good measure *the entire population of the United States*" (our emphasis added).[15] More remarkable, this total was for physical ailments only. It did not include the estimated 30 million with mental illnesses and psychiatric disorders, Koop says.

It should not be surprising, therefore, that the research assistant concluded that pretty "near everyone in this country is sick!" Some researchers might object that many of the people measured had multiple disorders that were counted singly. Even so, the great majority of Americans, says Koop, "are victims of chronic, crippling, or incapacitating diseases ranging from alcoholism to Alzheimer's. Sexually transmitted diseases alone have infected 40 million." (**Chronic** means of long duration or recurring, as opposed to an **acute** disorder, which is of short duration.)

However one may argue about numbers, the news from the health front is not good. For instance, Koop was also part of a commission of physicians and educators looking into what schools and communities might do to improve adolescent health.[16] The panel concluded that the United States is raising a generation of adolescents plagued by pregnancies, illegal drug use, suicide, and violence. Although you might not consider pregnancies, drunkenness, arrests, and homicides parts of the usual definition of ill health, they are indicative of frightening trends —signs of massive declines in the quality of American life. (*See ● Figure 2.2.*)

The Importance of Prevention It should be clear by now that a lot of ill health is *preventable*. Consider the age group you are in, which most likely is either ages 15–24 (adolescents and young adults) or ages 25–64 (adults).[17]

- *Adolescents and young adults:* There are two categories of preventable health problems found among people between the ages of 15 and 24.

  The first category consists of *injuries and violence* that kill and disable them while they are still young. Far and away the leading cause of death for young people is

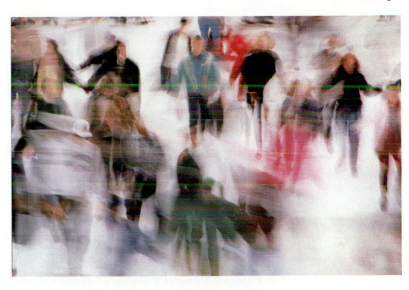

● **Figure 2.2 Life struggles.** The health status of Americans

Rank of U.S. in the world in infant mortality: 22

Percentage of teenage girls pregnant each year: 10

Percentage increase in teenage arrests since 1950: 300

Percentage of high school seniors who reported they had gotten drunk within the two previous weeks: 40

Rank of alcohol-related accidents as cause of death among adolescents: 1

Rank of suicide: 2

Percentage of increase in suicide among adolescents since 1968: 200

Percentage of teenage boys who have attempted suicide: 10

Of teenage girls: 20

Rank of murder as cause of death among minority youths ages 15–19: 1

Percentage change in income 1977–1988 in top fifth of American families: +27

Of bottom fifth: −13

Percentage of white Americans living below poverty line ($12,674 a year for a family of four): 10

Of blacks: 31

Years of life expectancy of whites: 75.2

Of blacks: 69.6

Heart disease deaths per 100,000 people for whites: 192

For minorities: 234

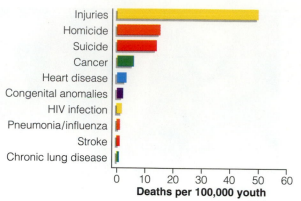

Leading causes of death for youth ages 15–24 (in 1987)

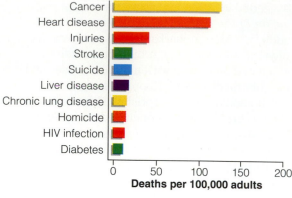

Leading causes of death for adults ages 25–64 (in 1987)

● **Figure 2.3 Leading causes of death for youth and adults**

The second category consists of *emerging lifestyles*, such as those having to do with diet, physical activity, use of alcohol and other drugs, safety, tobacco use, and sexual behavior. These are important because they affect one's health many years later.

- *Adults:* Many of the principal areas of ill health for people between the ages of 25 and 64 are also preventable, in whole or in part through changes in lifestyle, such as tobacco and alcohol use, diet, exercise, and safety.

  For adults in this age group, the leading causes of death are cancer and heart disease. Cancer is actually not one but many diseases, the significant ones being lung cancer, cancers of the colon and rectum, breast cancer, cervical cancer, and cancer of the mouth and throat. Other leading causes of death are heart disease and stroke (blood clot in the brain), and injuries, as from car crashes. (*Refer back to Figure 2.3.*)

Health and Personal Responsibility No doubt you know of someone who avoided all the standard advice for a healthy life and lived to a ripe old age. Or, conversely, you know someone who ate and did all the right things and still de-

veloped a severe illness. We need, then, to point out a fundamental fact: health-promoting habits *are not guarantees.* As health writer Jane Brody points out, "they do not offer 100% protection, like a vaccine against a disease. Good habits merely weight the odds in one's favor."[18]

Physician Gary Williams, director of medical sciences at the American Health Foundation, a health research organization, has ranked the value of various recommendations in preventing particular illnesses, based on thousands of studies. (*See ● Figure 2.4.*) Although his analysis is not all-inclusive, it does show that lifestyle matters do make a difference.

The lesson is clear: *Your habits matter.* The lifestyle choices you make today could have a tremendous influence on the quality of your life, both now and later. Thus, as we discuss throughout this book, taking responsibility for one's own health is a major part of the art of living.

1.11

Chapter 2
Health Status,
Personal
Responsibility,
and Mastering
Change

	No tobacco	Low-fat diet	High-fiber diet	Avoid alcohol	Avoid salted, pickled foods	Diet high in vegetables and fruits	Exercise, weight control
Cancer Lung Breast Colon Liver	✓✓✓	✓✓✓ ✓✓ ✓✓	✓✓✓	✓✓✓	✓	✓ ✓✓ ✓✓	✓ ✓
Heart attack	✓✓✓	✓✓✓				✓✓	✓✓
Stroke	✓				✓✓✓	✓✓	✓✓
Adult diabetes		✓✓✓	✓			✓✓	✓✓

Meaning of symbols:
✓✓✓ = Highly effective
✓✓ = Moderately effective
✓ = Somewhat effective

● **Figure 2.4 Preventing disease: a menu of health-saving tactics.** Dr. Gary Williams, of the American Health Foundation, has ranked various recommendations for healthy living as to their value in preventing certain cancers, heart attack, stroke, and adult diabetes. The analysis does not consider the harmful effects of high blood pressure, osteoporosis, and ulcers or the benefits of stress reduction, regular breakfast eating, and 7 hours of sleep a night.

Developing the Skills of Change

Response-ability **is the ability to respond flexibly and creatively to new events. Signs of inflexibility are the use of self-limiting words such as** *should* **and** *have to.* **When you freely choose your response to life (***willingness***), you live for inner satisfaction rather than outward gratifications. Once you know that you can change behavior, the next step is to become a positive risk-taker—have the courage to change.**

How do you approach any new situation—meeting someone new, a serious family illness, a failing grade? Many people simply let their "automatic pilot" take over and respond in old, set patterns. Particularly when they are feeling under stress, they behave in familiar ways rather than in ways that enable them to evaluate the situation and act appropriately in the present. Thus, many of us continue not only to eat, drink, and smoke out of habit but to respond rigidly and uncreatively to many other situations.

The Need to Develop a Flexible Response to Life Situations "In reality, life is never as it can be, should be, or as we hope it will be," says health education professor Janet Shirreffs. "Life just is. It doesn't care if we are ready for it or not, or if we think it is too difficult or unfair. Life just keeps coming."[19]

So how are we supposed to react when life, a series of new situations, "keeps coming" at us? Shirreffs suggests that what is needed is *response-ability*—the ability to respond flexibly and creatively to new events as they occur. The opposite of response-ability is *diminished response-ability,* in which people live their lives in set, patterned ways, responding to new situations as though they were situations they encountered in the past. This inflexibility means that one is closing off options that could offer opportunities for improved quality of life.

Self-Limiting Words How can you tell whether you are behaving with diminished response-ability? One way is to see how often you use the words *should*, *hope to*, *have to*, and *can't*, which, says Shirreffs, are expressions of self-limiting beliefs:

- *"I should . . .":* Should—as in "I should eat more vegetables" or "I shouldn't smoke"—implies being responsible to others rather than to oneself. In effect, "should" means you entrust others to assess the appropriateness of your health behaviors and to judge their rightness or wrongness. *Should* implies that you lack the freedom to direct your own life.

- *"I hope to . . .":* The word *hope* appears in statements such as "I hope to lose weight by summer" or "I hope to quit drinking when things get less stressful." The problem with *hope* is that it takes the individual out of the present and to some future time when things might get better. It implies that you will change when someone or something else changes.

- *"I have to . . .":* Have to—as in "I have to exercise three times a week" or "I have to eat fiber"—relates to the notion that if one doesn't do a certain activity, something bad will happen. *Have tos*, says Shirreffs, can yield feelings of anger and resentment because when we have to do something, we are not choosing it freely nor experiencing it joyfully.

- *"I can't . . .":* Can't appears in expressions such as "I can't seem to remember to put on my seat belt" or "I can't stay away from fatty food." It represents an attitude of depression and helplessness. Actually, when you say "I can't," it really means "I won't."

To begin to overcome these self-limiting thoughts, one must become aware of the kind of internal, nearly automatic perceptual processes that affect human behavior—and how you can modify those processes for yourself.

Gratification Versus Satisfaction: The Attitude of Willingness In opposition to the self-limiting beliefs of diminished response-ability is a health-affirming attitude called *willingness*. Says Shirreffs:

Willingness is an attitude and approach to life that is beyond guilt, fear, anger, and helplessness. Willingness requires letting go of the myth that life is a series of experiences and situations in which one should do, can't do, hopes to do, and has to do. It involves freely choosing what our response to life will be each moment.[20]

The most important way to develop the attitude of willingness is to clarify the distinction between *gratification* and *satisfaction* and their associated lifestyles.[21] *Gratification* comes from things, processes, and people outside yourself. Sex, drugs, and rock 'n' roll are gratifiers. *Satisfaction* comes from inside yourself, from living a life of healthy balance and high integrity. Specifically, satisfaction comes from the following primary activities:

- *Keeping agreements with yourself and other people:* If you make up your mind that you are determined to keep the "contracts" (agreements) you make, it will provide a solid foundation for making those behavioral changes important to you, whether losing weight, standing up for your rights, or becoming a peak performer.

- *Doing the best you can:* This means putting your full attention and intention into everything you do. *Intention* here means more than just having the intent to do something. It is an attitude, that of approaching your tasks with enthusiasm and zest—doing the very best you can.

- *Pressing beyond limits:* This means abandoning self-limiting beliefs, such as those represented by the words *should* or *have to*. The changes you make based on *should* probably won't last very long nor be very much fun.

Mastering Change: What and How Can You Change? Health depends on growth. Growth on change. Change on taking risks—provided the risks are not of the destructive kind.

A key question you have to ask yourself is: "What *can* I change?" We have said that a basic premise of this book is that you as an individual are responsible for much of your own health. However, in many instances, there are factors affecting your well-being—both outside of you

1.13

*Chapter 2
Health Status,
Personal
Responsibility,
and Mastering
Change*

and inside of you—that you have no control over or only limited control. What, after all, can *you* do about air pollution? about genetic problems? about how your parents raised you? Clearly, it's important to have a sense of what you can and cannot do something about. (*See* ● *Table 2.1.*)

Once you have determined what you can change, you need to have the courage to do it. In other words, you need to develop the skill for taking (nondestructive) chances. Taking chances implies loss, which implies failure.

What is risky for one person, of course, may be no risk at all for another. Only you know what is risky for you. In any event, learning to change is essential. Says psychiatrist Randy Cole, "It is almost a definition of mental health: that you can adapt and make necessary changes without being too upset and undone by them."[22] Fortunately, positive risk-taking and the ability to adapt to changes may be a skill that can be acquired—no matter what your age, occupation, or lifestyle.

Some ways to gain the confidence to become a risk-taker are as follows:

- *Prepare for the challenge:* Risk-takers who don't prepare for possible dangerous consequences are foolhardy, according to psychologist Sharon Hymer.[23] Don't make potentially disastrous moves, such as taking wild chances (a characteristic of gamblers and drug abusers) or entering an athletic or musical competition without preparation or practice. Do your homework and know what will happen if things don't work out as planned.

- *Expect to worry:* Be prepared to trade emotional or financial security for more stimulation and satisfaction. When you decide to change jobs, get out of an unhappy relationship, go from a salaried job to working for commissions, or start your own business, the change itself is a risk. There's nothing safer than leaving things as they are. However, what you hope to gain by taking risks is more satisfaction.

● **Table 2.1 How much can you control factors affecting your health?** Sometimes an individual has little control over health influences, such as pollution, but the community may have quite a bit of control. At other times, factors normally controlled by an individual, such as nutrition, may be quite beyond a person's control, as in the food served a prison inmate.

Generally extremely limited or no control	Generally limited control	Generally full control
Overall quality of environment	Peer pressure	Nutritional intake
Family social & economic status	Yearly income	Exposure to information
Genetic traits	General education	Religion
Culture	Access to health resources	Risk-taking behavior
Family	Role models	Lifestyle
Past family health status	Job	Seeking out health resources
Political factors	Access to food, water, etc.	Personal value system
Availability of resources	Safety level	General outlook on life
Community/governmental priority & commitment to good health	Health education	Ability to adjust
	Accidents	Activity level
	Personal health skills	Happiness
	Health provider(s)	Intake of mood modifiers
	Family	Attitude and beliefs

Source: Adapted from Eberst, R. M. (1984). Defining health: A multidimensional model. *Journal of School Health, 54*(3), table 2, p. 101.

• *Project confidence:* Even putting up a front—projecting confidence you don't feel—can pay off. Assuming an air of authority often makes one feel more confident and can hasten adjustment time, according to career counselor Doralee Schulman.[24]

The more chances you take, the easier such positive risk-taking becomes. Indeed, we believe it is *necessary* to learn to do what you feel is right for you rather than what others define as proper, that you learn to regard failures as small setbacks rather than barriers to achievement, that you not waste time on self-criticism and re-criminations but simply get ready for the next challenge. In fact, says psychologist Daniel J. Ziegler, if you don't learn to disregard the naysayers and forge ahead, it may be impossible for you to get anywhere in your career or personal life.[25]

How well do you handle being different from other people, coping with embarrassment, dealing with change? How willing are you to risk "making a fool of yourself" in order to accomplish something you know to be extremely worthwhile? These questions, which are basic to the art of living, are worth your reflection.

Looking at Your Life We spend much of our lives waiting—waiting for tomorrow to become today so that the goals we sought so avidly will pass into yesterday. For instance, perhaps you consider the course for which you are reading this book "just another course" to be checked off en route to the college degree. There is one important difference, however: This course is not just about giving you a well-rounded education, or teaching you how to think, or preparing you for a career, or for graduate or professional training. It is about your *life.* It is about learning how to analyze the way you live and learning habits of body, mind, and spirit that will affect you in important ways in all the years ahead.

Suggestions for Further Reading

Garfield, Charles (1986). *Peak performers: The new heroes of American business.* New York: Morrow. An interesting, well-researched book on personal high achievement and how to attain it.

U.S. Public Health Service (1990). *Healthy people 2000: National health promotion and disease prevention objectives.* DHHS Publication No. (PHS) 91-50213. Washington, D.C.: U.S. Department of Health and Human Services. National statement of purpose for American health by the end of the century.

Better Organization and Time Management

An essential part of the art of living is the art of learning. Both in college and thereafter, we are constantly involved in new situations that require us to take on new skills and habits. To see how well you understand the best approaches to learning, answer T (true) or F (false) to the following questions:

___ **1.** The best way to prepare for an exam is in one sustained session of studying the night before—in other words, cramming.

___ **2.** The most efficient system for getting information from lectures is to trade off attending classes with other students, then exchange notes later.

___ **3.** You should develop a knack for studying in as many areas and situations as possible, such as in the library, in the student union, in bed, and while watching television.

___ **4.** Constructing a study schedule is meaningless because things always come up to change your plans.

___ **5.** You can get good results by giving most textbooks just one close reading because most such books are designed to be read only once.

All the preceding statements are false. However, don't worry if you answered some incorrectly. Study skills are like any other activity: they can be learned.

The Art of Learning

How does one become a good learner? "Winning the game of higher education is like winning any other game," say learning experts Debbie Longman and Rhonda Atkinson. "It consists of the same basic process. First, you decide if you really want to play. If you do, then you gear your attitudes and habits to learning. Next you learn the rules. To do this, you need a playbook, a college catalog. Third, you learn about the other players—administration, faculty, and other students. Finally, you learn specific plans to improve your playing skills."[26]

Unfortunately, many students come to college with faulty study skills. They are not entirely to blame. In high school and earlier, much of the emphasis is on *what* is to be studied rather than *how* to study it.

"The secret to controlling time is to remember that there is always enough time to do what is really important," say Mervill Douglass and Donna Douglass. "The difficulty is knowing what is really important."[27]

What *is* important in college? Studying, going to classes, writing papers, and taking tests compete with social life, extracurricular activities, and perhaps part-time work. All must somehow fit into the same 24 hours available each day, yet—unlike in high school or many paying jobs—time in college is often very unstructured. For students, the clash of college demands can lead to several health-related problems: sleep disturbances, alcohol and drug abuse, eating disorders, money difficulties, procrastination, and other maladaptations. Let us discuss how to improve academic performance, which should be the top priority.

Developing Study Habits: Finding Your "Prime Study Time"

Here is a way you can use knowledge about your own body and mind to improve your academic performance: Devote the hours you *feel best* to *study best*. What is called *prime study time* is the time of day when you are at your best for learning and remembering.

Each of us has a different energy cycle. For example, two roommates may have different patterns. One (the "day person") may be an early riser who prefers to work on difficult tasks in the morning. The other (the "night person") may start slowly but be at the peak of his or her form during the evening hours.

The trick, then, is to effectively *use* your energy cycle, which tends to repeat itself from day to day, so that your hours of best performance coincide with your heaviest academic demands. If your energy level is high during the evenings, you should plan to do your studying then—especially for assignments requiring heavy concentration, such as writing papers or doing math problems. Yet you should recognize that evening hours are a time when others around you like to unwind or socialize or watch TV and that you will be tempted to join them. If, by contrast, your energy level is high during the mornings, you should hit the books then. But you may have to deal with the fact that others nearby are still sleeping or that most classes occur before noon. Probably most students will find that their energy levels are higher during the first part of the day and lower later on.

These different energy patterns and distractions suggest some important actions to take:

Make a Study Schedule First make a master schedule that shows all your regular obligations—classes and work, of course, but you may also wish to list meals and exercise times. This schedule should be indicated for the *entire school term*—semester, quarter, or whatever.

Now insert the times during which you plan to study. As mentioned, it's best if these study periods correspond to times when you are most alert and can best concentrate. However, don't forget to schedule in hourly breaks, since your concentration will flag periodically.

Next write in the major academic events—when term papers and other assignments are due, when quizzes and exams take place, any holidays and vacations.

At the beginning of every week, schedule your study sessions and write in the specific tasks you plan to accomplish during each session. It's best to try to study something connected with every class every day. If the subject is difficult for you (for example, language or math), try to spend an hour a day on it, which is more effective than 5 hours in one day.

In addition, rather than put off major projects, such as term papers, thinking you'll do them in one concentrated period of effort, you should realize that it's more efficient to break the task into smaller steps that you can handle individually. This prevents you from delaying so long that you finally have to pull an all-nighter to complete the project.

Find Some Good Places to Study Studying means first of all avoiding distractions. No doubt you know people who study while listening to the radio or watching television—indeed, maybe you've done this yourself. Still, most people *are* distracted by these activities.

Avoid studying in places that are associated with other activities, particularly comfortable ones. That is, don't do your academic reading lying in bed or sitting at a kitchen table. Studying should be an intense, concentrated activity.

You may wish to designate two or three areas as regular areas for studying. Assuming they are free of distractions, two good places are at a desk in your room or a table in the library. As these places become associated with studying, they will reinforce better studying behavior.[28]

Make sure the place you study is free of clutter, which can affect your concentration and make you feel disorganized. Your desktop should contain that which you are studying and nothing else.

Avoid Time Wasters, but Reward Your Studying Certainly it's much more fun to hang out with your friends or to watch television than to study. Moreover, these pleasures are real and immediate, whereas getting an A in a course, let alone getting a degree, seems to be in the distant future.

Thus, at the same time you must learn to say no to distractions so that you can study, you must also give yourself frequent rewards so that you will indeed be *motivated* to study. Thus, you should study with the notion that after you finish you will "pleasure yourself" with a walk, a snack, a television show, a video game, a conversation with a friend, or a similar treat.

Improving Your Memory

Memorizing is, of course, one of the principal requirements of being in college. Distractions are one of the main impediments to remembering as they are to other forms of learning. *External* distractions are those you have no control over—noises in the hallway, an instructor's accent, people whispering in the library. If you can't get rid of the distraction by moving, you might try to increase your interest in the subject you are trying to memorize. *Internal* distractions are daydreams, personal worries, hunger, illness, and other physical discomforts. Small worries can be shunted aside by listing them on a page for future handling. Large worries may require talking with a friend or counselor.

Beyond getting rid of distractions, there are certain techniques you can adopt to enhance your memory.

Space Your Studying, Rather Than Cramming Cramming—making a frantic, last-minute attempt to memorize massive amounts of information—is probably the least effective means of absorbing information, especially if it tires you out and makes you even more anxious before the test. Research shows that, in general, it is better to space out your studying of a subject on successive days rather than try to do it all during the same number of hours on one day.[29] It is *repetition* that helps move information into your long-term memory bank.

Review Information Repeatedly—Even "Overlearn" It By repeatedly reviewing information—what is known as *rehearsal*—you can usually improve not only your retention of it but also your understanding of it.[30] Overlearning—continuing to repeatedly review material even after you appear to have absorbed it—can improve your recall substantially. Thus, although "cramming" is not an effective way to learn, reviewing material right before an examination can help counteract any forgetting that may have occurred since the last time you studied the material.

Use Memorizing Tricks There are several ways to organize information so that you can retain it better. Longman and Atkinson mention the following methods of establishing associations between items you want to remember:[31]

- *Mental and physical imagery:* Use your visual and other senses to construct a personal image of what you want to remember. Indeed, it helps to make the image humorous, action-filled, sexual, bizarre, or outrageous in order to establish a personal connection.

  For instance, to remember the name of the 20th president of the United States, James Garfield, you could visualize your friend James holding a Garfield-the-cat doll while blowing out candles on a birthday cake with the number 20 written in frosting on the top. This mental image helps you associate James, Garfield, and 20.

  You can also make your mental image a physical one by drawing or diagramming. Thus, to learn the parts of the human gastrointestinal system, you could draw a picture and label the parts to assist recall.

- *Acronyms and acrostics:* An acronym is a word created from the first letters of items on a list. For instance, *Roy G. Biv* helps you remember the colors of the rainbow in order: *red, orange, yellow, green, blue, indigo, violet.* An acrostic is a phrase or sentence created from the first letters of items on a list. For example, *Every Good Boy Does Fine* helps you remember that the order of the five notes on a music staff (horizontal lines and spaces) is E-G-B-D-F.

- *Location:* Location memory occurs when you associate a concept with a place or imaginary place. For example, you could learn the parts of the gastrointestinal system by visualizing an imaginary walk across campus and associating each part with a building you pass.

- *Word games:* Jingles and rhymes are frequent devices used by advertisers to get people to remember their products. You may recall the spelling rule "I before E except after C or when sounded like A as in neighbor or weigh." To recall the difference between a stalactite (which hangs from the top of a cave) and a stalagmite (which forms on the floor of a cave), you might remember that the *t* in *stalactite* signifies "top." You can also use narrative methods, such as making up a story.

Successful students

Always or almost always in class	84%
Sometimes absent	8%
Often absent	8%

Unsuccessful students

Always or almost always in class	47%
Sometimes absent	8%
Often absent	45%

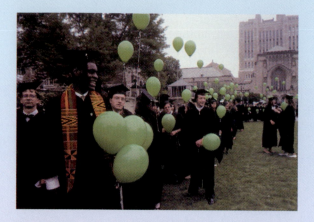

● **Class attendance and grade success.** Students who had grades of B or above were more apt to have better class attendance than students with grades of C− or below.

How to Benefit from Lectures

Are lectures really a good way of transmitting knowledge? Perhaps not always, but the fact remains that most colleges (and certainly most health courses) rely heavily on this method. Research has shown that students with grades of C− or below are more often absent from class compared to students who have of B or above.[32] (*See* ● *chart.*)

Most lectures are reasonably well organized, but you will probably attend some that are not. Even so, they will indicate what the instructor thinks is important, which will be useful to you on the exams.

Regardless of the strengths of the lecturer, here are some tips for getting more out of a lecture.

Take Effective Notes by Listening Actively
Research shows that good test performance is related to good note taking.[33] Good note taking requires that you listen actively—that is, participate in the lecture process. Here are some ways to take good lecture notes:

- *Read ahead and anticipate the lecturer:* Try to anticipate what the instructor is go-ing to say, based on your previous reading (text or study guide). Having background knowledge makes learning more efficient.

- *Listen for signal words:* Instructors use key phrases such as "The most important point is . . . ," "There are four reasons for . . . ," "The chief reason . . . ," "Of special importance . . . ," "Consequently . . . ." When you hear such signal phrases, mark your notes with an asterisk (*) or write *Imp* (for "Important").

- *Take notes in your own words:* Instead of just being a stenographer, try to restate the lecturer's thoughts in your own words. This makes you pay attention to the lecture and organize it in a way that is meaningful to you. In addition, don't feel you have to write everything down, just get the key points.

- *Ask questions:* By asking questions during the lecture, you necessarily participate in it and increase your understanding. Although many students are shy about asking questions, most professors welcome them.

Review Your Notes Regularly The good news is that most students, according to one study, do take good notes. The bad news is that they don't use them—that is, they wait until just before final exams to review their notes, when the notes have lost much of their meaning.[34] Make it a point to review your notes on a regular basis. We cannot emphasize enough how important this kind of reviewing is.

How to Improve Your Reading Ability: The SQ3R Method

We cannot teach you how to speed-read here, but perhaps we can help you make the time you do spend reading more efficient. The method we will describe here is known as the *SQ3R method*. "SQ3R" stands for *survey, question, read, recite, and review*.[35] The strategy for this method is to break down a reading assignment into small segments, each of which you master before moving on.

The five steps of the SQ3R method are as follows:

1. ***Survey* the Chapter Before You Read It** Get an overview of the chapter or other reading assignment before you begin reading it. If you have a sense of what the material is about before you begin reading it, you can predict where it is going, bring some of your own background experience to it, and otherwise become involved in it in a way that will help you retain it.

    Many textbooks offer some "preview"-type material, such as a list of objectives or an outline of topic headings at the beginning of the chapter. Other books offer a summary at the end of the chapter. In this book, for instance, when you first approach a unit, look at the topic headings on the first page. At the beginning of each chapter, look at the objectives. You may also wish to go through a chapter and read the summaries following each section heading.

2. ***Question* the Segment in the Chapter Before You Read It** This step is easy to do, and the point, again, is to get yourself involved in the material. After surveying the entire chapter, go to the first segment—section, subsection, or even paragraph, depending on the level of difficulty and density of information—and look at the topic heading. In your mind, restate the heading as a question. After you have formulated the question, go to steps 3 and 4 (read and recite), then proceed to the next segment and restate the heading there as a question.

    For instance, for the section heading in this unit that reads "The Five Dimensions of Health: Five Kinds of Well-Being," ask yourself, "What *are* the five kinds of well-being?" For the heading of the subsection "High-Level Wellness," ask: "What does the term *high-level wellness* mean?"

3. ***Read* the Segment About Which You Asked the Question** Now read the segment you asked the question about. Read with purpose, to answer the question you formulated. Underline or color-mark sentences you think are important, if they help you answer the question. Read this portion of the text more than once, if necessary, until you can answer the question. In addition, determine whether the segment covers any other significant questions and formulate answers to these, too. After you have read the segment, proceed to step 4.

    Perhaps you can see where this is all leading: If you approach your reading in terms of questions and answers, you will be better prepared when you see questions about the material on the examinations later.

4. ***Recite* the Main Points for the Segment** Recite means "Say aloud." Thus, you should speak out loud (or under your breath) the answer to the principal question about the segment and any other main points. Put these points in your own words, the better to enhance your understanding. If you wish, make notes of the principal ideas, so you can look them over later.

    Now that you have actively studied the first segment, move on to the second segment and do steps 2–4 for it. Continue this procedure through the rest of the segments until you have finished the chapter.

5. **Review the Entire Chapter by Repeating Questions** After you have read the

chapter, go back through it and review the main points. Then, without looking at the book, test your memory by repeating the questions.

Although the SQ3R method takes longer than simply reading with a rapidly moving color marker or underlining pencil, the technique is far more effective because it requires your *involvement and understanding.* This is the key to all effective learning.

How to Become an Effective Test Taker

The first requirement of test taking is, of course, knowledge of the subject matter, which is what the foregoing discussion has been intended to help you obtain. You should also make it a point to *ask* your instructor what kinds of questions will be asked on tests. Beyond this, however, there are certain skills one can acquire that will help during the test-taking process. Here are some suggestions offered by the authors of *Doing Well in College*.[36]

Reviewing: Study Information That Is Emphasized and Enumerated Because you will not always know whether an exam will be an objective or essay test, you need to be prepared for both. Here are some general tips.

- *Review material that is emphasized:* In the lectures, this consists of any points your instructor pointed out as being significant or important, or spent a good deal of time discussing, or specifically advised you to study.

  In the textbook, pay attention to key terms (often emphasized in *italic* or **boldface** type), their definitions, and the examples that clarify them. Also, of course, material that has a good many pages given over to it should also be considered important.

- *Review material that is enumerated:* Pay attention to any numbered lists, both in your lectures and in your notes, whether it is the 13 vitamins, the major schools of psychology, or the warning signs for heart dis-

ease. Enumerations often provide the basis for essay and multiple-choice questions.

- *Review other tests:* Look over past quizzes as well as the discussion questions and review questions given at the ends of chapters in many textbooks.

Prepare by Doing Final Reviews and Budgeting Your Test Time Learn how to make your energy and time work for you. Whether you have studied methodically or are only able to cram for an exam, here are some tips:

- *Review your notes:* Spend the night before reviewing your notes, then go to bed without interfering with the material you have absorbed (as by watching television). Get up early the next morning and review your notes again.

- *Find a good test-taking spot:* Make sure you go to the exam with any pencils and other materials you need. Get to the classroom early, or at least on time, and find a quiet spot. If you don't have a watch, sit where you can watch a clock. Again, review your notes and avoid talking with others, so as not to interfere with the information you have learned or increase your anxiety.

- *Read the test directions:* Many students don't do this and end up losing points because they didn't understand precisely what was required of them. Also, listen to any verbal directions or hints your instructor gives you before the test.

- *Budget your time:* Here is an important point of test strategy: Before you start, read through the entire test and figure out how much time you can spend on each section. The reason for budgeting your time, of course, is so that you won't find yourself with only a few minutes left and a long essay still to be written or a great number of multiple-choice questions to answer.

  Write the number of minutes allowed for each section on the test booklet or on a scratch sheet and stick to the schedule. The way you budget your time should correspond to how confident you feel about answering the questions.

Objective Tests: Answer Easy Questions and Eliminate Options Some suggestions for taking objective tests, such as multiple-choice, true-false, or fill-in, are as follows:

- *Answer the easy questions first:* Don't waste time stewing over difficult questions. Do the easy ones first and come back to the hard ones later (put a check mark opposite those you're not sure about). Your unconscious mind may have solved them in the meantime, or later items may provide you with the extra information you need.

- *Answer all questions:* Unless the instructor says you will be penalized for wrong answers, try to answer all questions. If you have time, review all questions and make sure you have recorded them correctly.

- *Eliminate the options:* Cross out answers you know are incorrect. Be sure to read all the possible answers, especially when the first answer is correct (because other answers could also be correct, so that "All of the above" may be the right choice). Be aware that the test may provide information pertinent to one question in another question on the test. Pay particular attention to options that are long and detailed, since answers that are more detailed and specific are apt to be correct. If two answers have the opposite meaning, one of the two is probably correct.

Essay Tests: First Anticipate Answers and Prepare an Outline Because there is only a limited amount of time during the test, there are only a few essay questions that your instructor is apt to ask during the exam. The key to success is to try to anticipate beforehand what the questions might be and memorize an outline for an answer. Here are some specific suggestions:

- *Anticipate 10 probable essay questions:* Using the principles we discussed above of reviewing lecture and textbook material that is *emphasized* and *enumerated*, you are in a position to identify 10 essay ques-

tions your instructor may ask. Write out these questions.

- *Prepare and memorize informal essay answers:* Write out each of the questions and list the main points that need to be discussed. Put supporting information in parentheses. Circle the key words in each main point, and below the question put the first letter of the key word. Make up catch phrases, using acronyms, acrostics, or word games, so that you can memorize these key words. Test yourself until you can recall the key words that the letters stand for and the main points the key words represent.

  For example, if the question you make up is "What is the difference between the traditional and the modern theory of adolescence?", you might put down the following answers:[37]

  1. *Biologically generated.* Universal phenomenon (Hall's theory: hormonal).

  2. *Sociologically generated.* Not universal phenomenon (not purely hormonal).
     BG SG   BIG GUY   SMALL GUY

  When you receive the questions for the essay examination, read all the directions carefully, then start with the *least demanding question.* Putting down a good answer at the start will give you confidence and make it easier to proceed with the rest. Make a brief outline, similar to the one you did for your anticipated question, before you begin writing.

The Peak-Performing Student

Good students are made, not born. They have decided, as we pointed out earlier, that they really want to play the college game, to learn the rules, the players, and the playing skills. We have listed some of the studying, reading, and test-taking skills that will help you be a peak-performing student. The practice of these skills is up to you.

Handling Stress: Hassles, Crises, and the Demands of Life

In These Chapters:

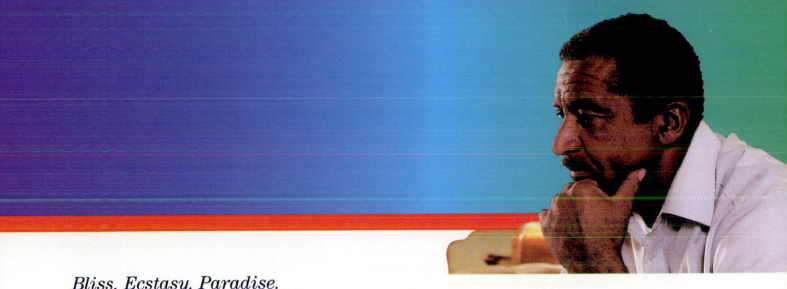

Bliss. Ecstasy. Paradise. Nirvana.

These and other names describe a condition to which we all aspire—a rarely experienced dream state of comfort, a zone beyond care and pain. It may help explain why people try to "lose themselves" through music, dance, athletics, massage, meditation, prayer, creative activity—or, less successfully, through television, overeating, alcohol, drugs.

But, of course, ecstasy is not what most of ordinary life is about. Everyday life is often filled with conflict, uncertainty, and difficulty—in a word, *stress*.

Usually we think of stress as being unpleasant. Some sources of uncomfortable stress occur on the physical level, from exposure to temperature extremes, to the common cold, to neighbors' radios, to air pollution, to earthquakes and hurricanes. Other sources of stress are people—roommates, lovers, families, landlords, coworkers, bosses, and so on.

For many people, ordinary life is apparently an anxious and exhausting experience. If you look around you, you can see that enormous industries exist because of the notion that stress is bad and should be prevented or alleviated. Aspirin and tranquilizers, for example, are among the world's most popular pharmaceuticals. Tobacco, alcohol, and other drugs legal and illegal continue to sell because millions of nervous people think they are the principal means of relaxing their tensions.

But stress is not always unpleasant. Sometimes stress is associated with *positive* events

and therefore challenges us and energizes us—as when we are competing at a sport or a video game or playing a musical instrument. Moreover, what we perceive as stressful and how we react to it are highly individual matters.

"The highest art," goes an old Tibetan saying, "is living an ordinary life in an extraordinary manner." Although stress cannot and probably should not always be avoided, you can learn to handle it—and perhaps handle it in an extraordinary manner.

3   How Stress Works: Body and Mind

▶ What are the definitions of *stress* and *stressor*?

▶ What are the differences between hassles and crises and strong stressors?

▶ What are the differences between "good" stressors and "bad" stressors?

▶ What are the three stages of physical stress, the General Adapation Syndrome?

▶ What are the different kinds of psychological stress reactions?

Here is an experience one of the authors had as a student in college on a Friday night: I had gone to bed early and lay in bed tossing and turning. I was behind in my studies in a course I felt I was not good at, with an exam coming up on Monday. I had invited a friend I was interested in to go to a party on Saturday and was hesitant to cancel. My parents had called to say that a family member was seriously ill and hinted I should come home for the weekend.

In the next room, my two roommates were drinking and talking. It's difficult to say whether they were being unusually loud. Nonetheless, at about 11:30, I'd finally had it. I stormed out into the living room. *"Shut up! Shut up! Shut up!"*, I screamed at the top of my lungs.

They looked at me aghast. Immediately I felt embarrassed. Maybe I had overreacted, I thought. "Got to get up early tomorrow," I mumbled, and left the room.

Sound familiar? Maybe I *did* overreact. Clearly, what was very stressful to me then— my roommates' talking—would not have been stressful to me on other occasions or stressful to other people in the same situation. And that is what is important to know about stress: its effect depends on one's *perception* of the source of stress. This is actually good news, because it means you can often alter your perceptions in order to reduce stress.

Stress and Stressors

Stress is the body's reaction; stressors are the source of stress. Stressors may be small irritating hassles, short-duration crises, or long-duration strong stressors. A source of stress may be negative and cause "distress" or be positive and cause "eustress."

Stress is the reaction of our bodies to an event. The source of stress is called a **stressor**. Stressors may be specific, ranging from a flat tire to a death in the family, but the physical reaction is nonspecific and generalized, being felt throughout the entire body.

Life and health in modern society require that we continually adapt to a variety of events. The human body constantly strives to maintain a state of balance known as **homeostasis**, in which physiological and psychological systems are stable, or in equilibrium. Stressors may disturb this homeostasis by causing one's body to become unbalanced and, if the stress is too great for too long, eventually causing illness and potentially death.

Stress has both physical and emotional components. Physically, according to Canadian researcher Hans Selye, a pioneer in this area, stress is "the nonspecific response of the body to any demand made upon it."[1] Emotionally, stress has been defined as the feeling of being overwhelmed, "the perception that events or circumstances have challenged, or exceeded, a person's ability to cope."[2]

Types of Stressors: Hassles, Crises, Strong Stressors There is probably no way to completely escape stress, whether it starts with small daily hassles or with unexpected one-time crises. Such negative sources of stress, when they become too cumulative or too powerful, eventually can lead to illness, depression, and even premature death. Let us consider the types of stressors, ranging in intensity and duration from hassles to crises to strong stressors.

Hassles Simply frustrating, **hassles** are irritants, but their cumulative effect can be significant and even hazardous to health. College students, says psychologist Richard Lazarus, are most hassled by (1) anxiety over wasting time, (2) pressure to meet high standards, and (3) feeling lonely.[3]

One of the authors took an informal poll: When I asked my students what the principal hassles were in their lives, they reported being worried about finding time to study, having relationship problems with roommates and partners, and conflicts over partying versus studying.

Lazarus contends that nearly everyone, regardless of age, complains about three kinds of hassles: (1) misplacing or losing things, (2) physical appearance, and (3) having too many things to do.

Of course we all have many other kinds of hassles, but their importance varies with one's age and situation in life. One study found that younger adults experienced significantly more hassles in the domains of finances, work, home maintenance, personal life, and family and friends than did older adults.[4] White, middle-class men and women of middle age had their own specific hassles. (*See* • *Figure 3.1.*)

Crises A **crisis** is an especially strong source of stress, one that may appear suddenly and be of short duration but have long-lasting effects. For instance, sudden occasions of overwhelming terror—a horrible auto accident, an incident of childhood abuse, a wartime experience—can have a tremendous biological impact. This is so whether the event is a one-time experience or repeated, according to Yale psychiatrist Dennis Charney, director of clinical neuroscience at the National Center for Post-Traumatic Stress Disorder.[5] Brain chemistry changes in response to the stress so that people are more sensitive to adrenaline surges even decades later, and people experience normal events as repetitions of the original trauma. Such people experience troubled sleep, irritability and rages, and recurrent nightmares and flashbacks that repeat the original horror.

Strong Stressors There are also strong sources of stress of continuing duration, called **strong stressors**, which can dramatically strain a person's ability to adapt. A strong stressor can be extreme mental or physical discomfort. For example, two years after Kay Bartlett suffered a neck injury from a fall in her kitchen

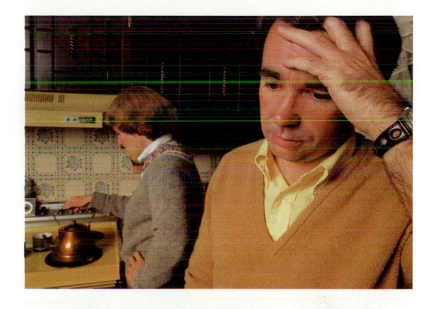

• **Figure 3.1 The hassles of middle age.** These are the top 10 annoyances for white, middle-class, middle-aged men and women studied during a 1-year period.

1. Concern about weight
2. Health of a family member
3. Rising prices of common goods
4. Home maintenance
5. Too many things to do
6. Misplacing or losing things
7. Yard work or outside home maintenance
8. Property, investment, or taxes
9. Crime
10. Physical appearance

she wrote that pain had become her constant companion. Pain, she stated, "regulates nearly every moment of my waking life, holding me captive to its savage dictates." Indeed, she said, "Pain has changed my life, narrowing it as old age will eventually do. But, at 49, I'm not old enough to be this old. I feel like in the last two years I have aged 30."[6] For Kay Bartlett, obviously, the stressor of chronic pain has significantly impaired the quality of her life.

Stressors, Good and Bad So far, we have mainly dealt with stress as though its sources were negative. However, stress researcher Selye

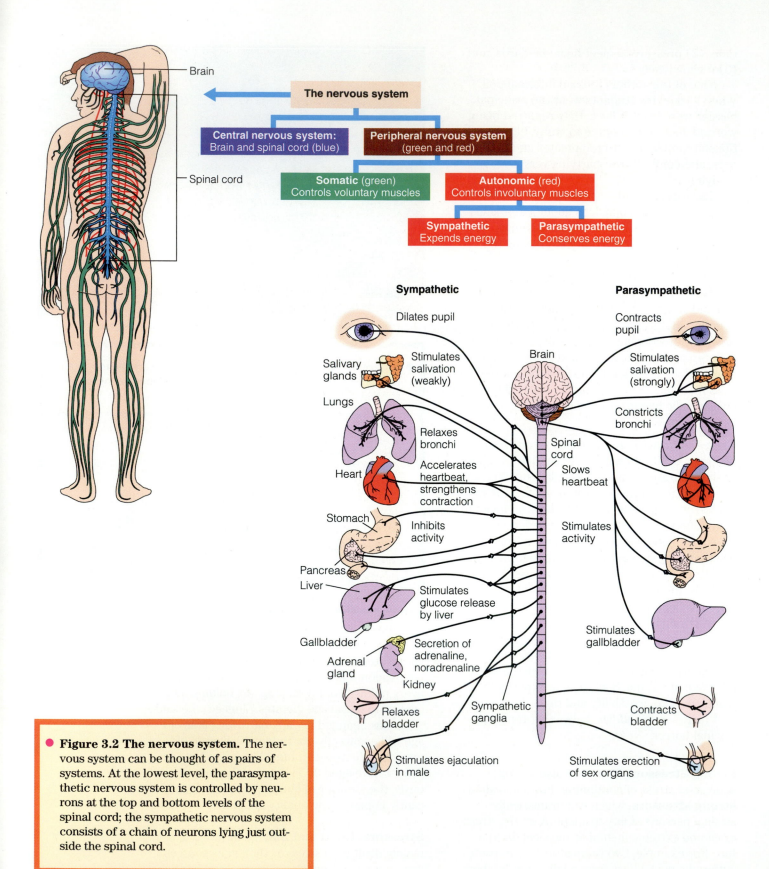

The nervous system

| Central nervous system: Brain and spinal cord (blue) | Peripheral nervous system (green and red) |

Somatic (green) Controls voluntary muscles

Autonomic (red) Controls involuntary muscles

Sympathetic Expends energy

Parasympathetic Conserves energy

● **Figure 3.2 The nervous system.** The nervous system can be thought of as pairs of systems. At the lowest level, the parasympathetic nervous system is controlled by neurons at the top and bottom levels of the spinal cord; the sympathetic nervous system consists of a chain of neurons lying just outside the spinal cord.

points out that stressors can be *both negative and positive*. He writes: "It is immaterial whether the agent or situation we face is pleasant or unpleasant; all that counts is the intensity of the demand for adjustment and adaptation."[7] Stressors, he says, are of the following types:

- *Distressors:* When the source of stress is a negative event (for example, being fired, being rejected in love), it is called a **distressor** and its effect is called **distress**. Although distress can be helpful when one is facing a physical threat, too much of this kind of stress may result in illness.

- *Eustressors:* When the source of stress is a positive event (for example, falling in love, being promoted), it is called a **eustressor;** its effect is called **eustress** (pronounced "*you*-stress"). Eustress can stimulate a person to better coping and adaptation. (Selye coined this word by adding the Greek prefix *eu*, for "good," to the word *stress*.)

We can't always prevent distressors, but we can learn to recognize them, understand our reactions to them, and develop ways of managing both the stressors and the stress. Eustressors, on the other hand, are what impel us to do our best—to become the "peak performers" we referred to in Chapter 1.

Physical Stress Reactions: The General Adaptation Syndrome

The physical response to stress has been described as a three-stage general adaptation syndrome. Stage 1, alarm, is the "fight-or-flight" response, in which the body's nervous system takes over. Stage 2, resistance, gives the body increased strength and endurance. Stage 3, exhaustion, is the wearing down from continuing stress.

As we mentioned, stress reactions have both physical and mental components, although the responses are intertwined. In this section, we consider the physical reactions. In the next section, we consider the psychological reactions.

As you might guess, one key player in stress is the nervous system. (*See* • *Figure 3.2.*) The nervous system consists of two principal parts:

- *Central nervous system:* The **central nervous system** is made up of the brain and the spinal cord.

- *Peripheral nervous system:* The **peripheral nervous system** consists of the nerves that carry messages from the sense organs to the central nervous system and from the central nervous system to the muscles and glands.

The peripheral nervous system in turn has two parts:

- *Somatic nervous system:* The **somatic nervous system** controls the voluntary muscles. When you do deep-breathing exercises to control stress, you are using muscles in the somatic nervous system.

- *Autonomic nervous system:* The **autonomic nervous system** controls the involuntary muscles. When you become frightened and begin to perspire and your heart begins to race, these activities are controlled by the autonomic nervous system.

The autonomic nervous system also has two parts:

- *Parasympathetic:* The **parasympathetic nervous system** *conserves* energy, decreases heart rate, increases digestive activities, and promotes body activities that are relaxing.

- *Sympathetic:* The **sympathetic nervous system** *generates* energy, increases the heart rate and breathing rate, and prepares the body for either fighting or fleeing when it perceives a threat.

Selye described the response to a stressor as a three-stage **general adaptation syndrome.**[8] The stages are *alarm, resistance,* and *exhaustion.* (*See* • *Figure 3.3.*) To various degrees, these reactions can occur whether you meet a mugger in an alley, get a terse "See me immediately!" note from the boss, hear the starting gun in a race, or are called upon to give a toast at a wedding. Before the first stage, there may be a conscious or unconscious evaluation in which a decision is made as to whether or not a threat exists.

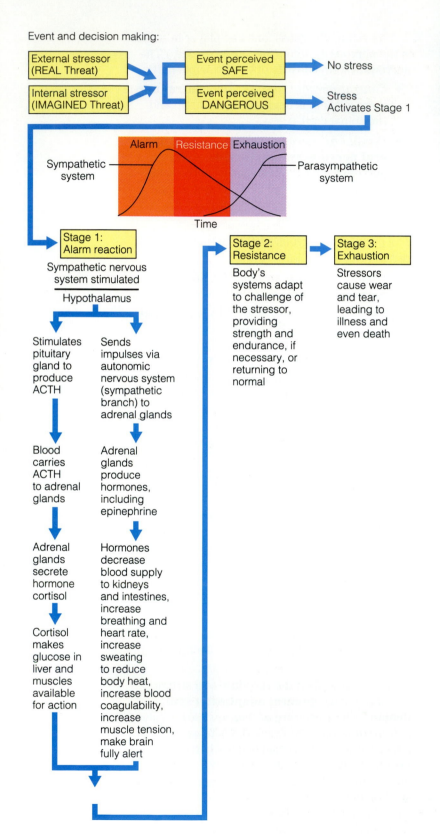

Stage 1—Alarm The alarm phase is often called the *fight-or-flight response.* This is the stage in which the brain rapidly and subconsciously perceives the stressor, which may be either external (real threat) or internal (probably imagined threat). The brain decides that the stressor is a disturbing event and almost instantly mobilizes your body's defensive forces to stand and fight or to turn and flee. Specifically:

- *The autonomic nervous system takes over:* The autonomic nervous system, which controls your movements and internal functions, operates largely without any conscious thought on your part.

- *The hypothalamus causes adrenal glands to release stress-response hormones:* The autonomic nervous system triggers the hypothalamus. The **hypothalamus** is a part of the brain that directs the flow of **hormones**, or chemicals, throughout the body. The hypothalamus stimulates the **adrenal glands**—specialized glands located on top of the kidneys. This stimulation comes about when two conditions occur:

  (1) The hypothalamus stimulates the **pituitary gland** (the "master gland" of the endocrine system) to produce **ACTH (adrenocorticotropic hormone)**, which is transmitted to the adrenal glands.

  (2) The hypothalamus sends impulses via the autonomic nervous system. The adrenal glands then release into the bloodstream hormones related to stress responses, among them **cortisol** and **epinephrine (adrenaline)**.

- *Cortisol and epinephrine "arm" your body to fight or flee:* The hormones cortisol and epinephrine (the "fear hormone") bring about a number of changes to enable your body to meet the stress. These hormones act to:

  (1) Reduce blood supply to your kidneys and intestines, making more blood ready for your brain and muscles.

  (2) Increase the intake of oxygen by the lungs and increase the supply of oxygen to muscles and brain.

  (3) Increase heart rate and blood pressure to increase blood circulation.

  (4) Release **glucose**, a type of sugar stored (as glycogen) in the liver, for use as energy for muscular exertion.

  (5) Increase perspiration to reduce the high body temperature caused by the speeding up of the body's functions.

  (6) Cause the pupils of the eye to expand (dilate), providing increased visual sensitivity.

  (7) Break down fat tissue (and, eventually, even muscle tissue) to provide additional fuel for energy, if needed.

  (8) Produce **antibodies**, specific chemical compounds to destroy disease-producing microorganisms, if the body is threatened by a specific disease.

Clearly, these include several of the reactions—thumping heart, rapid breathing, sweating—that one associates with fear or stress.

Stage 2—Resistance In this second stage of the general adaptation syndrome, your body's systems adapt themselves to the challenge of the stressor, giving the body increased strength and endurance, if necessary, or they return to a level of normal activity. In addition, during this phase, you begin to concentrate more on psychological coping mechanisms and defensive behavior to deal with the stressor rather than continuing the physical fight-or-flight response.

Stage 3—Exhaustion If the stress goes on long enough, your physical and psychological energy will be depleted, and your body will need to rest. When weeks and months pass with no letup in stress—as can happen with a work-ing parent short on money or a soldier exposed to constant combat—eventually you will show symptoms of exhaustion and may become ill. Indeed, if stressors cause wear and tear over a long period of time, they may even lead to death. *It's important, therefore, for you to find ways to counter long-sustained tension.*

Psychological Stress Reactions

Your psychological response to stress is affected by several factors. First are the number, kinds, and magnitude of stressors in your life. Also important are your emotional predisposition, or intensity of feeling, and your self-esteem. Your personality type, whether hurried and hostile "Type A" or unhurried "Type B," and the extent of your "psychological hardiness" are also major factors. Finally, your social support systems and other coping resources are critical.

How you respond psychologically to stress is an individual matter. Among the factors that influence your response are:

- The number, kinds, and magnitude of stressors in your life
- Your emotional predisposition and self-esteem
- Your personality type
- Your coping resources

Let us examine these categories.

Number, Kind, and Magnitude of Stressors
We have said that too many stresses can make you ill. Working from this proposition, in the early 1960s, physicians Thomas Holmes and Richard Rahe devised a "future illness" scale and tried it out on several medical students.[9] The scale, known as the Holmes-Rahe Life Events Scale, or the Social Readjustment Rating Scale, identifies certain stressors (life events), both positive and negative. Examples range from (at the most stressful end) death of a spouse, divorce, jail term, marriage, and sex difficulties to (at the least stressful end) change in sleeping habits, vacation, Christmas, and minor violations of the law. By adding up the values

assigned to the stressful events they have encountered in the past year, people can see how much adapting they have had to do and what the implications are for their health. In an improved version of the Holmes-Rahe scale, Irwin Sarason and his associates devised another test called the Life Experiences Survey.[10] (*See Self Discovery 3.1.*)

Emotional Predisposition and Self-Esteem
Emotional predisposition—your intensity of feeling—can influence how you perceive stressors and react to stress. Often, because the source of the stress is other people, your reactions can depend in part on how you feel about *yourself in relation to other people*—that is, the level of your self-esteem.

Emotional predisposition and level of self-esteem are, at least in part, learned behavior. If, in the past, a person learns from parents or others that expressing anger is "impolite" or "bad," or is unable to direct anger toward its source for fear of being criticized, that person may turn his or her anger inward. Lacking the self-esteem to direct the anger appropriately, such a person may express it in unhealthy ways: (1) by attempting to erase the stress with alcohol, drugs, binge eating, or similar escapist activities, or (2) by overreacting to the stress with expressions of fly-off-the-handle rage and even violence. We return to the subject of self-esteem in the next chapter.

"Type A" and Other Personality Types Do you become extremely irritated if you have to wait in line? Do you walk, talk, or eat rapidly? Do you always feel you should be working or studying when you're supposed to be relaxing? Do you often do two things at once—for instance, study while eating, pay bills while talking on the phone?

If you answered yes, you may belong to a hurried, deadline-ridden, and competitive group of people who have **Type A personalities**. If you answered no, you may be part of the relaxed, unhurried, and carefree group who have **Type B personalities**. Actually, Type A and Type B represent two ends of a range of hurried-unhurried behavior. Most of us fall somewhere between the two extremes. Nevertheless, the distinctions are useful.

In 1974, two San Francisco physicians, Meyer Friedman and Ray Rosenman, linked hurried, Type A behavior to stress-related heart disease.[11] The more laid-back Type B personalities, they suggested, seemed less prone to heart disease. Type A men between the ages of 39 and 49, research shows, are six times more likely to have heart attacks than Type B men. Type A women are three to seven times more likely to suffer from high blood pressure than less-hurried women. A 4½-year study of 862 people found that those who received counseling and were able to reduce their Type A behavior had half the number of heart attacks as those who received only advice about diet, exercise, and treatments.[12] It's important to note some qualifications about Type A behavior:

- *Hostility:* Hostility—especially an antagonistic, interactional style—seems to be a very important component in putting one at risk for heart disease.[13, 14] People with high ratings for potential for hostility are those who can be described as uncooperative, antagonistic, rude, disagreeable, unsympathetic, callous, and the like.[15]

- *Cigarettes and lack of exercise:* Both Type A men and women are more likely to smoke and less likely to exercise—and cigarettes and nonexercise are two important risk factors in heart disease.

- *Thriving on challenge:* Some Type A people seem to have learned to have directed their competitive, hurried attributes to their advantage and not suffered ill health.

The Type A theory tries to explain why some people react to stress more destructively than other people. The **hardy personality theory**, or **theory of psychological hardiness**, tries to explain why some people react to stress more positively than others do. Psychologist Suzanne Kobasa suggests that psychologically hardy people have these major traits:[16, 17]

- *Commitment:* People who are *committed* have high self-esteem, enthusiasm, and a sense of purpose in their lives.

- *Control:* Having the belief that they can *control*, or influence, events in their lives, people accept responsibility for their actions and make changes in harmful behaviors.

SELF DISCOVERY 3.1

The Life Experiences Survey:
Are Your Stressors Positive or Negative?

The Life Experiences Survey takes into account the notion that stress involves more than just change alone and that people differ in the way they assess stress. The survey also allows you to write in events that are personally important to you that are not included as "check-off" items on the scale. In addition, the version presented here includes a special section that applies just to students.

What to do

Check the events below that you have experienced in the past 12 months, using a ruler or paper edge to line up the event on the left with the numbers on the right. For each event that applies, you should do two things: (1) check the time period during which you experienced the event; (2) circle the plus or minus number indicating the extent to which you feel the event had a positive or negative impact on your life.

	0 to 6 mo	7 mo to 1 yr	Extremely negative	Moderately negative	Somewhat negative	No impact	Slightly positive	Moderately positive	Extremely positive
Section 1									
1. Marriage	__	__	−3	−2	−1	0	+1	+2	+3
2. Detention in jail or comparable institution	__	__	−3	−2	−1	0	+1	+2	+3
3. Death of spouse	__	__	−3	−2	−1	0	+1	+2	+3
4. Major change in sleeping habits (much more or much less sleep)	__	__	−3	−2	−1	0	+1	+2	+3
5. Death of a close family member:									
a. mother	__	__	−3	−2	−1	0	+1	+2	+3
b. father	__	__	−3	−2	−1	0	+1	+2	+3
c. brother	__	__	−3	−2	−1	0	+1	+2	+3
d. sister	__	__	−3	−2	−1	0	+1	+2	+3
e. grandmother	__	__	−3	−2	−1	0	+1	+2	+3
f. grandfather	__	__	−3	−2	−1	0	+1	+2	+3
g. other (specify)	__	__	−3	−2	−1	0	+1	+2	+3
6. Major change in eating habits (much more or much less food intake)	__	__	−3	−2	−1	0	+1	+2	+3
7. Foreclosure on mortgage or loan	__	__	−3	−2	−1	0	+1	+2	+3
8. Death of close friend	__	__	−3	−2	−1	0	+1	+2	+3
9. Outstanding personal achievement	__	__	−3	−2	−1	0	+1	+2	+3
10. Minor law violations (traffic tickets, disturbing the peace, etc.)	__	__	−3	−2	−1	0	+1	+2	+3
11. *Male:* Wife/girlfriend's pregnancy	__	__	−3	−2	−1	0	+1	+2	+3
12. *Female:* Pregnancy	__	__	−3	−2	−1	0	+1	+2	+3
13. Changed work situation (different work responsibility, major change in working conditions, working hours, etc.)	__	__	−3	−2	−1	0	+1	+2	+3
14. New job	__	__	−3	−2	−1	0	+1	+2	+3
15. Serious illness or injury of close family member:									
a. father	__	__	−3	−2	−1	0	+1	+2	+3
b. mother	__	__	−3	−2	−1	0	+1	+2	+3
c. sister	__	__	−3	−2	−1	0	+1	+2	+3
d. brother	__	__	−3	−2	−1	0	+1	+2	+3
e. grandfather	__	__	−3	−2	−1	0	+1	+2	+3
f. grandmother	__	__	−3	−2	−1	0	+1	+2	+3
g. spouse	__	__	−3	−2	−1	0	+1	+2	+3
h. other (specify)	__	__	−3	−2	−1	0	+1	+2	+3
16. Sexual difficulties	__	__	−3	−2	−1	0	+1	+2	+3
17. Trouble with employer (in danger of losing job, being suspended, being demoted, etc.)	__	__	−3	−2	−1	0	+1	+2	+3
18. Trouble with in-laws	__	__	−3	−2	−1	0	+1	+2	+3

(continued)

SELF DISCOVERY 3.1
(continued)

	0 to 6 mo	7 mo to 1 yr	Extremely negative	Moderately negative	Somewhat negative	No impact	Slightly positive	Moderately positive	Extremely positive
19. Major change in financial status (a lot better off or a lot worse off)	——	——	−3	−2	−1	0	+1	+2	+3
20. Major change in closeness of family members (increased or decreased closeness)	——	——	−3	−2	−1	0	+1	+2	+3
21. Gaining a new family member (through birth, adoption, family member moving in, etc.)	——	——	−3	−2	−1	0	+1	+2	+3
22. Change of residence	——	——							
23. Marital separation from mate (due to conflict)	——	——	−3	−2	−1	0	+1	+2	+3
24. Major change in church activities (increased or decreased attendance)	——	——	−3	−2	−1	0	+1	+2	+3
25. Marital reconciliation with mate	——	——	−3	−2	−1	0	+1	+2	+3
26. Major change in number of arguments with spouse (a lot more or a lot fewer arguments)	——	——	−3	−2	−1	0	+1	+2	+3
27. *Married male:* Change in wife's work outside the home (beginning work, ceasing work, changing to a new job, etc.)	——	——	−3	−2	−1	0	+1	+2	+3
28. *Married female:* Change in husband's work (loss of job, beginning new job, retirement, etc.)	——	——	−3	−2	−1	0	+1	+2	+3
29. Major change in usual type and/or amount of recreation	——	——	−3	−2	−1	0	+1	+2	+3
30. Borrowing for a major purchase (buying home, business, etc.)	——	——	−3	−2	−1	0	+1	+2	+3
31. Borrowing for smaller purchase (buying car or TV, getting school loan, etc.)	——	——	−3	−2	−1	0	+1	+2	+3
32. Being fired from job	——	——	−3	−2	−1	0	+1	+2	+3
33. *Male:* Wife/girlfriend having abortion	——	——	−3	−2	−1	0	+1	+2	+3
34. *Female:* Having abortion	——	——	−3	−2	−1	0	+1	+2	+3
35. Major personal illness or injury	——	——	−3	−2	−1	0	+1	+2	+3
36. Major change in social activities, e.g., parties, movies, visiting (increased or decreased participation)	——	——	−3	−2	−1	0	+1	+2	+3
37. Major change in living conditions of family (building new home, remodeling, deterioration of home or neighborhood, etc.)	——	——	−3	−2	−1	0	+1	+2	+3
38. Divorce	——	——	−3	−2	−1	0	+1	+2	+3
39. Serious injury or illness of close friend	——	——	−3	−2	−1	0	+1	+2	+3
40. Retirement from work	——	——	−3	−2	−1	0	+1	+2	+3
41. Son or daughter leaving home (due to marriage, college, etc.)	——	——	−3	−2	−1	0	+1	+2	+3
42. Ending of formal schooling	——	——	−3	−2	−1	0	+1	+2	+3
43. Separation from spouse (due to work, travel, etc.)	——	——	−3	−2	−1	0	+1	+2	+3
44. Engagement	——	——	−3	−2	−1	0	+1	+2	+3
45. Breaking up with boyfriend/girlfriend	——	——	−3	−2	−1	0	+1	+2	+3
46. Leaving home for the first time	——	——	−3	−2	−1	0	+1	+2	+3
47. Reconciliation with boyfriend/girlfriend	——	——	−3	−2	−1	0	+1	+2	+3

Other recent experiences that have had an impact on your life.
List and rate.

			Extremely negative	Moderately negative	Somewhat negative	No impact	Slightly positive	Moderately positive	Extremely positive
48. _____			−3	−2	−1	0	+1	+2	+3
49. _____			−3	−2	−1	0	+1	+2	+3
50. _____			−3	−2	−1	0	+1	+2	+3

Section 2. Students only

	0 to 6 mo	7 mo to 1 yr	Extremely negative	Moderately negative	Somewhat negative	No impact	Slightly positive	Moderately positive	Extremely positive
51. Beginning a new school experience at a higher academic level (college, graduate school, professional school, etc.)	——	——	−3	−2	−1	0	+1	+2	+3
52. Changing to a new school at same academic level (undergraduate, graduate, etc.)	——	——	−3	−2	−1	0	+1	+2	+3
53. Academic probation	——	——	−3	−2	−1	0	+1	+2	+3
54. Being dismissed from dormitory or other residence	——	——	−3	−2	−1	0	+1	+2	+3
55. Failing an important exam	——	——	−3	−2	−1	0	+1	+2	+3
56. Changing a major	——	——	−3	−2	−1	0	+1	+2	+3
57. Failing a course	——	——	−3	−2	−1	0	+1	+2	+3
58. Dropping a course	——	——	−3	−2	−1	0	+1	+2	+3
59. Joining a fraternity/sorority	——	——	−3	−2	−1	0	+1	+2	+3
60. Financial problems concerning school (in danger of not having sufficient money to continue)	——	——	−3	−2	−1	0	+1	+2	+3

Total Score _____

SELF DISCOVERY 3.1
(continued)

Scoring

You will wind up with three scores: *positive change, negative change,* and (the two combined) *total change.* To arrive at your scores, first add up the number of positive (+) impact ratings. Then total up your negative (−) impact ratings (e.g., −1, −2, and −3 would total up to −6). To get your total change score, subtract your minus score from your positive score (or the reverse, if your minus score is larger—it's possible you will wind up with a total score that is minus).

How to Evaluate Your Scores

Here's what the scores mean:

Positive change: A low score is 0–6, a medium score is 7–15, and a high score is 16 and above. Actually, positive scores have not been found to be a very good predictor of mental and physical health adaptations.

Negative change: (Drop the minus sign from your total.) A low score is 0–3, a medium score is 4–13, and a high score is 14 and above. This score is more crucial than that for positive change. Negative change scores have been related to a number of stress adaptations, including: nonconformity, athletic injuries, job dissatisfaction, menstrual discomfort, vaginal infections, psychological discomfort, anxiety, depression, and coronary disease.

Total change: A low score is 0–11, a medium score is 12–27, and a high score is 28 and above. *Note:* If you should score "high" on this scale (or on the negative change scale), you should not worry unduly. Despite all that you have heard about the relationship between stress and unhealthful kinds of adaptations, a lot depends on the individual. Many people put up with great levels of stress without developing problems. This seems to show that stress is only one factor in health; equally significant, perhaps, are genetic inheritance, psychological hardiness, social support systems, and individual coping techniques.

Source: Adapted from Sarason, I. G., Johnson, J. H., & Siegel, J. M. (1978). Assessing the impact of life changes: Development of the Life Experiences Survey. *Journal of Consulting and Clinical Psychology, 46,* 932–946.

- *Challenge:* Hardy people perceive changes in life as challenges, or as stimulating opportunities for personal growth, rather than as threats. The breakup of a relationship, for example, may be seen less as a sad event than as the end of a chapter in which one has learned lessons applicable to the next relationship.

Social Resources Social support systems, or their absence, may make a vast difference in how well one psychologically deals with stress.[18] Some examples:

- *Being single:* In men between the ages of 25 and 64, single men have a higher rate than married men of deaths from heart disease. Indeed, the single, the divorced, and the widowed have higher death rates in general than married people do.

- *Social isolation:* People who are uninvolved with other people or organizations are more vulnerable to chronic disease. Those who are more geographically mobile—and hence presumably less socially connected—tend to have higher rates of depression, heart disease, and lung cancer.

- *Altruistic egoism:* **Altruistic egoism,** according to Selye, is the process of cooperation in which you help others satisfy their needs and they in turn help you satisfy yours. In one study, students who scored high on a test for adaptive potential, which included altruism (as well as adaptivity and creativity), showed fewer physical problems than those who did not.[19]

How strong your ties are to others can have an important bearing on how well you handle stress. Belonging to a group of kindred spirits can go a long way toward helping one deal with the stressors and stresses in life.

Suggestions for Further Reading

Friedman, Meyer, & Rosenman, Ray H. (1974). *Type A behavior and your heart.* Greenwich, CT: Knopf.

Selye, Hans (1974). *Stress without distress.* New York: Lippincott.

Selye, Hans (1976). *Stress in health and disease.* Reading, MA: Butterworths.

4 What Stress Does to You

▶ What are some physical reactions to stress?

▶ What are some psychological reactions to stress?

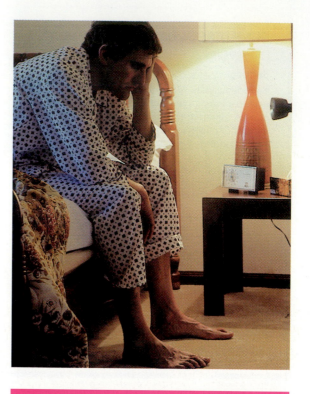

Would you admit that you occasionally suffer from **psychosomatic illnesses**—physical disorders caused by or worsened by psychological factors? Probably not, if you're like most people. Most of us will go to great lengths to avoid having others think that we are pretending sickness, called **malingering,** or that our illnesses are imaginary—**hypochondria**. "Our society has taught us not to be weak without a cause," says clinical psychologist Ivy Walker Wittmeyer.[20] (*See* ● *Figure 4.1*.)

Actually, we should take our "psychosomatic disorders" more seriously. Such symptoms as chronic headaches, abdominal pain, lower back pain, chest pain, and severe eyestrain often are stress-related conditions—and they affect almost everyone at one time or another. Let us consider these and other psychological and physical consequences of stress.

Physical Reactions: Your "Stress Site" and Other Matters

Physical reactions to stress may be expressed as particular problems in a particular part of one's body. Examples are skin problems, headache, gastrointestinal problems, ulcers, changes in the immune system, high blood pressure and heart disease, and difficulties during pregnancy.

All diseases, most stress experts seem to agree, are to some extent disorders of adaptation.[21] Often, however, the adaptation appears in a particular part of the body. Doctors sometimes talk about a person's *stress site* (or *stress*

● **Figure 4.1 The reality of psychosomatic illness**

"*Ask someone if he or she ever suffers from psychosomatic illness and bet on a flat-out 'no' for an answer.*

But people always seem to know someone else who experiences these so-called all-in-your-head diseases—conditions that make us feel awful even though doctors can't pinpoint why. Those ailments that seem to strike just when we're pressured to the limit.

Wary of being labeled hypochondriacs or malingerers, most of us closet our own psychosomatic aches and pains. . . .

Professionals who specialize in treating psychosomatic conditions hope this attitude will soon disappear. The ailments are as real as a clogged blood vessel or a wound, they say."

—Kathleen Doheny, Health & Fitness News Service. (1990, October 3). Illness "all in your head"? Maybe not. *San Francisco Chronicle*, p. B3.

organ)—the body part or area that is more prone to the effects of tension than others. Whatever the area—skin, head, stomach, bowel, and so on—pain in that place is often the first sign of stress. Respiratory conditions such as asthma, for example, can be excited by heightened stress. Muscle tension, felt as a knot in the neck or back, is a frequent stress reaction for many people. Some people grind their teeth. Others develop nervous tics or excessive perspiration.

Let's consider a few parts of the body apt to be affected by stress.

Skin If your skin takes a turn for the worse, it may be because of temperature, humidity, or cosmetics, but it may also be because of stress. Acne, hives, eczema, psoriasis, and herpes are among the stress-related skin conditions.

Head Headaches are of two major types:

- *Tension headaches:* The most common kinds of headaches are **tension headaches**, discomfort caused by involuntary contractions of muscles in the neck, head, and scalp.

- *Migraine headaches:* **Migraine headaches** have different causes. Blood vessels expand (dilate) in the brain, and chemicals leaked through the blood vessel walls inflame nearby tissues, sending pain signals. Migraine headaches often run in families.

Both types can be triggered by the kind of "hurry sickness" we have called Type A behavior, as well as by stress. While the tendency of most people is to treat themselves first, as with aspirin, visiting a physician is a good idea in order to rule out physical causes.

Gastrointestinal Tract The **gastrointestinal (GI) tract** consists of the stomach and large and small intestines. (*See* ● *Figure 4.2.*) The GI tract is the site of some common stress-related reactions, including **heartburn**, a burning discomfort in the lower part of the chest; **gastritis**, an inflammation of the membrane of the stomach; and **diarrhea**, frequent passage of unformed watery bowel movements.

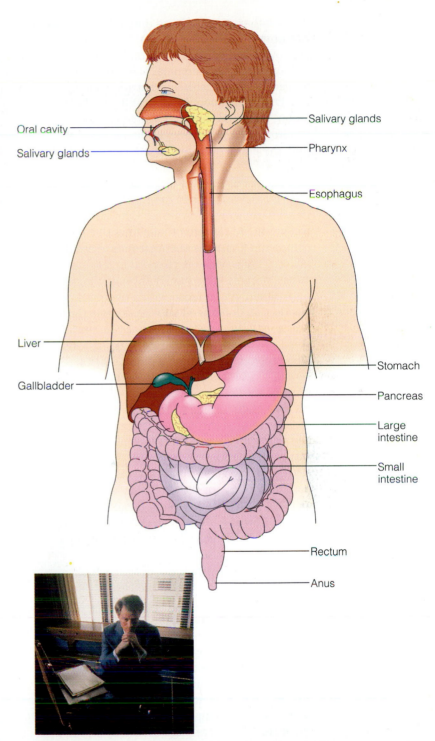

Oral cavity
Salivary glands
Salivary glands
Pharynx
Esophagus
Liver
Gallbladder
Stomach
Pancreas
Large intestine
Small intestine
Rectum
Anus

● **Figure 4.2 The gastrointestinal system.** The entire system includes the mouth, esophagus, stomach, and small and large intestines. Many people show stress-related reactions in the gastrointestinal system.

Another stress-related difficulty is **irritable bowel syndrome (IBS)**. IBS is characterized by chronic diarrhea or constipation accompanied by abdominal pain. According to a 4-year national health and nutrition survey, nearly 5 million people (almost 3% of the population) reported that they had irritable bowel syndrome.[22] Epidemiologist James Everhart puts the figure even higher, suggesting IBS afflicts 15–20% of the general population.[23]

The occurrence of IBS is linked to heightened stress rather than to physical abnormalities. Pharmacology professor Cynthia Williams has produced research that shows that a brain compound known as corticotropin-releasing factor (CRF), which is released in response to stress, propels food quickly through the colon.

"When you're faced with a tiger in the woods, you don't need your gastrointestinal functions," Williams says. "What you need, instead, is your heart pounding, sending a lot of blood to your muscles so you can quickly respond."[24] Eliminating food from the colon frees some of the body's blood supply so it can be used for "fight or flight." In addition, slowing the passage of food through the stomach makes you feel full, so you won't have to deal with hunger pangs while coping with danger.

For most people, however, meeting a tiger in the woods is not the problem—and thus IBS can be a highly inconvenient and embarrassing kind of distress. If this is an ongoing difficulty for you, you should definitely see a physician about it.

Many people still think of stomach ulcers as being stress-induced, as in the case of hard-driving business executives. Ulcers are open sores; **peptic ulcers**, caused by the action of digestive acids, develop in the lower esophagus, in the stomach lining, or in the first part of the small intestine (the duodenum) and create a burning pain in the upper abdomen. Ulcers may be associated with stress-*related* behavior, such as smoking, drinking, and taking aspirin-based painkillers. Ulcers are aggravated by stress, but they are not caused by stress itself.

More common reactions that stress produces in the stomach and digestive system are heartburn, stomach inflammation (gastritis), and diarrhea.

Immune System The **immune system** consists of the group of organs and tissues that protect your body against disease. It is still not clear why stress directly affects the immune system. Nevertheless, certain kinds of behavior and experiences can impair the immune system and make certain people more susceptible to disorders ranging from the common cold to cancer.[25, 26] For example, students faced with exam-related stress show a higher rate of infections than usual.[27, 28]

High Blood Pressure and Heart Disease
High blood pressure (hypertension), which affects perhaps 35 million Americans, is a serious risk factor in heart disease.[29] Although the causes of high blood pressure are not fully understood, some people appear to react to stress with a rise in blood pressure—sometimes several times a day.[30] In addition, cardiologist Meyer Friedman and other researchers have suggested a possible relationship between the stress associated with Type A behavior in some people and the development of heart disease.

Stress and Pregnancy Every pregnant mother experiences some stress, but pregnant women under severe stress may also affect the child they are carrying. A study led by psychology professor Christine Dunkel-Schetter reported that excessive stress during pregnancy may be related to premature birth.[31] There is also some evidence that maternal stress can lead to low birth weight, whether the birth is premature or the pregnancy is carried to full term.[32, 33]

Psychological Reactions to Stress

Among the emotional and behavioral reactions to stress are nervousness and anxiety, burnout, feelings of "personal victimization," and post-traumatic stress disorder.

Individual emotional reactions to stress cover such a wide range that we cannot describe them all. Eventually, if the stress is severe enough, frequent enough, and long enough, there can be various forms of mental illness. Among the emotional and behavioral reactions to stress are nervousness and anxiety, burnout, feelings of "personal victimization," and post-traumatic stress disorder. Let us consider these four types of reactions.

Nervousness and Anxiety When you feel constantly keyed up and irritable, are startled by small sounds, have trouble concentrating, feel a strong urge to cry or run away, or experience vague fears and feelings of dread without any obvious reason for them—these can be symptoms that you're suffering an unacceptable level of stress. Sometimes these feelings will express themselves in such behaviors as sleep disturbances (such as insomnia and nightmares), speech difficulties (such as stuttering), sexual problems, quarrels with family and friends, job mistakes and accidents, and various addictions—to television, to food, or to alcohol or other drugs.

Burnout Repeated emotional pressure can eventually cause **burnout**, a state of physical, emotional, and mental exhaustion. **Job burnout** is defined as a syndrome of emotional exhaustion, depersonalization of others, and a feeling of reduced personal accomplishment.[34] It is characterized by a loss of job satisfaction, confidence, performance, and morale, and by deteriorating productivity.[35]

Some researchers suggest that burnout evolves as a three-stage process, which somewhat reflects Selye's stages of stress:[36]

- *Stage 1—stress arousal:* In this early stage, the stress symptoms are increasing irritability and anxiety and sleep problems, such as insomnia.
- *Stage 2—energy conservation:* Here one experiences persistent tiredness and apathy, is often late for class or work, and may consume more coffee or alcohol than previously.

- *Stage 3—exhaustion:* In this late stage, people feel constant mental and physical fatigue and prefer isolation to social events. Depression is chronic, and some people have suicidal thoughts.

Burnout seems to be a modern disorder, afflicting a great many people. Students feel burned out at the end of final exams. Professional athletes burn out after years of intense competition. People in what are called the "helping professions"—people serving other people, such as teachers, psychologists, social workers, physicians, nurses, police officers, members of the clergy—are especially likely to experience burnout.

Burnout seems to be related to people's occupational conditions rather than to their psychological makeup, according to one study.[37] In terms of occupations, burnout seems to be associated with three external factors: repeated deadlines, too many demands, and too much responsibility. Burnout is reversible, but, more importantly, it is preventable.

Violence and Feelings of "Personal Victimization" Violence is a special kind of stressor—ugly, brutal, often sudden and terrifying. Besides physical consequences, violence—whether experienced or witnessed—can leave lifelong psychological effects.

Exposure to violence is more common than one might think, even among children.[38] For instance, on Chicago's violence-prone South Side, about one out of four middle-school and high-school students has seen someone killed and 35% have witnessed a stabbing.[39–41] Psychologist Rona Fields, who has studied children in war-torn areas such as Northern Ireland and southern Lebanon and troubled inner cities in the United States, finds a common thread in a progression from "fear to hate to violence."[42] That is, children learn to express their fear through terrorism or violence. (See ● *Figure 4.3.*) Boys exposed to violence, in fact, have a pattern of adjustment problems similar to those of abused boys.[43]

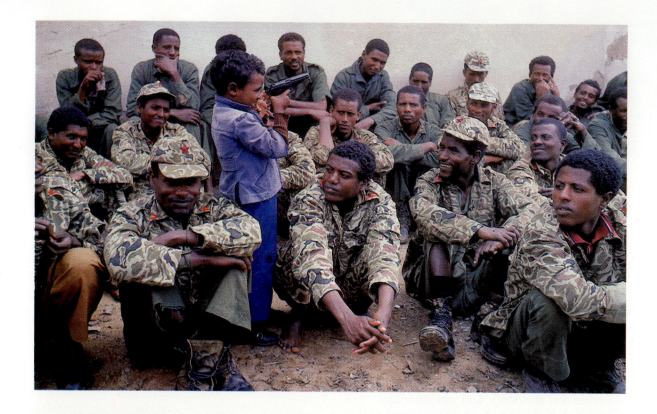

● **Figure 4.3 The children of violence.** For 25 years, psychologist Rona Fields has studied young victims in war-torn areas abroad and in ghettos in the United States.

" *The terror of children breeds many forms of terrorism. . . .*
Fear is sown in the brutalities children see every day, whether at the hands of occupying forces or in unpredictable street violence or beatings at home. Prejudicial hate grows when children objectify the source of their fear. In war-torn countries, that hate is turned toward the foreign oppressor. In the inner city, it is turned toward peers—'because if you don't see yourself as a viable human being, you don't see others as viable either,' Fields says. "

—Madeline Drexler (1990, July 1). Children of violence. *Boston Globe Magazine*; reprinted in *This World, The San Francisco Chronicle*, p. 23.

Spousal abuse is also commonplace. Perhaps 10–50% of all women who live with a male partner will be assaulted at least once during the relationship, according to some estimates.[44] Anxiety, depression, helplessness, living in constant fear, not knowing when the abuse will happen next, feeling that there's no escape—these are the feelings described by women battered by abusive men, according to Canadian Peter Jaffe, who has performed extensive studies of battered women.[45] These feelings, he found, were remarkably similar to those suffered by prisoners of war. As a result, Jaffe said, over time victims of abuse "visualize that the only way out is death—either their death or their captor's death."[46]

Researchers have discovered that victims of crime suffer adverse reactions far longer than anyone would have expected. "Victims of crime are ten times more likely than average to be severely depressed, even a decade or more later," says Dean Kilpatrick, director of the Crime Victims Research and Treatment Center at the University of South Carolina, "and they're two to three times more likely to have a phobia."[47] (A phobia is an exaggerated and persisting fear.) He found that depression lasting months or years occurred in about one out of ten victims of serious crimes like assault. One out of five rape victims later attempted suicide, and 40% had suicidal thoughts. Even nonviolent crimes can create considerable psychological damage because they alter a person's perception that the world is a secure place.

The term *personal victimization* has been proposed as a psychological diagnostic category by Stuart Kleinman, medical director of the Crime Victim Center, Brooklyn, N.Y. Kleinman lists the following as the principal emotional effects following a crime event.[48]

- *Sense of helplessness:* The world seems unsafe; victims lack confidence in their judgment and competence.

- *Rage at being a victim:* Intense anger is usually expressed toward family members and those who try to help; conversely, sometimes there is an inability to express any anger at anything.

- *Sense of being permanently damaged:* Rape victims, for example, may feel they'll never be seen as attractive again.

- *Inability to trust or be intimate with others:* This can include a loss of faith in institutions like the police or the court.

- *Persistent preoccupation with the crime:* Excessive concern with the crime and its details may reach the point of obsession.

- *Loss of belief that the world is just:* This may include self-blame—a sense of having done something to deserve being a victim.

The effects of crime and violence will probably grow: a 12-year-old American has an 80% chance of being the victim of a serious crime at some point, according to the National Institute of Justice.[49]

Post-Traumatic Stress Disorder Combat-related stress has had many names. In the Civil War it was called "nostalgia," in World War I "shell shock," and in World War II "combat fa-

tigue," although the true seriousness of this war-related condition may not have been fully recognized until after the Vietnam war.[50, 51] In 1980, the American Psychiatric Association, in its *Diagnostic and Statistical Manual of Mental Disorders*, Third Edition, finally named the behavioral disorder **post-traumatic stress disorder (PTSD)**.

It's important to note that PTSD is not just something that happens to combat victims. The disorder has also been found among rape victims, abused children, police officers involved in shooting incidents, terrorist-hijacking victims, parents of murdered children, mothers of AIDS victims, and others.[52–57]

PTSD is characterized by four conditions:[58]

- *Unusual violence:* The event the person has experienced is considered "outside the range of usual human experience and that would be markedly distressing to anyone," such as wartime events, rape, destruction of one's home.

- *Re-experiencing:* The traumatic event is relived through recollections, dreams, hallucinations, and symbols.

- *Avoidance:* The person avoids any stimuli associated with the event or experiences numbing, detachment, estrangement from others.

- *Arousal:* The person shows symptoms of increased arousal—sleep disturbances, irritability or anger, difficulty concentrating, hyperalertness, and jumpiness.

Getting Help Although the consequences of stress can be physically and emotionally severe, there are effective ways to cope with and manage stress. An important place to begin is to recognize that you do not have to manage alone. Instead, seek the assistance of a professional counselor, support group, physician, supportive friend, community mental health center, or other resource that makes sense to you. For the immediate management of a crisis, try a crisis hot line (listed in your telephone book, or check the toll-free numbers listed at the end of the following chapter).

5   The Art of Stress Management

▶ What are the principal stresses resulting from relationships and work?

▶ What stresses are created by economic differences?

▶ How do you handle stress now?

▶ What are five "strategies for living" that are ways of handling stress?

Which is more important—what happens to you or how you handle it? Try as we might, we can't always control what happens in our lives. Thus, learning how to manage stress—minimizing it, recovering from it—is more important. Indeed, the individuals called "peak performers" learn to make stress work *for* them.

The Stresses of Life

Two of the important pillars of life—love and work—are also two of the most important sources of stress.

The two hallmarks of a healthy maturity, Sigmund Freud thought, are the capacities to *love* and to *work*. Assuming our basic needs are taken care of, said the founder of psychoanalysis, for most of us the most important areas of life are (1) the people close to us and (2) the principal activity we work at. The domains of love and work certainly can and should be two sources of our greatest satisfactions. But precisely because they are so important, they can also produce our greatest stresses and crises.

The Stresses of Love: Communication and Miscommunication A lot of stresses occur because of miscommunication in our love relationships. Suppose you are a man driving along with your wife. "Would you like to stop for a drink?", she asks. "No," you answer truthfully, and continue driving. Later you become aware that your wife is quite irritated with you. Why? Because

she, in fact, had wanted to stop for a drink. Now you're feeling frustrated. "Why didn't she just say what she wanted?", you think. "Why did she play games with me?"

Recounting this incident, linguistics professor Deborah Tannen explains that the wife was annoyed not because she had not gotten her way but because her preference had not even been considered. "From her point of view," Tannen says, "she had shown concern for her husband's wishes, but he had shown no concern for hers."[59]

Such miscommunication can occur between members of the same sex too, of course. However, there are those such as psychologist Carol Gilligan who suggest that misunderstandings occur between the sexes because "men and women may speak different languages that they assume are the same. They are using similar words to talk about different experiences of self and social relationships."[60] Tannen, in fact, holds that male-female conversation is actually a kind of "cross-cultural" communication. It may have to do with how men and women see the world and derive meaning from it. For example, Tannen proposes that men think of life as a contest, a struggle to preserve their independence and to avoid failure. In this male world, conversations are "negotiations in which people try to achieve and maintain the upper hand if they can, and protect themselves from others' attempts to put them down and push them around." Women, on the other hand, feel that life is a community, a struggle to preserve intimacy and avoid isolation. In this female world, says Tannen, conversations are "negotiations for closeness in which people try to seek and give confirmation and support, and to reach consensus."[61]

If interacting with other people—both those close to us and others not so close—can be a great source of stress, so can being isolated from them. For instance, studies by Yale epidemiologist Leonard Syme and others found that those who were most isolated and had fewer feelings of being loved had coronary artery disease and death rates higher than did those with extensive social support networks.[62, 63]

The Stresses of Work It need hardly be pointed out that work-for-pay can be extremely stressful. On Sunday nights, after a weekend off, many people experience keen feelings of dread about going to work the next day. Stress at work may stem from tyrannical supervisors, unpleasant customers or coworkers, physical strains, boredom, constant deadlines, and many other difficulties. In addition, job stress may occur because many working Americans seem to be laboring at the wrong job: they are doing what they do only because of lack of choice, chance circumstances, or the influence of friends or relatives. Only 41% hold jobs that they had planned, according to a survey of 1350 people conducted for the National Occupational Information Coordinating Committee.[64] The poll also found that 25% of employed adults said job stress or pressure interfered with their off-the-job relationships, and 20% said such stress had affected their physical health.

If work is a major stressor, so is not working. When unemployment rises, it has been found that there are higher highway fatality rates, most likely due to stress.[65] There has also been found to be an increase in stroke deaths.[66] Suicide rates may also increase, according to research at Johns Hopkins University: every time unemployment rises by 1%, death rates have been noted to rise 1.9% and suicide rates by 4%.[67] However, other studies suggest that unemployment and suicide are not so closely connected.[68–70] For instance, some people may be so seriously depressed that they are unable to hold a job.

A great deal of toil—and consequent stress—is unpaid: housework, parenting, and schoolwork, for example. Domestic chores not only require a great deal of effort, they are one of the greatest sources of tension in a marriage, according to sociologist Arlie Hochschild.[71] Over an 8-year period Hochschild and others studied 52 couples as they cooked dinner, shopped, bathed their children, and the like. They found that these demands put a great deal of stress on a family. Housework produced stress not only because of the extra hours of work it entailed but also because of its effects on family relationships. Although men who *did* share the load at home seemed as pressed for time and as torn by the demands of work and children as did their wives, most men, Hochschild found, did not or were unable to share the housework load.

College, of course, is also a time of considerable stress. Alumni returning to campus may view with nostalgia students sunning themselves on the lawn while studying, but those students may be experiencing considerable anxiety. Indeed, there are many signs that the stress of college is very intense. One out of four students may be ready to drop out of school because of the effects of stress. Burnout is the largest single cause of students leaving school before receiving their degrees.[72]

The Stresses of Diversity

People of certain ages, abilities, economic levels, ethnic minorities, and from certain geographic areas experience more stress than others do.

All of us experience stresses quite apart from those produced by love and work. But members of some groups are more stressed than others. Some examples:

Age Certain time periods during one's life may be more stressful than others. According to one study, stress is particularly high during the following periods:[73]

- *Under age 25:* Some of the most significant decisions are made by young people, who deal with new relationships, colleges, marriages, pregnancies, and career choices. As previously mentioned, college itself, with its attendant deadlines and examinations, is a great source of stress.

- *Ages 40–44:* People in early middle age must cope with mortgage and other heavy expenses, changes in work responsibilities, deaths and illnesses of relatives, children moving out, and perhaps the beginning of menopause.

- *Over age 60:* People in later life may deal with financial changes caused by retirement, major illnesses and health changes, and death of a spouse.

Ability Being disabled produces stresses others might have no inkling of, according to several studies.[74, 75] For instance, one wheelchair-bound woman said her greatest difficulty is simply in getting around. Just because buses are equipped to pick up people in wheelchairs, she observed, doesn't mean that they do. "You get passed up by the drivers," she reported. "The equipment breaks down."[76] Because of such hindrances, independent disabled people often consider themselves "on time" to an appointment if they are half an hour early to half an hour late—but this is not a matter that gets much sympathy from many employers.

Economic Level As might be expected, the poor suffer great stress. Indeed, authors of a study of 140 of San Francisco's homeless people said that they found that the violence and harsh life caused many to display the same traumatic stress symptoms found in Vietnam combat veterans and survivors of airline crashes or earthquakes.[77] Their symptoms included nightmares or flashbacks of violent or disturbing experiences. Although the survey was criticized for its unscientific methodology, one of its authors nevertheless insisted that it indicated that homelessness should be treated as a mental health issue.

Minority Status Research indicates that blacks of all classes and ages continually experience more stress than whites do.[78, 79] If some of this stress may be associated with having low incomes, it has been shown that racism produces stress regardless of income. For instance, a nationwide study of 200 upper-income African-Americans by a University of Florida sociologist found they still face discrimination despite their economic advantages.[80] Blacks in the study reported numerous instances of hearing racial epithets and even of being suspected of being criminals. (A professor at a mostly white college described how she had been stopped by police because she was black and drove an older car.) Cultural differences have also been found to be a source of stress—for instance, among students on American campuses.[81, 82]

Geographical Area Where one lives geographically seems to relate to the pace of life, stress, and health. For example, a study of how rapidly or slowly people walk, talk, and work in four areas of the United States (Northeast, Midwest, South, and West) found that seven out of the nine fastest-paced cities were located in the Northeast. The West had the slowest pace overall. The pace of life within a given city and the rate of coronary heart disease were significantly related. For example, New York City had the highest rate of coronary heart disease and was the third fastest-paced city. The survey's principal author, psychology professor Robert Levine, suggests that fast-paced people both seek out and create time-urgent surroundings.[83]

Three-quarters of Americans live on just 1.5% of the land—that is, they live in urban or suburban areas. For many such people, there may be a fond nostalgia for an imagined rural life of simplicity and serenity. Others know better. "Farming," said economist John Kenneth Galbraith, who was raised on a farm in eastern Canada, "is the hardest kind of work there is." Rural life can be just as stressful as urban life. Indeed, farmers face the pressure of long hours, possible crop failure, and strong competition from large corporate farms.

How You Handle Stress Now: Are There Better Ways?

You can adapt to or cope with stress. Adaptation is not changing the stressor or stress. Some ways of adapting are escapes such as use of drugs, television watching, junk-food eating, or sleeping. Coping is changing the stressor or your reaction to it.

Regardless of your age—and stress certainly won't disappear after college—you are already finding ways to deal with stress in your life. The question is: Can your methods of reducing stress be improved?

Here are the two principal methods of dealing with stress:

- *Adaptation:* **Adaptation** is *not* changing the stressor or the stress.
- *Coping:* **Coping** *is* changing the stressor or changing your reaction to it.

Adaptations People sometimes adapt to stress through drug use and other self-indulgence. Coffee, cigarettes, and alcohol are all well-known legal drugs. Many people drink lots of coffee when under stress, although more

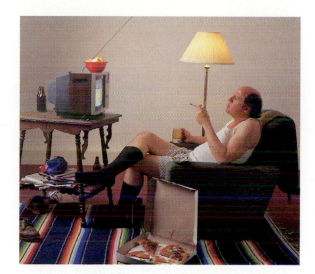

than four cups a day, depending on individual tolerance, can make you tense, "wired." Cigarettes also speed up your heart rate, may make it difficult to get going in the morning, and, of course, put you under the stress of always having to reach for another cigarette.

Alcohol seems to ease the strain of life temporarily, which is why it is so popular with so many people. The downside, however, is what too much drinking makes you feel like the next morning—jittery, exhausted, and depressed, all conditions that *increase* stress. Other drugs, such as tranquilizers, marijuana, and cocaine, may seem to provide relaxation in the short run, but ultimately they interfere with your ability to make realistic decisions about the pressures in your life and increase your stress.

The worry, anxiety, fear, anger, and depression that built-up stress creates can lead one to seek escapes other than drugs. Television is high on the list. The average American watches 4 hours of television a day.[84] Yet it has been found that television actually does *not* relax you.[85]

Overeating and junk-food snacking are favorite diversions of many people. The act of putting food in our mouths reminds us of what eased one of the most fundamental tensions of infanthood—hunger. Sleep, too, is often a form of escape from exhaustion and depression, and some individuals will spend more than the usual 6–9 hours required in bed. Withdrawal from the company of others is also usually an unhealthy form of adaptation.

Coping Let us now turn to five strategies for living that fight stress:

1. Reduce the stressors.
2. Manage your emotional response.
3. Develop a support system.
4. Take care of your body.
5. Develop relaxation techniques.

Strategy for Living #1: Reduce the Stressors

Reducing the source of stress is better than avoidance or procrastination.

"Reducing the stressors" seems like obvious advice, but it's surprising how long we can let something go on being a source of stress—usually because dealing with it is so uncomfortable. Examples: Falling behind in your work and having to explain your problem to your instructor or to your boss. Running up debts on a credit card or owing back taxes to the IRS.

It may not be easy, but all these problems are matters you can do something about, although getting the advice of a counselor may help. Avoidance and procrastination only make things worse.

Strategy for Living #2: Manage Your Emotional Response

You can't always manage the stressor, but you can manage your reactions. Techniques include understanding and expressing your feelings, feeling and acting positively, and keeping your sense of humor and having hope.

Learning how to manage your emotional response is crucial. Quite often you can't do anything about a stressor (being stuck behind a slow-moving truck on a mountain road, for example), but you can do something about your *reaction* to it (tell yourself that anger gets you nowhere, or choose to see a particular stressor as a challenge rather than a threat). Some techniques for managing your emotional response are the following.

Understand and Express Your Feelings

Understanding pent-up feelings is imperative. For instance, a study of students at Southern Methodist University found that those who kept a journal recounting traumatic events and their emotional responses had better immune function and reported fewer medical visits.[86]

Are you one who believes it's not becoming or appropriate to cry? Actually, crying helps. Widows who allowed themselves to cry over their husbands' deaths, according to one study, were not as apt to suffer stress-related diseases compared to widows who did not cry. In another study, 85% of women and 73% of men reported that crying made them feel better.[87]

Feel and Act Positively

To keep their spirits up, some people put up signs of positive affirmation on their bathroom mirrors or over their desks. For example:

- *Don't Sweat the Small Stuff.*
- *One Day at a Time.*
- *"Never Give Up."* —Winston Churchill.

Can you actually *will* yourself to feel and act positively and affirmatively? There is some evidence this is so.

Some studies have found that putting a smile on your face will produce the feelings that the expression represents. According to psychologist Robert Zajonc, "facial action leads to changes in mood."[88–90] Psychologists at the University of California, San Francisco, showed that when people mimic different emotional expressions, their bodies show changes in heart rate, breath rate, and other distinctive physiological patterns for each emotion.[91]

You can also make your "inner voice" a force for success. Positive "self-talk" can help you control your moods, turn back fear messages, and give you confidence.[92, 93] Positive self-talk, says clinical psychologist Harriet Braiker, is not the same as "mindless positive thinking, happy affirmations, or, even worse, self-delusion."[94] Rather, it consists of giving yourself positive messages—such as "You can do it. You've done it well before"—that correct errors and distortions in your thinking and help you develop a more accurate internal dialogue.

Braiker suggests there are three occasions when you should monitor your inner voice for negative thoughts, so that you can begin replacing your flawed ways of talking to yourself with better ways:

- *Event not as predicted:* When something happens to you that doesn't square with what you expected, it may be the result of negative self-talk. The example Braiker gives is when a newly divorced woman goes to a party expecting men to approach her but makes no effort to approach them; when no one comes up to her, that could be an opportunity for her to realize she was operating on the outmoded idea that "nice women don't start conversations with strangers."

- *Negative behavior toward others:* Ignoring the boss's orders or "forgetting" to attend meetings, for example, may be indicative of an employee's inappropriate self-talk.

- *Stressful life event:* A major personal transition or stressful life event may indicate the need to pay attention to self-talk. Crises may indicate old ways of looking at the world have become obsolete because of changing conditions in one's life.

These suggestions about self-talk represent some tenets of a school of psychology known as *cognitive therapy*. Cognitive therapy holds that beliefs and thoughts, as represented by one's words and assumptions, have the greatest impact on a person's emotions and behavior.

Keep Your Sense of Humor and Have Hope

Humor gained a lot of attention in the health profession when prominent magazine editor Norman Cousins published a 1979 book about his recovery from a painful connective-tissue disorder. Cousins discovered that by watching Marx Brothers films, old "Candid Camera" television episodes, and other funny movies, "10 minutes of genuine belly laughter had an anesthetic effect and would give me at least 2 hours of pain-free sleep."[95]

Since Cousins's revelations appeared, there has been a growing body of literature that *seems* to show that humor, optimism, and hope can help people conquer disease or promote their bodies' natural healing processes.[96, 97] For instance, one well-known champion of this view has been surgery professor Bernie Siegel, author of *Love, Medicine, and Miracles*, a book that is concerned not just with treating diseases but with healing lives.[98] Although there is some disagreement as to how much effect laughter and hope have on healing, so many accounts have been written of the positive results of these two qualities that they cannot be ignored.

Strategy for Living #3: Develop a Support System

Finding social support is vital for resisting stress. Sources of support are friends (in the true sense), counselors, and self-help and other support groups.

It can be tough to do things by yourself, so it's important to grasp a lesson that many people never learn: *You are not alone. No matter what troubles you, emotional support is available—but you have to reach out for it.*

Some forms of support are as follows.

Talk to and Do Things with Friends True friends are not just people you know. They are people you can trust, talk to honestly, and draw emotional sustenance from. (Some people you know quite well may actually not be very good friends in this sense because the way they interact with you makes you feel competitive, anxious, or inferior.) Friends can be people your own age or not, be related to you or not, be from groups of which you are a member—college, work, church, team, club—or not. Friends are simply those people you feel comfortable with. With a little training, people who are friends can learn to be counselors for each other.

In any case, it's vital to fight the temptation to isolate yourself. Studies show that the more students participate in activities with other students, the less they suffer from depression and the more they have feelings of health.[99]

Talk to Counselors You can get emotional support from counselors, paid or unpaid. Paid counselors may be psychotherapists, ranging from social workers to psychiatrists. Unpaid counselors may be clergy or perhaps members of the college health service.

Sources of free counseling that everyone should be aware of are telephone "hot lines," where, for the price of a phone call, callers can find a sympathetic ear and various kinds of help. (Hot lines are listed under the heading of *Crisis Intervention Service* in the telephone-book Yellow Pages. Other forms of stress counseling are listed under the heading *Stress Management and Prevention*.)

Join a Support Group This week an estimated 15 million Americans will attend one of about 500,000 meetings offered by some form of support group.[100] The number of these self-help organizations has probably quadrupled over the last decade, and the areas of concern they cover range from drug addiction to spouse abuse to compulsive shopping to stroke victims to various forms of bereavement.

In the true self-help group, membership is limited to peers; there is no professional moderator, only some temporarily designated leader who makes announcements and calls on people to share their experiences. This is in contrast with group-therapy groups, in which a psychologist or other therapist is in charge.

Support groups, whether self-help or group-therapy, don't just improve life, they may even prolong it. According to a 10-year study by psychologist David Spiegel and others, women with metastatic breast cancer who participated in group therapy (and instruction in pain control) added a year and a half of life.[101]

Strategy for Living #4: Take Care of Your Body

Taking care of the body helps alleviate stress in the mind. Techniques include eating, exercising, and sleeping right and avoiding drugs.

The interaction between mind and body becomes particularly evident when you're stressed: If you're not eating and exercising well, or are short on sleep, or are using drugs, these mistreatments of the body will only make the mind feel worse. In later chapters we show you in detail how to put the following "stress buster" techniques into effect, but we can get you off to an early start here.

Eat Right What is it about sugar and fat that makes them seem so desirable? Sugar not only tastes good—infants instantly become fond of it—but it *seems* to give you quick energy. Thus, when you're feeling run down, a candy bar, several cookies, or a couple of beers (alcohol contains sugar) seem to provide a pick-me-up. However, the lift that sugar gives you wears off very quickly.

Fat operates in a different way. Because fat takes a relatively long time to get through your digestive tract, it provides a satisfying feeling of fullness. But fat, such as that found in a meal of hamburgers, french fries, and ice cream, can also make you feel sluggish. Worse, a diet high in fat can put you in a high-risk category for heart attack and stroke.

If you only have time to follow a few pieces of health advice, let them be the following:

- *Reduce foods of animal origin:* Meat and dairy products are responsible for dietary fat, artery-clogging cholesterol, and a great many weight-adding calories. If you can revise your food choices so that your diet has less meat (particularly red meat), cheese (try lowfat cheese), greasy potato chips, ice cream, and the like, you not only will be healthier but also may lose weight.

- *Do yourself the fiber favor:* Whole grains, vegetables, and fruit not only have less sugar than candy bars (fruit has "naturally occurring" sugars, which are good) but also have fiber, which, it is thought, can help guard against the risk of colon cancer.

- *Drink water and juice:* Finally, drink water and juice rather than beverages such as coffee, sweetened soft drinks, or alcohol.

Exercise Right To those not used to it, exercise sounds like unexciting work, an expenditure of effort that simply makes one tired. Actually, once people become accustomed to exercise, they find it's a terrific stress reducer, energy enhancer, mental relaxant, sleep inducer, confidence builder, and, when done right, form of *fun*. Forty minutes of exercise can reduce stress for up to 3 hours afterward, whereas an equal period of rest and relaxation lowers stress for only 20 minutes, according to John Ragland of the University of Wisconsin sports psychology laboratory.[102]

Why does exercise seem not only to relax you but to re-energize you? One theory is that during exercise the body produces **endorphins**, opiate-like substances in the central nervous system that produce a mild euphoria resembling that produced by certain drugs such as morphine.

Different kinds of physical activity serve different purposes. Dancing or martial arts, for example, give you *flexibility*. Weight-lifting or mountain-climbing give you *strength*. Long-distance running, swimming, or bicycling give you *endurance*.

Exercise is a serious business, but if you don't make it interesting for yourself, you probably won't do it. It's best if you can commit yourself to 30 minutes four times a week of cardiovascular training (jogging, stair-climbing machine, stationary bike), plus some strength training.

Sleep Right We might envy the people we read about who supposedly need only 4 hours or less of sleep a night. (Generally, such people—Thomas Edison and Winston Churchill were among them—take frequent catnaps during the day.) However, if you sleep somewhere between 6 and 9 hours every night, you are within the normal range. Sleep is important because it is restorative: it helps you recover from the previous day's stresses and gives you energy to meet the stresses of the next day.

When you are under great stress you need even more sleep than usual. The *quality* of sleep is also important. Sleeping pills or alcohol may actually disrupt sleep so that you wake up in the morning feeling tired rather than energetic.

Avoid Drugs As we mentioned, the temptation of many drugs, whether legal or illegal, is that they *do* alleviate stress in the short run. In the long run, however, they not only come to have a powerful grip on your life (whether it is a "habituation" or a more serious "addiction") but they also damage the body. Alcohol, for instance, has extremely deleterious effects on the liver, brain, and nervous system—and thus greatly adds to the stress in one's life.

Strategy for Living #5: Develop Relaxation Techniques

Six relaxation techniques for de-stressing are (1) the "relaxation response," by slowing breathing and relaxing muscles; (2) progressive muscular relaxation, by tightening and relaxing muscle groups; (3) mental imagery, by visualizing a change; (4) meditation, by focusing on removing mental distractions; (5) mindfulness, by focusing on present thoughts; and (6) biofeedback, by monitoring and modifying physiological performance.

There is an entire body of activities *that most people in North America have never tried at all* that nonetheless have been found to be extremely effective stress reducers.[103] Several of these relaxation techniques were developed only within the last couple of decades or existed in other cultures but only recently have been tried on a wide scale in ours. These techniques are used to achieve the relaxation response.

The Relaxation Response As we have seen, the first stage of stress is a fight-or-flight response, a physiological reaction that is simply no longer appropriate for many of our day-to-day situations. The opposite of the fight-or-flight response, suggests cardiologist Herbert Benson, is what he calls the **relaxation response**—predictable, beneficial physiological changes that occur in both body and mind when one makes certain deliberate attempts to relax.[104, 105] Among these changes are slowed heart rate, lowered blood pressure, slowed and deep breathing, relaxed muscles—and (as shown by brain waves) a mind at peace. Once you have experienced the relaxation response, your body will be refreshed and have energy for several hours of work.

Deep Breathing One example of a relaxation technique is deep, slow breathing—useful when winding down from a tense telephone call, for instance. Try this technique now.

- *Breathe in:* Inhale through your nose, while gradually expanding first your abdomen and then your rib cage. (Imagine you're inflating a beach ball through your navel.)

- *Breathe out:* Release your breath through your nose, more slowly than you let it in, silently telling yourself "Relax." This technique takes only a few seconds to produce a calming effect.

Progressive Muscular Relaxation The technique of **progressive muscular relaxation** consists of reducing stress by tightening and relaxing major muscle groups throughout your body. Usually you start with your face and progress down to your toes (although some people do the reverse). (See ● *Figure 5.1.*)

An example of a quick (3-minute) version of the technique is as follows. (Try it now.)

- *Breathe in, hold, and tense:* Inhale, and hold your breath for 6 seconds. Simultaneously tense as many muscles as you can.

- *Breathe out, go limp, breathe:* Exhale quickly (with a whoosh). Let your body go limp. Breathe rhythmically for 20 seconds.

- *Repeat, relax, think peace:* Repeat twice. After the third cycle, relax for a few seconds and concentrate on a peaceful thought.

Mental Imagery Also known as **guided imagery** and **visualization**, **mental imagery** is a procedure in which you essentially *daydream* an image or desired change, anticipating that your body will respond as if the image were real. (See ● *Figure 5.2.*)

This technique has been used for:

- *Relaxation:* Mental imaging has been used very successfully for de-stressing and relaxation.

- *Habit change:* It has been used for changing habits, such as quitting smoking.

- *Healing:* It has been used to assist in healing (as in picturing one's immune system as sharklike cells eating up cancer organisms).

- *Improving performance:* It has been used for enhancing performance (imagining the outcome of a tennis serve or basketball shot, or the presentation of a speech).

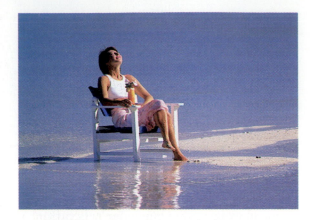

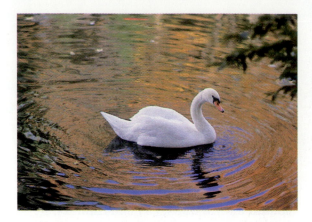

● **Figure 5.1 The progressive muscular relaxation technique.** It is recommended that you practice this technique for 10–20 minutes.

The progressive muscular relaxation technique is as follows:

- *Get comfortable and quiet:* Sit down or lie in a comfortable setting where you won't be disturbed. Close your eyes.
- *Become aware of your breathing:* Breathe slowly in through your nose. Exhale slowly through your nose.
- *Clench and release your muscles:* Tense and relax each part of your body two or more times. Clench while inhaling. Release while exhaling.
- *Proceed through muscles or muscle groups:* Tense and relax various muscles, from fist to face to stomach to toes. A good progression is: right fist, right biceps, left fist, left biceps, right shoulder, left shoulder, neck, jaw, eyes, forehead, scalp, chest, stomach, buttocks, genitals, and so on, down through each leg to the toes.

● **Figure 5.2 Mental imagery.** It's recommended you devote 10–20 minutes to this procedure, preferably daily or several times a week.

To practice mental imagery, do the following:

- *Get comfortable and quiet:* Remove your shoes, loosen your clothes, and sit down or lie in a comfortable setting, with the lights dimmed. Close your eyes.
- *Breathe deeply and concentrate on a word or phrase:* Breathe deeply, filling your chest, and slowly let the air out. With each breath, concentrate on a simple word or phrase (such as "One," or "Good," or a prayer). Focus your mind on this phrase to get rid of distracting thoughts. Repeat.
- *Clench and release your muscles:* Tense and relax each part of your body, proceeding from fist to face to stomach to toes.
- *Visualize a vivid image:* Create a tranquil, pleasant image in your mind—lying beside a mountain stream, floating on a raft in a pool, stretched out on a beach. Try to involve all 5 senses, from sight to taste.
- *Visualize a desired change:* If you're trying to improve some aspect of your performance, such as improving a tennis serve, visualize the act in detail: the fuzz and seam on the ball, the exact motion of the serve, the path of the ball, all in slow detail.

Meditation An age-old technique, **meditation** is concerned with directing a person's attention to a single, unchanging or repetitive stimulus as a way of quelling the "mind chatter" that goes on in the heads of all of us. Because meditation has a long history in Eastern religions (as in yoga), it has a reputation of being "strange" to people in North America. However, when the religious and philosophical connotations are stripped away, the act of meditation itself is not mysterious at all. Its purpose is simply to eliminate mental distractions and relax the body. (*See* ● *Figure 5.3.*)

A study done at Harvard University found that elderly people who were taught Transcendental Meditation (a technique that became popular in the 1960s and 1970s and that introduces a deep state of rest) lived longer than their peers.[106]

Mindfulness A state of active attention, **mindfulness** that involves focusing completely on the here-and-now. In this state, you focus on becoming aware of all *present* thoughts and sensations rather than the "mind chatter" judgmental thoughts ("I should," "What if," "I never") that the mind seems to generate. (*See* ● *Figure 5.4.*)

The purpose of mindfulness is to obsessively focus on the present so that you can clear your mind, which calms the body. This may begin with paying precise attention to your breathing, noticing each small aspect of it. Gradually, according to one writer, "you extend this attention to everything you do. As you walk, you notice each step with the same microscopic focus: the shift of weight from one leg to another, the contact with the ground."[107]

A study of elderly patients in nursing homes found that those who received mindfulness training had lower blood pressure and a better mortality rate than those who did not receive such training.[108]

Biofeedback The technique of **biofeedback** involves the self-monitoring and modification of one's own physiological performance. This form of de-stressing requires an electronic instrument that can detect internal changes in your body and communicate them back to you through a light, tone, or meter. (*See* ● *Figure 5.5.*)

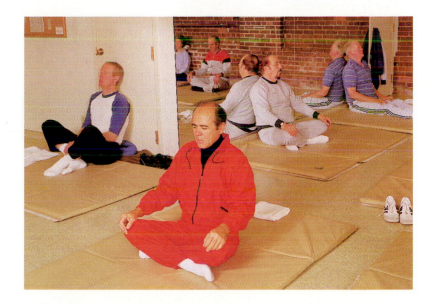

● **Figure 5.3 Meditation.** Meditation includes the repetition of a word, sound, phrase, or prayer. Whenever everyday thoughts occur, they should be disregarded, and you should return to the repetition. The exercise should be continued for 10–20 minutes and practiced once or twice daily.

"● *Pick a focus word or short phrase that is firmly rooted in your personal belief system. For example, a Christian person might choose the opening words of Psalm 23, "The Lord is my shepherd"; a Jewish person, "Shalom"; a nonreligious individual, a neutral word like "One" or "Peace."*

● *Sit quietly in a comfortable position.*

● *Close your eyes.*

● *Relax your muscles.*

● *Breathe slowly and naturally, and as you do, repeat your focus word or phrase as you exhale.*

● *Assume a passive attitude. Don't worry about how well you're doing. When other thoughts come to mind, simply say to yourself, "Oh, well," and gently return to the repetition.*"

—Herbert Benson, M.D. (1989). Editorial: Hypnosis and the relaxation response. *Gastroenterology, 96,* 1610.

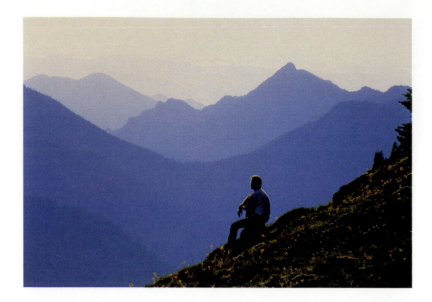

Biofeedback is a procedure in which a person is attached to a machine that monitors biological ("bio") processes such as blood pressure or heart rate. This information is then "fed back" electronically. Biofeedback techniques help people relax "by signaling lowered muscle tension, improved blood flow in the extremities, or reduced sweat gland activity," according to clinical psychologist Laurence Miller.[109]

A specialist in biofeedback is necessary to help people get connected to, and train them in the use of, a biofeedback machine. Training then proceeds as follows:

- *Developing body awareness:* You become familiar with the sensations and functions of your body—heart rate, muscle tension, body temperature, brain waves—and what kinds of thoughts and ideas increase or decrease them.

- *Learning to control body functions:* With practice, you learn how to slow your heart rate and relax other functions by adjusting your thoughts and images.

- *Learning to do without the machine:* In time, you can learn to produce the same physiological signs of relaxation without the assistance of a biofeedback machine.

> ● **Figure 5.4 Mindfulness.** Psychologist Jon Kabat-Zinn, director of the Stress Reduction and Relaxation Program at the University of Massachusetts Medical Center, offers seven "attitudes" that form what he calls *awareness/mindfulness.*
>
> *Seven attitudes for awareness/mindfulness—paying attention and seeing things as they are:*
>
> - *Nonjudging:* You become aware of the automatic judgmental thoughts passing through your mind.
> - *Patience:* You become open to each moment, knowing that some things cannot be hurried.
> - *Beginner's mind:* You try to see everything as if for the first time, to look at the familiar (even family and friends) with fresh eyes.
> - *Trust:* You try to learn to trust your own intuition, despite your mistakes, rather than to habitually look to outside authority for guidance.
> - *Non-striving:* Instead of always striving for results, you focus on accepting things as they are, so that movement toward your goals takes place by itself.
> - *Acceptance:* Denying and resisting what is already fact and trying to force situations to be the way you would like them to be often just add to the tension. While you need not be satisfied with things as they are (how you look, for example), by having the willingness to accept the picture of things as they are you are in a better position to change them.
> - *Letting go:* Letting go is like what you do when you go to sleep at night. The opposite is when your mind will not shut down.

Enhancing Your Performance: Making Stress Work for You, Not Against You

Stress can be made to work as a form of performance enhancement through such techniques as stress inoculation training.

Unquestionably, the recognition of stress as a commonplace feature of our lives has had some benefits. "Psychologists who specialize in treating workers who are resistant to traditional psychotherapy owe a lot to stress," writer Ronni Sandroff points out. "The enthronement of stress as a socially acceptable psychological problem has opened an avenue for therapy avoiders who wrestle with anxiety, depression, or addiction."[110]

One kind of therapy called **stress inoculation training**, developed by Donald Meichenbaum, consists of three phases:[111]

- *Conceptualization:* This is an education phase that emphasizes the development of a warm, collaborative relationship between a highly anxious individual and a therapist.

- *Skill acquisition and rehearsal:* In this phase, the anxious individual is trained in relaxation coping skills.

- *Application and follow-through:* In this final phase, the individual is rehearsed in role-playing, simulations, and imagery—for example, relaxation coping skills.

Equally important is the recognition of stress as key to *performance enhancement.* This area was first developed by sports psychologists to teach athletes how to psych themselves up or calm themselves down, so they can maintain the peak emotional context for their performance.

800-HELP

Crisis Line: 800-866-9600   Available 24 hours. Provides counseling on suicide, pregnancy, substance abuse, domestic violence, child abuse, sexual abuse, and other crisis situations. Also provides local referrals.

National Child Abuse Hotline: 800-422-4453 Available 24 hours. Provides phone counseling and local referrals.

National Domestic Violence Hotline: 800-333-SAFE   (For hearing impaired: 800-873-6363.) Available 24 hours. National organization of shelters and support services for battered women and their children.

Suggestions for Further Reading

American Health editors, with Daniel Goleman and Tara Bennett-Goleman. (1986). *The relaxed body book.* New York: Doubleday.

Benson, Herbert (1987). *Your maximum mind.* New York: Times Books.

Girdano, Daniel A., & Everly, George S., Jr. (1986). *Controlling stress and tension.* Englewood Cliffs, NJ: Prentice-Hall.

Kabat-Zinn, Jon (1990). *Full catastrophe living.* New York: Delacorte Press.

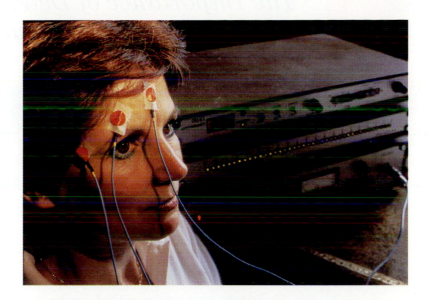

● Figure 5.5 Biofeedback. By attending to the feedback of this machine, people can change some functions, such as blood pressure, that were previously thought to be beyond a person's control.

"Imagine playing a video game blindfolded and earplugged. Such sensory deprivation would make it impossible to play well. It's the same with many signals from the body that are relevant to health and illness, such as blood pressure, skin temperature, or the level of contraction in various muscles. These subtle signals are below the threshold of normal awareness. And what you can't detect, you can't control.

Biofeedback makes that detection possible. . . . 'Bio' refers to an imperceptible physiological process, such as blood pressure. It's picked up by a special device and electronically amplified into a perceptible tone or other signal that is 'fed back' to the patient. The signal then guides him or her to increase or decrease activity in one of several of the body's systems."

—Laurence Miller (1989, November). What biofeedback does (and doesn't) do. *Psychology Today,* p. 22.

The Importance of Determining and Finding Meaningful Work

Work, we said, can be one of life's major stressors, both positive and negative. It's important, then, that we try to ensure that the work causing us such stresses is meaningful and work that we want to do.

Do you agree or disagree with the following statements about jobs and careers? Indicate "T" (True) or "F" (False).

__ **1.** Work hours have been going down and leisure hours have been going up during the last 20 years.

__ **2.** Despite occasional grumbling, most people enjoy their work.

__ **3.** However much they work, most people would rather spend more time with their families.

__ **4.** Clearly, most people make a conscious choice of their job or career, or they wouldn't be doing it.

1. Which Are Increasing— Work Hours or Leisure Hours?

Are we improving on the 8-hour day and 40-hour week for which the trade union movement fought earlier in the century? Consider:

- *More hours at work:* The average American employee works 42 hours a week (men 45, women 38), but many seem to be working even longer.[112] In 1989, among 88 million people with full-time jobs, nearly a quarter of them were working 49 hours a week or more, up from 18% 10 years previously, according to the Bureau of Labor Statistics.[113] Moreover, more people are working overtime or holding down second jobs, and the number of families with two or more wage earners has been steadily increasing.

- *The myth of leisure:* A 1987 Louis Harris survey found that the number of leisure hours for Americans aged 18 and over has dropped from 26.2 hours in 1973 to 16.6 hours in 1987.[114] The average U.S. worker gets only 14 paid vacation days, compared to 17½ paid vacation days for the hard-working Japanese, who don't tend to take them, and 6–7 *weeks* for the Germans (West Germans, at the time of the survey), who do.[115] "The leisure society in America is a myth," says Jerome Rosow, president of the Work in America Institute.[116]

Why work? Especially, why work so long and so hard? People give many reasons: Most say they must make ends meet; living standards have been eroded by taxes and inflation back to levels not seen in 5 years.[117] Others say they relish the hustle. Still others say they are scared of the competition or they are afraid they will be let go.

2. Are People Happier Working or Not Working?

As a child, how happy did you think you'd be when you grew up? In one survey, four out of five children ages 8–12 interviewed in 1989 thought they'd have as much or more fun when they became adults.[118] However, most grown-ups have to work for a living, of course, and what is it that today's adult workers feel? Some answers:

- *A preference for something other than work:* In general, 60% say they enjoy their *non*working time most, while only 18% say they prefer being at work.[119] Monday, say most people, is their least favorite day of the week, the morning hours are the least favorite hours of the day, and more than half would rather work a 4-day, 10-hour work week than the standard 5-day week (a change from 1971, when most preferred the 5-day week).

- *Stress and burnout:* The pace of work may be taking its toll in stress and burnout.

"They're in a time-compressed state," says psychiatrist Joseph Ruffin about some of his patients. "They've got more bellyaches and more headaches. They've got more diarrhea. I ask my patients: 'What if you were an automobile? What shape would you be in?' They say, 'I wouldn't last 3 weeks.' "[120]

- *The dissatisfaction of life at the top:* Even people in some of the more prestigious professions are unhappy with their work. Lawyers, for instance, are increasingly dissatisfied, and the number saying they are "very satisfied" with their work dropped 20% since 1984, according to an American Bar Association survey.[121] Clinical psychologist Steven Berglas, author of *The Success Syndrome*, has discovered that numerous high achievers—his patients include physicians, judges, venture capitalists, investment bankers, models, professional athletes, and executives—demonstrate that "life at the top can actually cause its own problems."[122] Many financially successful people, he found, were substance abusers, often depressed, given to self-destructive behavior, and had poor relationships.

Even young people have discovered that work is not all it's cracked up to be. Despite notions that after-school work "builds character," studies show that teenagers who "work long hours in today's routinized adolescent workplace of mostly dead-end jobs are more cynical about the value of hard work . . . than their peers who work less or not at all," say the authors of *When Teenagers Work*.[123] Moreover, contrary to public opinion, most student workers don't save their earnings for college but instead spend them on cars, fashions, stereo equipment, and alcohol and other drugs.

3. Is Family More Important Than Work?

What would most people rather do *instead* of work? Among those who are parents, nearly 40% of fathers and 80% of mothers answering a *Los Angeles Times*-commissioned survey said they would quit their jobs, if they could, to raise their children at home.[124] Parents are apparently motivated to join the rat race by what is one of the biggest concerns in raising children: money. But providing financial security and being around to pass on values to their children—the two top responsibilities of parenthood—seem to be on a collision course.

Women in particular have led the push for flexible work scheduling, part-time jobs, or switching to slower-paced careers, in an attempt to balance career and family life. Some work at full-time jobs but attempt to limit their business travel and daily schedules. Others quit to do consulting work from their homes. Says Judy Pesin, 38, a former Citicorp vice president who used to work 12-hour days but switched to part-time work after the birth of her child, "Unless I'm inventing a cure for AIDS, unless I'm really making a major social contribution, it's not worth missing my daughter growing up."[125]

Men, too, wish for such choices. More than half of 500 men polled by Robert Half International, an executive recruiting firm, said they'd be willing to cut their salaries by as much as one-fourth to have more family or personal time.[126] But the majority feel that cutting back is not an option. This does not mean they value their careers more: A survey for *Men's Life* magazine found that five of every eight men picked marriage as the top priority—above money, sex, fame, and career.[127]

How do men resolve the conflict of not doing right by their families yet wanting to hold down their jobs? Professor Robert Weiss, author of *Staying the Course: The Emotional and Social Lives of Men Who Do Well at Work*, has some ideas. "I think men resolve it by saying, 'I'm contributing to my family by knocking myself out at work. . . .' "[128] If they give more energy to their work than to their family, he suggests, "that's because work is so fundamental to everything else. It isn't that they care more for work than family. It's that work makes it possible for them to be the kind of person for their family they feel they ought to be."[129]

One element is most important in achieving a successful life, according to Aristotle: *balance.* Clearly, it's important that we somehow find a balance between work and the rest of our lives.

4. Do People Choose Their Work?

"Everyone wants a clear reason to get up in the morning," observes writer Dick Leider. "As humans we hunger for meaning and purpose in our lives. At the very core of who we are, we need to feel our lives matter . . . that we do make a difference."[130]

What is that purpose? "Life never lacks purpose," says Leider. "Purpose is innate—but it is up to each of us individually to discover or rediscover it. And, it must be discovered by oneself, by one's own conscience."

Unfortunately, for a great many people, work does not give them that sense of purpose. As we stated elsewhere, the majority of Americans may be working at the wrong job. That is, according to a Gallup Poll, only 41% of the respondents consciously chose the job or career they are in. Of the rest, 18% got started in their present job through chance circumstances, 12% took the only job available, and the remainder were influenced by relatives or friends. *Nearly two thirds said that, given a chance to start over, they would try to get more information about career options.*[131] Perhaps, then, you are in a good position to take advantage of others' hindsight: Get as much information as you can about careers and jobs. Avoid aimlessness.

The biggest-selling job-hunting book of the past 10 years (288 weeks on the *New York Times* best-seller list) is *What Color Is Your Parachute?*, which is revised annually.[132] Its author, Richard Bolles, a former Episcopal priest, offers several insights on finding that "lucky" job.[133] Luck, he says, favors people who:

- Are going after their dreams—the thing they really want to do most in the world.
- Are prepared.
- Are working hardest at the job-hunt.
- Have told the most people clearly and precisely what they are looking for.
- Treat others with grace and dignity, courtesy and kindness.

Why work?, we asked earlier. Most people *think* they know the answer. To earn money to put bread on the table. To support their families. To afford to do the things they want to do when they're *not* working.

Philosopher Jacob Needleman, author of *Money and the Meaning of Life*, disagrees.[134] In the seminars that he gives about people and money, he says, the most common question he hears is, "How do I engage in making a living and still keep my soul?"[135] To figure out the answer to "Why work?" is to begin to figure out the purpose of your life.

Suggestions for Further Readings

Bolles, Richard Nelson (1994). *What color is your parachute? A practical manual for job-hunters and career changers.* Berkeley, CA: Ten Speed Press. The classic career self-help book. Engagingly written, revised annually.

Needleman, Jacob (1991). *Money and the meaning of life.* New York: Doubleday/Currency. Using his experience in seminars given around the world, a philosopher examines how money influences our emotional and spiritual lives.

Electronic Resumes: On-Line Employment

Many of the jobs of the future will be found by going "on-line"—by posting your resume on an electronic database accessible by telephone-linked computer. Following are some services that, for a fee, will make your resume available to prospective employers. (Fees may have changed over time.)

1. CompuServe Information Service
   5000 Arlington Centre Blvd.
   P.O. Box 20212
   Columbus, OH 43220
   (800) 848-8199
   Offers Adnet Online database, specialized forums such as WORK (job listings and networking for people who work from home), JFORUM (job listings and networking for journalists) and PRSIG (job listings and networking for public relations people).
   Fee: No charge (apart from CompuServe's connect fee) for job seekers to search databases and forums; employers and job seekers placing ads on Adnet pay fees depending on length of listing and amount of time it stays in the system. Searchable by employers and job seekers.

2. Career Network
   Information Kinetics Inc.
   640 N. LaSalle St.
   Suite 560
   Chicago, IL 60610
   (800) 828-0422
   Fee: $50 for three-month enrollment ($150 a year); no extra connect charges; users get 30 free E-mail messages per month and pay 50 cents for each additional message. The company's KiNexus resume database service charges job seeker $19.95 for up to a year (free to recent and pending graduates through college placement center). Searchable by job seekers, employers and college placement officers.

3. Job Bank USA
   1420 Spring Hill Rd.
   Suite 480
   McLean, VA 22102
   (703) 847-1706 (phone)
   (703) 847-1494 (fax)
   Fee: Charges job seekers up to $30 for one-year enrollment in resume database; charges employers up to $100 for each database search. Searchable by Job Bank employees only.

4. National Resume Bank
   c/o Professional Association of Resume Writers
   3637 Fourth St. North
   Suite 330
   St. Petersburg, FL 33704
   (813) 896-3694 (phone)
   (813) 894-1277 (fax)
   Fee: Charges job seekers $25 for three-month listing; free to employers. Searchable by employers only.

5. Prodigy Interactive Personal Service
   445 Hamilton Ave.
   White Plains, NY 10601
   (800) 284-5933
   Offers Adnet Online, TPI Online Classifieds, databases.
   Fee: No charge (apart from $12.95 a month Prodigy subscription fee) for job seekers to search the databases; employers and job seekers pay fees to place ads. Searchable by employers and job seekers.

6. Resumes-on-Computer
   c/o The Curtis Publishing Co.
   1000 Waterway Blvd.
   Indianapolis, IN 46202
   (317) 636-1000 (phone)
   (317) 634-1791 (fax)
   Fee: No charge to job seekers (though resumes must be converted via special software to ASCII text file and sent to Curtis by a quick printer, trade association or other resume-preparation group); employers pay $1.20 per resume retrieved and $1.70 a minute to access the system. Searchable by employers only.

7. Resumes: On-Line
   3140 K South Peoria
   Suite 142
   Aurora, CO 80014
   (303) 337-4818 (modem)
   (303) 337-2420 (phone)
   Fee: $29.95 for job seekers, free to employers during service's introduction. Searchable by Colorado-area employers.

Source: Anonymous. (1992, October). Online information. *PC Today*, p. 41.

UNIT

3

Psychological Health:
The Power of the Mind

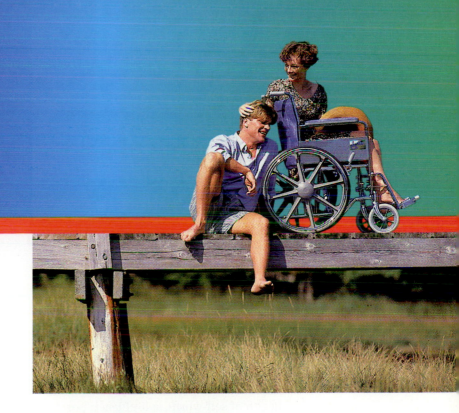

Are mind and body interrelated?

"Is there a split between mind and body?" a comedian asks. "And if so, which is better to have?"

The joke touches on one of people's most fundamental beliefs: we tend to think of mind and body as being separate. We even consult different medical specialties for different problems. For a heart pain we seek physical treatment; for what we call a "heartache" we seek psychological relief.

In fact, mind and body *are* interrelated. For instance, your body reacts the same whether a threat is real or imagined—whether you have that rush of terror as you swerve your car to avoid a collision or have that surge of anxiety that you might miss a deadline: both experiences can send your heart racing and blood pressure sky high.

Understanding the interconnectedness of mind and body is one of the most important lessons one can ever learn. Indeed, it is central to the art of living.

3.2

*Unit 3
Psychological
Health: The
Power of the
Mind*

6 In Search of Psychological Well-Being

▶ What is psychological health?

▶ What are the various views of how people develop their personalities?

▶ Describe the different views of Freud, Erikson, Piaget and Kohlberg, the trait theorists, the behaviorists, the social-learning theorists, and the humanists.

▶ Explain the importance to psychological health of self-worth, self-efficacy, personal control and responsibility, optimism, enjoyment and happiness, creativity, risk-taking and self-reinvention, and giving and receiving love.

Some days are diamonds, some days are duds. And some days are both, a roller coaster of moods.

You can go from terror on awaking late on the day of a test, to anxiety as you fight traffic jams to get to campus, to relief when you discover the test isn't as difficult as you had thought, to confidence that you "aced" the test when you leave the examination room. You can go from anger and resentment when your boss speaks harshly to you at your job, to happiness when a co-worker praises you, to gloom when someone breaks a date, to happiness when you are invited to a special celebration. If this is a normal range of emotions, how can we identify emotional and mental health?

The Meaning of Psychological Health

Psychological health includes mental (intellectual) health and emotional health. Mental or intellectual health refers to thoughts, emotional health to feelings. Psychological health may be thought of as being on a continuum of well-being.

One often hears the expressions "mental health" and "emotional health," but we prefer the term **psychological health,** which refers to the state of *both* mental and emotional well-being. In our usage, "mental" refers to *thoughts*. Having good **mental health** or **intellectual health** means one has the ability to think reasonably clearly and to avoid wildly distorting reality. The word "emotional" refers to *feelings*. Having good **emotional health** means one has the ability to be aware of and express one's feelings in an appropriate way.

As with physical health, perhaps the best way to think about psychological health is as a range or continuum. That is, as psychiatrist Karl Menninger has proposed, psychological states fall into a range, from severe psychological illness to optimal psychological well-being. (*See ● Figure 6.1.*)

Psychological difficulties are not at all uncommon. Indeed, at some point in their lives, one-third of all Americans feel they have what they perceive to be a shameful secret—namely, a problem related to psychological ill health or to drugs. At least this is what was found in a National Institute of Mental Health study of 18,571 people aged 18 and over, which was conducted in five geographical areas from 1980 to 1984.[1] With such 1-in-3 odds, you can see that it is not just possible but *quite likely* that you or someone you know has suffered or will suffer from some psychological ills. Unfortunately, very few people—only one in five—get help for their psychological health needs.

Your Personality

Such traits and attributes as motives, thoughts, emotions, and behaviors constitute your personality. Among the theories about how the human personality is developed are the Freudian view, Erikson's view, Piaget's and Kohlberg's views, trait theory, the behaviorist view, social-learning theory, and the humanistic view.

You have a certain amount of courage, patience, creativity, intelligence, and lovingness—as well as some less sterling traits, of course.

The combination of these and other characteristics and attributes constitutes your **personality,** the unique mixture of consistent motives, thoughts, emotions, and behavior that distinguish you from other people.

There are various theories about how the human personality is developed, many of which are based to varying degrees on the inter-play of hereditary and environmental influences. Among them are the theoretical notions of Freud, Erikson, Piaget, Kohlberg, the behaviorists, and the humanists, as well as trait theory and social-learning theory.

The Freudian View: Psychoanalysis Sigmund Freud (1856–1939), an Austrian physician, developed **psychoanalysis,** which is both a theory and a method of treatment. Psychoanalytic theory holds that the mind has dual levels: the **conscious** mind, of whose thoughts and feelings we are aware, and an **unconscious** mind, consisting of underlying motives, thoughts, and memories of which we are not aware. Psychoanalysis as a method of treatment is considered a "talking cure." Freud believed that if emotionally disturbed people could recall memories of early traumatic (strongly unpleasant) experiences, the resultant **catharsis**—the release of pent-up tensions—could help them gain relief from their irrational impulses.

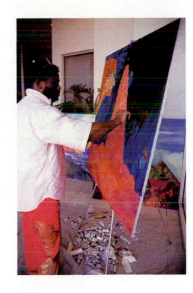

● **Figure 6.1 The hierarchy of psychological health.** Psychiatrist Karl Menninger has suggested that psychological states can be ranked in levels, according to increasing decline in coping ability.

Optimal mental health

Normal coping devices and ego control

Level 1

Hyperreactions

Anxiety

Nervousness

Minor physical symptoms

Level 2

Personality disorders

Phobias

Level 3

Social offenses

Open aggression

Violent acts

Level 4

Severe depression and despondency

Psychotic and bizarre behavior

Level 5

Severe psychological deterioration

Loss of will to live

Level of Dysfunction

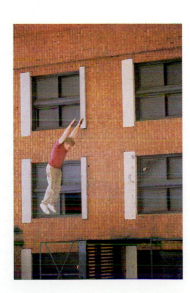

3.4

*Unit 3
Psychological
Health: The
Power of the
Mind*

Freud's theory also has a number of important ideas about how personality is developed:

- *Six stages of psychosexual development:*
Freud held that **psychosexual pleasure**—the pleasurable feelings that arise from stimulation of parts of the body—begins long before sexual maturity. Young children, he thought, respond in what he called a "sexual" way to stimulation of the mouth, the anus, and other body zones. Behind this lies a form of psychosexual energy that he called **libido,** which he felt provides the energy for much of our behavior. Freud believed that human behavior was formed by age 5. He also believed that human behavior was linked to conflict, especially conflict associated with aggressive and sexual impulses.

  Children go through six stages of **psychosexual development**, each with a characteristic sexual emphasis, ranging from the oral stage in the first year to the genital period at and following puberty. If normal development of one of these stages is frustrated, Freud theorized, it produces a **fixation**—the adult continues to be preoccupied with the pleasure area associated with that stage.

- *Parts of the psyche—id, ego, superego:*
One's personality, Freud proposed, consists of the **psyche,** the sum of all mental activity, including the conscious and unconscious. The psyche consists of three parts:

  (1) The **id** (the "I want"), which operates unconsciously, consists of all our biological instincts, such as hunger and sex. It constantly seeks pleasure and immediate gratification ("I want to eat that *now*!").

  (2) The **ego** (the "I will") is the rational, decision-making component. It controls and regulates the id's instinctual demands and is guided by what is realistic and socially acceptable ("You need to wait in line to get fed").

  (3) The **superego** (the "I should") consists of the internalized social standards of right and wrong—the rules and moral principles of our parents and society ("Nice people let others go first in

line"). Any internal voice that sounds like your conscience talking—that begins with such phrases as "You should" or "You shouldn't," or "You never" or "You always"—represents the superego.

- *Defense mechanisms against anxiety and frustration:* One's personality, according to Freud, is determined in great part by the way the unconscious mind handles anxiety. The conflict between the id and the superego may raise such anxiety that it causes the ego to force certain thoughts from the conscious mind into the unconscious. The mental processes that the self uses to cope with anxiety, frustration, and conflict are called **defense mechanisms.** (*See ● Figure 6.2.*) Often they are normal and healthy ways of dealing with difficulties; they become problems only if they prevent one from dealing with reality.

Some of Freud's century-old ideas, such as the notion of expressing unhealthy impulses in a healthy way through sublimation, or the idea of conflicting id, ego, and superego, continue to be debated. Nevertheless, the theory of the unconscious and the ideas of defense mechanism are very useful indeed.

Erikson's View: The Stages of Psychosocial Development Erik Erikson (born 1902), a pioneer in child psychoanalysis, built on Freud's work and identified eight stages of *psychosocial* development. He extended Freud's psychosexual stages of personality development into and through adulthood to cover the entire human life span.

Both Freud and Erikson theorized that the individual must resolve conflicts inherent in each phase, and that the lack of such resolution could lead to psychological problems later on. However, Erikson believed that society also contributes to personality development.[2]

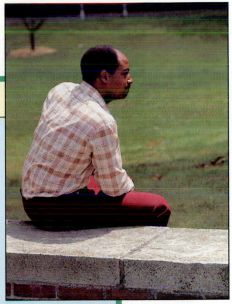

● Figure 6.2 Eight important defense mechanisms

Eight of the most important defense mechanisms are as follows:

- *Repression:* **Repression,** the master defense mechanism, is "motivated forgetting." We actively force unacceptable thoughts into the unconscious.

  Example: Victims of sexual abuse or incest during childhood may actually not remember any of the events that happened to them. On a lesser level, you might "forget" some criticism that a close friend or companion has made about you.

- *Denial:* The refusal to believe information that provokes anxiety is called **denial.** Instead of "forgetting," as in repression, one simply asserts that the information is incorrect.

  Example: Cigarette smokers who say the chances their habit will give them cancer are virtually nil are practicing denial ("My grandmother smoked all her life, and she's 85.").

- *Rationalization:* The assertion that the reasons for illogical behavior are "rational" and "good" is called **rationalization.**

  Example: Someone may be rationalizing dropping out of college because he or she hates the work with the supposed excuse that "No one is hiring college graduates these days anyway."

- *Displacement:* People who redirect their feelings from the true target to a less threatening substitute are practicing **displacement.**

  Example: Students who fail a test and blame everyone else—roommates for their distractions, parents for going through a divorce, professors for designing tests that are "too hard"—are displacing feeling.

- *Projection:* When you attribute your own unacceptable characteristics or impulses to other people, it is called **projection.** Often this takes the form of suggesting that one's own less desirable traits are actually widespread.

  Example: People who say "Everyone cheats" (on tests, on income taxes, on their spouses, or whatever) are probably doing some cheating themselves, or at least thinking about it.

- *Reaction formation:* **Reaction formation** occurs when people present themselves as the opposite of what they really feel. The notion is to somehow "prove" to the world that they can't possibly feel these unacceptable feelings because they are so obviously practicing the opposite.

  Example: A negligent adult child insists that every extraordinary life-saving measure possible be taken by physicians to prolong the life of a dying elderly parent.

- *Regression:* **Regression** is a relapse into a more child-like or juvenile form of behavior. The logic is that one adopts a more childish role to avoid the threat of the moment and perhaps to "return" to a phase of development that represents more security.

  Example: A child begins to wet the bed again or do thumb sucking after a new brother or sister is born or parents go through a divorce.

- *Sublimation:* Socially constructive behavior that is formed in order to disguise unacceptable behavior is known as **sublimation.**

  Example: Hostile impulses may be sublimated into seeking work as a police officer, sexual impulses into becoming a sculptor of nudes.

3.6

*Unit 3
Psychological
Health: The
Power of the
Mind*

Piaget's and Kohlberg's Views: The Development of Thought and Moral Reasoning

Swiss thinker Jean Piaget ("peah-*zhay*") (1896–1980) proposed that children are not simply inexperienced adults. Rather, he suggested, their cognitive processes are entirely different from those of adults: more intuitive and less logical.[3] (**Cognition** means the thought processes that enable us to imagine, to acquire knowledge, to reason, and to make judgments.) Children are also, he said, more **egocentric**—that is, they see the world centered on themselves and are unable to take another person's point of view. Piaget theorized that there were four stages of cognitive development, and only by the last stage (from about age 11 onward) are children able to deal with abstract, hypothetical situations.

Piaget laid the groundwork for ideas proposed by Lawrence Kohlberg, who argued that children's moral reasoning abilities developed in stages resembling those of Piaget's stages of intellectual development.[4,5] According to Kohlberg, children pass through three levels of moral reasoning, each indicating deepening moral responsibility. Only by the third stage are they able to operate according to whatever people have agreed is best for society—that is, laws—or, in special cases, according to a higher ethical principle that may violate human law.

The View of Trait Theory: Describing How We Differ
Do you consider yourself basically easygoing? pessimistic? changeable? peaceful? talkative? anxious? All these are called **traits,** characteristic behaviors that occur consistently under a variety of conditions.

Trait theory, pioneered by American psychologist Gordon Allport and his associate H. S. Odbert, does not try to explain behavior but rather to *describe* various relatively permanent personality tendencies.[6] Using procedures that test for such capabilities as reasoning ability or verbal skill, psychologists have been able to identify clusters of traits. For instance, a recent model has simplified human behavior into a model with five basic personality traits: emotional stability, extraversion, openness, agreeableness, and conscientiousness.[7] (*See ● Table 6.1.*)

● **Table 6.1 The five basic personality factors**

Trait	*Description*
Emotional stability	Calm versus anxious Secure versus insecure Self-confident versus self-conscious
Extraversion	Sociable versus retiring Talkative versus reticent Fun-loving versus sober Affectionate versus reserved
Openness	Daring versus conservative Conforming versus nonconforming Imaginative versus practical Preference for variety versus preference for routine
Agreeableness	Trusting versus suspicious Sympathetic versus unsympathetic Soft-hearted versus ruthless Cooperative versus uncooperative
Conscientiousness	Dependable versus undependable Organized versus disorganized Self-disciplined versus undisciplined

Source: Adapted from McCrae, R., & Costa, P. T., Jr. (1986). Clinical assessment can benefit from recent advances in personality psychology. *American Psychologist, 41,* 1002.

The Behaviorist View: Learning Theory
Behaviorists are concerned only with observable, measurable behavior. They believe that attempts to explain people's behavior by understanding emotions or mental states are not useful because, unlike behavior, feelings can never be observed and studied objectively. As the founding father of behaviorism John B. Watson said, "psychology must discard all reference to consciousness."[8] The behaviorists believe that human behavior is shaped by the learning that comes from experiences.

According to behavioral theory, human behavior is determined by the environment and human action consists of **conditioned responses**—learned reactions to stimuli in the environment. A **stimulus** is a factor in the environment that is able to evoke a response in an organism. For example, if you like ice cream, the sight of a bowl of ice cream (the stimulus) will make your mouth water (the response). Conditioned responses may be negative or positive, corresponding to punishments and rewards you have received for certain behavior. When applied repeatedly, rewards and punishments become **reinforcers,** events that strengthen the responses.

These concepts have been used with some success in *behavior therapies*, in which people are systematically desensitized to overcome fear of flying or of public speaking, to lose weight, or to quit smoking.

The View of Social-Learning Theory: Modeling and Imitation Behaviorists are concerned solely with how our environment determines us. Adherents of **social-learning theory** suggest that people can learn by observing and imitating the behavior of others and by imagining the consequences of their own behavior.[9] When people copy the behavior or customs of others, they are **modeling** or **imitating.** They do not have to experience something directly in order to learn.

What made you choose the college you are attending, the clothes you wear, the television you watch? The social-learning theorists think that such choices are influenced not only by environment but also by personal preferences, which are influenced by past experience. According to social-learning theorists, our behavior in any given instance, then, is determined by the interplay of different forces: our genetic inheritance, our personalities, our experiences, and our environment.

The Humanistic View: Self-Actualization **Humanism** emphasizes that people are unique beings who have the potential for personal growth and the ability to determine their own life course rather than being dominated by environmental or unconscious influences. According to humanists, people have the capacity to make choices about their lives and are able to live purposefully, to grow into the selves they are capable of becoming, and to lead lives that reflect important values. In contrast to psychoanalysts, who seem to focus on people's emotional problems, humanistic psychologists emphasize the human "potential" of people—their ability to realize themselves to the fullest.

The founding father of what has become known as the "human potential movement" was psychologist Abraham Maslow (1908–1970). In Maslow's view, people are essentially good but are often blocked by society from realizing their needs for self-fulfillment. Indeed, Maslow theorized that there is a **hierarchy of needs** to be realized—that only when physiological, safety, affection, and self-esteem needs are fulfilled can one concentrate on the highest need, self-actualization. (*See ● Figure 6.3.*) **Self-actualization,** according to one writer, is "the tendency of every human being . . . to *make real* his or her full potential, to become everything that he or she can be."[10] (*See ● Figure 6.4.*)

Key ideas stressed by humanistic psychologists include:

- *Importance of the individual:* Humanistic psychologists are interested in how individuals achieve their optimal potential. This is true whether the "self-actualized" person is as famous as Albert Einstein or a relatively unknown amateur athlete. Such individuals are problem-centered rather than self-centered, and they tend to concentrate their energies on important tasks that they regard as their mission in life.

- *Importance of beliefs:* What beliefs would you die for? Which do you live by? According to the humanistic psychologists, your beliefs shape your personality. Your convictions, your values, your spiritual experiences determine how you see and act in the world, and your personality can only be understood, they say, in terms of your interpretations of events in your life.

- *The value of "peak experiences":* Have you ever been moved by a moment of spirituality or ecstasy in which you feel truly fulfilled, serene, or "one with the universe"? This could be a religious experience—such as a "calling" or a strong inner impulse that moves one to a particular course of action

3.8

Unit 3
Psychological
Health: The
Power of the
Mind

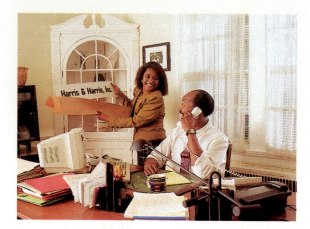

● **Figure 6.3 The hierarchy of needs.**
Once basic needs are satisfied, according to
Maslow, one can live to his or her full potential, achieving a state of wellness and fulfillment.

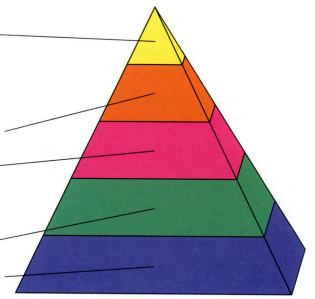

Self-fulfillment needs

Self-actualization need: Fulfillment of one's
potential, including satisfaction of creative
needs, needs for order and beauty, and
needs for knowledge and understanding

Psychological needs

Esteem needs: Achievement and gaining of
recognition

Belongingness and love needs: Social
interaction, affiliation, and acceptance

Basic needs

Safety needs: Long-term security, survival,
stability

Physiological needs: Hunger, thirst, shelter,
sleep, sex

—or it could be any other moment that sur-
passes ordinary consciousness, such as a
thrilling feeling of great accomplishment.
Such meaningful moments, called **peak experiences,** are of interest to humanistic
psychologists as important expressions of
our belief systems.

● *Importance of self-concept:* For Maslow
and for fellow humanist Carl Rogers
(1902–1987), an important aspect of personality is the **self-concept**—all the
thoughts and feelings that make up the image of who we think we are. According to
Rogers, as children we develop our self-
concept based on how we evaluate our actions, some of which we think are bad,
some good.[11] We weigh this self-concept
against the **ideal self**—the image of what
we wish we were. Psychological distress
arises, in this view, because of the disparity
between our self-concept and our ideal self.
It is the job of psychotherapy to overcome
this distress by adjusting one image to bring
the two into line with each other.

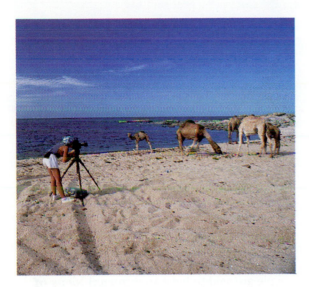

The Components of Psychological Health

Psychological health includes the following components: goal orientation, self-worth, self-efficacy, personal control and responsibility, optimism, enjoyment and happiness, creativity, risk-taking and self-reinventing, and giving and receiving love.

Psychologist Deane Shapiro analyzed studies of emotional wellness and concluded that emotionally healthy people share such qualities as a determination to be healthy, adaptability, affirmation of life, compassion, unselfishness, capability for intimacy, and a sense of control.[12] We will revise this list somewhat and consider the following components of psychological well-being:

- Goal orientation
- Self-worth
- Self-efficacy
- Personal control and responsibility
- Optimism
- Enjoyment and happiness
- Creativity
- Risk-taking and self-reinvention
- Love given and received

● **Figure 6.4 Qualities of self-actualized people.** Self-actualized people, according to Abraham Maslow, have several qualities, as follows.

1. *Sense of realism:* Self-actualized people are realistic. They know the difference between the world as it is and what they want, what they can change and what they can't. This point of view might be expressed in a famous axiom:

   Grant me the serenity
   To accept the things I cannot change,
   The courage to change the things I can,
   And the wisdom to know the difference.

   (This is known as the "serenity prayer" and is often recited by recovering alcoholics in Alcoholics Anonymous.)

2. *Self-acceptance and self-direction:* Self-actualized people accept themselves and are able to direct themselves. A key concept today is what is called "positive self-esteem." Self-actualized people, according to Maslow, have a positive self-concept, a realistic sense of their personal worth. This means they feel free to be themselves and to act autonomously.

   Another way of looking at this is to say that self-actualized people are *inner-directed*; they are guided by their own feelings and values, without being selfish or egocentric. *Other-directed* people, by contrast, don't find guidance from within but are directed by what they feel are outside pressures.

3. *Capacity for intimacy:* Self-actualized people are capable of deep feelings of intimacy, able to express their feelings and thoughts to others, to expose themselves to others in a sensitive way. They are comfortable enough to be able to express their feelings without fear of rejection or disapproval by others. (They are also comfortable being alone and indeed may find that solitude refreshes them for being in the company of other people.)

4. *Capacity for creativity and spontaneity:* Self-actualized people are creative and spontaneous. In this sense, they are like children. One quality that children have is *authenticity*, the quality of being genuine and spontaneous. Similarly, self-actualized people are able to express themselves without embarrassment, to be creative and open to new experiences. This need not mean creating great works of art or achieving spectacular athletic performance but simply being creative in everyday life, from cooking a meal to hunting for a job.

3.10

*Unit 3
Psychological
Health: The
Power of the
Mind*

Goal Orientation According to Maslow, an attribute of psychologically healthy people is a sense of self-direction.[13,14] A characteristic of peak performers, says psychologist Charles Garfield, is a sense of mission.[15] A key feature of good psychological health, then, is goal orientation—a sense of personal direction and purpose.

What is the goal of *your* life? If you admire those around you who seem to burn with serious purpose—to become a doctor, to travel the world, to excel in business or art or politics— observe also that there are many people who are serious *searchers* after meaning. A college or university is not designed solely (or even principally) to train people to make a living; it is also an arena for satisfying curiosity about how you and the world work. Here, for instance, one can study various belief systems, why people believe, and the history of belief.

Self-Worth To formulate a serious purpose for one's life, one must have a sense of self-worth. **Self-worth,** or **self-esteem,** is what psychologist Maslow called "self-acceptance." It may be defined as the extent to which one believes oneself to be significant, capable, and worthy.[16] (*See Self Discovery 6.1.*)

Self-worth comes in great part from one's upbringing. Learning academic subjects, for instance, requires basic emotional strengths that may be undercut in children whose families are unable to provide financial support and nurturing, according to self-esteem expert Leonard Schneiderman.[17] For example, divorce can be the cause of major disruption in nurturing and financial support for many children. Indeed, divorce is often the major crisis in some children's lives, according to psychologist Judith Wallerstein, who has studied divorced families for 20 years.[18] Half the children in her study lost the equivalent of at least a year in school.

Self-Efficacy A big part of self-worth comes from a sense of **self-efficacy**—your perception of your ability to perform certain tasks successfully. Self-efficacy stems from a belief in the possibility of success. This belief may arise from your previous successes. For instance, studying hard in the past has helped you raise your grades; therefore, you believe that studying

hard again will do the same in the future. Beliefs about self-efficacy are important because they give one the sense of empowerment to overcome obstacles. People who believe they can quit smoking have a good chance of succeeding; people who doubt their abilities often fail.[19]

Personal Control and Responsibility How much personal control do you feel you have over your destiny? The term **locus of control** refers to your beliefs about the relationship between your behavior and the occurrence of rewards and punishments. People who believe their rewards and punishments are controlled mainly by chance, fate, outside forces, or other people are said to have an **external locus of control.** Those who believe their rewards and punishments are due to their own behavior, character, or efforts are said to have an **internal locus of control.**[20] Studies have shown that people who have an internal locus of control are able to achieve more in school.[21] They are also able to delay gratification, are more independent, and are better able to cope with various stresses.[22] Some people may have both an internal and external locus of control, depending on their situation: they may feel they can control their lives at home but not in the workplace. Throughout this book, issues of locus of control are important because they translate into how you feel your lifestyle affects your health and whether you have any choices about that lifestyle.

Optimism "Mom, where are all the jerks today?" asks the young girl as she and her mother are driving along. "Oh," says the mother, slightly surprised. "They're only on the road when your father drives." Therapist Alan McGinnis tells this story to make a point: "If you expect the world to be peopled with idiots and jerks, they start popping up."[23]

Perhaps optimism is related to matters of self-efficacy and a sense of self-control. Pessimists may be overwhelmed by their problems, whereas optimists are challenged by them, according to McGinnis, author of *The Power of Optimism.*[24] Optimists "think of themselves as problem-solvers, as trouble-shooters," he says. This does not mean they see everything through rose-colored glasses; rather they have

Your Self-Image: How Do You Feel About Yourself?

This scale is designed to assist you in understanding your self-image. Positive attitudes toward oneself are important components of maturation and emotional well-being.

Self-image aspect	Strongly agree	Agree	Disagree	Strongly disagree
1. I feel that I'm a person of worth, at least on an equal plane with others.	A	B	C	D
2. I feel that I have a number of good qualities.	A	B	C	D
3. All in all, I am inclined to feel that I am a failure.	A	B	C	D
4. I am able to do things as well as most other people.	A	B	C	D
5. I feel I do not have as much to be proud of as others.	A	B	C	D
6. I take a positive attitude toward myself.	A	B	C	D
7. On the whole, I am satisfied with myself.	A	B	C	D
8. I wish I could have more respect for myself.	A	B	C	D
9. I certainly feel useless at times.	A	B	C	D
10. At times I think I am no good at all.	A	B	C	D

How to Score

Use the following table to determine the number of points to assign to each of your answers. To determine your total score, add up all the numbers that match the letter (A, B, C, or D) you circled for each statement.

Statement	A	B	C	D
1.	4	3	2	1
2.	4	3	2	1
3.	1	2	3	4
4.	4	3	2	1
5.	1	2	3	4
6.	4	3	2	1
7.	4	3	2	1
8.	1	2	3	4
9.	1	2	3	4
10.	1	2	3	4

Total: _____ This is your self-esteem score.

Interpreting Your Score

Classify your score in the appropriate score range.

Score range	Current self-esteem level
Less than 20	Low self-esteem
20–29	Below-average self-esteem
30–34	Above-average self-esteem
35–39	High self-esteem
40	Highest self-esteem

The higher your score, the more positive your self-esteem.

High self-esteem means that individuals respect themselves, consider themselves worthy, but do not necessarily consider themselves better than others. They do not feel themselves to be the ultimate in perfection; on the contrary, they recognize their limitations and expect to grow and improve.

Self-esteem is the most important variable in regard to human development and maturation. It is the master key that can open the door to the actualization of an individual's human potential.

Source: Rosenburg, M. (1986). *Society and the adolescent self-image.* Hanover, NH: Wesleyan University Press.

3.12

*Unit 3
Psychological
Health: The
Power of the
Mind*

several qualities that help them have a positive attitude while still remaining realistic and tough-minded. (*See ● Figure 6.5.*)

Are you an optimist or what some people like to call a "realist," when they actually mean a pessimist? (*See Self Discovery 6.2.*)

Enjoyment and Happiness Optimists are generally happier than pessimists, regardless of their actual circumstances. It almost seems like common sense: enjoying life produces psychological well-being.

An interesting discovery is that the *tendency* to feel unhappy may be genetic, but happiness is something you can develop yourself. In a study at the University of Minnesota, twins (raised together and raised apart) were tested for several personality traits. Identical twins who were separated soon after birth were less alike in terms of being happy (defined as the capacity to enjoy life) than twins raised together.

However, in terms of unhappiness, twins raised apart were as similar as those raised together. Unhappiness, then, is less influenced by environment. Why is this? According to psychologist Auke Tellegen, who designed the tests for the Minnesota twins study, "People in good moods tend to engage in pro-social behavior; in the absence of joy, people tend to cut themselves off."[25] Despite a potentially inherited disposition toward unhappiness, you can increase your happiness through your own activities. (*See ● Figure 6.6.*)

It's important to make pleasures (the good kind: touching, hot baths, music, food, good scents, naps, and the like) a personal priority, say psychologist Robert Ornstein and physician David Sobel, authors of *Healthy Pleasures*.[26] The reason: "Enjoying food, sex, work, and family is the innate guide to health . . . .. Good feelings and pleasures reward us twice: in immediate enjoyment and improved health."[27]

● **Figure 6.5 Optimist traits.** Optimism, which can be both born and bred in a person, is one of the attributes of psychological well-being.

"Twelve characteristics of tough-minded optimists are as follows. Optimists . . .

1. *Are seldom surprised by trouble.*
2. *Look for partial solutions.*
3. *Believe they have control over their future.*
4. *Allow for regular renewal.*
5. *Interrupt their negative trains of thought.*
6. *Heighten their powers of appreciation.*
7. *Use their imaginations to rehearse success.*
8. *Are cheerful even when they can't be happy.*
9. *Believe they have an almost unlimited capacity for stretching.*
10. *Build lots of love into their lives.*
11. *Like to swap good news.*
12. *Accept what cannot be changed."*

—Psychologist Alan Loy McGinnis (1990). *The power of optimism.* San Francisco: Harper & Row.

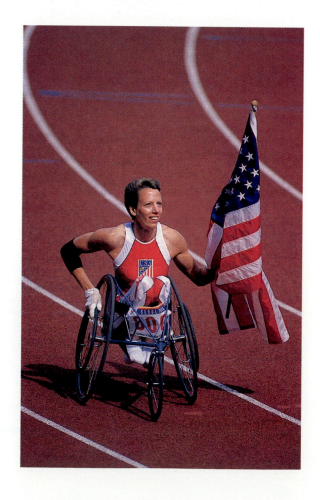

Creativity The capacity for creativity and spontaneity, Maslow held, was another attribute of the psychologically healthy person. This attribute is not limited to some supposed *artistic* class of people; it is built into all of us. **Creativity** refers to the human capacity to express ourselves in original or imaginative ways. It may also be thought of as the process of discovery. As Nobel Prize-winning physician Albert Szent-Györgyi expressed it, "Discovery consists of looking at the same thing as everyone else and thinking something different."[28]

Being creative means having to resist pressure to be in step with the world. It means looking for several answers, not the "one right answer," as is true of math problems. As Roger von Oech, founder of a creativity consulting company, puts it: "Life is ambiguous; there are many right answers—all depending on what you are looking for."[29] It means forgetting about reaching a specific goal, because the creative process can't be forced. One should, in von Oech's phrase, think of the mind as "a compost heap, not a computer," and use a notebook to collect ideas.

Risk-Taking and Self-Reinvention We are not endorsing the kind of risk-taking (such as drug taking or fast driving) that might jeopardize your health but rather that in which the main risk is to your pride, where the main consequences of failure are personal embarrassment or disappointment. This kind of risk-taking—having the courage to feel the fear and then proceeding anyway—is a requirement for psychological health.

Consider failure: None of us is immune to it. Some of us are shattered but bounce back quickly. Others of us take longer to recover, especially if the failure has changed our lives in a significant way. But what is failure, exactly? Carole Hyatt and Linda Gottlieb, authors of *When Smart People Fail,* point out that the word has two meanings. First, it is a term for an event, such as the loss of a job or nonattainment of promotion. Second, it is a *judgment you make about yourself*—"so that 'failure' may also mean not living up to your own expectations."[30] You may not be able to do anything about the event. The judgment, however, is something you can do something about. For instance, you can use your own inner voice—

your "self-talk"—to put a different interpretation on the event that is more favorable to you ("I didn't fit in there because I'm better suited to working alone than with a group").

One characteristic of many peak performers, according to Charles Garfield, is that they continually *reinvent* themselves. He says:

> *For example, look at Miles Davis, the jazz musician, and how he's constantly changed his musical direction to stay fresh and vital. Look at Bob Dylan.*

SELF DISCOVERY 6.2

The Life Orientation Test: Are You an Optimist?

In the following spaces, mark how much you agree with each of the items, using the following scale:

4 = strongly agree
3 = agree
2 = neutral
1 = disagree
0 = strongly disagree

1. In uncertain times, I usually expect the best. _____
2. If something can go wrong for me, it will. _____
3. I always look on the bright side of things. _____
4. I'm always optimistic about my future. _____
5. I hardly ever expect things to go my way. _____
6. Things never work out the way I want them to. _____
7. I'm a believer in the idea that "every cloud has a silver lining." _____
8. I rarely count on good things happening to me. _____

How to Score

For items 2, 5, 6, and 8, you will need to reverse the numbers. That is, if you strongly agree with the statement "I rarely count on good things happening to me," give yourself a score of 0 instead of 4. Now total up your score.

Interpreting Your Results

This test seems to demonstrate a relationship between a sunny or dismal outlook and physical well-being. When college students completed this test 4 weeks before final exams, the higher-scoring optimists (with 20 points and over) reported far fewer health problems. The pessimists complained of more dizziness, fatigue, sore muscles, and coughs.

Source: Adapted from Ornstein, R., & Sobel, D. (1989). *Healthy pleasures.* Reading, MA: Addison-Wesley, pp. 162–163. © 1990 Robert Ornstein/David Sobel. Reprinted with permission of Addison-Wesley Publishing Company, Inc.

3.14

*Unit 3
Psychological
Health: The
Power of the
Mind*

● **Figure 6.6 Seven steps to happiness.** Your genes may predispose you to unhappiness, but your personal choice can influence your moods.

" 1. ***Invest yourself in closeness:*** *Of all the circumstances happy people share, loving relationships seem the most characteristic and most important. So when you're setting your priorities, time for your loved ones should be No. 1.*

2. ***Work hard at what you like:*** *If love is most important to happiness, keeping busy at work you like may be second in importance. If your job doesn't fit that description now (or look like it will in the near future), search hard for ways to find work that satisfies your very real need to do something that is meaningful to you.*

3. ***Be helpful:*** *Altruism builds happiness in at least two ways. Doing good makes you feel good about yourself. In psychological terms, it enhances self-esteem. And there's evidence that altruism relieves both physical and mental stress—thus protecting the good health so important to most people's happiness.*

4. ***Make the pursuit of happiness a priority:*** *All things may indeed come to he (or she) who waits, but why wait to feel good? Discover what makes you happy and make time to do it.*

5. ***Energize yourself:*** *Run, play a sport, dance—the choice is yours, as long as you keep aerobically fit. Whether the feeling of well-being produced by exercise is due to the release of endorphins—the brain's natural painkillers—or something else, researchers agree that fitness is one reliable road to happiness.*

6. ***Organize, but stay loose:*** *It's good to know where you're going and to make plans for fun along the way. But since novelty makes us happy, be ready to seize an unexpected opportunity to try something different.*

7. ***Steady as she goes:*** *We all have our highs and lows, but strive for a sense of perspective. Emotional intensity can be costly. Those who hit the highest highs tend to reach the lowest lows as well.* "

—Diane Swanbrow (1989, July). The paradox of happiness. *Psychology Today,* p. 39.

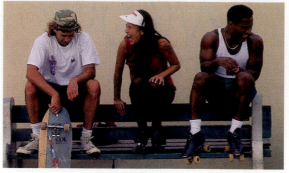

Critics say he's managed to redefine his old songs so that they and he seem new again. And look at James Michener, the novelist. Every book he writes takes him on a new adventure of travel and research. [31]

Love Given and Received We may hear or see the word *love* mentioned several times a day (usually in music), but what, in fact, *is* love? **Love** is "an act of full attention and giving that accepts and attaches to someone as he or she is, thereby enhancing the potential of what that person can become," according to one definition.[32] It's clear that we need to receive love, and if we have grown into complete human beings we also need to *give* love.

"Love" and "like" are, of course, part of the same emotional continuum. Why do some people seem to like us and some people not? The answer may lie in the observation that people whom we believe will like us generally will, and those whose rejection we fear will reject us.[33] The reason is that when we *believe* someone likes us, we respond to him or her warmly—are more disclosing and less disagreeable and speak in a more positive tone. These behaviors lead the other person to like us even more.

Suggestions for Further Reading

Hyatt, Carole, & Gottlieb, Linda (1987). *When smart people fail.* New York: Simon & Schuster. Our defeats are not only survivable, the authors say, they can be tools for renewed success.

Seligman, Martin E. P. (1990). *Learned optimism.* New York: Knopf. Discusses how cognitive therapy can replace a pessimistic outlook with an optimistic one.

7   The Art of Living Day by Day

▶ What are some strategies for overcoming loneliness, shyness, sadness, anxieties and fears, and anger and aggression?

Diane Keaton, the well-known actress, is also director of a film called *Heaven,* which contains interviews with people as to their thoughts about going to heaven. "I wish—as everyone wishes—for more than just nothing," Keaton said about the idea of heaven. ". . . It seems peculiar to want to live forever. Can you imagine? Forever with no conflict. What is life without conflict? What *is* it? It's almost as terrifying as being dead without anything [afterward]."[34]

We may not know what will happen after death, but we most certainly know that life itself is often filled with conflicts. Let us see what some of these are and how we may handle them. The principal areas we will consider are loneliness, shyness, sadness, anxieties and fears, and anger and aggression.

Loneliness

Loneliness is the feeling that arises from a mismatch between one's desire for social contact and the actual contact one has. People who feel lonely frequently have less healthy behaviors. Overcoming loneliness means taking chances.

All of us experience loneliness at one time or another. **Loneliness** is defined as the discomfort one feels because of a discrepancy between the social relationships one wishes or expects and the relationships one actually has. However, the feeling of loneliness varies from person to person. One person may feel lonely only when isolated from others, and another may feel lonely in a crowd.[35]

People who feel truly lonely most of the time have different health behaviors than do the not-lonely. For instance, a study of lonely adolescents found that they are more likely to use marijuana than not-lonely adolescents. Boys who are lonely are less likely to participate in aerobic exercise and be physically active and more likely to watch television than boys who are not lonely. Girls who are lonely are more likely than the not-lonely to smoke cigarettes, to be binge eaters, to be crash dieters, and to resort to vomiting to control their weight.[36] Clearly, here would seem to be a relationship between state of mind and state of health.

The Feeling of Loneliness   Lonely people tend to be self-conscious and lacking in self-esteem. College students, who may first experience the pangs of isolation when they leave home for college, may feel one of four types of loneliness. You might feel (1) *excluded* from a *community* you wish to be part of; (2) *unloved*—meaning uncared for—by people near you; (3) *constricted* about being able to share your feelings and worries with someone; or (4) *alienated from*—meaning isolated from—people in your group.[37]

Strategy for Living: Overcoming Loneliness   If you frequently or always feel lonely, do you tend to blame your isolation on your own inadequacies? If so, you may actually be on the right track to a solution: Lonely people find it difficult to participate in groups, introduce themselves, or make telephone calls—the very factors that can create loneliness.[38] Overcoming loneliness means beginning to take chances and giving the task of establishing friendly connections the same importance that you give to other priorities in your life. Thus, you might join groups with interests similar to yours or become a volunteer for a cause or activity you believe in. You can also pursue solo interests (music, photography, fishing, jogging) that are absorbing enough that you can be happy with your own company.

3.16

*Unit 3
Psychological
Health: The
Power of the
Mind*

Shyness

Shyness can range from occasional awkwardness in social situations to a complex condition that can disrupt a person's life. About 80% of people say they are shy at some point. Shy people need to overcome their extreme sense of perfectionism.

Some shy students stare down at their notebooks or desks to avoid making eye contact with the instructor, thus hoping to escape the instructor's attention. Sooner or later, however, most people are called upon to speak in public —and, for many, this can be an anxious, even terrifying, experience.

The Experience of Shyness Shrinking from public speaking is a form of shyness that most of us can relate to. For many, shyness is situation-specific. Situations that commonly result in temporary feelings of shyness include interactions with the other sex, meeting strangers, being the focus of attention, and interacting in large group settings. Some people, however, find themselves consistently tormented by feelings of shyness, regardless of the situation in which they find themselves. Shyness is often linked with loneliness, though the two do not necessarily go hand in hand.

Shyness, then, can range from occasional awkwardness in social situations to a complex and serious condition called social phobia that can completely disrupt a person's life. "To be shy is to be afraid of people," writes psychologist Philip Zimbardo in *Shyness,* "especially people who for some reason are emotionally threatening: strangers because of their novelty or uncertainty, authorities who wield power, members of the opposite sex who represent potential intimate encounters."[39]

Shy people may feel they are practically the only ones so afflicted, but the reality is quite different. According to one study, about 80% of those questioned reported they were shy at some point in their lives. Over 40% considered themselves presently shy. About 25% reported themselves chronically shy, now and always. A mere 7% of all Americans sampled reported that they have never, ever experienced feelings of shyness.[40]

Zimbardo has identified two types of shy people. The *publicly shy* are those who stutter, slouch, blush, avoid eye contact, and similarly show by their body language that they are unable to conceal their shyness. They are those whom we typically view as bashful, timid, or self-conscious. The *privately shy* cover up their shyness and may actually seem somewhat outgoing—or, alternatively, bored and aloof—but they suffer the same inhibitions and fearfulness as shy people. Whatever form it takes, shyness can be not just troubling but a disabling condition.

The causes of shyness include heredity, social skills, and personal experiences. About 10–20% of people inherit a predisposition to being inhibited and fearful in new situations, according to psychology professor Jerome Kagan.[41] This does not mean, however, that they necessarily are shy in adult life, particularly if their parents gently push them into new situations. Others develop shyness as a result of specific incidents, such as being criticized or rejected by parents or peers, falling behind in school, or having trouble adjusting to a new environment. Some people have not yet learned the social skills that can help them feel comfortable during social interactions.

Zimbardo suggests that those who are shy may unknowingly elicit the very criticism and rejection they fear. Because they are so preoccupied with being judged and rejected, and imagine that others will consider them stupid or inept, for example, they take the defensive action of withdrawing from social interaction. Their discomfort and withdrawal prompt people to avoid them. (See ● *Figure 7.1.*)

Strategy for Living: Overcoming Shyness
There are three key elements to coping with shyness:

- *Analyze your shyness.* Identify the situations in which you feel most shy and try to understand what is causing your anxiety.

- *Take steps to build self-confidence.* Making use of the college counseling center is a good way to start. Some of the techniques for conquering shyness consist of putting oneself directly into the situation that makes one uncomfortable. For instance, people who have difficulty with public speaking may go to a group such as Toastmasters to practice speaking to one another. People who have trouble with social encounters can expand their confidence and skills by introducing themselves to classmates or to other guests at a party.

- *Build your social skills.* Building communication skills will help here. Learn to be a great listener or to be an expert in one of your personal areas of interest. At least half of those who were once shy have been able to overcome their anxiety.

The main hurdle shy people have to overcome is the fierce perfectionism about themselves. As one woman who had difficulty with public speaking learned, the most important thing is "right before you get up [to speak], to mentally forgive yourself if you blow it. The degree to which you don't forgive yourself is the degree to which you [become anxious]."[42] In short, you have to give yourself permission not to be perfect.

Sadness

Ordinary sadness is experienced as the "blues," as opposed to more serious clinical depression, which can go on for 2 weeks or more. Dealing with sadness sometimes means changing your thinking and finding enjoyable distractions. It also means being able to recognize and acknowledge the need for additional help if symptoms persist or increase in intensity.

The word *depression* has a clinical meaning, as we shall discuss later. Here we are concerned simply with *sadness*—"the blahs," "the blues," the troubling thoughts and down moods that we all sometimes get.

Is It Sadness or Worse? It's important to distinguish between sadness (or disappointment or grief) and genuine clinical depression. According to the National Foundation for Depressive Illness, if you've gone at least 2 weeks experiencing the following symptoms, you should see a physician or therapist about the possibility of clinical depression.[43] The symptoms of clinical

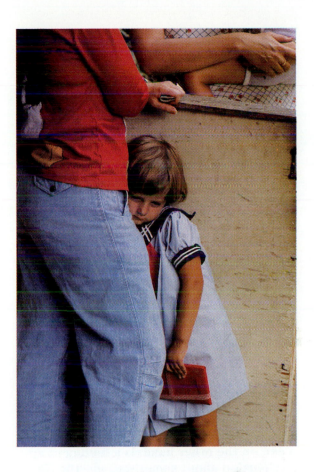

● **Figure 7.1 Shyness: the glass prison.** Psychologist Philip Zimbardo has called shyness a "glass prison" because of the way it traps people behind walls of anxiety, so that they prefer their present unhappy existence to unknown new experiences.

❝*At the root of many shy people's problems . . . is a compelling sense of inadequacy—a fear of being found wanting in the eyes of others. Coupled with this inferiority complex is a deeply ingrained tendency to be self-critical: Shy people are constantly telling themselves they will fail in any social encounter they attempt. They are so sure others won't like them that they go out of their way to avoid meeting new people or drawing attention to themselves.*❞

—Alison Bass (1990, September 24). Shyness doesn't have to be forever. *Boston Globe*, p. 29.

3.18

*Unit 3
Psychological
Health: The
Power of the
Mind*

depression include a change in your normal sleeping and eating habits; strong, persistent feelings of sadness and despair; difficulty concentrating or making decisions; feelings of worthlessness; fatigue; recurring feelings that life is not worth living and thoughts of death and suicide. In addition, feelings of sadness can be accompanied by physical symptoms such as a change in bowel habits, stomach aches, headaches, backaches, or a change in sex drive.

Strategy for Living: Overcoming Sadness
The best thing you can do is to break the pattern of negative thoughts that are bringing on the emotional lows. This means finding enjoyable distractions: being with people you like, going on outings that are fun, and engaging in pleasant exercise such as walking or bicycling. Seek the solace of talking to someone who cares.

Anxieties and Fears

Anxiety refers to generalized worry or apprehension that has no specific source. Fear, on the other hand, is a feeling of apprehension about something specific. In their mild forms, both can sometimes be alleviated by stress-reduction measures and "self-talk."

Are Sunday nights an agonizing time when you worry about what's in store for you on Monday? Are you sometimes so afraid that you don't even get out of bed the next day or answer the phone? Anxieties and fears can be so severe as to be incapacitating, as we describe elsewhere. Here, however, we are concerned about the kind of normal worries and apprehensions that are simply part of the process of being alive. It's important to note that anxiety can be adaptive when it signals the need for change but maladaptive when it is so low as to be nonmotivating or so high as to immobilize one. (*See Self Discovery 7.1.*)

Normal Worries Anxiety is *general;* you may have heard the term "free-floating anxiety." Fear, on the other hand, is *specific;* it is associated with something in particular, such as fear of examinations, of insects, of making a speech. Thus, Sunday-night anxiety (about returning to class or to work) may be manifested as a mild to almost paralyzing sense that something awful and unknown is about to happen to you. Or it may be expressed as mild to deep discomfort about a specific matter, such as giving a presentation to a group the next day. Both feelings of anxiety and fear may be accompanied by physical symptoms, such as sweating, a constriction in the chest, or a pounding heart.

Strategy for Living: Overcoming Normal Anxieties and Fears One of the most important strategies for coping with anxiety is to try to pinpoint its source and then apply steps in the problem-solving process. In addition, stress-reduction techniques, such as relaxation, meditation, physical exercise, distraction, and positive "self-talk," can be helpful.

Find a comfortable, dimly lighted place where you can sit and try to determine the feeling. Listen to your "Voice of Judgment," as it has been called.[44] This is your "mind chatter," your internal voice that broadcasts inhibiting pronouncements. If it's general (meaning that it's anxiety), the Voice of Judgment may send out messages that begin, "You never . . . ," "You always . . . ," "You should . . . ," or "You shouldn't . . . ." (Example: "You never do well in school.") If it's specific (meaning that it's a fear), you'll probably be able to attach the voice to a particular apprehension. (Example: "Your speech is going to bomb.")

As we explain later, changing your diet, cutting your drug intake (if any—and we include caffeine and nicotine here), and increasing your exercise level are all ways to lower your discomfort. If you feel particularly overwhelmed, you may need to seek professional help. However, you can also use your own inner resources to counter the Voice of Judgment. You can use positive self-talk to confront your anxiety or fear and lessen its effect. (See ●*Figure 7.2.*)

The Manifest Anxiety Scale: How Anxious Are You?

The statements below inquire about your behavior and emotions. Consider each statement carefully. Then indicate whether the statement is generally true or false for you. Check your answers in the spaces provided.

	True	False
1. I do not tire quickly.	___	___
2. I believe I am no more nervous than most others.	___	___
3. I have very few headaches.	___	___
4. I work under a great deal of tension.	___	___
5. I frequently notice my hand shakes when I try to do something.	___	___
6. I blush no more often than others.	___	___
7. I have diarrhea once a month or more.	___	___
8. I worry quite a bit over possible misfortunes.	___	___
9. I practically never blush.	___	___
10. I am often afraid that I am going to blush.	___	___
11. My hands and feet are usually warm enough.	___	___
12. I sweat very easily even on cool days.	___	___
13. Sometimes when embarrassed, I break out in a sweat that annoys me greatly.	___	___
14. I hardly ever notice my heart is pounding, and I am seldom short of breath.	___	___
15. I feel hungry almost all the time.	___	___
16. I am very seldom troubled by constipation.	___	___
17. I have a great deal of stomach trouble.	___	___
18. I have had periods in which I lost sleep over worry.	___	___
19. I am easily embarrassed.	___	___
20. I am more sensitive than most other people.	___	___
21. I frequently find myself worrying about something.	___	___
22. I wish I could be as happy as others seem to be.	___	___
23. I am usually calm and not easily upset.	___	___
24. I feel anxiety about something or someone almost all the time.	___	___
25. I am happy most of the time.	___	___
26. It makes me nervous to have to wait.	___	___
27. Soemtimes I become so excited that I find it hard to get to sleep.	___	___
28. I have sometimes felt that difficulties were piling up so high that I could not overcome them.	___	___
29. I must admit that I have at times been worried beyond reason over something that really did not matter.	___	___
30. I have very few fears compared to my friends.	___	___
31. I certainly feel useless at times.	___	___
32. I find it hard to keep my mind on a task or job.	___	___
33. I am usually self-conscious.	___	___
34. I am inclined to take things hard.	___	___
35. At times I think I am no good at all.	___	___
36 I am certainly lacking in self-confidence.	___	___
37. I sometimes feel that I am about to go to pieces.	___	___
38 I am entirely self-confident.	___	___

The scoring key is reproduced below. You should circle each of your true or false responses that *correspond to the keyed responses.* Add up the number of responses you circle. This total is your score on the Manifest Anxiety Scale.

1. False	9. False	17. True	25. False	33. True
2. False	10. True	18. True	26. True	34. True
3. False	11. False	19. True	27. True	35. True
4. True	12. True	20. True	28. True	36. True
5. True	13. True	21. True	29. True	37. True
6. False	14. False	22. True	30. False	38. False
7. True	15. True	23. False	31. True	
8. True	16. False	24. True	32. True	

Interpreting Your Score

Essentially this scale measures your tendency to experience anxiety in a wide variety of situations.

Low: 0–5   Intermediate: 6–15   High: 16–38

Source: Adapted from: Suinn, R. M. (1968). Removal of social desirability and response set items from the Manifest Anxiety Scale. *Educational & Psychological Measurement, 28,* 1189–1192. Suinn revised the Taylor Manifest Anxiety Scale in: Taylor, J. A. (1953). A personality scale of manifest anxiety. *Journal of Abnormal & Social Psychology, 48,* 285–290.

3.20

*Unit 3
Psychological
Health: The
Power of the
Mind*

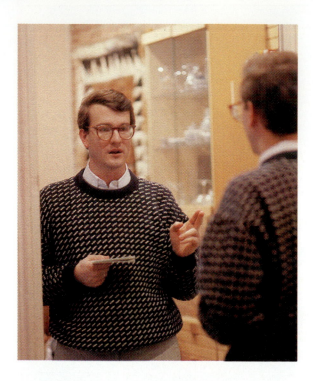

● **Figure 7.2 Using self-talk.** You can use positive "self-talk" to confront your fear and reduce its emotional significance.

"*Confront your fear.*

Once you locate your fear, say hello to it. Remember that you created it. You have invited it to live inside you. So get to know your guest. Talk to your fear, preferably out loud.

Say: Hello. Since you are staying here in my house, let's get clear what your chores are.

It is your job to make my life unpleasant. It is your job to give me an excuse not to try new things. It is your job to prevent me from feeling confident and free.

Thanks. You are doing a good job at this. Just remember, you are my guest. I can kick you out whenever I so choose."

—Psychologists Angela B. Miller & Richard Miller (1989, March 15). Phobias and free-floating anxieties. *San Francisco Chronicle*, Briefing section, p. 9.

Anger, Aggression, and Assertiveness

Anger can be ventilated by being expressed, but, depending on how you choose to express it, giving voice to anger can sometimes do more harm than good. Often not expressing anger, or expressing it in a civilized way, is best. Anger must be distinguished from aggression, which is behavior designed to inflict hurt, and assertiveness, which is simply standing up for one's rights.

How often do you get angry? In one study, most people who were asked to recall or keep careful records of such incidents reported becoming at least mildly angry several times a week, and some people were angry several times a day.[45] In more than half the cases, the anger was in response to the perceived wrongful act of a family member or friend. Anger was particularly prevalent when the incident was perceived to be avoidable and unjustified.

Clearly, anger is one of the most important and powerful emotions we ever have to learn to deal with. It can serve as an impetus for achieving important goals, as suggested by the work of many great leaders whose efforts have been fueled by outrage and indignation. It can also be a destructive emotion that can lead to destroyed relationships and violence in the form of abuse and homicide. If anger is suppressed, it can surface in unanticipated and often destructive ways. If it is managed and expressed appropriately, it can help us by signaling areas needing improvement.

Expressions of Anger Needless to say, expressing your rage is not a good idea under many circumstances. The work environment, for instance, is often a stimulus to anger, but it is also frequently an inappropriate setting for expressing it. "Men and women who are employed full time cited work twice as often as all other locations combined for occasions of feeling angry but remaining silent . . . ," writes Carol Tavris in *Anger: The Misunderstood Emotion.* "Conversely, the most popular location for screaming arguments and physical violence is—as you might expect—the home."[46]

But is an angry outburst a good way to handle your rage? Some people subscribe to the notion of catharsis—that expressing a feeling produces emotional release and a consequent reduction in that emotion. In the case of anger, this is sometimes true—provided the target deserved retaliation and the result doesn't leave you feeling guilty or anxious. However, expressing anger while you feel angry often makes you feel angrier and can be destructive to a relationship.

Even talking it out is risky. In one study, several laid-off aerospace engineers and technicians who were given the opportunity to vent their hostility toward their former employer were found to exhibit even more anger afterward.[47] In other words, even just talking about anger to a neutral party doesn't reduce it, it merely *rehearses* it.

Two quite different ways of expressing anger are with aggression and with assertiveness. We need to distinguish between these:

- *Aggression:* Although the word *aggression* can have a positive meaning (as in "an aggressive sales campaign"), in this case **aggression** refers to intentional acts of hostility and violence. Aggression here refers to physical or verbal behavior designed to inflict hurt on someone. Aggression is not the same as anger, for you may feel anger and express it in several ways, some of which may even be beneficial, such as cleaning the house energetically. You can also act aggressively without feeling anger, as professional soldiers do.

- *Assertiveness:* **Assertiveness** is simply behavior in which one stands up for one's rights, not by being angry or provocative but by simply stating one's feelings frankly and calmly. (We describe assertiveness, and assertiveness training, in more detail in a later place.)

Strategy for Living: Handling Anger How, then, should you best handle anger? Neither silent brooding and sulking (for the supposed sake of harmony) nor outspoken rage and cruelty (supposedly in the name of honesty) are useful. Sometimes the best response is nothing at all. "Let it go, and half the time it will turn out to be an unimportant, momentary shudder," says Tavris. "The other half of the time, keeping quiet gives you time to cool down and decide whether the matter is worth discussing or not."[48] Besides learning to nip your rising temper in the bud and disengaging from argument (perhaps by saying, "This is becoming a fight"), a second step is to learn to deal with anger with *civility.* Civility means knowing when to keep quiet about trivial irritations and when to discuss important matters clearly and assertively. Telling the other person how his or her aggravations make you *feel* ("I get upset when you leave the laundry for me to do") rather than leveling an accusation ("You *never* do anything about the dirty clothes") will invariably get better results.

Suggestions for Further Reading

Peplau, L. A., & Perlman, D. (1982). *Loneliness: A sourcebook of current theory, research and therapy.* New York: Wiley.

Tavris, Carol (1982). *Anger: The misunderstood emotion.* New York: Touchstone.

Zimbardo, Philip (1977). *Shyness: What it is; What to do about it.* Reading, MA: Addison-Wesley.

3.22

Unit 3
Psychological
Health: The
Power of the
Mind

8 Understanding Abnormal Behavior

▶ What is a psychological disorder?

▶ How can we distinguish between mood disorders, anxiety disorders, personality disorders, and schizophrenic disorders?

Many people aren't very sympathetic to problems of psychological illness because they don't believe that mental difficulties can happen to them. They have, as novelist William Styron observed about himself at a younger age, "a smug belief in the impregnability of my psychic health."[49] This notion is as unrealistic as the belief in the invulnerability of one's body. Psychological illness can occur as suddenly and be as devastating as any physical illness. Styron, for example, was well along in life when he experienced clinical depression, a disorder that affects 1 out of 20 Americans at some time in their lives.

Depression and other psychological illnesses are not moral weaknesses or defects of character, as some people seem to think. The far, dark place that Styron reached is simply the end of a continuum, or range, of joylessness or melancholy that we have all felt from time to time, and may feel again. The cliche that "Life has its ups and downs" is, like many trite expressions, true—although when one is in the depths of despair the notion that there may be a state of "up" may be inconceivable. One of the most important skills in the art of living, therefore, is learning *to appreciate that mental and emotional disorders are commonplace, that they are exaggerations of normal behaviors, that we can live through them—and that help is available.*

What Is a Psychological Disorder?

A psychological disorder is a pattern of behavior associated with distress; disability; risk of pain, death, or loss of freedom. Psychological disorders can have biological, early-life, and environmental causes.

Being naked sun-worshippers may be normal, even desirable behavior for some primitive peoples. It may also be considered positive activity among certain North American and European beach goers. But try doing it in the parking lot at the local mall and you will doubtless be arrested and held for psychiatric observation. Similarly, a lot of behavior that is permissible at a rock concert or at a showing of a cult horror film would be considered strange—even "sick"—at a college faculty meeting. Our point: what is considered psychologically healthy or unhealthy, or normal or abnormal behavior, can vary according to culture and according to situations within a culture.

What constitutes a **psychological disorder**? The American Psychiatric Association (APA) has defined it as a pattern of behavior that is associated with:

1. Distress—that is, pain

2. Disability—that is, impaired functioning

3. Risk of pain, death, or loss of freedom[50]

What are we to make, then, of San Francisco police officer Bill Langlois, who endured 256 vicious muggings and beatings during 10 years as a police decoy, smoking out attackers preying on the elderly? San Franciscans called him a hero and awarded him several medals for valor.[51] Under the APA definition, such bravery would be considered "crazy" behavior.

However a psychological disorder is defined, there are three possible causes, according to psychologist James Kalat:[52]

• *Biological causes:* Brain damage, biochemical abnormalities, faulty nutrition, disease, and various legal and illegal drugs may cause abnormal behavior. To this must also be added *heredity* as a possible cause, as it may be in schizophrenia, anxiety disorders, major depression, and bipolar mood disorder.

- *Early-life causes:* Distorted thinking may be caused by traumatic experiences in infancy and childhood, as Freud believed.

- *Environmental causes:* Instead of having causes originating from within the person, psychological disorders may be caused by reactions to difficulties in the environment, such as family or work difficulties, and the abnormal behavior may represent the person's attempt to cope.

Classifications of Psychological Disorders

Common psychological disorders are mood disorders, anxiety disorders, personality disorders, and schizophrenic disorders.

Because you may hear them often, it is worth defining two terms identifying two classes of psychological disorders, *neurosis* and *psychosis*. A **neurosis** is considered a relatively minor psychological disturbance, such as anxi-ety and depression. This is an exaggerated form of normal reaction to stressful events, but the individual remains in touch with reality and has no organic brain disorder. A **psychosis** is a severe psychological disturbance that grossly impairs contact with reality.

People still sometimes use these terms, but professional therapists have found them too vague to be useful. Thus, the most current classification of psychological disorders is that used by the touchstone of mental health professionals around the world, the American Psychiatric Association's *Diagnosis and Statistical Manual of Mental Disorders* (Third Edition—Revised), commonly known as **DSM III-R.** (A new edition, DSM IV, is expected in the near future.) This reference book lists symptoms characteristic of almost 300 different problems. It also describes the context in which psychological disorders exist, so that therapists can evaluate how severe the condition is and the best course of therapy. For example, two children might react entirely differently to their parents' divorce, with one suffering depression, sleeplessness, and difficulty concentrating more than

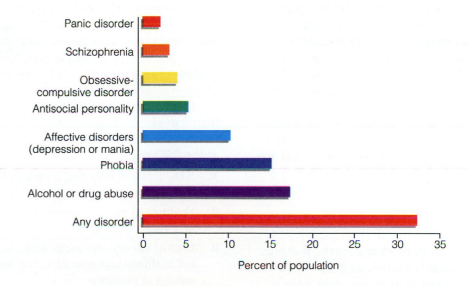

Percent of population

● **Figure 8.1 Prevalence of mental disorders.** Almost 20% of the people surveyed in three U.S. cities had some psychological disorder at some time during their lifetime. The total percentage for disorders (32%) is less than the total of the seven categories (49%) because some people had two or more disorders. The homeless were not surveyed.

3.24

Unit 3
Psychological
Health: The
Power of the
Mind

a year after the event while the other seems to have adjusted; the first one would probably be better served by having more therapy.

Among the many mental disorders described in DSM III-R, three that are *most* commonly experienced by Americans include anxiety disorders, alcohol and drug abuse, and mood disorders (such as depression). (*See* ● *Figure 8.1.*)In addition to anxiety and mood disorders, we will address personality disorders and schizophrenia in this chapter. Other commonly experienced problems, such as substance-use and eating disorders, are described in later chapters.

Mood Disorders

Mood disorders are characterized by severe depression, mania (elation), or swings between. Serious mood disorders include depression and suicide.

Are you one of those people who, when encountering hurt and disappointment, can find the strength to push on? Usually most of us can. But sometimes we are so despondent that it seems like nothing will help—and for some people this feeling endures for a long time.

Mood disorders are characterized by prolonged or severe depression or **mania**—elation—or swings between these extremes. Mood disorders are also called **affective disorders;** *affect* is the psychological term for "mood" or "emotion." The most common mood disorder is depression. DSM III-R also classes suicide as a mood disorder. We describe depression and suicide at length in the next few pages.

Depression

Depression refers to exaggerated feelings of sadness, hopelessness, and worthlessness. Several kinds of depression have been identified, including major depression, seasonal affective disorder, and bi-polar disorder. Numerous factors can predispose a person to depression. Regardless of the cause, depression can be effectively treated with psychotherapy and medication.

Being sad is part of the human condition. When someone close to us dies, when love ends, when we lose a job or suffer other major disappointment, sadness is the only legitimate way to feel. However, when sadness becomes one's constant outlook—when someone is lamenting a lost love, say, not just a year later but 5 or even 20 years after the loss—it has another name: depression.

As mentioned, about 1 out of 20 Americans suffer from a major depression at some point in their life.[53] In any given year, severe depression affects 15 million Americans, about 6% of the population.[54] Indeed, depression is so common it has been called the "common cold" of mental disorders. However, unlike the common cold, depression can become crippling and long-lasting. It can sap one's strength and spirit and destroy relationships, careers, and physical well-being. It can even destroy life itself: 30–70% of people who have committed suicide were previously identified as having major depression.[55]

What does it feel like to be in the grip of this disorder? According to novelist William Styron, in *Darkness Visible,* the word *depression* is inadequate for describing the experience. He calls it a "wimp of a word." Deep depression is a "howling tempest in the brain," a daily horror that rolls in "like some poisonous fogbank." A key aspect was the feeling of *loss*: "One dreads the loss of all things, all people close and dear. There is an acute fear of abandonment."[56]

Clinical depression generally lasts more than 2 weeks, impairs one's everyday ability to function, and is associated with such symptoms as the following:

1. Exaggerated, lingering feelings of sadness, hopelessness, anxiety, irritability, or despair

2. Feelings of worthlessness, low self-esteem, and guilt

3. Loss of energy and motivation; loss of interest in things and activities that were once a source of pleasure

4. Chronic, unrelenting fatigue and slowed speech and movement

5. Difficulty concentrating and problems with decision making and problem solving

6. Change in appetite, body weight, sex drive, and sleep; sleep disorders associated with depression may include insomnia, early morning awakening, or prolonged sleeping—that is, not being able to get out of bed

7. Thoughts of death and suicide

Anyone who has experienced these or similar problems for 2 weeks or longer should seek professional treatment.

Depression takes several forms. Some of the most important, described below, are the following:

- Major depression
- Seasonal affective disorder
- Bipolar disorder

Major Depression A **major depression** is a severe depression that lasts 2 weeks or longer. Some people suffer recurring major depressions throughout their lives. It has been suggested that depression may be *reactive,* occurring in reaction to a severe loss such as being fired or divorced, or *endogenous,* resulting from biological or biochemical causes. One biochemical problem that has been linked to depression is a deficiency of one or more chemicals in the brain. These chemicals, called *neurotransmitters,* carry information between neurons in the brain. However, the distinction between reactive and endogenous causes is often difficult to determine and is of little help in suggesting treatment. Indeed, sometimes depression appears for no apparent reason.

Seasonal Affective Disorder Why do so many New Yorkers go to Florida or Arizona for the winter? Why are December flights from Alaska to Hawaii sold out a year in advance? Are you more cheerful in the spring and summer than in the late fall and winter?

To some extent, seasonal fluctuations in mood are common among people living in the northern latitudes. However, the effect is exaggerated in people suffering from **seasonal affective disorder**—appropriately abbreviated **SAD**—a condition in which people become seriously depressed in winter and normal or slightly manic (excitable, the opposite of depressed) in summer. (*See* ● *Figure 8.2.*) Such

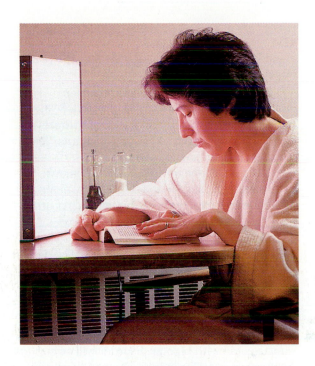

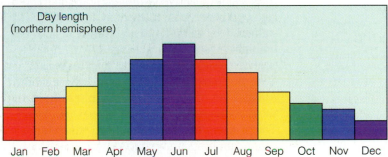

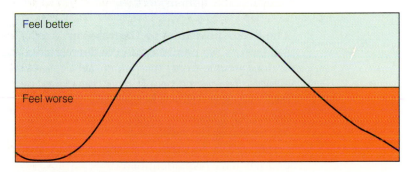

● **Figure 8.2 The SAD season.** People with seasonal affective disorder swing from severe depression in winter months to normal or manic (excitable) mood in summer months because of changes in daylight. Exposing SAD patients to 45–60 minutes of high-intensity light can relieve depression and carbohydrate craving after only 2–3 days of treatment.

3.26

*Unit 3
Psychological
Health: The
Power of the
Mind*

people are apparently more sensitive to sunlight; the earth's daily dark-light cycle influences the hormone melatonin, which affects mood and subjective energy levels.[57]

Those affected by SAD tend to sleep more and eat more when they are depressed.[58] They particularly show a craving for carbohydrate-rich foods, such as crackers or doughnuts. They also gain rather than lose weight.

The prevalence of SAD is not yet known.[59] Treatment consists of exposing SAD patients to high-intensity, broad-spectrum lights (not ordinary lights) for a period of time every day.

Bipolar Disorder Once known as *manic-depressive disorder,* **bipolar disorder** is marked by alternation between the two extremes, or poles (hence, "bipolar"), of depression and mania. *Mania* is characterized by constant, driven activity, excitability, and lack of inhibitions. Thus, people with bipolar disorder will swing from a slow, inactive, inhibited state characterized by a sense of helplessness and extreme sadness (depression) to an energetic, active, uninhibited state characterized by elation or anger (mania). Mood swings may take place over the course of a day or over several months. About 1 out of 100 American adults suffer from the disorder at some point during their lives.[60] The problem of bipolar disorder, which tends to run in families, can be treated with medication (most notably lithium) and psychotherapy.

The Predispositions to Depression Is a person born with a predisposition to depression or does it come from environmental circumstances? Depressed people have been found to have chemical changes in the brain, but it is not known if these are contributing factors to depression or the result of it.[61] Nevertheless, certain risk factors that predispose one to depression have been identified:

- *Family background and gender:* Apparently the most powerful risk factors for major depression are (1) having a family history of depressive illness and (2) being female. Depressed people are apt to come from families or have close relatives suffering from depression, which suggests a possible biological predisposition. For instance, depression is two to five times more common among close relatives of a depressed

person than it is among the rest of the population.[62] As for gender, the lifetime prevalence of a major depression is 5–9% for women as opposed to 2–4% for men.[63] The reasons for these differences are not clear.

- *Stress and life events:* Depressed patients tend to have an excess of negative events, particularly losses, in the 6 months before the onset of their disease. For children, the loss may be neglect or separation from a parent. For men and women, it may be loss of a relationship, whether by death or by decision; loss of a job; loss of health; or other problems.

- *Alcohol and drug abuse:* Substance abusers suffer high rates of depression. Many depressed people also turn to alcohol and drugs for relief.

- *Ill health:* People with incurable conditions such as Alzheimer's disease and terminal cancer are frequently depressed, although doctors often do not distinguish between the symptoms of depression and the symptoms of the disease.[64] Depression may also be a by-product of other serious, disabling disorders. Indeed, some studies indicate 5–32% of medical patients suffer from major depression, depending on the illness.[65]

- *"Toxin blue":* Some studies have proposed that depression and accompanying suicide have increased among the "baby boomers"—the large group of Americans born after World War II—compared with those born earlier. Is this difference the result of urbanization, drug abuse, and other stresses of modern civilization, or simply because there are possible differences between a large population and a small one? This difference, dubbed "toxin blue," has raised speculation about whether the causes are biological, environmental, psychosocial, or all of the above.[66]

The Learned-Helplessness Theory Another contributor to depression is suggested by the **learned-helplessness theory,** which says that people may develop depression when they perceive that they have no control over the major events affecting them. For instance, in one experiment, subjects were asked to perform tasks that were so difficult that they were bound to fail them, then asked to perform a second task that was only moderately hard.[67] Those who had been forced to fail on the first task did far worse on the second task than did subjects who never tried the first task. The failure at the hard task apparently decreased their self-confidence and made them somewhat depressed.

Of course, having just one failure is not usually enough all by itself to make a person feel depressed. What is important is that people become depressed if they think they are at fault. Depressed people tend to think that their successes are the result of luck but that their failures are the result of long-lasting deficiencies within themselves that apply to many situations.[68] Does depression precede the feeling of helplessness, or does the attribution of personal inadequacies precede the depression? Because often both events occur at the same time, it is difficult to know.

Strategy for Living: Fighting Depression

Depression is often treatable, but unfortunately doctors fail to recognize severe depression in half the patients who suffer it. According to a study of 650 severely depressed patients and 500 doctors, general medical doctors paid on a fee-for-service basis detected just 54% of depressed patients, and doctors working in prepaid health plans (who may be under more pressure to keep costs down) recognized only 42% of such people.[69]

Partly because many depressed people don't know how ill they are, or because they are too apathetic or despairing, only one of three seeks professional help.[70] Millions of people, however, are suffering needlessly. As we describe in the next chapter, psychotherapy, antidepressant medication (such as Prozac), and, finally, time can ease the pain of most sufferers. (See ● *Figure 8.3.*) Depression clinics and support groups are available in some metropolitan areas for those suffering from depression and for their families and friends.

For many depressed people, one study suggests, a way out is to break the cycle of their gloomy thoughts. Psychologist Richard M. Wenzlaff suggests that when depressed people try to distract themselves they tend to substitute other distressing thoughts.[71] To change this pattern, Wenzlaff suggests that depressed people do something enjoyable: "Force yourself

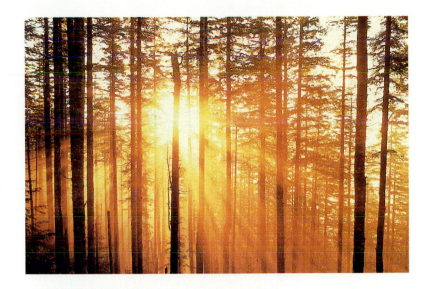

● **Figure 8.3 Behold the stars: delivery from depression.**
Eventually, after experimenting with a variety of kinds of healing, including "seclusion and time," novelist William Styron overcame his depression. He depicts the relief as resembling the emergence from hell of the poet in Dante's *Inferno*, with the evocation of hope in the last line of the poem.

"*For those who have dwelt in depression's dark wood, and known its inexplicable agony, their return from the abyss is not unlike the ascent of the poet, trudging upward and upward out of hell's black depths and at last emerging into what he saw as 'the shining world.' There, whoever has been restored to health has almost always been restored to the capacity for serenity and joy, and this may be indemnity enough for having endured the despair beyond despair . . . .*
And so we came forth, and once again beheld the stars."

—William Styron (1990). *Darkness visible: A memoir of madness.* New York: Random House, p. 84.

to get out, even if you feel like crawling into a hole. If you're obsessing about your rotten social life, for example, don't go to a bar if you hate that scene. Choose a comfortable activity that also holds the possibility of meeting someone."[72]

3.28

*Unit 3
Psychological
Health: The
Power of the
Mind*

Suicide: "The Forever Decision"

People who commit suicide are apt to suffer from severe depression, often combined with alcoholism and drug abuse. Clues to a person's likelihood of attempting suicide include changes in mood and habit, stressful life events, previous attempts, and talk of suicide. If you think someone may be suicidal, don't be afraid to get involved.

Choosing to take one's own life signifies not just the death of self. Before that, it means one has reached the death of hope.

It can be argued, as we explore in a later chapter, that some decisions to commit suicide are rational, as when an AIDS patient experiences progressive deterioration that severely interferes with the quality of his or her life. In other cases, however, depression, drug abuse, delirium, pain, illness, or other conditions can so cloud a person's thinking that it seems as though suicide is the only possible solution when in fact it is not.

Who Is Predisposed to Suicide? As we saw earlier, certain groups are more predisposed to the risk of suicide than others. The depressed make up a disproportionate share: according to one Cornell University psychiatrist, 30% of suicides suffered from pure depression, and another 30% suffered from depression combined with alcoholism and drug abuse.[73]

How do you know if someone will attempt suicide? The answer is that there are no dependably predictable patterns. Here are some considerations:

- *Look for changes in mood and habit:* We mentioned several of the signs for depression, including sadness, hopelessness, helplessness, apathy. In addition, studies of adolescents suggest looking for school problems, antisocial behavior, social isolation, running away, and preoccupation with death.[74] Another sign is when a person gives away valued personal possessions. An additional signal may be the occurrence of a suddenly positive outlook on life after a severe period of depression.

- *Look for changes in life events:* People experiencing very stressful life events are at a higher risk for suicide, such as a major loss associated with a death or relationship loss.[75]

- *Beware of previous attempts:* A prior suicide attempt is always significant: about one third of people who survive a suicide attempt eventually do kill themselves.[76]

- *Talkers may be doers:* If a person talks about suicide, always take it seriously: don't believe the myth that the people who talk about suicide are not the ones that commit it. Such talk may be about life not being worth living, about the suicide of someone else, or about how others will or will not miss them when they are gone.

- *Warnings versus no warnings:* Usually people contemplating suicide send out warning signals in advance. However, one study found that more than half the people who attempt suicide do so on the spur of the moment; that is, they make a decision less than 24 hours before making the attempt.[77]

Strategy for Living: Helping Prevent Suicide If you think that someone is contemplating suicide, don't be afraid to get involved.

- *Encourage talk, and listen.* Be direct: Ask, "Are you feeling really depressed? Have you had thoughts of suicide?" Don't be afraid that he or she is too fragile to hear the word "suicide." Encourage the person to talk, then *listen* to his or her response. You can't know the type or depth of that person's pain until that person is able to share it with you. Again, take any threat of suicide seriously.

- *Suggest solutions.* Be reassuring, but don't stop there. Suggest alternative solutions to the person's problems, if you can think of them. Most especially, urge him or her to get professional help. Offer to accompany the person to get help.

- *Show caring and be watchful.* Show you care by staying with the distraught person until you can get help. If you have to leave, make a pact with that person that he or she

- will do nothing in the way of self-harm without calling you—and when you are called, get to the person's side right away.
- *Get help.* If you feel events are beyond your control, call a suicide hotline, a counselor, or the police. Don't stop being involved until the person has the support and assistance of a trained professional.

Anxiety Disorders

Anxiety disorders include several conditions characterized by irrational fears and worries. General anxiety disorder is marked by excessive or unrealistic worries. Panic disorder is a moderate level of anxiety interspersed by panic attacks, episodes of intense fear. Phobias are specific fears so intense they interfere with normal living; they may be treated by gradual exposure (systematic desensitization) or sudden exposure (flooding). Obsessive-compulsive disorder consists of an unwanted, repetitive stream of thought (the obsession) or a repetitive, irresistible action (the compulsion).

Looking down from atop a high place you suddenly feel your mouth go dry, sweat breaks out, and you experience shortness of breath, clammy hands, racing heart, faintness, and trembling. Are these responses realistic? Perhaps, if you are treading a narrow trail along a wall of the Grand Canyon. Probably not, if you are in a glass elevator ascending the outside of a hotel. Certainly not, if you are simply looking at *pictures* of high-structure steelworkers.

Fear is a normal and, for survival reasons, even *necessary* part of life, a part of our built-in fight-or-flight response. However, fear is also a handicap when it no longer has a realistic basis. The results of irrational fear can be powerful, ranging from reliving wartime experiences and earthquakes in post-traumatic stress disorder to running parts of one's life according to superstitions—refusing to take a test or compete athletically or go on a job interview without wearing a "lucky" hat or rabbit's-foot charm. Irrational fears and worries comprise some common psychological disorders grouped under the term **anxiety disorders.** These include:

- Generalized anxiety disorder
- Panic disorder
- Phobias
- Obsessive-compulsive disorder

Generalized Anxiety Disorder A **generalized anxiety disorder** is characterized by excessive or unrealistic worries that extend over a period of 6 months or more. People suffering from this condition have no more basis for their concerns than anyone else, but they are constantly anxious that "I might flunk out of school," "I might run out of money," "My kids might get sick." This anxiety is often manifested in physical symptoms such as irritability, nervousness, sleeping difficulties, and concentration problems.

Panic Disorder **Panic disorders** involve recurrent attacks of severe anxiety that often occur suddenly and without provocation. People with panic disorder live constantly with a moderate level of anxiety that is interspersed by **panic attacks,** or episodes experienced as intense fear or terror, as in a fully aroused fight-or-flight response to a life-threatening event. This attack, which lasts from a few minutes to an hour or more, often occurs at night. The attack is manifested by such symptoms as pounding heart, racing pulse, shortness of breath, sweating, faintness, and fears about going crazy or dying.

Many people deal with anxiety by taking a couple of deep breaths, a useful way to calm oneself down. However, those who continue to do prolonged deep breathing—known as **hyperventilating**—on the theory that "more is better," may end up actually *increasing* their distress.[78] Hyperventilating expels carbon dioxide from the lungs, thereby lowering it in the blood. Then, if something increases the level of carbon dioxide, such as an experience that suddenly stimulates the nervous system, the surge of carbon dioxide stimulates signs of a panic attack: increased heart rate, trembling, sweating, and the like.

Strategy for Living: Coping with Panic Attacks There seem to be two strategies for combatting panic attacks. On the one hand, teaching people to do deep breathing but to

3.30

*Unit 3
Psychological
Health: The
Power of the
Mind*

avoid hyperventilation can help them deal with panic episodes.[79] On the other hand, people should be told to exercise regularly. Otherwise even slight physical activity can elevate the carbon dioxide in the blood and create a panic attack.[80] In addition, people suffering from panic attacks can benefit from psychotherapy and from medications such as antidepressants and antianxiety drugs.

Phobias Whereas anxiety is mild to immobilizing general apprehension, **phobia** is a *specific* fear associated with a particular person, place, or thing. It is not just a garden-variety fear, however, but an unrealistic, irrational, disproportionate fear, beyond the person's voluntary control. It is a fear so powerful that it interferes with normal living. People in the grip of a phobia suffer the kinds of reactions experienced in other anxiety disorders—sweating, rapid breathing, pounding heart, trembling—and often have the feeling that the fear itself may kill them with a heart attack. However, phobias differ from panic attacks in their intensity and in terms of what triggers them. The level of anxiety is so high in a phobia that it is immobilizing, preventing a person from doing something that could prove effective in alleviating the anxiety.

Phobias are the most widespread form of anxiety disorders, affecting 5–13% of all Americans.[81] The most common phobia is **agoraphobia**, the fear of being in open or public places or in crowds. **Simple phobias** are fears of specific objects, such as snakes or spiders, or situations, such as flying in planes or crossing bridges. Phobias of closed spaces (*claustrophobia*), public places, heights (*acrophobia*), lightning and thunder, animals (*zoophobia*), and illness are also common. (*See* ● *Figure 8.4.*)

Interestingly, nearly half the people with phobias have never had a difficult experience with the object of their fear.[82] Perhaps, it has been proposed, the reason is that over millions of years people have learned to perceive the more common objects of phobias, such as snakes, heights, and lightning, as threats. The human species has not yet had time enough to learn comparable fears of more recently invented threats such as guns.[83]

Strategy for Living: Coping with Phobias
The problem with phobias is that they keep one from discovering that his or her fear is exaggerated: if you stay away from *all* dogs, for example, you won't find out that your fear is disproportional to the threat. There are two kinds of treatment, both requiring therapeutic help, that are concerned with reversing this situation:

- *Systematic desensitization:* **Systematic desensitization** works to reduce fear by gradually exposing a person to the object that arouses the fear.[84] Example: People with a fear of snakes are first given training in relaxation, then are asked to lie on a couch while soft music plays and asked to imagine a black-and-white photo of snakes, then a full-color photo, then a real snake. Later they are given real photos and finally a real snake.

- *Flooding:* **Flooding** diminishes the fear by exposing the patient to the object of the phobia suddenly instead of gradually—the patient is "flooded" with fear. Example: People afraid of snakes are instructed to imagine themselves being crawled over and being bitten by snakes. Such images first stimulate the patients' breathing and heart rates to high levels, but they cannot remain high for long, and the patients begin to feel relaxed despite the continuing presence of the snake images.

Various kinds of programs are available for fighting specific phobias. (There is even a Phobia Society of America.) For example, for the estimated 12 million Americans who are dental phobics, dental phobia centers are available in large metropolitan areas.[85]

Obsessive-Compulsive Disorder "Everybody carries germs around with them," said anxiety-ridden billionaire Howard Hughes. "I want to live longer than my parents, so I avoid germs."[86]

With his insistence on elaborate hand-washing rituals and fear of being touched, Hughes presents an example of someone suffering from **obsessive-compulsive disorder,** a condition marked by repetitive thought patterns and actions. Actually, this disorder has two parts:

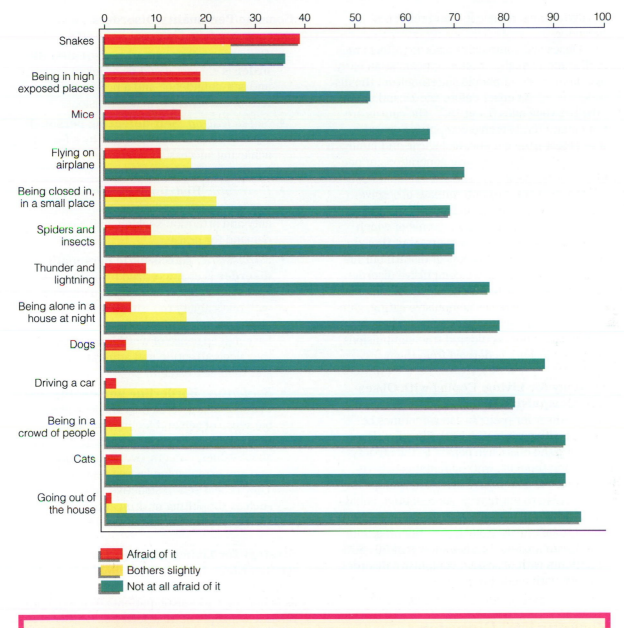

Legend:

- ■ Afraid of it
- ■ Bothers slightly
- ■ Not at all afraid of it

Figure 8.4 Fear levels. This national survey ranks the relative fear levels of Americans to some common sources of anxiety.

- *Obsession:* An **obsession** is a repetitive, unwanted stream of thought, as when you continue to hear a person's rebuke in your mind over and over years later.
- *Compulsion:* A **compulsion** is a repetitive, almost irresistible action, as when you constantly nibble on your fingernails or repeatedly wash your hands.

People with obsessive-compulsive disorder are often worried about the "right way" to do things. One frequent compulsion is cleaning, as was the case with Howard Hughes. Another is "double-checking," as with someone who repeatedly checks to see that a house is locked up before going to bed at night. Some believe that obsessive thoughts create anxiety, and com-

3.32

Unit 3
Psychological
Health: The
Power of the
Mind

pulsive actions reduce it—and reinforce the behavior.

Obsessive-compulsive disorder affects men and women equally. It often appears at an early age: about 60% of people suffering from the disorder report its onset before age 25 and about 30% between ages 5 and 15.[87] The causes are not clear, but obsessive-compulsive disorder may result from genetic, biological, and family factors. Some families have generations of people with the disorder.

It's important to differentiate obsessive-compulsive disorder from habits.[88] Most of us have habits of various kinds (some of which may seem peculiar to observers), but they do not cause us severe distress or disturb our life routines. Also, obsessive-compulsive disorders must be distinguished from so-called compulsive behaviors, such as compulsive eating, gambling, drinking, or sexual activities. These activities are not considered true compulsions, because pleasure is derived from them.

Strategy for Living: Coping with Obsessive-Compulsive Disorder Obsessive-compulsive disorder patients can sometimes be treated with systematic desensitization. By exposing the obsessive person to the anxiety-provoking thought, while simultaneously restraining the compulsive behavior, therapists may be able to extinguish the repetitive behavior. In addition, certain medications have been found to be effective, such as antidepressants that lessen anxiety. Studies show that 50–80% of patients with obsessive-compulsive disorder improve with medication.[89]

Personality Disorders

Personality disorders are maladaptive, inflexible ways of dealing with the world and other people. Examples are personality disorders characterized by excessive dependence on others or extreme self-centeredness.

A **personality disorder** is defined as a maladaptive (that is, poorly adaptive), inflexible way of dealing with the environment and other people. There are many personality disorders listed in DSM III-R.

Common Personality Disorders Some common ones are found in people who are:

- *Dependent:* **Dependent personality disorder** is characterized by a lack of initiative and self-confidence and a preference for letting other people make decisions.
- *Self-defeating:* **Self-defeating personality disorder** is characterized by a fear of achieving success, as expressed in self-handicapping symptoms.
- *Histrionic:* **Histrionic personality disorder** is characterized by excessive emotionality and attention-seeking, and a constant demand for praise.
- *Narcissistic:* **Narcissistic personality disorder** is characterized by an exaggerated self-centeredness that can interfere with one's ability to form attachments to others. People with this disorder actually have a deep sense of worthlessness, so that they need attention and admiration to bolster their self-esteem.
- *Borderline:* **Borderline personality disorder** is characterized by the lack of a stable sense of self and feelings of inadequacy. Such people have trouble making decisions about values, careers, even sexual orientation and establishing lasting relationships. They repeat self-destructive behaviors, such as shoplifting or drug abuse. They substitute empty lifestyles for real lives.

Strategy for Living: Therapy for Personality Disorders Individual psychotherapy may help treat some forms of personality disorders, as in helping narcissistic patients develop more realistic concepts of themselves as neither very special nor completely worthless.

Schizophrenic Disorders

Schizophrenia is characterized by personal deterioration, disturbed perceptions—including hallucinations, delusions of persecution, and delusions of grandeur—thought disorders, and inappropriate emotions. Causes are uncertain, and the disorder cannot be cured, although the condition can be alleviated with antipsychotic drugs.

In our dreams, we see ourselves acting heroically, hovering bird-like in the air, standing stark naked in a crowd, or being chased by phantom figures—and our minds leap from one event to another, defying time and space and logic. When we wake up, however, we know that we have been experiencing fantasy. Schizophrenics do not.

The Symptoms of Schizophrenia The word *schizophrenia* means "split mind"—not in the Jekyll-and-Hyde or "split personality" sense but rather as a "split from reality." According to DSM III-R, **schizophrenia** is characterized by various kinds of disturbed thinking, behavior, and feelings—particularly hallucinations, delusions, and thought disorder. If this definition seems a bit imprecise, it is because the symptoms of schizophrenia reflect a *range* of emotional and cognitive disorders. No one who has schizophrenia has all of the symptoms of the disease at a given time or even during the course of his or her illness.

The symptoms associated with schizophrenia include the following:

- *Personal deterioration:* Over 6 months' time, one's work performance, social relations, and personal appearance deteriorate. A schizophrenic finds he or she can't concentrate, relax, or sleep and withdraws from social relationships.

- *Disturbed perceptions:* Schizophrenics suffer from hallucinations and delusions.
  Hallucinations are sensory experiences—sights and sounds—that don't exist in reality. Sometimes they become exaggerated visual experiences.
  Delusions are unfounded beliefs. **Delusions of grandeur** refer to a person's false belief that he or she is supremely important ("I'm the Son of God"); **delusions of persecution** refer to the unrealistic belief that people are trying to harm him or her ("The CIA is after me"); **delusions of reference** are beliefs that many messages personally refer to oneself ("That TV announcer was talking about me").

- *Thought disorders:* The thoughts of schizophrenics often show a loose, bizarre association of ideas and difficulty in using abstract concepts. Indeed, psychologists of-

ten refer to the verbal thoughts of schizophrenics as "word salad."

- *Inappropriate emotions:* Schizophrenics generally display little emotion in their faces or display inappropriate expressions, such as laughter when the circumstances don't warrant it. Some patients fall into a state called **catatonia** ("kat-uh-*toh*-nee-uh"), consisting of being motionless or constantly in motion.

There are also several other kinds of schizophrenia. (*See* ● *Table 8.1.*)

The Causes of Schizophrenia One to two out of 100 Americans are affected by schizophrenia at some time in their lives.[90] The evidence seems to suggest an inherited vulnerability to the disease: the chances of being diagnosed with schizophrenia jump from

● **Table 8.1 Types of schizophrenia**

Type	Description
Catatonic	Bizarre physical movements, ranging from muscular rigidity to hyperactivity, sometimes with alternations between these extremes.
Disorganized	Incoherent speech and inappropriate emotion. Virtually complete social withdrawal. Aimless babbling and giggling.
Paranoid	Delusions of persecution or grandeur. Individuals believe that, because of their own greatness, they have many enemies.
Undifferentiated	People who cannot be placed into the previous categories but who show typical schizophrenic symptoms: delusions, hallucinations, and incoherence.

3.34

*Unit 3
Psychological
Health: The
Power of the
Mind*

about 1 in 100 for most people to 1 in 10 for people who have an afflicted sibling or parent and to about one in two for those who have an identical twin diagnosed with schizophrenia. (*See* ● *Figure 8.5.*) Of course, this does not mean inheritability is inevitable; after all, half the siblings of identical twins *don't* develop schizophrenia.

If genetic factors alone don't predispose people to schizophrenia, neither do environmental or psychological factors.[91] It is possible that stress may trigger the onset of schizophrenia among those genetically predisposed. Prenatal exposure to the illness may also play a role. Certain abnormalities in brain structure may also be a factor.

Strategy for Living: Treatment for Schizophrenia Schizophrenia cannot be cured. About half of all psychiatric hospital patients in the United States are schizophrenics. Still, with the help of antipsychotic drugs that reduce the thought disorders, disturbed perceptions, and tormenting voices, many schizophrenics can lead productive lives residing with their families and holding down jobs.

Suggestions for Further Reading

Mondimore, F. M. (1990). *Depression: The mood disease.* Baltimore: Johns Hopkins Press. A description of various treatments for this disease, including medicine, psychotherapy, and support groups.

Sheehan, Susan (1982). *Is there no place on earth for me?* New York: Vintage. This Pulitzer Prize-winning book chronicles a year in the life of a young woman who has struggled with schizophrenia since her late teens.

Styron, William (1990). *Darkness visible: A memoir of madness.* New York: Random House. Well-known novelist's absorbing account of his clinical depression.

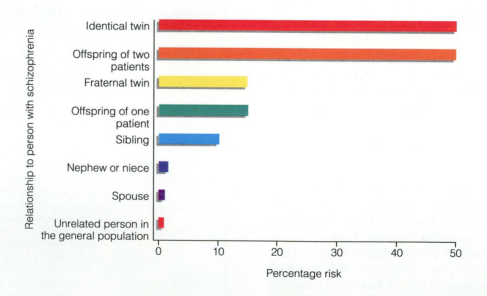

● **Figure 8.5 Schizophrenia—the lifetime odds.** The risks of being diagnosed with schizophrenia increase with one's relationship to certain biological relatives having the disorder. Those who have an identical twin who is schizophrenic or parents who are patients are at the highest risk.

9 Getting Help: Kinds of Therapy

▶ How can you determine when you need professional help?

▶ How can you find professional help, and how can you make it successful?

▶ What are the various kinds of individual psychotherapies, behavior therapies, group treatments, and medical therapies available?

If you can turn to family or friends for support when faced with the end of a relationship, loss of a job, depression, or other major problem, you will probably handle your problems more successfully than do people who try to cope on their own. However, anxiety, headaches, panic attacks, anger, loneliness, and other kinds of major distress may be too much to share with friends.

When Do You Need Professional Help?

You may need professional help if your present state is detrimental to yourself or others. Examples are depression and anxiety, a crisis, communication problems, addiction problems, and early-life problems.

Several kinds of trouble require professional help. All are essentially conditions that affirmatively answer the question: "Is my present condition damaging to me or others?"

- *Depression and anxiety:* Several weeks of feeling helplessness, hopelessness, despair, and a question if life is even worth living is solid evidence of depression that needs treatment. Worries that make it difficult to sleep, concentrate, or relax or fears so intense that you cannot function normally show the need for professional therapy.

- *Crisis:* The inability to cope with the loss or death of someone close to you, a major disruption or disappointment such as job loss or physical illness, or an abusive or destructive relationship is an occasion for seeking help.

- *Communication problems:* Problems with shyness, assertiveness, loneliness, or sex, or family or relationship conflicts are conditions that can be overcome through therapy.

- *Addiction problems:* The inability to stop drinking, smoking, abusing drugs, gambling, or shoplifting indicates an addiction that may be helped with treatment.

- *Early-life problems:* If you have been neglected or emotionally, physically, or sexually abused as a child, therapy may be able to help you come to terms with your experiences.

Getting Help

You can find a therapist through campus student services and through other services listed in the phone book—community services, crisis intervention services, and organizations set up to deal with specific problems.

The first thing most people want when they go to a therapist is to have someone relieve the pain—whatever it is. Here are some ways to connect with a therapist quickly.

- *Student services:* If you are a college student, campus student-health centers, health-education instructors, or the dean of student affairs can direct you to college and community health services.

- *Community services:* The telephone book is the place to start. Look at the following categories in the telephone book Yellow Pages: COUNSELING; ALCOHOL AND DRUG ABUSE; CHILD ABUSE AND FAMILY VIOLENCE; AIDS/ARC; HEALTH CARE; MENTAL HEALTH AND CRISIS INTERVENTION; MOTHER AND INFANT HEALTH; RAPE AND SEXUAL ASSAULT; SUICIDE PREVENTION.

Orientations Toward Seeking Professional Help: How Do You Feel About Psychotherapy?

Read each statement carefully and indicate your agreement or disagreement, using the scale below. Please express your frank opinion in responding to each statement, answering as you honestly feel or believe:

0 = Disagreement   2 = Probable agreement
1 = Probable disagreement   3 = Agreement

1. Although there are clinics for people with mental troubles, I would not have much faith in them. _____
2. If a good friend asked my advice about a mental health problem, I might recommend that he see a psychiatrist. _____
3. I would feel uneasy going to a psychiatrist because of what some people would think. _____
4. A person with a strong character can get over mental conflicts by himself or herself, and would have little need of a psychiatrist. _____
5. There are times when I have felt completely lost and would have welcomed professional advice for a personal or emotional problem. _____
6. Considering the time and expense involved in psychotherapy, it would have doubtful value for a person like me. _____
7. I would willingly confide intimate matters to an appropriate person if I thought it might help me or a member of my family. _____
8. I would rather live with certain mental conflicts than go through the ordeal of getting psychiatric treatment. _____
9. Emotional difficulties, like many things, tend to work out by themselves. _____
10. There are certain problems that should not be discussed outside of one's immediate family. _____
11. A person with a serious emotional disturbance would probably feel most secure in a good mental hospital. _____
12. If I believed I was having a mental breakdown, my first inclination would be to get professional attention. _____
13. Keeping one's mind on a job is a good solution for avoiding personal worries and concerns. _____
14. Having been a psychiatric patient is a blot on a person's life. _____
15. I would rather be advised by a close friend than by a psychologist, even for an emotional problem. _____
16. A person with an emotional problem is not likely to solve it alone; he or she *is* likely to solve it with professional help. _____
17. I resent a person—professionally trained or not—who wants to know about my personal difficulties. _____
18. I would want to get psychiatric attention if I was worried or upset for a long period of time. _____
19. The idea of talking about problems with a psychologist strikes me as a poor way to get rid of emotional conflicts. _____
20. Having been mentally ill carries with it a burden of shame. _____
21. There are experiences in my life I would not discuss with anyone. _____
22. It is probably best not to know *everything* about oneself. _____
23. If I were experiencing a serious emotional crisis at this point in my life, I would be confident that I could find relief in psychiatry. _____
24. There is something admirable in the attitude of a person who is willing to cope with his or her conflicts and fears *without* resorting to professional help. _____
25. At some future time I might want to have psychological counseling. _____
26. A person should work out his or her own problems; getting psychological counseling would be a last resort. _____
27. Had I received treatment in a mental hospital, I would not feel that it had to be "covered up." _____
28. If I thought I needed psychiatric help, I would get it no matter who knew about it. _____
29. It is difficult to talk about personal affairs with highly educated people such as doctors, teachers, and clergymen. _____

How to Score

Begin by reversing your response (0 = 3, 1 = 2, 2= 1, 3 = 0) for items 1, 3, 4, 6, 8, 9, 10, 13, 14, 15, 17, 19, 20, 21, 22, 24, 26, and 29. Then add up the numbers for all 29 items on the scale. The total is your score.

My score is: _____

Interpreting Your Score

Low score: 0–49   Medium score: 50–63
High score: 64–87

The scale measures how favorable your attitude is toward professional psychotherapy. The higher your score, the more positive your attitudes.

Source: From Fischer, E. H., & Turner, J. L. (1970). Orientations to seeking professional help: Development and research utility of an attitude scale. *Journal of Consulting & Clinical Psychology, 35*, 82–83. Copyright 1970 by the American Psychological Association. Reprinted by permission.

- *Crisis intervention:* If you are aware of a specific crisis in your life, there may well be a listing for a telephone hotline in the telephone book. Indeed, the word *crisis* no doubt has a telephone number for it. Other crisis lines are suicide prevention, violence prevention, sexual trauma, rape hotline, battered women, and the like.

- *Specific organizations for specific problems:* There are many kinds of self-help groups for specific ills, such as Alcoholics Anonymous, Narcotics Anonymous, Gamblers Anonymous, Women for Sobriety, and Adult Children of Alcoholics.

When you call, clearly state the nature of your complaint. Ask what services are provided, their cost, who is eligible, when and where your appointment is, how to get there, and what you should bring (such as addresses for medical records, medicine you are taking).

We are assuming that you are willing to consider getting help with what is clearly a difficult problem. However, many people have negative notions about therapy and are reluctant to pursue it. This is unfortunate, because such attitudes can prevent people from getting the very help they need. (*See Self Discovery 9.1.*)

Strategy for Living: Making Therapy Successful

Many kinds of therapy are available to treat psychological disorders. You can try individual psychotherapy, behavior therapy, group therapy, or other forms of assistance, including that offered by physicians. After determining the initial treatment that is best for you, try to promote the success of your treatment by establishing a level of comfort with your therapist, by setting goals for yourself, and by staying actively involved in your treatment.

Therapy for psychological disorders takes several forms:

- Individual psychotherapies
- Behavior therapies
- Group treatments
- Medical therapy

We consider these below.

Once your immediate distress is relieved, you need to explore the following two important issues:

- *Establish how comfortable you are with your therapist:* Find out what kind of methods your therapist uses, to see if you are comfortable with these techniques. (For example, if you think biofeedback will work better than hypnosis for relaxing you, then go to a therapist who practices biofeedback.) Also ask the therapist about credentials and experience—in particular, whether he or she has had experience with problems like yours.

  Listen to the answers to see if the therapist seems to take you seriously. After all, although this is a *paid* relationship, it is also a very *personal* relationship. Compatibility is important; you don't want to feel mistrustful or intimidated.

- *Establish short-term and long-term goals of therapy:* Setting measurable goals is *one* way to get the most out of therapy.[92] Otherwise, says therapist Paul Quinnett, "clients may waste time and money looking for help that doesn't exist, and therapists may waste the clients' time working on problems the clients don't consider problems." The early goals, Quinnett proposes, should arise out of a list of events, stresses, or relationships that are troubling you. The changes you want to make should somehow be measurable. (*See ● Figure 9.1.*) Long-term goals for change consist of goals for life: "success, rewarding relationships, creative expression, a sense of competence and confidence in handling conflict."

3.38

*Unit 3
Psychological
Health: The
Power of the
Mind*

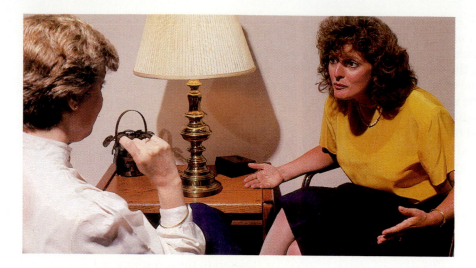

● **Figure 9.1 Early goals of therapy**

"Here's how to start deciding what you want your therapy to accomplish:

1. As best you can, jot down what you think is causing you distress. This list of events, relationships, or stresses can be long or short, but simply writing them down can help you understand better what has been going on, and going wrong.

. . . Your insight reveals a lot about how you think and how you understand the way life works. Left to their own devices and theories, therapists will come up with all sorts of reasons their clients are suffering. . . .

2. After the first visit, consider carefully how comfortable you felt. Will you and the therapist be able to work together week after week? . . .

3. As you work with your chosen therapist in setting early goals, try to make them measurable in some way. This isn't always easy, but when the changes you want can be measured, it's a lot easier to tell, down the road, how well the therapy is working."

—Psychotherapist Paul G. Quinnett (1989, April). The key to successful therapy. *Psychology Today,* p. 46.

Individual Psychotherapies

Psychotherapy is the interaction between therapist and patient to try to change psychological problems. Seven types of psychotherapies are described here. Psychoanalysis, the first of the "talking therapies," uses as tools free association of thoughts, dream analysis, and transference of emotions. Humanistic therapy tries to overcome a mismatch between patients' self-concepts and their ideal selves, focusing on the patients' self-insights. Gestalt therapy relies on body language as well as spoken language to help patients become aware of their feelings. Rational-emotive therapy tries to replace patients' irrational thoughts with rational thoughts. Cognitive therapy encourages patients to find evidence to support positive beliefs and overcome negative beliefs. Transactional analysis examines how three aspects of one's personality—"child," "parent," "adult"—transact, or communicate, with one another. Brief therapy uses a verbal contract between therapist and patient to achieve goals.

Psychotherapy, broadly speaking, is treatment designed to make changes by psychological rather than physical means, using persuasion, reassurance, and support. It is thought of as the interaction between a trained therapist and someone suffering a psychological difficulty. The principles of various kinds of individual therapy are also used in group therapy.

Psychotherapy is conducted by individuals whose professional training and experience vary widely. Some states enable anyone to call himself or herself a therapist or counselor. Other states require a professional license to practice. It is worthwhile to check the credentials and experience of any therapist with whom you are considering working. Most psychotherapy is now done by psychiatrists; clinical psychologists; clinical or psychiatric social workers; pastoral, marital, abuse, and school counselors; and psychiatric nurses. (See ● *Table 9.1.*)

There are perhaps 250 or more types of psychotherapy, some concerned with past emotions, others with current ones; some with changing behavior, others with understanding it; some with the individual, others with entire families. Here we consider only the most well-known therapies and will describe them in their purest form. However, it's important to point out that half of all therapists say they use a combination of methods and approaches—that is, they are **eclectic.**[93] We will describe the following types:

- Psychoanalysis
- Humanistic therapy: person-centered therapy
- Gestalt therapy
- Rational-emotive therapy
- Cognitive therapy
- Transactional analysis
- Brief therapy

Psychoanalysis Sigmund Freud's method of therapy, psychoanalysis, was the first of the talking therapies. In **talking therapies,** a patient interacts in a confiding way either individually with a trained therapist or in a group led by a therapist. The purpose of the talking is to help patients achieve insight into the reasons for their behavior. Therefore, talking therapies are often called *insight-oriented therapies.*

● **Table 9.1 Different types of therapists.**
Some therapists adjust their fees to a sliding scale, depending on the patient's income.

Type of therapist	Description
Psychiatrist	M.D. (medical doctor) degree required. Physician specializing in treating psychological disorders. Only therapist able to prescribe medications. Most expensive hourly rate.
Clinical psychologist or counseling psychologist	Ph.D. (doctor of philosophy) degree. Trained in therapy, testing, or research. Generally next highest hourly rate.
Psychoanalyst	M.D. or Ph.D. degree. Therapist trained in psychoanalytic (Freudian) methods. Hourly rate similar to preceding.
Psychiatric social worker	M.A., M.S., or M.S.W. (Master of Arts, Science, or Social Work) degree. Trained in individual and group therapy; may specialize in family therapy. Usually affordable hourly rate.
Other therapists	Other counselors include: (1) abuse counselors, (2) alcohol and drug counselors, (3) marriage and family counselors, (4) registered nurses, and (5) pastoral counselors. Hourly rates vary.

In **psychoanalysis,** therapy consists of focusing on the patient's unconscious motives and thoughts, releasing previously repressed thoughts in order to allow him or her to gain self-insight. Freud's psychoanalytic theory of personality is used to explain the interplay of conscious and unconscious forces. This method made famous the use of the psychoanalytic couch, in which the patient lies on a couch and the psychoanalyst sits out of view, behind the patient, in order to minimize distraction. The principal tools of psychoanalysis include:

3.40

*Unit 3
Psychological
Health: The
Power of the
Mind*

- *Free association:* In **free association,** the patient relaxes and reports everything that comes to mind, no matter how trivial or embarrassing. The therapist listens and tries to determine **resistances,** or blocks in the flow of the association, which may reveal the patient's unconscious mental life. The therapist then offers **interpretations**— that is, suggestions of hidden feelings and conflicts—to guide the patient toward self-insight.

- *Dream analysis:* Psychoanalysts also agree with Freud that dreams reveal the inner life but that the details have different meanings for different individuals.[94] The therapist can only establish what the hidden meanings of the details are by asking the dreamer what they mean.

- *Transference:* **Transference** is the transfer to the therapist of emotions linked with other relationships, such as feelings toward the father or mother. If the patient shows exaggerated dislike for or infatuation with the therapist, it may provide clues about old or current relationships.

Because the goal of psychoanalysis is to bring about a major reorganization of personality, it can require two or three expensive sessions a week for several years. Clearly, then, it is not affordable to a great many people.

Humanistic Therapy: Person-Centered The group of psychotherapies known as the *humanistic therapies* represent the point of view that people have the capacity for choice and growth. Humanistic therapists strive to overcome the **incongruence** or mismatch between patients' self-concept (the image of what they really are) and the ideal self (the image of what they wish they were). Unlike psychoanalysts, humanistic therapists tend to concentrate on the present instead of the past, the conscious rather than the unconscious, growth and fulfillment rather than illness, and "taking immediate responsibility for one's feelings and actions rather than uncovering the hidden obstacles to doing so."[95] Perhaps the most well known of the humanistic therapies is that known as *person-centered therapy.*

In **person-centered therapy,** which grew out of Carl Rogers's theories, the therapist focuses on the patient's own conscious self-insights rather than on the therapist's interpretations.[96,97] Person-centered therapy is also known as **nondirective** or **client-centered therapy,** and the person in therapy is called a **client** rather than a patient. On the theory that people already have the inner resources for growth and that these need only be encouraged, therapists attempt to exhibit *genuineness, acceptance,* and *empathy.*

The role of the therapist is nondirective: he or she does not guide or offer judgments but simply listens, like a loving parent. Indeed, Rogers called this technique **active listening;** the therapist echoes, restates, and clarifies the client's verbalizations and acknowledges the feelings being expressed. An example given by Rogers is that if a client says, "I just ain't no good to nobody, never was, and never will be," the therapist could say, "Feeling that now, hm? That you're just no good to yourself, no good to anybody. Never will be any good to anybody . . . . Those really are lousy feelings. Just feel that you're no good at all, hm?"[98]

Gestalt Therapy Another of the humanistic therapies is Gestalt therapy. Developed by Fritz Perls, **Gestalt therapy** tries to help patients to become aware of and to express their feelings, as well as to take responsibility for their feelings and actions.[99] In this, it combines the emphasis of psychoanalysis on making one aware of unconscious feelings with the humanistic emphasis on immediate experience and current behavior. In accordance with the notion of *Gestalt,* or "total environment," the Gestalt therapist pays attention to **body language**— the gestures and expressions patients make with their bodies—as well as spoken language. Thus, a therapist might point out, "You say your relations with your daughter are fine, but I notice whenever her name comes up you fold your arms across your chest."

Rational-Emotive Therapy Psychoanalytic therapy is concerned with revealing and interpreting the deep-down childhood experiences that lead to people's emotions. **Rational-emotive therapy** is concerned (1) with the *thoughts and beliefs* that lead to people's emotions and (2) with replacing *irrational* thoughts and beliefs with rational ones. The theory is called *rational-emotive* because it assumes that thoughts, or rationality, lead to emotions.

Rational emotive therapists, such as its creator, Albert Ellis, take the opposite view from that of the warm, caring person-centered therapists.[100,101] They believe that people are governed by self-defeating ideas about "musts" and "oughts" and "shoulds" and that the purpose of therapy should be to reveal the "absurdity" of these ideas. Rational-emotive therapists, therefore, do much more talking than their counterparts in humanistic therapy do, interpreting, instructing, and confronting patients with the "irrationality" of their beliefs. For example, if the patient says, "Oh, I'm always so stupid," the therapist might say, "It's always the same [nonsense]. Now if you would look at the [nonsense]—instead of 'Oh, how stupid I am! He hates me! I think I'll kill myself'—then you'd get better right away."[102]

Cognitive Therapy Like rational-emotive therapy, **cognitive therapy** assumes that our thinking influences our feelings and our reactions to events. To improve people's well-being, cognitive therapists encourage their patients to find evidence that supports positive beliefs and refutes negative beliefs. Unlike rational-emotive therapists, however, cognitive therapists don't try to tell their patients what to think; rather, they try to use gentle questioning to help people discover their irrationalities for themselves.

The best-known work in cognitive therapy has been that of Aaron Beck with depressed patients.[103] Beck found that depressed people held three negative forms of belief: (1) they feel themselves deprived or defeated ("I'm always left out"); (2) they see the world as full of obstacles ("Nothing works"); and (3) they see no hope in the future ("It'll never happen"). The therapist's goal is to get patients to see that these "hypotheses" are incorrect. For example, it has been found that depressed people usually blame themselves when things go wrong but attribute successes to external circumstances. In one attempt to change this kind of thinking, 235 depressed people were trained over a 10-week period to interpret events as normal people do (recording positive events, for example, and stating what they had contributed to each). Compared with depressed people who were not

so trained, the depressed people who went through the positive thinking exercises were much less depressed.[104]

Transactional Analysis Often mentioned by its abbreviation, **TA, transactional analysis** is a form of therapy that is concerned with how people communicate, or "transact," with one another. TA theory assumes we have three sides to our personality: instinctive child-like, rational adult-like, and judgmental parent-like. (These correspond to the Freudian notions of id, ego, and superego.) A transaction, or communication, is said to be "balanced" if one aspect of your personality is communicating with the same aspect of someone else's personality (such as adult to adult). However, the transaction is said to be "crossed" if one aspect of your personality is communicating with a different aspect of another's personality (for instance, child to parent), and this gives rise to problems in relationships. The purpose of therapy is to teach patients to be aware of how they are communicating with others so that they can keep their transactions from being crossed.

In *Games People Play,* Eric Berne, the creator of TA, has given some colorful names to the "scripts," or types of crossed transactions, that people find themselves repeating ("Ain't It Awful"; "If It Weren't for You, I Could"; "Let's You and Him Fight").[105]

Brief Therapy Transactional analysis and cognitive therapy are two types of treatment known as **brief therapy.** Instead of seeing a therapist in an open-ended way for several months (or even years, in the case of psychoanalysis), the patient makes a contract with the therapist in which both agree on how long treatment will last (generally 2–6 months) and what problems the two will concentrate on.

Psychotherapy: Does It Work?

Research shows that most psychotherapy patients improve compared with untreated people. Even though types of therapies differ, they may offer effective commonalities.

3.42

*Unit 3
Psychological
Health: The
Power of the
Mind*

Is psychotherapy really effective in treating patients? British psychologist Hags Eysenck reviewed available data from studies of various kinds of psychotherapy, and concluded that roughly two-thirds (about 66%) of those suffering neurotic disorders who were treated improved markedly—but so did two-thirds of "neurotic" patients who were *not* treated.[106] In other words, there was a significant rate of **spontaneous remission**—of improvement without treatment. A re-analysis of Eysenck's data found that the spontaneous remissions constituted only 43%, but that number is still surprisingly high.[107]

This is not the last word, however. An analysis of 475 investigations found that the average psychotherapy patient improves compared with 80% of untreated people on waiting lists. Said the authors, "The evidence overwhelmingly supports the efficacy of psychotherapy."[108] A different study of 240 patients found that psychotherapy works just as well as medication in the treatment of depression.[109] This does not mean that all psychotherapies are the same, nor that all problems are easily treated. In general, psychotherapy is *most* useful in treating specific, clear-cut problems.[110]

Despite their apparent differences, the various therapeutic methods may be effective because of commonalities, according to psychologists who have studied them.[111-113] Regardless of method, effective therapists offer patients *empathy*—understanding of their experiences—and are able to convey their care and concern in a way that earns the patients' trust. Psychotherapy also draws on the patients' own inner healing resources, possibly by drawing on the power of hope: depressed, anxious people seek out psychotherapy in the expectation that it will help them get better.

Behavior Therapies

Behavior therapies are based on the assumption that problem behavior is learned and therefore can be unlearned. Behavior modification makes changes by rewarding good behavior and withholding rewards for bad behavior. Aversion therapy substitutes a negative response for a positive response to undesirable behavior.

So far we have described so-called talking therapies. There are other forms of psychotherapy, however, in which it is assumed that psychological problems do not necessarily diminish with self-awareness. These are **behavior therapies,** so labeled because, instead of trying to get rid of psychological distress by searching out underlying problems, the therapy uses learning principles to change the troubling behavior. That is, the therapists assume that because the behavior is learned (such as smoking or fear of flying), it can be unlearned.

The behavior therapies work best for achieving very specific purposes, such as conquering phobias and eliminating certain habits such as bed-wetting or smoking. We already mentioned one type of behavior therapy, *systematic desensitization,* in our discussion of phobias. Other types include *behavior modification* and *aversion therapy.*

Behavior Modification In **behavior modification,** rewards are given for desirable behaviors and withheld for undesirable behaviors. For example, a women being treated in a hospital setting for a life-threatening condition of anorexia nervosa (self-starvation) was confined to a sparsely furnished room and was rewarded with privileges—reading materials, TV, the right to leave the room, the right to see visitors—only as a reward for gaining weight.[114]

Behavior modification is a five-step process:

1. Specify your target behavior, the behavior you want to change, such as smoking cigarettes or losing weight.

2. Gather baseline data describing your present behavior, such as how many cigarettes you smoke and under what conditions.

3. Design your program.

4. Execute and evaluate your program.

5. Bring your program to an end.[115]

Aversion Therapy Systematic desensitization attempts to substitute a positive reaction instead of a negative one; that is, a patient is taught to be relaxed instead of fearful around a harmless object such as a friendly dog. In **aversion therapy** or **aversive conditioning,** the reverse is true: a negative response is substituted for a positive response to an undesirable habit such as smoking. For example, someone who is trying to quit smoking may be instructed to smoke under very unpleasant conditions—in a small room, surrounded by overflowing ash trays, perhaps exposed to mild electric shocks whenever a cigarette is lifted to the lips. The idea, of course, is to create an aversion to the particular habit.

Hypnosis

Hypnosis uses the subject's susceptibility to suggestion to change certain habits.

Hypnosis is defined as a condition of heightened suggestibility that enables a hypnotist to instruct the subject to experience imaginary happenings as if they were real. Hypnotists put their subject into a "trance" by asking the subject to concentrate on a particular spot on the wall or on a moving object while the hypnotist states "Your eyelids are growing heavy . . . ."

Hypnosis does not work for everyone. Its power is present less in the hypnotist's skills than in the subject's susceptibility to suggestion.[116] However, it has had some success in reinforcing people who are resolved to change certain habits, such as eating too much, nail biting, smoking, or drinking too much. It has also helped some people to become more sexually responsive.[117,118] The device for doing this is the **posthypnotic suggestion,** in which the hypnotist suggests to the subject something the subject will do after coming out of hypnosis. The device seems to work quite well in helping to change behavior, although the effects generally wear off after days or weeks.

Group Treatments

For some psychological difficulties, group treatments are better than individual psychotherapy. Group therapy is less expensive and shows people they have similar problems. Couples or family therapy works well with relationship issues. Self-help and support groups are successful for people sharing the same problem.

The biggest advantages of individual psychotherapy are that it offers individual attention and privacy. However, for some kinds of psychological distress there are better results to be obtained in groups.

Group Therapy Group therapy, therapy given to a group of people at the same time, has the same aims as individual therapy, such as self-understanding and behavior change. Most of the individual psychotherapies we described are often practiced within therapist-led groups of 8–10 people. Such methods have the advantage of being less expensive than individual therapeutic sessions. They also show people they are not alone in the problems they have, whatever those problems may be.[119]

Couples or Family Therapy In couples therapy, also known as **marital therapy,** the treatment is concerned with the relationship problems between couples. **Family therapy** expands the treatment to include members of one family. Although the problems that bring the family to the attention of the therapist may be those of one individual, the therapy proceeds on the assumption that those problems may stem from problems of interaction within the family.

Self-Help and Support Groups Self-help groups have gained in popularity in recent years. A therapist may organize a group whose members all suffer from a similar problem (such as alcohol abuse). **Self-help groups**, however, are organized around a similar problem but are not led by a therapist. Such tasks as those of chair, secretary, and treasurer are generally rotated among the members. Fees are far less than those for conventional group therapy, often just the cost of the room rental and coffee (members of Alcoholics Anonymous, for example, each contribute a dollar at every meeting). Members are available to each other for help in ways that a professional therapist may not be after office hours. Finally, the members of the group are unified by a common understanding of and appreciation for each other's difficulties, in a way that may not exist between, say, a nonalcoholic therapist and a group of recovering alcoholics.

3.44

*Unit 3
Psychological
Health: The
Power of the
Mind*

We mentioned some examples of support groups in Chapter 5. Groups also exist for recovering gamblers, "sexaholics," former prisoners, current or former mental patients, and many others.

Medical Therapies

Medical therapies are useful when other therapies aren't enough. Drug therapies have been successful in treating anxiety, depression, and schizophrenia. Electroconvulsive therapy and psychosurgery are also sometimes useful.

Sometimes talking and behavior therapies aren't enough. The only hope is to alter the brain's functioning through direct medical intervention—by drug therapies, by electroconvulsive therapy, or by psychosurgery. All these require the supervision of a medical doctor.

Drug Therapies In the 1950s, the development of new drugs revolutionized the treatment of mentally disordered people, allowing the discharge of thousands of patients from mental hospitals. Some major categories of drugs are:

- *For anxiety:* Valium and Librium are among the most heavily prescribed drugs in the world. Originally used to reduce major anxieties, they are now prescribed, often wrongly, for even minor stresses.

- *For depression:* For patients suffering the mood swings of bipolar disorder, lithium has been found to level out the manias and depressions. In addition, three other classes of drugs have been found to bring relief to depressed people: tricyclic drugs (such as Elavil and Tofranil); monoamine oxidase inhibitors (MAOIs, such as Nardil and Parnate); and fluoxetine (Prozac).

- *For schizophrenia:* Schizophrenia cannot be cured. However, drugs known as *neuroleptic drugs* (chlorpromazine and haloperidol) can arrest the deterioration of behavior in schizophrenics. A new drug known as clozapine (brand name: Clozaril) relieves many negative symptoms and is free of the other drugs' side effects.

Although this pharmaceutical revolution has contributed to reducing the patient population of mental hospitals to a quarter of what it was in the 1960s, this has unfortunately not translated into freedom but into homelessness for many people. One study of homeless people in Chicago, for instance, found that 23% were psychotic and 47% were depressed.[120] Many such people are not taking their medication regularly or at all and thus suffer from a recurrence of symptoms. Nevertheless, these drugs have helped many other people live nearly normal lives.

Electroconvulsive Therapy Abbreviated **ECT, electroconvulsive therapy**—"electroshock therapy" or "shock treatment"—consists of administering a brief electrical shock to a patient's brain in order to induce a convulsion similar to epilepsy. Despite its connotations of horror movies and mad scientists, ECT has been found to be successful for treatment of severe depression that has not responded to drug therapy and for those with strong suicidal tendencies.[121,122]

Psychosurgery Probably the medical intervention of last resort, **psychosurgery** consists of attempting to change behavior through the surgical removal or destruction of brain tissue.

Strategy for Living: Deciding to Be in the Ballgame We cannot always avoid losses or guarantee successes. But we can try to develop the mental attitude that agrees with famous author James Michener: "I like challenges. I don't mind defeat. I don't gloat over victories. I want to be in the ballgame."[123]

800-HELP

National Mental Health Association. 800-969-6642. (In Virginia, 703-643-7722.) Gives information on depression, schizophrenia, and other psychological disorders. Provides local referrals.

The Will to Believe: The Search for Guides, Not Gurus

How well do you agree or disagree with the following statements? Indicate "T" (True) or "F" (False).

___ **1.** There is no God. You can believe only in yourself or your fellow human beings.

___ **2.** God exists. The Supreme Being is available to me through my organized religion.

___ **3.** I believe in Something—a Supreme Being or Life Force—but my form of worship or thinking does not exist within the framework of the usual forms of religion.

___ **4.** I don't know whether there's a Higher Power or not. I'm still searching.

Is there a correct answer? Only you can determine that. What remains true, perhaps, is what theologian Paul Tillich suggested: all of us have a *will* to believe, a *need* to have faith in something—an "ultimate concern" that we care about.[124] This Ultimate Concern may be a supreme being, a church, moral principles, one's country, one's family, one's support group, or one's self.

Over the last 25 years, religion in the United States has been changing. As philosopher-author Jacob Needleman says, among many people "There is a longing for a new world view, a new concept of God."[125] From 1952 to 1987, Protestant denominations shrank from the majority of 67% of American religious affiliations to 57% and Jewish from 4% to 2%. Catholics have increased 3% from 25% to 28%, according to Gallup Poll data.[126] However, the interesting news is that today 4% of the population claims a religion *outside* the major traditions, compared to only 1% in the 1950s. This includes Eastern mystical faiths, nature religions, Native American traditions, theosophical beliefs, goddess worship, and New Age practices.

Also significant: during the same period, the religiously *nonaffiliated* has grown from 2% to 9% today. According to religion professor Wade Clark Roof, of the University of California, Santa Barbara, their cultural characteristics have also changed: "No longer a small marginal group of atheists and social dissidents, nonaffiliates today are predominately young, white, well-educated, and socially mobile." Moreover, he says, many of those within this group are "perhaps better described as privately religious than as irreligious or antireligious."[127]

It seems, then, that people are determined to believe in something. The question is: what will we believe in next, now that the influence of some of the older beliefs has diminished for some people? For some young people, unfortunately, the answer is found among ardent religious sects that flourish on the edge of many college campuses—groups known as cults.

Cults and Cult Figures

According to the Cult Awareness Network, a nonprofit organization, 3 to 5 million Americans have been or are now involved in as many as 2500 "destructive" cults. A destructive cult, in the network's definition, is "a closed system or group whose followers have been recruited deceptively and retained through use of manipulative techniques of thought reform or mind control."[128] (*See* ● *accompanying figure on next page.*)

Many such groups are religious, some small and continually changing, with memberships ranging from half a dozen to several hundred, some large and stable, with groups near many college campuses. The groups may have great appeal to college freshmen, who are suddenly cut off from family ties, or to seniors, who may be insecure about their future. Converts may be drawn from devout churchgoers, but they may also be from atheists—or from neither. Rather than being deficient in social skills, converts may actually be open and personable. "It's no surprise that nice kids from nice families are picked up," says anthropology professor Laura Nader, who teaches a popular class on why people become vulnerable to ideological control.

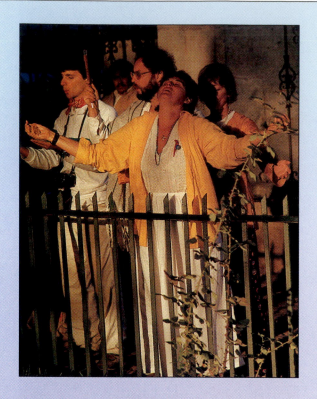

"The most altruistic kids are the most vulnerable to cults."[129] Although college years are a time when students often begin to distance themselves from their parents as part of the process of becoming adults, the effect of some religious cults is to *isolate* children from their families. Ginger Brown, for example, was midway through her sophomore year at the University of California, San Diego, when a friend invited her to a Bible study group called Ever Increasing Love Ministries. Before long, her family in northern California noticed a change in their daughter. She all but stopped calling, moved frequently without giving her parents her new address, became sullen and withdrawn, and began to treat the family with contempt. At the end of her sophomore year, she quit college, telling her father that she did so because Jesus Christ hadn't gone to school. The cult leader (who had a $60,000 Mercedes and other expensive assets purchased by the ministry's members) "ruled over his followers with fear, intimidation, and other tricks of the mind-control trade," according to former members. "He changed his followers' personalities so drastically that parents often didn't recognize their own offspring."[130] Eventually, Ginger's distraught parents had their daughter seized. They attempted to have her "deprogrammed" of her religious beliefs—a process that backfired when Ginger had them charged with kidnaping, although a jury later decided that Ginger was not believable.

The Six Stages of Faith

"What we need are guides, not gurus," says philosopher Needleman. "A guide is someone who helps you find the truth for yourself. A guru is someone who finds it for you."[131]

Most people, of course, start out being *directed*—by their parents and other adults—in their religious beliefs. However, according to James Fowler, these views don't just remain static.[132,133] Faith can be a developmental process, evolving to higher levels as people try to reconcile their faith—whether in religion or some other ultimate concern—with their daily living experience.

● **Recognizing cult involvement.**

Signs for students to watch for:
- *Authoritarian male figure*
- *High-pressure pitch*
- *Vows of a group's support and love for you before they know you*
- *Demands that you sever ties to family, friends, and religion*
- *Invitations to leave campus for a religious retreat*

Signs for friends and family to look for:
- *Abrupt personality change*
- *Cutting of ties with family and friends*
- *Total involvement with the group, excluding all else*
- *Quick involvement in proselytizing and fund raising*
- *Speech that begins to reflect the group's rigid dogma*

There are, Fowler proposes, six stages in the development of faith, progressing from simple and self-centered levels to complex and altruistic ones:

- *Stage 1: Intuitive-projective:* This stage, found in children ages 3–7, is filled with fantasy and magic, as about the power of God.

- *Stage 2: Mythic-literal:* Typical of children in middle childhood but also of many people in adulthood, the stage of mythic-literal faith is characterized by a literal belief in myths and symbols. Adherents also have a strong belief in reciprocity: those who follow God's laws are rewarded, those who don't are punished.

- *Stage 3: Synthetic-conventional:* In this stage of faith, people express a conformist, conventional outlook, holding beliefs and values because they "feel right" (for example, getting married in church rather than in a civil ceremony) and provide a sense of identity rather than because they make intellectual sense.

- *Stage 4: Individual-reflective:* This stage represents a break from the conventional, and it often happens because of the experience of college (when people question previous instances of authority) or because of a wrenching experience (job loss, divorce, death in the family) that leads one to question hitherto unquestioned beliefs. In the stage of individual-reflective faith, one begins to commit to goals (including, sometimes, those of religious cults) that differ from those of many other people.

- *Stage 5: Conjunctive:* This stage, which Fowler believes usually comes with middle age, involves the conjunction of Stage 2 beliefs in myths and symbols (such as the worshipper's belief in prayer) and Stage 4 intellectual independence (such as the conscientious objector's elevating the refusal to kill over other values). As might be apparent, people in this stage of faith are not only open to new truths but are also willing to live with and express contradictions.

- *Stage 6: Universalizing:* Mother Theresa, Martin Luther King, Jr., and Gandhi are among the handful of people who have reached the stage of universalizing faith, according to Fowler. All have undergone a transforming experience that produced a "universalizing" vision of justice and love that compelled them to radically alter their lives, often at tremendous self-sacrifice, so that they further cosmic values.

Clearly, most of us cannot expect to achieve the rarefied air of the stage of universalizing faith. However, Fowler does not actually say that we *should* advance from one stage to the next; instead, he says that each stage has its proper time for ascendancy. Indeed, he believes that each stage has the potential for "wholeness, grace and integrity, and for strengths sufficient for either life's blows or blessings." The task of any one stage is to realize and integrate "the strengths and graces" of that stage rather than to rush on to the next one.

Caffeine, Tobacco, and Alcohol: Common Mood-Altering Drugs

In These Chapters:

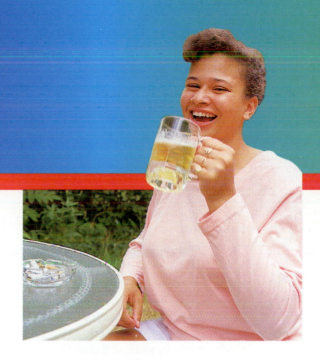

Is there a human need to alter consciousness?

No doubt lots of people you know—maybe you, too—feel that they need "something to get going" to start the day. It might be a cup of coffee or cup of tea, for some people even a Coke or Pepsi, all of which contain caffeine. Or it might be a cigarette, which contains nicotine. Then at day's end, many people feel they need "something to wind down"—a couple of beers maybe, a glass of wine or two, or something stronger though legal.

Caffeine and nicotine are *stimulants*—they stimulate the central nervous system, speed up brain activity, increase the level of arousal. Alcohol is a *depressant*—it slows down the central nervous system, makes one feel relaxed, sleepy, even anesthetized. No wonder sometimes we hear people talking about being on a "coffee-wine cycle": they drink coffee all morning and afternoon, and then they are so wound up they feel they have to have several glasses of wine or other drinks to calm themselves down.

Of course there are many other mind-altering substances of all sorts all around us, all the time, as part of our lives. Every day the newspapers and television are filled with news about drugs—about cocaine smuggling, marijuana busts, the upsurge in heroin use, and so on. But three drugs may have had a greater effect on human civilization than all the other mood-altering drugs combined: caffeine, nicotine, and alcohol.[1]

4.2

*Unit 4
Caffeine, Tobacco,
and Alcohol:
Common Mood-
Altering Drugs*

10 Caffeine: The National Wake-Up Drug

▶ What are the many sources of caffeine?
▶ What are the possible consequences of consuming too much caffeine?

What is extraordinary about our existence today," says medical school professor Peter Dews, "is that in order to function in society, you've got to be in synch. You've got to be ready to work at 8 o'clock—even though your own internal clock might not start until 10. I have speculated that caffeine helps you stay awake and alert throughout the mandatory eight hours of the working day."[2]

Caffeine, it has been suggested, may be the drug that keeps our industrialized society running, that gives people the lift that helps them fight boredom and fatigue. Consider coffee, which in the United States is what caffeine means to most people.[3] Although it is widely used all over the world, the United States, with one-twentieth of the world's population, drinks a third of the planet's coffee, some 360 million cups per day. Indeed, the amount of coffee imported is so costly (2 billion pounds costing $6 billion a year) that coffee ranks second only to petroleum in value.[4]

Caffeine: How You Get It, What It Does

Caffeine appears in coffee, soft drinks, tea, chocolate, some prescription and nonprescription drugs, and some processed foods. People often use caffeine to keep alert and to alleviate boredom. Too much caffeine can produce caffeinism—anxiety, headache, irregular heartbeat.

Caffeine, a bitter alkaloid, is the principal drug found in coffee. Until recently, coffee was the most significant source of caffeine for Americans, but now caffeine-containing soft drinks have overtaken coffee as primary sources of dietary caffeine, particularly among young adults aged 18–24.[5,6] Indeed, if you have switched to decaffeinated coffee, you may be surprised to learn that much of the caffeine *taken out of* coffee is used as an additive for soft drinks.[7]

It is hard to avoid this drug. Besides coffee and soft drinks, caffeine also appears in tea, cocoa, chocolate, a number of prescription drugs, and many nonprescription drugs used for staying alert (NoDoz), for minor pain relief (Anacin, Excedrin), for losing weight, and as decongestants. (*See ● Figure 10.1.*) Thus, people who take a pain reliever every day (to relieve arthritis, for example) may be getting a daily jolt of caffeine that they are not aware of. Moreover, those who drink a six-pack of Coca-Cola a day are getting the equivalent of four cups of instant coffee. Even those who swear off caffeine entirely may be unaware they are getting it in baked goods, puddings, and some other processed foods.

To get the usual lift that most people expect requires 150–250 milligrams (mg) of caffeine, which is equivalent to one or two cups of coffee. (*See ● Table 10.1 for an explanation of milligrams.*) On average, every American consumes caffeine from all sources in amounts equivalent to 4 or 5 cups of coffee a day. For most people, caffeine consumption in moderation does not present problems. Since it is possible to experience serious symptoms from high levels of caffeine, you need to assess how much caffeine you are really consuming every day. (*See Self Discovery 10.1.*)

The Effects of Caffeine Ninety-nine percent of the caffeine you consume is absorbed and distributed to all your body organs and tissues.[8] The effects of caffeine are similar to those of other stimulants such as amphetamines. Physiologically, caffeine works because the chemical somewhat resembles a brain chemical called **adenosine**, which depresses (slows down) the activity of the central nervous system and the brain. Caffeine fits into the brain's receptor sites intended for adenosine and blocks them, so that the adenosine can no longer do its work of slowing down nervous system activity; thus, one feels stimulated.[9]

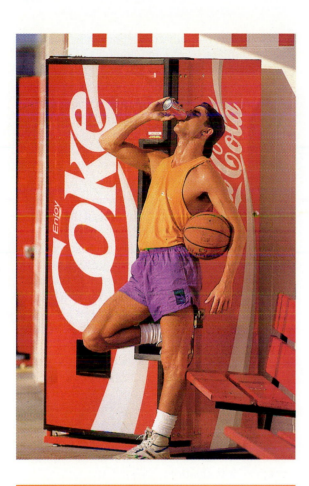

● **Figure 10.1 Caffeine content**

Food and beverages	Caffeine in milligrams
Coffee (5-oz. cup)	
Drip method	110–150
Percolated	64–124
Instant	40–108
Decaf	2–5
Instant decaf	2
Tea, loose or bags (5-oz. cup)	
1-minute brew	9–33
3-minute brew	20–46
5-minute brew	20–50
Tea Products	
Instant (5-oz. cup)	12–28
Iced tea (12-oz. can)	22–36
Chocolate Products	
Hot cocoa (6 oz.)	2–8
Dry cocoa (1 oz.)	6
Milk chocolate (1 oz.)	1–15
Baking chocolate (1 oz.)	35
Sweet dark chocolate (1 oz.)	5–35
Chocolate milk (8 oz.)	2–7
Chocolate-flavored syrup (2 tbsp.)	4
Soft Drinks, per 12-oz. serving, by flavor type	
Cola or pepper	30–48
Diet cola or pepper	0–59
Cherry cola	12–46
Citrus	0–64

Over-the-counter drugs	Caffeine in milligrams per tablet
Stimulants	
NoDoz	100
Vivarin	200
Pain Relievers	
Anacin	32
Excedrin	65
Excedrin P.M.	0
Midol (for cramps)	32
Midol P.M.S.	0
Plain aspirin	0
Vanquish	33
Diuretics	
Aqua-Ban	100
Cold Remedies	
Coryban-D	30
Dristan	0
Diet Pills	
Dexatrim	200
Dietac	200

● **Table 10.1 Metric Units**

Units of weight:

The meaning of 1 gram: 1 gram = 0.035 ounce, the weight of 2 paper clips or 1 shirt button

1 kilogram (kg) = 1000 grams (or 2.2046 pounds)
1 gram (g) = 1000 milligrams
1 milligram (mg) = 1000 micrograms (μg)

Units of liquid volume:

The meaning of 1 liter: 1 liter = 1.057 quarts, slightly more than a standard quart of milk

1 liter (l) = 1000 milliliters (ml)

4.4

Unit 4
Caffeine, Tobacco,
and Alcohol:
Common Mood-
Altering Drugs

SELF DISCOVERY 10.1

What's Your Caffeine Consumption?

How much caffeine do you drink, and what effect is it having on you? Take this test to find out.

	Yes	No
1. Does coffee drinking cause physical or psychological changes in your health?	_____	_____
2. Do you consume more than 250 milligrams of caffeine every day? (*See Figure 10.1.*)	_____	_____
3. Do you experience more than two of the recognized symptoms of caffeinism on regularly drinking one or more cups of coffee? The more you have, the more likely it is you're hooked. The symptoms include insomnia, irritability, depression, chronic fatigue, rapid pulse or heartbeat, jitteriness, lightheadedness, rapid breathing, diarrhea, stomach pains or heartburn, headaches, and anxiety.	_____	_____
4. Can you start the day without a cup of coffee?	_____	_____
5. Does it bother you if you ever miss your mid-morning coffee break?	_____	_____
6. Do you usually have a second cup?	_____	_____
7. Have you ever voluntarily gone a whole day without coffee or caffeinated soda or other caffeinated food and drink? Did you feel dramatically different? Did you drink more coffee the following day?	_____	_____
8. Do you get headaches when you try to stop for more than 18–24 hours?	_____	_____
9. Do you always choose a coffee, tea, or cola drink that has caffeine?	_____	_____
10. Do you depend on coffee every day to feel good?	_____	_____

Interpretation of Your Score

Answering yes to three to five of the questions calls for cutting back. If you answer yes to more than five questions, chances are that you are hooked on caffeine and should consider quitting.

Source: Adapted from: Goulart, F. S. (1984). *The caffeine book: A user's and abuser's guide.* Lexington, MA: Dodd, Mead.

How much stimulation a person feels depends on the person, including his or her age, use, level of tolerance, and use of other drugs.[10] An elderly person, for instance, tends to have a decreased tolerance to caffeine-containing drinks.[11] Cigarette smokers get rid of caffeine at twice the normal rate (which may be why smokers drink more coffee), but pregnant women take much longer to clear the caffeine, as do women taking oral contraceptives.[12]

Although people vary widely in their sensitivity to this drug—and caffeine *is* a drug—someone who drinks one or two cups of coffee in succession would likely notice an increase in attentiveness and a decrease in drowsiness. They might even notice that they can perform a task longer before getting bored. However, caffeine does not noticeably enhance one's ability to perform complex intellectual tasks.[13] In fact, perhaps the opposite is true: one study of college students showed an association between *high* intakes of caffeine and *lower* academic performance.[14]

As we explore later, the myth prevails that coffee can sober you up. Although coffee may arouse someone who has been drinking, it will not lower the amount of alcohol in the system or reduce intoxication.

Too Many Cups of Coffee: Caffeinism From time to time, a physician at a university health service told one of the authors of this book, students come to her complaining of anxiety, lightheadedness, breathlessness, headache, tremulousness, and irregular heartbeat. "The first thing I do," she said, "is ask them how much coffee they drink."

Sometimes it will turn out to be as many as 10 cups a day—more than 1000 milligrams of caffeine. However, instances of **caffeinism**—caffeine intoxication, sometimes called "coffee nerves," characterized by the aforementioned symptoms—have also been reported on smaller amounts.[15] Generally, 4–6 cups of coffee a day (containing 600 milligrams of caffeine) are considered enough to produce the symptoms of caffeinism.[16] But many coffee drinkers do not use the standard 5-ounce coffee *cups* found in restaurants. Rather, they favor 12-ounce coffee *mugs,* which hold as much liquid as a soft-drink can; clearly, it doesn't take many of these to deliver more than 1000 milligrams of caffeine.

Most people, it seems, have some internal mechanism that tells them when to stop drinking coffee, perhaps, so that they consume only enough caffeine to achieve a certain comfort level. There may also be some inherent differences in the way people process caffeine. Regardless of internal regulators, however, at one time or another most coffee drinkers have experienced caffeinism. High doses of caffeine can not only make people feel nervous, irritable, and unable to sleep, but also produce pronounced physiological effects: increased heart rate, respiratory rate, body temperature, blood pressure, urine production, and stomach acid secretions.

A study of college students revealed that moderate and high consumers of caffeine were more likely to be depressed and anxious compared to those who abstained.[17] In fact, the effects of too much caffeine may mimic the symptoms of anxiety disorders and may trigger a panic attack—with accompanying symptoms of breathlessness, sweating, and heart palpitations—in those who tend to suffer from this problem.[18-20]

Can you actually die from consuming too much caffeine? Probably only if you drink 50–100 cups of coffee, which is equal to 5–10 grams of caffeine. Fatal doses are rare, but they have occurred in adults who consumed such amounts.[21]

Caffeine Dependence and Withdrawal Caffeine use can lead to both psychological and physical dependence—an occurrence that might not be news to coffee drinkers but might surprise caffeinated soft-drink consumers. Stopping the drug after long-term heavy or even moderate use can result in a number of withdrawal symptoms: headache, nervousness, poor concentration, irritability, lethargy, restlessness, and nausea. If coffee is the primary culprit, withdrawal can even result in diarrhea. If tea, it may be constipation (because of the tannic acid in tea).

Headache is an especially common problem for people quitting caffeine, although caffeine withdrawal is sometimes overlooked as a cause of headache.[22] The headache usually begins about 18 hours after stopping the drug and gradually subsides within 2–6 days.[23,24] If you find yourself experiencing a headache owing to

caffeine withdrawal, keep in mind that many nonprescription pain relievers contain caffeine. Thus, use of these products may actually contribute to a continuing desire for caffeine.[25]

Risks: Has the Up Drug a Down Side?

It is not clear whether caffeine increases risk of heart disease, but it may be linked to infertility, low-birth-weight infants, and premenstrual syndrome. Pregnant women, nursing mothers, and those with a history of heart disease should avoid this drug.

What about long-term effects? Over the years there has been back-and-forth debate about the harmfulness of caffeine—whether, for instance, its long-term use may lead to increased risk of heart disease or to infertility or to birth defects. The results to date are as follows.

Possible, Unproven Link to Heart Disease
Caffeine is known to increase the heart rate and blood pressure, but it is not clear whether it is associated with long-term risk of heart and blood vessel disease. On the one hand, several major studies show an association of heavy caffeine consumption (5 or more cups per day) with heightened risk of heart disease.[26-29] On the other hand, a 1990 study of over 45,500 men ages 40–75 who were followed by Harvard researchers for 2 years revealed no association between total coffee consumption—even among men drinking 6 cups a day—and an increased risk of heart disease or stroke.[30,31]

Caffeine does not seem to be associated with high blood pressure (hypertension), which is considered a risk factor in heart disease, although blood pressure does go up with caffeine use.[32,33] Caffeine may promote heartbeat irregularities (arrhythmias), though moderate use of caffeine does not seem to increase the severity of the problem.[34-36]

It appears, then, that the question of the relationship of caffeine to heart disease is still undecided.

4.6

*Unit 4
Caffeine, Tobacco,
and Alcohol:
Common Mood-
Altering Drugs*

Possible, Unproven Link to Infertility The question of fertility, too, has different answers. One study found that women were much less able to become pregnant during 12 months of trying to conceive if they had the caffeine equivalent of 1 cup of coffee a day than were women who consumed less.[37] However, another study found no difference among the two groups regarding likelihood of conceiving.[38]

Possible, Unproven Link to Low-Birth-Weight Infants Like many kinds of drugs, caffeine crosses the placenta during pregnancy and enters the bloodstream of the fetus. Caffeine has also been found in breast milk. The good news is that caffeine does not seem to cause birth defects, but health professionals nevertheless worry that the drug may have some effect on fetal development, though the research findings have been inconclusive.[39] One study suggested that mothers who consumed caffeine fairly heavily (300 milligrams or more a day—3 cups of coffee or 6 cans of cola) produced low-birth-weight babies.[40,41] Other studies suggest it may not be caffeine use at all but rather *cigarette smoking* that is associated with the delivery of low-birth-weight infants.[42]

Because of the uncertainty, it would seem advisable that women who are trying to become pregnant, who are pregnant, or who are breast-feeding should avoid caffeine. Indeed, they might also consider avoiding even *decaffeinated* coffee, since the safety of this beverage has not been fully assessed.

Caffeine and PMS and Breast Changes No definitive relationship has been established, but there is some evidence that caffeinated beverages may aggravate **premenstrual syndrome (PMS),** a common disorder characterized by physical and psychological discomfort prior to menstruation.[43]

There appears to be no link between caffeine and breast cancer.[44,45] Women who have noncancerous (benign) breast lumps, a condition known as **fibrocystic breast disease,** might try eliminating caffeine to see if the condition improves.

Strategy for Living: Cutting Down and Quitting Caffeine

Cutting down caffeine is not difficult. Cutting it out, however, is a process that should be done gradually and with an eye on hidden sources of caffeine.

The advice experts give us regarding caffeine consumption is not very exciting, but there is no rule that says the truth always has to be spectacular and dramatic. The advice is, simply: use it in moderation—about 200 milligrams daily for most people, which is two or three 5-ounce cups of coffee. However, pregnant women and nursing women should avoid caffeine entirely; so also, probably, should people at risk for heart disease.

Cutting down on caffeine intake is usually not difficult; cutting *out* caffeine, however, takes more effort. Some suggestions:

- *Quit gradually, not outright:* Quitting "cold turkey" can lead to caffeine-withdrawal headache (often lasting days) and other problems, such as depression, lethargy, and nausea. It's best to ease off over a week or two—for instance, by half a cup less each day.

- *Watch out for hidden sources of caffeine:* Restaurants may sometimes pour regular coffee rather than decaffeinated. Soft drinks, candy, baked goods, and over-the-counter drugs also contain caffeine.

Many former coffee drinkers have switched over to decaffeinated coffee in hopes of avoiding the effects and hazards we've mentioned. However, concern has been raised about the decaffeination process itself: in the United States, at least, the removal of caffeine from coffee beans is often accomplished by means of an organic solvent that can leave some residue behind.[46] In addition, some studies suggest that decaffeinated coffee may be related to several health problems, including infertility, impaired fetal development, and heart disease.[47-49]

11 Tobacco: A Habit Under Fire

▶ Who smokes cigarettes, and why do they do it?

▶ What is in cigarette smoke, and what does it do to smokers?

▶ What are other tobacco products, and what do they do to people's health?

▶ What are strategies for quitting smoking?

It was just another average-selling cigarette brand until 1956. Then its makers began promoting the cowboy theme, and now Marlboro cigarettes have worldwide appeal, earning over $3 billion a year and controlling about 60% of the export cigarette market. "The leathery face and cowboy ways of the Marlboro man are equally compelling to hip magazine readers in New York City, television viewers in Buenos Aires, and billboard-watchers in Taipei," point out two journalists who have studied the still-powerful influence of the fantasy of the western frontier.[50]

Today, 100 years after the American frontier officially closed, the cigarette maker's image of manliness and personal freedom continues to lure smokers, mostly young men, to "go west by choosing Marlboro." Indeed, most Marlboro smokers—two-thirds are men, and 70% are ages 18–34—would be pleased to know that those are real cowboys that are recruited as models for Marlboro ads.[51] They would surely be uneasy, however, if they had to see the reality of an American cowboy whose smoking led to terminal lung cancer. This was vividly shown in a British documentary film, *Death in the West,* which contrasted the powerful image of cowboy manliness and personal freedom shown in cigarette ads with the scene of a cowboy with breathing apparatus strapped to his face, dying of cigarette-caused lung cancer and emphysema.

One of the authors of this book was once a Marlboro smoker. I began smoking in high school, and for many years smoked this and perhaps a dozen other brands. By the end, my consumption had risen to 50 cigarettes a day, the fingertips of my right hand were yellow, the smell of tobacco permeated my hair, skin, and clothing, and I had a hacking cough. Being any place I couldn't smoke (such as the library) for longer than an hour made me extremely uncomfortable. Every morning I had to jump-start myself with a cigarette practically upon getting out of bed. Every evening I went to bed with a sensation like moldy cotton in my mouth. I tried quitting on several occasions, using techniques ranging from toughing it out to self-hypnosis. In the end, when it became clear to me that tobacco was a true addiction, I was able to quit only by taking 6 months of classes in "unsmoking."

Who Smokes?

In North America, people making up the largest categories of smokers or fastest-growing numbers of smokers include children and teenagers, women, the poorly educated, those with lower incomes, people addicted to other substances, and the hard-core nicotine-addicted.

Today most smokers in North America have at least an inkling that what they are doing is unhealthy. They certainly are beginning to find that it is unpopular. You see them in restaurants holding their cigarettes at a distance, fanning the smoke away from their companions. In more and more "smoke-free" offices and public places they can be seen slinking off to bathrooms, lobbies, or outdoors in order to take deep drags that will hold them for the next 45 minutes.

At least we see such signs of tobacco's unpopularity in the United States and Canada, where cigarette smoking is declining. Indeed, only 29% of Americans now smoke, as opposed to 40% in 1965, the year after the U.S. Surgeon General issued his landmark warning against cigarettes. However, in Africa, Latin America, and Asia, tobacco use has jumped about 75% in the last 20 years, as tobacco companies have sought new markets. This explosion in tobacco use elsewhere in the world is a time bomb that could eventually kill 200 million people now under the age of 20.[52]

4.8

Unit 4
Caffeine, Tobacco,
and Alcohol:
Common Mood-
Altering Drugs

But if in North America smoking is, in fact, so unpopular these days, who's buying those 270 brands of cigarettes available? Let's consider this question.

Children and Teenagers Forty-five states prohibit the sale of tobacco to minors, but American young people ages 8–18 still consume around 1 billion packs of cigarettes every year. Although the use of other drugs by high-school students declined in the years 1984–1989, cigarette smoking did not.[53] Although there has been a general slumping of sales of cigarettes in the United States, the percentage of 13- to 15-year-olds who smoke went up 4% in just one year—from 7% in 1988 to 11% in 1989.[54] This fact is important because among smokers born since 1935, almost half started before age 18. Among 24-year-old smokers, 68% began smoking before age 18.[55] Thus, more cigarette ads are placed in youth-oriented (and women's) magazines than in magazines aimed at other segments of the population.[56] The good news is that the number of 20- to 24-year-olds who smoke is down a great deal from 25 years previously; even so, a third of this group still smokes.[57]

Women Catching Up to Men In the United States, more men (31%) smoke than women (26%), but today's female smoker is a heavier smoker than yesterday's and women are now starting to smoke at younger ages. Among high-school seniors, more females than males smoke.[58] "Some may say they've 'come a long way, baby,' " said U.S. Surgeon General Antonia Novello, blasting tobacco ads aimed at women, "but I say they are digging an early grave for themselves and the generation they will bear."[59]

Poorly Educated and Lower-Income People Typical smokers resemble users of other drugs: they tend to be less educated and to earn lower incomes than nonsmokers do. College students are less likely to smoke than other people of the same age.[60] So also are college graduates: only 18% of college graduates smoke, compared with 34% of those who never went to college.[61] Of people living in households earning more than $40,000, only 22% smoke, compared with 29% in households earning a quarter that amount or less.[62]

People Addicted to Other Substances People who are heavy users of alcohol, cocaine, and similar substances are likely to smoke cigarettes as well.[63] Smokers are also more likely than nonsmokers to drink while they drive and consequently to have more traffic violations and auto accidents.[64] As some experts on addiction observe, "smoking is very often a sign of heedlessness toward health and safety. Cigarette addicts are more antisocial and less concerned for their physical well-being than nonsmokers."[65]

The Hard-Core Addicted A proportion of people who smoke could be considered "the diehards"—hard-core smokers addicted to nicotine. Says physician David Sachs, who treats smoking addiction: "With all the health warnings, the people for whom it has been easy to quit have already quit. What we're left with is a group of more addicted smokers."[66]

Why Smoke?

The reasons for smoking include stimulation, handling, and relaxation; tension reduction; the wish to be different; a desire to be slim; and finally the addiction process itself.

The cartoony billboards shout "Party with the Wild Pack!" The magazine ads of people frolicking in the surf cry "Alive with Pleasure!" Cigarette smoking occupies a place in society unlike that allowed other addictive substances. Despite their clear hazards, cigarettes are not only a legal drug, they are also aggressively promoted: the tobacco industry spends $2.7 billion a year (tax deductible) on advertising and promotion. A good part of that promotion, of course, is concerned with giving people reasons to smoke—whether to start, to continue, or to switch to a different brand (although only 10% of smokers switch brands every year).[67]

Some of the reasons for smoking behavior are as follows.

Stimulation, Handling, and Relaxation Because nicotine is a stimulant (depending on the dose), smokers often begin to depend on the lift of the drug to get going in the morning, to ease boredom on the job, to keep them going through the day. Cigarettes (and pipes particularly) also give one a "prop" to handle or manipulate, something to toy with in social and work situations. Smokers say that cigarettes also provide people with a means of pleasurable relaxation, as when completing a job well done or ending a delicious meal.[68]

Tension Reduction: Maintaining Emotional Balance According to psychologist Paul Nesbitt, smokers are more anxious than nonsmokers, but they feel more calm when they are smoking.[69] Stress has also been cited by the U.S. Surgeon General as a reason for increased cigarette consumption among smokers.[70] Researchers suggest that smoking masks the tension a smoker would otherwise feel. That is, by using nicotine to maintain their internal stimulation, smokers seem to protect themselves from the ups and downs of external stimulation.[71]

Adolescents in particular find cigarettes a tension reducer. As British researcher Alan Marsh says about teenagers who take up smoking: "A cigarette covers embarrassment, lifts depression, restores youthful cool. What the smoking adolescent never has the chance to learn is that, like his nonsmoking friends, he would have acquired that knack of affect [emotional] control anyway. It is called growing up and nearly everyone does it, with or without the help of cigarettes."[72] (See ● *Figure 11.1.*)

The Desire to Be Different Advertisements try to appeal to smokers' sense of being adventurous, independent, and otherwise different from others. That's why, of course, so many cigarette ads show people in race cars or speedboats, climbing mountains, and performing other risky activities. "Research indicates that smokers are more often risk-takers, extroverted, defiant, and impulsive," writes Jean Kilbourne. "It is no coincidence that cigarette companies are the leading sponsors of events that appeal to risk-taking and rebellious teenagers: races of motorcycles, dirt bikes, hot rods, [and] rodeos and ballooning."[73]

The Desire to Be Slim Many advertisements aimed at women use the slimmest models to try to reinforce the idea of cigarettes as a form of weight control. This pitch is a major reason,

probably, why cigarette smoking is on the increase among teenage females, a group especially susceptible to concerns about weight.[74] Cigarettes may, in fact, act as an appetite suppressant, deadening the taste buds, decreasing hunger contractions in the stomach, and slightly increasing the body's blood sugar level. In addition, cigarette smoking seems to speed up the oxygen consumption in the body, producing a higher metabolic rate and consequent weight control.

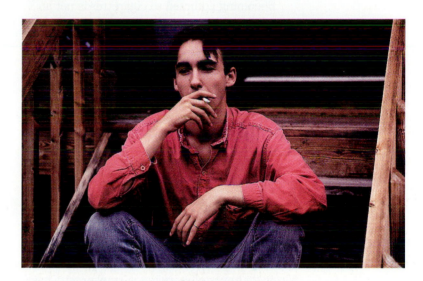

● **Figure 11.1 Smoking: the artificial means of emotional regulation**

"*All people experience fear, insecurity, discomfort, weariness. More is expected of us than we can fulfill, and our energy and attention levels are not always up to the demands of our jobs or families. We are not blessed with ideally fulfilling lives. For some, smoking has been a device for negotiating the gap between human frailty and a fast-paced, sometimes emotionally draining world. The more a person relies on artificial means of emotional regulation, however, the less practiced he or she becomes at regulating tension and anxiety naturally. Thus begins the cycle of dependence on nicotine, parallel to that which people experience with alcohol or drugs, in which the psychoactive [mood-altering] effects of a substance become for a time an essential means of gaining a desired emotional state.*"

—Stanton Peele, Ph.D., Archie Brodsky, with Mary Arnold. (1991). *The truth about addiction and recovery.* New York: Simon & Schuster, p. 102.

4.10

*Unit 4
Caffeine, Tobacco,
and Alcohol:
Common Mood-
Altering Drugs*

The Process of Addiction Cigarettes are highly addictive, or at least the nicotine in them is. Indeed, the 1988 report by the U.S. Surgeon General, *Nicotine Addiction*, states that cigarette smoking is as addictive as alcohol, cocaine, and heroin.[75] A 1989 Toronto study of a thousand people seeking to overcome their dependency on alcohol or other drugs reported that 57% thought that cigarettes would be harder to kick than the substance that they were presently trying to give up.[76]

Becoming addicted to cigarettes is not an immediate process; one has to work at it. Most people inhaling on their very first cigarette in an alley or behind the garage experience dizziness, palpitations, coughing, sweating, even nausea and vomiting. It usually does not take long, however, for a person to become a seasoned smoker; many people reach a pack a day in only a few weeks. Indeed, it has been found that 85% of teenagers who occasionally smoke more than two or three cigarettes go on to become dependent on nicotine.[77] People who are "puffers"—who smoke only occasionally or only a couple of cigarettes a day—are rare, making up only 2% of all smokers.

As with other mood-altering drugs, smoking cessation produces withdrawal symptoms. Within 24 hours of stopping, a smoker who has become dependent typically experiences irritability, anxiety, difficulty concentrating, restlessness, increased appetite, impatience, insomnia—and, of course, a strong craving for tobacco.[78] No wonder one of the most powerful incentives to smoke is to prevent the unpleasantness of withdrawal. Indeed, one reason why some smokers find the first cigarette of the day so pleasurable is that it helps them begin to overcome the 8 hours of tobacco withdrawal they underwent while asleep.

The Inside Story of Tobacco: What Goes In

The principal constituents of tobacco are nicotine, tar, and carbon monoxide. Nicotine, the addictive element, can seriously damage the heart and blood vessels. Tar can cause cancerous growths. Carbon monoxide interferes with the transport of oxygen.

It would be almost impossible to create tobacco in a laboratory. There are over 4000 chemical compounds in tobacco smoke. Benzene, for example, is not a chemical one associates with cigarettes, but cigarettes are said to have over 2000 times as much benzene as the Perrier water that was recalled in 1990 for contamination.[79] Benzene is a poison that is prohibited by law in paint thinners, presumably so people who sniff thinners to try to get high won't kill themselves.

Let us consider the principal constituents of cigarettes: nicotine, tar, and carbon monoxide.

Nicotine A colorless, oily compound, **nicotine** is the principal and addictive element in tobacco, whether cigarettes, cigars, or snuff. Actually, nicotine is a poison, one of the most toxic of all drugs. The nicotine in an average cigar, in fact, could kill several people, provided the cigar was soaked in water and people could be made to drink the liquid.[80] How quickly nicotine is absorbed into the body depends on how it is delivered. Smoking, or inhaling through the lungs, is the most efficient way to absorb the drug. Nicotine can reach the brain from the lungs in only 7 seconds—twice as fast as heroin can reach the brain when injected into the arm. When people simply take smoke into their mouths, 20–30% of the nicotine is absorbed into the body, but when they inhale, 90% of the nicotine in the smoke is taken in. Thus, pipe and cigar smokers, who generally do not inhale, take in less nicotine than do cigarette smokers, although they do take in some.

Nicotine is a **stimulant,** which means that it stimulates the central nervous system, producing an aroused, alert mental state. Although unlike amphetamines, it is considered a *minor* stimulant (like caffeine), it nevertheless has a variety of effects. It speeds up the heart rate 15–20 beats a minute, raises blood pressure, increases the respiration rate, and stimulates the adrenal glands to produce adrenaline. Nicotine also constricts the blood vessels, thereby causing the heart to have to work harder to pump the blood. As a result, there can be serious damage to the heart and blood vessel system.

Tar A sticky, dark fluid produced when tobacco is burned, **tar** is made up of several hundred different chemicals, many of them poisonous. The chemicals in tar are apt to damage the bronchial tubes, the branchlike tubes in the lungs, so that they are less able to remove unwanted foreign materials. These chemicals are also responsible for the development of cancerous growth in the respiratory system.

Carbon Monoxide The same gas that comes out of a car's exhaust, **carbon monoxide** is an odorless, colorless gas that is a by-product of burning tobacco. Smokers who find themselves short of breath are feeling the effects of carbon monoxide, which interferes with the blood's ability to transport oxygen. Carbon monoxide in tobacco smoke is found in concentrations 400 times that considered safe by the Environmental Protection Agency.

What Smoking Does to Smokers

One-fifth of all deaths in the United States are attributable to smoking. Cigarette smoking raises the risk for developing any number of disorders: lung cancer, chronic obstructive lung disease (pulmonary emphysema and chronic bronchitis), heart and blood vessel disease and stroke, wrinkled skin, diminished sexuality in men, cervical cancer in women. Cigarette smoking is also related to hazards during pregnancy and to healthy fetal development. Many of the same hazards affect nonsmokers exposed to cigarette smoke.

Smoking causes more preventable illness than any other form of drug addiction.[81] Throughout the world, an estimated 2.5 million premature deaths occur every year owing to tobacco use, according to the World Health Organization.[82] In the United States, smoking is a leading cause of premature death.[83] One-fifth of all deaths in the United States are attributable to smoking. Or, as epidemiologist Thomas Novotny put it, "It's as if each year, the city of Atlanta, Oklahoma City, St. Louis, or Kansas City were eliminated through the use of tobacco."[84]

In personal terms, what it comes down to is this: if you are a deep-inhaling smoker who

started before age 15, you are essentially giving up a minute of life for every minute you smoke. Many people—more than 400,000 a year—have not gotten the message soon enough, or found the force of the addiction too strong, and are dying prematurely from smoking-related diseases. The good news, however, is that although smoking-related deaths are presently rising, they are expected to fall in the next few years because of the decline in Americans who smoke—29% now, down from 30% in 1985 and 40% in 1964.[85]

Many smokers think of themselves as risk takers. But do they *know* what their risks are? One of the finer arts of living is knowing when the risks you're taking with your life are acceptable and when they are not.

Smoker's Odds Many smokers simply don't ever see themselves as being statistics. There are all kinds of excuses and rationalizations: "It'll never happen to me, I'm the lucky type." "I have a lot of years left to kick it." "I could get hit by a bus before I get cancer." "Grandma's still smoking, and she's all right." How true are these statements?

If you commute by car 27 miles a day—as a great many people do—the odds of death from an accident are quite high: 1 in 4000 in a year, or 1 in 60 over a lifetime.[86] What about smoking? Here the odds are *much* higher. If you smoke a pack a day, the odds of death within a given year are 1 in 200.[87] If you smoke a pack a day for 50 years, the odds are equivalent to those of playing Russian roulette with a six-shot revolver: 1 in 6.[88]

Lung Cancer Everyone seems to have heard that there is an association between smoking and lung cancer. Actually, smokers are more likely to die of heart disease than of lung cancer, but cancer of the lung is a serious matter for a very important reason: when smokers quit, their risk of heart disease decreases very quickly, but the relative risk of lung cancer remains high for 10–20 years compared to the risk of people who have never smoked.[89]

Stark revelations like this, which came out of a 1990 study of 12,866 male smokers ages 35–57, provide one of the best reasons there is for never taking up smoking. Of course, they are also apt to make any smoker throw up his or her

4.12

Unit 4
Caffeine, Tobacco,
and Alcohol:
Common Mood-
Altering Drugs

hands and say, "Why bother to quit? What difference could it make now?" As we shall show, however, it is never to late to stop. In fact, the 1990 U.S. Surgeon General's report on smoking states that the risk for lung cancer drops year by year after one quits smoking.[90] (*See ●* *Figure 11.2.*)

Lung cancer is the leading kind of cancer death in the United States. The great majority of such deaths could be avoided if people did not smoke.[91] Male pack-a-day smokers who do not quit, according to the Surgeon General's report, are 22 times more likely than nonsmokers to die of lung cancer. Among women pack-a-day smokers, the risk is 12 times that for nonsmokers. Indeed, lung cancer has surpassed breast cancer as a primary killer of women.[92]

One problem for anyone hoping that an X ray or physical checkup will spot lung cancer in time is that the disease is difficult to detect early enough to treat it effectively. Symptoms do not appear until the cancer has progressed. Thus, despite technological advances in methods of treatment, the survival rate for people who are alive 10 years after detection has not changed appreciably over the years.[93]

Recently, there has been some evidence that genetic factors make some patients more apt to develop lung cancer than others. If this is true, it would account for the fact that the known cancer-causing chemicals in cigarette smoke apparently do not themselves have the ability to cause lung cancer in humans. This gene would explain why some people are more likely than others to get lung cancer if they smoke.[94]

Respiratory Disorders: Chronic Obstructive Lung Disease With all the efforts being made nationally to improve the quality of the air we breathe—through smog-control devices on cars, and other measures—it's important to know that smoking is more dangerous than any air pollution, at least in most parts of the United States. (Together, however, air pollution and cigarette smoking are far more harmful than each activity alone.) Even young people are apt to be aware of some effects of smoking on their breathing, causing shortness of breath or chronic cough.

Among the principal respiratory disorders are *pulmonary emphysema* and *chronic bronchitis,* which are often seen together and

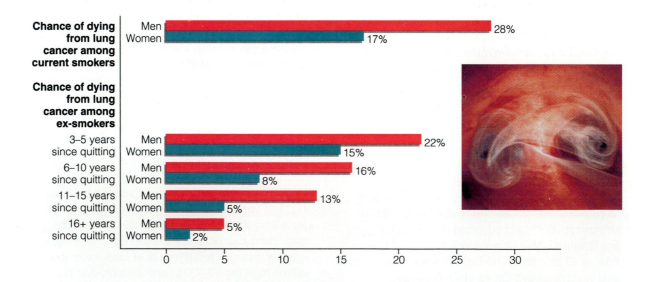

● **Figure 11.2 Lessened lung cancer risks.** The 1990 U.S. Surgeon General's report concludes that smokers who quit significantly reduce their risks of dying from lung cancer. Photo shows cigarette smoke swirling down the windpipe.

which are referred to jointly as **chronic obstructive lung disease,** abbreviated COLD. COLD, of which cigarette smoking is the most important cause, is characterized by the slow, progressive interruption of air flow within the lungs.

- *Pulmonary emphysema:* Occasionally you may see someone on the street who is suffering from pulmonary emphysema. They are recognizable by the plastic tubes protruding from their nostrils and running to an oxygen tank on a cart. **Pulmonary emphysema** is one of the sadder consequences of smoking, because the person has such great difficulty breathing. (*See* ● *Figure 11.3.*)

Over the years, cigarette smoke causes the *alveoli,* the tiny air sacs of the lung, to lose the elasticity that normally allows them to expand and contract. In time, many of the air sacs are stretched to the point that they rupture and are destroyed. In addition, the chest cage becomes enlarged as it tries to accommodate the overstretched lungs, which makes the diaphragm work less efficiently, which in turn interferes with the lungs' ability to exchange oxygen and carbon dioxide. This leads to continual shortness of breath and an overworked heart.

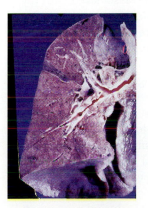 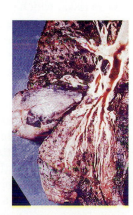

● **Figure 11.3 Healthy and unhealthy lungs.** *Left:* Normal lung tissue. *Right:* Lung taken from person with emphysema.

- *Chronic bronchitis:* The bronchial tubes, or bronchi, are the large passageways that deliver air into the lungs. The bronchi become smaller passageways; the smallest are called bronchioles. **Chronic bronchitis** consists of inflamed bronchi and increased mucus production, which narrow the air passages.

Cigarette smokers not only suffer from COLD, chronic bronchitis, and other chronic lung diseases such as pneumonia but also take longer to recover from respiratory infections. Quitting seems to reduce the risk of dying from these lung diseases and other disorders that afflict smokers.

Heart Disease and Stroke It isn't hard to see why inhaling tobacco smoke would affect the lungs, but it is less obvious why smoking affects the heart and blood vessels. Apparently, nicotine stimulates the heart rate, constricts the blood vessels, and raises the blood pressure, all of which force the heart to work harder.

The result is that heart disease, not cancer, is the number 1 cause of death among smokers. Smokers are two to three times as likely to die of heart disease as nonsmokers. Indeed, even smoking one to four cigarettes a day is associated with a twofold risk of fatal heart and blood vessel disease.[95] For smokers consuming more than 25 cigarettes a day, the risk of heart attack is 10-fold compared with nonsmokers.[96] Moreover, compared with nonsmokers, smokers are two to three times more likely to have a **stroke,** an interference with the blood circulation in part of the brain.[97]

There is good news, however: According to the 1990 Surgeon General's report, the risk for heart disease drops in half within a year after smokers quit and it keeps dropping the longer they abstain.[98] This is true even for people who have been smoking for decades. The risk of stroke is also reduced to only slightly more than that for nonsmokers. Even people who already have heart disease benefit by quitting, because the risk of recurrent heart attacks is reduced.[99]

Smoking is in such a class by itself when it comes to heart disease that cigarette smoking alone is estimated to be more dangerous—four times greater—than either of the other two leading risk factors for heart disease, high blood pressure and high blood cholesterol level.[100]

4.14

Unit 4
Caffeine, Tobacco,
and Alcohol:
Common Mood-
Altering Drugs

Diminished Sex Appeal and Sexuality To judge by the advertising, smokers like to think they look sexy. Unfortunately, the evidence is all the other way. Consider:

- *Increased facial wrinkles:* If you think appearance is an important part of sexual attraction, you should know that smoking can ultimately affect your looks. Or, as one writer put it, "Caution: Cigarette smoking may be hazardous to your face."[101] A study by dermatologists found that people who smoke are more susceptible to premature facial wrinkling than nonsmokers. Smokers who are heavily exposed to the sun show the most wrinkles, apparently because smoking multiplies the wrinkling effects of sunlight.[102]

- *For men—decreased sexual arousal and possible damage to sperm:* Smoking is sexy? Men who smoke may find they have a problem with sexual arousal. Smoking can reduce sexual motivation and performance by constricting the blood vessels, thus slowing the body's response to sexual stimulation, and by reducing testosterone (the male sex hormone) levels in the blood.[103]

    Men who smoke also have an increased risk of fathering children with brain cancer and leukemia, because smoking may damage their sperm, according to a study led by Anne Berg.[104]

Special Risks for Women Cigarettes are not sexy and certainly not healthy for women, either. In particular, smoking increases the risk of early **menopause,** the end of monthly menstrual cycles, which under normal conditions generally occurs between the ages of 45 and 55.[105] It may also be a risk factor in the development of **osteoporosis,** called *brittle-bone disease,* in which loss of bone density results in easily broken bones.[106]

Cervical cancer risk for smokers is difficult to evaluate because it is influenced by the number of sexual partners a woman has had and her exposure to sexually transmitted diseases, as well as the number of cigarettes smoked. In any case, evidence suggests that cigarette smoking increases a woman's risk of cervical cancer, particularly among those who are current smokers.[107–109]

Finally, sexually active women ages 18–44 who smoke and use oral contraceptives ("The Pill") should be aware they are at vastly increased risk for heart and blood vessel diseases (such as heart attack) and stroke.[110] Indeed, the risk is so serious that women over 35 are strongly advised to stop using one or the other —get rid of cigarettes or use other kinds of contraceptives.

Smoking and Pregnancy Smoking presents a significant risk to pregnancy, to the growing fetus, and to the newborn. Infant mortality is already a tremendous problem in the United States, far higher than a developed nation should have. Experts estimate that the elimination of smoking by pregnant women would reduce infant mortality by 10%, or 2500–3000 deaths per year.[111]

Women who have been smoking at the time of conception have been found to have twice the risk of nonsmokers of a potentially fatal pregnancy complication known as **ectopic pregnancy.** The problem involves the implantation of a fertilized egg somewhere other than the lining of the uterus, such as the fallopian tubes. A growing embryo that is implanted in a fallopian tube may rupture the tube and blood vessels within it, putting the woman at risk of bleeding to death.[112] In addition, smoking women are more apt to experience spontaneous abortion, fetal death, and premature birth.[113] These risks, which may be associated with the number of cigarettes smoked every day, are even greater for older pregnant women.

Even if the fetus survives, negative effects of the mother's smoking may show up at birth in the infant's low birth weight and reduced body length—probably the result of poor development because of reduced availability of oxygen during pregnancy. This does not mean merely a smaller baby. Cigarette smoking deprives the fetus of essential growth of *all* its body organs, including the brain, which can lead to permanent developmental delays in children.[114] The more cigarettes a woman smokes during pregnancy, the more the baby's weight is reduced. Conversely, the earlier a woman quits smoking during her pregnancy, the more positive the impact on her baby's birth weight.[115]

It's clear that smoking is bad for babies, but there's something that's even worse: smoking combined with other drugs. The combination of cigarette smoking during pregnancy with either alcohol or caffeine, for example, decreases the infant's birth weight even further.[116,117]

Other Hazards The depressing list goes on. Smokers experience less pain relief from painkilling drugs because the constituents of tobacco interact negatively with other drugs.[118] Smokers need more time to recover from anesthesia after surgery than nonsmokers do.[119] Smokers are more apt to develop oral cancer.[120] Female smokers who take oral contraceptives are more apt to develop inflammatory bowel disease.[121] Male smokers with the deadly human immunodeficiency virus (HIV) are more apt to develop full-blown AIDS than HIV-infected men who are nonsmokers.[122] Finally, there are the great number of smokers who fall asleep with a cigarette in their hands and set fire to themselves and others.[123,124]

Other Tobacco Products

Greater awareness of the hazards of cigarette smoking has led many people to switch to other tobacco products, which offer their own sets of problems. Pipes and cigars lead to oral cancers. Smokeless tobacco—snuff and chewing tobacco—leads to nicotine effects and dependency, oral and dental problems, and various cancers. Clove cigarettes—which are 60% tobacco and generate even more nicotine, tar, and carbon monoxide than all-tobacco cigarettes—produce respiratory illnesses.

Public health awareness campaigns about smoking have had an impact. Sales of cigarettes are down. Smoking is being banned in more and more places. Does this mean that tobacco in general no longer occupies the prominence it used to? To answer this, let us examine the use of some other tobacco products—pipe tobacco and cigars, smokeless tobacco, and clove cigarettes.

Pipes and Cigars Smokers who *start* smoking by using pipes or cigars rather than cigarettes are less likely to develop lung cancer and heart disease than cigarette smokers—for the simple reason that most pipe and cigar smokers don't inhale. They are, however, putting themselves at risk for an assortment of oral cancers—cancer of the mouth, larynx, throat, and esophagus. This is because the drug nicotine, along with its associated dangers, is present in all tobacco products.

Cigarette smokers who *switch* to pipes and cigars, on the other hand, are likely to continue to inhale, and so not only suffer the same risks but also bring on the aggravations of inhaling the more throat- and lung-irritating tobaccos found in pipes and cigars.

According to the 1988 Surgeon General's report, use of pipes and cigars has decreased 80% since 1964.[125]

Smokeless Tobacco: Snuff and Chewing Tobacco Some people think that switching to smokeless tobacco—snuff and chewing tobacco—can give them some of the pleasures of cigarettes without the risks. **Snuff** is finely shredded or powdered tobacco that is sold in cans or tea-bag-like packets that allow the user to absorb nicotine through the mucous membranes in the nose or the mouth. Most American users "dip" snuff out of the can and place it between their lower lip and gum. **Chewing tobacco** consists of loose-leaf tobacco mixed with molasses or other flavors and pressed into cakes (called *plugs*) or twisted into ropelike strands. A portion of loose-leaf tobacco, plug, or strand can be chewed or placed between the gum and cheek or lower lip. The nicotine is absorbed through the mucous membranes in the mouth.

Although smokeless tobacco does not precipitate the deadly heart and lung diseases that cigarettes do, it still poses a high risk of oral cancer. Sales of snuff and chewing tobacco have increased because many Americans perceive them to be a safer alternative to smoking, yet smokeless tobacco is so risky that its use has become a national health concern. In addition, users can become as effectively dependent on snuff and chewing tobacco as they can on cigarettes, with all the difficulty that quitting entails.

4.16

*Unit 4
Caffeine, Tobacco,
and Alcohol:
Common Mood-
Altering Drugs*

An estimated 10 to 12 million Americans use smokeless tobacco.[126] Although a picture of the average user would show a 17- to 19-year-old white male living in the South, there are all sorts of users of varied ages, genders, races, and geographical locations.[127] Many begin using smokeless tobacco as children or teenagers. In fact, one study found that many college student users began using it before age 10.[128] College student use of smokeless tobacco is not unusual, particularly among males. One national survey found that 22% of college males and 2% of college females reported that they currently use smokeless tobacco.[129]

The major smokeless tobacco risks, which tend to increase as dose and frequency increase, are (1) nicotine effects and dependency, (2) oral and dental problems, and (3) cancer, especially oral cancer.[130]

- *Nicotine effects and dependency:* If it weren't for the nicotine in smokeless tobacco, it might have no more effect than soap bubbles. Interestingly, however, some researchers say smokeless tobacco has even *more* of an effect on the heart and blood vessel system than does cigarette smoking. Holding tobacco in the mouth results in nicotine exposure that is twice that of cigarette smokers.[131] Nicotine absorbed into the bloodstream through the membranes in the mouth acts on the central nervous system and increases the heart rate and blood pressure.

    The addictive potential of smokeless tobacco is significant. In one study, adolescent male smokeless-tobacco users were found to be more addicted than male cigarette smokers.[132] Some users increase their risks by using progressively stronger types of smokeless tobacco, and others combine their chewing or snuff habit with cigarette smoking.

- *Oral and dental problems:* The use of smokeless tobacco has long been associated with baseball, as you can see in the moving jaws of players when you tune in the World Series. However, one study of National League ball players found that 48% of the 386 smokeless tobacco users had developed leukoplakia.[133]

Leukoplakia consists of white, thick, hardened, wrinkled patches on the mucous membrane lining of the mouth. It usually occurs in the area where the smokeless tobacco product is held against the cheek or gum. Leukoplakia is a precancerous lesion, which means that the tissue changes leukoplakia signify may develop into cancer. The risk of leukoplakia in those who have used snuff has been observed to be 50 times that for nonusers.[134]

In time most smokeless tobacco users develop other problems that snuff and chewing tobacco manufacturers don't tell you about. These problems include bad breath, tooth discoloration, tooth loss, excessive wearing away of enamel on teeth, and an impaired ability to smell and taste.[135]

- *Cancer:* Even though smokeless tobacco products are not burned, they still contain powerful **carcinogens**—cancer-causing agents.[136] Indeed, the most potent, called *TSNA* (for *Tobacco-Specific-N-Nitrosamines*), have been found in snuff to exceed that in any other consumer product known to contain carcinogenic nitrosamines.[137] Some of the newer products on the market contain the highest levels of TSNA ever found in smokeless tobacco.

    In the end, smokeless tobacco is associated with most of the nicotine-related health hazards linked to smoking, including cancer. Long-term use of snuff and chewing tobacco has been associated with increased risk of cancer of the mouth, larynx, throat, and esophagus.[138] Long-term snuff users have a 50-fold increased risk of oral cancer.[139] Smokeless tobacco may also be related to other upper digestive tract cancers, such as cancer of the pancreas, kidneys, and bladder.[140,141] On the bright side, precancerous lesions in the mouth have been observed to heal quickly when people stop using smokeless tobacco.[142]

Clove Cigarettes In the 1980s, cigarette smokers began to take up Indonesian-produced **clove cigarettes** in the mistaken belief that they were safer than regular cigarettes. Clove cigarettes (also called *kretek cigarettes*) contain about 60% tobacco and 40% shredded clove buds.[143] Clove is the spice taken from the dried flower buds of East Indian evergreen trees.

Actually, clove cigarettes not only produce all the problems associated with all-tobacco cigarettes, they generate even *more* nicotine, tar, and carbon monoxide than American cigarettes do.[144,145] They can cause serious lung injury and respiratory illnesses in some users. Indeed, for users with early, nonspecific symptoms of respiratory illness, smoking clove cigarettes may lead to the development of pneumonia, bronchitis, and bloody fluid in the lungs.[146]

Some lung problems also occur in those who have normal respiratory tracts and no signs of respiratory illness. These are caused in part by a chemical in cloves called *eugenol,* which acts as a throat anesthetic. The eugenol in clove cigarettes diminishes the gag reflex and increases the risk of pneumonia and other problems because smokers can unintentionally inhale fluid into their lungs.

What Smoking Does to Nonsmokers: Passive Smoking

Passive smoking, when nonsmokers inhale surrounding cigarette smoke, is responsible for thousands of deaths. Children are especially at risk. Separating smokers from nonsmokers in the same air space helps but does not eliminate the risk.

Maybe you don't smoke yourself; but have you lived with or are you living or working closely with a smoker? If so, you should be aware that you don't own the air you breathe—that you are engaging in **passive smoking.** That is, you are breathing **secondhand smoke,** also known as **environmental tobacco smoke (ETS).**[147] A smoker who inhales **mainstream smoke**—the smoke drawn directly from the cigarette—may take in smoke for only about half a minute. However, everyone else in the room may be breathing in what is known as **sidestream smoke** for the entire 12 minutes or so that the cigarette is burning. Although sidestream smoke is more diluted, it happens that it contains a larger number of carcinogens than does mainstream smoke, perhaps because mainstream smoke is filtered.[148]

Should you treat this as just another annoyance in your life, or are you right to think that you are being put at risk?

Here's what the research says:

- *Cigarette smoke kills nonsmokers too:* Secondhand smoke is responsible for thousands of deaths.[149] According to one draft federal report, it kills 53,000 nonsmokers in the United States every year—3700 from lung cancer, 37,000 from heart disease.[150,151] It may also increase breast cancer risk.[152] If these figures are true, secondhand smoking would be the third leading cause of preventable death, behind active smoking and alcohol abuse. It also means that cigarette smoking is causing *the death of one nonsmoker for every eight deaths of smokers.*[153]

- *Children are especially at risk:* Researchers strongly recommend that contact be limited between smokers and children, particularly newborn infants.[154] The children of parents who smoke, compared with children of nonsmoking parents, have increased frequency of respiratory infections and increased respiratory symptoms.[155] Passive smoking is associated with pneumonia, wheezing, and middle-ear disease in children. Children of mothers who smoke have impaired lung growth and development.[156]

- *Separation helps only slightly:* The simple separation of smokers from nonsmokers within the same air space—as within an office—may reduce the exposure of nonsmokers to secondhand smoke, but it does not eliminate it.[157]

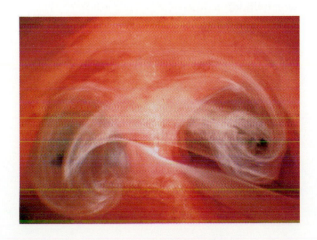

4.18

*Unit 4
Caffeine, Tobacco,
and Alcohol:
Common Mood-
Altering Drugs*

Strategy for Living:
Quitting Cigarettes

It is never too late to quit smoking, even for older people. Although cigarette smoking is one of the toughest of drug addictions, it can be beaten with a combination of motivation and selection of the right quit-smoking techniques. Methods of cessation include tapering off, "cold turkey" (the most successful way), stop-smoking groups, nicotine gum and patches, hypnosis, aversion therapy, acupuncture, and inpatient groups.

More than 50 million Americans are smokers today. However, an estimated 40 million others are ex-smokers.[158] "Almost half of all living adults in the United States who have ever smoked have quit," the U.S. Surgeon General pointed out in her 1990 report on smoking and health.[159]

What is encouraging about this news is that so many people have quit even though cigarettes have been called the very toughest drug addiction—even more addictive than heroin. The reason the smoking habit is so strong, point out addiction experts Peele and Brodsky, is that:

> (a) *it fits easily into an ordinary, productive lifestyle and* (b) *commercial cigarettes are an unparalleled delivery system for getting the drug into the blood and to the nervous system in the most efficacious way possible.*[160]

Before people can begin the work of quitting, however, they need to believe that it is worthwhile.

Is It Too Late? If you are a smoker now, and have been smoking for some time, you may feel that you're just too far along to give it up. In fact, however, it is almost never too late to quit. A study of elderly smokers—people in their 60s, 70s, and beyond—contradicts the widely held belief that by the time smokers reach old age the habit has either already taken its toll or those who survive that long have somehow become immune to the dangers of cigarettes.[161] Smoking is a killer at any age, and the study showed that no matter how long people smoked, there were real benefits to giving up cigarettes and the benefits began to appear very quickly.

"Older people who smoke can still do their health a lot of good by quitting," said researcher Andrea LaCroix, who directed the study. "A lot of older people believe that once you've smoked 40 or 50 years, you have nothing to gain from quitting. That's clearly not true."[162]

Telling people that they have an addiction is like telling them they have no control over their behavior, and so they think there is no way to quit. We do not mean to imply that the task of quitting cigarettes is simple and easy. Relapse rates for smokers who quit are high. Of the approximately 1.3 million smokers a year who quit between 1974 and 1985, 75–80% resumed smoking within 6 months of stopping.[163] Eventually, however, many smokers do quit. The keys to stopping are these:

- Motivation and persistence
- Finding the right technique that works for the person
- Developing ways to cope with the difficulties of quitting, including relapse

Understanding Yourself: How Badly Do You Want to Quit? The first order of business is to establish why you smoke, then attempt to determine how much you want to change your smoking habits. (*See Self Discovery 11.1.*) It's important to know that change will also entail a fair amount of discomfort, so you should try to ascertain how prepared you are to endure this difficulty and look for resources and support to help you.

As you might imagine, people quit for all kinds of reasons. Sometimes it has to do with what psychologists call "maturing out"—when a particular life stage or life event is reached and substance abuse is simply outgrown. For instance, a new father, feeling the responsibilities of parenthood, might finally quit when his first child is born. Some quit when the stresses of life level off. Others stop because of signals they cannot possibly disregard: comedian Jerry Lewis and Governor John Brown of Kentucky gave up their four-pack-a-day habits after they had open-heart surgery. The health movement in North America has probably also helped motivate many to quit.

SELF DISCOVERY 11.1

Why Do You Smoke?

Here are some statements made by people to describe what they get out of smoking cigarettes. How often do you feel this way when smoking? Choose one number for each statement.

| 5 = always | 4 = frequently | 3 = occasionally | 2 = seldom | 1 = never |

A. I smoke cigarettes in order to keep myself from slowing down. _____

B. Handling a cigarette is part of the enjoyment of smoking. _____

C. Smoking cigarettes is pleasant and relaxing. _____

D. I light up a cigarette when I feel angry about something. _____

E. When I have run out of cigarettes, I find it almost unbearable until I can get more. _____

F. I smoke cigarettes automatically without even being aware of it. _____

G. I smoke cigarettes to stimulate me, to perk myself up. _____

H. Part of the enjoyment of smoking a cigarette comes from the steps I take to light up. _____

I. I find cigarettes pleasurable. _____

J. When I feel uncomfortable or upset about something, I light up a cigarette. _____

K. I am very much aware of the fact when I am not smoking a cigarette. _____

L. I light up a cigarette without realizing I still have one burning in the ashtray. _____

M. I smoke cigarettes to give me a "lift." _____

N. When I smoke a cigarette, part of the enjoyment is watching the smoke as I exhale it. _____

O. I want a cigarette most when I am comfortable and relaxed. _____

P. When I feel "blue" or want to take my mind off cares and worries, I smoke cigarettes. _____

Q. I get a real craving for a cigarette when I haven't smoked for a while. _____

R. I've found a cigarette in my mouth and didn't remember putting it there. _____

How to Score

1. Enter the numbers you have selected for the test questions in the spaces below, putting the number you have selected for question A over line A, for question B over line B, etc.
2. Total the three scores on each line to get your totals. For example, the sum of scores over lines A, G, and M gives you your score on Stimulation. Scores 11 or above indicate that this factor is an important source of satisfaction for the smoker. Scores of 7 or less are low and probably indicate that this factor does not apply to you. Scores in between are marginal.

_____ (A)	+	_____ (G)	+	_____ (M)	=	_____ Stimulation
_____ (B)	+	_____ (H)	+	_____ (N)	=	_____ Handling
_____ (C)	+	_____ (I)	+	_____ (O)	=	_____ Relaxation
_____ (D)	+	_____ (J)	+	_____ (P)	=	_____ Crutch
_____ (E)	+	_____ (K)	+	_____ (Q)	=	_____ Craving
_____ (F)	+	_____ (L)	+	_____ (R)	=	_____ Habit

(continued)

4.20

Unit 4
Caffeine, Tobacco,
and Alcohol:
Common Mood-
Altering Drugs

Once you have determined that you do, in fact, want to quit, you can choose among several methods. As one former smoker writes, "Conventional wisdom dictates that there's only one way to approach quitting smoking: do whatever it takes. Almost all those stop-smoking techniques you see and read about are useful for some people, useless for others."[164] Some smokers can successfully quit regardless of the techniques they use, others have great difficulty quitting regardless of what they try.[165]

The methods include:

- Tapering off
- Quitting cold turkey
- Stop-smoking groups
- Other methods—nicotine gum or patches, hypnosis, aversion therapy, acupuncture, and inpatient treatment

Self-Quitting: Tapering Off Gradual reduction may be a good way to start. For one thing, it can help you understand when and why you smoke. You discover what are known as your *conditioned association triggers,* the particular triggers that you have learned to associate with lighting up, such as talking on the telephone or drinking a beer, and then learn to perform each of these activities without a cigarette.

(*See* ● *Figure 11.4.*) This cutting down can also help you through the first few days of withdrawal symptoms.

Some smokers experience no withdrawal symptoms, but for many withdrawal is unquestionably difficult. The withdrawal pains may range from drowsiness and difficulty concentrating to nervousness, anxiety, and irritability. Physical symptoms may include headaches and constipation. Withdrawal symptoms usually peak within 1–3 days after quitting, although for some people they may linger up to 6 weeks, and craving for the drug may continue for a much longer period of time.

Tapering off works well for some people down to the range of 10–15 cigarettes per day, says disease-prevention researcher Stephen Fortman. However, people may not only find it difficult to reduce their consumption beyond a certain level but also tend to inhale more deeply, making each remaining cigarette so precious that it becomes even harder to quit completely.[166]

Self-Quitting: Cold Turkey Some smokers prefer to try quitting by tapering off because they feel they might set themselves up for failure if they go "cold turkey" and stop outright. In fact, one analysis of 13,000 people discovered that, of the people who succeeded in quitting, 85% did so with the cold-turkey approach; the rest gradually decreased the number of cigarettes they smoked, switched to low-tar and low-nicotine cigarettes, or substituted other tobacco products.[167]

Quitting smoking by abstinence—going cold turkey—seems to work better than participating in formal stop-smoking programs, according to the same survey. Among those who had smoked in the decade before the survey was done, 48% of those who tried to quit on their own succeeded, compared with 24% of those who sought assistance, including counseling, hypnosis, and acupuncture.[168] This conclusion affirms those of earlier studies.[169]

One reason that self-quitting cold turkey seems to have a higher success rate than that of smoking cessation clinics is that smokers who enter cessation programs may be those who are unable to quit on their own.[170] In addition, it seems that those who are able to quit on their own are those who have not been smoking long or as much as those who participate in treatment programs.[171]

Stop-Smoking Clinics and Self-Help Programs If a smoker is motivated to quit but is having trouble doing so, he or she may need to try a treatment program—and to keep trying different programs until one turns up that works.

The most successful programs are those that use a variety of approaches. Such programs may use a mixture of group support, behavior modification techniques, and counseling to help wean smokers of their habit. Some programs are nonprofit, such as those sponsored by the American Cancer Society, the American Lung Association, or the Seventh-Day Adventist Church. Others are profit-oriented groups, such as SmokEnders. Most programs involve a fee. In some localities there are also meetings of Smokers Anonymous, which has no dues or fees and which is a self-help program based on the Twelve Steps of Alcoholics Anonymous.

Daily Cigarette Count

Instructions: Attach a copy of this form to a pack of cigarettes. Complete the information each time you smoke a cigarette (those from someone else as well as your own). Note the time and evaluate the need for the cigarette (1 is for a cigarette you feel you could not do without; 2 is a less necessary one; 3 is one you could really go without). Make any other additional comments about the situation or your feelings. This record helps you understand when and why you smoke.

Time	Need (1 to 3)	Feelings/Situation

● **Figure 11.4 Daily cigarette count**

4.22

*Unit 4
Caffeine, Tobacco,
and Alcohol:
Common Mood-
Altering Drugs*

Other Methods There are at least six other methods that people can try in conjunction with giving up smoking, as follows:

- *Nicotine gum:* Although currently available nonprescription smoking-cessation aids have not proven effective, a prescription drug, nicotine gum (such as Nicorette), has been effective in helping some people ease withdrawal symptoms and stop smoking, according to one study. This is particularly true for smokers who are highly nicotine-dependent, who are motivated to quit, and who are involved in a support program.[172] However, another study found that use of gum was minimally effective or had no effect at all.[173]

  The theory is that chewing the gum (and it needs to be chewed in a particular way and replaced often) will release nicotine into the body. Since the nicotine level of the blood rises, the use of the gum alleviates withdrawal symptoms. The smoker can then taper off the dose until there is complete cessation. Any short-term risks from the nicotine are considered acceptable in view of the ultimate goal of helping someone stop smoking.[174]

- *Nicotine patch:* Also available by prescription are nicotine patches (Nicoderm, Habitrol), which are applied daily to the skin anywhere on the upper body. Over several weeks, the amount of nicotine that seeps into the bloodstream decreases. Treatment is typically 10–12 weeks.

  The use of the patches has met with some success. One study found that successful abstinence occurred for 31% of smokers who used the nicotine patch for 6 weeks, compared with 14% of those wearing a similar-looking patch (a placebo) that contained no nicotine.[175]

- *Hypnosis:* Hypnosis may well be an effective smoking-cessation technique for motivated quitters. The ex-smoker-to-be meets with a psychiatrist, psychologist, or social worker who is a licensed hypnotherapist and learns to practice self-hypnosis to give strength to the idea that smoking is a poison and the body deserves more respect. In one study involving 226 heavy smokers, psychiatrist David Spiegel and colleagues

were able to achieve a 2-year abstinence rate of 23% after only a single session of hypnosis.[176]

- *Aversion therapy:* **Aversion therapy** tries to teach smokers to associate smoking with unpleasantness. Sometimes this involves forcing the smoker to inhale so many cigarettes in rapid succession that he or she feels nauseous. Sometimes it involves administering mild electric shocks in conjunction with smoking. Needless to say, this approach is so unpleasant that it should not be considered the method of first choice, and anyone contemplating it—especially anyone with heart disease, diabetes, or respiratory problems—should first consult a health-care professional.

- *Acupuncture:* **Acupuncture** is an ancient Chinese technique in which a needle or a staple is inserted in a specific part of the body, often the outer ear. The results of this technique, too, are mixed.

- *Inpatient treatment:* Just as people with other forms of drug dependencies are admitted to hospitals or treatment centers (such as the famous Betty Ford Center in Rancho Mirage, Calif.) to overcome their dependences, some smokers now have the option of inpatient treatment for nicotine addiction. Such programs follow the models of other drug-treatment programs in offering 7-day courses in group therapy, individual counseling, exercise, nutritional guidance, and meditation. They may be somewhat expensive.

Some additional strategies can be used with most of these stop-smoking techniques. (*See ● Figure 11.5.*) Although relapses may occur, those who are ex-smokers just have kept trying and trying different methods until they finally were successful.

Worries About Weight Gain A great many people worry they will gain weight when they quit smoking. According to a survey of over 9000 people, the average smoker who gives up cigarettes gains only 6–8 pounds over a 5-year period after quitting. Those who stop smoking may continue to gain weight at a faster rate than smokers for at least 7 years after they stop. Nevertheless, the study concluded, the health benefits of giving up cigarettes far exceed any risk from gaining the few extra pounds.[177]

Actually, weight gain should be viewed as a sign of *success,* one study found. Those who put on 20 pounds or more after they quit are less likely to light up again. As Keilli Skoog, a co-author of the study put it, "Abstinent smokers—those who quit—who gained more weight were less likely to relapse than others."[178] Incorporating lifestyle changes, such as a low-fat diet and an exercise program, in addition to quitting smoking may decrease one's risk for weight gain and increase one's overall state of health and well-being.

The Addiction Can Be Treated No one says that quitting smoking is easy. Indeed, many patients questioned at a drug-addiction treatment facility in Toronto said they thought that cigarettes would be harder to give up than the other drug or drugs for which they were seeking treatment. Yet they also said they found cigarettes less pleasurable than alcohol or drugs.[179] Whether you are a smoker or simply know people who smoke, it's important to understand the power that tobacco holds but realize that the addiction can be broken.

Suggestion for Further Reading

Farquhar, J. W., & Spiller, G. A. (1990). *The last puff: Ex-smokers share the secrets of their success.* New York: Norton. Unlike the usual stop-smoking books, this one is a collection of over 30 interviews of smokers from truck drivers to poets to models for cigarette ads who tell how they kicked their habit.

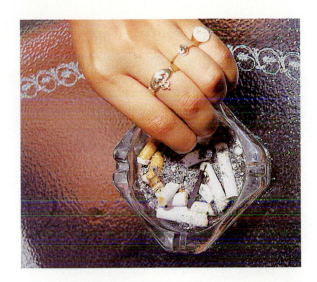

● **Figure 11.5 Tips for quitting smoking**

- *Make a contract:* Analyze your personal commitment to change and state it in writing. A signed contract enhances your chances of success.
- *Set a Quit day:* Determine the day you will stop—then do it.
- *Determine your resources:* Identify your personal resources and support for your plan. Tell people what you're trying to do. Going public with your intentions helps you activate your plan and enables others to support you.
- *Develop healthy habits:* Encourage healthy lifestyle behaviors such as exercising and relaxation techniques.
- *Don't despair:* View a relapse as a learning opportunity, not cause for despair. If you are among the four out of five smokers who have already quit at least once, you can draw on your quit-smoking experiences and resources for the next try. Remember that you stopped before and you can stop again.
- *Prepare for danger spots:* Identify high-risk situations—those that trigger a craving for a cigarette. Prepare by practicing how to deal with such occasions. Even after several years of not smoking, a personal crisis can make you want to reach for a cigarette.

4.24

Unit 4
Caffeine, Tobacco,
and Alcohol:
Common Mood-
Altering Drugs

12 Alcohol

▶ What is considered a standard alcoholic drink, and how many drinks does it take to make one intoxicated?

▶ What does alcohol do in the body?

▶ What are the kinds of things one should know about alcohol and oneself to make decisions about drinking?

▶ What does heavy drinking do to people in the short run? In the long run?

▶ What effect does alcohol have on other people involved with a heavy drinker?

▶ What is alcoholism, and what kind of help is available for an alcohol-dependency problem?

W ine, beer, and liquor are considered by many to be the center of some of life's most pleasurable and important activities. Someone probably lifted a glass when they learned you came into the world, and people will probably do so again when they learn of

your passing. And in between there will be many other times of celebration when a bottle will be produced—graduations, weddings, promotions, victories and joyful occasions of all sorts. Drinking, then, is not just a peripheral activity for many of us; it is so much a part of our culture that people almost cannot imagine being without it.

How Alcohol Works: "Magic" in a Glass?

A can of beer, glass of wine, or shot glass of whiskey are all equivalent to a "standard drink," or a half ounce of pure alcohol. Intoxication is determined by blood alcohol concentration (BAC), or ratio of alcohol to blood. Increased BACs, which are usually higher in women than in men for similar amounts, can eventually produce comas and be fatal. Hangovers, caused by high BACs and fermentation by-products or additives called congeners, are mainly alleviated by time.

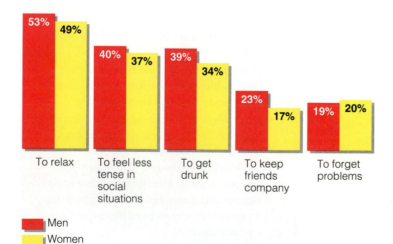

	Men	Women
To relax	53%	49%
To feel less tense in social situations	40%	37%
To get drunk	39%	34%
To keep friends company	23%	17%
To forget problems	19%	20%

■ Men
■ Women

● **Figure 12.1 Why college freshmen drink.**
Survey respondents could choose more than one reason.

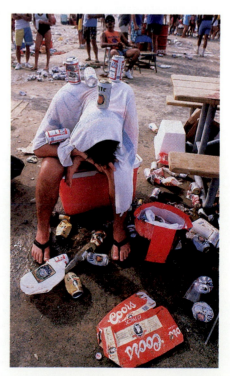

People tend to equate drinking with relaxation, good times, fellowship, and the easing of pain and problems. (*See ● Figure 12.1.*) In fact, we may attribute such properties to alcohol because drinking really *does* change behavior. We stop feeling shy or tense or anxious. As we begin to feel less tongue-tied and awkward, we find ourselves bolder and presumably wittier, quicker, and more inspired. At the same time, the people we are drinking with become more relaxed and thus apparently more receptive to us, our jokes, our astute opinions about almost everything. If one or two drinks make us feel this good, we think, another—and another—would be even better.

Unfortunately, several thousand years of human experience say this idea isn't so. We can show what happens to thinking and behavior after we explain (1) what a "drink" is, and (2) what blood alcohol concentration means.

What a Drink Is Although the major types of alcoholic beverages—beer, wine, distilled spirits—have different alcohol concentrations, a typical *serving* of any such beverage contains about the same amount of alcohol. That is, a **standard drink** is defined as ½ ounce of pure alcohol. This is equivalent to:

- *One beer:* one standard-size can or bottle (12 ounces) of beer that is 5% alcohol; or

- *One glass of table wine:* one standard wine glass (4 ounces) of table wine, such as chablis or burgundy, that is 12% alcohol; or

- *One glass of fortified wine:* one small glass (2½ ounces) of fortified wine that is 20% alcohol, such as sherry or port; or

- *One shot of distilled spirits* ("*hard liquor*"): one shot glass (1 ounce) of distilled spirits, such as whiskey, vodka, gin, rum, brandy, or tequila, that is 50% alcohol.

If you think of certain drinks as being "stronger" or "harder" than others (whiskey more than beer, for instance), you may be surprised that all of the above contain about the same amount of alcohol. That is, if you multiply the percentage of alcohol by the number of ounces, you will arrive at approximately the same thing: the equivalent of a ½-ounce glass of straight 100% pure alcohol. (*See ● Figure 12.2.*)

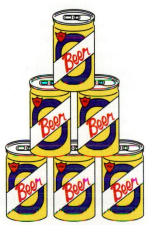

6 beers (12 oz)

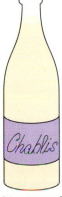

15 ounces of fortified wine

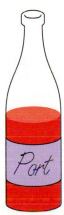

24 ounces of table wine

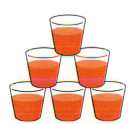

6 glasses of liquor (1.3 oz 80 proof)

● **Figure 12.2 Six equivalent drinks.** These containers all have the same amount of alcohol, equivalent to 3 ounces of pure alcohol. When consumed within a 2-hour period, they would cause a 160-pound person to be considered legally intoxicated in most places. (Mixed drinks or poured drinks may have more alcohol than those in bottles or cans.)

4.26

*Unit 4
Caffeine, Tobacco,
and Alcohol:
Common Mood-
Altering Drugs*

Pure alcohol of the kind used in alcoholic beverages is known as **ethanol** or **ethyl alcohol.** Other types, such as methyl (wood) alcohol or isopropyl (rubbing alcohol), are poisonous and should not be consumed. The alcohol percentage contained in "one drink" is based on fairly standard measures. However, alcohol content can range from 0.5% to 80%, and container sizes can also vary quite a bit. For instance, a tall, 16-ounce can of malt liquor with 9% alcohol is a more powerful "drink" than a standard can of "three-two" beer (3.2% alcohol). Table wines can vary from 10% to 13.5% alcohol. Fortified wines, such as certain dessert wines, are so called because the wines have been "fortified" (made stronger) by adding alcohol. Distilled liquors or spirits can range from 40% to 75% alcohol. The alcohol content of distilled spirits is expressed in terms of **proof,** a number that is twice the percentage of alcohol. Thus, a 100-proof bourbon or rum contains 50% alcohol. Indications of proof are found on the labels of alcoholic beverages.

Intoxication: Blood Alcohol Concentration and Its Effects If a car is stopped at a checkpoint by the highway patrol a few hours past New Year's Eve, the police may try to determine if the driver is legally fit to drive by determining how much alcohol is in his or her bloodstream. This can be assessed on the spot through a breathalyzer test. A breathalyzer is a device used to measure breath alcohol. Alcohol is one of the few addictive substances that appears in exhaled air in direct and precise proportion to the level of the drug in the blood. Or, if the driver refuses the breathalyzer, the police may take him or her back to the station to determine the alcohol amount with a blood or urine test.

What the police are looking for is the **blood alcohol concentration (BAC).** The BAC is the amount of alcohol in the blood, which is usually expressed as a ratio of milligrams (mg) of alcohol per 100 milliliters (ml) of blood. Thus, 10 drops of alcohol, which is about 10 mg, in 1000 drops of blood, which is about 100 ml, is a BAC of .10. This is the legal level of intoxication in most places (in some places it is lower), although many people are significantly impaired at a lower BAC than this. (See ● *Figure 12.3.*)

Let's assume you are of legal age and have gone to a party and are having some drinks. Is there any way you can tell—short of falling down, of course—whether you are in a condition to drive home? To some extent, there is, if you're capable of keeping track of the number (and kinds) of drinks you're having and the number of hours you've been drinking. To see this, you need to know how much you weigh and the number of drinks you've consumed in a 1- or 2-hour time period. (See ● *Table 12.1.*) Find your weight in Table 12.1 and then look down the column to see what your approximate (repeat: this is only *approximate*) blood alcohol concentration would be for a given number of drinks. For example, if you weigh 160 pounds and within 2 hours you have six drinks—a six-pack of beer, for example—you will have a BAC of .10%, which will make you legally intoxicated in most places. An important note, however: in general, for men and women of equal weight, *women* will experience a higher BAC after the same number of drinks, as we explain shortly.

Drinking Rituals and Hangovers Looking at the pints of whiskey on the shelf behind the clerk in the liquor store, you might wonder how many people can drink these in only an hour. Unfortunately, there are too many people who seek oblivion this way—and who run the real risk of stopping breathing (perhaps permanently) when they do so. More dangerous for college drinkers, perhaps, is the ritual of "chug-a-lugging." Every year a number of deaths result from this "Let's see who can drink the most" activity. Normally, the body has a built-in safety mechanism in which too much alcohol produces gastric irritation and consequent vomiting and a spasm (called pylorospasm) that closes the valve between the stomach and small intestine. However, for some people if alcohol is consumed rapidly, as happens in drinking contests, the safety valve may not work, with possibly fatal results.

Hangovers—morning-after headache, fatigue, upset stomach, irritability, anxiety, and thirst—are believed to be the result of alcohol withdrawal, the body's reaction to excessive alcohol intake. Two factors contribute significantly to hangovers:

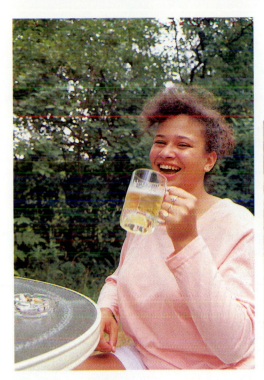

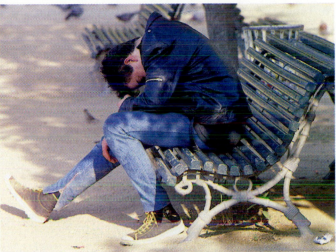

● **Figure 12.3 Effects of blood alcohol concentrations**

- *.02% BAC:* You feel a bit relaxed and loosened up. Your mood is heightened, but there is little behavior change.
- *.04% BAC:* You feel more relaxed. Your muscular coordination is slightly decreased, but there is no intoxication.
- *.06% BAC:* Your judgment begins to be impaired. You may become louder and boisterous. Your speech begins to slur. You have difficulty making decisions about ability to drive or operate machinery.
- *.08% BAC: You are considered legally drunk in many places.* This is the equivalent of the BAC found in a 160-pound male drinking 4 drinks in an hour. Your balance, vision, and hearing are slightly impaired. You are talkative and noisy. Your muscular coordination and driving skills are affected. Four hours will be required for alcohol to disappear from your system.
- *.10% BAC: You are legally drunk in most places.* Your mental facilities and judgment are distinctly impaired. Five hours will be required for all alcohol to disappear from your system.
- *.12% BAC:* This is equivalent to the BAC a 160-pound male would have if he drank a six-pack of beer in an hour. You will be distinctly clumsy and show serious lack of judgment. Vomiting may occur.
- *.14% BAC:* You're staggering, your speech is highly slurred, your vision quite blurred.
- *.16% BAC:* This is equal to a half pint of whiskey, or 8 drinks, for a 160-pound male consumed in an hour. You might as well go to bed, since it will take 8 hours for the alcohol to be metabolized through your system.
- *.20% BAC:* You'll be highly confused and will need assistance moving about. If you stop now, you'll still be legally drunk 6 hours from now.
- *.30% BAC:* This is equal to the BAC produced by a pint of whiskey consumed by a 160-pound male in an hour. Judgment and coordination are gone; the senses don't register anything and you may lose consciousness.
- *.40% BAC:* This is equal to 1¼ pints, or 20 shots, of whiskey for a 160-pound male consumed in an hour. You will lose consciousness and be in a coma. You will also be dangerously close to death—perhaps even dead. At a blood alcohol level of *.40%–.50%,* a person is usually in a coma. At *.60%–.70%,* death occurs.

4.28

Unit 4
Caffeine, Tobacco,
and Alcohol:
Common Mood-
Altering Drugs

● **Table 12.1 Calculating the percentage of alcohol in your bloodstream.**
This table presents the approximate blood alcohol concentration (BAC) according to your body weight and the number of drinks consumed during 1 or 2 hours.

	Body weight, pounds							
Number of Drinks	100	120	140	160	180	200	220	240
For 1 hour of drinking:								
1	0.03	0.03	0.02	0.02	0.02	0.01	0.01	—
2	0.06	0.05	0.04	0.04	0.03	0.03	0.03	0.02
3	0.10	0.08	0.07	0.06	0.05	0.05	0.04	0.04
4	0.13	0.10	0.09	0.08	0.07	0.06	0.06	0.05
5	0.16	0.13	0.11	0.10	0.09	0.08	0.07	0.07
6	0.19	0.16	0.13	0.12	0.11	0.10	0.09	0.08
7	0.23	0.19	0.16	0.14	0.13	0.11	0.10	0.09
8	0.26	0.22	0.18	0.16	0.14	0.13	0.12	0.11
For 2 hours of drinking:								
1	0.01	0.01	—	—	—	—	—	—
2	0.04	0.03	0.02	0.01	0.01	0.01	—	—
3	0.08	0.06	0.04	0.03	0.03	0.02	0.02	0.01
4	0.11	0.09	0.07	0.06	0.05	0.04	0.03	0.03
5	0.15	0.12	0.10	0.08	0.07	0.06	0.05	0.04
6	0.18	0.14	0.12	0.10	0.09	0.08	0.07	0.06
7	0.22	0.18	0.15	0.12	0.11	0.09	0.08	0.07
8	0.25	0.20	0.17	0.15	0.13	0.11	0.10	0.09

- *High BAC:* Too much alcohol consumed the night before—that is, a high blood alcohol concentration—produces alcohol withdrawal symptoms the next morning.

- *Type of alcoholic beverage:* Alcoholic beverages contain substances called **congeners,** which are additives or by-products of fermentation and preparation. Distilled spirits such as bourbon are more frequently associated with hangovers than are beer or vodka. Bourbon and scotch have more congeners (.1%–.2%) than do gin and wine (.04%), which in turn have more than vodka and beer (.01%).

Here are some of the symptoms of a hangover—and some things that can be done about them. (See ● *Figure 12.4.*)

- *Headache:* Caused by alcohol's expansion of the blood vessels in the head, headaches can be alleviated with aspirin and, perhaps, coffee and a hot shower. Note: Taking aspirin *before* you start drinking is *not* a good idea because research has shown that aspirin significantly lowers the body's ability to break down alcohol in the stomach.[180]

- *Nausea:* Caused by irritation to the stomach, nausea can be eased by antacids and bland foods, such as toast.

- *Thirst:* Brought on by dehydration because of frequent urination while drinking, thirst can be abated with fluids, especially slightly salty ones.

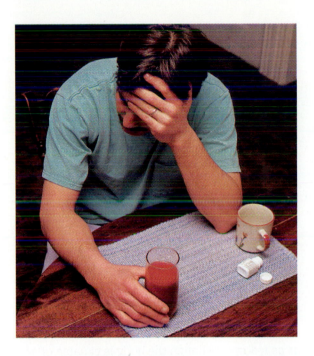

The only way to get alcohol out of the body is by the slow, steady, one-speed rate of metabolism of the substance by the liver, as we discuss next. For an adult, the average rate of metabolism for four cans of beer (or 4 ounces of whiskey) is 4–6 hours. Hangovers occur because the liver works at one speed to metabolize the alcohol. Any extra alcohol continues to circulate and accumulates in the bloodstream. Depending on the amount taken in, it may take the better part of the day for the body to recover from excess alcohol intake. During this period, the strongest of mortals may be laid low by the effects of a hangover.

What Happens When You Drink: How Alcohol Affects You

Alcohol can be absorbed, or consumed, at a fast rate, but it can be metabolized, or processed by the body, at the rate of about only one drink an hour. Alcohol sedates and depresses the central nervous system, eventually dulling the senses, distorting perception, and interfering with sexual performance, creative activity, sleep, and memory.

● **Figure 12.4 Any hangover remedies?**

> *Uncle Charlie's 'surefire miracle medicine' notwithstanding, there is no known cure or palliative for the morning-after miseries. . . . There seems little doubt, though, that the condition is an inherent part of the 'sobering up' process for some individuals. In that respect, although solid food, bed rest, and aspirin will make the discomfort somewhat more bearable, time and time alone will do the job. . . .*
>
> *Folklore dies hard, to be sure, but the fact remains that neither black coffee nor cold showers nor breaths of pure oxygen will hasten the sobering-up process. 'Give a drunk black coffee and a cold shower,' I've heard it said, 'and you end up with something really special—a wide-awake, soaking-wet, shivering drunk!'*

—Jack B. Weiner (1976). *Drinking.* New York: W. W. Norton.

Absorption Alcohol is a unique substance in that it does not need to be digested. Unlike food or pills, a small portion of alcohol begins to be absorbed as soon as it is swallowed, being taken into the tiny blood vessels called *capillaries* as it passes through the mouth and esophagus. Although about 20% is absorbed into the bloodstream through the stomach walls, the majority of alcohol is absorbed from the small intestine. (See ● *Figure 12.5.*) The bloodstream delivers the alcohol throughout the body, including liver, heart, and brain. Indeed, alcohol is distributed so quickly that it can be detected in the bloodstream only 2 minutes after being swallowed.

How fast alcohol is absorbed depends on four factors over which you have some control and four factors that may be less controllable. The four things that you can do something about are:

4.30

*Unit 4
Caffeine, Tobacco,
and Alcohol:
Common Mood-
Altering Drugs*

1. Strength of the drinks

2. Amount of alcohol and kind of alcoholic beverage consumed. The more concentrated an alcoholic beverage, the faster it is absorbed. Those that are carbonated speed absorption, because they tend to move quickly out of the stomach into the small intestines, where more rapid absorption takes place.

3. Speed of drinking

4. Whether there is food in your stomach—especially milk products and foods high in protein—that delays the absorption of the alcohol

Less controllable, perhaps, are:

1. *Your gender:* Compared to men, women tend to have reduced amounts of stomach enzymes that serve to break down some of the alcohol before it is absorbed. In addition, menstrually related hormonal changes can affect alcohol absorption.

2. *Your weight:* Heavier people have more body fluids in which the alcohol is diluted.

3. *Your body chemistry and emotions:* Such matters as condition of stomach tissues and presence of negative emotions affect emptying time of the stomach.

4. *Drinking history:* Long-term heavy drinkers develop tolerance—they require more alcohol to produce intoxication than less experienced drinkers.

Metabolism An important fact to be aware of is as follows: although the body is capable of *absorbing* (consuming) alcohol at a very fast rate, it can *metabolize* (process) it at a fixed rate—about only one drink per hour (equivalent to ½ ounce of pure alcohol). This means that if a person drinks a six-pack of beer in an hour, the body needs another 5 or more hours to get rid of all the alcohol. Alcohol, then, is metabolized at a relatively slow, constant rate that is independent of the amount you take in.

About 95% of the alcohol is metabolized by the liver. A small portion may be metabolized by the stomach (particularly for males). Less than 5% is expelled in breath, urine, and sweat.

Effects on the Central Nervous System

Many people look forward to winding down with a drink or two after work or school or when they're tired. The expression "winding down" is apt: alcohol is one of a class of drugs known as central nervous system *depressants.* These drugs (as we show in Chapter 13) depress the activity of the nerve cells (neurons) in the brain, gradually dulling or repressing—winding down—their responses. Thus, at low dosages, one feels looser, less inhibited, relaxed.

At higher dosages, however, there is a progressive reduction of central nervous system activity. At first, this is experienced as loss of concentration, discrimination, and motor control. Later there are mood swings and memory loss. Eventually, there is sleep, general anesthe-

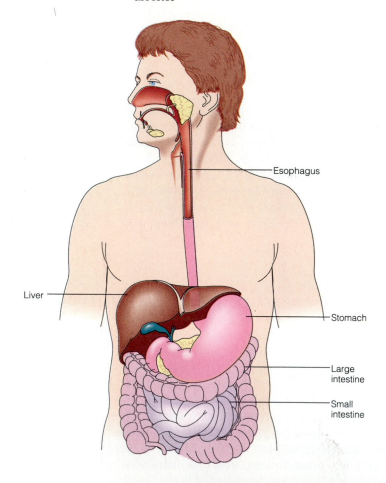

— Esophagus

Liver —

— Stomach

— Large intestine

— Small intestine

● **Figure 12.5 How alcohol is absorbed and metabolized.**
Some alcohol is absorbed into small blood vessels as it passes through the mouth, esophagus, and stomach. Most of it passes through the small or upper intestine before it is absorbed into the bloodstream.

sia, and, eventually, coma and death. Two primary reasons that people die from alcohol overdoses are that they stop breathing or suffocate on their own vomit.

What happens to your sensations and behavior as the sedative and dulling consequences of alcohol take effect? Consider some of the things that might happen to people during an evening's drinking:

- *Hearing:* On arriving late at a party, you notice that the noise level is high. This is because people who drink alcohol lose their inhibitions and so talk and laugh more loudly. In addition, alcohol has affected their hearing: people's ability to judge the direction of sound and distinguish between sounds is impaired.

- *Taste and smell:* At first alcohol stimulates the taste but later, on being called to dinner, drinkers may notice their interest in food is reduced. Their hunger may have been partly satisfied by snacks during the cocktail hour, but after awhile alcohol interferes with the senses of taste and smell.

- *Time and space:* Drinkers may find themselves sitting in one place for several hours without knowing it, because alcohol distorts perceptions of time and space.

- *Touch, temperature, and pain:* Leaving the party, a drinker may step outside into freezing weather but be unaware of it. This can pose a real danger, because drinkers have been known to die of *hypothermia*, a reduction in body temperature. In part this is because alcohol expands the blood vessels in the skin. Although one feels warmer, alcohol actually reduces body temperature.

    The sense of touch is also affected, so that the drinker may not be able to distinguish between hot and cold. In addition, alcohol diminishes the perception of pain, increasing the risk of harm.

- *Vision:* If the drinker has been so unwise as to get behind the wheel of a car, here's what alcohol may have done to that person's vision: He or she has "tunnel vision" (the visual field is narrowed), blurred vision, and difficulty adjusting to the glare of oncoming headlights. The sensitivity to color is also reduced, so that one sees a red light less quickly.

- *Motor skills and judgment:* Alcohol slows down control of muscles and interferes with reaction time and coordination, the principal reason why drunken drivers have difficulty staying in their lane and why police officers often ask those suspected of being intoxicated to walk a straight line. Alcohol also affects one's judgment, making a drinker more inclined to take risks, such as passing cars with insufficient room to spare. It also seems to unleash hostile, aggressive, or violent behavior. Many murders and other acts of violence are associated with heavy drinking.

- *Sexual performance:* If drinkers managed to arrive home without being jailed or causing an accident and approach their sexual partner, they may, if male, discover what Shakespeare pointed out about alcohol: "It provokes the desire, but it takes away the performance." That is, in men it increases the interest in sex but reduces the ability to achieve or maintain an erection. Recent evidence suggests that women, too, continue to perceive sexual arousal and pleasure but experience a decrease in physiological response.[181]

- *Creative activity:* If a drinker has decided to devote the rest of the evening to working on a term paper, he or she will doubtless find the next morning that the work is superficial, sloppy, and poorly organized. As with sex, so in art and in work: alcohol may release one from inhibitions but does nothing constructive for imagination and productivity.

- *Sleep:* Alcohol may help a drinker get to sleep, but it does not give truly restorative sleep. Alcohol interferes with normal sleep rhythms.

- *Memory and blackouts:* A drinker may wake up the next morning and have no recollection about some of the evening's events—including where he or she parked the car—even though no loss of consciousness occurred during that time. This kind of amnesia is called a **blackout**, and it is thought to result from an alcohol-induced interference in ability to transfer information from short-term to long-term memory.

4.32

Unit 4
Caffeine, Tobacco,
and Alcohol:
Common Mood-
Altering Drugs

Strategy for Living: Deciding What to Do About Drinking

Learning how to drink or not drink means knowing who you are—how your individual character, biological basis, and ethnic, family, and economic background affect your ability to consume alcohol. The "drinker's toolkit" shows how to drink without getting drunk.

Knowing Who You Are: Choice and Responsibility In our society, you almost have to make a choice *not* to drink. About 77% of men and 60% of women drink alcohol; that is 67% of the adult population.[182] This means that about one-third of Americans do not use alcohol at all. Actually, fewer Americans drink now than in the past. Despite the country's overall population growth, the number of drinkers dropped by 10 million people from 1985 to 1990 (from 113.1 million to 102.9 million), or from 59% down to 51% for those aged 12 and over.[183]

How much drinking is problematic? The Addiction Research Foundation in Toronto has suggested the following standards:[184]

- *Risk to good health:* more than 2 drinks a day

- *Hazardous:* 5–6 drinks a day

- *Harmful:* 7–8 drinks a day

- *Extremely dangerous:* 9 or more drinks a day

The difficulty with these guidelines is that they seem to perpetuate the notion that the problem is *daily* drinking, when in fact there are many alcohol abusers who go for long stretches without drinking. According to the American Psychiatric Association's *Diagnosis and Statistical Manual of Mental Disorders* (Third Edition—Revised, known as *DSM III-R*), alcohol abuse can be evaluated according to the answers to the following questions:

1. Have you ever continued to use alcohol despite negative consequences?

2. Have you ever used alcohol in situations in which drinking is physically hazardous?

3. Have you had symptoms associated with #1 or #2 for 1 month or more?

4. Have you ever met the criteria for dependence?

(We discuss dependence in Chapter 13.) These criteria differentiate between alcohol abuse and dependency.

People are considered alcohol abusers who answer yes to *either* 1 or 2 *and* 3 but no to 4, which indicates dependency, not abuse. (The DSM III-R criteria for alcohol dependency are presented later in the chapter in Figure 12.9.)

Knowing Who You Are Biologically Not all drinkers are created equal. People differ in their ability to handle alcohol. Some of the factors that affect this ability include the following:

- *Larger people can drink more than smaller people:* As we suggested earlier, a heavier person can handle more alcohol in a given period of time than a smaller person can. In an hour's time, a 100-pound person can attain .10% BAC after three drinks whereas a 200-pound person may require five to six drinks. One reason for this is that larger people have more water within their bodies (adult males are 55% water, adult females 45%), which dilutes the alcohol they drink.

- *Men have lower BACs than women for the same amount of alcohol:* Women can handle less alcohol than men can, but the fact that most women weigh less is only one reason. Even when members of the two sexes are of the same weight and are drinking the same amounts, women will reach a higher BAC sooner.

A partial reason is that women's bodies contain a higher proportion of fat and less water, and thus have less water with which to dilute the alcohol. Also, because alcohol is not very fat-soluble, women have more alcohol in their bloodstreams. In addition, women have less of a protective enzyme (alcohol dehydrogenase) that breaks down alcohol in the stomach.

Yet another difference is that hormonal changes associated with women's menstrual cycles influence the absorption and/or metabolism rate of alcohol. Prior to their menstrual periods, women absorb alcohol faster than at other times during their menstrual cycles. In addition, women who take birth-control pills may also absorb alcohol faster.[185]

- *Younger people tend to have lower BACs than older people:* Younger people have more water in their bodies with which to dilute alcohol than older people do. Thus, a 20-year-old and a 50-year-old trying to match drinks will find that the older person reaches a high BAC sooner than the younger person does. However, young people may experience more impairment than those who are older, despite similar BACs.

Knowing Your Ethnic, Economic, and Family Background Some people believe that some ethnic and economic groups are more vulnerable to alcohol abuse than others. Let us consider this.

- *Some ethnic groups have more history of drinking problems than others.* We do not suggest that there is a genetic or racial basis that predisposes some ethnic groups to alcoholism. Nevertheless, some groups have higher alcoholism rates than others and this may be due, in part, to cultural norms and expectations.

    Although African Americans and Hispanics are more likely to abstain than whites are, African Americans and Hispanics who drink have higher rates of alcohol dependency than do whites who drink.[186,187] Irish Americans and Native Americans (Indians and Eskimos) have very high rates. (Among Native Americans, however, drinking practices differ significantly among tribal groups.) People of English and Slavic descent and some other American Protestant groups also have somewhat high rates. People of Italian, Jewish, Greek, and Chinese extraction have very low rates.[188]

    Interestingly, high-alcoholism groups also show a high number of abstainers. If you should happen to be of one of these ethnic backgrounds, it does not mean that you personally are more disposed to develop or avoid a drinking problem, only that you may have been raised in the kind of environment that shows this kind of profile.

- *Economically deprived groups have a history of more drinking problems than affluent groups.* A 40-year study has found that members of an inner-city working class population were more than three times as likely to become alcoholic as those who were in a middle-class, college-educated population.[189] This may explain why some ethnic groups are more disposed to develop drinking problems than others: many minorities have a history of economic deprivation.

- *Groups of males have a history of more drinking problems than do groups of females.* College fraternities, the armed forces, construction crews, and other groups of males have a history of heavy drinking. Even in those ethnic and socioeconomic groups that show more alcoholism, there are fewer female alcoholics than males. As Peele and Brodsky point out, being part of a hard-drinking social circle is difficult because the group is more powerful than the individual. "If you want to drink healthily," they suggest, "the best single thing you can do is to associate exclusively with people who drink moderately."[190]

Because of the rise of the "Children of Alcoholics" movement, many people are worried that being offspring of alcoholics may somehow cause them to be alcoholics themselves. Alcoholism does indeed seem to run in families. The typical finding suggests that the offspring of alcoholics have a *four times greater risk* of developing the disease.[191] This may not mean it is inherited, however, any more than learning to speak English in North America is inherited. Still, current thinking is that heredity plays a significant part in the development of alcoholism—in some people.

Reducing Risk: How to Drink Without Getting Drunk A lot of what happens to drinkers develops out of their own expectations. For instance, people who believe they are drinking alcoholic drinks but in fact are consuming non-alcoholic drinks may be more talkative and relaxed—simply because they expect to be affected by alcohol in certain ways.

Many people, of course, deliberately drink to get drunk—to wipe out major pain, to really celebrate, or just to "party," because that's their idea of the best way to have a good time. Unfortunately, for some people, even getting inebriated *once* can be disastrous, perhaps fatal. If

4.34

Unit 4
Caffeine, Tobacco,
and Alcohol:
Common Mood-
Altering Drugs

you do choose to drink, the following will help you reduce your risks:

- *Don't mix alcohol with other drugs.* This rule is primary above all others, because it is literally a matter of life or death. Alcohol in combination with another mood-altering (psychoactive) drug—particularly another depressant, such as a tranquilizer, pain-killer, or sleeping pill—has several times the effect of each used alone. Thus, be sure to check with your pharmacist and to read the warnings on any prescription or non-prescription drugs you are taking to make certain they will not cause you harm.

- *Eat before and while drinking.* Food in the stomach—particularly protein and fat, such as cheese, milk, and meat—slows down alcohol absorption in the stomach and small intestine by coating the areas through which the alcohol is absorbed. There's a good reason, therefore, to attack the cheese dip while you're at a party.

- *Avoid fizzy drinks.* Carbonated beverages, such as champagne, cola, club soda, tonic, and ginger ale, help speed the absorption of alcohol and thus the delivery of alcohol through the bloodstream to the brain. Avoid bourbon-and-beer combinations ("boiler-makers," "depth charges"), since they are a surefire way to get drunk fast.

- *Measure drinks, use ice, drink slowly.* These actions enable you to control the amount of alcohol you consume. Using a bartender's shot glass to measure the amount of alcohol added to a mixed drink (instead of just splashing in liquor), letting ice melt in your glass, and sipping rather than gulping drinks—all these are ways to slow down the alcohol consumption.

- *Take care of your friends.* If you're hosting a party, you are responsible for your guests, and you can help everyone by measuring drinks, pushing snacks but not drinks on people, and making nonalcoholic alternatives available.

    In recent years, breweries and a handful of wineries have been making nonalcoholic, or de-alcoholized, beers and wines available, some of which have even less alcohol than fruit juices and soft drinks (for example, Kaliber nonalcoholic beer is only

.01% alcohol). Some of these nonalcoholic alternatives have been found in taste tests to be the equal of their alcoholic counterparts.[192,193] (*See* ● *Figure 12.6.*)

You are not out of place in setting drinking limits, politely expressing your concern for your guests, and offering coffee or nonalcoholic drinks. Above all, don't let an inebriated guest get behind the wheel of a car. Besides the threat to life—to your guest and to other people on the road—there is the risk that you (or your parents) can be sued for negligence.

What Alcohol Does to People: Alcohol and Abuse

Alcohol *in moderation*—one or two drinks a day—may actually lower risk of heart disease. However, heavy drinking has unfortunate consequences at different stages of life: younger drinkers suffer injuries, peaking at age 24; older drinkers suffer chronic diseases, peaking in the 60s.

Can alcohol in fact be good for you?

It has been reported that people who have less than two alcoholic drinks a day actually have less heart disease than people who are either abstainers or heavy drinkers. For instance, a 1988 Harvard University study found that women who regularly take a drink or two a day reduce their risk of heart attacks and some kinds of strokes compared to nondrinkers.[194] Researchers at Harvard's School of Public Health studied 44,000 men ages 40–75 over 2 years and found that those who drank light to moderate amounts of alcohol had a 25–40% lower chance of developing heart disease compared to their counterparts. "Moderate" drinking was defined as one to two drinks a day of a standard drink.[195]

Indeed, says one writer, "If you control your drinking, and aren't pregnant, a glass or two of wine, a couple of beers, even two shots of rye, appear to be reasonable indulgences."[196] He means, of course, two drinks of *any* of these, not all of these. The limitation is important: *more* than two drinks begins to cause medical complications, including an increased problem with heart disease.

Still, the studies showing that moderate drinking is good for you may rest on some shaky assumptions. One trio of alcohol and drug experts question whether many light or moderate daily drinkers in fact exist. In their opinion, "Most light drinkers do not drink every day, and most people who drink every day do not drink lightly." Also, they point out, more than twice as many of the people who were classified as abstainers in the studies were poor, and it is known that poor people have worse health than those with economic advantages.[197]

What happens if you take three or four or more drinks a day? That is, what outcome can we foresee for a career of chronic heavy drinking? In general, according to one study performed for the national Centers for Disease Control and Prevention, heavy drinking tends to be fatal in two different stages of life:

- In early adulthood, peaking at about age 24, due to injuries

- Later in life, peaking in the 60s, due to chronic disease

When victims' life expectancies were figured in, the study found alcohol had cheated them of *about 26 years apiece.*[198] (*See* ● *Figure 12.7.*)

Short Young Lives: Accidents, Suicides, and Homicides

Among young people, alcohol has been heavily implicated in accidents, particularly car accidents, as well as suicides and homicides.

Car accidents account for the overwhelming majority of alcohol-related deaths. For instance, in 1989, about 7000 persons ages 15–24 died in alcohol-related crashes.[199] Injuries were responsible for killing 30,205 Americans, or 28.7% of alcohol-caused deaths in 1987. Accidents involving alcohol among the young cause more deaths than any single chronic disease does among the middle-aged or older alcohol victims. Deaths from alcohol-related injuries, mainly automobile accidents, rise sharply through adolescence and peak at 6000 a year at ages 20–24, then fall off rapidly.[200]

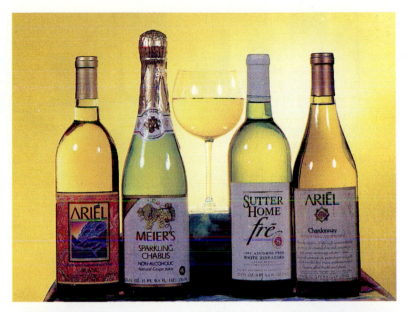

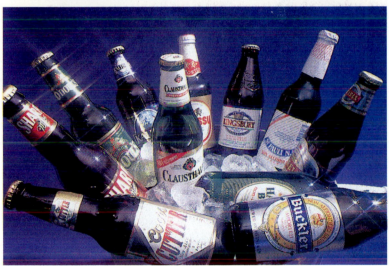

● **Figure 12.6 Nonalcoholic beers and wines.** These are available mostly nationwide or in major urban areas. Other brands, both domestic and foreign, are also available.

4.36

Unit 4
Caffeine, Tobacco,
and Alcohol:
Common Mood-
Altering Drugs

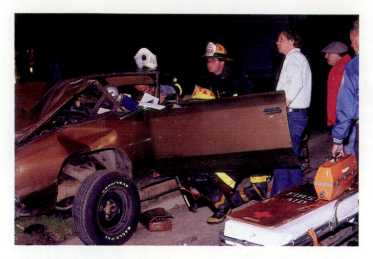

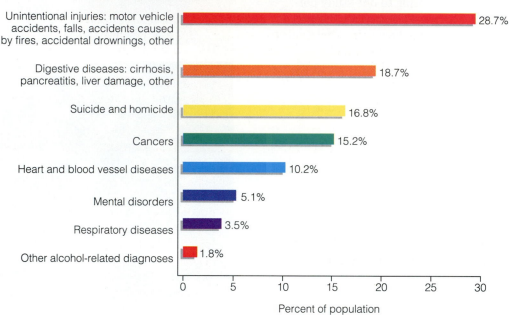

Unintentional injuries: motor vehicle accidents, falls, accidents caused by fires, accidental drownings, other — 28.7%

Digestive diseases: cirrhosis, pancreatitis, liver damage, other — 18.7%

Suicide and homicide — 16.8%

Cancers — 15.2%

Heart and blood vessel diseases — 10.2%

Mental disorders — 5.1%

Respiratory diseases — 3.5%

Other alcohol-related diagnoses — 1.8%

Percent of population

● **Figure 12.7 Alcohol-related deaths**

To be sure, increasing public awareness and stiffer penalties—especially for people under 21 found driving even with low BACs (generally .01–.05% BAC)—have reduced drunk driving deaths somewhat. Another important factor is probably the increase in the minimum drinking age in 37 states from 1982 to 1988, so that now in all 50 states and the District of Columbia the minimum drinking age is 21.[201] Yet in a 4-year study of over 1500 tavern and nightclub goers, researcher Barry Caudill found that many heavy drinkers still report feeling confident that they can drive safely when intoxicated. According to his findings, 87% had driven while intoxicated an average of 30 times and 75% said they might be able to, or definitely could, drive safely while intoxicated.[202]

Alcohol also figures in accidents other than motor-vehicle fatalities. In deaths caused by fire, alcohol is involved in at least half the cases. It is also involved in half of home accidents and nearly 70% of drownings.[203]

Intentional injuries, primarily suicides and homicides, ran a close second in alcohol-related deaths to car crashes in 1987, having killed over 17,600 people, or 16.8% of the total.[204] In four out of five suicide attempts, the individual has been drinking; half of all successful suicides are alcoholics. In 67% of all homicides, either the killer or the victim or both had been drinking.[205]

Although these statistics are disconcerting, one study suggests that alcohol is even deadlier than we might think. That is, oftentimes official cause-of-death data listed on death certificates do not reflect the true culprit. Research into the deaths of 450 young Army veterans found six times as many alcohol-related deaths occurred as were reflected on death certificates. Motor-vehicle injuries were the leading cause of death (with alcohol playing a role 40% of the time), but suicides and homicides ranked second, with alcohol a factor 30% of the time for each.[206]

Reduced Life Spans:
Alcohol-Related Diseases

A lifetime of heavy drinking leads to sexual problems; brain problems such as Wernicke's Syndrome and Korsakoff's Syndrome; liver problems such as acute fatty liver, hepatitis, and cirrhosis; gastrointestinal problems such as pancreatitis, heart and blood vessel problems; and cancers, especially breast cancer.

The death toll from chronic alcohol-related diseases (such as cirrhosis of the liver and hepatitis) rises slowly from age 20 to age 60. At that age, however, it accounts for three times as many deaths as accidents do. Cancer of the esophagus accounts for under 10% of total alcohol-related deaths, stroke for less than 10%, and cirrhosis for about 7%.[207]

Disorders that relate to heavy drinking are as follows.

Sexual and Reproductive Health Problems
Heavy drinking affects the male sex hormones,

producing a loss of sexual desire, difficulty in sexual performance (including impotence), formation of breasts in men (gynecomastia) because of sex hormone imbalance, decreased sperm production, sterility, and risk of conceiving defective offspring.[208] In women, heavy drinking may produce impaired sexual functioning, different menstrual disorders, and halting of the menstrual period.[209] Finally, drinking is associated with poor judgment and high-risk sexual behavior, making it a risk factor for unintentional or forced sex, unplanned pregnancy, and sexually transmitted diseases, such as HIV.[210]

Brain Problems After a while, heavy drinkers begin to show, even when sober, remnants of the neuropsychological problems they experience when under the influence: memory loss, impaired motor skills, and difficulty in solving problems and learning. In general, however, such impairments can be almost completely reversed (though some problems remain) if drinkers become abstinent.[211]

One consequence of chronic alcoholism is nutritional and vitamin deficiency, especially thiamine (vitamin B_{11}). This and the accompanying heavy drinking may lead to **Wernicke's syndrome,** which is characterized by paralysis of eye nerves, mental confusion, loss of memory, and staggering gait. **Korsakoff's syndrome,** which may also have a nutritional basis but is mostly due to alcohol, is characterized by memory and learning dysfunction, mental confusion, and hallucinations.

Liver Problems Some parts of the body regenerate if they are damaged. The liver, however, is not one of them; at some point alcohol can cause irreversible damage. As the "detox center" of the body, the liver is the major metabolic site for alcohol.

Alcohol dependence can cause three progressively serious kinds of damage to this essential organ:

- *Acute fatty liver:* This is characterized by fat accumulating in the liver. The condition can be reversed by stopping alcohol consumption.

- *Alcoholic hepatitis:* This is characterized by inflammation of liver cells and by **jaundice,** in which the skin appears yellow,

4.38

Unit 4
Caffeine, Tobacco,
and Alcohol:
Common Mood-
Altering Drugs

caused by the liver's inability to remove a yellow pigment called bilirubin. This condition too can be reversed with abstinence and medical treatment, although it can be fatal if not treated.

- *Cirrhosis:* **Cirrhosis,** characterized by irreversible scarring of the liver, is the ninth leading cause of death in the United States.[212] A cirrhotic liver is unable to metabolize various toxins and drugs. These toxins accumulate in the body, resulting in death.

Although cirrhosis is a serious and irreversible condition, only about 10% of alcohol-dependent people develop it.[213]

Gastrointestinal Problems Besides liver disease, chronic alcohol use can cause irritation of the stomach lining. As a result, heavy drinkers often experience loss of appetite, morning nausea, frequent belching, and diarrhea alternating with constipation. Sometimes they also experience abdominal pain and even bleeding from the gastrointestinal tract.

Pancreatitis, inflammation of the pancreas, the gland that manufactures digestive juices, is experienced as nausea, vomiting, diarrhea, and upper abdominal pain. The disorder, which can result from chronic alcohol use, reduces the ability of the pancreas to produce insulin, possibly leading to diabetes.

Heart and Blood Vessel Problems Heavy drinkers suffer increased risk of premature death from heart and blood vessel diseases. Indeed, many alcohol-dependent people have shown raised blood pressure (hypertension), which has been linked to higher risk of strokes and heart attacks. Alcohol also elevates blood fat levels of a kind that may be linked to the development of atherosclerosis, or hardening of the arteries. In addition, irregularities in heartbeat (arrhythmias) and an enlarged heart are associated with heavy alcohol.

Cancers—Especially Breast Cancer There is a whole laundry list of cancers associated with heavy alcohol use, running, as it were, from beginning to end of the body: oral cavity, tongue, pharynx, larynx, esophagus, stomach, liver, lung, pancreas, colon, and rectum.[214]

Some of these may be related to cigarette smoking, since many heavy drinkers are also smokers. Indeed, alcohol may actually *increase* the cancer-causing effects of cigarettes.

Women who are heavy alcohol users have a special concern: breast cancer. A study of more than 89,000 female nurses found that women who have more than one drink a day have a higher risk of breast cancer.[215] In general, it seems that, as an added risk from drinking, women with a family history of breast cancer or who are obese should be particularly alert for signs of breast cancer.[216]

The Effects on Others

Problem drinkers harm others, not just themselves. Pregnant women who drink may produce offspring suffering from fetal alcohol syndrome or fetal alcohol effects. Alcoholism is a family disease that tends to have an impact on all family members. Children and even grandchildren of alcoholics show difficulties in many areas. Society at large also suffers from the behavior of alcoholics.

One might argue that since alcohol-dependent persons are only doing damage to themselves, why not simply let them alone? Unfortunately, there are a great many other unwilling and even unknowing participants in a heavy drinker's life. Let us look at them.

Unborn Children: Fetal Alcohol Syndrome and Fetal Alcohol Effects How much alcohol should you allow yourself if you're pregnant? The answer: none.

The leading known cause of preventable mental retardation and birth defects in the United States is **fetal alcohol syndrome (FAS).** A baby born with FAS is characterized by a common pattern of physical and behavioral abnormalities and mental retardation. The principal features are as follows:[217]

- *Mental retardation and other central nervous system problems:* Although the most common dysfunction is mental retardation, other problems of the central nervous system include poor motor coordination and muscle tone and hyperactivity. FAS children show delayed language development and low I.Q. scores.

- *Growth deficiency and facial abnormalities:* Newborns are often only about 38% of normal birth weight and 65% of normal birth length. FAS children have small heads, small eyes, and abnormal facial features, including an underdeveloped midface. (*See* ● *Figure 12.8.*)

- *Other malformations:* FAS offspring usually display malformations of various organ systems—heart, urinary, genital, and skeletal.

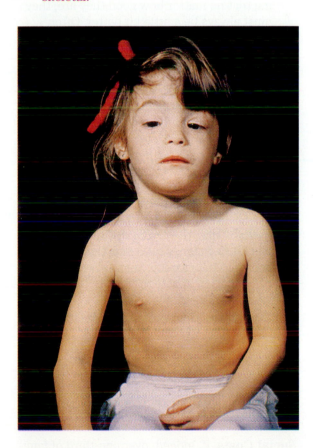

● **Figure 12.8 Child with fetal alcohol syndrome.** Children with FAS, which is characterized by mental retardation and physical deformities (including underdeveloped midface, as shown here), are the offspring of alcohol-dependent mothers who drank during pregnancy.

About 1 in every 750 babies born has the characteristic symptoms of FAS. Many more children, however, are affected by alcohol during pregnancy and don't have FAS. This condition is known as **fetal alcohol effects (FAE).** A woman does not have to be alcoholic to place her unborn baby at risk for alcohol-related problems. The symptoms of FAE include low birth weight, abnormalities of the mouth and the genital and urinary systems, and altered behavioral patterns.[218]

Perhaps 30–40% of the children of chronic alcoholic mothers who were drinking during pregnancy will have FAS, but even more children whose mothers were abusing alcohol during pregnancy can be at risk for various learning problems even without FAS.[219] As the FAS child grows into adolescence and adulthood, he or she will experience major psychosocial problems and life-long adjustment problems.[220]

Fortunately, many women seem to be getting the message that alcohol and pregnancy don't mix. Researchers from the Centers for Disease Control found that in the 1980s drinking during pregnancy became steadily less common. For instance, in 1988, among the oldest and most educated pregnant women—women who were college graduates—only 19% said they drank, down from 41% in 1985.[221]

Codependents and COAs: Families and Children of Alcoholics Until recently the problems of family members of alcoholics were ignored by health professionals and denied by the families themselves. However, this was a huge population that was overlooked: there are an estimated 28 million children of alcoholics in the United States, 7 million of whom are under age 18.[222] A 1988 national survey found that an astonishing number of people, 43% of American adults—76 million people—have been exposed to alcoholism in the family. They grew up with an alcoholic or problem drinker, married one, or had a blood relative who was one.[223]

Thus, alcoholism is now considered to be a *family illness*, which signifies the tremendous impact that alcoholics have on those around them. As families react to alcoholic behavior with anger, confusion, and bewilderment, their behavior becomes as impaired as that of the alcoholic. Accordingly, health professionals are

4.40

Unit 4
Caffeine, Tobacco,
and Alcohol:
Common Mood-
Altering Drugs

now giving increasing attention to treating members of the alcoholic's household.

Several terms have emerged to describe two groups greatly affected by alcoholics:

- *Codependents:* **Codependents,** or **co-alcoholics,** were originally considered to be spouses of alcoholics, although now the term has been extended to children and others close to an alcoholic family member. The chief characteristic of codependents is that they tend to accommodate themselves to the alcoholic. At first they may attempt to control the alcoholic, initially being "understanding," then being angry, then trying to ignore the situation, but eventually they give up and try to work around the alcoholic. Gradually they may take over many of the drinker's usual responsibilities, such as meal preparation or bill-paying. Indeed, they become **enablers,** protecting the alcoholic from the negative consequences of his or her addiction.

  The term *codependents* has been extended to people in families troubled by other addictions or compulsions such as drugs, gambling, or food. We should note, however, that the widespread adoption of "codependency" terminology bothers some treatment professionals because of the indiscriminate application of the concept to all family members.[224]

- *Children of alcoholics:* "Please send me some pamphlets," says the letter. "I am twelve-and-a-half years old. Please hurry. I can't stand it anymore. My father's drinking."[225]

  This kind of pain and anguish is often experienced by **children of alcoholics (COAs)**, those who grow up in a family in which one or both parents is an alcoholic. As might be imagined, children of alcoholics must frequently weather marital conflict, spousal abuse, and divorce more than other children. In fact, such children are more likely than other youngsters to have emotional, social, physical, and chemical-dependency problems.[226] Children of alcoholics are three to four times more likely to become alcoholics themselves.

  COAs demonstrate why alcoholism is often called a "family disease." Because alcohol interferes with the parents' ability to give their offspring the attention that is important for emotional growth, the children often go to great lengths to gain attention from others or withdraw into a world of their own.[227] In hopes of coping with and surviving their dysfunctional families, some may strive to be responsible for everyone in the family, such as taking care of the other children and cleaning and cooking. Some may exhibit poor academic performance and behavior problems. Many, however, are often successful in school and in other areas of life, but tend to go through life feeling that no matter how good they are, they must always be a little bit better. Often COAs marry alcoholics, continuing the roles they developed in childhood.

Adults raised in alcoholic families report difficulties in several areas: expressing their needs to others, identifying and expressing their feelings, putting themselves first, trusting people, and dealing with issues of dependency and intimacy in relationships.[228] If you suspect you are a COA, try taking the accompanying survey. (*See Self Discovery 12.1.*)

The problems of codependency can carry on not only into adulthood but also to the next generation. Thus, the **grandchildren of alcoholics (GCOAs)** may not know that there is alcoholism in their family, but because their parents are often unable to express feelings and are uncomfortable about asking for help, they may pass on negative behaviors to their children. According to Ann Smith, author of *Grandchildren of Alcoholics,* "the absence of unconditional love, openly expressed feelings, and other necessary ingredients for emotionally healthy lives leave grandchildren of alcoholics without adequate preparation for life."[229]

Social Costs If, indeed, over one-third of families are struggling with someone with alcohol dependency, this can only begin to hint at the magnitude of the problem to society. As we have already suggested, alcohol is a factor in half of motor-vehicle fatalities and suicides and homicides, and in about a third of homicides, drownings, and boating deaths victims are intoxicated. Alcohol figures in a large number of spouse and child abuse cases and in more than

SELF DISCOVERY 12.1

Are You an Adult Child?

Give yourself 10 points for each of the following statements if it is often true of you or sounds like you as a child.

	Yes	No
1. I take care of other people, but no one takes care of me.	___	___
2. No matter what happens, I feel I get blamed for it.	___	___
3. Usually it's best when no one notices me.	___	___
4. I'll do almost anything to get a laugh.	___	___
5. It's really hard for me to figure out what I want in a relationship.	___	___
6. People praise me for all I've done but I never feel I've done enough.	___	___
7. I think I'm just no good.	___	___
8. I'm more comfortable with computers than people.	___	___
9. I usually change the subject when people get excited about something.	___	___
10. I'm not sure what people want me to say when they ask about my feelings.	___	___
11. It's hard for me to be close to people.	___	___
12. It's probably my fault my family has so many problems.	___	___
13. People say I could achieve more, but I don't have the self-confidence.	___	___
14. Sometimes I wish someone would just tell me what to do.	___	___
15. I work hard at getting approval.	___	___
16. I always try to do the correct thing.	___	___
17. Most of my friends get in trouble.	___	___
18. My animals are my best friends.	___	___
19. I'm really attracted to strong people.	___	___
20. Angry people scare me.	___	___
21. My job involves teaching or healing other people.	___	___
22. As soon as I am old enough I'm leaving home.	___	___
23. I procrastinate a lot.	___	___
24. It's hard for me to sit still—I'm usually hyper.	___	___
25. I feel different from other people.	___	___
26. People think I'm a nice person, but my spouse complains I won't get close.	___	___
27. If everyone would leave me alone, I'd be okay.	___	___
28. It's hard for me to relax with someone else around.	___	___
29. When I was a kid, I was the class clown.	___	___

Scoring

If you answered yes to 1, 6, 11, 16, 21, and 26 you are probably the oldest child, the only child, or the oldest girl or boy in your family.

If you tended to agree with 2, 7, 12, 17, 22, and 27 you are more likely to be the second child or the second sister or brother child in your family.

A predominance of yes answers to 3, 8, 13, 18, 23, and 28 would indicate that you are the middle child.

Identifying with answers 4, 9, 14, 19, 24, and 29 suggests the likelihood that you were the last born.

Overall Score

An overall score of over 100 indicates a strong identification with typical traits of adult children of alcoholics, though you may find you are not in the birth order indicated. If you find you don't agree with many statements, you may still recognize the behavior of someone close to you.

Source: Developed by Stephanie Abbott, President, National Foundation for Alcoholism Communications.

four-fifths of police arrests. It is the principal contributor to cirrhosis, the ninth leading cause of death in the United States. Its use during pregnancy is the leading preventable cause of birth defects. Alcohol also costs our society a great deal economically—$70 billion a year, mainly in reduced productivity.[230] With all this, no wonder it has been said that if alcohol were invented today it would immediately be put on the government's list of controlled substances.

4.42

*Unit 4
Caffeine, Tobacco,
and Alcohol:
Common Mood-
Altering Drugs*

Alcoholism

Alcoholism is a chronic, progressive, and potentially fatal disease characterized by a growing compulsion to drink and loss of control. The development of the disease may be influenced by genetic, pychosocial, and environmental factors. Alcoholism increases in severity through several stages. Some alcoholics "hit bottom" and voluntarily seek treatment. Others may require intervention.

Many readers of this book may need to address a fundamental question: how badly do you need alcohol to change your mood? The belief that it is necessary as a basic pleasure in your life or as a stress and pain reliever may be central to alcohol becoming a difficulty, as you may be able to determine from the accompanying self-survey. (*See Self Discovery 12.2.*) If asked whether they have (1) ever felt they should cut down on their drinking, (2) been annoyed by people criticizing their drinking, (3) felt guilty about their drinking, or (4) had to have an "eye-opener" first thing in the morning to steady their nerves, most nonalcoholics would answer yes to just one or none of these. Answering yes to two or more, however, might indicate a likelihood of alcoholism.

What Is Alcoholism? People have all kinds of misguided notions about what an alcoholic is—for instance, someone who is homeless, who panhandles, who drinks in the morning, who drinks alone, who drinks all day, who drinks every day. Such preconceived notions about the characteristics of an alcoholic make it difficult to recognize alcoholism in a friend or family member.

Consider the stereotypical view of homeless people as society's castoffs who have failed in the competitive world and have sunk into alcoholic squalor. In fact, however, only some of the homeless have alcohol problems, although more than in the general population. Since the turn of the century, surveys of the homeless—who represent all ages, ethnic groups, and degrees of ability and employability—have found an alcohol abuse rate averaging only 30–33%, as opposed to about 10% in other groups. The problem, however, is that, unlike people who

may drink in the privacy of their own homes, homeless people who drink are highly visible.[231] In actuality, alcoholics come from every social class, from students to college professors to priests to airline pilots. (Indeed, in 1990, three professional pilots of a major U.S. airline were fired for flying a jetliner while under the influence of alcohol.[232] Surveys have found the incidence of heavy drinking among private and professional pilots to be similar to that in the general population.[233])

Alcoholism is defined as a chronic, progressive, and potentially fatal disease characterized by a growing compulsion to drink. *Control* is an important aspect of the disease. As psychiatrist George Vaillant writes, you may consider yourself an alcoholic when "you're not in control of when you begin drinking and when you stop drinking."[234] Continuing to drink despite the negative consequences associated with drinking is another important aspect of the disease.

In a recent expanded definition agreed upon by the American Society of Addiction Medicine (ASAM) and the National Council on Alcoholism and Drug Dependence (NCADD), alcoholism is "characterized by continuous or periodic impaired control over drinking, preoccupation with the drug alcohol, use of alcohol despite adverse consequences, and distortions in thinking, most notably denial."[235] **Denial** is the defense mechanism whereby one simply refuses to admit or to face unpleasant realities. It is a major characteristic of those who are alcoholic. The American Psychiatric Association's *Diagnostic and Statistical Manual of Mental Disorders* (Third Edition—Revised, called *DSM III-R*) has published criteria for diagnosing alcoholism. (*See ● Figure 12.9.*)

People wonder how there can actually be a "disease" of alcoholism when drinkers must voluntarily lift a glass to their lips to initiate the act of intoxication. Indeed, for centuries, alcoholism—until recently called drunkenness—has been viewed as simply a lack of willpower, a weakness of character, a vice that drinkers choose but could stop if they really wanted to. Only recently has the majority view come around to regarding alcoholism as a chronic *disease,* resembling diabetes, say, or sickle-cell anemia. Although the disease concept is still criticized by some (as we discuss in the Life

SELF DISCOVERY 12.2

What Kind of Drinker Are You?

Answer each of the following questions by placing a check in the appropriate column.

	Yes	No
1. Do you feel you are a normal drinker? (If you are a total abstainer, check "Yes.")		
2. Have you ever awakened the morning after some drinking the night before and found that you could not remember a part of the evening before?		
3. Does your spouse (or a parent) ever worry or complain about your drinking?		
4. Can you stop drinking without a struggle after one or two drinks?		
5. Do you feel bad about your drinking?		
6. Do friends or relatives think you are a normal drinker?		
7. Do you ever try to limit your drinking to certain times of the day or to certain places?		
8. Are you always able to stop drinking when you want to?		
9. Have you ever attended a meeting of Alcoholics Anonymous (AA)?		
10. Have you gotten into fights when drinking?		
11. Has drinking ever created problems with you and your spouse?		
12. Has your spouse (or other family member) ever gone to anyone for help about your drinking?		
13. Have you ever lost friends or dates because of drinking?		
14. Have you ever gotten into trouble at work because of drinking?		
15. Have you ever lost a job because of drinking?		
16. Have you ever neglected your obligations, your family, or your work for two or more days in a row because you were drinking?		
17. Do you ever have a drink before noon?		
18. Have you ever been told you have liver trouble? Cirrhosis?		
19. Have you ever had delirium tremens (DTs) or severe shaking, heard voices or seen things that weren't there after heavy drinking?		
20. Have you ever gone to anyone for help about your drinking?		
21. Have you ever been in a hospital because of drinking?		
22. Have you ever been in a psychiatric hospital or on a psychiatric ward of a general hospital where drinking was part of the problem?		
23. Have you ever gone to a psychiatric or mental health clinic or to a doctor, social worker, or clergyman for help with an emotional problem in which drinking had played a part?		
24. Have you ever been arrested, even for a few hours, because of drunk behavior?		
25. Have you ever been arrested for drunk driving or driving after drinking?		

(continued)

4.44

*Unit 4
Caffeine, Tobacco,
and Alcohol:
Common Mood-
Altering Drugs*

SELF DISCOVERY 12.2
(continued)

Scoring

Give yourself points for your answers as follows:

Question	Yes	No		Question	Yes	No
1	0	2		14	2	0
2	2	0		15	2	0
3	1	0		16	2	0
4	0	2		17	1	0
5	1	0		18	2	0
6	0	2		19	2	0
7	0	0		20	5	0
8	0	2		21	5	0
9	5	0		22	2	0
10	1	0		23	2	0
11	2	0		24	2	0
12	2	0		25	2	0
13	2	0				

Interpretation

0–3	You are most likely a nonalcoholic.
4	You may be an alcoholic.
5 or more	You almost definitely are an alcoholic.

Source: Michigan Alcoholism Screen Test, adapted from Selzer, M. L. (1971). The M-A-S-T. *American Journal of Psychiatry, 127,* 1653. Copyright 1971, the American Psychiatric Association. Reprinted by permission.

Skill box at the end of this chapter), it has been accepted by the American Medical Association since 1957 as well as by 88% of the American public, according to a 1988 Gallup poll.[236,237]

The Causes of Alcoholism No one knows exactly what causes alcoholism. The ASAM-NCADD definition above notes that it has "genetic, psychosocial, and environmental factors influencing its development and manifestations." These are worth considering.

- *The possible genetic basis:* Over the years, there have been theories—none of them proven—that alcoholism has a biological basis: metabolic, biochemical, glandular, or allergic. Alcoholism may or may not be inherited. In 1990, a study indicated that inheriting a common version of a gene may place people at risk for alcoholism.[238,239]

Later studies suggest that the gene is only one of many genes that may increase an individual's susceptibility to alcoholism.[240]

Family studies also show that offspring of alcoholics are four times more likely to develop the disease themselves compared to people whose parents are not alcoholic. Adopted children of alcohol-dependent biological parents also show more alcohol problems, even when they are raised in homes without alcohol problems.[241] Such studies strengthen the argument for a genetic or biological predisposition to alcohol dependence.

- *The psychosocial basis:* Some researchers have tried to identify an "alcoholic personality" that might predispose people to alcohol dependence. The closest research has found in this respect is an "antisocial personality," which is characterized by "impulsivity, intensity of mood, unstable self-esteem, and alternating dependence on and independence from others."[242] Such traits *might* predispose people to dependence on alcohol and other drugs. By and large, however, the idea of an alcoholic personality is not accepted. Such traits seem to follow, rather than precede, the onset of alcoholism.

- *The environmental basis:* As we mentioned earlier, some cultural groups seem to be more disposed toward alcoholism than others. For instance, there seems to be a reduced likelihood of alcohol abuse in cultures characterized by clear messages regarding how and when to drink as well as those that have significant sanctions against intoxication. (See ● *Figure 12.10.*)

The Stages of Alcoholism The emergence of alcoholism has been described by Vernon Johnson, in *I'll Quit Tomorrow,* as a four-stage process along a pain–euphoria continuum.[243] (See ● *Figure 12.11.*)

- *Learning stage:* Stage 1 is *learning the mood swing,* in which people learn that if they are feeling "normal" and then have a drink, their mood will shift toward euphoria, then swing back to normal when the alcohol wears off.

- *Seeking stage:* Stage 2 is *seeking the mood swing,* when people learn that, when they feel down, alcohol can be counted on to enhance their mood; drinking now has a particular purpose, to make one feel better.

- *Harmful-dependence stage:* Stage 3 is *harmful dependence,* in which people are unwilling to stop using alcohol to alter their moods. They begin to rationalize their reasons for using alcohol and find that when the alcohol wears off it leaves them in a more uncomfortable place than before.

- *Drinking-to-feel-normal stage:* In stage 4, people (who are by now alcoholic) *drink to feel normal;* they no longer drink to achieve euphoria but to escape the weight of the negative feelings oppressing them from the "pain" end of the mood scale.

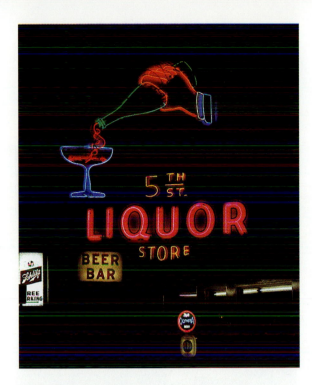

● **Figure 12.9 The diagnosis of alcoholism**

Any person with THREE or more of the following is considered "alcohol dependent":

1. Alcohol is often taken in larger amounts or over a longer period of time than the person intended.

2. There exists a persistent desire or one or more unsuccessful efforts by the individual to cut down on or control his or her alcohol use.

3. A great deal of time is spent in activities necessary to get alcohol, taking the substance, or recovering from its effects.

4. Frequent intoxication or withdrawal symptoms occur when the person is expected to fulfill major role obligations at work, school, or home (such as performing child care when intoxicated, not going to work because of being hung over, going to school intoxicated) or when alcohol use is physcially hazardous (driving drunk, for example).

5. Important social, occupational, or recreational activities are given up or reduced because of alcohol.

6. Continued alcohol use occurs despite a knowledge of having a persistent or recurrent social, psychological, or physical problem that is caused by or exacerbated by the use of the substance.

7. A marked tolerance exists. The person experiences a need for markedly increased amounts of the substance (at least a 50% increase) in order to achieve intoxication or the desired effect, or a markedly diminished effect with continued use of the same amount.

8. Characteristic withdrawal symptoms occur when the person ceases to ingest the substance.

9. Alcohol is often taken to relieve or avoid withdrawal symptoms.

4.46

Unit 4
Caffeine, Tobacco,
and Alcohol:
Common Mood-
Altering Drugs

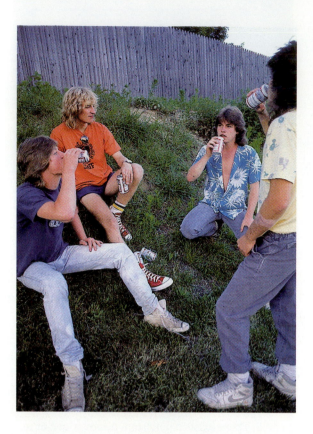

The Recognition of Alcoholism: "Hitting Bottom" How do alcoholics get to the point of recognizing that they *are* alcoholics and accept treatment? Quite often it simply doesn't happen, which is why the death rate from alcohol-related disorders is so high. Moreover, because alcohol problems fall along a continuum that ranges from occasional misuse by social drinkers to continual misuse by the alcohol-dependent, it is easy for denial—the refusal to face reality about one's problems—to persist. Indeed, as the disorder worsens, alcoholics are increasingly impaired in their judgment, losing touch with their emotions and viewing all attempts to interrupt their drinking as meddling.

Recovering alcoholics use the phrase "hitting bottom" to describe the point where they finally realized that they were in the grip of a terrible affliction and must seek treatment. Usually the recognition is brought about by outside events that the alcoholic can no longer ignore. For some alcoholics the moment may come with the departure of a spouse, loss of a job, arrest, hospitalization, or the like. Other alcoholics may develop this realization before their lives have reached this level of destruction.

Among recovering alcoholics are those who have been reached through a process called **intervention.** Vernon Johnson describes intervention as "presenting reality to a person out of touch with it in a receivable way."[244] That is, a team of concerned family members and friends, sometimes accompanied by an alcohol counselor or mental health professional, confronts the sufferer with specific objective facts and observations or descriptions of that person's behavior in a nonjudgmental and caring way. The goal is to compel that person to seek recovery from chemical dependency. The process of intervention must be researched and rehearsed carefully, and the team must assemble a list of local treatment options to share with the alcoholic.

● **Figure 12.10 Cultural practices predictive of alcoholism**

In a review of the medical literature, the following cultural norms and practices have been identified as predictive of alcohol problems:

1. Solitary drinking
2. Overpermissive norms of drinking
3. Lack of specific drinking norms
4. Tolerance of drunkenness
5. Adverse social behavior tolerated when drinking
6. Utilitarian use of alcohol to reduce tension and anxiety
7. Lack of ritualized and/or ceremonial use of alcohol
8. Alcohol use apart from family and social affiliative functions
9. Alcohol use separated from overall eating patterns
10. Lack of child socialization into drinking patterns
11. Drinking with strangers, which increases violence
12. Drinking pursued as a recreational activity
13. Drinking concentrated among young males
14. A cultural milieu that stresses individualism, self-reliance, and high achievement

Stage 1: Learning about the mood swing
One learns that alcohol is a drug and if one is feeling "normal," alcohol will produce euphoria. After the alcohol wears off, one's mood returns to normal.

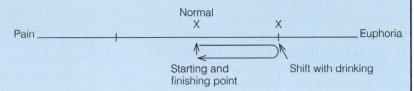

Stage 2: Deliberately seeking the mood swing
One learns to drink to make things better, so that when a person is "feeling a little down," alcohol will help. After drinking, one's mood returns to normal. Most people who experience a hangover or other unpleasantness will learn to avoid alcohol in excess in the future. However, alcohol-dependent persons will not, and will progress to Stage 3.

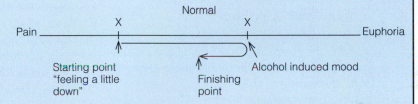

Stage 3: Developing harmful dependence
One becomes unwilling to stop using alcohol to achieve euphoria and begins to rationalize reasons for needing alcohol. When the alcohol wears off, the drinker is left in a more uncomfortable place than before.

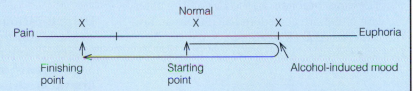

Stage 4: Drinking to feel normal
One drinks not to achieve euphoria but to escape negative feelings, such as withdrawal pangs, and to feel "normal." After a drinking experience, one's mood is at an even lower state than before. By now the drinker is an alcoholic in chronic pain.

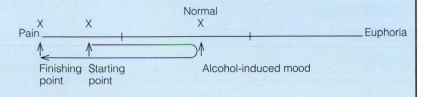

● **Figure 12.11 Four stages in the development of an alcohol-dependent person.** Vernon Johnson has described these four changes in the drinker's relationship to alcohol on a pain–euphoria scale.

4.48

Unit 4
Caffeine, Tobacco,
and Alcohol:
Common Mood-
Altering Drugs

Getting Help for an Alcohol Problem

There are several kinds of treatment available for alcoholism, some of which may be available through employers. There are programs for detoxification, individual rehabilitation, and family rehabilitation. Also available are self-help programs such as Alcoholics Anonymous for the alcoholic and his or her family members.

There seem to be two degrees of alcohol abuse that require attention, according to reports by the Institute of Medicine:[245,246]

- *Mild or moderate alcohol problems:* These are the concern of the 60% of the population that drinks lightly or moderately. Just by the weight of their numbers, these drinkers are responsible for the greater share of personal and societal alcohol-related problems.

- *Substantial or severe alcohol problems:* These are problems of the 10% of the population that are considered alcoholics and require specialized treatment.

Those with mild or moderate alcohol problems, the institute suggests, could be helped by brief treatment such as short-term counseling, discussions with clergy or family, or simply reading self-help materials. They may also benefit from prevention strategies, such as programs that teach students to cope with peer pressure. Those with substantial or severe alcohol problems may be helped with more specialized treatment, as is described below.

Employee Programs With many alcoholics, the job is one of the last things they lose, after the driver's license and after the spouse. Many employers are aware of the work-related problems caused by substance abuse and have found that taking action can increase productivity and decrease job-related accidents significantly. (*See ● Figure 12.12.*) Employers have discovered that, when threatened with firing, alcoholic employees can also be reached and persuaded to attend a treatment program. Many for-profit and nonprofit organizations offer employee alcohol counseling and treatment programs.

Detoxification Programs Alcoholics who suddenly stop drinking develop withdrawal symptoms within 6–24 hours and may require 3–10 days of "drying out." The **alcohol withdrawal syndrome** is a cluster of symptoms that may include tremulousness, seizures, and hallucinations. **Detoxification** consists of hospitalizing alcoholics, preventing them from getting alcohol, and helping them get through any withdrawal symptoms (which can range from the unpleasant to the life-threatening). A minority of alcoholics may have **delirium tremens (DTs)**—trembling, fevers, hallucinations, and delusions.

Individual Rehabilitation Programs Whether or not they require detoxification, alcoholics have several inpatient and outpatient rehabilitation program options available. Inpatient residence programs are located in a hospital or alcohol rehabilitation facilities and provide 2–6 weeks of treatment, including various kinds of counseling and psychotherapies, drug therapy, and alcohol education. Following inpatient treatment, recovering alcoholics are directed toward various kinds of outpatient

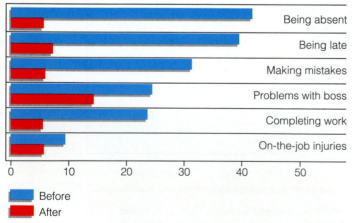

Percent of substance abusers with work-related problems before and after treatment.

Before
After

● **Figure 12.12 Substance abuse and work productivity.** Substance abusers create many problems on the job. Employers who take action can help employees get the help they need.

treatment programs, allowing them to resume their lives while continuing their recovery.

Both inpatient and outpatient rehabilitation programs offer the following kinds of therapies:

- *Individual therapy:* Psychotherapy, or conversation between the patient and a specially trained therapist, is valuable in helping alcoholics understand their feelings, although psychotherapy alone may be insufficient.

- *Group therapy:* Small groups consisting entirely of alcoholics led by a trained therapist are useful because members can reinforce for each other the truth about addiction.

- *Drug therapy:* Used in conjunction with other kinds of therapy, drug therapy principally consists of using the drug disulfiram (trade name: Antabuse), which comes in tablet form and is taken by the alcoholic every day. Disulfiram acts as a deterrent to drinking because when alcohol is consumed it makes one nauseated.

  Other kinds of drug therapy involve the use of tranquilizers to help alcoholics overcome withdrawal symptoms and depression. If alcoholics suffer from malnutrition (as those in advanced stages often do), they may also be treated with vitamin supplements. Preliminary studies have found that a drug called naltrexone can help drinkers quit by lessening the pleasurable effects of alcohol.[247]

  A drug that could significantly decrease the time it takes to lower a person's blood alcohol content is currently under development. The drug could be useful for those who are hospitalized and for life-threatening situations.[248]

- *Behavior therapy:* Behavior therapy, or behavior modification, attempts to change alcoholic behavior so that people will not be as likely to drink. For instance, aversion therapy puts drinkers through a 10-day course of taking drugs that make them vomit after several drinks. According to one study, 35–60% of those with such conditioning were abstinent after a year.[249]

Family Rehabilitation Programs We mentioned that alcoholism is thought of as a "family disease." One writer, Sharon Wegscheider-Cruse, describes the family as similar to a mobile, which is designed to hang in delicate balance. Like a mobile, the family may be disrupted by the winds of alcoholic crises, but the family comes back to rest when the storms subside. Alcoholic families maintain this kind of equilibrium as long as everyone supports the alcoholic's drinking, but when that person begins to recover, the system is stressed and all family members must shift their position.[250]

Sobriety in itself will not transform a family relationship; indeed, sobriety brings a whole new set of problems. Family therapy aims at helping both alcoholics and their families to live together in new ways. In addition to counseling by trained family therapists, there are several self-help organizations dedicated to helping members of alcoholic families deal with their special problems. Perhaps the three most well-known organizations are:

- *Al-Anon:* Al-Anon was founded as an adjunct to Alcoholics Anonymous and now has more than 28,500 groups meeting in 100 countries. Anyone whose life has been affected by an alcoholic may join, particularly family and friends. Like AA, Al-Anon is a nonprofit, nonprofessional fellowship. Recovery consists of attending meetings and following a twelve-step program similar to that in Alcoholics Anonymous. (The Twelve Steps are presented in the Life Skill section at the end of this chapter.) Open meetings feature Al-Anon speakers and may be attended by nonmembers.

- *Alateen:* Alateen was formed for the teenaged children of alcoholics, but now many groups are open to preteens through 20-year-olds. As with Al-Anon and AA, all members are anonymous. At meetings, members focus on themselves, not on the alcoholic in their family, trying to separate themselves from the alcoholic's behavior.

- *Adult Children of Alcoholics:* Some adult children of alcoholics affiliate themselves with Al-Anon groups, which offers close to 1500 adult children meetings. Others join groups of Adult Children of Alcoholics (ACOA), which was founded in 1984 and

4.50

Unit 4
Caffeine, Tobacco,
and Alcohol:
Common Mood-
Altering Drugs

which has more than 1350 meetings in five countries, including the United States and Canada. In both organizations, adult children try to work through their feelings and experiences about living with an alcoholic parent.

Alcoholics Anonymous and Other Self-Help Programs Most alcoholism recovery programs are based on a policy of long-term, usually lifelong abstinence from drinking. However, because alcoholism is characterized by a strong tendency toward relapse, no program can claim to be entirely successful.

The principal self-help programs are these:

- *Alcoholics Anonymous:* The world's oldest alcoholism recovery program, begun in 1935 by two alcoholics, Alcoholics Anonymous (AA) today has almost 2 million members in 63,000 groups in 114 countries. About half of all members are in the United States.[251] AA is a self-help organization, or "fellowship," of men and women whose aim is to help each other maintain sobriety. People who wish to begin to solve their drinking problems can call Alcoholics Anonymous by looking up the number in any phone book. In recent years, more young people have poured into the organization, many of whom are addicted to other drugs as well as alcohol. In some areas, there are special-interest meetings: women only, men only, gays and lesbians, Spanish-speaking, and so on.

  The program consists of the following: trying to remain sober "one day at a time" (because it's easier than trying to think of quitting drinking for life); attending meetings, which take place in nearly every city in the country, where recovering alcoholics share their experiences; enlisting the help of a "sponsor," another member who has been longer in sobriety whom one can call during difficult times; and "working the steps" of the famous Twelve Steps program, the first of which is: "We admitted we were powerless over alcohol—that our lives had become unmanageable."

- *Women for Sobriety/Men for Sobriety:* Established in 1975, Women for Sobriety (WFS) today has 5000 members in 300 chapters throughout the United States. Although nearly a third of AA members are women—half in urban areas—WFS was founded on the premise that women alcoholics have different problems than male alcoholics. The WFS "New Life Program" is based on Thirteen Statements of Acceptance aimed at building self-confidence and self-responsibility. (*See ● Figure 12.13.*) Groups are limited to 6–10 women and are led by a moderator certified by WFS.

  The WFS New Life Program has been adapted for men, Men for Sobriety.

- *Save Our Selves:* Founded in 1986, Save Our Selves, also called *Secular Organizations for Sobriety* (*SOS*), consists of 300 groups in the United States, Canada, Europe, and Asia. SOS was formed to provide a "nonspiritual" alternative, or supplement, to AA for agnostics, atheists, and others who have difficulty with the spirituality of the AA program. Instead of believing in a "higher power," members are encouraged to credit themselves for their sobriety and build their self-esteem through group support.

Many self-help recovery groups are available for alcohol- and drug-dependent professionals. Examples are Lawyers Concerned for Lawyers, Social Workers Helping Social Workers, and International Nurses Anonymous. Additional resources are available for young people, women, gays and lesbians, African Americans, Hispanics, Native Americans, and people of the Asian/Pacific American community.

800-HELP

Alcohol Abuse Emergency. 800-ALCOHOL. Available 24 hours

Alcoholism and Drug Addiction Treatment Center. 800-477-3447. Available 24 hours. Provides phone counseling and local referrals

American Council on Alcoholism. 800-527-5344. Available 24 hours. Provides referrals and treatment information

Drug and Alcohol Abuse (Canada). 800-387-2916

National Institute on Drug Abuse. 800-662-HELP. Drug information and treatment hotline

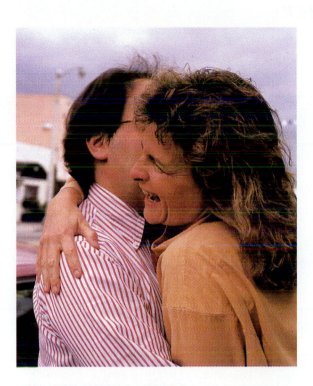

Suggestions for Further Reading

Ackerman, Robert (1986). *Growing in the shadow: Children of alcoholics.* Pompano Beach, FL: Health Communications. Addresses children of alcoholics from childhood to adulthood.

Cermak, Timmen (1985). *A primer on adult children of alcoholics.* Pompano Beach, FL: Health Communications. Identifies issues and steps to recovery for adults who have grown up in alcoholic families.

Johnson, Vernon E. (1980). *I'll quit tomorrow: A practical guide to alcoholism treatment.* New York: Harper & Row.

Kasl, Charlotte Davis (1992). *Many roads, one journey: Moving beyond the Twelve Steps.* New York: HarperCollins. An addiction expert offers a new look at addiction and codependency that goes beyond Twelve Step programs.

● **Figure 12.13 Thirteen statements of acceptance.** These statements constitute the "New Life" program of Women for Sobriety, which has also been adapted for Men for Sobriety.

1. I have a drinking problem that once had me.
2. Negative emotions destroy only myself.
3. Happiness is a habit I will develop.
4. Problems bother me only to the degree I permit them to.
5. I am what I think.
6. Love can be ordinary or it can be great.
7. Love can change the course of my world.
8. The fundamental object of life is emotional and spiritual growth.
9. The past is gone forever.
10. All love given returns twofold.
11. Enthusiasm is my daily exercise.
12. I am a competent woman and have much to give life.
13. I am responsible for myself and my actions.

Addiction and Recovery: Are Twelve Steps and a "Higher Power" Necessary?

Which of the following describes how you feel about alcoholism?

Alcoholism is a . . .

___ **1.** Disease or illness

___ **2.** Mental or psychological problem

___ **3.** Problem caused by a lack of will power

___ **4.** Moral weakness

In a 1988 Gallup poll, 88% of Americans agreed with the statement that "Alcoholism is a disease" (78% agreed "strongly," 10% agreed "somewhat"). However, they split markedly over what precise definition applies to the condition: 60% thought it a disease or illness; 31% a mental problem; 23% a lack of will power; 16% a moral weakness; and 6% had no opinion.[252]

The differences of opinion—some people chose more than one answer, so the total is more than 100%—reflect the confusion about what alcoholism is, its causes, and its treatment. The disease concept of alcoholism is currently most accepted and used as a basis of treatment. The definition of alcoholism as a disease has not only been accepted by the American Medical Association since 1957 but also lies at the basis of the principal alcoholism self-help recovery program, that pioneered by Alcoholics Anonymous. AA's principal program of recovery is the famous Twelve Steps, five of which make reference to God or a "higher power." (*See* ● *figure on next page.*) The Twelve Steps have been adopted as a program by many other self-help organizations trying to help people in the grip of other addictions and problems. (*See* ● *table on page 4.54.*)

The Difficulty of Changing Addiction

Few would deny that alcoholism is an addiction. "Addiction is an ingrained habit that undermines your health, your work, your relationships, your self-respect, but that you feel you cannot change," write drug and alcohol experts Stanton Peele and Archie Brodsky.[253] And addictions are difficult to change, they point out, because you have relied on them for years "as ways of getting through life, of gaining satisfaction, of spending time, and even of defining who you are."

What is the best way to change the addiction of alcoholism? The one course of treatment on which the majority of alcoholism counselors are likely to agree is that of complete abstinence: give up drinking entirely. However, treatment programs face several difficulties:

- *The relapse rate is high.* The attrition, or relapse, rate is extremely high in all forms of treatment—probably over 50%, perhaps as high as 90% in some programs.[254,255] Evaluating treatment programs is difficult: No one knows what happens to alcoholics who drop out. Self-reports by drinkers about their habits are notoriously unreliable. Short-term follow-up studies may not be accurate because people who quit drinking may resume later, and those who resume drinking may quit again later.

- *No one treatment program works better than others.* One official of the National Institute on Alcohol Abuse and Alcoholism (NIAAA) says that the goal has been to find a "magic bullet" that will work with all or most alcoholics, based on a unitary concept of alcoholism as a disease.[256] Yet the course of the disorder is by no means uniform or predictable and no one treatment program seems to be more successful than others. For instance, full-time inpatient treatment centers for alcoholism may be up to 21 times more expensive than part-time outpatient programs, yet they have been found to be no more effective in enabling alcoholics to maintain abstinence.[257]

- *Some problem drinkers may be able to resume controlled drinking.* It is the wish of probably every drinker whose life has been damaged by alcohol to moderate his or her consumption. Is this possible? In an 8-year follow-up of 140 problem drinkers who had been taught self-control drinking strategies, alcoholism researcher William Miller found that of the 99 who could be traced, 14 were controlling their drinking. (Of the rest, 23 were abstinent, another 22 were improved but still had some alcohol problems, and 5 were deceased; the remaining 35 were doing poorly.) Miller says that of 28 studies of controlled drinking treatment of milder alcoholics, findings from 23 show similar favorable results.[258]

Because of the fear that this notion will give recovering alcoholics an excuse to relapse, there has been limited research on controlled drinking. Yet in Europe, points out Miller, controlled drinking is widely accepted. "They consider our black-or-white, abstinence-or-abuse attitude too rigid," he says. In general, however, it seems that only persons suffering from milder alcoholism—and persons without a family history of the disorder—have the best chance of success at controlled drinking.

The Twelve Steps and the Role of Spirituality

Controlled drinking does not seem to be much of an option for alcoholics whose disorder is so advanced that they have sought treatment at a medical facility. Of 1200 such subjects studied by medical researcher John Helzer, only 13 were able to drink without problems.[259] What, then, is required to relieve the addiction of those more severely afflicted?

Alcoholics Anonymous insists that alcoholics must make fundamental changes in their attitudes and relationships, as outlined in AA's Twelve Steps. The Twelve Step program was originally adapted from a Christian conversion process by former stockbroker Bill Wilson, an advanced alcoholic who founded AA in 1935. In essence, the program seems to come down to

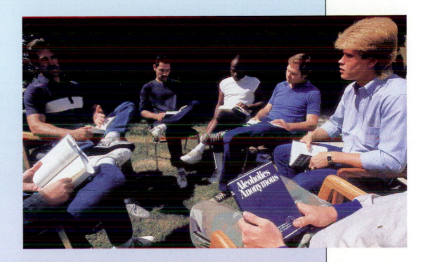

● **The Twelve Steps of Alcoholics Anonymous**

" 1. We admitted we were powerless over alcohol—that our lives had become unmanageable.
2. We came to believe that a Power greater than ourselves could restore us to sanity.
3. We made a decision to turn our will and our lives over to the care of God, as we understand God.
4. We made a searching and fearless moral inventory of ourselves.
5. We admitted to God, to ourselves, and to another human being the exact nature of our wrongs.
6. We were entirely ready to have God remove all these defects of character.
7. We humbly asked God to remove our shortcomings.
8. We made a list of all persons we had harmed and became willing to make amends to them all.
9. We made direct amends to such people wherever possible, except when to do so would injure them or others.
10. We continued to take personal inventory, and when we were wrong, we promptly admitted it.
11. We sought through prayer and meditation to improve our conscious contact with God, as we understand God, praying only for knowledge of God's will for us and the power to carry that out.
12. Having had a spiritual awakening as the result of these steps, we tried to carry this message to alcoholics and to practice these principles in all our affairs. "

—*Alcoholics Anonymous* (Third Edition) (1976). New York: Alcoholics Anonymous World Services, Inc., pp. 59–60.

this: Admit you have no control over alcohol and can't go it alone. Do a "fearless and searching" inventory of your faults. Make amends to the people you have hurt. Reach out to help other alcoholics.

The part of the Twelve Steps that some people find controversial, however, is the notion of spirituality. Alcoholism is "generally defined as a disease of the body, mind, and spirit," as one alcoholic put it.[260] Several steps suggest that the alcoholic accept help from a "higher power," defined however one wishes—God need not be the Christian God or the deity of any organized religion. Some people derive comfort from using prayer to ask for God's help.

Others are repelled by what they perceive to be the religious emphasis of Twelve Step meetings (including most meetings' closing collective recitation of the Lord's Prayer) and by the notion of renouncing self-reliance and surrendering oneself to a higher power. Still others who are secularly inclined choose to define their "higher power" as the association with other recovering alcoholics. Finally, some invoke a piece of AA advice—"Take what you like, and leave the rest"—ignoring religious/spiritual matters and going for the group support.

In their book *The Truth About Addiction and Recovery,* Peele and Brodsky suggest that for some people Twelve Step programs do more harm than good. Even when the group refrains from emphasizing a higher power, they say, it is wrong to force people into conversion experiences where they must adopt a new self-concept, that of addict.[261] In being told that they have no power over themselves and must give up their own outlook in favor of group policy, individuals may have their self-confidence undermined and find themselves obliged to attend meetings where members focus on their own and each others' weaknesses.

On the other hand, we have defined *spirituality* as one dimension of health. For many people, it is difficult to know what spirituality is, although it is promoted by organized religions. Alcoholism and drug use may be epidemic because, in the opinion of one writer, our culture "offers so few sustainable, non-drug opportunities for interconnection, self-expression, and spiritual meaning."[262] Twelve Step meetings may at least offer people the opportunity to begin to explore the meaning of spirituality for themselves.

Handling Relapses

A problem that all recovery programs must—or should—address is that of relapses, when an addict "slips" (to use the AA term) and resumes drinking. Roughly 60% of alcoholics relapse within three months of treatment.[263] However, according to relapse-prevention experts Alan Marlatt and Judith Gordon, who have interviewed many ex-addicts, relapse is not generated by physical cravings, even in substance

● **Self-help organizations using AA's Twelve Step program**

Adult Children of Alcoholics
Al-Anon
Alateen
Anorexics/Bulimics Anonymous
Cocaine Anonymous
Co-Dependents Anonymous
Codependents of Sex Addicts
Codependents Anonymous for Helping Professionals
Families Anonymous (for families of drug addicts)
Gam-Anon (for families of compulsive gamblers)
Gam-A-Teen (for teenagers of compulsive gamblers)
Gamblers Anonymous
Incest Survivors Anonymous
Marijuana Addicts Anonymous
Marijuana Anonymous
Nar-Anon (for people involved with drug addicts)
Narcotics Anonymous
O-Anon (for people involved with compulsive overeaters)
Overeaters Anonymous
S-Anon (for people involved with sex addicts)
Sex and Love Addicts Anonymous
Smokers Anonymous
Workaholics Anonymous

addictions such as cigarettes and alcohol. Rather, it is in response to negative emotions: stress, fear, anxiety, frustration, anger, depression.[264]

Psychologist Emil Chiauzzi, who trains professionals in relapse-prevention techniques, says his research suggests that most people relapse because of a combination of biological, psychological, and social "weak spots" that lead to destructive patterns of thought and behavior. The four major trouble spots that cause people to resume their addictions are as follows:[265]

- *Troublesome personality traits:* Compulsiveness, dependency, passive-aggressiveness, narcissism, and antisocial traits frequently interfere with recovery. Compulsiveness causes people to be perfectionistic and inexpressive, making it difficult for patients to admit the powerful role of addiction in their lives. Dependency makes people want to lean on others and on drugs. Passive-aggressive people shift blame to others. Narcissists find it hard to accept constructive criticism. Antisocial people resist societal norms and obligations.

- *Substitute addictions:* Sometimes people will take up a "replacement addiction"—workaholism, addictive relationships, compulsive spending, eating disorders, caffeine abuse—that, Chiauzzi says, signals a step back toward alcohol or drug dependency. The substitute addiction leads to a false, temporary sense of security and when that wears off, the momentum toward relapse may build until it becomes inevitable.

- *Narrow view of recovery:* Many relapsers take a limited view of their recovery. Some, for example, may equate recovery with abstinence or AA attendance alone. Although avoiding alcohol is clearly important, Chiauzzi says, people engaged in successful recovery are also aware of the importance of self-understanding and such necessary components of healing as positive feelings, coping skills, and personal growth.

- *Failure to see warning signals:* Addicts may also relapse because they overlook the danger signs of negative emotions, such as irritability, depression, uncertainty; poor

physical functioning, such as headaches, fatigue, or insomnia; or loss of structure in their daily routine. Unable to handle such negative reactions, they turn to their previous "problem-solving" method—drinking.

Alcohol- and other drug-dependent people should realize that the first attempt to quit is not necessarily the last. As Peele and Brodsky point out, "relapse is a common experience on the road to a stable nonaddict identity."[266] Relapse, they say, should not be interpreted as meaning one has totally lost control (otherwise it becomes a self-fulfilling prophecy, and one likely *will* lose control); rather, it should be viewed as "just one moment in a seesaw process."

Marlatt and Gordon have recommended a relapse-prevention strategy consisting of the following steps:[267]

1. *Stop, look, and listen.* Stop the rush of events or behavior and pay attention to your situation. If possible, retreat to a quiet place to contemplate what you are doing.

2. *Keep calm.* It doesn't pay to become guilty or to chastise yourself, since these reactions only prompt more addictive behavior. Nor will panic help you get back on track.

3. *Renew your commitment.* Instead of giving up on your plan to stay nonaddicted, now is the time to reassert your desire and your commitment to be free of the addiction. Remind yourself of your success up to this point.

4. *Make an immediate plan.* You had a plan for licking your addiction from which you temporarily departed. Start right now to map out how you will proceed from here on with your plan.

5. *Ask or look for help.* Look for support from whomever you count on. Now is the time to turn to friends and helpers. In doing so, you will let them know that you are serious and that you don't want to let them down.

6. *Review the relapse situation.* After a relapse, instead of punishing yourself, analyze the elements in the situation that created your slip. There is much to learn from a relapse, and what you learn may help you immeasurably in your recovery process.

Drug and Other Dependencies: Lifestyles and Gratifications

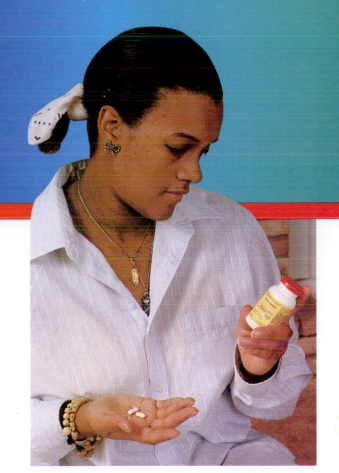

Are drugs an inevitable part of life?

People have been using and abusing substances for a long time. The European explorations of the world have in great part been driven by the search for profits from drugs—tea, tobacco, rum. We no longer hear the terms *Indian hemp* and *coca*, popular drugs in the mid-1800s, but that's only because they are better known today as *marijuana* and *cocaine*.

Society's drugs of choice seem to come in cycles. In the view of the late Harvard psychiatrist Norman Zinberg, for instance, the United States has recently gone through four major waves of drug use, beginning with LSD in the early 1960s, marijuana in the mid- to late-'60s, heroin from 1969 to 1971, and cocaine in the late '70s and '80s.[1] In addition, choices about drug use vary from region to region. Some drugs of choice are frequently found within a particular social class structure, and some drugs will piggyback on others, as cocaine and alcohol became associated or amphetamines and heroin were linked to each other.[2]

Whatever their patterns, it seems that drugs have always been with us. "History teaches that it is vain to hope that drugs will ever disappear and that any effort to eliminate them from society is doomed to failure," write physician and addiction researcher Andrew Weil and his co-author.[3] The same might be said of other addictive habits, such as addiction to gambling, eating, sex, spending, and other compulsions. If indeed such strong areas of addiction are here to stay, the best defense is an understanding of how they work—and how you are affected. In this unit, then, we describe two principal areas of dependence—those of *substances*, such as drugs, and those of *processes*, such as gambling or spending.

5.2

*Unit 5
Drug and Other
Dependencies:
Lifestyles and
Gratifications*

13 Drugs and Dependence

▶ What is the magnitude of the "drug problem" and who is using drugs now?

▶ What are the factors in drug use that determine their effect?

▶ Describe the differences among the main types of mood-altering drugs: stimulants, depressants, cannabis, hallucinogens, opiates, and designer drugs.

▶ What are some treatment programs for overcoming drug dependency?

What are the two following descriptions about?

Experience #1: "Time no longer seems to pass the way it ordinarily does," writes a psychologist about the experience. "The objective, external duration we measure with reference to outside events like night and day, or the orderly progression of clocks, is rendered irrelevant by the rhythms dictated by the activity. Often hours seem to pass by in minutes. . . ."[4]

Experience #2: "Your mind starts to race," writes another psychologist about a different experience. ". . . You're able to capture images and ideas one after the other with a clarity that you've never known before. . . . You find yourself coming up with solutions to problems that have been bugging you for as long as you can remember. Or at least this is the way things seem. . . ."[5]

We hope that you have from time to time had the first experience. This is part of what psychologist Mihaly Csikszentmihalyi calls *flow*. Flow, he says, is "the state in which people are so involved in an activity that nothing else seems to matter; the experience itself is so enjoyable that people will do it even at great cost, for the sheer sake of doing it."[6] Examples he gives are climbers focusing their attention on the irregularities of the rock wall, solitary sailors feeling the boat as an extension of themselves, and violinists wrapped in the stream of sound they help to create. Flow is the *optimal experience* that we can achieve—and it is an experience we can *make* happen.

The second experience, described by psychologist and drug researcher John Flynn, is one person's experience after using cocaine. The drug operates directly on the brain's pleasure centers, and the feelings of intense pleasure that result explain why cocaine is so highly addictive. This is precisely the reason, Flynn states, why cocaine is "the most destructive drug of abuse in human history."[7]

Knowing the difference between the life-*enhancing* possibilities of one experience and the life-*threatening* possibilities of the other has a profound bearing on one's future. The first allows you to attain some of the most meaningful moments humans are capable of realizing. The second can lead to the deepest kind of despair.

The Status of Drug Use Today

Use of illicit drugs—controlled substances—has declined significantly among many groups. The assertion that some "psychologically healthy" young people experiment with drugs is suspect.

It is estimated that Americans spend $110 billion a year to buy cocaine, marijuana, heroin, and other illegal drugs. More than a third of Americans—74 million people—ages 12 and over have used an illicit drug at least once.[8] If to this are added the number of users of legal drugs—alcohol, cigarettes, caffeine, and tranquilizers—it seems that most people have at one time or another tried to find chemical ways to transcend ordinary consciousness and stresses. The largest group of users is ages 18–25. (See ● *Table 13.1.*)

The Decline in Drug Use Concern about drug use is pervasive. By now the amount of antidrug information that has poured from educators, the mass media, politicians, and other sources cannot have escaped the attention of very many people. And the evidence is that in many ways the message has gotten through:

● **Table 13 .1 Who uses drugs?** The largest proportion of people who have used or are presently using drugs is in the 18–25 age group.

	Percent age 12–17		Percent age 18–25		Percent age 26 & up	
Drug Type	Ever Used	Now Use	Ever Used	Now Use	Ever Used	Now Use
Alcohol	55.9	31.5	92.8	71.5	89.3	60.7
Cigarettes	45.3	15.6	76.0	37.2	80.5	32.8
Cocaine	5.2	1.8	25.2	7.7	9.5	2.1
Hallucinogens	3.2	1.1	11.5	1.6	6.2	***
Heroin	***	***	1.2	***	1.1	***
Inhalants	9.1	3.6	12.8	1.0	5.0	.6
Marijuana	23.7	12.3	60.5	21.9	27.2	6.2
Sedatives	4.0	1.1	11.0	1.7	5.2	.7
Stimulants	5.5	1.8	17.3	4.0	7.9	.7
Tranquilizers	4.8	.6	12.2	1.7	7.1	1.0

*** Less than 0.5 percent

Source: National Institute on Drug Abuse. *National household survey on drug abuse: Main findings 1988.* DHHS Pub. No. (ADM) 90-1682. Washington, DC: U.S. Department of Health and Human Services.

- *More awareness of drugs as a problem among young people:* According to one Gallup Organization poll, 58% of people ages 16–24 said they thought the biggest problem facing the youth of today was drugs. No other issue was named as the biggest problem by more than 5% of those interviewed.[9] Among parents and teachers surveyed in 1991 in another Gallup poll, fewer mentioned drug use as a problem in the public schools than in previous years (from a high point of 38% in 1990 to 22% in 1991).[10] A 1988 study of U.S. public high-school administrators also found decreasing alcohol and drug use problems among students during the 1980s.[11]

- *Less drug use among high-school seniors:* For the first time since 1975, fewer than half (47.9%) of American high-school seniors say they have tried an illegal drug, down from 64% in the early 1980s.[12]

- *Less college student drug use:* In a study of college seniors conducted in 1989, students reported strikingly lower frequencies of virtually all kinds of drug use than in 1969 and 1978.[13] (*See* ● *Figure 13.1.*)

- *Less drug use among workers:* The number of workers and job applicants among American transportation workers who have been tested for drug use and found positive has declined from 18.1% to 13.8% in 4 years. The federal government requires such testing of airline and railroad employees, bus drivers, and others in the transportation industry.[14]

With such good news about the decline in drug use, what is there to worry about? Perhaps the next few paragraphs will help explain why drugs are such a complicated issue.

Is There a Well-Adjusted Drug User? Researchers Jonathan Shedler and Jack Block created a real uproar when in 1990 they released a 15-year study that showed that teenagers who had experimented casually with drugs appeared to be better adjusted than adolescents who either abstained or regularly abused drugs.[15,16] The teenagers the researchers labeled "experimenters" used no drug more than once a month, and no more than one drug other than marijuana. The frequent users used marijuana regularly, at least once a week, and had tried

5.4

*Unit 5
Drug and Other
Dependencies:
Lifestyles and
Gratifications*

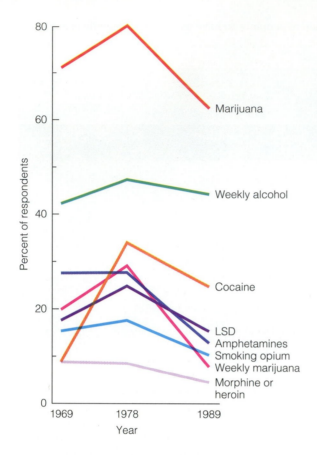

● **Figure 13.1 Decline in college drug use.**
Groups of college seniors reporting use of
various drugs in 1969, 1978, and 1989. All
rates represent the percentage of students
who had ever used a given drug in their lifetime, except for the categories of weekly
marijuana and weekly alcohol, which represent the percent of students reporting
current weekly use of these substances.
Cocaine, morphine, and heroin were combined as one category in 1969; therefore,
rates for these drugs cannot be computed
separately. The significance of the difference in rates of morphine and heroin use in
1989 versus 1969 also cannot be calculated.

several stronger drugs such as cocaine. The frequent users showed evidence early in life of
psychological maladjustments, emotional mood
swings, inattentiveness, stubbornness, insecurity, and other signs of emotional distress.
Shedler and Block insisted that their research
absolutely did not mean that they were advocat-
ing drug experimentation or that using drugs
could possibly be beneficial. Nevertheless, many
drug counselors were horrified. One questioned
the validity of the conclusions, pointing out that
the study was somewhat dated because the 101
boys and girls surveyed went through their developing years before the explosion of crack, a
cheap and highly addictive form of cocaine.[17]

Perhaps three conclusions may be drawn:

- *Drug experimenters are not necessarily
  healthier:* Young people who experiment
  with drugs aren't necessarily psychologically healthier. Rather, the healthiest people
  can survive the drug-experimentation years
  and are flexible enough to right themselves
  if they do experiment.

- *Drug experimentation CAN lead to addiction:* Unfortunately, some beginning
  users are unable to be "casual experimenters." For reasons not clearly known,
  though heredity and environmental factors
  play a role, some people become dependent
  on the chemicals they use. No one knows
  beforehand that dependency is *not* a risk
  for them. After all, how do you *know* you're
  "psychologically healthy" when you begin
  using potentially addictive drugs? Many
  people who start out exploring life by experimenting with "gateway drugs" such as
  alcohol and marijuana get caught in the
  trap of addiction. Finally, even "psychological health" may not be enough: some people
  are vulnerable to chemical dependency owing to biological, cultural, and other factors.

- *Drug experimentation is unnecessary:* It
  is not necessary to explore drugs in order
  to explore life or to combat stress. Techniques for achieving the "optimal experience" and for escaping tension are available
  without drugs.

Types of Drugs

Drugs are chemical substances that alter an organism's function or structure. Psychoactive drugs are those that alter thinking, mood, and/or behavior. Categories of drugs are prescription drugs, over-the-counter drugs, and drugs both legal and illegal available for nonhealth purposes.

What, exactly, *is* a drug? Consider this definition: **Drugs** are chemical substances other than those required for the maintenance of normal health, such as food. The administration of these chemical substances alters a living organism's function or structure.[18] The terms "medication" and "drug" are often used interchangeably. **Medications** (or **medicines**) are drugs used for the purpose of diagnosing, preventing, or treating disease, or to help in the care of an individual during illness, such as drugs used to relieve pain.[19]

Clearly, the basic definition of a drug includes medication such as prescription drugs and nonprescription drugs, as well as illegal drugs, cigarettes, alcohol, food additives, and industrial chemicals and can, in fact, even include food. All drugs are risky for some people under some circumstances at some dosage levels. Some drugs are more hazardous than others. Importantly, some individuals are more susceptible to the effects of some drugs than they are to others.[20]

Drugs may be classified in a variety of ways, including their origin, their effects, and their chemical structure. In this chapter, however, we are concerned primarily with **psychoactive drugs**—those mind-altering substances that are capable of altering people's moods, thinking, perceptions, and behavior.

Psychoactive and other drugs are obtained in several ways:

- *Prescription drugs:* **Prescription drugs** are substances that require a physician's prescription and are obtained from a pharmacy. Examples are tranquilizers, major pain relievers, and antibiotics. Some of these drugs are considered psychoactive because they are mind-altering.

- *Over-the-counter drugs:* **Over-the-counter drugs,** or **nonprescription drugs,** are substances that can be legally obtained without a prescription and are available in pharmacies, supermarkets, and convenience stores. Examples are aspirin, sunscreens, laxatives, and some cold remedies.

- *Legal psychoactive drugs for nonhealth purposes:* These are drugs that are marketed to people for no other reason than supposedly to help them have fun or be more alert or relaxed. Some, such as chocolate, tea, and coffee, are available in stores even to minors. Some, such as tobacco and alcohol, are legally available only through licensed sellers to those over age 18 or 21 (depending on the state). Though legal, some of these drugs are capable of doing great harm.

- *Illegal psychoactive drugs for nonhealth purposes:* These are the drugs that people think about when they hear about "the drug problem." The government has determined that these drugs are harmful and has declared their cultivation, manufacture, sale, and use illegal. Examples are psychoactive drugs such as marijuana, cocaine, LSD, amphetamines, and heroin.

How Psychoactive Drugs Work Psychoactive drugs work by altering chemicals in the **central nervous system**, which in turn alter one's ability to monitor, interpret, and respond to stimuli. A vast network of specialized cells called **neurons** make up the complex communication system that is our nervous system. When the communication system is unimpaired, messages can be sent and received and the person is able to function in anticipated ways.

Although there are millions of neurons in the brain, they are not directly connected. Messages are transmitted from one neuron to another by means of chemical messengers. The space between any two neurons that these chemical messengers must cross is called a **synapse**. The messengers themselves are called **neurotransmitters**. About 50 different chemicals serve as neurotransmitters, but each neuron is responsive only to one or a few of them. [The neurotransmitters affected by the psychoactive drugs include dopamine, serotonin, endorphins, GABA (y-aminobutyric acid),

5.6

Unit 5
Drug and Other
Dependencies:
Lifestyles and
Gratifications

acetylcholine, and norepinephrine.] Psychoactive drugs modify the transmission of nerve impulses and thus behavior, mood, perception, and thought processes by affecting these neurotransmitters in some way.

The Dynamics of Drug Use: Basic Training

Besides its chemical composition, the effect of a drug depends on many factors, including its site of action, toxicity, tolerance, means of administration, level and kind of personal experience, interactions with other drugs, individual human factors, and setting.

All of us are exposed to a tremendous number of messages from the mass media, family, or friends that invite or entice us to use legal and/or illegal drugs. It is one thing to use a drug, however, and quite another to misuse or abuse it. Consider these distinctions:

- *Drug use:* The Food and Drug Administration, or FDA, the main government regulator of drugs, restricts the term **drug use** to the use of a legal drug for the purposes and in the amounts for which it was intended or prescribed.

- *Drug misuse:* **Drug misuse,** according to the FDA, means a drug is not used in accordance with the purpose or ways it was intended or prescribed—for example, in too great amounts or too frequently. This applies whether the drug is a vitamin, an aspirin, or a tranquilizer.

- *Drug abuse:* **Drug abuse,** or **illicit drug use,** is what the FDA calls the circumstances of a drug being used in violation of legal restrictions or for other nonmedical reasons.

    The American Psychiatric Association defines drug abuse as a maladaptive pattern of psychoactive drug use, as indicated by at least one of the following over a period of at least 1 month: (1) Continued use despite problems associated with use. Such problems may be psychological, physical, occupational, or social. (2) Recurrent use in

situations that are physically hazardous (such as operating machinery, driving a car, or placing oneself in socially risky situations).

The action of a drug on the body is called a **drug effect.** The use of marijuana, for example, increases the heart rate and causes dryness in the mouth. Besides its chemical composition, the effect of a drug depends on several factors:

- Method of administration
- Site of action
- Dosage
- Toxicity
- Tolerance
- Dependence
- Interaction with other drugs
- Individual human factors
- Setting

Method of Administration Drugs can be taken into the body in a variety of ways. The principal methods of administration are:

- *Ingestion:* **Ingestion** is taking a drug by swallowing it. This method is also called *oral administration.*

- *Inhalation:* **Inhalation** is breathing or sniffing a drug into the lungs.

- *Injection:* **Injection** is using a hypodermic needle to insert a drug directly under the skin (*subcutaneously*), into a muscle (*intramuscularly*), or into a blood vessel (*intravenously*).

- *Absorption:* One kind of **absorption** is placing a drug in contact with the skin (*topical* or *dermal*) or mucous membrane lining. Another way is via *suppositories* placed in the vagina or rectum. Some drugs are absorbed after placement under the tongue (*sublingual*) or on the conjunctiva of the eye.

The two fastest routes of administration are by inhalation and injection. (*See Figure 13.2.*) The best or most effective method of administration depends on the specific drug. Some drugs, for example, are inactivated when swallowed; others cannot be injected. Some drugs can be effectively administered by several routes. Marijuana, for example, can be adminis-

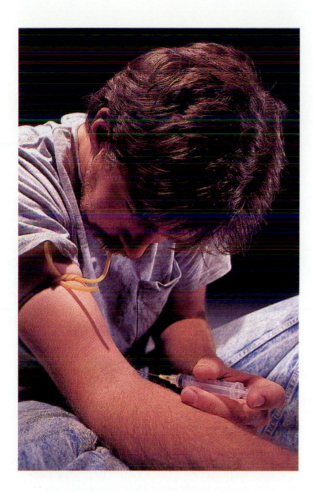

tered by inhalation and ingestion. Cocaine can be administered by injection, absorption, or inhalation.

Site of Action Once inside the body, a drug can affect the body to various extents:

- *Locally:* A drug can act **locally,** as when the dentist uses novocaine to deaden pain in one part of your mouth but not others.

- *Generally or systemically:* A drug can act **generally**—also called **systemically**—as when a patient is rendered unconscious with an anesthetic prior to surgery.

- *Selectively:* A drug can act **selectively,** as when it affects one organ or body system more than others, as in drugs used to control the speed of a person's heartbeat.

The main site of action for psychoactive drugs is the nervous system: the brain, spinal cord, and the peripheral nervous system.

Some drugs act **cumulatively.** That is, they accumulate when they are taken in faster than the body can process and excrete them. Alcohol is one such drug: the faster you drink, the more it accumulates in your body.

Dosage The **dosage** or amount of a drug dictates its effects. Some drugs have multiple effects, depending on dosage.

Toxicity The level at which a drug causes temporary or permanent damage to the body is referred to as **toxicity.** The damage may be minor, such as the wakefulness caused by certain cold tablets. Or it may be major, as in some of the effects on the liver from alcohol. The toxicity of a drug is influenced by several factors, including the amount of the drug used and how the drug is taken.

Tolerance The word **tolerance** refers to the diminished effect of a drug as a person continues its use. Tolerance occurs as a result of different mechanisms:

- *Dispositional tolerance:* **Dispositional tolerance** means that the user's metabolism rate for a drug—the body's ability to break down and get rid of the drug—increases. Thus, greater quantities of the drug are required to maintain a given level of the substance within the body.

● **Figure 13.2 How fast drugs work**

"*Cleopatra may have been one of the first to realize that a drug taken orally is slower to act than one that is injected through the skin.*

The relatively slow onset of an orally administered drug is partially because the medicine must first travel into the stomach and then usually pass through the lining of the small intestine before it enters into the circulation. That takes time.

A drug injected under the skin, as Cleopatra's snake demonstrated, has a much faster action simply because it avoids the barriers of the gut wall."

—Kenneth Jon Rose (1988). *The body in time.* New York: Wiley.

5.8

Unit 5
Drug and Other
Dependencies:
Lifestyles and
Gratifications

- *Functional tolerance:* **Functional tolerance** means that the user's brain and central nervous system become less sensitive to a drug's effect. Over time, for instance, some people may find they have to drink a six-pack of beer in order to achieve the effects they formerly achieved with three cans of beer.

- *Cross tolerance:* **Cross tolerance** (or **cross addiction**) means a tolerance for one drug results in tolerance to other drugs within that category. For example, a tolerance to alcohol also results in tolerance to tranquilizers. Both alcohol and tranquilizers belong to the drug category of depressants.

Chemical Dependency Dependence on a drug refers to reliance on or need for a chemical substance. Drug or chemical dependence is sometimes called *addiction.* It is characterized by a drive to use a drug in order to experience the psychoactive effects and, in some cases, to avoid symptoms associated with withdrawal.

The dependence may be physical, psychological, or both:

- *Physical dependence:* **Physical dependence** is characterized by (1) increased tolerance that requires increasing doses of the drug in order to achieve the same effect, and (2) withdrawal symptoms if the drug is discontinued.[21]

- *Psychological dependence:* **Psychological dependence** refers to a craving for a drug and a compulsive drive to use it. The focus of activity by the person is on obtaining and using the drug. With psychological dependence, the person experiences no withdrawal symptoms when drug use ceases.

Psychoactive drugs such as tranquilizers, cocaine, or heroin can produce physical dependence—that is, addiction. Marijuana may create psychological dependence but does not seem to lead to physical dependence.

Interaction with Other Drugs There is a reason why so many prescription drugs carry a warning not to use them in conjunction with other drugs, including alcohol. When mixed together, drugs that are safe individually can become harmful.

There are four possible ways drugs can interact with each other:

- *Additive:* In an **additive interaction,** the effect is the same as the sum of the effects of the drugs used.

- *Synergistic:* In a **synergistic interaction,** the effect of two drugs together is *greater* than the effect of each drug used alone. For instance, the combination of alcohol and barbiturates has *four times* the depressant effect of either used alone.

- *Potentiating:* In a **potentiating interaction,** one drug can increase the effect of another. For example, a drug called probenecid is given with penicillin to enhance the effects of the penicillin.

- *Antagonistic:* In an **antagonistic interaction,** one drug neutralizes the effects of another. The drug naloxone, for instance, will neutralize the effects of the heroin.

Who You Are: Individual Human Factors
There are, to be sure, physical and biological differences that determine how a drug will affect you. Among them:

- *Weight:* A person who weighs 100 pounds may experience greater effects from a certain amount of a drug than someone who weighs 200 pounds.

- *Gender:* For some drugs, the dosage given to a woman produces greater effects than it does when administered to a man. This is because women generally have a higher percentage of body fat, which results in a drug being active in their bodies longer.[22]

- *Age:* The very young and very old are more sensitive to drugs. Children are more sensitive because the enzyme systems that metabolize drugs may not be fully developed, whereas an older person's system may be impaired.

- *Inherited characteristics:* Inherited differences may explain why some people are more apt to become dependent on drugs than others. This question has been particularly investigated with reference to alcoholism.

- *General physical health:* A drug may affect you more intensely when you're weakened by flu or some other health problem.

- *Emotional disposition:* One's mood influences the effects of a drug. If you already feel depressed, for instance, a depressant such as alcohol may make you feel worse.
- *Expectation:* **Drug expectancy**—what one expects to occur when using a drug—is an important factor in drug use, whether it derives from personal experience or exposure to friends' experiences, advertising, or other factors.

Setting In terms of drug effects, not only is your inner state of mind (called your *mindset*) important, so are the external influences. The **setting,** the immediate environment in which you take drugs, can profoundly alter the results. This includes the physical environment, such as the size of the room; the attributes of the setting, such as music, lighting, temperature, furnishings, or cost of drinks; and companions present in the setting.[23]

The Classes of Psychoactive Drugs Psychoactive drugs—both legal and illegal—are classified according to the primary effects they produce:

- *Stimulants*—for example, caffeine and nicotine (mild stimulants); amphetamines and cocaine (major stimulants)
- *Depressants*—for example, alcohol and sedative-hypnotics
- *Cannabis*—marijuana and hashish
- *Hallucinogens*—LSD, mescaline, psilocybin, phencyclidine (PCP)
- *Opiates* (narcotics)—opium, morphine, codeine, heroin
- *Inhalants*

The accompanying table summarizes these categories. (See Table ● 13.2)

Stimulants: Drugs That Arouse

Stimulants speed up brain activity, increasing arousal. Mild stimulants include caffeine and nicotine. Major stimulants include amphetamines and cocaine, both highly addictive. Amphetamines in small doses increase attention and counter sleep, but in repeated large doses lead to stimulant psychosis, including hallucinations. Cocaine acts like amphetamines but is shorter-acting and is considered an extremely destructive drug. Types of cocaine are cocaine hydrochloride, freebase, and crack.

Stimulants excite the central nervous system. That is, they speed up brain activity and body processes, thereby increasing excitement and alertness. The stimulating characteristic of these drugs raises people's level of arousal so that they feel "up"—more responsive to the world inside and outside.

Stimulants can be classified into two categories of drugs:

- *Mild stimulants:* **Mild stimulants** are those that are easily available commercially. They include caffeine and nicotine.
- *Major stimulants:* **Major stimulants** are either closely regulated by the government or are illegal. Examples are amphetamines and cocaine.

We described the mild stimulants of caffeine and nicotine (in tobacco) in Chapters 10 and 11. We discuss the major stimulants of amphetamines and cocaine below.

Amphetamines Considered a major central nervous system stimulant, **amphetamines** (street names: "uppers," "speed") are laboratory-made (synthetic) drugs whose effects are impaired judgment, impulsiveness, decreased fatigue, improved concentration, and exaggerated feelings of well-being, self-confidence, and elation. They can be administered by ingestion, injection, or inhalation. The prescription drug is marketed under a variety of names, and their illegal distribution has given rise to several street names:

- *Amphetamine*—brand name Benzedrine, street name "bennies"
- *Dextroamphetamine*—brand names Dexedrine and Miphetamine, street names "dexies," "black beauties," "Cadillacs"
- *Methamphetamine*—brand names Methedrine and Desoxyn, street names "meth," "crank"; methamphetamine crystals are called "ice" or "crystal meth"

5.10

Unit 5
Drug and Other
Dependencies:
Lifestyles and
Gratifications

● **Table 13.2 Categories of psychoactive drugs**

Drugs	Often-Prescribed Brand Names	Medical Uses	Dependence Potential Physical/Psychological
Narcotics			
Opium	Dover's Powder, Paregoric	Analgesic, antidiarrheal	High/high
Morphine	Morphine	Analgesic	High/high
Codeine	Codeine	Analgesic, antitussive	Moderate/moderate
Heroin	None	None	High/high
Meperidine (Pethidine)	Demerol, Pethadol	Analgesic	High/high
Methadone	Dolophine, Methadone, Methadose	Analgesic, heroin substitute	High/high
Other narcotics	Dilaudid, Leritine, Numorphan, Percodan	Analgesic antidiarrheal, antitussive	High/high
Depressants			
Chloral hydrate	Noctec, Somos	Hypnotic	Moderate/moderate
Barbiturates	Amytal, Butisol, Nembutal, Phenobarbital, Seconal, Tuinal	Anesthetic, anticonvulsant, sedation, sleep	High/high
Glutethimide	Doriden	Sedation, sleep	High/high
Methaqualone	Optimil, Parest, Quaalude, Somnafac, Sopor	Sedation, sleep	High/high
Tranquilizers	Equanil, Librium, Miltown, Serax, Tranxene, Valium	Anti-anxiety, muscle relaxant, sedation	Moderate/moderate
Other depressants	Clonopin, Dalmane, Dormate, Noludar, Placydil, Valmid	Anti-anxiety, sedation, sleep	Possible/possible
Stimulants			
Cocaine*	Cocaine	Local anesthetic	Possible/high
Amphetamines	Benzedrine, Biphetamine, Desoxyn, Dexedrine	Hyperkinesis, narcolepsy, weight control	Possible/high
Phenmetrazine	Preludin	Weight control	Possible/high
Methylphenidate	Ritalin	Hyperkinesis	Possible/high
Other stimulants	Bacarate, Cylert, Didrex, Ionamin, Plegine, Pondimin, Pre-Sate, Sanorex, Voranil	Weight control	Possible/possible
Hallucinogens			
LSD	None	None	None/unknown
Mescaline	None	None	None/unknown
Psilocybin-psilocyn	None	None	None/unknown
MDA	None	None	None/unknown
PCP†	Sernylan	Veterinary anesthetic	None/unknown
Other hallucinogens	None	None	None/unknown
Cannabis			
Marijuana Hashish Hashish oil	None	Antinausea for cancer patients; experimental for glaucoma	Unknown/moderate

*Designated a narcotic under the Controlled Substances Act.

†Designated a depressant under the Controlled Substances Act.

Source: Drug Enforcement Administration, *Drugs of abuse*

Tolerance	Usual Methods of Administration	Possible Effects	Effects of Overdose	Withdrawal Syndrome
Yes	Oral, smoked			
Yes	Injected, smoked	Euphoria, drowsiness, respiratory depression, constricted pupils, nausea	Slow and shallow breathing, clammy skin, convulsions, coma, possible death	Watery eyes, running nose, yawning, loss of appetite, insomnia, irritability, tremors, panic, chills and sweating, cramps, nausea
Yes	Oral, injected			
Yes	Injected, sniffed			
Yes	Oral, injected			
Yes	Oral, injected			
Yes	Oral, injected			
Probable	Oral	Slurred speech, disorientation, drunken behavior without odor of alcohol	Shallow respiration, cold and clammy skin, dilated pupils, weak and rapid pulse, coma, possible death	Anxiety, tremors, delirium, convulsions, possible death
Yes	Oral, injected			
Yes	Oral			
Yes	Oral			
Yes	Oral			
Yes	Oral			
Yes	Injected, sniffed	Increased alertness, excitation, euphoria, dilated pupils, increased pulse rate and blood pressure, insomnia, loss of appetite	Agitation, increase in body temperature, hallucinations, convulsions, possible death	Apathy, long periods of sleep, irritability, depression, disorientation
Yes	Oral, injected			
Yes	Oral			
Yes	Oral			
Yes	Oral			
Yes	Oral, injected	Illusions and hallucinations (with exception of MDA); poor perception of time and distance	Longer, more intense "trip" episodes, psychosis, possible death	Withdrawal syndrome not reported
Yes	Oral, injected			
Yes	Oral			
Yes	Oral, injected, sniffed			
Yes	Oral, injected, smoked			
Yes	Oral, injected, sniffed			
Yes	Oral, smoked	Euphoria, relaxed inhibitions, increased appetite, disoriented behavior, amotivational syndrome	Fatigue, paranoia, possible psychosis	Insomnia, hyperactivity, and depressed appetite reported in a limited number of individuals

5.12

*Unit 5
Drug and Other
Dependencies:
Lifestyles and
Gratifications*

Related stimulants are methylephenidate (Ritalin), phenmetrazine (Preludin—"bam"), and diethylpropion (Tenuate and Apisate).

Amphetamines have a cocaine-like effect that lasts for several hours after they have been taken orally. Some people have begun taking amphetamines after discovering that in the short run they improve performance by counteracting fatigue and boredom. At one time, they were prescribed medically as appetite suppressants for people wanting to lose weight. The amphetamine-like drug Ritalin has been used to control hyperactive children because, for unknown reasons, it acts to calm them rather than stimulate them. In 1970, the Food and Drug Administration restricted amphetamines to treatment of three problems: narcolepsy, attention-deficit hyperactivity disorder, and short-term weight reduction for patients who are obese.

Amphetamine use may begin as an attempt to control pressures in one's life—for instance, efforts by students straining against exhaustion to meet deadlines or long-haul truck drivers on tight schedules. In small amounts, amphetamines increase attentiveness and counter sleep, although they may also produce increased blood pressure, dizziness, and headaches. In larger amounts—especially when "mainlined" (injected intravenously) rather than taken in pill form—amphetamines can give people a momentary highly pleasurable feeling that is often described as a euphoric "rush." Because the "rush" lasts only a few minutes, the user craves another one, and a series of injections often follows. Because amphetamines not only prevent sleep but also suppress appetite, the user may go for several days without sleep and with little food, repeatedly doing injections until the drug runs out or he or she finally has to "crash" (fall asleep for a long period).

When taken repeatedly, particularly in high doses, amphetamines can produce a **stimulant psychosis,** characterized by paranoid delusions, hallucinations, and disorganized behavior. Repeated use of these drugs leads to rapid tolerance and strong psychological dependence.

Crystal methamphetamine ("ice") can be smoked or injected. When smoked, its effects are felt in less than 10 seconds. Unlike other forms of amphetamine or cocaine, crystal methamphetamine has effects ranging from 8 to 14 hours. Chronic use can result in insomnia, restlessness, irritability, and nervousness. Dangers associated with use include the development of a schizophrenia-like psychosis and severe depression. In addition, overdoses may result in convulsions, coma, and death. Research findings suggest an association between chronic use and depletion of neurochemicals.

In the 1970s, law-enforcement efforts put a substantial dent in the diversion of legally produced amphetamines to illicit street use. This had two principal results: (1) A multitude of home-grown laboratories called *speed labs* sprang up to manufacture the drug illegally. (2) Users unable to find amphetamines discovered another stimulant drug whose effects have had the profoundest results for the nation and even the world: cocaine.

Cocaine Over a decade ago, one could write that cocaine "has emerged as a recreational drug of the upper-middle classes, perhaps partly because it costs a lot and so has been considered a status symbol."[24] Clearly, this is no longer the case. Over the past several years, cocaine (street names: "coke," "snow," "blow"), in different forms, has become widely available to people in all levels of society.

As psychologist John Flynn points out in his book *Cocaine,* this drug is not to be taken lightly:

> *Even among drugs of considerable addiction potential, cocaine stands apart. It is, in its various forms, the most destructive drug in human history. Not heroin, not LSD, not marijuana, not alcohol, not PCP—none of these drugs is as capable as cocaine of grabbing on and not letting go. . . .*
>
> *The reason that cocaine can exert this powerful hold on people is the unique relationship of the drug to the pleasure centers of the brain. Cocaine acts, in effect, as a "key" that opens up these parts of the brain as no other drug can do.*[25]

Unlike other drugs, cocaine is so addictive because it *directly* stimulates the pleasure circuits, or reward centers, in the brain. The brain's reward areas exist for a biological purpose—to make us feel good about food, sex, perhaps even the care of offspring, so that we will do those things that will ensure our survival and the survival of the human species. However, the important thing about direct brain stimulation—as when laboratory rats are stimulated by electricity through electrodes attached directly to the brain—is that it is a great deal more powerful than other rewards. Hungry laboratory rats will ignore food and water and repeatedly self-administer electrical stimulation to the point of physical exhaustion in order to receive the pleasures of brain stimulation. The same is true of people who are addicted to cocaine: they will ignore their other primary needs—food, sleep, sex—in pursuit of the ultimate "feel-good" feeling.

What is so pleasurable about cocaine that it would make people ignore food, sleep, or sex? Flynn says that sexual pleasure "gets very close to the type of experience that cocaine provides to the user of the drug. Sexual pleasure is, of course, one of the most intense of human experiences."[26] Another way that cocaine users describe the experience is as a burst of energy—they feel an astonishing surge in their physical and mental powers, that anything is possible and almost any task can be accomplished. In this respect, the euphoria produced by cocaine resembles amphetamines, although the duration is somewhat shorter, and in fact a cross tolerance exists between cocaine and amphetamines. One difference, however, is that cocaine has local anesthetic effects and indeed has been used in nose and throat surgery.[27] Cocaine can be administered by ingestion, injection, inhalation, and absorption.

Cocaine is extracted from the coca plant (not to be confused with the cacao plant, from which chocolate is derived), which the South American Indians have long used as a stimulant, chewing the leaves to alleviate fatigue. The crude cocaine available in coca leaves, however, has nowhere near the addictive power of the products chemically extracted from them: cocaine hydrochloride, freebase, and crack. (*See* ● *Figure 13.3.*)

- *Cocaine hydrochloride:* **Cocaine hydrochloride,** a white, crystalline powder, is what most people call simply "cocaine." This was the form most used in the 1970s. The two principal means of administering this form of cocaine are inhalation and injection. Users who inhale ("snort") the

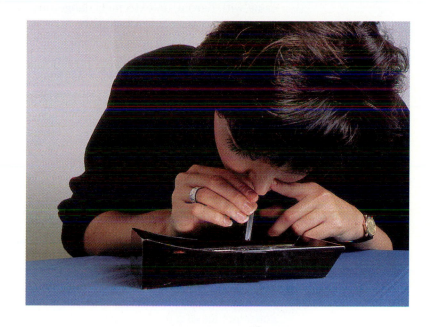

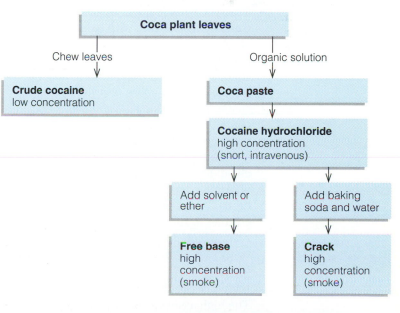

Coca plant leaves	
Chew leaves	Organic solution
Crude cocaine low concentration	**Coca paste**
	Cocaine hydrochloride high concentration (snort, intravenous)
	Add solvent or ether / Add baking soda and water
	Free base high concentration (smoke) / **Crack** high concentration (smoke)

● **Figure 13.3 Forms of cocaine.** Various forms of cocaine obtained from the coca plant, and typical methods of use.

5.14

Unit 5
*Drug and Other
Dependencies:
Lifestyles and
Gratifications*

powder through the nose experience intense effects within 10–15 minutes. Users who inject the drug using a hypodermic syringe and needle (the powdered drug is mixed with water) experience a much quicker effect, beginning within 30 seconds. (Some users combine an injection of cocaine with heroin, an extremely dangerous practice known as "speedballing.")

- *Freebase:* **Freebase cocaine** is obtained chemically from cocaine hydrochloride crystals. An acid (hydrochloric acid) is removed, leaving what chemists call a *base.* Unlike cocaine hydrochloride, freebase cocaine can be smoked, which delivers the drug to the body's system much more quickly than inhalation, producing a much more intense euphoria.

  Note: To "free the base," the cocaine hydrochloride must be treated with solvents, some of them highly flammable, such as ether. If the ether is not completely removed from the powder before one smokes it, it can literally blow up in one's face—as Richard Pryor discovered. The comedian was badly burned in 1980 allegedly as a consequence of a freebase accident.

- *Crack:* **Crack** is made by dissolving cocaine hydrochloride with baking soda or another alkaline solution, producing small, hard lumps, or "rocks," which may be smoked in a pipe. Compared to making freebase, this is a less volatile, less expensive way of producing a smokable, cocaine-containing substance that will nevertheless produce quick and intense euphoria.

  Unfortunately, the appearance of this cheap form of cocaine has made the drug affordable to nearly anyone (including children). When smoked, crack quickly delivers cocaine to the brain, producing a powerful rush, which is followed 10–20 minutes later by a crash—and the beginning of a craving for more crack. Dependency develops rapidly with crack cocaine use.

The high associated with cocaine is fleeting, followed by a severe depression (a "crash"), followed by anxiety, fatigue, shakiness, and withdrawal ("cocaine blues"). The quickest perceived solution to this unhappiness? More cocaine, though the cycle begins again. However,

as one uses cocaine more and more in an attempt to recover the feelings of ecstasy, repeated and higher doses are required. As the use gets heavier, the highs get higher but the valleys get deeper. (*See* • *Figure 13.4.*)

Cocaine is one of the most devastating and destructive drugs known to humankind. As with amphetamines, repeated use at increasingly high doses of cocaine can produce stimulant *psychosis*—paranoid delusions, hallucinations, compulsive rocking, hyperactivity. High dosages can also cause seizures, heart attack, heart muscle damage, hypertension, and stroke. Many people recall the cocaine overdose deaths of University of Maryland basketball star Len Bias, Cleveland Browns pro football star safety Don Rodgers, and comedian ("The Blues Brothers") John Belushi.

Even if cocaine is not lethal, repeated use can produce a host of health problems: headaches, shakiness, nausea, lack of appetite, loss of sexual interest, depression. People who "snort" (inhale through the nose) the substance suffer from a chronically inflamed runny nose, because of the irritation to their nasal passages, and may develop a perforated nasal septum. Freebasers and crack users may suffer lung damage from smoking. Cocaine users who share hypodermic needles risk hepatitis and, more seriously, HIV infection. Freebase users risk setting themselves on fire. Finally, whatever the method of administration, addiction is an extremely serious problem.[28]

The Cocaine Age is leaving a legacy from which recovery may take years. Pregnant cocaine users have an increased risk of miscarriage (spontaneous abortion), birth defects, premature babies, low-birth-weight babies, and babies who die from sudden infant death syndrome (SIDS, or "crib death"). Some offspring are also affected by the drugs used by their mother in addition to cocaine. "Crack babies," infants born addicted to cocaine because their mothers continued to use the drug during pregnancy, suffer lifelong and potentially life-threatening disabilities.[29] Their disabilities may range from respiratory and kidney disorders to mental damage caused by oxygen deprivation. In addition, these children are at increased risk for neglect and abuse.

Crack has had a major impact on the crime rates not just of large cities but of small towns as well, as drug gangs have widened their influence and violence. The rise in criminal activity has put great pressure on law-enforcement agencies and politicians in turn to push for the suspension of civil liberties. Finally, entire countries in Latin America have been corrupted by the enormous industry of cocaine, to which the United States has responded by involving itself in the domestic affairs of other nations.

Depressants: Drugs That Take You Down

Solvents and inhalants, sedatives/hypnotics, and tranquilizers are classes of drugs known as depressants, which slow down or sedate brain activity. Solvents are chemicals found in cleaning products and adhesives, and inhalants are found in aerosols and many anesthetics. Sedatives induce relaxation, and hypnotics induce sleep; barbiturates and nonbarbiturates are sedatives/hypnotics prescribed as sleeping aids and tension relievers. Tranquilizers, or anti-anxiety drugs, are minor and major. Minor tranquilizers are used to ease minor anxieties, muscle tension, and sleeplessness. Major tranquilizers are used to treat serious mental disorders.

Unlike the stimulants that arouse the central nervous system and speed up brain activity, **depressants** ("downers" in street language) are drugs that slow down or sedate it. All depressants act in similar ways as the dosage is increased: a feeling of relaxation progresses to a lessening of inhibitions and drowsiness. Depending on the dosage, sedation can lead to anesthesia, then to coma and eventually death from respiratory failure. The most widely used depressant drug is alcohol. Here we discuss three classes of depressants:

1. Solvents and inhalants
2. Sedatives/hypnotics
3. Tranquilizers

Solvents and Inhalants There is a vast world of highly dangerous depressants classed as solvents and inhalants. **Solvents** are chemicals found in many cleaning products and adhesives.

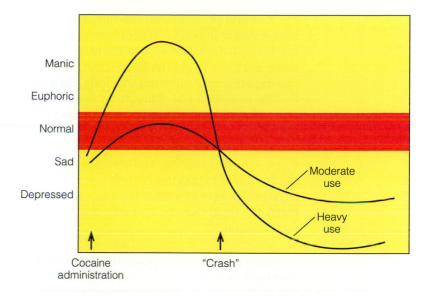

● **Figure 13.4 Cocaine highs and lows.** The relationship between cocaine dose and mood.

Inhalants are found in aerosols and many anesthetics. When inhaled, both kinds of chemicals act as depressants and produce delirium.

Examples of these chemicals show just how readily available they are: gasoline, glue, paint, varnish, kerosene, butane, paint thinners, cleaning fluids, spot removers, rubber cement, nail polish remover, typewriter correction fluid, and aerosol propellants. Clearly, it would be hard to try to remove these products from the control of anyone who wants to use them for purposes for which they were not intended.

Other inhalants include:

- *Butyl nitrate:* An over-the-counter drug, butyl nitrate (brand names: Locker Room, Rush) produces a brief period of euphoria.

- *Amyl nitrate:* A drug prescribed for heart patients, amyl nitrate (street names: "poppers," "snappers"), which is used to widen (dilate) the blood vessels and increase the heart rate, has also found its way to the street, where it is used to produce brief euphoria.

- *Nitrous oxide:* Nitrous oxide (laughing gas) is another inhalant that has a valid medical use as a dental anesthetic but has been diverted to illicit purposes.

5.16

Unit 5
Drug and Other
Dependencies:
Lifestyles and
Gratifications

The first problem with solvents and inhalants is that common to all depressants: regular use leads to tolerance, so that the user requires more and more to get the same effect. Initially, one experiences a euphoria that feels like a floating sensation and delirium. As more substances are inhaled, users begin to experience not just excitement but also confusion and headaches. Eventually, these chemicals can cause nausea, coughing, and abnormal heart rhythms. More importantly, their use can lead to hepatitis, liver or kidney failure, possible coma and brain damage, and even death by asphyxiation.

Sedatives/Hypnotics: Barbiturates and Nonbarbiturates Depressants are chemical substances that can produce muscular relaxation and relief from tension and anxiety. They can also produce a calming effect and, as such, are called **sedatives**. At larger doses, some depressants, called **hypnotics**, are capable of inducing sleep or a trancelike state. The sedatives/hypnotics include five classes of drugs:

1. Some inhalants
2. Barbiturates
3. Nonbarbiturate sedatives/hypnotics
4. Minor tranquilizers
5. Major tranquilizers

Barbiturates are chemical compounds dispensed by prescription in pill or liquid form to be used as sleeping aids, tension relievers, or to control epileptic seizures. Barbiturates can also be used as general anesthetic agents, in which case they are injected intravenously. Barbiturates may be short-acting or long-acting:

- *Short-acting:* Short-acting barbiturates rapidly penetrate into the brain and can induce sleep very quickly. Examples are pentobarbital (brand name Nembutal, street name "yellow jackets") and secobarbital (Seconal; "reds").
- *Long-acting:* Longer-acting barbiturates take longer to be absorbed by the brain and can lead to sedation for several hours. Examples are amobarbital (Amytal; "blues") and phenobarbital (Luminal; "phennies").

In moderate doses, barbiturates act like alcohol and produce staggering, slurred speech, loss of motor coordination, euphoria, and disinhibition—in short, the characteristics of drunkenness. Indeed, like alcohol, they produce hangovers. Increased doses lead to sedation and sleep, which is why barbiturates were once prescribed medically as sleeping pills. Higher doses produce anesthesia, and barbiturates are still prescribed for this purpose as well as to control seizures, such as those caused by epilepsy.

Barbiturate use causes so many problems that their medical use has been greatly reduced. Tolerance develops rapidly and withdrawal from barbiturates after regular use produces a syndrome similar to that found among those withdrawing from alcohol—shakes, perspiration, confusion, even delirium and convulsions. Indeed, barbiturates are one of the most dangerous drugs for withdrawal. In addition, there is the danger of drug overdose, particularly—and this cannot be stressed enough—when barbiturates are used with another depressant such as alcohol, because these drugs potentiate each other. Barbiturates have often played a role in suicides and unintentional deaths, including the case of film star Marilyn Monroe.

Some nonbarbiturate sedatives have been introduced for treating sleep disorders and anxiety. Perhaps the best known is methaqualone, marketed under such names as Quaalude (street name: "ludes") and Sopor ("sopors"). Methaqualone became known as "the love drug" because it was thought to enhance sexuality, but there is no evidence that it has any more qualities as an aphrodisiac than any other depressant.

Methaqualone and other nonbarbiturates have not lived up to their promise as a safe alternative to barbiturates. They are quite toxic at high doses, lead quickly to dependence, and produce withdrawal symptoms similar to those of alcohol and the barbiturates.

Minor and Major Tranquilizers Also called *anti-anxiety drugs*, **tranquilizers** are marketed under such brand names as Valium and Librium, the most widely prescribed drugs in the United States. Tranquilizers may be classed as minor and major:

- *Minor tranquilizers:* Minor tranquilizers include benzodiazepines and nonbenzodiazepines and are used primarily for three purposes: (1) to treat minor anxieties, (2) to ease muscle tension, (3) to induce sleep.

- *Major tranquilizers:* Major tranquilizers, such as chlorpromazine (Thorazine) and haloperidol (Haldol), are used to treat people with serious mental disorders in institutional settings. Although major tranquilizers allow patients to remain conscious and will reduce hallucinations, they may also cause confusion and stupors.

Those minor tranquilizers called the *benzodiazepines* have had an enormous impact on our society, with four of them being among the top 30 most prescribed drugs in America. These are diazepam (Valium), flurazepam (Dalmane), lorazepam (Ativan), and clorazepate (Tranxene).[30] The group of minor tranquilizers called the *nonbenzodiazepines* include meprobamate (brand name Equanil) and buspirone (BuSpar).

The benzodiazepines have become the drugs of choice for alleviating anxiety and insomnia.[31] However, using these drugs as the sole treatment for anxiety disorders, especially over the long term, merely masks the patients' symptoms; they do not cure anxiety or affect its origins. The main adverse effects of most minor tranquilizers are drowsiness and interference with memory—that is, blackouts. In addition, tolerance develops, albeit slowly, and there is cross tolerance with other depressants, particularly alcohol. The effects of benzodiazepines can last for several days. Withdrawal from these drugs is similar to that for barbiturates and for alcohol—insomnia, anxiety, tremors—although not as severe.

Cannabis: Marijuana and Hashish

The hemp plant produces marijuana and hashish, both of which contain the psychoactive agent THC. THC may be smoked or ingested. There are several harmful long-term effects from the drug.

The effects of marijuana depend upon the dosage. At lower doses, the drug typically produces mild analgesia and sedation, but hallucinations are possible at higher doses.

How commonly used is marijuana? The following statistic is revealing: in 1985, one-third of all Americans over age 12 had tried it at least once, according to the National Institute on Drug Abuse.[32] Still, its popularity has declined significantly since the 1960s and 1970s, especially among youths and young adults. For example, the number of users decreased from a high of 51% in 1979 to a low of 37% in 1987.[33] Why this decline? In part it may be for economic reasons, but it may also have to do with health concerns.

Marijuana and hashish are both derived from the hemp plant cannabis (*Cannabis sativa*), which grows freely throughout the world and which has been widely used to provide fibers (hemp) for rope and clothes. **Marijuana** ("pot," "grass," "weed") is the leafy top portion of the plant. **Hashish** is made from gum-like secretions (resin) produced by the hemp plant, which are dried and compressed. Although marijuana is comprised of at least 400 chemicals, the principal psychoactive agent is **THC** (short for delta-9-tetrahydrocannabinol), whose content can range from near zero to 8%, depending on the plant. Hashish is the more potent form of marijuana and is more likely to produce hallucinogenic effects.

In general, the most efficient way to absorb THC is by inhalation, by smoking it in a hand-rolled cigarette ("joint") or pipe. The effects vary depending not only on the particular plant (its concentration of THC and the part of the plant used) but also on how long a person can hold the inhaled marijuana in the lungs. Thus, cigarette smokers or experienced marijuana smokers tend to feel the effects more intensely than inexperienced users do. Peak drug concentrations occur 30–60 minutes after the first "toke" (inhalation), and the effects are experienced for about 2–4 hours. However, even non-smokers sitting in the same room with pot smokers can experience some drug effect, a "contact high," with THC showing up in non-users' urine tests hours and even days after the event.[34] In addition, complete elimination of a large dose of marijuana in users may take 2–3 weeks.

THC can also be administered orally, as when it has been baked in the form of marijuana brownies and ingested, but requires a dose about three times greater than when smoking. The onset of the high may be as long as 1 hour; however, the drug effects may last 4–6 hours.

5.18

*Unit 5
Drug and Other
Dependencies:
Lifestyles and
Gratifications*

THC is also available on the street in the form of **hash oil,** a concentrated liquid extract that is even more potent (up to 60% THC) than marijuana or hashish.

In the short run, marijuana acts somewhat like alcohol or some tranquilizers, producing feelings of relaxation and tranquility and, for some people, a heightened sense of perception, and impaired psychomotor performance. Although marijuana can produce feelings of being carefree and relaxed, it can also produce anxiety and paranoia, particularly among inexperienced users.[35] In addition, users also report headaches, nausea, and muscle tension. Often the negative effects are transitory and alternate with the positive states. Heart rate and blood pressure increase, eyes become reddened, and the throat and mouth feel dry. Nausea and dizziness are often reported. Some users experience panic attacks. It is unsafe to drive a car while under the influence of marijuana since the drug affects reaction time, concentration, and balance. Although users develop tolerance to the drug, the question of physical dependence on marijuana remains open, particularly since there do not seem to be significant withdrawal symptoms. There may, however, be some psychological dependence: heavy users who stop show such signs as sleep disturbance, irritability, and nausea.[36]

Cannabis may actually have some medical uses. It has been shown to reduce pressure in the eye (intraocular pressure), which is a cause of glaucoma, the leading cause of blindness in the United States. It also has been found to reduce the nausea and vomiting associated with chemotherapy and some radiation treatments for cancer. Cannabis and THC synthetics have been used to treat pain, convulsions, hypertension, asthma, and depression, although the results are inconclusive.

That's the good news. The bad news is that, particularly when used frequently and in heavy doses, marijuana smoking has been linked to respiratory disorders, such as chronic bronchitis and pulmonary disease. Marijuana cigarettes have more tar than those made with tobacco, and the cannabis tar seems to contain more cancerous substances than tobacco tar.[37] Still, the long-term effects are unknown and are complicated by the fact that many cannabis smokers are also cigarette smokers. The short-term ef-

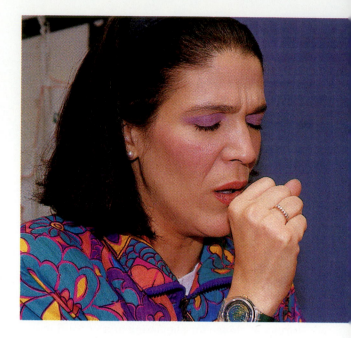

fects of increased heart rate and slight to moderate elevation in blood pressure seem to hold no danger for healthy people, but they might be detrimental to people with existing heart and blood vessel problems. Cannabis use has been found to decrease the activity of the immune system in animals, but there seems to be no long-range effect in human beings.

An additional area of concern regarding this drug is in its reproductive effects. Men who are heavy marijuana users have been found to have decreased testosterone and sperm production. Women who are continual users have been found to have nonovulatory menstrual cycles. Several studies have reported lower birth weights in babies born to mothers who smoke marijuana. The results from many of these studies, however, have been inconsistent and the significance unclear; the impact on fertility remains inconclusive.[38] As with nearly all drugs, however, pregnant women should abstain from cannabis use because of possible significant effects on the fetus.

At one point, some scientists reported an **"amotivational syndrome,"** in which people who were chronic, heavy marijuana users showed such behaviors as apathy, difficulty concentrating, learning problems, lost ambition, and decreased sense of goals.[39] It is not clear, however, that cannabis is necessarily a cause of these behaviors, since this syndrome has not been found among heavy marijuana users in other countries. Since marijuana remains in the body for a long period of time, some researchers suggest that amotivational syndrome is actually the result of chronic marijuana intoxication.

Hallucinogens

Hallucinogens, or "psychedelics," profoundly alter consciousness, producing hallucinations, scrambling of senses, depersonalization, and flashbacks. The most potent is LSD. Other hallucinogens are mescaline from the peyote cactus, psilocybin from several mushrooms, and morning glory seeds. The extremely dangerous drug phencyclidine, or PCP, is classified as a hallucinogen, although it seldom causes visual hallucinations.

Hallucinogens are drugs that can alter consciousness in profound ways. In the 1960s, they were also called **"psychedelics,"** because of their supposed "mind-expanding" or "mind-revealing" properties. Whatever their name, their effect is to alter consciousness so that it produces not only the sensory disturbances that people call hallucinations but also significant changes in thinking, mood, and physiological processes as well.

Although we have discussed it separately, marijuana is sometimes classified as a hallucinogen. Other hallucinogens are LSD and PCP (lysergic acid diethylamide and phencyclidine, synthesized in laboratories) and mescaline and psilocybin (derived from natural sources), which we describe below.

Among the principal effects of hallucinogens are the following:

- *Hallucinations:* Hallucinations are the vivid images that users have reported when under the influence of these drugs. Examples are spiral explosions, vortex patterns, lattice patterns, flashing lights, and sense of movement around objects.

- *Scrambled senses:* **Synesthesia** is the perception of a stimulus in a sense other than the one in which it was presented—for example, "seeing music," "touching a taste," "hearing colors."

- *Depersonalization:* **Depersonalization** is the distortion in how people see their bodies and themselves. Examples of this phenomenon: one's legs appear to be wriggling out of one's trousers or a person feels "a oneness with the universe."

- *Flashbacks:* **Flashbacks,** unexpected re-experienced parts of a hallucinogenic episode or perceptual distortions, can occur weeks, months, or even years after the drug was used. One study reported that 53% of LSD users reported flashbacks.[40]

Unlike other drugs we've discussed, hallucinogenic drugs do not seem to cause physical dependence or addiction or their withdrawal symptoms. On the other hand, tolerance develops quickly, so that users find a drug's effects reduced after a few days of use. Moreover, with many of these drugs (LSD, mescaline, and psilocybin) people also develop cross-tolerance, so that they cannot switch from one hallucinogenic drug to another in hopes of changing their level of tolerance.

LSD One class of hallucinogenic drugs (*serotonergic hallucinogens*) includes LSD, mescaline, psilocybin, and morning glory seeds, all of which cause vivid visual hallucinations. We will describe the most potent of the hallucinogens first.

First synthesized in the laboratory in 1938, **LSD** (lysergic acid diethylamide, street name "acid") was originally derived from ergot, a fungus that infests grain; now it is synthetically produced. Its discoverer, Swiss chemist Albert Hoffman, reported on the bizarre results of one of his initial experiences. (*See* ● *Figure 13.5.*)

5.20

Unit 5
Drug and Other
Dependencies:
Lifestyles and
Gratifications

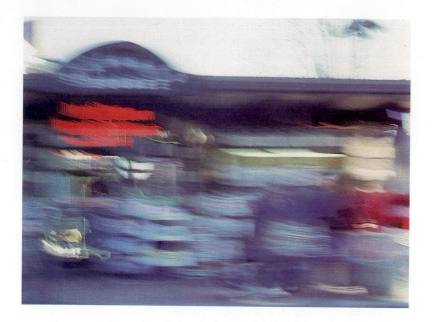

● **Figure 13.5 One of the first LSD trips.** The discoverer of LSD reported the following experience as the result of ingesting a mere 250-microgram dose.

" *After 40 minutes, I noted the following symptoms in my laboratory journal: slight giddiness, restlessness, difficulty in concentration, visual disturbances, laughing. . . . Later: I lost all count of time. I noticed with dismay that my environment was undergoing progressive changes. My visual field wavered and everything appeared deformed as in a faulty mirror. Space and time became more and more disorganized and I was overcome by a fear that I was going out of my mind. The worst part of it being that I was clearly aware of my condition. My power of observation was unimpaired. . . . Occasionally, I felt as if I were out of my body. I thought I had died. My ego seemed suspended somewhere in space, from where I saw my dead body lying on the sofa . . . . It was particularly striking how acoustic perceptions, such as the noise of water gushing from a tap or the spoken word, were transformed into optical illusions.* "

—Albert Hoffman, Swiss discoverer of LSD

By the early 1960s, a great many people had tried the drug, from British author Aldous Huxley to Time-Life publisher Henry Luce, lured by the promises that it would open "the doors of perception" or spiritual enlightenment. Some psychotherapists experimented with the drug on the theory that it would help break down patients' defenses and facilitate the therapeutic process, although this has not been verified. One influential voice during the 1960s was that of former Harvard psychologist Timothy Leary, who exhorted people to "Turn on, tune in, drop out." Eventually word extolling its use spread to the larger world. Then reports surfaced about the possibility of chromosomal damage and insanity, murder, and suicide, and its popularity began to wane. In addition, as some authors point out, "perhaps equally important was a loss of faith in the LSD mystique, the recognition that spiritual enlightenment produced by LSD was a false hope."[41]

LSD is odorless, tasteless, and colorless. Because it is so much more potent than other drugs, extremely small doses of the drug are needed to produce effects. The drug is sold in a variety of forms, including on paper, in a gel, or in a sugar cube or tablet. The effects begin within 20–60 minutes of ingestion and last for 8–12 hours. During an "acid trip," heart rate and blood pressure increase slightly, the pupils dilate, and nausea, vomiting, sweating, and chills may occur. The qualitative nature of the hallucinatory experience varies, with some people reporting numerous pleasurable, ecstatic experiences followed by an occasional "bummer" or bad trip, associated with acute panic and paranoia. Setting, companions, and one's own feelings seem to greatly influence the character of the drug experience. So does the nature of the drug actually used, since adulterated street drugs lead to uncertain effects and potential dangers.

The effects of LSD are unpredictable; they not only vary from person to person but also from one drug-taking experience to another. Hazards include flashbacks, the recurrence of initial effects days to months after LSD was taken. Their occurrence is unpredictable and they most often occur prior to sleep, during periods of emotional stress, and while driving. Other problems include fear of losing one's mind, accidental injury, and panic reactions.

Pregnant women should not take the drug because LSD causes contractions of the uterus, although there is no evidence it causes chromosomal damage or other birth defects.

The long-range effect of prolonged LSD use is not clear. Despite concerns that it might cause cancer, this has not been authenticated. There is speculation that heavy LSD use may produce psychiatric disorders, but this, too, has not been proven.

Mescaline, Psilocybin, Morning Glory Seeds Originally these LSD-like hallucinogens were obtained from natural substances, although mescaline and psilocybin are now synthesized in laboratories. All these were used by native peoples in the New World for rituals of healing and worship. All produce vivid hallucinations, including bright colors and lights.

Mescaline is the major psychoactive ingredient found in the small crown or button of the peyote cactus, a spineless cactus of Mexico and the Southwest United States. Members of the Native American Church have used peyote since the 19th century. Peyote buttons are eaten, boiled and drunk as peyote tea, or smoked in cigarettes or pipes. When eaten, the effects of mescaline begin within 30–90 minutes and may last 8–12 hours. Although mescaline causes altered perceptions and other effects similar to LSD, it is only about 1/3000 as potent as LSD. Although no delirium or amnesia has been reported, the drug may produce nausea.

Psilocybin is found in several kinds of "magic mushrooms" throughout the world. The drug is only about 1% as potent as LSD and is eaten or drunk in a tea. Its effects last about 4–6 hours. Psilocybin is known for the strong visual distortions it produces.

Morning glory seeds, pulverized seeds of the morning glory plant, contain a psychoactive substance that is similar to LSD but less potent, being only about 5–10% as strong as LSD. In order to discourage use of the seeds as a psychoactive drug, commercial morning glory seed producers apply a poisonous substance to the seeds that causes nausea, vomiting, diarrhea, and dizziness.

Phencyclidine Called, on the street, "PCP," "angel dust," "love boat," "lovely," and "hog,"

phencyclidine has stimulant, depressant, hallucinogen, and anesthetic properties. It has been classed as a hallucinogen, although visual hallucinations seldom occur with its use. Instead, users experience perceptual changes or distortions in body image. They may feel, for example, as though parts of their bodies are extremely large or detached. The effects also resemble those of alcohol intoxication: euphoria, slurred speech, numbness, lack of motor coordination, and double vision.

One of the serious problems with this drug is its unpredictable effects: users sometimes exhibit bizarre and, rarely, aggressive or violent behavior. Phencyclidine was originally developed in the 1950s as a surgical anesthetic, but because people often developed psychotic symptoms as they recovered from anesthesia, its use was discontinued in 1965. The drug can be injected, but it is usually sprinkled as a powder on a cigarette and smoked. The drug effects generally take place 5–15 minutes after smoking and last 4–6 hours or even days with high doses.

PCP is an extremely dangerous drug, in part because its effects are unpredictable. It seems to produce a higher rate of negative reactions with frequent use than other psychoactive drugs.[42] Overdoses may result in seizures, coma, or death from respiratory failure. Bad trips may occur in 50–80% of PCP users.[43] The drug may also produce paranoia and violence lasting several days and long-term psychotic episodes and depression. "In many cities," experts write, "PCP is responsible for more psychiatric emergencies than any other drug, and in some hospitals PCP psychoses exceed schizophrenia and alcoholism as a cause of psychiatric admission."[44]

Opiates

Opiates, or narcotics, are drugs derived from the opium poppy plant that provide pain relief and sedation. Major opiates include opium, morphine, codeine, heroin, and other synthetic opiates. All are addictive. Opium serves as a source of morphine, codeine, and heroin.

5.22

*Unit 5
Drug and Other
Dependencies:
Lifestyles and
Gratifications*

Opiates, also known as **narcotics,** include several drugs derived from the Oriental poppy plant that produce numbness, relieve pain, and induce sleep. These sleep-inducing **analgesic,** or pain-killing, effects give the opiates important, legitimate medical uses. They have also been used medically to treat diarrhea and coughing. What makes them popular as illicit drugs, however, is the euphoria they produce. The opiates include opium, morphine, codeine, heroin, meperidine, and methadone. These drugs are called *opiates* because they can be derived naturally from the opium poppy plant (opium, morphine, or codeine), made by modifying the chemicals in opium (heroin, Diladid, or Percodan), or synthesized in the laboratory (Meperidine, methadone, or Darvon). Opium-like substances called **endorphins** or **enkephalins** have also been found naturally in the body. Tolerance, cross tolerance, and physical as well as psychological dependence characterize chronic use of the drugs in this category.

Opium Smoked in a pipe (although it may also be taken orally or injected), opium produces vivid dream-like experiences, which have given rise to the expression "pipe dreams." **Opium** consists of dark brown chunks or powder that is the dried sap from the seedpod of the Asian poppy plant. In the 19th century, it was widely used both medically, in numerous patent medicines in the United States, and recreationally, as when it was smoked in China. Opium is still used in some parts of the world, but today it is principally important because it provides morphine, codeine, and heroin.

Morphine **Morphine** is the active ingredient in opium. It is an extremely effective analgesic, or painkiller, that can be taken orally or smoked, but is principally administered by injection. Morphine's effects last about 4–5 hours. Analgesics like morphine act on the central nervous system, blocking out the pain messages sent to the brain. Thus, morphine does not actually remove pain but changes a person's awareness of the pain so that he or she no longer cares about it. A person under the influence of the drug feels drowsy, tranquilized, and often euphoric.

Although euphoria is an attraction of the drug for many people, some people actually experience anxiety and fear. Other possible side effects include nausea and vomiting. Morphine depresses respiration; too large a dosage can cause death because people stop breathing. The drug is extremely addicting, and tolerance develops after only a few injections—indeed, after a while, tolerance builds to the point that no amount of the drug will provide the desired effects. Withdrawal symptoms can be very unpleasant: chills, sweating, shaking, cramps, and nausea, to name a few.

Codeine The analgesic **codeine,** found in opium, is principally derived from morphine. Codeine is a less effective painkiller and sedative than morphine, but it is also much less addictive. It is found in many medications, both prescribed and over-the-counter, such as cough medicines and combined forms of aspirin (Empirin and a form of Tylenol). Codeine is one of the most effective cough suppressants currently available.

Heroin A semi-synthetic drug derived from morphine and four times as potent, **heroin** ("horse," "junk," "smack," "scag") is one of the most addictive drugs available. "It's so good," one young middle-class addict said about it, "don't even try it once."[45]

Discovered in 1874, heroin was promoted as a nonaddictive substitute for morphine, just as morphine was once hailed as a nonaddictive substitute for opium. It was used medically in the United States as an analgesic early in the 20th century but eventually was banned for any nonmedical use. In Great Britain, however, physicians are allowed to administer a preparation called *Brompton's cocktail*, a mixture of heroin and cocaine, to ease the pain of the terminally ill.[46]

When injected, heroin produces euphoria and analgesia lasting 3–4 hours. Addicts experience the injection as a "rush" of ecstasy, although it may actually be simply the relief of withdrawal symptoms, which resemble those of morphine withdrawal: sweating, chills, cramps, nausea, shaking, restlessness, and anxiety. Goose bumps appear, perhaps the basis for the expression "going cold turkey." Tolerance to heroin increases rapidly. Indeed, the tolerance develops so quickly that users often speak lyrically of their first dose and keep trying to find stronger blends of the drug in an attempt to recreate that experience. This escalation in turn increases the risk of overdose and death.

During the 1960s and 1970s, heroin, then principally administered by injection, became the scourge of the American streets. Its use dropped markedly in the 1980s as cocaine and crack became more available. In the early 1990s, however, as the cocaine market received heavy law-enforcement attention, heroin sellers began packaging the drug in potent blends that could be snorted or smoked rather than injected.[47,48] An even more potent combination, heroin and crack ("moon rock," "speedball," "parachute"), also became available.[49] It was an injection of a speedball that caused the death of comedian John Belushi. Heroin and depressant drugs such as alcohol have also been found to potentiate one another. Rock singer Janis Joplin's death in 1970 was attributed to an injection of heroin following an evening of heavy drinking.

Other Synthetic Opiates Besides codeine, several other legal opiates less powerful than morphine are available for the relief of pain: propoxyphene, meperidine, oxycodone, hydromorphone, and methadone.

Propoxyphene (Darvon) is actually less effective than aspirin in pain relief and half as potent as codeine, yet in the past has been widely prescribed for all kinds of pain, from menstrual cramps to cancer. However, because people rapidly develop tolerance to this drug, they are apt to increase the dosage. It has been implicated in numerous deaths and suicides.

Meperidine (Demerol; street name "demies"), a frequently used painkiller whose effects last 2–4 hours, is as potent as codeine and quite addictive. **Oxycodone** (Percodan; "perkies") has a drug action of 4–5 hours. Somewhat less potent than morphine, it is slightly more potent than codeine. **Hydromorphone** (Dilaudid; "Little D") has about five times the potency of a similar amount of morphine. Its action lasts about 4–5 hours.

Methadone (Dolophine; "meth," "dollies") is equal in potency to morphine and is used principally as a substitute drug to treat heroin addiction. However, whereas the duration of action is 4–5 hours for morphine and 3–4 hours for heroin, the effects of methadone last 24–48 hours. Sometimes methadone is given in decreased doses over a 2-week period in order to wean someone off narcotics; sometimes in regular doses over a 6-month period or even indefinitely as a maintenance dose—enough to reduce heroin withdrawal pains but not enough to produce much euphoria. The danger, however, is that methadone itself is addictive.

Some opiates are even more powerful than heroin. **Fentanyl** (Sublimaze, "China white") is *80 times* as potent as morphine and *20 times* as potent as heroin. This drug is used to produce anesthesia in surgery, but from time to time it has been sold on the street. In early 1991 in the greater New York City area, several heroin addicts died after buying heroin that was apparently laced with fentanyl.

Designer Drugs: More Dangerous Than Heroin

Designer drugs are drugs that are chemically similar to other controlled substances, which were originally designed to circumvent the law banning dangerous addictive drugs. Designer drugs are highly unpredictable and dangerous.

Far more dangerous than heroin are the so-called **designer drugs,** also called **analog drugs.** In the 1970s and early 1980s, back-room chemists began to try to circumvent the law by

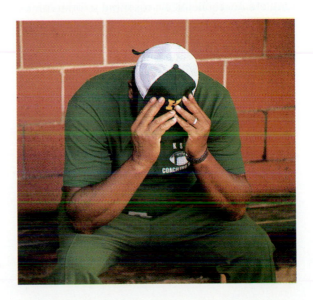

5.24

Unit 5
Drug and Other
Dependencies:
Lifestyles and
Gratifications

making drugs that were closely related in chemical structure to regulated or banned drugs (such as amphetamines). Thus, they were able to manufacture drugs that produced similar effects in the body, but they could not be prosecuted under the law at the time, which required that the exact chemical nature of illegal drugs had to be specified.[50] Producers wanted to avoid the legal problems of distributing a controlled substance by manufacturing drugs that were not legally restricted because they were slightly different chemically. The synthesis of MDMA, for example, was based on methamphetamine. In 1986, however, the Controlled Substance Analogue Act was passed, which banned drugs similar to those classified as controlled substances.

The earliest designer drugs to appear on the street belonged to a class of drugs called *methylated amphetamines,* which produced mild euphoria and a sense of openness. One of these was *MDA* ("Love drug," "Mellow Drug of America"), which supposedly helped users develop loving or positive feelings toward others. This was succeeded by *MDMA* ("Ecstasy," "Adam"), which some psychotherapists said could help patients achieve insight breakthroughs, although no carefully controlled studies have supported this contention. MDMA, DOM, and MDA are considered hallucinogenic amphetamines. Concerns associated with these drugs include fatal or nearly fatal toxic reactions that may be related to hypersensitivity to the drug or an overdose. The drugs may also deplete neurochemicals essential to brain function. These drugs in turn were followed by *MDE* ("Eve").

A form of "designer heroin" known as *MPPP* or *MPTP* has been found to produce brain damage and associated neurological disorders that have left people seriously impaired. Derivatives of the above-mentioned fentanyl have been developed that may be 10–1000 times more potent than heroin, posing a great risk of death from overdose. The greatest danger is that in the future makers of designer drugs will be able to develop substances that are even more addicting or have more serious side effects than those around today.

Strategy for Living: Managing Drug Use and Abuse

Overcoming drug dependency means first admitting the problem—overcoming denial. This may require intervention by others to confront the addicted with his or her abuse. Mild or moderate drug problems may be handled with brief treatment and identification of goals in life. Severe drug problems may require detoxification, treatment in a hospital milieu, and/or outpatient treatment in a therapy or other self-help program. Families of recovering addicts often need treatment, too.

We live in a society that offers constant inducements to medicate oneself to escape life's pain: aspirin, alcohol, tranquilizers, and then—the logical next step for many people—illegal drugs. People may go for months or years using drugs moderately, then immoderately as continued use of these addictive substances leads them to dependence. Progression to drug dependence is often gradual, but there may come a time when the drug use begins to interfere with sleep, memory, peace of mind, interest in sex, and performance levels. Family members may be the first to notice the signs of addiction. There may be conflicts in relationships, absences from work or school, and trouble with the law. If any of these events are happening in your life or in the life of someone you know, the next step is to get help. (*See Self Discovery 13.1.*)

Admitting the Problem: Overcoming Denial At some point there may occur what alcoholics call "hitting bottom"—the point when drug users finally realize that they are in the grip of an addiction and must change. Sometimes this is a natural development in people's lives as people mature and come to realize that their drug use is no longer satisfying but rather life-disturbing. Sometimes the realization may come about through **intervention,** as family members or friends, often accompanied by a trained counselor, confront the drug user with specific facts about his or her behavior in an effort to help him or her recognize the possibility of dependency.

In any case, before addicts can change their behavior, they must first overcome (or be made to overcome) their denial of abuse. Nearly all people with drug-related problems deny that they have a problem. Indeed, because their initial drug use resulted in positive effects, they continue to seek those positive feelings even when drug use can no longer offer that possibility. This may explain why the relapse rate is high for addicts initially entering treatment. As Herbert D. Kleber of the Office of National Drug Control Policy put it, addicts don't enter treatment the first time to get rid of their habit. Rather, they want "to get back to that honeymoon when the drug felt great and [they] could control it."[51]

Nevertheless, acknowledging addiction to a drug is the first step. Giving it up is the next.

Getting Help for Mild or Moderate Drug Problems Some drugs produce only mild or moderate withdrawal symptoms, and users are able to overcome their habits without great difficulties. If you think this might apply to yourself, there is much that you can do yourself. You should consider where you stand in your life, how extensive your drug use is, what the drug does *for* you, and what your reasons are for giving up drugs. (See ● *Figure 13.6*.) In addition, you might try the following:

- *Get treatment:* Brief treatment includes such things as short-term counseling, discussions with family or friends, or simply reading self-help materials.

- *Identify goals and methods:* Set your goals for drug use, such as the extent to which you will limit your use, and the methods for controlling it. For example, you might make a contract with a friend listing goals, deadlines, rewards, and punishments.

- *Identify how you will strengthen your life:* Indicate how you will change your environment and otherwise strengthen your life to help you break the habit. For example, you might indicate drug-related social situations you will avoid, self-help groups you will join, exercise programs you will take up, and other pleasures you will seek out in lieu of drugs. Some healthy activities that people take up as alternatives to drugs include athletics, music, art, the outdoors.

SELF DISCOVERY 13.1

Are You an Addict?

The following questions were written by recovering addicts in Narcotics Anonymous.

	Yes	No
1. Do you ever use alone?	❑	❑
2. Have you ever substituted one drug for another, thinking that one particular drug was the problem?	❑	❑
3. Have you ever manipulated or lied to a doctor to obtain prescription drugs?		
4. Have you ever stolen drugs or stolen to obtain drugs?	❑	❑
5. Do you regularly use a drug when you wake up or when you go to bed?	❑	❑
6. Have you ever taken one drug to overcome the effects of another?	❑	❑
7. Do you avoid people or places that do not approve of you using drugs?	❑	❑
8. Have you ever used a drug without knowing what it was or what it would do to you?	❑	❑
9. Has your job or school performance ever suffered from the effects of your drug use?	❑	❑
10. Have you ever been arrested as a result of using drugs?	❑	❑
11. Have you ever lied about what or how much you use?	❑	❑
12. Do you put the purchase of drugs ahead of your financial responsibilities?	❑	❑
13. Have you ever tried to stop or control your using?	❑	❑
14. Have you ever been in a jail, hospital, or drug rehabilitation center because of your using?	❑	❑
15. Does using interfere with your sleeping or eating?	❑	❑
16. Does the thought of running out of drugs terrify you?	❑	❑
17. Do you feel it is impossible for you to live without drugs?	❑	❑
18. Do you ever question your own sanity?	❑	❑
19. Is your drug use making life at home unhappy?	❑	❑
20. Have you ever thought you couldn't fit in or have a good time without using drugs?	❑	❑
21. Have you ever felt defensive, guilty, or ashamed about your using?	❑	❑
22. Do you think a lot about drugs?	❑	❑
23. Have you had irrational or indefinable fears?	❑	❑
24. Has using affected your sexual relationships?	❑	❑
25. Have you ever taken drugs you didn't prefer?	❑	❑
26. Have you ever used drugs because of emotional pain or stress?	❑	❑
27. Have you ever overdosed on any drugs?	❑	❑
28. Do you continue to use despite negative consequences?	❑	❑
29. Do you think you might have a drug problem?	❑	❑

Are you an addict? This is a question only you can answer. Members of Narcotics Anonymous found that they all answered different numbers of these questions "yes." The actual number of yes responses isn't as important as how you feel inside and how addiction has affected your life. If you are an addict, you must first admit that you have a problem with drugs before any progress can be made toward recovery.

5.26

*Unit 5
Drug and Other
Dependencies:
Lifestyles and
Gratifications*

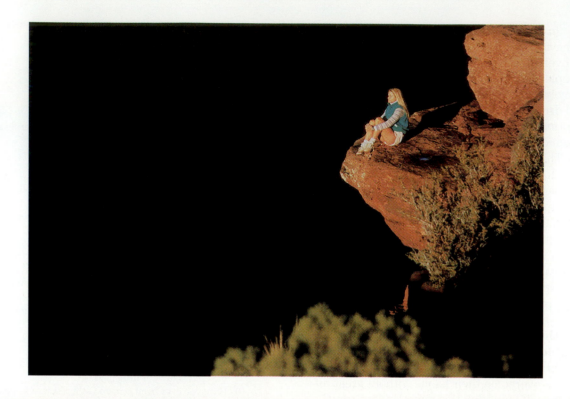

● **Figure 13.6 Peace of mind.** Some benefits of quitting illegal drugs.

❝*People who give up illegal drugs cut a lot of unnecessary risk and tension out of their lives. They no longer have to fear getting busted for possession or losing a job because of a positive drug test. They don't have to worry about getting the money for their next fix, rock, or pill, and they don't have to waste energy trying to look clean when they're using. They can stop associating with unsavory characters and quit aligning themselves with a system of greed and violence. Through abstinence they can resign from the rat race and rejoin the human race. Recovery brings them many gifts, not the least of which are the simple peace of sobriety and the welcome renewal of self-respect.*❞

—Barbara Yoder (1990). *The recovery resource book.* New York: Fireside, p. 186.

Getting Help for Substantial or Severe Drug Problems People who are drug-dependent may require specialized treatment, as follows:

- *Detoxification:* **Detoxification**—ridding the body of the drug—may require hospitalization or a stay in a health-care facility, where withdrawal symptoms can be monitored and treated.

- *Milieu treatment:* Inpatient residence programs, known as **milieu treatment,** are lo-

cated in a hospital or drug rehabilitation facility and provide 2–6 weeks of treatment, including various kinds of counseling and psychotherapies, drug-withdrawal therapy, and drug education. Some of the most famous treatment centers for chemical dependency are Hazelden in Center City, Minnesota, and the Betty Ford Center in Rancho Mirage, California.

- *Outpatient treatment:* Following inpatient treatment, those recovering from chemical dependency are directed toward various kinds of outpatient treatment programs. In fact, many drug-dependent people may skip the inpatient phase and go directly to an outpatient program. Sometimes outpatient treatment includes drug therapy, such as methadone maintenance for recovering heroin addicts.

- *Self-help groups:* Newly abstinent addicts are urged to join Twelve Step programs, which follow the model pioneered by Alcoholics Anonymous. Examples are Narcotics Anonymous, Pills Anonymous, Marijuana Anonymous, Marijuana Addicts Anonymous, Cocaine Anonymous, and Cokenders.

Family Rehabilitation Programs Chemical dependency, including alcoholism, affects not only the individual who is drug-dependent but also the people with whom he or she has close relationships. Drug dependency of any kind, therefore, is considered a "family disease." Family therapy helps the chemically dependent and their families learn new ways of communicating with one another. In addition to counseling by trained family therapists, there are several self-help organizations, such as Families Anonymous, Nar-Anon, and ToughLove, which are dedicated to helping family members with their problems.

800-HELP

Alcoholism and Drug Addiction Treatment Center. 800-477-3447. Available 24 hours. Provides phone counseling and local referrals.

National Council on Alcoholism and Drug Dependence Hotline. 800-475-HOPE. Available 24 hours

National Institute for Drug Abuse. 800-662-HELP. (In Spanish: 800-66-AYUDA.) Available M–F 9 a.m.–3 p.m., Sat.–Sun. 12 p.m.–3 a.m. Gives counseling over the phone. Refers callers to local support groups and treatment programs.

800/Cocaine Hotline. 800-COCAINE. Available 24 hours

Suggestions for Further Reading

Goode, Erich (1989). *Drugs in American society.* New York: McGraw-Hill.

Peele, Stanton (1985). *The meaning of addiction.* Lexington, MA: Lexington Books.

Washton, Arnold (1991). *Cocaine addiction: Treatment, recovery, and relapse prevention.* New York: W. W. Norton.

Weil, Andrew. (1973). *The natural mind.* Boston: Houghton Mifflin. Discusses how altered states of consciousness can be achieved without drugs.

5.28

Unit 5
Drug and Other
Dependencies:
Lifestyles and
Gratifications

14 Non-Drug Forms of Dependence

▶ Can the definition of addiction be expanded beyond drug dependency?

▶ Distinguish between substance addictions and process addictions.

▶ Discuss the following dependencies: gambling, spending and debt, work, and codependency.

The words *dependence* and *addiction* have become broadly generalized to behavior other than drug use in recent years. Indeed, the word *addictive* has been used to characterize our society itself. For instance, psychotherapist Anne Wilson Schaef writes, in *When Society Becomes an Addict,* "the society in which we live is an addictive system. It has all the characteristics and exhibits all the processes of the individual alcoholic or addict."[52] Addictive systems are built on self-centeredness and dishonesty, she says, and we live in a society "in which we are expected to cheat on our taxes and get away with as much as we can."[53] The notion that our society is an addictive system can stir up a good deal of debate, but let us consider some of the problems that now come under the heading "addictions."

Can the Definition of *Addiction* Be Expanded?

Some propose that the meaning of *addiction* be expanded to cover two categories: (1) substances, including drugs and food and (2) processes, including "mood-altering events" such as gambling, spending money, and workaholism. Many health experts disagree that addiction should be broadened beyond drug dependence.

Dependence means reliance on or need for something and can be physical, psychological, or both. It may be for food, for another person, for exercise, for cigarettes, or for cocaine. However, in recent years the term *addiction* has been given wider meaning. (See ● *Figure 14.1.*) For instance, Schaef says that an **addiction** "is any process over which we are powerless. It takes control of us, causing us to do and think things that are inconsistent with our personal values and leading us to become progressively more compulsive and obsessive."[54] Schaef divides addictions into two major categories— *substance addictions* and *process addictions:*

- *Substance addictions:* **Substance addictions** are addictions to mood-altering substances that are usually artificially refined or produced. According to Schaef, these substances include *drugs*—caffeine, nicotine, alcohol, and more powerful mood-altering chemicals, such as tranquilizers, marijuana, cocaine, and heroin—and *food.* (We describe food-related disorders, such as overeating, anorexia, and bulimia, in Chapter 16.)

- *Process addictions:* **Process addictions** consist of any specific series of actions or interactions, or "mood-altering events," on which one becomes extraordinarily dependent. Some prominent examples include "addictions" to gambling, spending money, and work, which we describe below. Exercise can become an "addiction" (we discuss that in Chapter 18). Sex and love can also become an addiction (as we discuss in Chapter 20). Even excessive television watching has been called "addictive." Finally, there is codependency, described as "an addiction to another person's addiction."[55]

Are "process addictions" true addictions? One study found that gambling, for instance, produced a euphoria that was similar to the euphoria produced by psychoactive drugs.[56] Another study found gamblers scored similarly to heroin addicts on an addiction scale.[57] However, other studies report different results. One found that gambling was not perceived to be characterized by the underlying construct of dependence, a dimension associated with the abuse of illicit substances.[58] A second concluded that the concept of addiction involves physiological processes that do not appear to be present in cases of excessive gambling.[59]

Whatever one may think about this new category of addiction, it represents dependencies that ultimately limit personal freedom. "Dependencies become problems," write Andrew Weil and Winifred Rosen, "when they take up vast amounts of time, money, and energy; create guilt and anxiety; and control one's life."[60]

In the following sections, we examine four activities that can become process addictions or dependencies:

- Gambling
- Spending and debt
- Work
- Codependency

Gambling

Gambling's popularity has surged and is greater among high school and college students than among the general population. Pathological gamblers are unable to resist impulses to gamble, despite the dismal chances of winning, and the gambling disrupts their lives.

Gambling is a major industry in the United States. Thirty-two states and the District of Columbia have lotteries.[61] Forty-eight of the 50 states allow some form of legal gambling (Hawaii and Utah are the exceptions). Then there is the $20-billion-a-year *illegal* sports-betting market. All together, an estimated $253 billion is legally and illegally wagered in the United States each year ($2.5 billion on the Super Bowl alone).[62]

Compulsive Gamblers Compulsive gambling is a significant problem. Perhaps 3–4% of those who gamble are unable to control their betting and seem especially vulnerable to the aura of hype that surrounds gambling. An additional 10–15% gamble more money than they can afford. However, according to one authority on compulsive gambling, these two groups may account for nearly *half* of all money wagered.[63] In states where gambling is legal 24 hours a day, such as Nevada and New Jersey, the number of compulsive gamblers jumps to about 2½ times the national rate.[64]

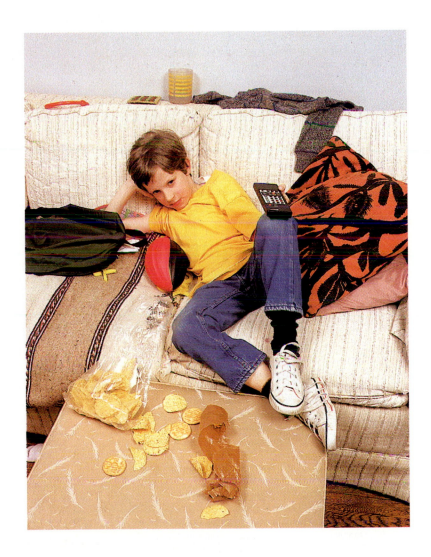

● **Figure 14.1 The broader meaning of addiction.** In recent years, the meaning of the word *addiction* has been expanded to include dependence on far more than alcohol and drugs, although many professionals do not agree with this widened definition.

"*It's possible to become addicted to almost any ingestible substance or mood-altering event: Work. Money. Booze. Pills. Computers. Exercise. Sex. Religion. Sports. Television. Crossword puzzles. Cocaine. Tobacco. Food.*

Any repeated use of a substance or event to numb pain or enhance pleasure, to take us out of our senses, away from ourselves, has the potential to become an addiction."

—Barbara Yoder (1990). *The recovery resource book.* New York: Fireside, pp. 2–3.

5.30

Unit 5
Drug and Other
Dependencies:
Lifestyles and
Gratifications

Gambling by high school and college students has surged—and the rates seem to be higher than among the adult population. A study by sociology professor Henry R. Lesieur of New Jersey high school students found that 86% had gambled in the past year and 32% had gambled at least once a week.[65] About 5% of the teenage population had lost control of their gambling activity and had become "pathological" or "compulsive" gamblers; this compares with 2–3% of the adult population. A survey by William C. Phillips of 2000 college students in six states found that 87% had gambled, 25% had gambled weekly, and 11% had gambled more than $100 in one day, with amounts ranging to $50,000 in one week.[66] About 5.7% were described as having pathological gambling behavior, including repeatedly betting in hopes of winning big to make up for losses and continuing to gamble despite inability to pay debts. The study found that several students frequently gambled money set aside for college tuition.[67]

Compulsive gambling has been officially recognized as a psychiatric illness by the American Psychiatric Association since 1980. **Pathological gambling** has been defined, in the *Diagnostic and Statistical Manual of Mental Disorders* (Third Edition—Revised), as a chronic and progressive failure to resist impulses to gamble, resulting in disruption of or damage to family, personal, and vocational pursuits.[68,69] Originally, gambling was categorized as a disorder of impulse control, like the need to steal or to start fires. Indeed, some experts regard it as purely psychological. As one compulsive gambler put it, "People don't smell dice on your breath or see card marks on your arm."[70] However, researchers led by Alec Roy found pathological gambling to be linked to low levels of brain chemicals (by-products of norepinephrine) that regulate arousal, thrills, and excitement. It is speculated that the deficit can lead to a need to engage in risky, exciting activities, such as gambling, that will stimulate the brain to secrete more of these chemical substances.[71,72]

Compulsive gambling has all the hallmarks of an addiction, says psychologist Valerie Lorenz, who directs the National Center for Pathological Gambling in Baltimore. "It follows the classic course for an addiction: It becomes chronic and progressive, tolerance levels increase, and you lose all regard for the consequences of the habit."[73] (*See Self Discovery 14.1.*)

Pathological gamblers generally share certain characteristics:[74]

- *They are intelligent:* They often have above-average or superior intelligence.

SELF DISCOVERY 14.1

Are You a Compulsive Gambler?

Only you can decide. Compulsive gamblers are those whose gambling has caused continuing problems in any facet of their lives. The following questions may be of help to you.

	Yes	No
1. Do you ever lose time from work because of gambling?	❑	❑
2. Has gambling ever made your home life unhappy?	❑	❑
3. Has gambling ever affected your reputation?	❑	❑
4. Have you ever felt remorse after gambling?	❑	❑
5. Do you ever gamble to get money to pay debts or otherwise solve financial difficulties?	❑	❑
6. Does gambling cause a decrease in your ambition or efficiency?	❑	❑
7. After losing, do you feel you must return as soon as possible and win back your losses?	❑	❑
8. After winning, do you have a strong urge to return as soon as possible and win more?	❑	❑
9. Do you often gamble until your last dollar is gone?	❑	❑
10. Do you ever borrow to finance your gambling?	❑	❑
11. Have you ever sold anything to finance gambling?	❑	❑
12. Are you reluctant to use "gambling money" for normal expenditures?	❑	❑
13. Does gambling make you careless of the welfare of your family?	❑	❑
14. Have you ever gambled longer than you had planned?	❑	❑
15. Have you ever gambled to escape worry or trouble?	❑	❑
16. Have you ever committed, or considered committing, an illegal act to finance gambling?	❑	❑
17. Does gambling cause you to have difficulty sleeping?	❑	❑
18. Do arguments, disappointments, or frustrations create within you an urge to gamble?	❑	❑
19. Do you ever have an urge to celebrate any good fortune by a few hours of gambling?	❑	❑
20. Have you ever considered self-destruction as a result of gambling?	❑	❑

Scoring

Most compulsive gamblers will answer yes to at least seven of these questions.

Source: Reprinted from Gamblers Anonymous *Combined pamphlet* by permission of Gamblers Anonymous.

- *They are competitive and energetic:* They are strongly competitive, are industrious workers, have high energy level, often have outstanding athletic ability, and generally have shown good academic performance.

- *They seek challenge:* They thrive on challenges, don't tolerate boredom well, and don't finish tasks they find dull.

- *They prefer skill games:* They prefer games of skill, such as those found in casinos (craps, blackjack, sportsbook), rather than games of chance, such as lotteries.

- *They have had a "big win":* Compulsive gamblers usually have had a history of a big win that equals or exceeds several months of salary. This establishes in their minds that it could happen again.

- *They "chase" to recoup losses:* As losing becomes intolerable, they "chase," or bet more money, to recoup losses. They borrow heavily to cover losses.

- *They go into debt:* They borrow until their own resources are exhausted, then turn to bookies and loan sharks for more. Eventually they may turn to writing bad checks, forgery, or embezzlement.

Strategy for Living Are any gamblers, even the noncompulsive ones, getting rich? Not very many. Among the 97 million Americans who wager on state lotteries, for instance, those who win $1 million are only .000008% of those who participate.[75] It is said that the odds of your winning a lottery grand prize are 1 in 5.2 million; you are much more likely to appear on the "Tonight Show" (1 in 490,000) or to be struck by lightning (1 in 600,000).[76] Casino gambling has better odds for gamblers, but the odds are always best for the house.

Yet few players seem to pay attention to the dismal chances of winning. The reason, according to Dutch psychologist Willem Wagenar, is faulty thinking: a trick of memory helps gamblers recall their wins more than their losses, preserving the illusion that their chances are far better than they really are.[77]

Compulsive gamblers may find help through organizations such as Gamblers Anonymous.

Spending and Debt

Compulsive spenders repeatedly engage in impulse buying to find self-assurance, escape anxiety, and achieve excitement. Compulsive spenders often become compulsive debtors who continually borrow money.

Over the last decade, many people have been spending beyond their means. As a result some 30 million Americans have financial troubles, according to the National Foundation for Consumer Credit. Personal bankruptcy increased

---

SELF DISCOVERY 14.2

Are You a Compulsive Shopper?

	Yes	No
1. Do you "take off for the stores" when you've experienced a setback or a disappointment, or when you feel angry or scared?	❏	❏
2. Are your spending habits emotionally disturbing to you and have they created chaos in your life?	❏	❏
3. Do your shopping habits create conflicts between you and someone close to you (spouse, lover, parents, children)?	❏	❏
4. Do you buy items with your credit cards that you wouldn't buy if you had to pay cash?	❏	❏
5. When you shop, do you feel a rush of euphoria mixed with feelings of anxiety?	❏	❏
6. Do you feel you're performing a dangerous, reckless, or forbidden act when you shop?	❏	❏
7. When you return home after shopping, do you feel guilty, ashamed, embarrassed, or confused?	❏	❏
8. Are many of your purchases seldom or never worn or used?	❏	❏
9. Do you lie to your family or friends about what you buy and how much you spend?	❏	❏
10. Would you feel "lost" without your credit cards?	❏	❏
11. Do you think about money excessively—how much you have, how much you owe, how much you wish you had—and then go out and shop again?	❏	❏
12. Do you spend a lot of time juggling accounts and bills to accommodate your shopping debts?	❏	❏

Scoring

If you answered yes to more than four of these questions, the chances are you're a compulsive shopper.

Source: Reprinted from Damon, J. (1988). *Shopaholics*. Los Angeles: Price Stern Sloan. Copyright © 1988 by Janet Damon.

5.32

Unit 5
Drug and Other
Dependencies:
Lifestyles and
Gratifications

10% between 1988 and 1990.[78] Some of this was caused by job loss, illness, divorce, or career setbacks or family problems. However, many financial problems are caused by out-of-control spending.

Compulsive Spenders All of us occasionally make impulsive purchases for reasons that have nothing to do with the specific objects purchased, such as to cheer us up when we're feeling down. But **compulsive spenders** (also called *compulsive shoppers* or "shopaholics") repeatedly engage in impulse buying. Buying things becomes an activity used to provide feelings of self-assurance and self-worth and to help the buyer escape feelings of anxiety and despair. One particular hallmark of compulsive spending is making unnecessary purchases,

sometimes of luxury items, that end up unused or hidden away, because the *process* of buying is more important than the purchase itself. A shopping expedition that begins with feelings of euphoria and reckless excitement, however, often ends with feelings of self-recrimination and depression.

Not surprisingly, compulsive spenders often become **compulsive debtors,** who continually borrow money from institutions, family, and friends to pay their bills. Both compulsive spenders and compulsive debtors follow an "addiction cycle" similar to that of substance abusers: They resort repeatedly to their activity in order to obtain relief from depression and anxiety, but develop a craving for the activity, and eventually lose control. (*See Self Discoveries 14.2 and 14.3.*)

Compulsive spenders make up about 6% of the population, and the problem cuts across all income levels, according to a 1989 study by Thomas O'Guinn and Ronald Faber. They estimate that about 60% of compulsive spenders are women.[79] Because shopping is used to bolster feelings of low self-worth, the relationship with salespeople becomes quite important, since clerks make shopaholics feel good about themselves.

Some characteristics of compulsive spenders are as follows:[80]

- *They are very anxious and depressed.* Many compulsive spenders use shopping to alleviate their depressed feelings. Thus, they may go on shopping binges when their feelings are hurt.

- *They often buy for other people.* Because many compulsive shoppers have a desperate need for approval, they buy things not for themselves but for other people.

- *They may be "binge buyers," "daily shoppers," or "multiple buyers."* Compulsive shoppers do not all act the same way, according to O'Guinn and Faber. People who are "binge buyers" may go off on a shopping binge only occasionally, perhaps triggered by an upsetting event. "Daily shoppers" go shopping every day and become upset if they do not. "Multiple buyers," a less common type, repeatedly buy several of the same item (perhaps because they like the sales clerk).

SELF DISCOVERY 14.3

Are You a Compulsive Debtor?

	Yes	No
1. Do you find yourself borrowing money to meet basic expenses month after month?	☐	☐
2. Do you often write checks for amounts greater than your account balance and expect to make a deposit to cover them later?	☐	☐
3. Do you avoid balancing your checkbook for weeks or months at a time?	☐	☐
4. Are you often focused obsessively on how much money you have and how much you owe?	☐	☐
5. Have you charged your credit cards up to the maximum limit?	☐	☐
6. Do you open new credit card accounts when you spend the limit on existing accounts?	☐	☐
7. Do you believe it's okay to borrow money from anyone who's willing to lend it?	☐	☐
8. Have you ever borrowed money from a "loan shark"?	☐	☐
9. Have you concealed the extent of your debt from family members?	☐	☐
10. Does the anxiety of being in debt create conflicts within your family?	☐	☐
11. Do you worry that you'll never have enough cash to pay your bills?	☐	☐
12. Do you believe that you'll never enjoy prosperity?	☐	☐

Scoring

If you answered yes to four or more of these questions, you may have a problem with compulsive debt.

Source: Yoder, B. (1990). *The recovery resource book.* New York: Fireside, p. 248.

Strategy for Living People who are deeply in debt feel "helpless, angry, and confused," says former debtor Jerrold Mundis. "They become fearful, depressed, even suicidal. They live with a daily sense of impending disaster."[81]

How does one avoid or recover from this state of affairs? The obvious action is to rein in expenses, stay within a budget, and otherwise inject rationality into the shopping process. For example, one can draw up plans for shopping, ask others to do the shopping, or shop only when feeling calm. One can also destroy all credit cards, even those (such as American Express or department-store cards) that are supposed to be paid off every month.

Resources for those who believe themselves to be compulsive debtors include support groups such as Debtors Anonymous and counseling.

Work

Workaholism is work addiction. Workaholics would rather work than play, are driven and perfectionistic, and let work interfere with their lives. Ultimately they may suffer from "burnout."

What is considered more socially productive than work? This thought is precisely the reason that so many people have difficulty understanding that work can be a compulsion or another "process addiction." Many people who work long hours are *not* compulsive workers: they like what they do, but they take time out to relax and to be with their families. Some people, however, are focused on and driven by work-related activities to the exclusion of other aspects of their lives.

Workaholics Work addicts, or **workaholics,** are people who are self-destructively obsessed with their career and making a living. (*See Self Discovery 14.4.*) How do you tell a work addict from someone who finds fulfillment in his or her work? Here are some characteristics associated with workaholics:[82,83]

- *They would rather work than play:* Workaholics often work anywhere and anytime. They don't take much time off to play (and may not take vacations or may take work with them on vacation) and don't have much of a personal or love life. A great deal of their socializing and interpersonal relationships involves co-workers.

- *They are driven and perfectionistic:* Work-addicted people labor extremely hard in part because they have such great self-doubts. They often constantly strive for perfection. As one writer describes it, "Nothing you produce at the office seems good enough, so you compulsively revise and polish each memo, letter, and presentation."[84] They tend to be perfectionists in their relationships and regard their spouse or partner and children as extensions of their own egos.[85]

- *Their work interferes with their lives:* Their long hours at the job cause workaholics problems with others: "Your family resents the amount of time you devote to your job and lets you know it. In addition, your co-workers are fed up with your unreasonable demands and expectations."[86] In the end, workaholism leads to such signs of stress as general exhaustion, fitful sleep, and headaches.

Strategy for Living At some point—perhaps after many years—work stops providing the workaholic the rewards it did: avoidance of intimacy, heightened self-esteem, perfection, total control. This is often known as "burnout." When this "hitting bottom" occurs, the work addict is in a position to begin to recover—not to give up work completely (since most people need to work to support themselves), but to learn to work less, to work for fulfillment, and to lead a more balanced life.

If you suspect you might be a workaholic, the first thing to do is to determine where your time goes. If you sleep 8 hours a day, that leaves 16 hours a day (112 hours a week) for everything else. Keep a diary of the time you spend preparing for work, commuting, working, unwinding from work, doing housework, and engaging in play or leisure activities. Then ask yourself if you are comfortable with the balance of time between work and play, how much more time you would like to spend with family and friends, and what leisure activities you would like to schedule into your week.

5.34

Unit 5
Drug and Other
Dependencies:
Lifestyles and
Gratifications

SELF DISCOVERY 14.4

Are You Addicted to Work?

Read each of the 25 statements below and decide how much each one pertains to you. Using the rating scale of 1 (never true), 2 (seldom true), 3 (often true), and 4 (always true), put the number that best fits you in the blank beside each statement. Once you have responded to all 25 statements, add up the numbers in the blanks for your total score.

_____ 1. I prefer to do most things myself rather than ask for help.

_____ 2. I get very impatient when I have to wait for someone else or when something takes too long, such as long, slow-moving lines.

_____ 3. I seem to be in a hurry and racing against the clock.

_____ 4. I get irritated when I am interrupted while I am in the middle of something.

_____ 5. I stay busy and keep many "irons in the fire."

_____ 6. I find myself doing two or three things at one time, such as eating lunch and writing a memo, while talking on the telephone.

_____ 7. I overly commit myself by biting off more than I can chew.

_____ 8. I feel guilty when I am not working on something.

_____ 9. It is important that I see the concrete results of what I do.

_____ 10. I am more interested in the final result of my work than in the process.

_____ 11. Things just never seem to move fast enough or get done fast enough for me.

_____ 12. I lose my temper when things don't go my way or work out to suit me.

_____ 13. I ask the same questions over again, without realizing it, after I've already been given the answer once.

_____ 14. I spend a lot of time mentally planning and thinking about future events while tuning out the here and now.

_____ 15. I find myself continuing to work after my co-workers have called it quits.

_____ 16. I get angry when people don't meet my standards of perfection.

_____ 17. I get upset when I am in situations where I cannot be in control.

_____ 18. I tend to put myself under pressure with self-imposed deadlines when I work.

_____ 19. It is hard for me to relax when I'm not working.

_____ 20. I spend more time working than on socializing with friends, on hobbies, or on leisure activities.

_____ 21. I dive into projects to get a head start before all phases have been finalized.

_____ 22. I get upset with myself for making even the smallest mistake.

_____ 23. I put more thought, time, and energy into my work than I do into my relationships with my spouse (or lover) and family.

_____ 24. I forget, ignore, or minimize birthdays, reunions, anniversaries, or holidays.

_____ 25. I make important decisions before I have all the facts and have a chance to think them through.

_____ = Total

Scoring

A total score of 25–54 points means you are not work addicted; 55–69 means you are mildly work addicted; 70–100 means you are highly work addicted.

Source: Adapted from: Robinson, B. E. (1989). *Work addiction: Hidden legacies of adult children.* Deerfield Beach, FL: Health Communications.

The principal self-help recovery program is Workaholics Anonymous, whose slogans are: "Work smarter, not harder" and "If everything else fails, lower your standards."

Codependency

Codependents are family members or others close to a substance-dependent or process-addicted person who tend to accommodate their lives to the addict.

As we discussed in Chapter 12, **codependents** were originally considered to be spouses of alcoholics, but the term was expanded to include others close to an alcoholic family member. The chief characteristic of codependents is that they tend to accommodate themselves to the alcoholic.

In the last few years, however, the term *codependents* has been extended to people in families troubled by other addictions or compulsions, such as compulsive gambling or workaholism. Some critics complain that codependency is less a psychological disorder than it is "a business, generating millions of book sales [and] countless support groups . . ."[87] If, as asserted by some self-proclaimed experts (many of whose credentials are simply those of self-described "recovering codependents"), 96% of all Americans suffer from codependency, then the category may be so wide as to be meaningless. Nevertheless, the idea may be useful because it helps us consider how our selves are formed within the fabric of family life.

People in Families of Addicts Codependency rests on the idea that the *family* is more important than the *individual* within that family. Alcoholism and other addictions are considered family illnesses because of the tremendous impact that addicts have on those around them.

Physician Timmen Cermak views codependency as a type of personality disorder. He advocates the use of codependency as a clinical diagnostic category, using diagnostic criteria found in the American Psychiatric Association's DSM III-R.[88] (See ● *Figure 14.2.*) In general, it may be said that codependent family members become concerned with others to the point of neglecting themselves and their needs; they

also learn to not take responsibility for their own lives. (*See Self Discovery 14.5.*)

Some of the characteristics associated with codependents are as follows:

- *They become addicted to the addict:* People living with a person who is dependent

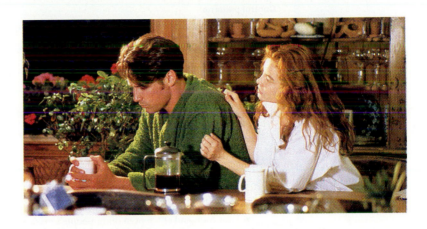

● **Figure 14.2 Codependency: Suggested criteria for diagnosis.** Physician Timmen Cermak advocates the use of codependency as a clinical diagnostic category, using diagnostic criteria found in the American Psychiatric Association's DSM III-R.

- *Investment in others:* Continued investment of one's self-esteem in the ability to control oneself and others in the face of serious adverse consequences.
- *Excluding one's own needs:* Assumption of responsibility for meeting other's needs to the exclusion of one's own.
- *Anxiety about separation:* Anxiety and boundary distortions around intimacy and separation.
- *Involvement with ill individuals:* Enmeshment in relationships with personality disordered, chemically dependent, other codependent, and/or impulse-disordered individuals.
- *Other difficulties:* Three or more of the following: (1) excessive reliance on denial; (2) constriction of emotions; (3) depression; (4) hypervigilance; (5) compulsions; (6) anxiety; (7) substance abuse; (8) the past or current victim of physical or sexual abuse; (9) stress-related medical illnesses; (10) remaining in a primary relationship with an active substance abuser for at least 2 years without seeking help.

—Timmen Cermak, M.D., cited in Kinney J., & Leaton, G. (1991). *Loosening the grip: A handbook of alcoholism* (4th ed.). St. Louis: Times Mirror/Mosby, pp. 177–178.

5.36

Unit 5
Drug and Other
Dependencies:
Lifestyles and
Gratifications

SELF DISCOVERY 14.5

Are You Codependent?

Mark the items that apply to you "always," "usually," "sometimes," or "never."

Control patterns

_____ I must be "needed" in order to have a relationship with others.

_____ I value others' approval of my thinking, feelings, and behaviors over my own.

_____ I agree with others so they will like me.

_____ I focus my attention on protecting others.

_____ I believe most other people are incapable of taking care of themselves.

_____ I keep score of "good deeds and favors," becoming very hurt when they are not repaid.

_____ I am very skilled at guessing how other people are feeling.

_____ I can anticipate others' needs and desires, meeting them before they are asked to be met.

_____ I become resentful when others will not let me help them.

_____ I am calm and efficient in other people's crisis situations.

_____ I feel good about myself only when I am helping others.

_____ I freely offer others advice and directions without being asked.

_____ I put aside my own interests and concerns in order to do what others want.

_____ I ask for help and nurturing only when I am ill, and then reluctantly.

_____ I cannot tolerate seeing others in pain.

_____ I lavish gifts and favors on those I care about.

_____ I use sex to gain approval and acceptance.

_____ I attempt to convince others of how they "truly" think and "should" feel.

_____ I perceive myself as completely unselfish and dedicated to the well-being of others.

on a mood-altering substance or activity take on a certain way of behaving. They base their self-esteem on what others think of them and organize their lives according to others' expectations of them. They become supporting actors to the major player, the addict. Their urge to help others becomes subsumed in an obsession with other people, so that they lose their own identity and self-worth.

- *They become enmeshed in a cycle of pain:* Assuming responsibility for family well-being, they attempt to manage the addict's life. Failing to control the addiction itself, they become obsessed with protecting

the family and the addict from intervention or knowledge by others outside the family. By becoming "enablers" of the addict and sparing him or her from the consequences of addiction, they actually allow the cycle of pain to persist.

- *They remain stuck in codependent behavior:* Even after they leave the family or after the addict leaves the family, codependents remain locked in a pattern of living their lives through other people. Thus, they may continue to look for other dependent or addicted people to take care of. They continue to deny their feelings of pain.

Compliance Patterns

_____ I assume responsibility for others' feelings and behaviors.

_____ I feel guilty about others' feelings and behaviors.

_____ I have difficulty identifying what I am feeling.

_____ I have difficulty expressing feelings.

_____ I am afraid of my anger, yet sometimes erupt in a rage.

_____ I worry how others may respond to my feelings, opinions, and behavior.

_____ I have difficulty making decisions.

_____ I am afraid of being hurt and/or rejected by others.

_____ I minimize, alter, or deny how I truly feel.

_____ I am very sensitive to how others are feeling and feel the same.

_____ I am afraid to express differing opinions or feelings.

_____ I value others' opinions and feelings more than my own.

_____ I put other people's needs and desires before mine.

_____ I am embarrassed to receive recognition and praise, or gifts.

_____ I judge everything I think, say, or do harshly, as never "good enough."

_____ I am perfectionistic.

_____ I am extremely loyal, remaining in harmful situations too long.

_____ I do not ask others to meet my needs or desires.

_____ I do not perceive myself as a lovable and worthwhile person.

_____ I compromise my own values and integrity to avoid rejection or others' anger.

If you see a pattern emerging from your answers and if you're concerned about the health of your relationships, you can find help and understanding at meetings such as Co-Dependents Anonymous.

Source: Co-Dependents Anonymous pamphlet, *What is co-dependency?*

Strategy for Living Despite criticisms of the whole notion of codependency, the positive side of the movement is that it helps many people discover they don't have to live their lives through someone else—that they need to nurture and take care of themselves. The goal of any relationship should be *inter*dependency, or mutual dependency, usually a constantly changing task in which one tries to maintain independence within the confines of the relationship.

It's highly likely that nothing can change in the family system of someone who is dependent on chemicals or activities until the codependent realizes that rescuing the addict isn't really helping either of them. Once the codependent stops making excuses and stops trying to protect the person from the consequences of his or her behavior, the addict will have to face his or her own problem.

Some codependents may be able to establish their independence by themselves, but many will need to reach out and get help. The principal self-help Twelve Step group is Co-Dependents Anonymous (CoDA). Other groups, such as Al-Anon, Nar-Anon, and Gam-Anon, are designed for codependents involved with specific types of addicts and addictions.

Coming to Terms with "the Drug Problem"

Forget the stories about crack-addicted babies, swelling jail populations, dealers swapping automatic-weapons fire, and turmoil in South American cocaine-supplier nations. To begin to clarify what you think about "the drug problem"—and what it means in your life—you need to think about your own drug use.

Which of the following describes how you feel about using drugs yourself?

It's all right for me to use drugs . . .

___ **1.** Only for medical purposes, such as to alleviate pain, and only if they are legal.

___ **2.** For recreational as well as medical uses, provided the drugs are legal.

___ **3.** For medical and recreational uses, regardless of whether the drugs are legal or illegal, provided they are not addictive and harmful.

___ **4.** For medical and recreational uses, regardless of whether the drugs are legal or illegal—no matter how addictive. It's no one else's business what I do with drugs.

Whatever the nature of society's problem with drugs, you have to consider yourself a part of it: that is the place to start. Consider the meaning of the opinions expressed above.

1. It's All Right to Use Drugs for Medical Purposes Only, Provided the Drugs Are Legal

Do you use a legal drug such as aspirin or a decongestant or a prescription drug sometimes to relieve pain? Then you clearly believe in the medical efficacy of drugs. If you were suffering from glaucoma (an eye disorder that can cause blindness) or spasticity or, as a cancer patient, chemotherapy-induced nausea, would you want to be able to be treated with THC?

THC is the principal active ingredient in marijuana. The smokable form of marijuana is currently prohibited for medical use because the drug does not undergo chemical analysis for quality control and there are health problems associated with inhalation. THC *is* available in pill form as Marinol, a prescription drug processed by a large pharmaceutical company and subject to testing by the Food and Drug Administration. Note: Just like illegal marijuana, it may also have a psychoactive effect.

But here's the point we want to make: Suppose you, as a cancer patient suffering from nausea, respond better to illegal smoked marijuana than to legal Marinol. For a number of people, this is in fact the case: according to a 1988 study by Vincent Vinciguerra, some patients who did not respond to oral THC *did* respond to smoked marijuana.[89] Why is this? According to another study, reported in 1979 by Alfred Chang of the National Cancer Institute, inhaled marijuana acts on the brain almost immediately, whereas pills taken orally and requiring absorption may leave a cancer patient with nausea to suffer for several hours.[90]

Should marijuana in smokable form be legalized for medical uses? According to a 1991 study by Richard Doblin and Mark Kleiman of oncologists (physicians specializing in cancer), 48% said they would prescribe marijuana to some patients if it were legal, 54% said they thought smoked marijuana should be available by prescription, and 44% said they had recommended marijuana to a patient even though it was illegal.[91]

In 1988, administrative law judge Francis L. Young ruled that the ban on prescription marijuana was "unreasonable, arbitrary, and capricious." So far, however, the government has not reclassified the drug, probably because of political reasons. Government officials apparently worry that the act would "send a signal" that marijuana is acceptable for recreational use. What do you think?

2. It's All Right to Use Drugs for Recreational as Well as Medical Purposes, Provided the Drugs Are Legal

From time immemorial, people have used drugs to "get high," and some observers believe there is some basic human inclination to use drugs to alter consciousness. For instance, before the Spanish conquest of the Inca civilization in South America in the 16th century, the natives used the coca plant, from which cocaine is now obtained, in conjunction with rituals and ceremonies. Indeed, in earlier times, the plant was restricted to the use only of the emperor and his royal family—a case of making a drug "legal" for some and "illegal" for a great many others.[92]

Today, many psychoactive drugs are legally available for medical uses only, and a handful of others—caffeine, tobacco, alcohol—are allowed for public consumption without a prescription. The picture of drug use that many politicians seem to favor is this: drugs are strictly a legal issue, and "the drug problem" consists of dealing with people who sell or use substances in violation of the law.

But another real issue, of course, is that some legal drugs create grave ill health: cigarettes and alcohol are among the leading killer substances the world over. Indeed, in the case of alcohol, the highway deaths and injuries, health care, and associated problems far exceed any social benefits. If the purpose of declaring a substance illegal is to safeguard people's health and well-being, then a substance such as alcohol should have been outlawed long ago. Indeed, this has been tried—during Prohibition, "the Noble Experiment," as it was called—and it actually produced some positive results.

The Volstead Act, which took effect in 1920 and prohibited the manufacture, sale, and transport of "intoxicating liquors" in the United States, lasted until 1933. The popular notion of Prohibition is of an era of hip flasks, speakeasies, and gangsters with machine guns fighting each other and alcohol-control agents—that is, a time of widespread illegal consumption and law-breaking. In fact, however, Prohibition *did*

reduce drinking: annual per capita consumption of all forms of alcohol stood at 2.60 gallons before the Volstead Act took effect and was down to 0.97 gallons in 1934, the year after the act was repealed. Chronic or acute alcoholism went from 7.3 cases per 100,000 people in 1907 to 2.5 in 1932; deaths from cirrhosis of the liver (one cause of which is alcohol abuse) went from 14.8 per 100,000 in 1907 to 7.1 in 1920.[93] Clearly, then, a case can be made for restricting availability.

As for an increase in law-breaking, Prohibition did not create criminal organizations. In Chicago, points out one writer, the gangs were already there, profiting from other vices; "Prohibition simply gave them new markets." Yet, he concludes, Prohibition finally was abandoned in part "because it did contribute to hypocrisy, graft, and disrespect for the law."[94]

Today the government's approach to legal recreational drugs is decidedly mixed—and influenced by political considerations. While on the one hand the U.S. Department of Agriculture hands out subsidies to tobacco farmers, on the other hand the U.S. Surgeon General strives mightily to alert the public to the dangers of smoking. Alcohol use is encouraged informally, with even the White House responding to pressure from wine-producing states by serving California and New York wines at official functions, while at the same time health authorities attempt to educate teenagers, drivers, pregnant women, and others to the dangers of alcohol.

And, of course, as modern chemistry continues to produce more and more drugs that must be put on the government's list of controlled substances, law enforcement efforts must increase proportionately. Under the Bush administration, $10 billion a year was spent on the war on drugs—three quarters of it on law enforcement—and victory still seems to be a long ways away.

3. It's All Right to Use Legal or Illegal Drugs for Recreational and Medical Purposes, Provided They Are Not Addictive or Harmful

One might argue that adults, at least, should be allowed to consume whatever mind-altering drug they desire so long as it is not addictive. Unfortunately, most such drugs, both legal and illegal, can be addictive, but some are more harmful than others.

Let's consider legal drugs first. Alcohol was once used by battlefield surgeons as an anesthetic, but it is rarely recommended by doctors today. Do you see anything wrong with self-medicating your anxiety with alcohol, which is certainly highly addictive to many people? If you were feeling extremely anxious, would you (or do you) use the tranquilizer Valium? Valium is a legal drug, of course, a controlled substance. It is also quite addictive, and millions of addicted patients do "doctor shopping" or obtain illegal prescriptions to continue their habits. Controlled substances such as the tranquilizers Valium and Xanax as well as several sedatives and amphetamines—all legal, all addictive—are responsible for a third of all drug overdoses that turn up in emergency rooms, about three times the rate of heroin overdoses.[95] Some drugs, then, have addictive properties that we might tolerate for medical use for a short while but not for recreational use.

Now let's consider illegal drugs. Are there any illegal mind-altering drugs that are not addictive? Perhaps a distinction must be made between "soft drugs" and "hard drugs," as is done in Holland. Possession of the soft drugs marijuana and hashish has been decriminalized in Holland, and small amounts are legally sold in certain cafes. This gives the Dutch government a certain amount of credibility when it warns about the dangers of hard drugs, such as cocaine and heroin, in the opinion of one American observer.[96] (Cocaine and heroin smugglers face lengthy prison terms in Holland if caught.) Indeed, he quotes a Dutch secretary of drug policy who stated that cannabis used to be attractive to young people because it was forbidden; "Our aim was to turn it into an unsensational item." As a result the use of marijuana has dropped from 12% a decade ago to 1%.[97]

The experience of Alaska was somewhat different. Owning small amounts of marijuana for personal use was decriminalized in 1975. (Marijuana is no longer legal in that state, beginning March 3, 1991.) Health sciences professor Bernard Segal found in a 1988 study of school-age children in Alaska that marijuana had "become well incorporated into the life style of many adolescents" and that it could no longer be considered an experimental drug for them. Indeed, he found that overall marijuana use among minors rose slightly from 1983 to 1988; in Anchorage, it was 16 percentage points above the national average. The good news, however, was that during the same period, cocaine use among Anchorage teenagers "declined dramatically," well below national rates, according to a separate study by the Anchorage school district.[98] This fact has been suggested as evidence that people seem less inclined to use the more addictive cocaine when marijuana is easy to obtain.

Do you think the use of drugs, legal or illegal, is permissible for medical or other purposes provided the drugs are not addictive or harmful? Consider the following:

- *Support of illegal gangs:* If you buy an illegal drug such as marijuana, you may be helping to support a criminal organization whose other antisocial activities may run from tax evasion to corrupting officials to bringing terror to people who threaten its business. (How would you like to go hiking in a national park and step in a steel trap protecting a marijuana farmer's illegal patch?)

- *Damage to self and friends:* You run the risk of bringing tremendous harm to yourself and your friends if the government finds your drug cache. For example, in March 1991, narcotics agents, determined to show there are "no safe havens" for users of prohibited substances, swept down upon several fraternities at the University of Virginia. They found no cocaine, amphetamines, or other hard drugs, just a small quantity of marijuana and psychedelics. But that was enough for the U.S. Justice Department to seize the three fraternities (under asset forfeiture laws) and charge 11 students with crimes that could keep them in prison for the rest of their lives.[99,100]

Note: Under mandatory federal sentencing laws, judges are no longer allowed to easily deviate from certain sentencing formulas. Thus, a *first-time* offender found guilty of possessing 5 grams of crack cocaine must serve 5 years in prison, with no parole.[101]

4. It's All Right to Use Drugs, Legal or Illegal, No Matter How Addictive, for Medical and Recreational Purposes

Some people may think the government should not be regulating drugs at all, no matter how addictive they are. Or perhaps, they think, the government should regulate drugs for medical uses (as the Food and Drug Administration does), but it has no business outlawing drugs for personal consumption. Either stance is against the official war on drugs.

The war has gone on now for several years. To be sure, there seems to have been progress. According to government studies, the casual use of cocaine and marijuana has declined, particularly among students, the middle class, and the affluent. However, critics say that progress is far slower among the homeless and African Americans and other minorities.[102] And the price of the drug war has been high, not only in money but also in other ways. In the United States, it can be argued, using criminal law to try to reduce demand has caused more harm than it prevents. Among the results:

- *More AIDS cases:* The prohibition on drugs not only prohibits marijuana's being used for medical purposes, as we described above. It also has led to bans on the distribution of clean hypodermic needles to intravenous drug users, who otherwise are apt to transmit AIDS to each other by sharing needles. Other countries, such as Holland, Switzerland, England, and Australia,

have adopted a clean needle policy, but the United States has not. As a result, the number of drug-related AIDS cases jumped from 2000 in 1985 to 14,000 in 1990.[103] In Holland, where clean needles are exchanged for used ones, only 9% of intravenous drug users have AIDS as opposed to 26% in the United States.[104]

- *More homicides:* Drug trafficking—cocaine in the early 1980s, crack in recent years—has played a crucial role in the rise of violent crime. Even as overall drug use has declined, murders have increased, including those of innocent bystanders caught in disputes between rival drug gangs.[105,106]

- *More criminals:* Attempts to shut off the flow of drugs drive up the price of drugs, enrich criminal cartels both at home and abroad, and create economic opportunities for ghetto youth that lure them into the drug trade and a life of violence. As one writer points out, "How do we tell kids with no realistic economic opportunity, 'just say no' to $300 or more a day?"[107]

- *More people in courts and jails:* Drug cases have overwhelmed the criminal justice system, clogging courts, delaying civil cases, and overcrowding jails. For example, in 1990 it was reported that the number of people convicted in state courts of drug-related felonies increased 69% in just 2 years.[108] There are fewer trials on the civil (as opposed to criminal) side because no one can afford to wait.[109] The flood of drug offenders boosted the U.S. jail population to a record 400,000 inmates in 1989—a 77% increase over 1983, the last time a similar U.S. Justice Department study was conducted.[110]

- *Damage to civil liberties:* The confiscation of the three University of Virginia fraternity houses (worth $1 million) as drug-related assets means those fraternity members became rent payers to the U.S. government. Indeed, at that time, the Seized Asset Division of the U.S. Marshals Services held more than 30,000 homes, cars, airplanes, yachts, businesses, and other items.[111] Until seizure of drug assets was blocked by the

Supreme Court in 1993, civil liberties were rapidly being eroded, with valuable property being taken by the government for minor offenses. Similar threats still exist with urine testing of innocent employees, airport and train-terminal searches based on supposed profiles of drug couriers, and more frequent police targeting of low-income blacks and Latinos for searches and arrests.[112–114] Even the Postal Service and the Defense Department have been forced to enter aggressively into the drug-interdiction effort.[115,116]

- *Damage to foreign relations:* In our relations with Latin American countries, points out one writer, the American war on drugs has had the appearance of the real thing.[117] Troops invaded Panama in December 1989 to bring Manuel Noriega to justice for allegedly being a drug trafficker, although reportedly private drug cartels took over narcotics trading afterward.[118] U.S. Marines engaged smugglers on the Mexican border. In Peru and Colombia, U.S.-backed military interdictions may have driven peasants (who can make eight times as much from coca as any other crop) to support leftist guerrillas. Some believe the military option is misguided, and it might be better to help Latin American farmers grow other crops besides coca and to develop their rural economies.[119]

- *Erosion of drug-treatment programs:* Although the budgets for the drug war have been rising, most of the money has been spent on law enforcement. Meanwhile, drug treatment programs in the United States have been neglected and have been eroding for more than a decade, according to medical and drug treatment experts.[120] Some people believe federal spending priorities should be reversed, so that 70% of federal funds are spent on treatment, education, prevention, and research instead of law enforcement.[121]

Many people would take the preceding evidence as reasons for legalizing illicit drugs. Calls for legalization have come from all points on the political spectrum: conservative writer William F. Buckley and economist Milton Friedman and former Secretary of State George Shultz on the one hand and liberal former U.S. Attorney General Ramsey Clark and American Civil Liberties Union director Ira Glasser on the other. What do you think?

Should Illicit Drugs Be Legalized?

Professor Stephen Jay Gould points out that our current drug crisis arises from having arbitrarily divided a group of nonfood substances into two categories—namely, substances purchased legally for supposed pleasure, such as alcohol; and illicit drugs. "The categories were once reversed," Gould writes. "Opiates were legal in America before the Harrison Narcotics Act of 1914; and members of the Women's Christian Temperance Union, who campaigned against alcohol during the day, drank their valued 'women's tonics' at night, products laced with laudanum (tincture of opium)."[122]

Should we erase these differences? The arguments *in favor* of legalization are suggested by the current problems described above. Many advocates of legalization qualify their endorsement in various ways. Drugs should be made off-limits to children. Drugs should be *decriminalized* rather than simply legalized: the use of addicting substances would be declared not illegal and the price, quality, and distribution would be strictly controlled by the government; drugs would not be commercialized, as are beer and cigarettes today.[123] Because there might be a rise in the number of users and addicts under this system—nobody knows how many—education and treatment programs should be expanded.

The arguments *against* legalization are suggested by the following questions about legalization: What products would be for sale? How would they be sold—through private shops or state-run stores? Would taxes be imposed? Would advertising be allowed? Would legalizing drugs multiply the deaths of adults and, in particular, infants? Is it morally right to make dangerous drugs *more available* to everyone? After all, alcohol use soared when Prohibition was repealed in 1933, and it would be expected that the demand for drugs would climb as the market price fell.[124] Wouldn't legalization, like that in Britain in which heroin addicts are required to register with the government, simply represent a transfer from the dependency on illegal drugs to a dependency on the government's drugs? What about the fact that the effects of heroin are short-lasting (6 hours), and crack even less so (15 minutes); wouldn't addicts have to live near a dispensary?[125] Even Britain abandoned experiments with heroin maintenance because it proved difficult to stabilize legally registered addicts on heroin. (It now uses methadone, as the United States does in treatment for heroin addicts, because a methadone dose, while similar to heroin in many ways, lasts 24 hours and so is easier to manage.)[126]

When all is said and done, you have to decide for yourself. Does prohibiting substances really limit their availability? Think how easy it is for minors now to get cigarettes and alcohol. Might confiscating a driver's license for drunken driving improve the drinker's behavior? Maybe you know people who have lost their licenses and simply continue to drive anyway—but they drive carefully because they are worried about getting caught.[127] Finally, consider that ultimately the solution to the drug problem rests not so much with *supply* as with *demand:* the solution is not with restriction or availability but rather within ourselves.

"The most profoundly important truth about drugs," says one commentator, Charles Murray, "is not that drugs are evil but that drugs are unsatisfying."[128] This is the reason, he suggests, why drug use has dropped among the middle and upper classes. For those whose lives are limited to a drab and despairing existence in the streets compared with the unattainable and glamorous life shown on the television screen, drug use may stop when other options appear that give them the opportunity to make their lives satisfying. What do you think?

Nutrition and Weight Management

In These Chapters:

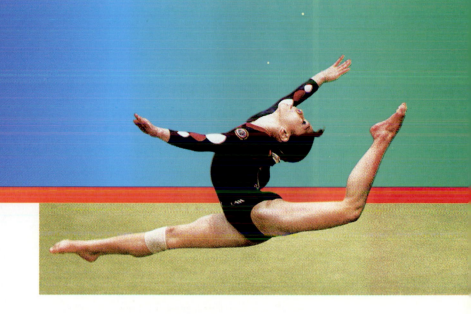

Don't eat this. Don't drink that. Do more of this, do less of that.

We are beset by conflicting messages influencing how and what we eat. Some of these messages seem to be unhealthy, such as the dazzling advertising campaigns urging us to greater consumption of wonderful-taste, awful-nutrient foods. Some of the messages seem to be healthy, such as the advice offered by recognized scientists and health experts—but the trouble is, *their* advice often seems to be contradictory:

- One expert says cholesterol levels should be kept low to avoid heart disease. Another says the level of cholesterol in your blood doesn't seem to matter.

- One week decaffeinated coffee is heralded as healthy. The next week we're told it raises cholesterol levels.

- One study says moderate alcohol use may help prevent heart disease. Another says it may elevate the risk.

What, then, are we to believe?

15 Right Eating for Right Living

▶ What nutrients and other substances does food consist of?

▶ Explain the two types of carbohydrates; the types of protein and fat; their uses; and the best sources for each. Discuss some of the controversies about sugar, sugar substitutes, fiber, protein, and vegetarianism and about fat and heart disease and cancer.

▶ Explain the different types of vitamins and minerals, their uses, sources, and controversies about megadoses, vitamin C, and sodium, and the importance of calcium, iron, and fluoride.

▶ Describe the uses and sources of water and controversies about tap water versus bottled water and water substitutes.

▶ Discuss recommended nutrient and energy intakes; how to read food labels; and controversies over additives, irradiation, and processed versus "organic" food; and the basic food groups.

▶ Discuss guidelines for healthful eating.

Perhaps, like one out of five Americans, you know you could improve the way you eat but feel it's just too much work and sacrifice to do anything about it.[1] After all, it's hard to give up favorite foods or to keep track of the kinds or amount of food you eat. Or perhaps, like so many of us, you're confused by all the dietary advice: there's *so much* information about how to eat that it's difficult to keep it all straight.

Despite messages from the media reporting on nutritional controversies and despite conflicting findings from ongoing research studies, a great deal of agreement exists about many aspects of nutritional health. However, the knowledge base about nutrition is continually evolving. Nutrition scientists may not be united on everything, but then what fields are free from disagreement?

. In addition, there *is* a consensus of nutritional advice, and it is based on two things: (1) studies from *available data,* and (2) the *probabilities* suggested by that data.

Although the data presently in our possession may suggest certain conclusions, other data may surface to change those conclusions. Moreover, the present state of knowledge allows us only to suggest probabilities: certain health and lifestyle habits *probably* will produce well-being and longevity. However, there can be no guarantees: only the uninformed and misinformed can make guarantees.

Since eating is something you will do all your life—and since what you eat has a major impact on your health and well-being—you might as well become good at it. Eating right will not extend your life beyond what your heredity has determined, but it can help you live a healthier and more active life. In the following pages we try to help you make sense of some of the nutritional controversies so that you can make positive choices about what you eat.

What Food Is: Nutrients and Other Substances

Food consists of six essential nutrients for the body's growth and maintenance: carbohydrates, proteins, fats (lipids), vitamins, minerals, and water. Energy-yielding nutrients, measured in Calories, are carbohydrates, proteins, and fats. In addition, food consists of nonnutrients, microorganisms, additives, and other chemicals. Foods rich in nutrients are said to have "high nutrient density."

Our bodies are constantly changing. Enzymes may last hours, hormones only minutes. Both must be renewed, and the only way to do that is by eating food. **Food** is that material—solid, liquid, or both—that you take into the body and that provides the *nutrients* you need to keep yourself alive. Besides nutrients, food contains other substances, including nonnutrients, microorganisms, and contaminants. Processed foods may also include additives, such as added colors or nutrients. Some of these other substances give the food flavor, odor, and texture. Some are helpful, some detrimental, and some of no benefit to human beings but also of no harm.

Let us describe food according to three principal categories:

- *Essential nutrients*—carbohydrates, proteins, fats, vitamins, minerals, and water.
- *Energy-yielding nutrients*—carbohydrates, proteins, and fats.
- Other food substances—nonnutrients, microorganisms, environmental toxins, and additives.

The Essential Nutrients **Nutrients** are the substances obtained from food that the body uses to promote its maintenance, growth, and repair. Some nutrients are called essential nutrients. In nutrition, the word **essential** means a substance that the body requires for growth and maintenance but cannot make by itself in amounts sufficient to meet its needs. Thus, **essential nutrients** are those chemicals your body needs to promote its growth, maintenance, and repair but that it cannot make itself and must obtain from food.

How many essential nutrients do you think you need just to survive? Fifteen? One hundred and fifteen? In fact, present research suggests that the number of essential nutrients is just . . . 46. (There is some dispute about this, but this seems to be the figure accepted by most scientists.) These 46 essential nutrients, none of which can be produced by our own bodies, fall into six major categories: *carbohydrates, proteins, fats* (also called *lipids*), *vitamins, minerals,* and *water.* (See ● *Figure 15.1.*) Any single mouthful of food will contain something from at least one major category.

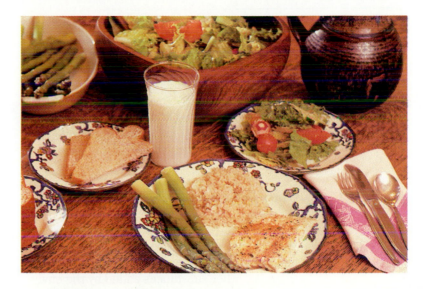

Categories of essential nutrients	Major food sources
1. Carbohydrates	Cereals, fruits, milk, some vegetables
2. Proteins	Meats, fish, legumes, nuts, eggs, dairy products, cereals
3. Fats (lipids)	Fats, oils, meats, fish, dairy products, some seeds & nuts
4. Vitamins	Variety of foods
5. Minerals	Variety of foods
6. Water	Liquids and water-containing solid foods

● **Figure 15.1 The essential nutrients**

Energy-Yielding Nutrients and Calories
Three of the six categories of essential nutrients—carbohydrates, proteins, and fats—are **energy-yielding nutrients.** They yield energy when they are used (oxidized or burned) by the body for movement, heat, or growth. Some may also be stored in the body for later use.

Energy is defined as the capacity to do work. The cells in our bodies can survive only with a fairly constant and adequate supply of energy. The energy potential of food is measured in units of heat called *Calories:*

- *Calorie* (*kilocalorie*): A **Calorie** (capital *C*), actually **kilocalorie** (abbreviated **kcalorie**), is a measure of the heat potential of food. The technical definition is that a Calorie is the amount of heat required to raise the temperature of 1 kilogram of water 1 degree Celsius.

- *calorie:* The word **calorie** (no capital *C*) is one-thousandth of a *Calorie* (*kilocalorie*).

You can hardly escape the word *calorie;* it is one of the major themes in current food advertising ("Low in calories!"). Most adults in the United States and Canada consume between 1500 and 3000 Calories a day. To give you an idea what that means in food, consider the restaurant luncheon plate once advertised as the "dieter's special": ground sirloin, cottage cheese, and tomato slices. Depending on the sizes and quantities, that meal could well generate up to 730 Calories—nearly half of some people's daily needs!

Other Food Substances A bite of food contains many naturally occurring substances called nonnutrients. (An order of scrambled eggs, for instance, consists of 15 chemicals that are naturally present in food.) In addition, there are other substances added by the environment, by food producers, or during food processing.

Some of the substances found in food include nonnutrients, microorganisms, environmental toxins, and additives:

- *Nonnutrients:* **Nonnutrients** are not required by the body for its growth, maintenance, and repair, but some may serve other healthful purposes. An example is *fiber,* found in plant foods, which is so avidly promoted in conjunction with whole-grain breads and breakfast cereals. One type of fiber serves the purpose of helping digestion and elimination, but it is not in itself required by the body. *Alcohol* is another example of a nonnutrient. It does not help the body with growth or maintenance, but it can contribute energy in the form of empty Calories. Other examples of nonnutrients are naturally occurring chemicals that provide the color, odor, and flavor of food.

- *Microorganisms:* **Microorganisms** are molds, fungi, and bacteria. These also occur naturally if a food is stored long enough to develop them or under conditions that encourage them. Some of these microorganisms are desirable; indeed, we would not have yogurt, cheese, or wine without them. Others are undesirable, such as salmonella, which causes food poisoning. Still others, like botulism, are lethal.

- *Additives:* **Additives** are various chemicals that may be added during food production to change color, to enhance flavor, or to en-

sure a longer storage life. One of the oldest known additives is salt. Salt is frequently used as a preservative.

- *Environmental toxins:* Food contains naturally occurring toxic agents. However, as a result of human carelessness, high levels of **environmental toxins,** certain contaminants, have crept into some foods. Examples are mercury in fish and lead in water. Even radioactive particles are found in some foods, such as those that appeared in the milk supply throughout Europe after the 1986 Chernobyl nuclear reactor calamity in the Soviet Union sent radiation skyward.

Nutrient Density An important concept in selecting foods is **nutrient density.** This is a *measure of the nutrients provided per Calorie of food.*

Suppose two people go out to dinner and have two different kinds of meals, both of which provide the same number of Calories of energy. The first person has a dinner that is low in fat and high in carbohydrates—fish, vegetables, and nonfat milk. The second person has a meal high in fat—from red meat, sour cream, butter, and blue cheese salad dressing. The first meal is considered to have a *higher nutrient density* because it provides several more essential nutrients relative to Calories taken in. Thus, paying attention to nutrient density enables people to control their caloric intake while obtaining an adequate diet.

In general, the more unprocessed a food is—that is, the more it resembles its farm-grown origin or natural state—the higher its nutrient density. The more it is processed, with sugar, salt, and fat added, the lower its nutrient density. Thus, the Calories produced by a baked potato (which is unprocessed) are of a higher nutrient density because they deliver more vitamin C (among other nutrients) than the equivalent number of Calories produced by potato chips (which are processed). Some processed foods are practically *nutrient-empty.*

Now let us take a closer look at the six essential nutrients: carbohydrates, proteins, fats, vitamins, minerals, and water.

Carbohydrates: Energy Providers

Carbohydrates provide energy, help elimination, aid fat metabolism, allow protein to do its work, and provide energy for nerve tissue. Derived mostly from plants, carbohydrates are either simple (sugars) or complex (starches and fibers). Half our daily energy should come from carbohydrates, preferably complex. Sugar has few benefits, fiber has many.

The principal nutritional function of carbohydrates is simple: to provide energy. Indeed, carbohydrates usually satisfy half of a person's energy needs.

Types of Carbohydrates: Simple and Complex The class of nutrients known as **carbohydrates** are of two types: *simple carbohydrates* and *complex carbohydrates.* (See ● *Figure 15.2.*)

Simple carbohydrates provide the body with short-term energy and consist mainly of *sugars.* They are found primarily in fruits, maple sugar, honey, corn syrup, and molasses. Simple carbohydrates include two kinds of sugars:

- *Monosaccharides:* The **monosaccharides,** or "single sugars," are the basic units into which most carbohydrates break down and include the common sugars *glucose, fructose,* and *galactose.*

- *Dissacharides:* The **dissacharides,** or "double sugars," include the sugars *sucrose, lactose,* and *maltose.*

Types of carbohydrates	Common food sources
SIMPLE CARBOHYDRATES	
Monosaccharides (single sugars)	
Glucose (dextrose)	Fruits, honey, molasses, maple sugar, traces in most plant foods
Fructose	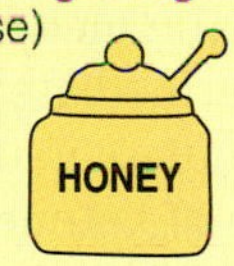 Honey, fruits, berries, corn syrup, traces in most plant foods
Galactose	Found mainly as lactose (milk sugar)
Disaccharides (double sugars)	
Sucrose	Table sugar, fruits, maple sugar
Lactose	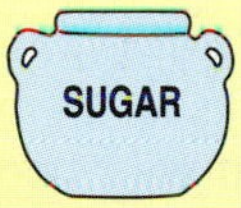 Milk and other dairy products
Maltose	Sprouted seeds; produced in digestion of starch
COMPLEX CARBOHYDRATES (POLYSACCHARIDES)	
Starches and dextrins	Starchy plants, grains
Glycogen	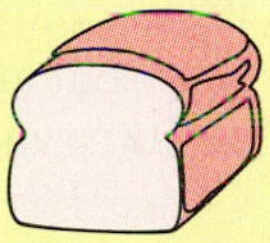 Liver (in very small amounts)
Fiber	
Cellulose	Wheat bran, part of plant-cell walls, whole-grain products
Hemicellulose	Part of plant-cell walls
Pectins and gums	Fruits, oat bran, legumes

● **Figure 15.2 Carbohydrates.** Foods containing carbohydrates

The monosaccharide *glucose* (also known as dextrose or "blood sugar") is *the* central carbohydrate. Why is it more important than any other carbohydrate? The answer is that glucose is your body's main energy source. If you don't get glucose from carbohydrates in the food you eat, your body will have to start using fat and protein to make the glucose. Diverting the body's fat and protein this way in order to provide energy is not, as we shall see later, a way you want to try to lose weight. Glucose is found, in greater or smaller amounts, in nearly all plant foods. In peaches, for instance, it makes up about 10% of total sugars; in cherries, it is 53%.

The **complex carbohydrates** provide the body with sustained (rather than short-term) energy and may be thought of as principally being *starches.* Complex carbohydrates are found mainly in fruits and grains and in the seeds, roots, stems, and leaves of vegetables. Complex carbohydrates are **polysaccharides** (*poly-* means "many"), very large molecules made of hundreds or even thousands of monosaccharides linked together. The polysaccharides include *starches and dextrins, glycogen,* and *cellulose.*

Sugars are sweet. *Starches and dextrins* (which are formed from starch) are not. Starch is found in cereals and other plant foods: grains, legumes (peas, peanuts), tubers, nuts, and seeds.

Whether simple or complex, most carbohydrates come from plants. An exception is the complex carbohydrate *glycogen,* which is found only in animal tissue, such as oysters or liver. Glycogen in the body is mobilized to provide glucose for the body's cells, such as the muscle cells.

Cellulose, the woody part of a plant, provides the structural framework of plants. Cellulose molecules cannot be broken down by human digestive enzymes (although they can be digested by bacteria that *reside* within the human digestive tract), and so glucose from this source is unavailable for energy use. Nevertheless, cellulose is important as a *fiber.*

Different plants have different kinds of fiber. Fibers are found in the walls and skins of plants, the peels of fruits, and the outer layer—called the **bran** layer—of whole grains. They are also found as *pectin,* a water-soluble fiber, in some fruits, such as apples, and vegetables and gums from some tropical plants. By and large, vegetables have more cellulose and fruits have more pectin.

The Uses of Carbohydrates Carbohydrates have several functions in the body.

- *They are a major source of energy.* As mentioned, the principal function of many carbohydrates—sugars and starches, although not fiber—is to provide the body with energy. Each gram of carbohydrate, whether from sugar, spaghetti, milk, pizza, apple, or some other source, yields 4 Calories of energy.

- *They stimulate movements of the gastrointestinal tract and aid in elimination.* The kinds of carbohydrates popularly known as fiber or "roughage" provide little energy. They do, however, function as "nature's broom." That is, they absorb water, thus stimulating peristaltic movements in the gastrointestinal tract. (**Peristalsis** consists of involuntary intestinal contractions that move food along.) Thus, fiber acts as a "natural laxative."

- *They aid fat metabolism.* Some carbohydrates are essential for the biochemical process of turning fat into energy. Without carbohydrates, the metabolism of fat is diverted, and intermediate products called **ketones** accumulate in the blood. Excessive production of ketones produces **ketosis,** which results in dehydration and loss of energy.

- *They allow protein to do its work.* Protein has its own tasks in the body, as we shall see. However, if your body is short on carbohydrates, protein will be diverted to the task of energy production. An adequate carbohydrate intake means that proteins can perform their primary and most useful work. To spare protein and prevent ketosis, we need at least 100 grams of carbohydrate each day.

- *They provide energy for nerve tissue.* Carbohydrates are a source of glucose, a chemical that is an indispensable source of energy for nerve tissue. A constant supply of glucose is therefore needed and can be obtained from the food, from the body's stores, or from the conversion of other compounds.

Controversy: How Bad Is Sugar? People have always liked sweets—there is evidence that 3000 years ago people chewed sugar cane for its sweet taste—but sweets were not always as readily available as they are now. Today Americans eat about 128 pounds of sugar per person per year—more than three times as much as a century ago.[2] More than 70% of this is sucrose—table sugar—found in processed foods of all kinds.

Two problems with sugar consumption have been suggested—one real, one not.

- *True: It leads to cavities.* Sticky-sweet foods that adhere to tooth enamel make teeth a target for mouth-dwelling bacteria.[3] As these bacteria metabolize sugars in the mouth, they produce acids that gradually destroy tooth enamel. Eventually these lesions become pockets of decay known as tooth **cavities** or **dental caries.** The worst sugar offenders are sucrose and glucose, followed by fructose, maltose, and lactose.

  Three other factors also contribute to the likelihood of developing cavities. First, some people are simply more disposed because of genetic susceptibility; the crystal structure of their teeth may not be strong. Second, children growing up in communities without fluoridated water supplies are apt to have more dental caries than those with fluoridation. Finally, because bacteria continue to produce acid in the mouth for about 20 minutes after each last swallow, people who eat frequently expose their teeth to more bombardment with cavity-producing acid.

- *False: It produces "sugar blues"—hypo-glycemia—in some people.* The condition that results when blood glucose concentration falls too low is called **hypoglycemia,** or low blood sugar. Once called "sugar blues," hypoglycemia was thought to occur in some people when the pancreas reacted to the consumption of simple carbohydrates, such as sugar. It was believed the pancreas produced so much insulin—the hormone that regulates how the body uses sugar—that blood sugar levels plummeted. The idea of a sugar-hypoglycemia link is as much a myth as that sugar causes criminal behavior.

The notion that eating sugar can cause diabetes is a myth. Actually, the cause of diabetes can be two problems: insufficient insulin produced by the pancreas or an increased insensitivity by body cells to the presence of insulin.[4]

Controversy: Are Sugar Substitutes Safe? If too much sugar is a problem, could better health result from using sugar substitutes? In the last two decades, an array of artificial sweeteners has come on the market that have accounted for sweeping changes in food products. Many of these are called *high-intensity sweeteners,* because their sweetness is so much more intense than sucrose. For example, *saccharin* is 500 times as sweet as sucrose. (*See ● Figure 15.3.*) Why the craze for such sugar substitutes?

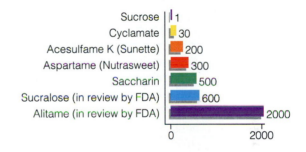

Sucrose	1
Cyclamate	30
Acesulfame K (Sunette)	200
Aspartame (Nutrasweet)	300
Saccharin	500
Sucralose (in review by FDA)	600
Alitame (in review by FDA)	2000

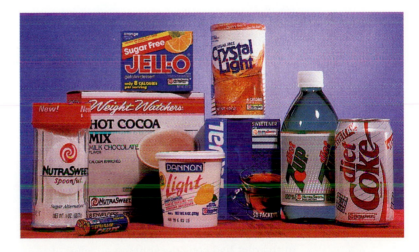

● **Figure 15.3 How sweet it is.** Sweetness ratings of high-intensity sweeteners

The answer: they provide more taste for fewer Calories. Our national obsession with weight loss and being slim continues to fuel an interest in low-Calorie foods.

But are such artificial sweeteners safe? The answer is yes. Consider:

- *Saccharin:* Approved for use in more than 80 countries, saccharin is stable in a variety of products under extreme processing conditions. Because many people detect a bitter aftertaste when saccharin is used in high concentrations, some products, such as Sweet 'N Low, contain saccharin modified with other ingredients, such as dextrose and cream of tartar. The Food and Drug Administration has found saccharin safe for use in a variety of foods, although it has been tentatively linked to bladder cancer in laboratory rats.[5]

- *Aspartame:* Saccharin yields no Calories, whereas aspartame (marketed under the brand name NutraSweet) produces 4 Calories per gram. However, since aspartame is 300 times sweeter than sucrose, only tiny amounts are used. Some questions have been raised about whether aspartame poses health risks, such as headaches or seizures.[6] However, the present evidence suggests it is safe. (The exception is for individuals suffering from *phenylketonuria.*)

Controversy: The Fervor over Fiber You can survive without fiber in your diet, for it is not an essential nutrient. However, in recent years the importance of fiber began to be recognized when it was argued—though by no means proved—that the lack of "roughage" in the diet might be linked to gastrointestinal disorders common in North America and Europe.

You need only scan the cereal and bread shelves in a supermarket to see how food manufacturers have jumped on the fiber bandwagon. Numerous claims have been made in the wake of a 1970 medical report by a British physician that nations with large amounts of dietary fiber in the diet had considerably fewer cases of colon cancer and intestinal diseases. Some of the health benefits of fiber consumption are believed to be the following:[7]

- *Fiber diminishes the risk of colon cancer.* It has been hypothesized that, because of

the water-holding capacity of dietary fiber, the contents of the intestine move along faster. Consequently, cancer-causing substances spend less time in the colon.

- *Fiber diminishes diverticulosis.* **Diverticulosis** is a condition in which the intestinal wall develops outpouchings called *diverticula.* Fiber may exercise the muscles of the intestinal tract so that these pockets are less likely to develop.

- *Fiber reduces constipation and hemorrhoids.* **Constipation** is the condition of hard, dry, and sometimes painful bowel movements. **Hemorrhoids** are swollen, hardened veins in the rectum often caused by the pressure resulting from constipation. Fibers attract water into the digestive tract, thereby softening the stools and easing pressure on the bowel.

- *Fiber helps to keep weight down.* Foods containing dietary fiber are low in fat, and their bulking effect in the stomach helps to ease hunger and give a sense of fullness, thus aiding weight-loss efforts.

But does fiber lower cholesterol? Can it prevent gallstones? Does it help to manage diabetes by affecting blood glucose? Unfortunately, we do not yet know the impact of fiber on these health problems.

Strategy for Living: Getting the Right Kind of Carbohydrates For people in the United States and Canada, the problem is not so much getting the right amount of carbohydrates as getting the right *kind.* We tend to eat too much sugar and sweeteners and not enough grain products, fruits, and vegetables. It is recommended that people get at least half their Calories from carbohydrates, eat more foods with starch and fiber, and consume less sugar. (*See* ● *Figure 15.4.*)

Protein: Of Prime Importance?

Protein is important to the structure of the body, helps growth and maintenance, regulates body processes helps build important compounds, and provides a source of energy. Protein consists of amino

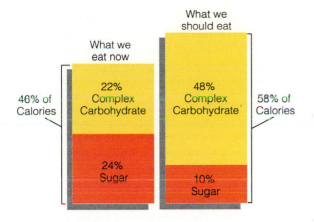

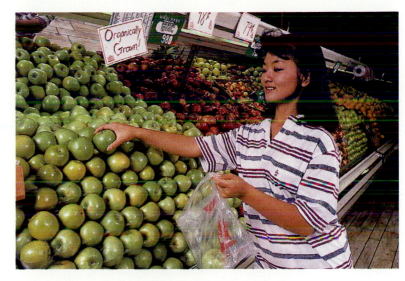

● **Figure 15.4 How much carbohydrate should we eat?** We are advised to increase our intake of complex carbohydrates—starch and fiber—and decrease our intake of sugar.

acids—9 are essential and derived from the diet; 11 are nonessential and are made by the body. Most people get too much protein or too little of the right kind. Too much protein can lead to increased body fat, obesity, calcium loss, and dehydration.

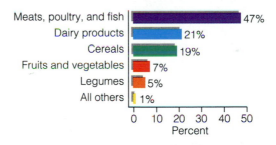

● **Figure 15.5 Sources of protein in the United States.** Most Americans get their protein from meats and dairy products— both sources often high in fat.

Think of all those ads showing steak on the barbecue, the chicken being taken from the oven, the roast on the dining room table. Consider how many meals are planned with meat or fish or fowl—in a word, *protein*—as the central dish. When you picture prime rib, think of the words "of prime importance"—that is the meaning of the Greek word (*protos*) from which *protein* is derived.

Is protein, in fact, really more important than other nutrients? Many people in North America seem to think so. No wonder the average middle-aged American man eats 60% more protein than is required and the middle-aged woman 25% more. No wonder infants and children in the United States consume about twice the protein they need. Even many athletes erroneously think that beefing up means, literally, eating beef.

Indeed, in the United States, nearly two-thirds of the protein in our diet comes from meat (including poultry and fish) and dairy products, although there are acceptable alternatives, such as pasta, beans, and peas (legumes). (*See ● Figure 15.5.*) Unfortunately, some meats and dairy products are also high in fat: ground beef, for instance, may be more than 20% fat.

The Types of Proteins: Essential and Nonessential Amino Acids **Proteins** comprise thousands of different combinations of amino acids. **Amino acids,** which are building blocks found in all living things, are of two types, essential and nonessential:*

- *Essential:* The nine **essential amino acids** are indispensable to life and growth and must be supplied by the diet. In general, you need to get protein that will give you the *nitrogen* you need so that your body can synthesize its own amino acids.

- *Nonessential:* The eleven **nonessential amino acids** are the ones the body can manufacture itself—assuming you are eating an adequate diet in general.

The Uses of Protein Your body contains, on average, 24 pounds (11 kilograms) of protein. Although two-fifths of it is in your muscles, it is a constituent of every cell in your body.

Protein has some important purposes:

- *It provides structure, growth, and maintenance in the body.* Protein gives the body structure and helps it grow. Maintenance of the body is an ongoing activity. For instance, the types of protein making up the wall of that hardworking organ the intestine must be replaced every 4 to 6 days.

- *It affects and regulates body processes.* Protein is important in affecting and regulating several body processes. Specifically, it helps provide **enzymes,** catalysts that help speed up chemical reactions in cells, and **hormones,** substances produced in one part of the body that affect processes in another part. It also helps defend against infection, maintain water balance and mineral balance, and affect the generation and transmission of nerve impulses.

- *It helps build some important compounds.* Protein helps the body manufac-

ture such compounds as **hemoglobin,** which carries both oxygen and carbon dioxide in the blood; substances that are responsible for blood clotting; and substances that transport nutrients into tissues.

- *It provides a backup source of energy.* Many people think protein provides energy. Indeed, like carbohydrates and fats, protein can be metabolized for energy, providing 4 Calories per gram of protein. However, here is an important fact to know: *the body first uses carbohydrate and fat for energy.* Protein in the body is used for energy only when a person (1) has eaten more protein than the body needs (the excess protein is often stored as fat) or (2) is starving and there is not enough carbohydrate and fat in the diet to meet the body's energy needs.

Thus, we might agree the Greeks were right: protein *is* of prime importance.

Controversy: What's So Bad About Too Much Protein? While many people in the world struggle just to get food, let alone enough protein, in industrialized countries the problem is quite the opposite. In North America, we suffer from the results of *overindulgence* in our diet. Recommended protein intake is about 15% of Calories consumed. The health consequences of taking in protein well above the recommended nutritional levels—more than twice as much, for the average American—can be quite serious:

- *Extra protein leads to more body fat.* If you take in more Calories of protein than you need, you will convert extra protein to body fat. Interestingly, the process of converting extra protein into fat requires more energy than converting *fat* into fat.

- *Meat and dairy products can produce high fat intake.* Protein-rich foods tend also to be high-fat foods, which can lead to problems with weight control and obesity. Moreover, people who tend to have diets high in meat and dairy products often eat less from other food groups: vegetables, fruit, and fiber. Of course, if you get most of your protein from non-animal sources, fat may not be a problem.

- *Too much protein may produce a loss of calcium.* This point is still debatable, but

*The nine *essential* amino acids are histidine, isoleucine, leucine, lysine, methionine, phenylalanine, threonine, tryptophan, and valine. The eleven *nonessential* amino acids are alanine, arginine, asparagine, aspartic acid, cysteine, glutamic acid, glutamine, glycine, proline, serine, and tyrosine. One essential amino acid you may have heard of is *tryptophan.* Tryptophan, which is contained in milk, may promote sleepiness—which is why folklore suggests that drinking warm milk before bedtime may help you sleep.

some researchers believe that if your dietary protein intake is more than twice the recommended dietary allowance (over 112 grams of protein for men, 88 grams for women, on the average), it can lead to calcium loss, because the protein causes an increase in the excretion of calcium. The loss of bone calcium ultimately can lead to *osteoporosis*—that is, decrease of bone mass—in older adults, as we describe later.

- *High protein consumption can lead to dehydration.* If you consume a lot of protein, you also need to consume a lot of water. Indeed, protein requires about *seven times* more water for metabolism than does carbohydrate or fat. The reason is that excess protein is broken down into amino acids, which, when used for energy, also produce urea. Urea is excreted in the urine. This explains why high-protein weight-loss diets and high-protein athletic programs— neither of which are recommended—stress that you must drink a lot of water. If you don't, you may be in danger of dehydration and consequent fluid imbalance.

Controversy: Vegetarian Diets Popular singers Michael Jackson and Madonna are vegetarians. So are track star Edwin Moses and actress Daryl Hannah. There is really nothing unusual about a diet that does not include meat. Indeed, 2 billion people in the world are vegetarians, 10 million of them in the United States. Some have been influenced by the Eastern religions such as Hinduism and Buddhism, which emphasize reverence for life and thus prohibit eating of meat. Others follow the example of certain Western religions; for Seventh Day Adventists, vegetarianism is recommended, though not required. Some vegetarians do it for reasons of principle or conscience, feeling it is wasteful or abhorrent to slaughter animals. Finally, many people are concerned about health issues, such as dietary cholesterol and saturated fat intake.

People who are nonvegetarians, who eat meat as well as other food, are called *omnivores;* they put few or no restrictions on the meat they eat. Some omnivores, called **semivegetarians,** avoid red meat (meat from four-footed animals) but eat fish and poultry. Vegetarians may be classified as follows, ranging downward in the amount of animal protein in their diets:

- **Lacto-ovovegetarians:** Eat no meat, fish, or poultry, but do eat eggs and dairy products.
- **Lacto-vegetarians:** Eat no eggs, but do eat dairy products.
- **Vegans:** Eat foods of plant origin only.
- **Macrobiotic vegetarians:** After progressing through a series of 10 dietary stages, in which they gradually limit vegetables, legumes, fruits, and nuts, they arrive at a very restricted diet consisting principally of grains (perhaps rice only). *At its extreme, this diet is unsafe.*
- **Fruitarians:** Eat fruits, nuts, honey, and olive oil. *This diet is definitely unsafe.*

Vegetarians such as vegans, who avoid all foods of animal origin, including milk and milk products, may find themselves short on certain amino acids, unless they plan their food intake carefully and eat complementary proteins. For instance, they may lack lysine, which is not found in grains, and methionine, which is missing in legumes. The solution, then, is to apply the **principle of complementation,** which means that two or more plant foods are eaten together—and *at the same time* (this is important for chemical reactions to take place)—in order to provide the essential amino acids needed by the body. Thus, combining corn (a grain) with beans (a legume) will provide both methionine and the lysine. This is why a Mexican meal of corn tortillas and refried beans is a successful complementary protein combination.

Complementary protein combinations generally involve *legumes plus grains* or *legumes plus nuts and/or seeds.* (See ● *Figure 15.6.*) Some other complementary protein combinations well known in North America are peanut butter on whole-wheat bread sandwiches, macaroni and cheese, pizza, and (in the southern United States) rice and black-eyed peas.

Vegetarians must also take care to avoid other deficiencies. Most important are shortfalls of vitamin D, riboflavin, and calcium (especially for children). Women of childbearing age must be careful to get enough iron. Zinc and iodine deficiencies are possible as well. A potentially serious problem for vegans, who eat no animal protein at all, is a deficiency of vitamin B_{12}.

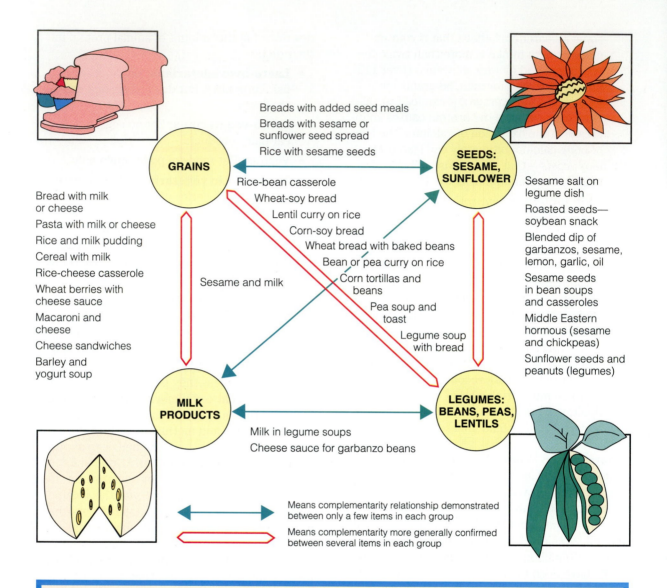

Breads with added seed meals
Breads with sesame or
sunflower seed spread
Rice with sesame seeds

GRAINS

**SEEDS:
SESAME,
SUNFLOWER**

Rice-bean casserole
Wheat-soy bread
Lentil curry on rice
Corn-soy bread
Wheat bread with baked beans
Bean or pea curry on rice
Corn tortillas and
beans
Pea soup and
toast
Legume soup
with bread

Bread with milk
or cheese
Pasta with milk or cheese
Rice and milk pudding
Cereal with milk
Rice-cheese casserole
Wheat berries with
cheese sauce
Macaroni and
cheese
Cheese sandwiches
Barley and
yogurt soup

Sesame and milk

Sesame salt on
legume dish
Roasted seeds—
soybean snack
Blended dip of
garbanzos, sesame,
lemon, garlic, oil
Sesame seeds
in bean soups
and casseroles
Middle Eastern
hormous (sesame
and chickpeas)
Sunflower seeds and
peanuts (legumes)

**MILK
PRODUCTS**

**LEGUMES:
BEANS, PEAS,
LENTILS**

Milk in legume soups
Cheese sauce for garbanzo beans

Means complementarity relationship demonstrated
between only a few items in each group

Means complementarity more generally confirmed
between several items in each group

● **Figure 15.6 The great peanut-butter sandwich and other complementary proteins.** People who
don't eat animal proteins must ensure they have enough meals in which legumes are combined with either grains or with nuts and/or seeds in order to provide essential amino acids.

With careful planning to provide adequate amino acids, vitamins, and minerals, a vegetarian diet can be safe and produce health benefits by reducing obesity and high cholesterol levels. The key to success in being a vegetarian can be summed up in one word: diversity. When any group of foods is eliminated from the diet, special care must be taken to ensure that nutrient requirements are met from alternate foods.

Strategy for Living: Getting the Right Kind of Protein In general, the more Calories one takes in a day, the more protein. Most of us, however, don't need to take in more protein. Increased amounts of protein are needed only for the following: pregnant women, to help the growth of the fetus; lactating women, to help manufacture milk for breast-feeding; infants and children, to help them with the development and growth of bones and tissue; and people recovering from malnutrition or injuries, whatever their age.

For the rest of us, what's important to realize is not how *much* protein we eat but *what kind*. The finest quality sources of essential amino acids are foods of animal origin. Plant foods are low in one or more of the essential amino acids. However, this does not imply that a meatless diet is a deficient diet. After all, many people in the world do not eat meat, and in some countries such as India a major part of the population is vegetarian. Moreover, protein-rich foods such as meat and dairy products are not only more expensive than cereals, fruits, and vegetables but are also higher in fat content—which leads to the third of the six categories of nutrients.

Fat: What Good Is It?

Fat provides energy, body protection, and essential fatty acids and carries vitamins A, D, E, and K. Fatty acids, the basic chemical units of fat, may be saturated (harmful in excess), monounsaturated (mostly beneficial), or polyunsaturated (both). How hard a fat is at room temperature tells you how saturated it is, but the presence of fat in food is sometimes not obvious. High levels of cholesterol, considered harmful, are found only in foods of animal origin.

Fat makes food taste good—makes it more palatable, flavorful, juicy. No wonder the sound of a steak sizzling or the aroma of bacon cooking is enough to stimulate the appetite. No wonder so many people—perhaps yourself included—prefer a hamburger that is 30% fat rather than the lean ground meat containing 5–10% fat. (*See Self Discovery 15.1.*)

However, if we are to believe what the researchers tell us, nearly everyone holds these truths to be self-evident: "Eating fatty foods is bad." "They make you put on weight." "They may lead to heart disease and cancer." Despite these sentiments, most people in the United States and Canada don't practice what is preached. On the average American adults currently consume about 36% of their total

SELF DISCOVERY 15.1

How Do You Score on Fat?

Do the foods you eat provide more fat than is good for you? Answer the questions below, then see how your diet stacks up.

How often do you eat:	Seldom or never	1–2 times a week	3–5 times a week	Almost daily
1. Fried, deep-fat fried, or breaded foods?	____	____	____	____
2. Meats such as bacon, sausage, luncheon meats, and heavily marbled steaks and roasts?	____	____	____	____
3. Whole milk, cheese, and ice cream?	____	____	____	____
4. Desserts such as pies, pastries, and cakes?	____	____	____	____
5. Cream sauces and gravies?	____	____	____	____
6. Oily salad dressings or mayonnaise?	____	____	____	____
7. Whipped cream, table cream, sour cream, and cream cheese?	____	____	____	____
8. Butter or margarine on vegetables, dinner rolls, and toast?	____	____	____	____

What the Results Mean

If you checked several responses under "3–5 times a week" or "Almost daily," you may have a high fat intake. It's time to cut back on foods high in fat, starting today.

Source: Adapted from *Home and Garden Bulletin*, no. 232–3 (April 1986), pp. 1, 8. Published by Human Nutrition Information Service, U.S. Department of Agriculture.

Calories from fat—including 13% from saturated fat. However, most health authorities recommend limiting fat to about 30% of our total intake and some experts suggest even less.[8]

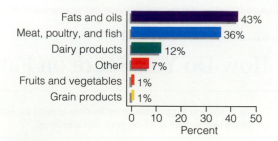

Fats and oils 43%
Meat, poultry, and fish 36%
Dairy products 12%
Other 7%
Fruits and vegetables 1%
Grain products 1%

Percent (0 10 20 30 40 50)

● **Figure 15.7 Sources of fat in the U.S. diet.** Contribution of different food groups to the fat content in the American diet

Most of us know what fat is. Some obvious dietary sources are butter, margarine, shortening, cheese, and salad dressings. Fat also comes from the "marbling" (white streaks) in meat such as steaks and from chicken and turkey skin, ice cream, and baked products. (*See* ● *Figure 15.7.*)

Types of Fat: Saturated, Monounsaturated, Polyunsaturated What we commonly just call "fat" may be divided into **fats,** which are solid fatty substances at room temperature (such as a cube of butter), and **oils,** which are fats in liquid form (such as corn oil). Both are called **lipids,** the general term for fatty substances.

When people talk about fats, they tend to use some specialized terms. Some of these words are already part of the vocabulary of food merchandisers: "Low cholesterol!" "No saturated fats!" "High in *unsaturated* fats!" Let us clarify what these phrases mean.

There are several types of lipids (*fatty acids, triglycerides, cholesterol,* and *phospholipids*); however, here we are principally concerned with fatty acids. **Fatty acids** are the basic chemical units of fat. Fatty acids are of two types—*saturated* and *unsaturated. Un-*saturated fatty acids in turn are of two types—*monounsaturated* and *polyunsaturated.* (*See* ● *Figure 15.8.*) Let us see what these three kinds of fatty acids (or simply "fats") look like.

- *Saturated fats:* **Saturated fats,** which are considered harmful if eaten in excess, generally come from foods of animal origin—meat, milk, and cheese—although they also come from palm and coconut oil. Research shows that saturated fat elevates blood cholesterol, an indicator for high risk of heart disease in some people.

- *Monounsaturated fats:* **Monounsaturated fats,** which are largely beneficial, come from foods of both animal and plant origin, such as peanut butter, many margarines, and olive oil.

- *Polyunsaturated fats:* **Polyunsaturated fats** (or *polyunsaturated fatty acids,* abbreviated *PUFAs*) may be both good and bad—good for a healthy heart but possibly bad in that they have been implicated in the development of breast cancer.[9] Polyunsaturated fats come from vegetable oils, such as safflower, soybean, and corn oils, and from some fish.

Two forms of beneficial polyunsaturated fats are particularly important:

1. **Omega-3 fatty acids,** found in fish oils, Chinook salmon, and albacore tuna, may decrease the risk of heart and blood-vessel disease and cancer.

2. **Omega-6 fatty acids,** found in plant oils such as corn and peanut oil, are important for growth.

We said that the basic chemical units in fats are fatty acids. Most (95%) of the fats and oils in our bodies and in our foods consist chemically of three fatty acids joined to a molecule of glycerol to make a type of fat known as **triglycerides.** The significance of triglycerides is this: according to some research, high triglyceride levels in people's blood may be a warning that a person is at risk for cardiovascular (heart and blood) vessel disease, the No. 1 killer disease in the United States.

Cholesterol Another kind of fat, which appears in the class of fats and oils known as sterols, is that often-mentioned substance cholesterol. One point should be clarified that confuses many people—the word *cholesterol* has two meanings:

Type of fat	Food source	Effect on heart	Effect on breast
Saturated fats	Meat Milk Cheese Butter Egg yolk Vegetable shortening Coconut and coconut oil	Bad 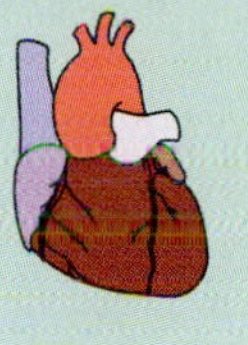	Bad
Unsaturated fats			
Monounsaturated fats	Peanut butter Peanuts and peanut oil Olives and olive oil Avocado Cashews Many margarines	Good	Good 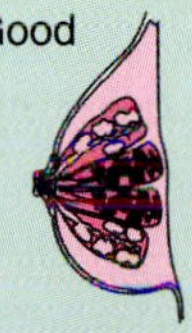
Polyunsaturated fats	Fish oils Corn oil Safflower oil Soybean oil Albacore tuna Chinook salmon	Good	Probably bad

Figure 15.8 Fat. Foods containing fat. Saturated fats have been implicated in both heart disease and breast cancer, polyunsaturated fats in breast cancer but not heart disease.

- *Dietary cholesterol is found in food.* **Dietary cholesterol** is a type of fat found principally in eggs (actually egg yolks) and in organ meats such as liver. It is not found in foods of plant origin, such as fruits and vegetables.

- *Serum cholesterol is produced by your body.* **Serum cholesterol,** or **blood cholesterol,** is a compound produced by our own bodies. It is needed to form bile acids (which aid in the digestion and absorption of fats), hormones (such as sex hormones), cell membranes (which selectively allow the entry and exit of materials), and other body substances.

High blood cholesterol levels have been implicated in heart disease, as we will describe. *It is important to note that the most significant factor in food that affects blood cholesterol is saturated fat, rather than dietary cholesterol.*

The Uses of Fat Does fat do you any good? Surprisingly, considering its negative image, the answer is yes—at least in reasonable amounts. Besides making food more palatable and satisfying, fat does the following:

- *It provides energy.* There is one area in which fat is better than carbohydrate and protein: it delivers more energy. Indeed, a gram of fat provides more than twice as much energy (9 Calories) as a gram of either of the other two major nutrients (only 4 Calories). When carbohydrate, protein, and fat are consumed beyond body needs, they are stored as fat. This assures that we are able to provide our body with a constant supply of energy without having to eat constantly. The disadvantage, however, is that because fat is the most efficient way to consume a lot of Calories, this ease of consumption can be a problem if the energy is not needed. If we are not physically active, the fat ends up being added to our waistlines, abdomens, or hips.

- *It provides body protection and insulation.* If you ever take a long-distance bicycle trip, you'll be glad you have fat on your body. Fat protects your internal organs from shocks and bruises. It also provides insulation against extremes in outside temperature and holds in your body heat. Indeed, one consequence of extreme weight loss is that a person feels cold all the time. (The reverse of that, however, is that very overweight people are less comfortable in hot weather.)

- *It provides essential fatty acids.* A needed substance is declared "essential" if our bodies can't make it at all or can't make it at a rate sufficient to meet our needs. For example, if for some reason you had no fat at all in your diet, you would be missing at least one essential nutrient, the fatty acid known as linoleic acid. If you did not get linoleic acid as a child, your growth would be below normal. If you go several months without it as an adult, your skin will become scaly and you will experience higher than usual water loss through it.

- *It carries fat-soluble vitamins.* Some fat in the diet is needed to enable you to more easily absorb what are known as fat-soluble vitamins—vitamins A, D, E, and K—all of which are carried in fat.

- *It provides building materials for several important compounds.* Along with proteins, fats provide the primary structure of all membranes in cells. Fats also form compounds that help blood clotting and form complex molecules that make up part of our brains.

Controversy: Fat, Cholesterol, and Heart Disease Heart disease kills more Americans than all other causes of death combined— about one person every minute, or half of all deaths. There are several risk factors for heart disease, including smoking, heredity, lack of exercise, personality characteristics, and more, as we discuss elsewhere in the book. Here, however, we describe the possible link of heart disease with diet—particularly fat.

What is it we mean when we say "heart and blood-vessel disease"? Impairment of the heart and blood vessels is called **cardiovascular dis-**

ease. When the impairment is so severe that it interrupts the blood flow, it may cause either of two life-shattering events:

- *Heart attack:* A **heart attack** is the consequence of impaired blood flow to the heart muscle, depriving the heart of oxygen and nutrients and eventually killing the tissue.

- *Stroke:* A **stroke** is the interruption of blood to the brain, resulting in the death of brain tissue.

Several factors can cause these events, including the appearance of a blood clot, which obstructs the flow of blood through blood vessels. The blockage may come about because of the collection of fatty material, cholesterol, and other matter on the inside of a blood vessel. Although it is not entirely clear what role fat and dietary cholesterol play in heart and blood vessel disease, all the major health agencies support reducing these substances in our diet.

Controversy: Fat and Cancer Studies of laboratory animals suggest that fat in the diet can raise the risk of certain cancers, particularly cancers of the breast, colon, and prostate. Other evidence comes from **epidemiological** studies—that is, comparisons of various human populations.[10] For example, until recently the Japanese have not been exposed to the fat-heavy diet found in the United States, and cancers of the breast, colon, and prostate—so common in Americans—have been less commonly found among the Japanese. Interestingly, however, the children and grandchildren of Japanese immigrants to Hawaii and California reportedly have breast cancer rates similar to those of white Americans and significantly higher than those of native Japanese. In addition, since 1949, there has been a dramatic increase in deaths from breast and ovarian cancers in Japan. At the same time, there has been a change in the Japanese diet, with more consumption of fat, animal protein, and American-style foods such as ham, sausage, butter, and dairy products.[11]

Can we say, then, that a Westernized, fat-heavy diet causes cancer? Not necessarily, for the Japanese are also heavy smokers. Yet the United States and Canada show correlations between consumption of fat and cancer deaths. For example, since 1900 in the United States, the intake of fats, both animal and vegetable, has gone up by 40%, and rates of breast, colon, and prostate cancer have gradually increased.[12]

Still, the correlation between cancer and diet remains controversial because cancer rates in other countries have been similar to U.S. rates despite varying levels of fat consumption.

Controversy: Do Fish Oils Reduce Heart Disease? Once upon a time, traveling medicine shows peddled snake oil as a cure-all for people's ills. More recently, to look in the windows of some health-food stores, you might think the cure-all being peddled is fish oil.

Following the discovery in the 1960s that Greenland Eskimos had low rates of heart and blood vessel disease *despite* a high-fat diet, researchers began to explore the possibility that fish and fish oils offer healthful properties. Eskimos have been found to eat an average of three-quarters of a pound of fish a day, whereas Americans eat only 13 pounds a year.[13] A closer look at the fish intake by Eskimos revealed that polyunsaturated fats called omega-3 fatty acids in the fish oil changed the chemistry in the blood and reduced the risk of heart disease.[14] A 20-year study of 852 middle-aged men found that those who ate an ounce of fish a day had half the rate of heart disease of men who ate little or no fish. Moreover, the more fish these men consumed, the less they were apt to suffer fatal heart attacks.[15]

How do fish oils accomplish this? Research shows that apparently they alter the relationship between "bad" and "good" cholesterol (called lipoproteins). That is, they lower the "bad" cholesterol, which blocks arteries, and possibly raise the "good" cholesterol, which reduces such blockages. In addition, certain fish oils produce substances that make the blood less likely to clump together and form clots. They also reduce triglycerides, which have been implicated in heart disease.[16]

Fish-oil supplements have become a popular item in health-food stores. However, it takes many pills, perhaps 15–20 a day, to get the blood-cholesterol-lowering effects that the Eskimo studies have shown. Of significant concern is the unknown long-term effects of omega-3 fatty acids. In addition, the anti-clotting effects could be potentially dangerous. Rather than taking fish-oil supplements, consider simply increasing the number of servings of fish in your weekly diet.[17]

Strategy for Living: Getting the Right Kind of Fat Different foods have different amounts of fat. In general, fat is low or nonexistent in fruits, vegetables, and grain products and high in foods of animal origin. Unfortunately, the presence of fat in foods is not always obvious. That is, a lot of fat is *invisible.* If you really want to reduce the amount of fat in your diet, you need to know how to identify sources of invisible as well as visible fat.

- *Visible fats:* Visible fats are fairly easy to spot: they are almost anything greasy—butter, margarine, shortening, and cooking and salad oils.
- *Invisible fats:* Invisible fats are harder to identify, although nowadays people in North America get more fats from this source than from visible fats. The major sources of invisible fats are meat, poultry, fish, and dairy products.

Fat is frequently added during the preparation of food. If you often eat at restaurants, remember that fat is frequently used in the preparation and presentation of food. Examples are fried foods, butter on baked potatoes, foods in cream sauces, or anything deep-fried in batter. Order foods that are broiled or baked. Ask to have sauces and dressings served on the side. Ask questions if you are not sure about how a dish is prepared.

When shopping for food, read labels to help you identify products with fat added. When cooking, avoid fried foods and cream sauces. Also avoid using cooking oils; use nonstick pans or a spray instead. Remove the skin from chicken before cooking. Some dishes can be cooked ahead of time, chilled so that fat can be skimmed off the top, and then reheated in a microwave when ready to serve.

Vitamins: Mighty Micronutrients

There are 13 known vitamins, four of which are fat-soluble (A, D, E, and K) and nine of which are water-soluble nutrients (eight B-complex vitamins and C). Vitamins put major nutrients to use in the body, help growth, and maintain many body activities. To ensure adequate vitamin intake, eat a variety of foods. Avoid vitamin supplements. Megadosing is not advised.

Vitamins are organic substances derived from animals and plants. Vitamins work primarily by facilitating the action of enzymes in the body to enable the use of other nutrients. We frequently hear that we can get all the vitamins we need from a balanced diet. Yet at the same time the media are filled with messages about the importance of vitamin supplements and "vitamin-enriched" foods. Which interpretation is correct? We consider this question in this section.

First we need to distinguish between macronutrients and micronutrients:

- *Macronutrients:* A **macronutrient** is a food substance that is generally required in large quantities every day—2–5 grams or more. (A gram is 0.035 ounce.) Generally speaking, we need carbohydrates, proteins, and fats in macronutrient quantities.

- *Micronutrients:* A **micronutrient** is an organic compound that is essential in very small (trace) amounts every day and that does not supply energy. *Vitamins* and *minerals* (such as iron and calcium, discussed in the next section) are micronutrients.

Although vitamins are derived from animals and plants, they are not always usable in the form in which they are consumed. Some need to be converted from **precursors**—compounds that are not nutrients but from which a nutrient can be formed. Vitamin precursors are called **provitamins.** For example, a substance known as beta carotene is the provitamin for vitamin A.

Types of Vitamins: Fat-Soluble and Water-Soluble To look at the ads from a vitamin store you might think there are hundreds of vitamins.

Actually, there are just 13 on which experts can agree, and they are classified as *fat soluble* and *water soluble.* (See ● *Figure 15.9.*)

- *The only fat-soluble vitamins are A, D, E, and K.* They are called **fat-soluble vitamins** because they are just that: soluble in fat. **Soluble** means they can be dissolved. Fat-soluble vitamins, then, are absorbed into the body through the intestinal membranes with the aid of fats in the diet or bile produced by the liver. Cooking makes some fat-soluble vitamins more available to the body, but overcooking reduces the availability of these substances.

  In addition, a significant fact about fat-soluble vitamins is that you do not have to consume them every day—unless your diet is unbalanced—because the vitamins are stored in your liver. Fat-soluble vitamins are found in fatty foods: meat, fish, dairy products, vegetable oils. In addition, certain precursors (called carotenoids) are found in green and yellow vegetables.

  An important characteristic of the fat-soluble vitamins, especially A and D, is that, because they are stored in the body, they can build to toxic levels if you consume too much of them. People who take exceptionally large doses (megadoses) of vitamins risk toxicity or unpleasant side effects.

- *The water-soluble vitamins include the eight B-complex vitamins and vitamin C.* The eight B or B-complex vitamins were so named because they were originally thought to be one vitamin. Scientists several years ago gave up identifying the B's numerically, and they now go principally by names other than letter names: *thiamin, riboflavin, niacin, pantothenic acid, folacin, biotin,* and *vitamin B_6* and *vitamin B_{12}.* Vitamin C, the other water-soluble vitamin, is also called *ascorbic acid.*

  The chief characteristic of **water-soluble vitamins** is that they do not need fat or bile to be absorbed by the body. Moreover, the body has only small reserves of them— hence, such vitamins are more perishable. In general, you should take in these vitamins every day (for example, drink a glass of orange juice for vitamin C), since they are constantly disappearing from your body in urine and sweat.

Fat-soluble vitamins
Vitamin A
Vitamin D
Vitamin E
Vitamin K
Water-soluble vitamins
B-complex vitamins
Thiamin
Riboflavin
Niacin
Pantothenic acid
Biotin
Vitamin B$_6$
Folacin
Vitamin B$_{12}$
Vitamin C

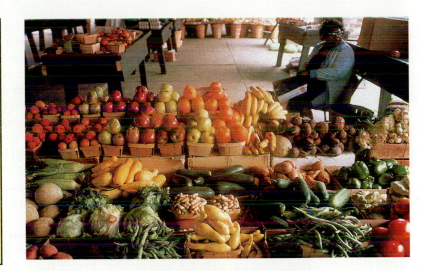

● **Figure 15.9 The vitamins**

In addition, because the eight B vitamins and C are soluble in water, they may be washed out or disappear during food processing, preparation, or storage. If you overcook green beans, for instance, you destroy vitamins. If you pour out the cooking water, you pour out the vitamin C with it. Vitamin pills or capsules are also likely to become less powerful after sitting on a shelf or being exposed to light or air.

The Uses of Vitamins Vitamins perform many tasks, as follows:

- *They help macronutrients release energy.* Some vitamins aid carbohydrates, proteins, and fats in the metabolism of the body by helping to release energy.
- *They help growth.* Some are involved in the formation of cells, bones, and teeth.
- *They help regulate body functions.* Some act with the enzymes in the body to help regulate chemical functions. Some help maintain eye function, neuromuscular function, and blood clotting.

By discovering the function of each vitamin, scientists have been able to determine how to treat disorders resulting from too little or too much of a vitamin. Too little vitamin D, for instance, will produce poor bone formation, resulting in a bone deformity called rickets in children. Too much vitamin D retards growth and damages kidneys. However, not all disorders are reversible with vitamin therapy. For instance, the blindness caused by a vitamin A deficiency cannot be cured.

Controversy: Is Vitamin C a Miracle Vitamin? Before the mid-1700s, the voyages of British ships could not last longer than 3 months, because crews on long trips often experienced **scurvy,** the devastating effects of a vitamin C deficiency. Scurvy is a particularly gruesome, painful disease that is ultimately fatal. It is characterized by severe weakness, bleeding gums, painful joints, loss of teeth, and damage to bone and muscle. In 1747, a British naval surgeon discovered that eating oranges and lemons, which were later found to contain vitamin C, would prevent scurvy. In a few years, ships' stores routinely included citrus fruits such as limes, as a result of which British sailors came to be known as "limeys." Vitamin C is also known as **ascorbic acid;** *ascorbic* means "without scurvy."

Some people today have attributed special powers to vitamin C. Indeed, Americans take vitamin C more often than any other vitamin. In 1970, Linus Pauling, twice winner of the Nobel Prize (for chemistry and for peace), suggested that high doses of vitamin C would help fight the common cold.[18] Taking megadoses of 1–3 grams—or even up to *10 grams*—a day, Pauling asserted, would prevent colds or diminish cold symptoms. Numerous studies have failed to demonstrate this, but the sales of vitamin C supplements show the continuing belief in this idea.[19]

People have taken extra doses or megadoses of vitamin C for other reasons as well—to try to alleviate stress, allergies, arthritis, and diabetes and to reduce blood cholesterol levels. Unfortunately, the vitamin does not seem to be the miracle drug that will do these things. Some scientists think that vitamin C builds the body's defenses against cancer or that it prolongs the survival rate of cancer patients, but this, too, has not been confirmed.[20–22]

Controversy: Do Megadoses Work? The term **megadose** refers to a vitamin dose that is more than 10 times the recommended dietary allowance (RDA). The problem with megadoses is that they are often either wasteful or dangerous. Megadoses of water-soluble vitamins (the B's and C) are wasteful because they are simply flushed out rapidly by the body, and thus they don't stay around long enough to provide long-term results, as fat-soluble vitamins do. On the other hand, fat-soluble vitamins (A, D, E, and K) are dangerous because they can build up to toxic levels when taken in megadoses.

In the past, because vitamin C is water-soluble and rapidly excreted, people assumed that the risk of toxicity was low. But that was back when people thought of megadoses in terms of several hundred milligrams a day rather than *grams* a day. An intake of 5–10 grams a day is another matter. Such huge megadoses can cause diarrhea, kidney stones, gout, iron overload, and burning sensation during urination. Nevertheless, if you decide to take extra vitamin C—say, several hundred milligrams rather than grams a day—you should be aware that there is no need to take pills. You can obtain this amount by including many vitamin C-rich vegetables and fruits in your diet.

Another instance of the "more is better" idea occurred in the 1980s, when vitamin B_6 became the vitamin of the decade. Some studies implicated vitamin B_6 deficiency in premature aging of the brain, in *premenstrual syndrome* (characterized by depression, mood swings, water retention, sore breasts, fatigue, and other symptoms), *"Chinese restaurant syndrome"* (characterized by burning sensations, chest and facial flushing, pain, and other adverse reactions to the flavor enhancer monosodium glutamate, or MSG, used in Asian cooking), and other problems.[23–25] However, it is irresponsible for anyone to treat—or self-treat—these disorders by giving megadoses of vitamin B_6 without first having their symptoms assessed by a health care professional. More importantly, people who take megadoses (200 milligrams or more) of B_6 report numbness in the hands, difficulty walking, and other symptoms.[26]

Strategy for Living: The Best Sources of Vitamins Health writer Jane Brody points out that vitamins are required in such tiny amounts that all the vitamins you need together add up to about *an eighth of a teaspoon a day.*[27] Indeed, over a year's time, the recommended dietary allowance for vitamin C, for instance, is only about 22 grams—less than an ounce. In theory, healthy adults consuming the average requirement of 2000–3000 Calories of food a day should get all the vitamins they need, particularly in North America, where a variety of foods are available, including vitamin-fortified cereals and breads. Indeed, extreme vitamin deficiency in the United States is rare. But some Americans and Canadians simply don't eat enough of the right foods, or they have special nutritional needs. In particular, these individuals include the elderly, pregnant or nursing mothers and their infants, those in low-income families (particularly children), cigarette smokers, alcoholics, and users of certain legal and illegal drugs.

The best way to get the amount and kinds of vitamins you need is by eating a variety of foods. (*See* ● *Figure 15.10.*) You cannot rely on vitamin pills or vitamin-fortified foods (such as breakfast cereals) to make up for faulty nutrition. Nevertheless, let us consider vitamin supplements.

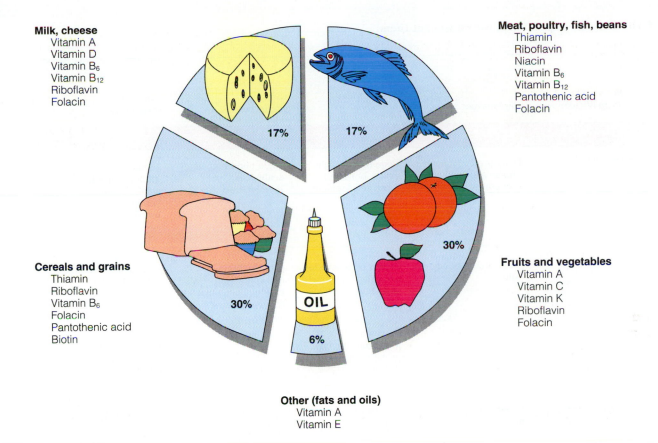

Milk, cheese
Vitamin A
Vitamin D
Vitamin B₆
Vitamin B₁₂
Riboflavin
Folacin

Meat, poultry, fish, beans
Thiamin
Riboflavin
Niacin
Vitamin B₆
Vitamin B₁₂
Pantothenic acid
Folacin

Cereals and grains
Thiamin
Riboflavin
Vitamin B₆
Folacin
Pantothenic acid
Biotin

Fruits and vegetables
Vitamin A
Vitamin C
Vitamin K
Riboflavin
Folacin

Other (fats and oils)
Vitamin A
Vitamin E

● **Figure 15.10 Best dietary sources of vitamins**

Vitamin supplements are usually found in the form of tablets or capsules, but are also available as powders and liquids for people unable to swallow solid forms. Because water-soluble vitamins cannot be stored long in the body, manufacturers now market them as **time-release supplements,** so that the vitamin is slowly released into the bloodstream over a 6- to 12-hour period. Certain breakfast cereals are also classified as vitamin supplements because they are heavily fortified with vitamins.

Vitamins are organic (rather than inorganic) substances because they contain carbon and are derived from living material. However, health-food enthusiasts sometimes try to promote "natural" vitamin supplements as being somehow better than the synthetic vitamins produced in laboratories. But is vitamin C made from rose hips (a "hip" is the ripened fruit of the rose) better than vitamin C made in a test tube? Actually, your body can't tell the differ-

ence. Moreover, manufacturers of supposedly "natural" vitamins often have to add synthetically derived ascorbic acid (vitamin C) to their tablets because not enough of the chemical can be extracted from a rose hip. Be sure to read the label on the bottle of any vitamin supplements you are considering buying.

In the end, vitamin supplements are not needed or recommended for people who eat a healthy diet. Obtain your vitamins naturally—change your diet rather than opt for vitamin supplementation. Supplementation is not without its risks—it should not be used during the first trimester of pregnancy without the guidance of a physician.

The Food and Nutrition Board of the National Academy of Sciences/National Research Council has established recommended dietary allowances (RDA) and estimated safe and adequate dietary intake for the 13 vitamins. (*See* ● *Table 15.1.*)

● **Table 15.1 Vitamins: What you need, where you get them**

Vitamin	Recommended daily allowance	Best sources	Some known functions	Signs of deficiency	Signs of megadoses
Fat soluble					
A	5000 IU*	Dairy products; liver; orange and deep green vegetables	Required for night vision, bone and tooth development	Night blindness; dry, scaling skin; poor immune response	Damage to liver, kidney, bone; headache, irritability, vomiting, hair loss, blurred vision; yellow skin
D	400 IU	Dairy products, egg yolk	Promotes absorption and use of calcium and phosphorus	Rickets (bone deformities) in children; osteomalacia (bone softening) in adults	Gastrointestinal upset; cerebral, kidney damage; fatigue
E	30 IU	Vegetable oils and their products; nuts, seeds	Prevents cell membrane damage	Possible anemia	May be fatal if premature infants given it in intravenous infusion
K	Not established	Green vegetables; tea, meats	Aids blood clotting	Severe bleeding on injury: hemorrhage	Liver damage and anemia from high doses
Water Soluble					
Thiamin (B₂)	1.7 mg	Dairy products, meats, eggs, enriched grain products, green leafy vegetables	Used in energy metabolism	Skin lesions	
Riboflavin (B₁)	1.5 mg	Pork, legumes, peanuts, enriched or whole-grain products	Used in energy metabolism	Beriberi (nerve changes, sometimes edema, heart failure)	

*IU = International Units. Less accurate than RE values; to be used only until food composition tables are converted to RE values.

Table 15.1 (*continued*)

Vitamin	Recommended daily allowance	Best sources	Some known functions	Signs of deficiency	Signs of megadoses
Water soluble (*continued*)					
Niacin	20 mg	Nuts, meats, and other proteins	Used in energy metabolism	Pellagra, skin disorders, diarrhea	Flushing of face, neck hands; liver damage
B$_6$	2.0 mg	High protein foods in general, bananas, some vegetables	Used in amino acid metabolism	Nervous and muscular disorders	Unstable walk, numb feet, poor hand coordination, abnormal brain function
Folacin	0.4 mg	Green vegetables, orange juice, nuts, legumes, grain products	Used in DNA and RNA metabolism	Gastrointestinal disturbances; a form of anemia	Masks vitamin B$_{12}$ deficiency
B$_{12}$	0.6 mg	Animal products	Used in DNA and RNA metabolism; single carbon utilization	Nervous system damage; some kinds of anemia	
Pantothenic acid	4–7 mg	Widely distributed in foods	Used in energy metabolism	Fatigue, sleep disturbances, nausea, poor coordination	
Biotin		Widely distributed in foods	Used in energy metabolism	Dermatitis, depression, muscular pain	
C	60 mg	Fruits and vegetables, especially broccoli, cabbage, cantaloupe, cauliflower, citrus fruits, green pepper, strawberries	Maintains collagen; is an antioxidant; aids in detoxification; still under intense study	Scurvy (skin spots, bleeding gums, weakness); delayed wound healing; impaired immune response	Gastrotinestinal upsets; possible decreased immunity; interferes with some lab tests

Sources: Adapted from Christian, J. L., & Greger, J. L. (1991). *Nutrition for living* (3rd ed.). Redwood City, CA: Benjamin/Cummings; Hegarty, V. (1988). *Decisions in nutrition.* St. Louis: Times Mirror/Mosby; Whitney, E. N., & Hamilton, E. M. (1987). *Understanding nutrition* (4th ed.). St. Paul: West.

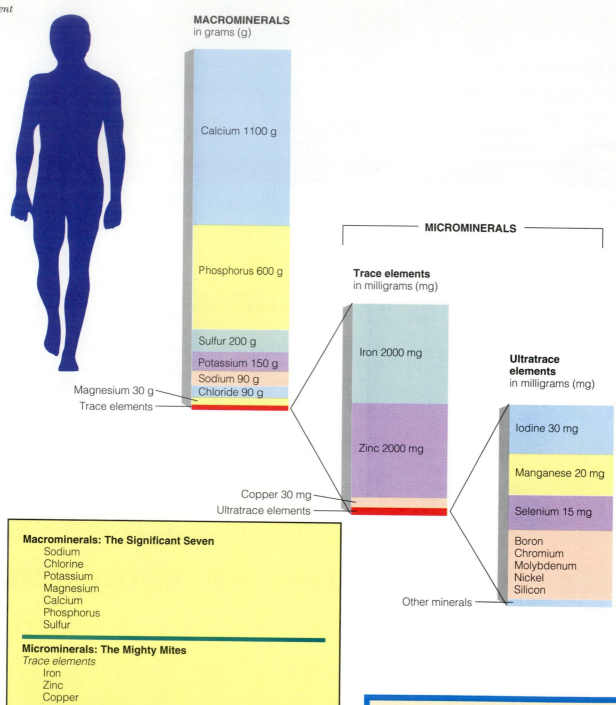

MACROMINERALS
in grams (g)

Calcium 1100 g

Phosphorus 600 g

Sulfur 200 g

Potassium 150 g

Sodium 90 g

Chloride 90 g

Magnesium 30 g

Trace elements

MICROMINERALS

Trace elements
in milligrams (mg)

Iron 2000 mg

Zinc 2000 mg

Copper 30 mg

Ultratrace elements

**Ultratrace
elements**
in milligrams (mg)

Iodine 30 mg

Manganese 20 mg

Selenium 15 mg

Boron
Chromium
Molybdenum
Nickel
Silicon

Other minerals

Macrominerals: The Significant Seven
  Sodium
  Chlorine
  Potassium
  Magnesium
  Calcium
  Phosphorus
  Sulfur

Microminerals: The Mighty Mites
Trace elements
  Iron
  Zinc
  Copper

Ultratrace elements
  Fluoride
  Iodine
  Manganese
  Selenium
  Chromium
  Molybdenum
  Cobalt
  Silicon
  Tin
  Vanadium
  Nickel
  Others: Arsenic, Boron, Bromine, Cadmium, Lead, Lithium

● **Figure 15.11 Macrominerals and microminerals.** This is the approximate mineral composition of a 132-pound (60-kilogram) person. About 50% of a person's mineral composition is calcium and 25% is phosphorus. Values vary depending on bone mass and stores of minerals such as iron. Some ultratrace elements (boron, chromium, and so on) are present in such small amounts that good estimates are not available.

Minerals: The "Significant Seven" and the "Mighty Mites"

Minerals are inorganic substances classified as seven macrominerals (calcium, phosphorus, sulfur, potassium, sodium, chloride, magnesium) and 14 microminerals. Macrominerals help maintain fluid balance in the cells and assist with the growth of bones and teeth. Microminerals—divided into trace elements (iron, zinc, copper) and ultratrace elements (all others)—are essential components of enzymes and help the body handle oxygen. We tend to get too much sodium (salt), but many women do not get enough iron and calcium.

People often think of "vitamins and minerals" as if they were one nutrient group. There are, however, differences between vitamins and minerals. The basic distinction is that vitamins are *organic* compounds; they contain carbon. **Minerals,** on the other hand, are *inorganic.* They are chemical elements *other than* carbon, hydrogen, oxygen, and nitrogen—the "big four" that make up your body. The big four elements constitute 96% of your body weight, and minerals account for the remaining 4%. Nevertheless, minerals are far more important than their proportion suggests.

Types of Minerals: Macrominerals and Microminerals Minerals are classified as *macrominerals* and *microminerals,* organized according to the amounts in the body, from large to small. (*See ● Figure 15.11.*) Microminerals in turn include *trace elements* and *ultratrace elements.* Let us describe these.

- *Macrominerals—the "significant seven":* **Macrominerals** consist of seven elements that should be consumed in amounts *greater than 100 milligrams per day.* These elements are *calcium, phosphorus, sulfur, potassium, sodium, chloride,* and *magnesium.*

   About half of all the minerals you should take in is calcium, about a quarter is phosphorus. The other 25% is distributed among the several other minerals.

- *Microminerals—"mighty mites":* **Microminerals** are minerals for which it is recommended you take in *less than 20 milligrams each day.* There are about 14 microminerals (although there is some disagreement as to that number). Microminerals may be categorized as two types:

  (1) The **trace elements** consist of *iron, zinc,* and *copper.*

  (2) The **ultratrace elements** are all other microminerals, the best known of which are iodine, manganese, and selenium.

The Uses of Minerals As you might suspect, even though some minerals are present in minuscule amounts, their presence is important. Indeed, as we shall describe, their absence or their surplus can cause all kinds of havoc within the body.

Among the tasks the seven *macrominerals* perform are the following:

- *Sodium, chloride, and potassium help maintain fluid balance among the body's cells.* The body is made up of cells that contain water and are surrounded by water. The water in and around the cells contains many dissolved minerals called **electrolytes**—such as sodium, chloride, and potassium—that regulate the distribution of the water.

- *Calcium, phosphorus, and magnesium help build bones and teeth.* The macrominerals calcium, phosphorus, and magnesium also help maintain fluid balance, but they are especially important as builders of calcified tissues—bones and teeth.

- *Sulfur helps form joint lubricants.* Sulfur helps to form lubricants for joints, among several other functions.

Among the tasks the 14 *microminerals* perform are these:

- *They assist enzymes.* Many microminerals are part of enzymes or need to be present in enzymes for them to work. (Recall that enzymes are catalysts that help speed up chemical reactions in cells.)

- *They help the body use oxygen or protect it from oxygen damage.* Many microminerals, such as iron and copper, are involved with helping the body use oxygen. Others

—copper, zinc, and selenium—protect the body against damage by forms of oxygen.

- *They may substitute for other minerals.* Some microminerals may even serve in place of others, albeit temporarily and imperfectly, for certain purposes.

Controversy: Is Sodium Linked to Heart Disease? Next time you find yourself filling up on potato chips or beer nuts, you might want to remember the powerful craving that some people develop for salt, or sodium. In one study, a researcher gave subjects higher than normal levels of salt in their food, or they took salt tablets or **placebos**—nonactive pills that looked like salt tablets but contained no salt, so their principal effect was psychological. The results were telling: only subjects who ate the highly salted foods started to crave more salt.[28]

Human beings' preference for salt seems to result from both innate factors and early experience. For instance, at about age 4 months, infants show a distinct shift from indifference to salt to a preference for it. Children between ages 3 and 6 have been found to prefer salted to unsalted soup—and indeed like it more salty than adults do. Nevertheless, reducing the amount of salt in the diet results in people having less and less a desire for it.[29]

Sodium definitely has important uses. As an electrolyte, it serves to regulate blood pressure; it helps in the transmission of nerve impulses; it is involved in protein and carbohydrate metabolism. Despite its importance, you do not need very much of this mineral. The safe and adequate intake per day for adults is considered to be 1.1–3.3 grams (1100–3300 milligrams). To get an idea what this means, consider that just a teaspoon of salt provides 2 grams of sodium. Most Americans take in 6–18 grams a day—way too much. People in the United States and Canada get most of their sodium from **table salt,** which is 40% sodium and 60% chloride.

In recent years, sodium has received a bad press because of a suspected link between salt-heavy diets and high blood pressure, or hypertension. Hypertension is considered an important risk factor in heart and blood-vessel disease. Although sodium is often restricted for people with hypertension, we now know that controlling blood pressure is more complicated than was previously thought. Some people are not salt sensitive at all. In addition, other minerals (chloride, potassium, calcium), hormones, and other factors also play a role in regulating blood pressure.

Because sodium occurs naturally in some foods and is added to so many others during processing, you generally do not need to add any salt to your food. By and large, there is more sodium in meat than in vegetables and grains. Fruits contain little or no sodium. Many nonprescription drugs also contain significant amounts of sodium.

All About Iron Iron is the body's principal oxygen handler; one of its most important purposes is to transport and distribute oxygen to the cells. Nearly three-quarters of the iron in your body is found in **hemoglobin,** the blood protein, which, apart from water, is the major component of blood. Hemoglobin picks up oxygen inhaled into the lungs and transports it through the bloodstream to the body's cells. Hemoglobin also transports carbon dioxide through the bloodstream to the lungs, where it is exhaled.

An insufficient amount of iron can produce a type of **anemia.** Anemia refers to a decreased oxygen carrying capability of the blood due to reduced numbers of red blood cells or lower than normal hemoglobin levels. In people with iron deficiency anemia, less oxygen is transported to the cells, and carbon dioxide is not removed as efficiently. The result is continual fatigue, lack of appetite, shortness of breath, and cold fingers and toes. School children who are anemic show reduced learning ability, although their achievement test scores go up once iron supplements are administered to correct the deficiency.[30] People who complain of feeling "run down" may suffer from anemia.

Iron-deficiency anemia is second only to obesity as the leading nutritional disorder in the United States. Among children ages 1–3 in low-income families, about 60% have low iron intakes that put them at risk for iron deficiencies. More than three-quarters of women ages 19–34 have low iron intakes.[31]

The adult recommended daily intake for iron is 10 milligrams for men, 18 milligrams for women. The reason it is higher for women is that they experience iron loss during menstruation and childbirth.

Dietary iron can be obtained from both animal and plant sources. The best animal sources are liver—pork liver is best, followed by calf, beef, and chicken liver. Other sources include fish, poultry, red meats, kidneys, and eggs. The best sources from plant foods are dried beans and peas; nuts; green, leafy vegetables; and enriched and whole-grain cereals. People who consume only nonmeat sources of iron should also consume vitamin C (ascorbic acid) in the same meal in which they eat iron because the vitamin C enhances absorption.

Because it is difficult to get more than 6–7 milligrams of iron per 1000 Calories, people who routinely eat only 1200–1800 Calories a day—infants, children, many premenopausal women—may find an iron supplement useful. Pregnant women are routinely advised to take an iron supplement.

All About Calcium Calcium is the most abundant mineral in the body. About 99% of the calcium is found in the bones and teeth. Bones are not like the wood of a dead tree; they are constantly in the process of building or renewal. Among children and adolescents, of course, bones must enlarge as the person grows, but even in adults the nutrients going to the bone must be continually replenished. Calcium and other minerals are delivered via the blood and crystallize around the connective framework of bone.

Many women do not get enough calcium. Among low-income women, between half and two-thirds have low intakes that would put them at risk for calcium deficiencies.[32] This may lead to **osteoporosis**—"porous bones" or "brittle bones" among post-menopausal women. Beginning at age 30 or 40, many women (and some men) lose bone mass because of calcium deficiency. After a while skeletal strength cannot be maintained, and the slightest impact can produce bone fractures. Many elderly women suffer hip fractures (150,000 a year in the United States alone) owing to osteoporosis.[33]

The best dietary sources of calcium are milk and milk products: yogurt, cheddar cheese, ice cream, and cottage cheese. Calcium may also be obtained from eggs, shrimp, sardines, canned salmon eaten with bones, clams, and oysters. Some dark-green, leafy vegetables and citrus fruits are also calcium sources.

For adults, the recommended daily intake for calcium is 800 milligrams; for adolescents, it is 1200 milligrams. Today a man on the average consumes 1143 milligrams of calcium, but many women and adolescents have low intakes. In general, pregnant and breast-feeding women have a higher need for calcium and should take calcium supplements.

Controversy: Who Needs Fluoride? Tooth decay (dental caries) still affects many children and some adults. The 1988 Surgeon General's report recommends that community water systems contain the mineral fluoride (fluorine) at optimal levels for the prevention of tooth decay.[34] If such water is not available, other appropriate sources of fluoride should be used, such as fluoride tablets, especially during the years of primary and secondary tooth formation and growth. Brushing teeth with fluoride-containing toothpaste also helps.

Strategy for Living: The Best Sources of Minerals Despite the number of breakfast cereals and other processed foods that are promoted for their minerals, some believe we are exposed to *fewer* varieties of food than our ancestors were (for instance, most people don't eat bone marrow these days). Consequently, we probably get less exposure to the range of minerals available. If we eat a reasonable diet, most of us probably won't develop mineral deficiencies. However, we also probably won't consume the optimal amounts of minerals. The best source of minerals is a diet that includes a variety of foods. (See ● *Table 15.2.*)

Many people are "at risk" for developing certain mineral deficiencies because of their low intakes over long periods of time. Infants and young children are at risk for not getting enough iron and zinc; so are women of childbearing years. Women in general are at risk for not getting enough calcium. People with low incomes may have calcium and iron deficiencies and also not get enough zinc, which can lead to mental or physical retardation in children. The elderly may have some general mineral deficiencies, owing to past eating habits or physiological changes with age.

● **Table 15.2 Minerals: What you need, where you get them**

Mineral	Recommended daily allowance	Best dietary sources	Some known functions	Signs of deficiency	Signs of megadoses
Major minerals					
Calcium	800 mg	Milk, cheese, dark green vegetables, beans or peas	Aids in bone and tooth formation; blood clotting; nerve transmission	Growth problems; in adults bone loss	Drowsiness; impaired absorption of iron, zinc, manganese
Phosphorus	800 mg	Milk, cheese, meat, poultry, whole grains	Bone and tooth formation; acid-base balance; part of enzymes	Weakness; loss of mineral from bone	Decreased absorption of some minerals
Magnesium	300–350 mg	Whole grains, green leafy vegetables	Part of enzymes; building bones	Neurological disturbances	Neurological disturbances
Potassium	1875–5625 mg*	Meats, milk, many fruits and vegetables, whole grains	Water balance; assists in nerve function	Muscular weakness	Muscular weakness; heart rhythm problem, heart attack
Sulfur		Foods containing protein	Part of cartilage, tendons, and proteins; acid-base balance		Poor growth; liver damage
Sodium	100–3300 mg*	Salt, soy sauce, cured meats, pickles, canned soups and vegetables, processed cheese, frozen meals	Water balance; assists in nerve function	Muscle cramping; appetite decreased	High blood pressure in people genetically predisposed
Chloride	1700–5100 mg*	Salt, many processed foods	Figures in acid-base balance; formation of stomach juice	Muscle cramping; decreased appetite; poor growth	Vomiting

* Estimated safe and adequate daily dietary intake

Sources: Adapted from Christian, J. L., & Greger, J. L. (1991). *Nutrition for living* (3rd ed.). Redwood City, CA: Benjamin/Cummings; Hegarty, V. (1988). *Decisions in nutrition*. St. Louis: Times Mirror/Mosby; Brody, J. (1982). *Jame Brody's nutrition book*. New York: Bantam Books.

Table 15.2 (*continued*)

Mineral	Recommended daily allowance	Best dietary sources	Some known functions	Signs of deficiency	Signs of megadoses
Trace minerals					
Iron	Males: 10 mg Females: 18 mg	Meats, eggs, beans, peas, whole grains, green leafy vegetables	Part of hemoglobin and enzymes	Iron deficiency anemia, weakness, impaired immune function	Acute: shock, death; Chronic: liver damage, heart failure
Copper	2–3 mg*	Seafood, nuts, beans, peas, organ meats	Enzyme formation	Anemia; bone and cardiovascular changes	Liver and neurological damage
Zinc	15 mg	Meats, seafood, whole grains	Enzyme formation	Growth failure; reproductive failure; impaired immune function	Acute: nausea; vomiting, diarrhea; Chronic: adversely affects copper metabolism and immune function
Iodine	150 mg	Marine fish and shellfish; dairy products; iodized salt; some breads	Part of thyroid hormones	Goiter (enlarged thyroid)	Goiter
Fluoride	1.5–4.0 mg*	Drinking water, tea, seafood	Maintenance of tooth (and maybe bone) structure	Increased tooth decay	Mottling of teeth; skeletal deformity
Selenium	0.05–0.2 mg*	Seafood, meat, whole grains	Enzyme formation; works with vitamin E	Muscle pain; maybe heart muscle deterioration	Hair and nail loss
Cobalt		Vitamin B_{12} (animal products)	Part of vitamin B_{12}	Not reported except as vitamin B_{12} deficiency	With alcohol: heart failure
Chromium	0.05–0.2 mg*	Brewer's yeast, liver, seafood, meat, some vegetables	Glucose and energy metabolism	Impaired glucose metabolism	Lung, skin, and kidney damage from occupational exposures
Manganese	2.5–5.0 mg*	Nuts, whole grains, vegetables and fruits	Enzyme formation	Abnormal bone and cartilage	Neuromuscular effects
Molybdenum	0.15–0.5 mg*	Beans, peas, cereals, some vegetables	Enzyme formation	Disorder in nitrogen excretion	Inhibition of enzymes; adversely affects cobalt metabolism

*Estimated safe and adequate daily dietary intake

Water: The Life Fluid

Water acts as a transporter and lubricant and regulates the body's temperature. Water quality varies in many areas. Bottled water may be no better than tap water. Milk is superior to water in some ways, not in others. Soft drinks and coffee provide water but don't advance health. Fruit juices are the best substitute for water.

Think how much we take water for granted. Your morning shower can take 25 gallons, a washing machine load 60 gallons. And how much water does your *body* consume? On average, it is about 2½–3 quarts a day, perhaps 4 quarts if you live in a hot climate and are very active. However, the range is broad: one researcher found it stretched from a pint to 6 quarts daily.[35]

Sources and Losses of Body Water Outside sources of water consist principally of *fluids,* then of *food,* then of *water generated during metabolism* of energy nutrients. (*See* ● *Figure 15.12.*) Let us consider these.

- *Fluids:* About 6 cups (1.5 liters) of water a day come from fluids—not just tap water but also such beverages as soft drinks, coffee, juice, milk, beer, and wine.

- *Foods:* About 2–4 cups of water are acquired from solid foods. Some foods have more water content than others. Pure fats, such as vegetable oils, have none. Lettuce is 95% water, when measured by weight. Meat and fish are more than half water, and bread is a third water.

- *Metabolism:* A small amount of water comes from within the body itself, perhaps 1–2 cups a day. This *water of metabolism* is produced during many chemical reactions in the body and is used in the same ways as water obtained from drinks or food.

Once water has been used by the body, it must be disposed of. This is accomplished mainly in the urine, through the skin and lungs, and in the feces. (*Refer back to Figure 15.12.*)

You can lose water almost without knowing it. On a 3½-hour plane flight, for instance, the dry air in the cabin can cause you to lose up to 2 pounds of water. On a marathon run (about 26 miles), a person might lose up to 10 pounds of water. **Dehydration**—abnormal depletion of body fluids—occurs when not enough water is taken in to compensate for the amount lost. A loss of only 10% of the body's usual water intake can cause severe disorders; a loss of 20% may cause death.

The Uses of Water A newborn baby can be as much as 75% water, by weight. An adult male is 60%, an adult female 55%, with the water located in every part of one's body. Among the functions this "life fluid" performs are the following:

- *It transports nutrients and wastes.* Water helps transport dissolved substances throughout the body—in the blood and in the urine, to name two "waterways."

- *It lubricates.* Water acts as a kind of oil can for the body—a lubricant. As you move your eyes across this page, they are helped by fluids around the eyeballs in their sockets. Fluids in the joints help you bend knees and elbows. In the digestive system, saliva facilitates chewing and swallowing, and digestive juices move food particles through the gastrointestinal tract.

- *It regulates temperature.* Water helps dissipate heat from the body and thereby regulate the body's temperature. Normally, body temperature is around 98.6° Fahrenheit (37° Celsius). If it exceeds the range of about 80°–107°F (37°–42°C), death may result.

There are two ways by which water in the body controls temperature:

(1) *Blood circulation:* About 85% of the body's heat is lost through the skin. When your body begins to gain heat—because of exercise, fever, or the heat of the day—your blood circulates nearer the cooler air on the surface and releases excess body heat to the outside. When you're cold, less blood is circulated beneath the skin, reducing body heat losses.

(2) *Perspiration:* Perspiring (sweating) does not itself cool the body, but the evaporation of water off the skin gets rid of the surplus heat—at least up to a certain point. This suggests why

it is dangerous to exercise when the weather is high in temperature *and* humidity: The high water content of the air will not allow the water on your skin to evaporate. The result may produce **heat stroke,** with body temperatures soaring past 107°F (42°C), which may lead to irreversible cell damage and death.

Controversy: Is Bottled Water Better Than Tap Water? Tap water quality varies in many areas. Since 1908, chlorine has been added to water supplies in the United States to kill disease-causing bacteria and viruses. Nevertheless, contaminants do enter the water supply—whether from decay of vegetation or collection of chemicals from agricultural runoffs and industrial wastes.

Bottled water, many people believe, is healthier than tap water. However, a great deal of bottled water is probably no better than your local tap water, and certainly more expensive. Indeed, the majority of the bottled water sold in the United States and Canada is not natural spring water but simply reprocessed water from local community water supplies. Some bottled waters contain considerable amounts of minerals. The worst of these is sodium, which may raise blood pressure in certain people, thus increasing the risk of heart disease. (*See* ● *Figure 15.13.*)

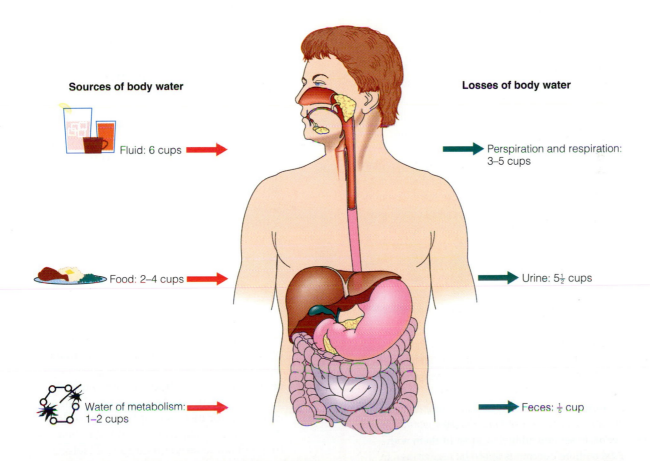

Sources of body water

Fluid: 6 cups

Food: 2–4 cups

Water of metabolism: 1–2 cups

Losses of body water

Perspiration and respiration: 3–5 cups

Urine: $5\frac{1}{2}$ cups

Feces: $\frac{1}{5}$ cup

● **Figure 15.12 Sources and losses of body water**

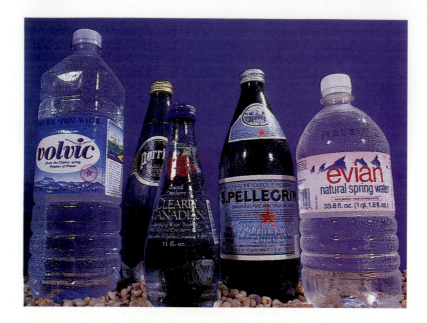

● **Figure 15.13 Types of bottled water**

- **Distilled:** This is simply pure water that has been freed of impurities by evaporation and recondensing. Distilled water is tasteless, which makes it unpalatable to many people. It is frequently used when ironing clothes to avoid leaving stains.

- **Natural spring water:** If the word "natural" appears on the label, it means the water is unprocessed and has come directly from a protected spring. Whether or not a spring water can be called *mineral water* depends on the amount of minerals it contains and the definitions under various state laws. The mineral content varies, but most natural spring waters contain calcium, magnesium, potassium, and sodium. Waters labeled "low-sodium" or "no salt added" must specify the amount of sodium on the label.

  A bottled water is *not* spring water if its label says "spring pure" or "spring fresh." It is simply processed—that is, filtered and sterilized—well water or tap water.

- **Naturally carbonated:** This kind of water is often described as "effervescent" or "sparkling," but it's important that the word "natural" be present on the label, which indicates that the carbonation ("bubbliness") is present in the water at the source.

- **Artificially carbonated:** Water may be artificially carbonated with carbon dioxide, as are club soda and seltzer water. Club soda tends to contain several additives, most of them with sodium; thus, the sodium content is apt to be higher than in other kinds of water. Seltzer, which is filtered three times and then has carbonation added, is low in sodium and has no other additives.

Controversy: Can Other Beverages Replace Water? Water itself is no longer the biggest source of liquid for most of us. Is this a healthy development? Let's consider some of the replacements.

- *Soft drinks:* Today Americans drink more *soft drinks* than they do water. (In 1986, they consumed an average of 30.5 gallons of soft drinks per person.[36]) Most soft drinks contain Calories and no nutrients.

  Although it could be argued that they help the body meet its fluid intake requirements, it's not that simple. During periods of physical growth, when people need all the nutrients they can get, soft drinks may simply displace more nutritious foods. Moreover, because so many have artificial sweeteners and caffeine, they may have some negative effects on health. Finally, the sweetened drinks, at least, don't really quench your thirst: indeed, they actually increase the body's need for water.

- *Caffeine drinks:* Coffee, tea, cocoa, and many cola drinks contain **caffeine,** a mild stimulant that provides the "pick-me-up" property that keeps us awake and alert. However, caffeine is also a **diuretic,** which means it causes you to actually *lose* fluids. Thus, when you drink coffee, you aren't replenishing your body fluids but in fact are further dehydrating yourself.

- *Milk:* There is no doubt that—with the exception of fruit and vegetable juices—milk is the most healthful alternative to water. Milk is high in protein, high in calcium, a good source of riboflavin and (when added as fortified vitamins) the vitamins A and D.

  Despite the milk industry slogans, not Every Body Needs Milk. After the age of 2, a great many of the peoples of the world—two-thirds of them, in fact—are unable to digest the milk sugar lactose. Eighty percent of Asian and Middle Eastern peoples and 70% of African Americans and American Jews, for instance, suffer a great deal of discomfort—gas, cramps, and diarrhea—if they consume large quantities of lactose.[37]

  However, many people can consume small amounts of milk and milk products, particularly with meals, as well as milk products specially developed to meet their needs. The problem with discomfort associated with consuming milk and dairy products is called *lactose intolerance.*

- *Fruit juices and fruit drinks:* Probably the best alternative to plain water is a fruit juice, which is apt to be low in sodium and high in potassium.[38] Oranges and other citrus fruits provide juices with high amounts of vitamin C. (Orange-juice concentrates now account for nearly three-quarters of the orange juice market in the United States.) Tomato juice is a good source of vitamins A and C, and moreover contains only 35 Calories in a 6-ounce glass.

    You must be careful, however, to distinguish between a fruit *juice* and a fruit *drink.* Fruit drinks include fruit juices, but they may also include sugar and usually are not as nutritious because they have been diluted. Still, they do provide water—something many people have trouble getting enough of.

Strategy for Living: Getting the Right Kind of Fluids Do you regularly drink enough water? Most people don't give much thought to this: they just drink when they're thirsty. Although this automatic trigger usually works fairly well, it doesn't always lead a person to replenish the water needed, particularly if one is sick or is performing strenuous physical activity. (Older people are also less likely to feel thirsty.) Indeed, the thirst mechanism may cause only 60–70% of the water needed to be replaced.[39] Thus, it's recommended—particularly if you are physically active—that you drink *beyond* the point of quenching thirst. Any excess water will simply be excreted from the body.

If you are an athlete or otherwise physically active, you should drink fluids not only during and after workouts and competitions but also before. Because the stomach can empty out only about 1 quart of fluid an hour, athletes often sweat faster than their stomachs are able to accept replacement fluids. Thus, to prevent heat disorders, you should drink 2 or more cups of water 2 hours before an event and another 2 cups 15 minutes before. During the activity, depending on how vigorous it is, you should then drink ½ to 1 cup of water about every 15 minutes. Exercise physiologists usually recommend

water rather than sports beverages, such as Gatorade, because sports beverages often have a high concentration of sugar, which tends to keep the fluid in the stomach rather than speeding it to the areas of the body needing replenishment.[40] If sports drinks are used, they should be diluted by adding equal parts water.

In general, to make sure you're getting the water your body needs, nutritionists recommend that you drink at least *six* 8-ounce glasses of liquids a day. *Eight* glasses is even better. An 8-ounce glass is equivalent to 1 cup.

Recommended Nutrient and Energy Intakes: What and How Much Should You Eat?

The RDAs (RNIs in Canada), ESADDIs, and recommended energy intakes state average nutrients and quantities people should consume to maintain good health.

Most developed countries have standards known as *nutrient allowances*—the recommended intakes of nutrients. Here we consider two kinds of allowances that apply in the United States and Canada:

- Nutrient intakes
- Energy intakes

Nutrient Intakes: RDAs (RNIs) and ESADDIs The standards used for expressing nutrient intakes are the *Recommended Dietary Allowances,* or *RDAs* (and their counterpart in Canada, the *Recommended Nutrient Intakes,* or *RNIs*), and the *Estimated Safe and Adequate Daily Dietary Intakes* (*ESADDIs*).

In the United States, the **Recommended Dietary Allowances (RDAs)** state the amount of each nutrient that scientists on the Food and Nutrition Board (a part of the National Research Council of the National Academy of Sciences) believe that healthy Americans should consume—on the average—every day. The latest RDAs appear in the front of this book. (*See Table 1, inside front cover.*) Canada uses the **Recommended Nutrient Intakes (RNIs),** a table prepared by the Department of National Health and Welfare.

Important note: As we shall discuss in the next section, these RDAs *are not the same* as the U.S. RDAs found on many food labels. In addition, the old term "minimum daily requirement," which some people still confuse with the RDA, is no longer used.

RDAs are given for six groups: infants (to age 1), children (to age 10), male adults, female adults, pregnant women, and lactating (breast-feeding) women. Most of these groups are further broken down into different age levels with corresponding average weights and heights.

The RDA table shows the amounts recommended every day for protein and important vitamins (vitamins A and C, for example) and minerals (calcium and iron, for instance). Not all the essential nutrients appear in the RDA table because scientists don't know enough about them to make firm recommendations. Most of the amounts in the table are expressed in metric units:

- **gram (g):** There are about 30 grams in an ounce.
- **milligram (mg):** 1 milligram is a thousandth of a gram.
- **microgram (μg):** 1 microgram is a millionth of a gram, or one thousandth of a milligram.

Estimated Safe and Adequate Daily Dietary Intakes (ESADDIs) are used in the United States to represent a range of "safe and adequate" amounts for nutrients that scientists are less than certain are essential. (*See Table 2, inside back cover.*) Examples are minerals such as biotin, copper, and manganese. Nutrition scientists say the upper levels in the safe and adequate range should not be habitually exceeded, because toxic levels may be reached.

Recommended Energy Intakes Recommendations for *nutrients* and recommendations for *energy* are two different things. The Food and Nutrition Board was concerned that people get enough nutrients—protein, vitamins, and minerals—to maintain good health. Therefore, the requirements are *higher* than necessary. That is, the RDAs for nutrients are actually *overestimates* for the nutrients we really need. Indeed, the RDAs are designed to cover "practically all healthy persons" in the United States; thus, they cover 97.5% of the people in this country.

Recommended intakes for *energy*, as opposed to nutrients, are established in a different manner. (*See Table 3, inside back cover.*) Whereas the recommendations for nutrients (RDAs) address the needs of "practically all" healthy people in the United States, the intakes for energy, as measured in Calories, reflect the *average* (mean) population requirement for each age group. The reason for this difference is that the scientists setting the standard were concerned that establishing an additional RDA allowance to cover individual variations in energy requirements might lead to obesity in a person with average requirements.

Recommended energy intakes are given for average individuals in the same six groups described above for the RDAs for nutrients: infants, children, male adults, female adults, pregnant women, and lactating women. For example, if you are 19–22 years old and a 5′4″, 120-pound female, you should consume an *average* of 2100 Calories a day. A 5′10″, 154-pound male the same age should consume an *average* of 2800 Calories a day. If you are different from this imaginary "average person" in this age group—shorter, taller, lighter, heavier, less active, more active—your daily requirements will vary. Again, the point of these recommendations is to ensure that people get enough food to meet their energy needs without gaining additional weight.

When you sit down to eat, you need not—and probably would not—think about whether you are consuming all the right amounts of nutrients. Indeed, you would probably only be concerned about the RDAs of specific nutrients if you suspected that you had some sort of dietary problem—for instance, an iron or calcium deficiency. However, even nutritionists don't think in terms of nutrient allowances when they eat. Rather they think in terms of *foods*—for example, whether they are getting enough iron-rich or calcium-rich foods. Let us see, then, how nutrient requirements are applied to foods.

The U.S. RDAs and Food Labels

U.S. RDAs, which appear on food package labels, express the percentage of nutrients that a food supplies to meet a person's

daily needs. Food labels must provide nutritional information if any nutritional claims appear on a package.

U.S. RDAs are simplified versions of the RDAs so that people can see at a glance on a food package the nutrients that a serving of food contains. Let us see how this works.

The U.S. RDAs U.S. RDA stands for **U.S. Recommended Daily Allowances.** These are the figures you see on food labels that indicate nutritional values for healthy people. In particular, the U.S. RDA expresses a food's nutrient contents *as a percentage of a person's daily needs.* Most food labels assume the person is over age 4 and is not pregnant or breast-feeding. Thus, if a nutrition label states that a serving of cornflakes includes 25% of the U.S. RDA for vitamin A, this means that most people will get *at least* 25% of their daily vitamin A requirement from a single serving. (The serving size is defined on the label.)

Note two things here:

- The U.S. RDAs are *based on* the RDAs.
- The "D" in RDA stands for *Dietary,* whereas the "D" in U.S. RDA stands for *Daily.*

How to Read a Food Label The U.S. government has some specific requirements for the kinds of data that must be presented on a food label. There are two sets of requirements—*legal requirements* and *nutrition information.*

Legal Requirements Every food label, whether it makes nutritional claims or not, must state the following:

- The product name (such as "Wheaties")
- The name and address of the manufacturer, packer, or distributor
- The net contents, stated in terms of weight, measure, or number of units
- The ingredients, listed in *descending* order by weight

The last requirement—listing ingredients in descending order—is not necessary for certain foods (such as ketchup or mayonnaise) that the federal government says meet its *standards of identity.* Standards of identity have been devised for common foods (for example, bread) that at one time were often prepared at home, so it was presumed that everyone understood the basic recipe.

Nutrition Information According to the law, if any nutrition claims are made on the label of a food package, then it must have the heading "Nutrition Information" and contain certain specific details. (*See ● Figure 15.14.*) These details include the following:

- Serving or portion size.
- Number of servings or portions in the container.
- Food energy per serving, stated in Calories.
- Protein per serving, stated in grams.
- Carbohydrate per serving, stated in grams.
- Fat per serving, stated in grams.
- Sodium, stated in milligrams.
- The U.S. RDA percentage for eight specific nutrients: protein, vitamin A, vitamin C, thiamin, riboflavin, niacin, calcium, and iron. (These values need not be stated if the product contains less than 2% of the U.S. RDA for five or more such nutrients.) To protect themselves, most food processors understate the amount on the labels.
- Ingredients listed in order of weight, from heaviest to lightest.

The law also has certain restrictions about what terms may be used on food labels and what the terms mean. (*See ● Figure 15.15.*) Although the present system of nutrition labeling could be improved, food labels offer valuable health information.

Controversy: Are Additives Safe? A food **additive** is a substance that you would not normally eat as food by itself but that is added to food during growing, processing, packaging, or storing. For instance, chemicals may be added during food production to change color, to enhance flavor, to ensure longer storage life, or to enhance nutritive value. (*Contaminants,* such as lead, are discussed in Chapter 36.) The agency charged with approving an additive's use as safe is the Food and Drug Administration. No additives are permanently approved; all are periodically reviewed.

● **Figure 15.14 Reading a food label.** Besides meeting certain legal requirements (such as giving name and address of manufacturer), a food container that makes nutrition claims must also state certain nutrition information.

Serving size: Size of portion, portions in container, and Calories (kilocalories) per serving. *Note:* Products may use *different* serving sizes, so it's not always easy to compare portions.

Protein, carbohydrate, fat, and sodium: For each serving size, the grams of protein, carbohydrate, and fat and milligrams of sodium. (Carbohydrates are broken down further below.) *Note:* The label need not state what percentage of Calories come from fat or whether the fat is saturated or unsaturated.

U.S. RDA: This part lists percentage of U.S. Recommended Daily Allowances in each serving for eight specific nutrients: protein, vitamin A, vitamin C, thiamin, riboflavin, niacin, calcium, and iron. (Others are optional.)

Ingredients: Listed in order by weight from heaviest to lightest. *Note:* Different kinds of sugars (sugar, brown sugar) may obscure the fact that the product is heavy on sugar.

Carbohydrate information: Not required by the Food and Drug Administration.

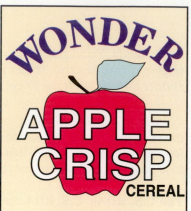

WONDER APPLE CRISP CEREAL

NUTRITION INFORMATION PER SERVING

SERVING SIZE ....1 OUNCE (1/2 CUP)	
SERVINGS PER PACKAGE.................14.5	
CALORIES.................110	
PROTEIN, g 2	
CARBOHYDRATE, g...................21	
FAT, g....................2	
SODIUM, mg.................170	

PERCENTAGE OF U.S. RECOMMENDED DAILY ALLOWANCES (U.S. RDA)

PROTEIN.....................2	
VITAMIN A....................25	
VITAMIN C.....................*	
THIAMIN.....................25	
RIBOFLAVIN.....................25	
NIACIN.....................25	
CALCIUM.....................4	
IRON.....................10	
VITAMIN D 10	
VITAMIN B$_6$.....................25	
FOLIC ACID 25	

*Contains less than 2 percent of the U.S. RDA of this nutrient.

INGREDIENTS: ROLLED OATS, RICE, APPLES, SUGAR, BROWN SUGAR, ALMOND PIECES WITH FRESHNESS PRESERVED BY BHT, COCONUT OIL, HONEY, SALT, CEREAL MALT SYRUP, CALCIUM CARBONATE, VITAMIN C (SODIUM ASCORBATE), ARTIFICIAL AND NATURAL FLAVORS, A B VITAMIN (NIACIN), IRON (A MINERAL NUTRIENT), VITAMIN A (PALMITATE), VITAMIN B$_6$ (PYRIDOXINE HYDROCHLORIDE), VITAMIN B$_2$ (RIBOFLAVIN), VITAMIN B$_1$ (THIAMIN MONONITRATE), A B VITAMIN (FOLIC ACID) AND VITAMIN D.

CARBOHYDRATE INFORMATION

COMPLEX CARBOHYDRATES, g............12	
SUCROSE AND OTHER SUGARS g ‡.......9	
TOTAL CARBOHYDRATES, g.................21	

VALUES BY FORMULATION.
‡ 4 OF THE 9 GRAMS OF SUGAR OCCUR NATURALLY IN APPLES

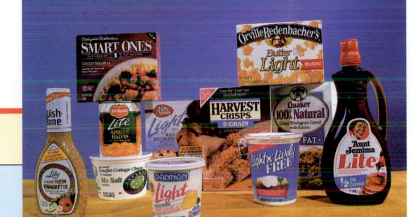

● **Figure 15.15 What some of those label terms mean**

Here are some common food labeling definitions:

- **Diet, Dietetic:** These terms can be used only if the item meets the requirements for a *low-Calorie* or *reduced-Calorie* food (see below), or if the item is intended to meet a special dietary need. A *diet* food contains no more than 40 Calories per serving or one-third fewer Calories than the regular product. A *dietetic* product is the same, but some dietetic products are low or reduced in sodium only, not necessarily low in Calories.

- **Low-calorie, reduced-calorie:** Food items described as *low-calorie* must have no more than 40 Calories per serving or 0.4 Calories per gram. *Reduced-calorie* foods must contain at least one-third fewer Calories than the product for which it substitutes and must compare standard and reduced Calorie versions on their labels. Food naturally low in Calories, such as lettuce, can only be labeled, for example, "lettuce, a low-calorie food," not "low-calorie lettuce."

- **Light/lite:** For meat and poultry products, *light* (or *lite*) means there is a 25% reduction in sodium, Calories, breading, or fat. For other foods there is no legal definition. Currently it signifies versions of regular foods that can contain less sodium, Calories, fat, sugar, or alcohol. It may also refer to color or texture and not fat or Calorie content.

- **Imitation, substitute:** The term *imitation* is required when a product resembles another product but is not as nutritious as the real thing. *Substitute* is a term that may be used when a product is not the real thing but is nutritionally equivalent to the food it is imitating.

- **Natural:** For meat and poultry, *natural* means no artificial flavors, colors, or preservatives, or synthetic ingredients. The food must also be minimally processed. There is no legal meaning for *natural* when used with baked goods, beverages, or processed foods. A natural food can contain artificial ingredients.

- **Naturally flavored:** The government requires flavoring by the essential oil, extract, or other derivative of a juice, spice, herb, root, leaf, or other natural source. There's no guarantee there are no artificial colors, preservatives, or other additives.

- **Organic:** Like natural, organic has no legal meaning or definition. The government does not allow the word *organic* to be used on meat or poultry.

- **Reduced sodium:** This term is permissible on foods that have had the usual level of sodium reduced by at least 75% from the regular version.

- **Salt-free, unsalted, no salt, without added salt:** All these terms mean no sodium or salt was added during processing. However, the food may still contain sodium. Check the sodium content per serving. Also, check the list of ingredients for sodium sources such as baking soda or any chemical with the word *sodium* or *salt* in it.

- **Sugar-free/sugarless:** These terms means that no table sugar (sucrose) was added to the food. However, there may be other sweeteners, such as fructose, corn syrup, high-fructose corn syrup, honey, or molasses, which are as caloric and cavity-causing as table sugar.

One recurring question that people have about food is, Can some additives cause cancer? A controversial part of the 1938 Food, Drug, and Cosmetic Act has been the **Delaney clause,** which prohibits the inclusion of carcinogenic (cancer-causing) additives in food. Certainly having no cancer-producing substances is a worthwhile goal, but the clause is so worded that it implies *zero tolerance* for any potential carcinogen. The difficulty, however, is that the techniques of chemical analysis are so refined—capable of determining parts per billion—that even carcinogenic additives that appear in foods *naturally* may be considered illegal.

The law was complicated further when another amendment was passed in 1960 that a food could be considered adulterated if it contained even natural toxicants in high enough levels to injure the health of the public. As a result, new varieties of foods have been kept out of the marketplace because higher levels of natural toxicants have been detected in them.

Next time you eat a hot dog or other cured meat, think about whether you would prefer that they not be made with sodium nitrite. This is an important additive, for which there is presently no useful substitute, that has caused controversy because it converts in the human body to nitrosamines—and nitrosamines cause cancer in laboratory animals. Yet sodium nitrite preserves a hot dog's color (pink), enhances its flavor (by slowing the rate at which it becomes rancid), and protects against bacterial growth (especially the deadly toxin that produces *botulism,* a form of food poisoning). Such trade-offs are typical of certain food additives, although we should note that, because there are over 3000 different substances commonly added to food, it is difficult to make generalizations about additives.

Controversy: Is Irradiation Safe? A fairly recent form of food processing, **irradiation** consists of exposing food to low doses of ionizing radiation, ultraviolet light, gamma rays, or high-energy electrons. It does not make the food radioactive (just as exposing yourself to an X ray machine does not make *you* radioactive). However, because of public concerns about safety, at present irradiation in the United States is approved for only a handful of uses: killing insect eggs in wheat grain and flour; pre-venting insect growth on fruits and vegetables; and sterilizing spices, herbs, and similar dehydrated foods. It has also been used to inhibit sprouting in grains and in root crops such as carrots, onions, and potatoes.

Irradiation is currently classified in the United States as a food additive under the Food, Drug and Cosmetic Act, and so irradiated foods must be tested for toxicity. All irradiated products must be labeled as such ("Treated with radiation" or "Treated by irradiation"), and they must carry the international symbol for irradiated foods. Other countries, including Canada, are more accepting of irradiated foods.

Is irradiation really safe? As a technical process, it seems to be.[41] It appears, however, that in the United States so many Americans have fears about irradiated products that they will not be accepted in the marketplace. Still, even if irradiated foods are accepted, the process still has its limitations—an important one being undesirable taste changes.

Controversy: Processed Food and Fast Food Versus "Natural" or "Health" Food
There are currently no legal definitions of "natural foods," or "health" foods. **Health food** is simply a term often used on labels to imply that that the food (usually organic or natural) has some sort of superior power to advance health. **Natural food** is also used on labels to imply the same healthful properties, but the term means only that the food has been altered as little as possible from its farm-grown state. **Organic food** seems to mean that the food is produced without chemical fertilizers, pesticides, or additives—also misleadingly suggesting that it is safe or has unusual power to promote health.

However, processed foods may not be necessarily worse than "natural" food. A **processed food** is food that has gone through a process in which it is cooked, mixed with additives, or altered in texture. During processing, milk is **pasteurized** (sterilized to destroy objectionable organisms) and **fortified** (enriched with vitamins and minerals), and loses Calories. However, recalling our discussion of nutrient density, nonfat milk is probably more nutrient-dense than, say, potato chips, which lose nutrients, gain fat and salt, and gain Calories during processing.

Fast foods usually refer to the convenience foods that one buys in drive-in or drive-through restaurants, ranging from McDonald's to KFC to Pizza Hut. Fast foods are often high in Calories, fat, sugar, and salt, but they need not be. Pizza, for instance, provides a reasonably balanced meal, and many fast-food restaurants are putting in salad bars and attempting to provide offerings with reduced fat. Thus, one *can* eat reasonably healthily in fast-food restaurants by avoiding high-Calorie, high-fat foods.

Many people are concerned about the pesticides used by modern farmers to control crop-destroying pests, since the same poisons that kill insects may also be harmful to people. This is one reason why it is *imperative* that you wash vegetables and fruits before cooking and eating them. Yet even organic foods sold in health-food stores have been found to contain as much pesticide residue as the foods in regular grocery stores, perhaps because of pesticide runoffs from neighboring farms. Thus, "organic" or "natural" foods may be more expensive but not chemically superior to conventional produce. Organic foods are often grown using "natural" fertilizers such as manure and compost instead of chemical ones, although the plant can't tell the difference. In addition, organic foods undergo less processing than usual (as in the case of whole-grain flours, for instance) and so have fewer additives. Whether this gives them any nutritional or even safety advantages has not been shown.

Probably a more useful distinction than that between natural and conventional grocery-store foods are those between *whole foods* and *partitioned foods.*[42] **Whole foods** are unaltered from their farm-grown state. **Partitioned foods** are composed of only *parts* of the plant and animal tissues we need to eat to obtain nutrients. They are foods that have been altered from their farm-grown state and packed in boxes, bags, bottles, or cans. An apple is a whole food; a jar of apple juice or apple jelly (whether labeled "natural" or not) is partitioned. Rolled oats (such as those found in Quaker Oats oatmeal) are whole food; rolled oats that take the form of oatmeal cookies or sugar-coated breakfast cereal are partitioned food. In general, it is best to choose foods that are from the whole-foods category than from the partitioned-foods category, regardless of any health-promotion labels such as "natural" or "organic."

The Basic Food Groups: The "Food Guide Pyramid"

The basic food groups consist of five categories: (1) breads and cereals; (2) fruits and vegetables; (3) milk, yogurt, and cheese; (4) meat, poultry, fish, and eggs; and (5) fats, oils, and sweets. These are expressed graphically in the "Food Guide Pyramid."

A **food group plan** tells what kind of food to eat and how much of each kind. There are many such plans, including some designed for different ethnic and religious groups. However, the ones for the general public in the United States and Canada are based on five principal food groups:

- Bread, cereal, rice, and pasta group
- Fruit and vegetable group
- Milk, yogurt, and cheese group
- Meat, poultry, fish, dry beans, eggs, and nuts group
- Fats, oils, and sweets group

These five food groups, which in 1992 replaced the old four food groups, are expressed in a Food Guide Pyramid. (*See Figure 15.16.*) The old standard charts visually presented four food groups in pie-chart-like form so that each group appeared to be an equal part of the diet. The Food Guide Pyramid, however, presents five food groups in a way that emphasizes the importance of some categories over others, based on government nutrition guidelines developed over a decade. For example, the top of the pyramid gives less graphic space, and therefore supposedly less emphasis, to dairy products, meat, and high-protein foods than it does at the bottom to bread, cereal, rice, and pasta. (Some think the pyramid violates a tenet of graphic design by being upside down: it sends the wrong message by suggesting that those foods at the top are *better* to consume than those at the lowly bottom.[43])

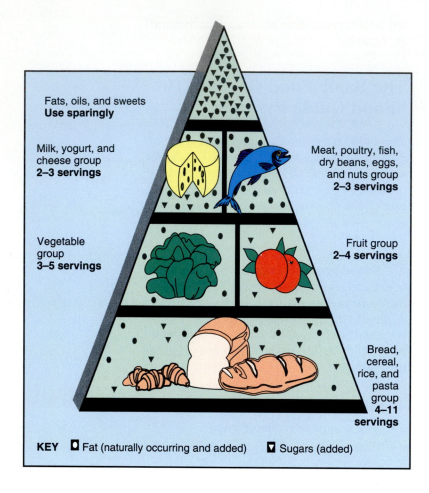

KEY ☐ Fat (naturally occurring and added) ▽ Sugars (added)

● **Figure 15.16 The Food Guide Pyramid.** The pyramid emphasizes the importance of making fruits, vegetables, and grains the basis of the diet.

1. Bread, Cereal, Rice, and Pasta Group
This group includes breads, cereals, and pasta. Enriched and whole-grain breads and cereals are sources of protein, B vitamins, and iron.

The U.S. Department of Agriculture (U.S.D.A.) offers the following recommendations.

- Eat breads, but avoid spreads, such as butter and jams, that are high in fat and sugar.

- Eat breakfast cereals, but add little or no sugar. Try raisins, grapes, or bananas instead.

- Eat rice and pasta, but watch out for sauces (especially cream sauces), which tend to be heavy in fats and sugars.

2. Fruit and Vegetable Group Besides being low in fat and high in fiber, fruits and vegetables are important sources of vitamins A and C and many minerals, including iron, calcium, and magnesium.

USDA suggestions are:

- Eat any fruits you like—except avocados and olives, because they are high fat. (You didn't know avocados and olives were considered "fruit"?) Don't add sugar or whipped cream to fruits.

- Eat any vegetables, except those that are fried. Go easy on butter, margarine, and other sauces or toppings that are high in fat.

3. Milk, Yogurt, and Cheese Group This group includes milk, cheese, yogurt, and ice cream and contributes protein, calcium, riboflavin, and vitamins A, B_6, and B_{12}.

Some suggestions:

- Drink nonfat or low-fat milk. Eat low-fat cheeses.

- Eat low-fat, plain yogurt.

4. Meat, Poultry, Fish, Dry Beans, Eggs, and Nuts Group This group includes not only beef, veal, lamb, pork, fish, shellfish, chicken, turkey, and eggs but also all kinds of beans: dry beans, dry peas, soybeans, lentils, seeds, nuts, and peanuts. These foods are good sources of protein, vitamin B_6, and such minerals as iron, zinc, and phosphorus.

You need to be cautious about consuming too much meat and eggs. Suggestions:

- Eat only the lean parts of meat. Eat poultry only without the skin. Fish is preferable to either meat or poultry.

- Avoid fried or breaded meat dishes. Meat is best broiled, roasted, or simmered.

- Substitute good alternatives to meat, such as dried beans, dried peas, and tofu.

- Eat eggs sparingly.

5. Fats, Oils, and Sweets This group also includes alcohol. Watch out for the foods in this group. Fat in particular can be a health liability. Fats, oils, and sweets provide Calories, which add weight but very little else. Suggestions:

- Eat fresh fruit as an alternative to sweet snacks and desserts.
- Eat baked products made with less fat and sugar, such as angel-food cake.
- Avoid eating anything greasy—butter, margarine, shortening, and cooking and salad oils—as well as fried foods, deep-fried foods, and cream sauces.

Defensive Eating: What the Experts Say

Experts suggest we eat a variety of foods, including more vegetables and fruits; consume less fat, sugar, salt, and alcohol; and maintain desirable weight.

In the last two decades especially, there has been more official concern about our nutritional health and more attempts made to educate us to do better, as reflected in numerous reports.[44–48] Let us try to summarize their advice.

1. Eat a Variety of Foods The key word here is *variety*. A varied diet, according to the report *Nutrition and Your Health,* consists of foods from each of the following groups each day.

- Fruits—2–4 servings
- Vegetables—3–5 servings
- Breads, cereals, or other grain products—6–11 servings
- Meat, poultry, fish, or alternates such as beans—2–3 servings, totaling 5–7 ounces lean meat
- Milk, cheese, or yogurt—2 servings (3 for teenagers and women who are pregnant or breast-feeding)

The variety that is desirable might be achieved more easily if more kinds of foods were available. As it stands now, however, four crops—wheat, rice, corn, and potatoes—contribute more to the North American diet than 26 other species of plant foods combined.[49]

Nevertheless, the important thing is to eat as many different *kinds* of foods as possible. The 1989 report *Diet and Health* adds some specific suggestions to reinforce this point:[50]

- Eat 5 or more daily servings of a combination of vegetables and fruits—especially green and yellow vegetables and citrus fruits.
- Eat 6 or more daily servings of a combination of breads, cereals, and legumes (such as beans and peas).

Stepping up the intake of these kinds of foods will help us get sufficient quantities of essential vitamins and minerals. It will also reduce the percentage of our diet that is high in sugar and fat, which are thought to increase our risk of cancer and cardiovascular disease.

2. Avoid Too Much Fat, Saturated Fat, and Dietary Cholesterol This advice offered by all reports is especially important for people who are at risk for heart and blood-vessel disease, such as high blood pressure. Some recommendations in *Nutrition and Your Health* are:[51]

- Eat less meat and more lean poultry and fish.
- Trim meats, use leaner cuts, and prepare them by roasting or broiling.
- Steam or bake vegetables instead of cooking them in oils.

Diet and Health is quite specific: Americans should reduce their total fat intake to 30% or less of Calories.[52] The present average intake of protein is 1.6 grams per kilogram of body weight for American adults—twice what they need—and diets high in meat have been associated with increased risks of certain cancers and heart disease.

To lower our fat and protein consumption, the report suggests, we should do the following:

- Substitute fish, poultry without skin, lean meats, and low-fat or nonfat dairy products for fatty meats and whole-milk dairy products.
- Choose more vegetables, fruits, cereals, and legumes.
- Limit oils, fats, egg yolks, and fried and other fatty foods.

3. Eat Foods with Adequate Starch and Fiber The term *dietary fiber* refers to those parts of plants that human beings do not digest. High-fiber foods may be helpful in preventing and alleviating constipation and certain intestinal disorders, such as diverticulosis (inflammation of the colon). Most Americans need to increase their fiber consumption, suggests *Nutrition and Your Health,* although it is not clear how much is desirable.[53] Some recommendations are:

- Eat more whole fruits and vegetables with edible skins.
- Eat bran, whole wheat, or rye muffins, bread, or pancakes.
- Eat pasta and rice.

4. Avoid Too Much Sugar and Salt (Sodium) Sugar provides energy but not many nutrients other than carbohydrate. Moderate sugar intake with meals is all right; however, most of it should come not from high-sugar foods such as candy but from "natural sugar" sources, such as fruits. The three reports *Nutrition and Your Health,* the 1988 Surgeon General's report, and *Diet and Health* all suggest reducing sugar consumption.[54–56] Some recommendations are:

- Eat fresh fruit for snacks or desserts.
- In recipes, cut down on sugar and use spices instead to add flavor.

Too much salt may raise blood pressure, especially in certain sodium-sensitive people, although there is presently no way of telling who they are. High blood pressure is an indicator of potential heart disease. All reports agree you should limit your salt intake, most recommending your total daily intake should be about 6 grams or less.[57]

Some recommendations for salt control are:

- Taste your food before you salt it; it may already be salty enough.
- For seasoning, try using pepper and/or herbs instead of salt.
- When shopping, check the nutrition label and buy low-sodium versions of processed foods.
- Use fresh rather than canned vegetables and soups.

5. Drink Alcohol in Moderation, If at All How moderate is "moderate"? The current thinking is: probably about 1–2 drinks a day, depending on gender. Heavy drinkers may suffer from nutritional deficiencies, and they also run the risk of certain cancers (especially if they smoke) and other serious diseases, such as cirrhosis of the liver. Pregnant women should avoid all alcohol.[58]

6. Avoid Excess Vitamin or Mineral Supplements, but Watch Calcium and Iron Intake Some vitamin and mineral supplements that exceed the RDA and other supplements (such as protein powders, single amino acids, fiber, and lecithin) "not only have no known health benefits for the population," says *Diet and Health,* "but their use may be detrimental to health. The desirable way for the general public to obtain recommended levels of nutrients is by eating a variety of foods."[59]

Two cautions:

- *Women should increase their calcium intake.* To avoid the weakening of the bone disorder known as *osteoporosis,* both the Surgeon General's report and *Diet and Health* recommend that adolescent girls and adult women increase consumption of foods high in calcium, the mineral that strengthens bones. Calcium is found in many low-fat dairy products.
- *Increase sources of iron.* To forestall anemia, *The U.S. Surgeon General's Report on Nutrition* recommends that children, adolescents, and women of childbearing age eat foods that are good sources of iron. These include lean meats, fish, certain beans, and iron-enriched cereals and whole-grain products. This issue is of special concern for low-income families.

7. Maintain Desirable Weight In this context, "desirable" means "appropriate for your height and build." In the United States, more people need to lose weight than to gain it. According to *Nutrition and Your Health:*[60]

- To *lose* weight: Eat more fruits, vegetables, and whole grains; to eat less fat and fatty foods; to reduce sugar and sweets; to drink fewer alcoholic beverages; and to increase their physical activity.

- To *gain* weight: People should increase their caloric intake but not their intake of fat. They should not give up exercise.

It is important to maintain appropriate body weight by balancing food intake and physical activity. Excess weight is associated with increased risk of several chronic disorders, among them high blood pressure, heart and blood-vessel disease, gallbladder disease, and types of bone and joint arthritis.[61]

Does Everyone Agree on These Guidelines? The guidelines above represent a compilation of dietary wisdom from the most influential government reports released during the last few years. These recommendations were made after a good deal of consultation among many health experts and organizations. Thus, the guidelines reflect various compromises. That does not mean they are wrong—only that other guidelines in these matters may be stricter or more lenient.

Consider cholesterol. The American Heart Association guidelines severely limit both sodium and cholesterol intake. On the other hand, the guidelines of organizations in other countries assume that as the consumption of saturated fats declines, so will the intake of cholesterol, and so they do not include specific recommendations. Several years ago, the Canadian government guidelines dropped prohibitions on cholesterol altogether.[62] In other respects, however, nutrition recommendations for Canadians are much the same as those for Americans.

800-HELP

American Institute for Cancer Research Nutrition Hotline. 800-843-8114. Registered dietitians answer questions on how diet affects health.

Food Allergy Center. 800-937-7354. Offers advice on reactions to various foods.

National Center for Nutrition and Dietetics. 800-366-1655. Hotline to correct misconceptions and myths about nutrition and diet.

Suggestions for Further Reading

Applegate, Liz (1991). *Power foods: High-performance nutrition for high-performance people.* Emmaus, PA: Rodale. The nutrition editor of *Runner's World* magazine offers a guide to food for the semi-active and athletic, based on her "60-15-25 Power Diet," which takes 60% of its Calories from carbohydrates, 15% from protein, and 25% from fat to provide an ideal amount of energy and nutrients.

Brody, Jane (1987). *Jane Brody's nutrition book* (rev. ed). New York: Bantam. Written by the "Personal Health" columnist for *The New York Times*, this well-researched, well-written book offers valuable information on eating for health and weight control.

Jacobson, Michael F., Lefferts, Lisa Y., & Garland, Ann W. (1991). *Safe food: Eating wisely in a risky world.* Los Angeles: Living Planet Press. The executive director of the Washington, D.C.–based advocacy group Center for Science in the Public Interest and two co-authors attempt to present an even-handed evaluation of the risks related to what we eat.

Saltman, Paul, Gurin, Joel, & Mothner, Ira (1987). *The California nutrition book*. Boston: Little, Brown. Written by a professor of biology at the University of California, San Diego, along with two editors from American Health magazine, this book covers current data about nutrients, digestion, weight control, and the role of nutrition in disease.

16 Weight Management

▶ What are some of the myths and concerns about attractiveness in our society?

▶ Describe how much weight and body fat is desirable and the ways to measure them.

▶ Discuss obesity and its treatment.

▶ Describe the eating disorders: anorexia, bulimia, and bulimarexia.

▶ Discuss the pros and cons of various kinds of weight-loss diets and describe a safe, effective strategy for losing weight and reducing body fat.

Appearances can be deceiving, you hear. Beauty is only skin deep. Certainly these cliches are true. Yet, as all those gorgeous people on magazine covers and in television and movies attest, our culture attaches tremendous importance to physical attractiveness.

Good Looks, Good Luck?

People attribute exceptional qualities to handsome people. Although standards for attractiveness vary over time, most women are self-critical of their looks, men are less so. Size and weight are important factors in body image.

Are looks important? Of course they are, said most of the 1220 American adults responding to a 1990 telephone poll by Princeton Survey Research Associates.[63] If you had an opportunity to change your body, would you? Yes, said most respondents; only 13% said they would stay as they were.

Is the importance of good looks in our society what lies behind the growth of diet programs, the increase of eating disorders, and the surge in cosmetic surgery? Let us briefly consider the focus on physical appearance in North America today.

The Advantages of Attractiveness Even babies seem to prefer attractive faces to unattractive faces, to judge by their gazing times.[64] Other evidence also shows that beautiful people enjoy advantages that others do not:

- *Association with desirable traits:* Physically attractive people are thought to have more desirable traits than unattractive people have.[65] They are believed to be happier, kinder, more successful, more socially skilled, and more sensitive.[66] They are also seen as more interesting, independent, exciting, and sexually warm than unattractive people.[67] We even think that handsome people are smarter and nicer.[68,69]

- *More favorable treatment:* As if anyone needed additional proof that life is unfair, it has been shown that attractive people generally are treated better than unattractive people. Teachers have higher expectations of them in terms of academic achievement.[70] Potential employers are more apt to view them favorably.[71] Attractive employees are generally paid higher salaries than unattractive ones.[72]

- *Marital satisfaction and sexual interest:* Studies show that physical appearance is important in determining satisfaction in marriage and sexual interest, especially for men.[73] Moreover, in midlife, physical changes related to age are perceived more critically when they affect women than when they affect men.[74]

As far as finding a life partner, does this mean there's no hope for those of us who are not blessed with exceptional good looks? Actually, people generally tend to match up with partners who are about as attractive as they are, in part because they tend not to approach those they consider to be in a class beyond or beneath them.[75] Or a less-attractive partner may have compensating assets, such as intelligence, wealth, or status.

Who *Are* the Beautiful People? Standards of attractiveness change over time, particularly for women. For example, as Phyllis Bronstein-Burrows observes, the plump and buxom female "who was a Victorian romantic ideal today is eating cottage cheese and grapefruit, and weighing in every Tuesday at Weight

Watchers."[76] Ideas about beauty also vary among cultures, as a look at photos in *The National Geographic* will illustrate.

Standards can change significantly within a person's lifetime. In the 1960s, the ideal of Jane Russell or Marilyn Monroe was replaced by the thin, narrow-shouldered look of high-fashion models like Twiggy. A generation ago, reports writer Naomi Wolf in *The Beauty Myth*, models weighed 8% less than the average American woman. Today they weigh 23% less. Put another way, the average model—and dancer and actress—is thinner than 95% of women.[77]

Recently, standards have changed again. According to a 1988 Gallup Poll of 1037 American adults, the new desirable look—among both women and men—is no longer thinness.[78] As writer A. G. Britton states, "skinny is passe; muscular and fit is the new silhouette of choice."[79] (See ● *Figure 16.1.*)

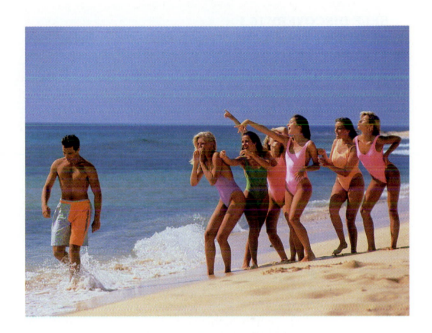

● **Figure 16.1 How we are, and how the other sex wants us to be**

The average man is:	Women want a man to be:	The average woman is:	Men want a woman to be:
5'10"	5'11"	5'3½"	5'4"
172 pounds	171 pounds	134 pounds	121 pounds
Medium width shoulders and chest	Medium to broad shoulders and chest	Soft body tone	Same
33-inch waist	Same		
Lean build	Muscular build	Average body type	Same
Half hairy chest, half smooth	Hairy chest	Average-sized breasts	Same
Brown eyes	Half say brown eyes, half say blue	Brown eyes	Blue eyes
Short, straight, dark hair	Short, curly, dark hair	Short, straight, brown hair	Long, wavy hair (half say blond, half say brown)
Clean-shaven	Same	Some wrinkles, blemishes, freckles	Smooth-skinned
Half tanned, half untanned	Tanned	Not tanned	Tanned

How Much Does Appearance Matter?

Please read the following statements and indicate how strongly you agree or disagree with each.

1. A man would always prefer to go out with a thin woman than one who is heavy.

Strongly agree	Agree somewhat	Agree	Neither agree nor disagree	Disagree	Disagree somewhat	Strongly disagree
☐	☐	☐	☐	☐	☐	☐

2. Clothes are made today so that only thin people can look good.

Strongly agree	Agree somewhat	Agree	Neither agree nor disagree	Disagree	Disagree somewhat	Strongly disagree
☐	☐	☐	☐	☐	☐	☐

3. Fat people are often unhappy.

Strongly agree	Agree somewhat	Agree	Neither agree nor disagree	Disagree	Disagree somewhat	Strongly disagree
☐	☐	☐	☐	☐	☐	☐

4. It is not true that attractive people are more interesting, poised, and socially outgoing than unattractive people.

Strongly agree	Agree somewhat	Agree	Neither agree nor disagree	Disagree	Disagree somewhat	Strongly disagree
☐	☐	☐	☐	☐	☐	☐

5. A pretty face will not get you very far without a slim body.

Strongly agree	Agree somewhat	Agree	Neither agree nor disagree	Disagree	Disagree somewhat	Strongly disagree
☐	☐	☐	☐	☐	☐	☐

6. It is more important that a woman be attractive than a man.

Strongly agree	Agree somewhat	Agree	Neither agree nor disagree	Disagree	Disagree somewhat	Strongly disagree
☐	☐	☐	☐	☐	☐	☐

7. Attractive people lead more fulfilling lives than unattractive people.

Strongly agree	Agree somewhat	Agree	Neither agree nor disagree	Disagree	Disagree somewhat	Strongly disagree
☐	☐	☐	☐	☐	☐	☐

8. The thinner a woman is, the more attractive she is.

Strongly agree	Agree somewhat	Agree	Neither agree nor disagree	Disagree	Disagree somewhat	Strongly disagree
☐	☐	☐	☐	☐	☐	☐

9. Attractiveness decreases the likelihood of professional success.

Strongly agree	Agree somewhat	Agree	Neither agree nor disagree	Disagree	Disagree somewhat	Strongly disagree
☐	☐	☐	☐	☐	☐	☐

These items test how much you believe that appearance matters. Score your responses as follows:

For items 1, 2, 3, 5, 7, and 8, give yourself a zero if you said "strongly disagree"; a 2 for "disagree"; up to a 6 for "strongly agree."

Items 4, 6, and 9 are scored in reverse. In other words, give yourself a zero for "strongly agree" and a 6 for "strongly disagree."

Add together your points for all nine questions. A score of 46 or higher means that you are vulnerable to being influenced by the great importance that current society places on appearance.

Source: Rodin, J. (1992, January/February). Body mania. *Psychology Today*, pp. 56–60.

Now, according to the Gallup Poll, the preferences seem to be as follows:

- *What women want in men:* Women prefer some muscularity, but are not much more demanding than that: they seem satisfied with medium-to-broad chests and shoulders and a more or less average height of 5'11" and weight of 171 pounds. In addition, they like dark hair (though curly is desired over straight) and prefer men to be clean-shaven—which most men are. The Princeton survey, mentioned above, also found that women were attracted to men of average height and musculature and preferred men to be clean-shaven rather than to have beards and long hair.[80]

- *What men want in women:* Men say they like blue eyes in women—although most women have brown—and brunette or blonde hair, with long hair preferred. Men say they prefer smooth skin, but, unfortunately, according to Britton, "skin problems are a concern for many women; about half are struggling with wrinkles, freckles or blemishes."[81] The Princeton survey found that men preferred dark-hair women to blondes and were divided almost equally in their appreciation of thin (preferred by 42%) and more "generous" (44%).

Interestingly, both men and women find a tan attractive in the other sex—although exposure to sun may create skin problems and wrinkling in later life and increase the risk of skin cancer.

How People Feel About Their Looks Do you have the kind of specifications that make you as highly attractive as the attributes outlined above? Very few of us are so lucky, of course. If you're like most people, you think you're less than perfectly attractive. Indeed, even handsome people are dissatisfied with their physical attributes. (*See Self Discovery 16.1.*)

When asked about their bodies, women in particular are highly self-critical, especially about their thighs, hips, and weight. (*See ● Figure 16.2.*) Men, by contrast, are less critical of women than women are of themselves. Indeed, men prefer women who are heavier than women think is attractive.[82,83]

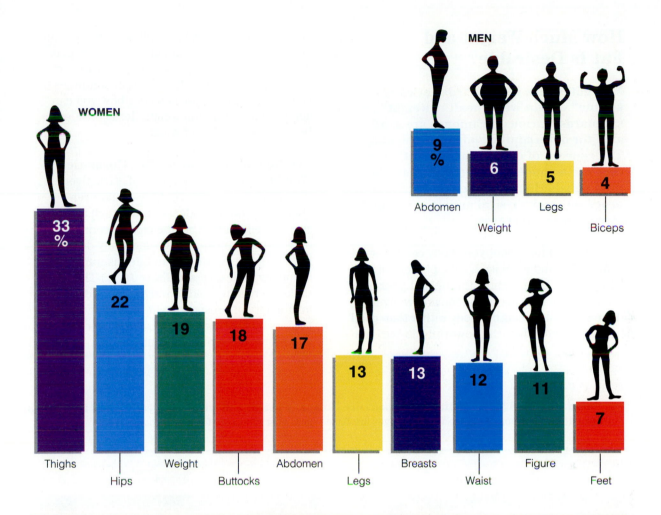

● **Figure 16.2 Negative feelings about parts of the body.** This chart shows the percentage of respondents in a sampling of college students who reported very strong negative feelings about specific parts of their bodies. Women reported negative feelings at a significantly higher rate.

Men also tend to overestimate their own attractiveness or are relatively tolerant of their physical drawbacks, such as being overweight. (*Refer back to Figure 16.2.*) The exception is men who describe themselves as homosexual, according to a study by UCLA psychiatrist Joel Yager.[84] Whereas straight men tend to prefer a toned, "hunky" physique, gay men are more concerned with being slim and, in fact, are more likely to feel fat in spite of others' perceptions.

There are a great many other areas of sensitivity—baldness, eyeglasses, teeth—that bear on the matter of body image. However, it is very

clear that *size and weight* are considered important—indeed, almost overriding—issues for many people, especially women. A late 1990 Gallup survey revealed that *half* of all Americans, particularly women, view themselves as overweight, compared to 25% of males and females who are actually considered so.[85] In a study of 850 young women, ages 12–23, more than two-thirds were unhappy with their weight and more than half with their shape—although most of those who wanted to lose weight were not even overweight.[86]

How Much Weight and Fat Is Desirable?

New guidelines replace "cosmetically desirable" weight with "healthy weight" standards. Various techniques are available for determining body fat percentage. The concept of energy balance is that either the amount of energy consumed in food equals that expended in metabolic processes and physical activity or weight increases or decreases.

How you feel about your body can influence your eating and exercise habits, particularly in adolescence but probably throughout your life. No doubt about it, for both men and women, the pursuit of a beautiful body rather than good health is what drives the powerful $33-billion-a-year diet industry, the $20 billion cosmetics industry, and the $300-million cosmetic surgery industry.[87] Ironically, however, even with 1 of 4 Americans now dieting, the nation continues to gain weight. Before we consider how you can achieve your optimum weight, let's consider how much you *should* weigh.

The New Ideal: Healthy, Not Cosmetic Weight From the standpoint of attractiveness, there is probably some elusive—and ever-changing—cultural ideal of how much a person should weigh. Probably the closest codification of what was considered "cosmetically desirable" have been the Metropolitan Life Insurance Company tables. (*See* ● *Table 16.1.*) These tables were supposed to roughly predict the insurability of prospective life-insurance policyholders by relating their weight to their height and frame size (small, medium, large).

● **Table 16.1 1983 Metropolitan Life Insurance Company height and weight tables.** Weights and heights are without clothes or shoes. Weight ranges are based on lowest mortality for people ages 25–29.

Men					Women				
Height		**Small Frame**	**Medium Frame**	**Large Frame**	**Height**		**Small Frame**	**Medium Frame**	**Large Frame**
Feet	**Inches**				**Feet**	**Inches**			
5	2	128–134	131–141	138–150	4	10	102–111	109–121	118–131
5	3	130–136	133–143	140–153	4	11	103–113	111–123	120–134
5	4	132–138	135–145	142–156	5	0	104–115	113–126	122–137
5	5	134–140	137–148	144–160	5	1	106–118	115–129	125–140
5	6	136–142	139–151	146–164	5	2	108–121	118–132	128–143
5	7	138–145	142–154	149–168	5	3	111–124	121–135	131–147
5	8	140–148	145–157	152–172	5	4	114–127	124–138	134–151
5	9	142–151	148–160	155–176	5	5	117–130	127–141	137–155
5	10	144–154	151–163	158–180	5	6	120–133	130–144	140–159
5	11	146–157	154–166	161–184	5	7	123–136	133–147	143–163
6	0	149–160	157–170	164–188	5	8	126–139	136–150	146–167
6	1	152–164	160–174	168–192	5	9	129–142	139–153	149–170
6	2	155–168	164–178	172–197	5	10	132–145	142–156	152–173
6	3	158–172	167–182	176–202	5	11	135–148	145–159	155–176
6	4	162–176	171–187	181–207	6	0	138–151	148–162	158–179

Source: Reproduced with permission of Metropolitan Life Insurance Company. Source of basic data: *1979 Build Study*, Society of Actuaries and Association of Life Insurance Medical Directors of America, 1980.

In November 1990, however, the U.S. Food and Drug Administration and the Health and Human Services Department came out with a new set of guidelines to suggest what constitutes "healthy weight." (*See ● Table 16.2.*) Unlike the Metropolitan Life tables, these new guidelines combine both sexes into one table, with higher weights generally applying to men and lower weights to women. They also allow for weight gain as one grows older.

Body Composition: Measures of Fat Percentage Number of pounds isn't the only critical number. Another is the *percentage of fat in*

your body, which should be in the range of 15–19% for men and 22–26% for women. You'll note from this that women are, in fact, supposed to have more fat than men. This is because women naturally store fat in the hips and abdomen for extra energy needs during pregnancy and breast-feeding.

Following are six ways of determining your percentage of body fat, described in increasing order of sophistication and accuracy. The first three you can easily do yourself.

- *Pinch test:* In the **pinch test,** you simply extend an unclothed arm to the side and pinch the loose skin on the underside of your upper arm between thumb and forefinger. (*See ● Figure 16.3.*) If you can pinch more than an inch of skin, you have too much body fat.

- *Waist-hips ratio test:* The **waist-hips ratio test** can help you determine if you have an unhealthy amount of abdominal fat. Using a tape measure, measure your waist circumference near your navel, not pulling in your stomach. Then measure around your hips, over the buttocks, where they are largest. To determine your waist-hips ratio, divide the waist measure by the hip measure. Ratios above a certain number are linked to greater risk of disease. For men the ratio is .95. For women the ratio is .80.

- *Girth test:* The **girth test** was developed by exercise physiologist Jack Wilmore. Men may measure their waist circumference and women their hip circumference to arrive, via Wilmore's tables, at an indicator of their percentage of body fat. If you have a tape measure, this, too, is a test you can perform yourself. (*See Self Discovery 16.2.*)

- *Fatfold test:* In the **fatfold test,** formerly known as the **skinfold test,** a pincer-like instrument called a **skin caliper** is used to measure the percentage of body fat. (*See ● Figure 16.4.*) As in the pinch test, the thickness of skin may be measured on the underside of the upper arm, or it may be taken below the shoulder blade, at the waistline, or in several places, and the different fatfolds may be averaged out to determine the total body fat.

- *Body-density test:* One way to determine the percentage of body fat is by the **body-**

● **Table 16.2 1990 guidelines for suggested weight.** Weights and heights are without clothes or shoes. Higher weights generally apply to men, lower to women. These guidelines allow for weight gain as you grow older.

Height	19–34 Years	35 Years and over
5'0"	97–128	108–138
5'1"	101–132	111–143
5'2"	104–137	115–148
5'3"	107–141	119–152
5'4"	111–146	122–157
5'5"	114–150	126–162
5'6"	118–155	130–167
5'7"	121–160	134–172
5'8"	125–161	138–178
5'9"	129–169	142–183
5'10"	132–174	146–188
5'11"	136–179	151–194
6'0"	140–184	155–199
6'1"	144–189	159–205
6'2"	148–195	164–210
6'3"	152–200	168–216
6'4"	156–205	173–222

Source: U.S. Food and Drug Administration and U.S. Department of Health and Human Services. Reprinted in: Anonymous (1991). Great bodies come in many shapes. *University of California, Berkeley Wellness Letter, 7,* 1–2.

density test, also known as *underwater weighing,* or *hydrodensitometry.* The purpose is to determine the body's density—that is, a comparison of body mass with body volume. Lean tissue in your body is denser than fat tissue; thus, the more dense your body is, the more lean tissue it contains. Your weight is determined by a scale. The volume is determined by submerging your whole body in a large tank of water, then measuring the amount of water displaced. From the density, the percentage of body fat is estimated.

- *Bioelectrical-impedance test:* In the **bioelectrical impedance test,** electrodes are attached to the person's wrists and ankles. A tiny electric current is sent through the body. How the current moves through the body indicates how much lean tissue the person has.

The Concept of Energy Balance A **Calorie** is the unit of heat used to measure the energy potential of food, energy being defined as "the capacity to do work." (A Calorie is the amount of heat required to raise the temperature of 1 kilogram of water 1 degree Celsius.)

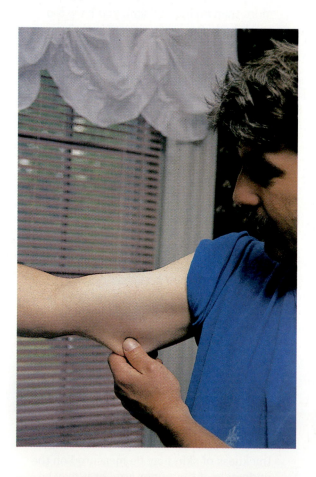

● **Figure 16.3 The pinch test.** If you can pinch more than an inch of skin beneath your upper arm, you may have too much body fat.

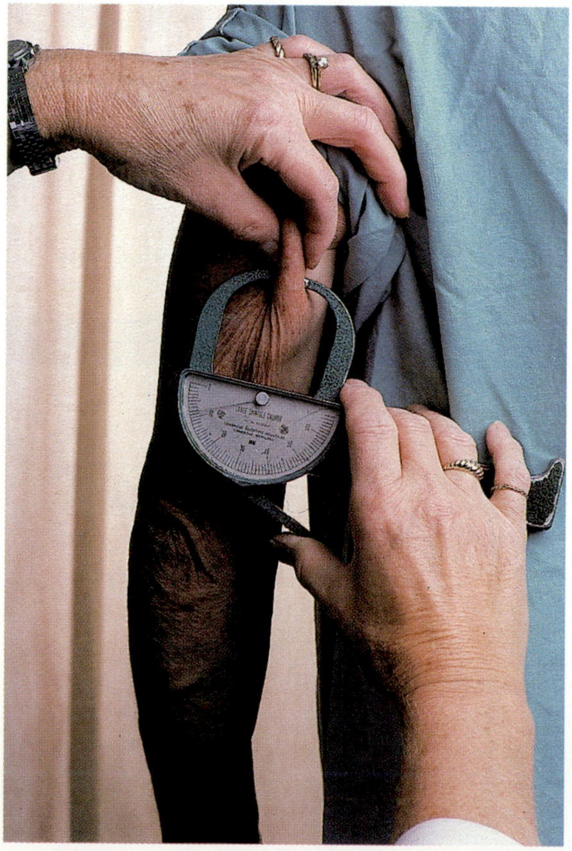

● **Figure 16.4 The fatfold test.** Skin calipers are used to measure the thickness of fat on the underside of the arm, below the shoulder blade, or elsewhere on the body.

The U.S. Committee on RDA and the Canadian Ministry of Health and Welfare have set certain recommended energy (Calorie) intakes for people of both sexes and various ages and populations. The Calories you need depend on your sex, age, frame, percentage of body fat, and level of activity; it is difficult to determine energy needs without knowing the individual and his or her lifestyle. Two examples of U.S. recommendations for 20-year-olds are:

- *For women:* If you are 5′4″ tall, weigh about 120 pounds, and generally engage in only light activity, you need 1700–2500 Calories a day to maintain your weight.

- *For men:* If you are 5′10″ tall, weigh about 154 pounds, and engage in only light activity, you need 2500–3300 Calories a day.

"Light activity" means that you spend 2 hours a day in light physical activity, ranging from putting on your clothes to fixing dinner. Beyond that, it is assumed you walk for 2 hours a day, stand for 5, sit for 7, and sleep or lie down for 8. People who are more active will need more Calories than the above; so will people who are taller. Shorter people will need less; so will older people.

It is helpful to try to compute the number of Calories you *consume* in your daily intake of food and compare it to the number of Calories you *expend*. If the Calories expended are the same as those consumed, you have what is called **energy balance.** If the Calories you eat are not expended in activity, you will gain weight; if you don't consume enough Calories for the energy you expend, you will lose weight.

Actually, energy expenditure is affected by two factors, not just physical activity:

- *Metabolic processes:* About two-thirds of the energy you expend each day is devoted to involuntary metabolic processes, the basic work of your body's cells. The **basal metabolic rate** refers to the energy spent to sustain your life when you are in a resting position. This includes the Calories you expend performing such basic functions as keeping your heart beating, lungs inhaling and exhaling, nerves generating impulses, and cells conducting metabolic activities. The metabolic rate is highest when you are young and decreases about 2% per year after you stop growing.

SELF DISCOVERY 16.2

The Girth Test: What Is Your Percentage of Body Fat?

This self-evaluation requires a tape measure.

Directions for Men

Measure your waist at your navel, keeping the tape level. In the chart below, draw a straight line from your "Body Weight" (left) to your "Waist Girth" (right). At the point where it crosses the "Percent fat" line, read your body-fat percentage. You are fit if the figure is between 12 and 17.

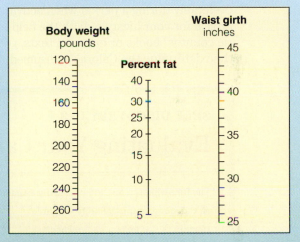

Directions for Women

Measure your hips at the widest point, keeping the tape level. In the chart below, draw a straight line from your "Hip girth" (left) to your height (right). At the point where it crosses the "Percent fat" line, read your body-fat percentage. You are fit if the figure is between 19 and 24.

Source: Adapted from Wilmore, J. H. (1986). *Sensible fitness* (2nd Ed.). Champaign, IL: Leisure Press.

- *Voluntary physical activity:* About one-third of the energy you expend daily is in voluntary physical activity, mostly using your muscles, whether it is writing a paper (little energy expenditure) or lifting bar-bells (great energy expenditure). In general, heavier people require more energy to perform an activity than less heavy people because they must move more body weight in the course of accomplishing the task.

To compute your *energy consumption,* you can keep a "food diary" for a week or two, in which you accurately record all the food and beverages and the amounts that you consume, preferably during a period when activities are typical for your lifestyle. With the help of "calorie counter" books or nutrition texts, you can then determine the Calories consumed. Com-

puting your daily *energy expenditure* is a little easier, because you can use formulas to gain a rough approximation of your basal metabolic rate and your voluntary physical activity. (*See Self Discovery 16.3.*)

The Heavy, the Overweight, the Obese

Being overweight (10% over normal weight) is not unhealthy, but obesity is. Obesity is a condition of being 20% or more over normal body weight. Among the theories of obesity are fat-cell, setpoint, and external cue, but lack of activity is certainly a contributor.

SELF DISCOVERY 16.3

Evaluating Your Calorie Needs

The following is a method of roughly estimating caloric needs for healthy, nonpregnant adults 18–50 years old.

A. Calculate your ideal body weight.

Height: _____ feet _____ inches

Women: Allow 100 pounds for first 5 feet of height
plus 5 pounds for each additional inch

Men: Allow 106 pounds for first 5 feet of height
plus 6 pounds for each additional inch

Example:
Woman 5'2"

	100
+ _____	+10
Ideal body weight _____	110

Man 5'7"

	106
	+42
Ideal body weight _____	148

B. Classify yourself by lifestyle and activity level.

Sedentary _____   Active _____   Very active _____

C. Determine your energy needs.

Multiply your ideal body weight by your activity level:

Sedentary = 13   Active = 15   Very active = 17

$$\underline{\hspace{4cm}} \times \underline{\hspace{4cm}} = \underline{\hspace{4cm}} \text{ Calories/day}$$
(Ideal body weight)   (Activity level)

D. Adjust for weight gain or weight loss.

$$\underline{\hspace{3cm}} - 500 = \underline{\hspace{4cm}} \text{ To LOSE 1 pound a week}$$
(Calories from section C)

$$\underline{\hspace{3cm}} + 500 = \underline{\hspace{4cm}} \text{ To GAIN 1 pound a week}$$

E. DAILY CALORIC GOAL = _____ Calories

Source: Zaret, B. L., Moser, M., Cohen, L. S., & Subak-Sharpe, G. J. (Eds.) (1992). *Yale University School of Medicine heart book.* New York: Hearst Books, p. 58.

Can you be simply "heavy" rather than overweight? From the standpoint of *attractiveness,* some people—such as members of the National Association to Advance Fat Acceptance—say there is no difference, that the real point is simply learning to accept your looks whatever the number of pounds you carry around. From the standpoint of the *body frame,* physiologists have identified three sizes—heavy, medium, and light—which can be determined using elbow measurements. (*See Self Discovery 16.4.*) From the standpoint of *health,* the new weight tables shown in Table 6.2, which represent the United States' official nutrition policy, allow for a certain amount of overweight—provided one does not have hypertension, diabetes, or other weight-aggravated health problems.

Weight and Health Even health officials, however, don't agree on the point at which healthy weight becomes unhealthy overweight. In general, health professionals use the following definitions:

- *Underweight:* If you are 10% below the Metropolitan Life tables shown in Table 16.1, you are **underweight.**

- *Overweight:* If you are 10% above the Metropolitan Life tables, you are **overweight.**

- *Obese:* If you are 20% above the life insurance tables, you are **obese.** *Mild obesity* is 20–40% above the ideal weight; *moderate obesity* is 41–100% above; *severe obesity* is more than 100% above.

Weight by itself, however, is not all that useful for determining health risks. As we've suggested, at least equally important is the percentage of body fat one has. And in point of fact, as one nutritionist observes, "it is actually more dangerous to be too thin than to be 20% overweight, which is the borderline for obesity."[88] Still, obesity *is* a highly serious matter, as we discuss next.

Obesity Being a few pounds overweight or having moderate amounts of body fat seems to pose no real threat to long-term health.[89] Obesity, however, is a devastating risk factor. The dangers include not only back and knee problems and hernias but a host of other troubles.[90–92] Obesity seems to contribute to or fur-

---

SELF DISCOVERY 16.4

What Is Your Body-Frame Size?

The following tells you how to estimate your frame size from your elbow breadth. For the most accurate measurement, you should ask a physician to measure your elbow breadth with a caliper, but for this activity you may use a ruler or tape measure.

1. Extend right your arm and bend the forearm upwards at a 90-degree angle.
2. Keeping your fingers straight, turn the inside of your right wrist away from your body.
3. Place the thumb and index finger of your left hand on the two prominent bones on either side of your elbow.
4. Using a ruler or tape, measure the space between your fingers on your left hand.
5. Compare the measurements with those given below.

Women		Men	
Height	Elbow breadth, inches	Height	Elbow breadth, inches
4'9"–4'10"	2¼–2½	5'1"–5'2"	2½–2⅞
4'11"–5'2"	2¼–2½	5'3"–5'6"	2⅝–2⅞
5'3"–5'6"	2⅜–2⅝	5'7"–5'10"	2¾–3
5'7"–5'10"	2⅜–2⅝	5'11"–6'2"	2¾–3⅛
5'11"	2½–2¾	6'3"	2⅞–3¼

The elbow measurements above are given for medium-framed men and women of different heights. Measurements *lower* than those given indicate that you have a small frame. Measurements *higher* than those given indicate that you have a large frame.

Source: Adapted from Metropolitan Life Insurance Company tables. Reprinted courtesy of the Metropolitan Life Insurance Company.

---

ther aggravate high blood pressure, heart and blood vessel problems, liver disorders, gallbladder disease, arthritis, respiratory problems, diabetes, surgical complications, and certain types of cancer—of the breast, uterus, and cervix for women, and of the colon, rectum, and prostate for men. In addition, there are dangers that derive from misguided diets. The bottom line is that the obese tend to die at a younger age. In addition, they experience social and psychological problems as a result of rejection and self-concept problems. (*See ● Figure 16.5.*)

With all these hazards, one might think obesity is uncommon. We need only look around to see that it is not. In the United States, *15%* of adolescents are obese and, astonishingly, *26%* of adults are also obese.[93] Among people with high blood pressure, the prevalence of overweight is significantly higher—about two out of five men and half the women.

Possible Causes of Obesity Despite the bad news about obesity, the good news is that, for many people, it can be reversed. Indeed, when it is, the mortality risk for the formerly obese is no more than that for those who have never been obese. In order to better focus on treatment, however, it may help to understand the possible causes. The principal question is, Is obesity caused by circumstances inside the body, outside the body, or both? Actually, there are probably many causes, and there may also be different types of obesity. Let us consider these possibilities.

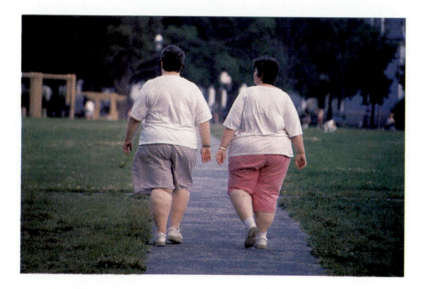

• *The fat-cell theory:* Is there such a thing as inheriting fat genes from one's parents? Perhaps. Still, the environment is important in accentuating or prohibiting the development of obesity. Obesity does tend to run in families, but such families may encourage overeating habits in childhood that persist in later life. In any event, studies show that obese people have more fat cells than other people do.[94,95]

The **fat-cell theory** suggests that overfeeding in early childhood increases the numbers of fat cells. When this happens, the number of fat cells becomes fixed and these cells then cause the person to be abnormally hungry as an adult. The theory has been disputed, because it is hard to determine numbers of fat cells. Even so, once people become obese, they have a tendency to remain so.

• *The setpoint theory:* Does the body "set points" so that, like a thermostat, there is a point below which it tends to gain weight and a point above which it tends to lose weight? This is the reasoning behind **setpoint theory,** which assumes that the body instinctively "chooses" its weight range, that the **setpoint** represents the body's natural point of stability in body weight.[96]

In this theory, every person has a built-in "control system dictating how much fat he or she should carry," according to the authors of *The Dieter's Dilemma.*[97] The reason may be that the body's metabolism compensates for increases or decreases in eating or physical activity. Thus, someone who overeats on a given day may expend that energy faster than normal, and someone who does not eat enough may "conserve" that energy. Setpoint theory may explain why people tend to get stuck at certain plateaus when losing weight.

• *The external cue theory:* Some scientists theorize that the body eats in response to *internal cues*—**hunger,** the physiological need to eat, and **appetite,** the desire to eat. Proponents of the **external cue theory,** on the other hand, believe the body eats in response to *external cues*—such as the time of day (noon signifies lunch) or the presence of food (chance offerings of potato chips provide an impetus to eat).

The external cue theory suggests that food is its own reward. Because of its pleasurable taste, soothing effects, and appetite-enhancing nature, the presence of food induces people to eat more and reduce their activity level, so that they gain weight. This is shown by the fact that obese people often show signs of "stress eating"—they try to alleviate anxiety by eating more.

The jury is still out on which cues—internal or external—are strongest in causing obesity. The debate shows, however, some of the principal areas that must be considered in why one eats.

Obesity and Lack of Activity No doubt, some people are obese because they eat too much. But that's only half the story. As we saw from the concept of energy balance, the Calories expended are as important as the Calories consumed. Not being physically active enough, in fact, may be *the* most important reason that one out of four adults in the United States is obese.[98]

We describe exercise and activity at length in the next chapter. Many people may wonder how much activity may be required to do any good in terms of weight loss. Energy-expenditure requirements necessarily will vary for each person. Nevertheless, a study of Harvard alumni found those expending 2000 extra Calories per week were healthier and lived longer than their more inactive counterparts.[99] This kind of activity level can be worked into your life without undue difficulty. Using a mixture of physical exercise (such as walking and cycling) and doing chores (gardening and housecleaning) for 5 hours over the course of a week, a 150-pound person could burn an extra 1500–2000 Calories per week. (See ● *Figure 16.6.*)

Treating Obesity Losing weight by fasting is not generally recommended. Instead, a slow reduction in weight through diet modification and exercise is advised. Reducing dietary fat and increasing exercise may play key roles in weight reduction.

The treatment for obesity depends on how mild or severe the obesity is.

- *For mild obesity: Mild obesity* is 20–40% above the ideal weight in the Metropolitan Life Insurance tables. (*Refer back to Table 16.1.*) This level of overweight can be treated by following some of the activities we describe below. Essentially, it calls for changing eating and exercise habits so that you can *maintain* your desirable weight once it is achieved. Among the useful weight-reduction techniques are those emphasizing behavior change and support groups, such as those offered by Weight Watchers, Take Off Pounds Sensibly (TOPS), or Overeaters Anonymous.

- *For moderate obesity: Moderate obesity* is 41–100% above ideal weight in the Metropolitan Life tables. This kind of weight loss may be treated in the same way as mild obesity, with the addition of nutritional education, counseling, and support groups to help people practice assertiveness and raise their self-esteem levels.

- *For severe obesity: Severe obesity* is more than 100% above ideal weight in the Metropolitan Life tables. This condition may be so threatening to health that a health care professional must be consulted. Extraordinary measures may have to be taken. One radical solution is *bypass surgery,* which involves shortening the small intestine to reduce absorption. Another is *gastric stapling,* in which the stomach is stapled to make it smaller.

We describe a course of weight loss in another few pages.

Eating Disorders: Anorexia, Bulimia, and Bulimarexia

Eating disorders consist of anorexia, or self-starvation; bulimia, or binge-eating and purging; and bulimarexia, a combination of both.

Christine Alt is 28 years old, 5′10½″ tall, blond, and blue-eyed, and for much of her 10-year modeling career she managed to keep herself to a size 4. Despite her terrific looks, she has what she perceives to be some embarrassing secrets. "I have a spastic colon, I have colitis," she confessed. "I throw up a lot. If I'm not throwing up, I either have diarrhea or constipation." Food is a major problem. "I don't have

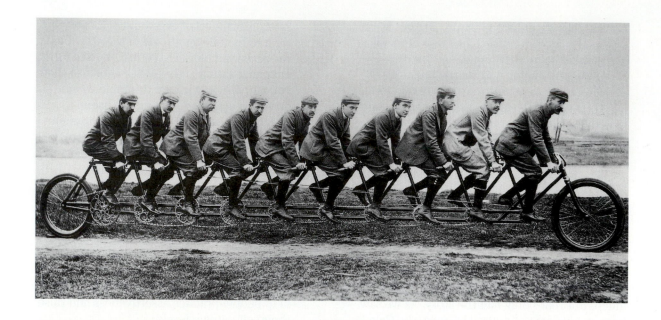

● **Figure 16.6 Fitting in fitness.** Fitness can be worked into your daily life. A 150-pound person following a program that mixes physical activity with chores can expend an extra 1500–2000 Calories per week.

Activity	Calories
Monday	
Brisk walking, to and from work, 30 minutes	160
Stair climbing, 5 minutes	35
Tuesday	
Cycling, stationary, 15 minutes	
(10 mph)	105
Wednesday	
Brisk walking, to and from work, 30 minutes	160
Thursday	
30 minutes at gym:	
Stair climbing, fast, 10 minutes	85
Rowing, on machine, 10 minutes	65
Running, treadmill, 10 minutes	95
Friday	
Swimming, 20 minutes	180
Cycling, 20 minutes	135
Saturday	
Brisk walking, 30 minutes	160
Gardening, 20 minutes	110
Housecleaning, 20 minutes	80
Sunday	
Brisk walking, 15 minutes	80
Mowing lawn, 20 minutes	150
Raking grass and yard work, 20 minutes	135
Washing car, 20 minutes	65
GRAND TOTAL	1800 (in about 5 hours)

normal eating habits," she told an interviewer. "I'm afraid if I sit down and eat three meals—like somebody could eat eggs and toast for breakfast and a sandwich for lunch and go out for a steak and baked potato for dinner and be fine—if I ate that, I know I would gain weight. I just know I would."[100]

Christine Alt has been lucky to survive fashion's ideal of female beauty. During most of her career, she suffered from anorexia, or self-starvation, which has rates of mortality of 15–21%—among the highest levels recorded for psychiatric disorders.[101] She also suffered from bulimia, which is characterized by cycles of binge eating alternating with purging and which afflicts half the people with anorexia.

Alt is a casualty of the myth that "thinner is better," and she is far from being the only one. With our culture's emphasis on thinness and physical fitness as a symbol of attractiveness and success, the malady has become increasingly widespread. (*See Self Discovery 16.5.*)

Alt suffers from what are called **eating disorders,** which often involve hazardous food consumption behaviors. In this section, we discuss three types of eating disorders:

- Anorexia nervosa, or self-starvation
- Bulimia nervosa, or binge eating and purging
- Bulimarexia, or both binge eating with purging and self-starvation

Anorexia Nervosa The term **Anorexia nervosa** originated from the Greek word meaning "nervous lack of appetite." However, anorexics don't lose their appetites—at least not until the final stages of the disorder; rather, to be thin they simply refuse to eat. Their self-imposed starvation leads not only to weight loss but also to potential problems with malnutrition and even to death.

Less than 1% of all women suffer from anorexia, perhaps only 1 in 250.[102] But it *is* mainly women who have it: females comprise 94–95% of those afflicted.[103] Why mainly women? Perhaps, suggests one article, because men may be less subject to mood disorders, less concerned about body shape, and more apt to exercise—perhaps excessively, as in compulsive running—than women are.[104] Middle-aged men who severely restrict their food consump-

---

SELF DISCOVERY 16.5

Eating Disorders: Are You at Risk?

How do you think about eating, dieting, and your body? To find out, see if these statements are true for you:

1. A day rarely passes that I don't worry about how much I eat.
2. I am embarrassed to be seen in a bathing suit.
3. There are many foods I always feel guilty about eating.
4. Most attractive people I see are thinner than I am.
5. I usually begin the day with a vow to diet.
6. My thighs are too fat.
7. I feel uncomfortable eating anything fattening in front of people.
8. It makes me nervous if people can watch me from behind.
9. After I eat a lot, I think about ways of getting rid of, or burning up, calories.
10. I hate seeing myself in a mirror.
11. I feel terrible about myself if I don't do a lot of exercise every day.
12. I find my naked body repulsive.
13. If I eat too much, I sometimes vomit or take laxatives.
14. My worst problem is the appearance of my body.

The odd-numbered questions tell whether your eating and exercise patterns have gone awry. The even ones tell if you're overly critical of your body. Add up the number of "true" answers. Your score is interpreted as follows:

2–4: You're typical, and probably not at risk.
5–8: You're overly concerned with your weight. Watch your attitudes and behavior carefully.
9–14: You may well be developing an eating disorder. Consider professional psychological help.

Source: Anonymous (1986, October). To be sure you're not at risk. *American Health*, p. 72.

---

tion and increase their physical activity, however, have been likened to young adolescents with anorexia nervosa.[105]

Anorexia characteristically develops during the teen years or the twenties, although it is even being encountered among people in their fifties and sixties.[106] The principal symptoms are the following:

- *Refusal to maintain normal body weight:* Anorexics often starve themselves to produce weight loss, often to 15% or more below minimal normal weight for their height and age.

- *Fear of fatness or weight gain:* Even anorexics who are *underweight* express a fear of being fat.

- *Distorted body image:* Anorexics show a disturbed perception about their body size so that they claim to "feel fat" and see themselves as fat even when they are emaciated.

- *Absence of three menstrual cycles:* Women show **amenorrhea**—abnormal absence or suppression of the menstrual discharge—for at least three consecutive monthly menstrual cycles that would otherwise be expected to occur.

Anorexics are often rigid and perfectionistic, are often model students and daughters, and tend to be highly achievement-oriented. They tend to fear loss of control in any area of their lives. The anorexia may develop when they go on a diet and find that weight loss gives them a sense of control and achievement. Thereafter the weight control becomes a dominant focus of their lives.

Many anorexics develop eccentric behaviors about food. They may eat only a narrow range of foods, eat only alone, secretly throw food away, hoard small amounts of food to eat later, and in general show an obsessive interest in food and Calorie-counting. In addition, they may exercise compulsively and force vomiting (particularly after eating binges, when large amounts of food are consumed in a short time). They may also use **laxatives,** drugs that stimulate evacuation of the bowels, or they may use **diuretics** (called "water pills"), drugs that increase the flow of urine.

Because anorexics frequently deny their symptoms, there is often powerful resistance to treatment. With therapy, about 70% of patients recover or are improved. Unfortunately, the disease may be fatal for those who are not able to seek treatment or don't respond to treatment.[107,108] Clearly, an important goal of treatment is to improve nutrition. Other therapies include psychotherapy and behavior therapy to control food-consumption behavior. Some drug

therapy has been successful, including the use of antidepressants and antipsychotic drugs.

Bulimia Nervosa Derived from the Greek term meaning "ox hunger," which suggests the enormous quantity of food involved, **bulimia nervosa** (or simply bulimia) consists of episodes of binge eating alternating with purging —that is, repeated attempts to lose weight by self-induced vomiting or use of laxatives or diuretics. (*See ● Figure 16.7.*)

Bulimia seems to be more in evidence than anorexia. Estimates run 2–19% among college women—the group at greatest risk—and as high as 5% for men, although in actuality for both sexes it may be a good deal less.[109–111] Like anorexia, bulimia is found mostly among women in their teens and twenties, although it is being encountered among females in middle age and later.

The main symptoms are as follows:

- *Recurrent binge eating:* Great amounts of food are consumed in short amounts of time. Bulimics may eat three to five times the normal quantities of a meal. One writer says that food intake can reach 166 Calories per minute.[112]

- *Feeling of lack of control over eating behavior:* This is particularly true during eating binges. "After a substantial dinner," writes one former bulimic, "I'd drive to the grocery store and buy all kinds of high-calorie junk foods. . . . The next night, I'd shop at a different grocery store and do the same thing. I'd often go to three or four drive-in restaurants—Burger Kings and McDonalds—in one evening. . . ."[113]

- *Frequent vomiting, use of laxatives, or intense exercise:* Bulimics regularly engage in self-induced vomiting, use of laxatives or diuretics, strict dieting or fasting, or vigorous exercise to prevent weight gain. Some bulimics build up a tolerance to laxatives and need increasing quantities. Exercise addiction may be hard to detect as a component of an individual's problem because it is considered "healthy."

- *Three months of two eating binges a week:* Bulimics engage in a minimum of two binge-eating episodes a week for at least 3 months.

- *Overconcern with body shape and weight:* Bulimics show depressive symptoms and express self-deprecation about their weight and their looks.

Binge eating alone does not make a bulimic. After all, some athletes trying to "make weight" may stuff themselves with great quantities of food (particularly carbohydrates) during a short period of time. But bulimics also experience dental decay, gum damage, and tooth enamel erosion (from stomach acid); strange body odor (from vomitus); and scars on the knuckles (from pushing one or more fingers down the throat). There may be other signs: One college student said, "We had one bathroom. I was renowned for my long showers. The water ran forever. My two roommates never knew I was vomiting."[114]

Does binge eating have a biochemical basis? It has been suggested that both binge eaters—people who go through episodes of overindulgence in food—and bulimics tend to crave and binge on sugars and starchy foods—that is, simple carbohydrates.[115] Laboratory animals have been observed to overeat and become obese when offered highly palatable foods that are high in sugar and fat and low in fiber, and perhaps the same is true with some humans.[116–118] A possible explanation is that simple carbohydrates elevate the level of the brain chemical serotonin, which affects mood and emotion and which may be low in compulsive overeaters and bulimics. In other words, people with eating disorders may be self-medicating themselves against depression by responding to carbohydrate cravings.

There may also, however, be some psychological bases for bulimia. Like anorexics, bulimics may come from traditional families with "old-fashioned" parents—mothers who do not work outside the home and fathers who do and who are emotionally distant. There may also be a family history of depression or substance abuse. Bulimics are inclined to be people-pleasers who do not deal easily with their feelings.[119]

Bulimics wait an average of 5½ years before seeking help, according to some research.[120] Some never seek help, and as a result the prospects for bulimics are less optimistic than those for anorexics. Death may occur because

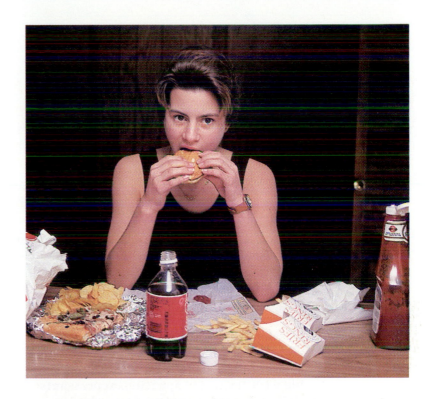

● **Figure 16.7 The bulimia cycle.** Bulimia is a cycle of binge-eating and purging.

❝*The pain in my left side was so severe I couldn't stand straight. I made my way to the bathroom, pushed my finger down my throat, and forced myself to vomit out the enormous amount of food I had just eaten—a box of sugared cereal, a half-gallon of milk, a loaf of bread, a jar of peanut butter, a dozen donuts, and a package of Oreos.*

When I finished vomiting, the pain in my side was gone, but my throat burned, my abdominal muscles ached, and I felt hot, sweaty, smelly, dizzy, and exhausted. I wanted to die, yet I still felt driven to eat and vomit disgusting amounts of food night after night.❞

—Dianne-Jo Moore (1989, November/
December). I invented bulimia. *Medical Self Care*, p. 30.

of the higher likelihood of fluid imbalances and because the concomitant depression that goes along with the disorder may pose a higher risk of suicide.[121,122]

In extreme cases, hospitalization may be required to isolate the bulimic from opportunities for binge eating. Antidepressant drugs may also be helpful. Behavior-modification techniques may be required to help bulimics relearn healthy eating patterns. Psychotherapy is particularly important, although it is suggested that patients work with therapists experienced in treating eating disorders.[123]

Bulimarexia Some experts do not separate bulimia and anorexia, saying that anorexics often show bulimic binge-and-purge behavior and bulimics go through periods of self-starvation. This combination of symptoms is called **bulimarexia.** Perhaps 40–50% of anorexics show bulimic behaviors.[124]

Diets and Beyond Diets

Types of diets include fasting, partial fasting with the use of appetite suppressants or liquid supplements, and two classes of weight-loss programs that should be avoided—high-protein diets and food-combining diets. "Yo-yo," or repetitious, dieting is especially harmful. We describe seven steps to permanent weight loss.

You've made up your mind that you want to be thinner. What's the quickest way to get there? Fasting? Appetite suppressants? Liquid supplements? Gimmick diets? Group programs?

No doubt any number of these will help you lose weight, although some methods are risky. The problem with these methods is not only that they pose a physical health risk but also that afterwards most people simply put their old weight back on again. Dieting, then, is not the answer. The real answer is something people are reluctant to hear: improve physical fitness.

Before we discuss that, however, let us describe some principal areas of dieting.

Fasting **Fasting** or **semistarvation**—eating nothing or very little for a certain length of time—is advocated by those who think it will not only help them lose weight but also perform a kind of "spring cleaning" of the body, getting rid of worn-out cells. Besides the fact that it

takes a long time to lose weight with this method—because the body's metabolism slows down to conserve energy—fasting has some important hazards. Although in fasting the body supposedly uses up its fat for energy before it draws on its muscle, it may result in loss of lean body mass. It may also produce heart-rhythm abnormalities that can be fatal. Finally, once your weight-reduction program is over, your metabolism will continue to remain slowed down, using up fewer Calories, so that you may actually gain weight while eating little.

Modified Fasting: Appetite Suppressants
At one time, amphetamines were prescribed as appetite suppressants. However, it has been found that they not only were dangerous but also were largely ineffective—they helped people lose only about 10 pounds, which subsequently quickly returned. Even the chemically similar appetite suppressants now available by prescription (mazindol, phentermine, diethylproprion), though somewhat safer than amphetamines, can cause dizziness, palpitations, hypertension, nausea, insomnia, irritability, and other adverse side effects.[125]

Nonprescription appetite suppressants are considered safer, but they are not necessarily more effective. They include:

- *Diet candies and gum:* These contain a local anesthetic (benzocaine) that numbs the taste buds. There is no evidence they work.

- *Diuretics:* Diuretics, or "water pills," may help you take weight off quickly, but it's mainly water. After you stop taking the pills, the weight is gained back almost immediately.

- *Fiber fillers:* When taken in large enough doses, agents containing fiber (methylcellulose, glucomannan) may produce a feeling of fullness in the stomach.

Other appetite suppressants (thyroid hormones, starch blockers) have been taken off the market by the Food and Drug Administration.

Modified Fasting: Liquid Supplements
Wouldn't it be ironic, indeed terrible, if you went on a diet to avoid the very risk factor, obesity, that increases chances of heart disease—and then had a heart attack? The low-calorie, liquid-supplement formulas can increase the

risk of heart attack by altering one's fluid (electrolyte) balance or damaging the heart muscle.

The principle of liquid (or powder) supplements is that they include vitamins and minerals and essential nutrients, both protein and carbohydrates, in 600 Calories to prevent the body from using its own muscle tissue for energy. These may be useful for *medically supervised* diets for moderate or severe obesity, or even to help get other weight-loss programs off the ground. However, you should be aware that in October 1991 the Federal Trade Commission charged the marketers of three liquid diets—Optifast 70, Medifast 70, and Ultrafast—with making deceptive claims that their programs are safe and effective over the long term.[126]

Diets to Avoid There are so many diets that we have not the space (nor probably you the time) to look at them all. However, since most new diets are simply variations on old diets, we can make a few general assertions.

- *Avoid low-carbohydrate, high-protein diets:* Dr. Atkins' Diet Revolution, the Complete Scarsdale Medical Diet, and the Magic Mayo Diet (Grapefruit Diet) are all examples of low-carbohydrate, high-protein diets. Such diets seem to work fast because they cause one to rapidly lose water and hence weight—at least at first. In addition, the lack of carbohydrates makes food so unappetizing that people tend to eat less (like cheeseburgers without the buns—how many could you eat?).

  Ultimately, however, surplus protein (amino acids), even if it derives from lean meat, cannot be stored in the body in that form; it is converted into fatty acids and thence stored as body fat.

- *Avoid food-combining diets:* Food-combining diets claim, with no evidence, that eating certain foods at certain times or in combination with other foods can produce weight loss. For instance, the Beverly Hills Diet instructs you to eat meat and fruit at separate times during the day, and the fruits are varied from day to day. The Fit for Life Diet calls for eating only fruit before noon and vegetables with a little protein and starch from noon until evening.[127]

Again, there is no scientific basis for such diets, and the eating of too much fruit, for instance, can produce diarrhea.

The Dangers of Yo-Yo Dieting The thinness obsession has come to this: At any given time, 50% of American women—half of whom are not overweight in the first place—and about 25% of American men are dieting to lose weight.[128] A Gallup poll revealed that nearly a third of American women aged 19–39 diet *at least once a month.*[129] If these figures are true, then a significant proportion of the rest must be *putting* on weight, because up to 95% of dieters are unable to keep their weight off.

This cycle of weight loss and weight gain, called the **yo-yo syndrome,** is bad news. According to one study, repeated changes in weight (regardless of a person's initial weight) are linked to an increased death rate overall and to as much as twice the chance of dying of heart disease.[130] Indeed, the harmful effects of yo-yo dieting may be equal to the risks of simply remaining obese, which also doubles the chance of early death.

Not only do frequent cycles of weight loss/weight gain pose hazards to health, but yo-yo dieters tend to have more difficulty losing weight on subsequent tries. For example, one study found that yo-yo dieters lost an average of 2.3 pounds a week the first time but only 1.3 pounds a week the second time. In addition, yo-yo dieters lose fat from one part of the body and gain it back somewhere else.[131]

Strategy for Living: The "Beyond Diets" Diet There are so many new diet gimmicks and gimmick diets every year that it's hard not to believe that surely one of them is the ultimate key to weight loss. Unfortunately, as we have suggested, most are simply flashy variations on old ideas. Let us therefore propose a program that reflects the latest consensus among health care professionals about taking weight off. It involves a combination of physical exercise and modifying food-related choices (especially fats) and behavior. In order to give it the kind of come-hither title with which many diet programs are named, we shall call it The "Beyond Diets" Diet—because one must look beyond dieting for a successful program.

The first thing to realize is that it is not impossible to lose weight and keep it off. Weight-control specialists say that, instead, it's important not to diet at the wrong time for the wrong reasons. Too many people apparently rush into diets under circumstances that make lasting success unlikely. What's important is how well you can assess your *diet readiness*—your state of mind, your motivation, your commitment, and your life circumstances, as well as your attitude toward exercise and your reasons for eating at various times.[132] How realistic your assessment is can significantly increase your chances of lasting weight loss—regardless of the weight-loss program you follow. Indeed, your reasons for losing weight may be even more important than the diet you choose.

Here, then, is a seven-step program recommended by psychologist Kelly Brownell for losing weight that will also initiate attitude changes and a way of life that will keep you from regaining those pounds.[133]

1. *Set reasonable goals:* Compare your weight with the height/weight tables. (*Refer back to Table 16.1.*) Bear in mind, however, that the tables focus on weight, not fat, and that some muscular individuals, for instance, may weigh in as too heavy even though they are not carrying excess fat. Determine your body fat, using some of the techniques previously described. If you can, you might attempt to go through a college health center or fitness club to find an expert to ascertain your percentage of body fat.

2. *Do a reality check:* Your expectations should be realistic. Many people who start a diet want the pounds off next week. However, rapid weight loss produces mainly losses of water and muscle than of fat and so is easily regained. People who expect quick weight loss are setting themselves up for a fall. Slow and gradual weight loss is better—no more than 1 or 2 pounds a week.

   To compute how long you should diet, Brownell suggests that (a) you take the number of pounds you want to lose and calculate the number of weeks it will take to reach that goal if you lose 1 pound a week, then (b) do the same calculation for losing

2 pounds a week. Look ahead to the number of weeks it will take for both figures, then set a date for reaching your goal that is midway between those two dates.

3. *Follow a balanced, low-fat diet:* Whatever diet program you follow, good nutrition is essential. Eat a variety of foods to ensure you get the vitamins and nutrients you need (including calcium, iron, and protein), while limiting Calories. To lose 1 pound a week, you need to take in about 500 Calories a day less than the amount you expend. Avoid fat and eat fruits, vegetables, and grains to provide both fullness and nutrition.

   Limiting fat is particularly important. Refer back to the section on fats in the previous chapter so that you can learn to recognize both "visible" and "invisible" fats.

4. *Reshape bad eating habits:* Get an understanding of your eating patterns by keeping a 2-week record of what you eat (amount and Calories), the time, location, what you are doing, and how you feel. This will suggest to you the conditions under which you eat too much. From these you can devise strategies for lifestyle change—for instance, avoiding situations that cause eating. It's important to become aware of the link between eating and feelings.

5. *Exercise:* Exercise can help control your appetite. In addition, dieters who exercise are more apt to lose weight and keep it off than those who do not. Brownell says exercise gives people the confidence to make positive changes.

   The trick is to find an exercise program you enjoy so you will stay with it. Begin by making small changes (such as walking instead of riding and climbing stairs instead of taking the elevator). Explore a variety of activities to find ones that you enjoy. Begin doing physical activities on a regular basis, exercising 3–5 times a week. Vary your workout routine to avoid boredom and monotony.

6. *Track your progress:* You should weigh yourself probably no more than once a week, so that transient changes will even

out. Or, using a tape measure, you can measure your thighs, hips, and waist every 3–4 weeks.

7. *Celebrate your success:* Brownell points out that rewarding yourself for your achievements is an important part of all programs that produce lasting change. Thus, when you reach the midway point of your weight loss, you should give yourself something you want (Brownell's examples: a new book, tickets to a show, a weekend away). For the end of the program you should do something really special (for example, give all your old clothes to charity, then "indulge in new ones that show you off as you now are").

Onward: Life Without Dieting The key to permanent weight control is simple in principle. It consists of four concepts:

- *Be positive:* Wanting to lose weight because you dislike how you look or want to be more successful at work are not great motivators for holding your weight down. Instead, think of the positive things: self-esteem, energy, health, sexual vitality.[134] Relapsers, according to one survey, were by and large unhappy with their bodies; most maintainers viewed themselves as thin or of average weight.[135]

- *Actively confront problems:* Relapsers are more likely to try to escape from dealing with stressful or troubling issues by eating, sleeping more, or wishing problems will go away. Maintainers usually seek social support or professional help and actively try to confront and solve their problems.[136]

- *Limit sugar and fat and eat complex-carbohydrate foods:* There is nothing that says you have to give up Haagen-Dazs ice cream and Big Macs forever. However, you should know that sugary and fatty foods may promote weight gain not only because of the Calories but because of their effects on appetite and metabolism. For instance, sugar (though not artificial sweeteners, as was once thought) may increase hunger by raising insulin levels.[137,138] Sugar is also the principal flavoring used with fat, so eating more of one may lead to eating more of the other.

On the other hand, foods high in complex carbohydrates—fruits and vegetables, grains, legumes, and pasta, for example—can help keep weight off for two reasons: (a) they provide a feeling of fullness; (b) they provide fewer digestible Calories. This does not mean you should go overboard on complex carbohydrates (as the Pritikin diet does), which could prove boring.

- *Get exercise:* Exercise does a number of things:[139]
  (1) It burns off Calories while you're active and, even more important, it *keeps burning Calories after you've stopped exercising.* Indeed, with enough exercise, you may be able to eat *more* than you did before and stay slim.
  (2) Exercise burns fat, not muscle. Indeed, exercise helps build muscle.
  (3) Exercise—particularly aerobic exercise (such as running, cycling, or swimming) can keep lost weight from returning.

The main thing is to make exercise an integral part of your life—for the rest of your life.

800-HELP

Bulimia/Anorexia Self-Help Hotline. 800-227-4785. M–F 10 A.M.–5 P.M. Eastern time.

National Food Addiction Hotline. 800-872-0088. For people with eating disorders.

Suggestions for Further Reading

Bennett, William, and Gurin, Joel (1982). *The dieter's dilemma: Eating less and weighing more.* New York: Basic Books. Discusses weight loss from the standpoint of the "setpoint" theory.

Wolf, Naomi (1991). *The beauty myth: How images of beauty are used against women.* New York: William Morrow. Proposes thesis that male-dominated society retards the advance of feminism by putting pressure on women to look thin and gorgeous.

Power Eating—Premium Fuel

Can you develop a high-energy power diet? To get to that point, you first need to deal with any concerns about your present eating behavior. Check which of the following areas are of concern to you. (You may check more than one.)[140]

My main worries about my daily diet are . . .

___ **1.** Fat and cholesterol

___ **2.** Weight gain

___ **3.** Foods I like aren't good for me

___ **4.** Guilt about eating foods I like

___ **5.** Confusion about what foods are healthy

Dealing with Your Present Food Worries

The five concerns expressed in the list above were all voiced by people in a survey of 772 adults conducted by The Gallup Organization. The percentages responding to each concern are given below. (The total exceeds 100% owing to multiple responses.)

1. I Worry About Fat and Cholesterol. This concern led the list in the Gallup poll, with 56% saying they worried about the fat and cholesterol in their daily diet. Despite the concern, many of us continue to nourish our cravings—often in the name of convenience—by consuming increasing amounts of take-out food, headed by hamburgers and french fries.[141] Although fat intake has decreased over the past 4 years from 40% to 36% of the average American's Calories, that's still too high: most health authorities recommend we get 30% or fewer of our Calories from fat.[142] As for cholesterol, the number of people reporting changes in their diet to lower their cholesterol levels actually took a turn for the worse, going from 19% in 1986 to 15% in 1990.[143] Although men are three times more likely than women to have a heart attack and al-

though more than half of men ages 20–74 have too-high blood cholesterol levels, only 14% of 506 men questioned in a 1991 survey said they are eating less fat.[144] Finally, it's especially worth noting that, in one 1991 survey of 1004 Americans, a third had the mistaken notion that eating food low in *cholesterol* was the best way to lower their blood cholesterol. Less than a quarter have gotten the message that *saturated fat*—prevalent in meat and dairy products—is most likely to raise blood cholesterol.[145]

What you can do: If you're worried about fat and dietary cholesterol, you should probably try to get your blood cholesterol tested. Don't do it at a local shopping mall with a quickie finger-stick test, which can be vastly inaccurate. Get it done through a physician, who should send you to have blood drawn at a lab certified by the Centers for Disease Control and Prevention. The physician may also ask you to get more than one test to ensure a correct reading. Regardless of the result, you should work *actively* to reduce your consumption of saturated fats. (See ● *table below and* ● *table on next page.*)

● **Blood cholesterol count and risk of heart disease.** Levels are in milligrams per deciliter of blood.

Age	Moderate risk	High risk
2–19	170 or higher	185 or higher
20–29	200 or higher	220 or higher
30–39	220 or higher	240 or higher
40 and up	240 or higher	260 or higher

Source: National Institutes of Health.

2. I Worry About Weight Gain. If you're concerned about this, you're worrying about the same thing that half (50%) of the people in the Gallup poll were concerned about. And at least you're on the right track: the number of overweight Americans may now be nearly two out of three—but almost a third of those who are too heavy do not admit it, according to a Louis Harris and Associates survey for *Prevention* magazine. Overweight men were nearly twice as likely as overweight women to feel they were "at about the right weight."[146] Another survey found that most people (81%) eat a lot more than they think they do—maybe as much as 25% more.[147]

What you can do: While being mindful that many people worry about their weight *unnecessarily,* take a look at the weight tables, assess your body fat, and then make an honest assessment of what you need to do. (The key word here is "honest.")

3. I Worry That the Foods I Like Aren't Good for Me. This, too, is a reasonably commonplace anxiety, with 45% of the respondents in the Gallup poll reporting this concern. In another survey, by the American Dietetic Association, it was found that almost 40% of Americans surveyed are dissatisfied with the way they eat, but many think it's too much work and sacrifice to do anything about it.[148] The same survey found that 79% of the people questioned thought nutrition was important, but only 44% believed they were doing all they could to eat a healthy diet.

What you can do: This concern seems to have two bases: (a) A person knows what foods are healthy or unhealthy but isn't motivated to change eating habits. (b) A person is not aware of the foods that are considered healthy or unhealthy. You may be able to determine which category you're in by seeing how (or if) you responded to questions #4 and #5 below, which deal with these two matters. In any case, the time to take action is *now.* Don't try to change all of your nutritional habits at once, but begin today to make the change.

● **How to lower your blood cholesterol count.** The following diet guidelines will help to achieve the American Heart Association recommendation of a diet in which 30% or fewer of your Calories are in fat.

Food	Guidelines
Beef or pork	Limit servings of lean beef or pork (3.5 ounces each) to three times a week
Poultry, fish	Eat skinless poultry and fish
Fats	Use polyunsaturated oils made from corn, soy beans, and olives
Eggs	Limit egg yolks to two or three a week
Milk	Drink nonfat milk
Fruits, grains	Eat in unlimited amounts: vegetables, fruits, pasta, grains, and beans
Avoid	Animal fats such as butter and cheese, tropical fats such as nuts and peanut butter, heavy sauces, organ meats, and mayonnaise

Source: Adapted from Gladstone Foundation Laboratories, San Francisco General Hospital, San Francisco, CA.

4. I Feel Guilty Over Eating Foods I Like. Thirty-six percent of the Gallup poll respondents agreed with this statement. At bottom, this seems to indicate, as an American Dietetic Association survey found, that people believe—erroneously—that there are "good" and "bad" foods and that the "bad" foods taste best.[149] However, nutritionists point out that any food can be part of a healthy diet—provided it is eaten in moderation.

What you can do: This is a question of motivation. Guilt feelings about eating sugar- or fat-laden food may not translate into behavior change until something inspires you or frightens you. The rest of this essay may give you some reasons for change, if the earlier discussion about the relationship of food to heart disease and cancer has not. Again, you need not *completely* give up those foods that make you feel guilty.

5. I Am Confused About What Foods Are Healthy. You might think more people would share this concern—after all, there is a great deal of information out there about how to eat, and much of it is conflicting—but only 35% did so, according to the Gallup poll. Perhaps this low response is because most Americans believe, contrary to the facts, that they *do* eat a healthful mixture of foods and see no reason to change.[150] In addition, people hate to admit ignorance, even though studies have found a great deal of confusion about what is and is not all right to eat. For example, when asked to identify the chief health problem in the American diet (as singled out by the U.S. Surgeon General), only 39% knew that the most dangerous thing in our food is fat, linked to heart disease, cancer, and weight problems.[151] Six out of 10 Americans seem not to have heard this, one of the most important health messages of our time.

What you can do: This may be a question of knowledge. Reading this chapter, learning how to read nutrition labels, learning what it actually *means* when a pizza label states it has 10 grams of fat (how does that compare with the daily recommended amount of fat?)—such knowledge can give you the skills to both eat for pleasure and eat for health. It may also be a question of motivation, always a strong factor in health matters.

Developing a Power Diet

Are you tired all the time? Do you slow down after lunch? Or do you feel well enough but seek premium fuel that will boost productivity or athletic performance? Getting more energy does not depend just on food. As we discuss elsewhere, you need to avoid shorting yourself 1½ hours of sleep a night (as many people evidently do, but don't recognize it), participate in a regular program of exercise (you'd be surprised how little investment is required), and manage stress and depression. But food is important. What follows are some high-performance eating suggestions for high-performance people.

1. Don't Eat Too Much Protein. Unfortunately, even athletes, both amateurs and professionals, mirror the excessive fat-and-protein diet of the general population, proving just how difficult eating habits are to change. (San Francisco 49er Bubba Paris, for instance, was barred from football practice after showing a blood cholesterol level in the 280–400 range, putting him at risk for heart disease. Paris reportedly often skipped the healthy training-table meals in favor of take-out fried chicken.[152]) "The steak-and-eggs breakfast on game day is purely psychological," says Kathy Heyl, vice president of a dietary consulting firm in Boulder, Colorado. "Eight-ounce filets are 50–70% fat, and there's no reason at all for bacon—it's all fat."[153]

Recently, however, athletes and others interested in high performance have begun to shift to a leaner diet. This has some bonuses. As sports nutritionists point out, the dietary changes that best improve athletic performance "are exactly those that also support better preventive health and long-term body control."[154]

Athletes need only slightly more (perhaps only 10% more) protein than anyone else, but this is taken into account in the normal protein recommendations. Even building muscle doesn't require extra protein. Some sports nutritionists recommend a high-performance diet as follows:[155,156]

- *Protein:* 15% of Calories
- *Fats:* 25% of Calories
- *Carbohydrates:* 60% of Calories

2. Eat Complex Carbohydrates to Provide Glycogen, the Performance Fuel. Why would being a race-car driver require any special kind of diet? Driver Emerson Fittipaldi, who won the 1989 Indianapolis 500 at age 42, was able to beat younger competitors in large part as a result of his diet and exercise regimen. (*See • chart on next page.*) Driving an Indy-car race, after all, isn't like just commuting to work: going through a corner exerts a lateral pull on the driver's head and arms that is up to three times the force of gravity. Drivers thus need muscular endurance and flexibility to survive three hours or more in a cramped cockpit for a 500-mile race.

Besides weight training, Fittipaldi has a year-round high-energy diet that consists of 70–75% complex carbohydrates: whole grains, barley, whole-wheat pasta, vegetables, and fruit. The rest is split between protein—specifically beans and some fish and poultry—and fat, in the form of grains, fish, and poultry.[157]

A race-car driver's performance requirement of endurance and flexibility may be slightly different from that of a football player, which is speed and power, or of a marathon runner, which is mainly endurance, or of a weight lifter, which is strength. Still, the reason athletes of all sorts need large quantities of carbohydrates is to produce *glycogen*, which is mobilized to provide glucose, the body's main energy source and the fuel that enables the body to sustain intense physical activity. Fat and protein do not produce glycogen; carbohydrates do. During low or moderate activity, the body principally uses fat as fuel, but as the intensity of the activity increases, it switches to glycogen.

This concept has led to the idea of *glycogen loading* or *carbohydrate loading* for marathon runners, an overstock-and-starve strategy for getting the muscles to store more glycogen than usual. The idea is to provide extra glycogen so that the runner can continue to perform past the normal "hitting the wall" point of exhaustion. In the old-fashioned extreme approach, which involved a wildly fluctuating pattern of eating and exercise the week before a race, glycogen loading was found to be dangerous to runners' health. Some people passed out, and others injured themselves. Today's modified strategy involves these steps:[158]

- The athlete exercises rigorously until 7 days before the race.

- In the next 3 days, the training is less strenuous, and the runner eats about half his or her Calories in carbohydrates.

- On the last 2 days before the race, the training is light. However, carbohydrate intake increases to 70% of Calories.

- On the day before the race, the athlete rests but maintains the high carbohydrate intake.

- **A race-car driver's diet.** Indianapolis 500 winner Emerson Fittipaldi is a near–vegetarian. Between meals, Fittipaldi snacks on organic fruit and roasted seeds.

A typical day's meals for Fittipaldi during racing season:
- *Breakfast:* Granola with soy milk
  - Whole-wheat toast with apple jam
  - Herb tea
- *Lunch:* Brown rice vegetable sushi (norimaki)
  - Vegetable salad with arame sea vegetable
  - Garbanzo beans
- *Dinner:* Broiled salmon
  - Vegetable medley
  - Rice pilaf
  - Salad
  - Apple oatie crumb crisp

Although few readers of this book may be marathon runners, everyone can still take advantage of a high-complex-carbohydrate diet to achieve maximum performance.

3. Eat a Diet That Provides All the Vitamins and Minerals. What vitamin pills should you take for high-performance activity? It's tempting to think that gobbling great amounts of vitamin and mineral supplements will transform you, but that is reflective of our society's belief in the magic of pills. However, unless you've decided that the five food groups are named McDonald's, Wendy's, Burger King, Carl's Jr., and Jack in the Box—that is, you've elected not to get a balanced diet—you probably won't need, and shouldn't take, vitamin and mineral supplements, except as noted below. (Even then, a lopsided, fat-heavy diet cannot be counteracted with a daily dose of multivitamins.)

Of course athletes and other high-energy individuals need micronutrients, such as the B vitamins, to activate the fuel reserves in their muscles. And a person who expends 4000–6000 Calories a day, as some football players do, needs two or three times more B vitamins than someone who expends 2000 Calories. Even so, you can get these vitamins, plus vitamins A, C, and E, which are important in oxygen-carrying red blood cells, from a low-fat, high-complex-carbohydrate, *balanced* diet. Even sodium, potassium, and zinc losses from frequent heavy perspiration can be restored from a regular balanced diet—particularly one containing fruit juices, fruits, and vegetables—rather than from supplements. Salt tablets are seldom necessary for sodium replacement; you can get the sodium you need from your regular food. Zinc, which promotes wound healing, can be obtained from lean beef, turkey, cereals, and beans.

One instance where a supplement may be required is in cases of women who have an iron deficiency. Many women must pay special attention to consuming foods that are iron sources (meats, dark green vegetables, legumes) to avoid iron depletion through menstruation. Those who are diagnosed as iron-deficient may benefit from iron supplements. So may women who are pregnant.

4. Get *More* Fluids Than You Need to Satisfy Your Thirst. This is critical for athletes. We have stated that the thirst mechanism is a faulty indicator of your liquid requirements—that it does not cause you to replenish all the water you need, particularly if you are physically active. Thus, it's recommended that you drink *beyond* the point of quenching thirst and drink before athletic workouts and competitions as well as during and afterwards. (An indication that you have drunk enough water before an event is that your urine is clear.) Specifically, to prevent heat disorders, you should drink 2 or more cups of water 2 hours before an event and another 2 cups 15 minutes before. During the activity, depending on how vigorous it is, you should then drink ½ to 1 cup of water about every 15 minutes. Because dehydration may continue several days past an athletic event, you should continue to drink extra amounts of water in the days that follow.

Despite their popularity, most sports beverages such as Gatorade have a high concentration of sugar, which tends to keep the fluid in the stomach rather than speeding it to the areas of the body needing replenishment. Exercise physiologists recommend water because it is absorbed faster. If sports drinks are used, they should be diluted by adding equal parts water. Next to water, juices are the best form of fluid. Caffeine and alcohol should be avoided because they act as diuretics and thus speed the excretion of fluid.

5. Eat Frequently, If You Like, but Avoid Junk Diets. If you are so active as to expend 5000–6000 Calories a day, it may be difficult for you to consume the food required at three sit-down meals. Thus, if you expend this much energy, it is permissible, in fact desirable, to have five or six smaller meals or to have frequent nutritious snacks—"grazing," as it is called. You should be aware that what we *do not* mean by snacks are chips, pretzels, ice cream, cookies, and the like, which are not low-fat and not nutritious.

Even those whose Calorie requirements aren't that high can benefit from snacking. A series of mini-meals instead of a big lunch may help avoid that drowsy afternoon letdown, says sports nutritionist Liz Applegate.[159] A midafternoon snack, she says, will also help you do a physical workout in late afternoon and enhances your memory and alertness, perhaps because it boosts the energy supply to the brain. Frequent snacking on low-fat, nutritious foods may even lower blood cholesterol levels.

By now, perhaps, it should be apparent that snacking won't work if it consists of sugar- and fat-laden candy bars, cookies, potato chips, or ice cream. Better are fruit, vegetables, yogurt, bread sticks, unbuttered popcorn, juices, unsalted nuts, whole-grain crackers, and similar high-complex-carbohydrate items. Apples, for instance, are particularly good for helping you to bounce back.

Three further suggestions:

- *Eat often:* Eat every few hours and eat before you get too hungry. This will keep you from being overwhelmed by hunger and gorging.

- *Avoid large containers:* Don't eat food directly out of a large container. A box of crackers can disappear before you know it.
- *Try reaching for a sport bar instead of a candy bar:* A sport bar, available in supermarket health-food sections or health-food stores, looks like a candy bar but is fortified with carbohydrates, protein, vitamins, and minerals. The important point is to make sure you're not getting a high-fat candy bar in disguise. Read the labels carefully to make sure your snack choice has less than 30% of its Calories from fat and more than 60% from carbohydrates (particularly complex carbohydrates), which break down more slowly than simple sugars—thus providing a steady flow of energy.[160]

Examples of sport bars are Alena Energy Bar, Cross Trnr., Energize, Exceed Sports Bar, Meal on the Go, Pure Power Energy Bar, and Quigley's Alpha 1 Nutri-Bar. They are best washed down with water during and after exercise.

6. Avoid Phony Body-Building Products, Such as Protein Supplements. Significantly increasing your performance should not significantly decrease the content of your wallet. In other words, athletes can get most of what they need from a normal, varied diet rather than from the products of the health promoters out there promising all kinds of marvelous outcomes from using their products.

For instance, if the average adult needs only 0.8–1.2 grams of protein per 2.2 pounds of body weight, then the typical North American diet probably furnishes all the protein you need. Even most athletes and heavy-duty exercisers don't need to increase their protein intake. The makers of amino-acid-containing protein supplements, however, promise their products will build muscles and bulk. But, as one writer points out, protein supplements "may hurt more than help in your efforts to improve your strength, endurance, and appearance."[161] Protein not burned for energy will be converted to body fat. Products billed as "smart drinks" (some brand names: Focus, Go For It) also contain amino acids, but there is no evidence they produce any benefits.

In These Chapters:

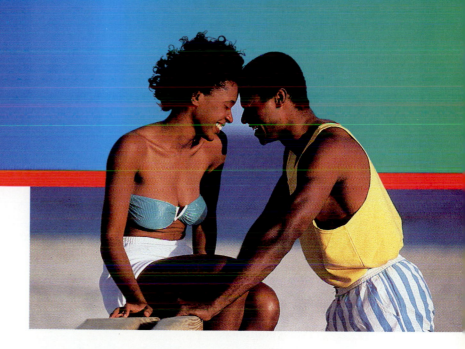

Are there an ideal man and an ideal woman?

Let us consider a couple of stereotypical ideas about males and females and exercise.

First consider men. No doubt you've seen them—the muscular, tattooed, heavy-smoking, hard-drinking embodiments of supposedly manly attributes. They lift washing machines or packing boxes or stacks of lumber for several hours straight. Their diet consists of soft drinks, cigarettes, burgers, and fries. Their relaxation after hours is beer and television. Aside from heavy lifting, they get almost no exercise. They treat their bodies as though they would last forever. How do they do it?

The answer is: we have not seen the end of their story yet. These rugged types are walking time-bombs, almost certain to self-destruct prematurely from heart disease or cancer, if they are not side-lined first by bad backs or other crippling injuries. While a new generation of men was learning new behaviors, these stereotypes of the Old Male Ways were buying into a myth of indestructibility. As one writer describes it, "They're still in the thrall of every old cowboy movie they've ever seen, still living in some sort of Health Time Warp from the 1950s."[1] Yet perhaps, as the author points out, it is the examples of these gritty he-men that makes it so hard for some other males to take seriously the idea of taking care of themselves.

Now let us consider the stereotypical woman. According to psychologist Marilyn Mason, many women are not socialized to be physical.[2] When growing up, she says, few females are complimented on their strength or height or speed or athletic ability. In addition, of course, women must deal with society's powerful messages about the desirability of being thin, so that they may be highly fearful of being overweight—and hence afraid of appearing un-

gainly in athletics. Thus, many women have much to discover about self-confidence and esteem regarding their bodies.

In the struggle to "improve" themselves, women often concentrate on areas other than physical activity, such as makeup, dieting, or cosmetic surgery, according to the St. Paul-based Melpomene Institute for Women's Health Research. Even some of those who become serious about exercise and begin to tone up their muscles and smooth out their torsos are not able to accept their bodies, so distorted is their ideal body image.[3] Fortunately, these reactions are exceptions rather than the rule. "For most women," the Melpomene authors write, "taking up exercise helps them to put less importance on the issue of weight."

A stereotype by definition is an oversimplified, uncritical, standardized mental picture. Needless to say, it is unfair to portray many working men as abusing their bodies or many women as not having been socialized to be comfortable with the physical. Yet these myths linger in the minds of many people. Let us consider the place of physical activity in our lives, one of the most underrealized of the arts of living.

17   Physical Fitness

▶ What is a major risk factor in heart
disease?

▶ Describe several benefits of physical
activity.

▶ Discuss the importance of motivation in
exercise and describe three principal areas
of physical fitness.

▶ Discuss the benefits and activities that increase each of the following: flexibility, aerobic endurance, and muscular strength and
endurance.

▶ What are some principal methods for
avoiding injuries and pain?

How do you keep yourself healthy as the
years go by? One means is psychological:
you stay interested in and intellectually
engaged with the world. This engagement will
be reflected in the way you move—purposefully and energetically, rather than downtrod-
den and hunched forward, as if everything were
hopeless, says William Nagler, professor of
physical and rehabilitation medicine.[4] The other
means is physical: most people by age 40 have
lost 30–35% of the range of motion in their
hips, but if one merely walks 10 or so minutes a
day and stretches the hips, says Nagler, this loss
of motion most likely will never happen.

And so we come to the first question people
have about exercise: Do you have to push hard,
get sweaty, run, or do high-impact aerobic
dance in order to deliver benefits to the body?
The answer is simple: no, you don't. Even a little exercise goes a long way. But, as the expression goes, you have to use it or lose it.

The Sedentary Society

**Inactivity, not high cholesterol, is one of
the most important risk factors for heart
attacks. Unfortunately, only a third of
Americans engage in a regular program of
physical activity. One enemy of fitness is
television: people who watch 4 or more
hours of TV a day are more apt to be fat.
Some healthy people are not necessarily
athletic but engage in a great deal of daily
physical activity anyway.**

In the 1970s and 1980s, people by the millions throughout North America began adopting
healthier ways of living. They gave up smoking,
started eating less cholesterol-rich eggs and red
meat, and began exercising regularly. By now,
one would think, these healthy habits must
really be catching on. Is it true they have been
adopted by most Americans?

The Enemy Is the Easy Chair The fitness
movement may have peaked recently, according
to evidence from an annual survey conducted
by the Harris Poll. Since 1983, the survey has
shown steady advances on 21 key health behaviors, but the 1991 survey suggests these improvements may have slowed or stopped.
Indeed, some health gains that did occur in recent years came from changes in technology,
legislation, and government. A notable lack of
progress occurred in areas having to do with
lifestyle or self-discipline, such as nutrition,
weight control, and exercise. Most significant,
for our present discussion, the percentage of
adult Americans who exercise regularly was
found to be unchanged since 1983—just 34%.[5]

This is a tremendously important fact, for
this reason: despite all the publicity about cholesterol being a cause of coronary heart disease,
it turns out that this fatty substance is not the
most important factor in deaths from heart attacks in the United States. Rather, the principal
cause is **sedentary living,** a way of life characterized by little or no physical activity—defined
as being physically active fewer than three
times per week and less than 20 minutes per
session.[6] (*See ● Figure 17.1.*)

The moral: A regular program of physical
activity won't just help you look better or feel
better. It may save your life.

**TV or Not TV: Does Television Make You
Fat?** How do you spend your time? For most
American adults, watching television is second
only to working for a living in the hierarchy of
waking activities. For children it's even worse:
watching TV is their *primary* waking activity—
only sleeping consumes more of their time.[7,8]

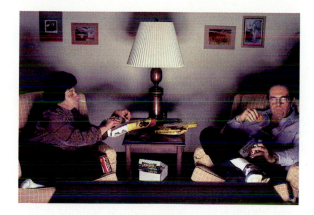

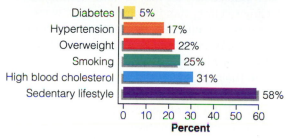

Ninety-nine percent of American homes have at least one TV set (14% of homes have four or more), and 98% of Americans watch some TV every day. Women ages 18–34 watch an average of 25 hours of TV a week, men of the same age 22 hours. Television viewing tends to increase with age.[9] When teenagers today reach the age of 70, most will have watched *7 years* worth of television.[10] Think of all that one could do with those 7 years: develop a talent, become an A student, write a novel, build a business, see the world, help the less fortunate, and so on.

Are you a television addict? Forty-two percent of Americans say they think they watch too much TV, and 13% consider themselves addicted.[11] (*See Self Discovery 17.1.*)

SELF DISCOVERY 17.1

Are You a TV Victim?

Check yes or no for each question.

	Yes	No
1. Do you watch more than 2 hours a day of television?	___	___
2. Do you cease to communicate with others while you are viewing TV?	___	___
3. Do you become unhappy or irritated when you must turn the television off to do something else?	___	___
4. Do you feel extremely tired during a regular day's schedule?	___	___
5. Do you frequently eat unhealthy snack food when you sit down to watch television?	___	___
6. When you experience insomnia, do you use TV as a means of distraction during your sleeplessness?	___	___
7. On a pleasant day, are you more likely to stay indoors and watch television than to do something outside?	___	___
8. Is it difficult for you to share and communicate your feelings and experiences with others?	___	___
9. Are you actively involved in fewer than two hobbies, clubs, or sports at least 4 hours a week?	___	___
10. Do you frequently turn on the television and search the stations without having a specific program in mind to watch?	___	___

Grading your quiz

For every odd-numbered question you answered yes, give yourself 2 points. These factors were determined by *Prevention* magazine experts to be indicators of too much TV watching.

For every even-numbered question you answered yes, give yourself 1 point. These factors, in conjunction with poor viewing habits, signal possible trouble.

Tally your score, then use the following scale as a rating guide:

3 points or less—No problem
4–6 points—Potential trouble brewing
7–9 points—Excessive television viewing
10 points or more—Your brain is becoming fused to your TV's circuitry

Source: Adapted from: Anonymous (1991, November). Better health with a twist of the wrist. *Prevention, 43*, pp. 41–43, 116.

With so much time being spent before the tube, perhaps we can begin to understand why so many people are overweight and out of shape. Indeed, the evidence seems pretty clear that many hours of TV viewing increases one's risk of obesity. In one study of 6000 working middle-aged men, those who spent more than 3–4 hours a day watching television had twice the risk of obesity—that is, having 20–30% or more body fat—as men who watched less than 1 hour.[12] A similar study of 5000 working women, average age 35, found that those who watched 3–4 or more hours a day were twice as apt to be obese.[13] A 1990 study of nearly 800 adults found that only 4.5% of those who watched an hour or less of TV a day were obese; however, for those watching 4 or more hours, obesity shot up to 19.2%.[14]

Of course it's not the light waves from the TV that cause obesity. Larry Tucker, who co-authored two of these studies, suggests that there is a cyclical relationship between TV viewing and obesity, with one behavior reinforcing the other. That is, as TV viewing time increases, exercise decreases and snacking increases. And as people become less physically fit, they are more likely to engage in passive recreation such as TV viewing.[15]

Breaking TV-aholism is like breaking other strong habits that have a grip on your life: you have to *think about what you're doing*. If you decide that you are pouring too much of your time into television watching, there are a number of things you can do:[16]

- *Plan your viewing:* You may dislike this idea because it takes away the spontaneity, but if great hunks of time are disappearing into the TV, one has to start somewhere. Take Sunday's TV log and mark the programs you want to watch that week. *Watch only those programs, and turn off the set when they are over.*

- *Avoid channel hopping:* When you're looking at one of your prearranged programs, don't change channels. Nearly two-thirds of people who watch television "graze" or "channel surf"—flick through the channels to other stations. This leads to mindless viewing.

- *Get away from the TV set:* Avoid sitting around. When you're not following your prearranged viewing plan, get out of the room where the TV is located. In fact, get out of the house if you can and take a walk, see friends, or do something else that's active. If you have to stay near the TV, replace TV viewing with another activity you like, such as reading. Of course you can always go study, too.

Are You Fitter Than You Think? Maybe you lead what you think is an essentially unathletic life. You may, however, be physically active in ways that you don't normally regard as "exercise." Such activities may include walking or bicycling to class, standing or moving at work, taking care of children, doing housework or gardening, and similar physical tasks. (*See Self Discovery 17.2.*)

In their book *Healthy Pleasures,* psychologist Robert Ornstein and physician David Sobel suggest that a lot of people have *exercise* and *physical activity* confused. They write: "Exercise is usually a deliberate, sometimes odious, sweat-soaked endeavor that can take time away from life, whereas physical activity can be any daily undertaking, work or play, that involves movement."[17]

Although exercise need not be "odious," Ornstein and Sobel have an important point: the physical activity you do can either be part of your regular daily exertions or it can be something you elect to do for *fun.* Either way, you're more apt to do it if you don't consider it an unpleasant chore.

The Benefits of Physical Activity

Physical activity can enhance your mood, energy, and creativity; keep weight down; reduce heart disease risk; perhaps reduce risk of cancer and diabetes; protect against bone loss in women; make you sexier; and slow aging.

Perhaps many of us have come of age with some misguided ideas about physical activity. In North America, the essential yardstick for measuring physical fitness is *competitive sports*. People often grow up thinking it is better to learn how to accurately throw a football, dunk a basketball, or hit a hockey puck than to develop strength and endurance. Indeed, many exercise

SELF DISCOVERY 17.2

Could You Be Fitter Than You Think?

Even if you are seemingly unathletic, you may get more physical activity than you think. To find out, take the following quiz. (Score zero for any questions that don't apply.)

1. In an average day, I climb _____ flights of stairs (approximately 12 stairs per flight).
   - A. 1–5   1 point
   - B. 6–10   2 points
   - C. More than 10   4 points
   - D. None of the above   0 points

2. My job or my daily work- or school-related activity requires that I be on my feet and moving _____ hours a day. Count actual time moving only—usually about half the time on the job.
   - A. 1 hour   2 points
   - B. 2 hours   3 points
   - C. 3 hours   4 points
   - D. 4 hours or more   6 points
   - E. None of the above   0 points

3. My job or daily work- or school-related activity requires that I be on my feet _____ hours a day, but I move around very little.
   - A. 4 hours   1 point
   - B. 6 hours   2 points
   - C. 8 hours   3 points
   - D. None of the above   0 points

4. In an average day I walk about _____ miles without stopping.
   - A. 1 mile   2 points
   - B. 2 miles   4 points
   - C. 3 miles   6 points
   - D. 4 miles or more   10 points
   - E. None of the above   0 points

5. I spend about _____ hours a week tending a garden or lawn. (Points assume year-round activity. If seasonal, cut points in half.)
   - A. 1 hour   1 point
   - B. 2 hours   2 points
   - C. 3 hours   3 points
   - D. 4 hours   4 points
   - E. 5 hours or more   5 points
   - F. None of the above   0 points

6. I am a parent who assumes primary responsibility for a preschool child. (Add 50% of points for each additional child.)
   - A. child and parent at home all day   5 points
   - B. half day in day-care center   3 points
   - C. full day in day-care center   1 point
   - D. I am not a parent   0 points

7. My job is physically demanding (lifting, carrying, shoveling, climbing) for _____ hours a day. (Consider only the time you are actually involved in vigorous activity.)
   - A. 1 hour   3 points
   - B. 2 hours   5 points
   - C. 3 hours   7 points
   - D. 4 hours   9 points
   - E. 5 hours or more   12 points
   - F. None of the above   0 points

8. I engage in light sports (doubles tennis, softball) or dancing _____ hours a week. (Year-round activity is assumed, even though the sports may change. If the activity is seasonal, divide the points earned accordingly.)
   - A. 1 hour   1 point
   - B. 2 hours   2 points
   - C. 3 hours   3 points
   - D. 4 hours or more   5 points
   - E. None of the above   0 points

(continued)

SELF DISCOVERY 17.2
(*continued*)

9. I perform household chores (laundry, cleaning, cooking) an average of _____ hours a week.
   A. 1 hour   1 point
   B. 2 hours   2 points
   C. 3 hours   3 points
   D. 4 hours   4 points
   E. 5 hours or more   6 points
   F. None of the above   0 points
10. I have a desk job, but I leave my desk regularly to run errands, greet visitors, attend meetings, and so on, at least _____ times an hour.
   A. 6 or fewer   0 points
   B. more than 6   1 point

Scoring

11 or more points: Even though you are not engaged in a formal exercise/fitness program, chances are good that you are getting a sufficient amount of physical activity each day. This is a plus, especially if you are covering health bases in terms of stress control, body weight, and diet.

5–10 points: You're probably in a little better shape than you think, but can do much better.

0–4 points: You're a couch potato all-star, and your health could be suffering for it. Try to build more activity into your life, no matter how trivial it may seem.

Source: Adapted from Stamford, B. A., & Shmer, P. (1990). *Fitness without exercise.* New York: Warner Books.

researchers are concerned that school physical-education programs tend to devote attention and resources to sports that enable comparatively few students to play or participate, such as football, basketball, and baseball. There is little attempt, they say, to emphasize running, swimming, bicycling, and similar activities that people can rely on for the rest of their lives.[18]

As we shall show, physical fitness can be derived from a wide range of activities. The important point is to realize that the benefits of physical activity are substantial. Among them are the following.

Enhance Mood, Energy, and Creativity

"I've never treated a depressed patient who was physically fit," claims psychiatrist and medical professor Robert S. Brown. Indeed, when he sits down with a new patient, his first question is not "What's on your mind?" Rather, it is "How much do you exercise?"[19]

Physical activity or exercise can improve happiness in several ways. (*See ● Figure 17.2.*)

- *It releases "feel good" brain chemicals—endorphins and serotonin:* You may have

heard of a euphoria called the "runner's high" that is said to energize long-distance runners.[20] This euphoria can be achieved in activities (such as dancing) that don't require the runner's kind of heavy training, although it may take 20–30 minutes of sustained activity for the experience to develop. The positive feeling seems to have something to do with chemicals in the brain.[21] Exercise delivers the release of two substances in particular that seem to promote good feelings:

(1) *Endorphins:* **Endorphins** are naturally occurring painkillers (opiates) that make the mind feel anywhere from mildly better to ecstatic. Endorphins are produced in the brain and spinal cord to minimize pain in the body. However, researchers believe these chemicals also produce the runner's high—the feeling similar to (but certainly safer than) the euphoria that heroin and morphine addicts get.[22]

(2) *Serotonin:* **Serotonin** is a brain chemical that is associated with a sense of

well-being and impulse control. Depletion of serotonin results in depression. Serotonin is one of the brain's principal neurotransmitters. (A *neurotransmitter* is a chemical that transmits nerve impulses.)

- *It can prevent or alleviate depression:* Although we don't mean to suggest that physical activity will *always* keep one from feeling depressed or cure depression, nevertheless exercise can help alleviate the blues. For instance, in one experiment, a group of mildly and moderately depressed patients were assigned randomly to one of two groups—those who received psychotherapy and those who began running. The runners felt better after only a week, and were declared "virtually well" within 3 weeks, with the benefits lasting at least a year. The runners were reported to do as well as the patients receiving short-term psychotherapy and better than those receiving long-term psychotherapy.[23–26]

- *It can relieve anxiety and tension:* Exercise may provide a way to release anger, anxiety, and physical tensions.[27–29] One study of men and women ages 30–49 who walked at slow, medium, fast, and self-selected paces showed "immediate and significant decrease in anxiety and tension." Each group showed improved moods up to 2 hours after the workout ended. Most interesting, the benefits occurred at all paces; the intensity of the exercise did not matter.[30]

- *It can dramatically increase your energy level:* When you are depressed, you may have less energy. But even if you are just feeling run down, exercise can boost your energy level. For instance, a brisk 10-minute walk can increase energy and decrease fatigue for as long as 2 hours.[31] Thus, when you have an afternoon slump in energy, you will probably find a short, vigorous walk is a better picker-upper than, say, a candy bar.[32]

- *It can distract you and stimulate creative thinking:* Some people who exercise experience *disassociation*—the ability or tendency to take one's mind off the task at hand and let the brain "take a vacation."[33]

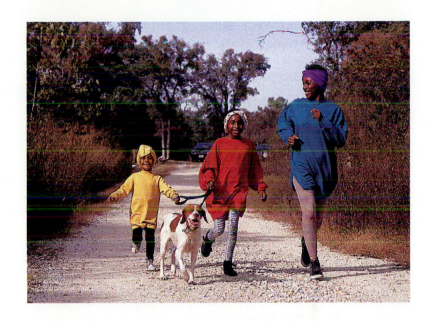

● **Figure 17.2 Feeling great.** Regular physical activity seems to make us happy.

> ❝*Gentle exercise can make you feel terrific. When you begin an exercise program you improve mood, happiness, confidence, and body image, and achieve a sense of self-mastery. It doesn't take much exercise to make a difference: walking a mile or two substantially reduces your anxiety level. And it doesn't seem to matter whether you walk slowly or fast.*❞
>
> —Robert Ornstein, Ph.D., & David Sobel, M.D. (1989). *Healthy pleasures.* Reading, MA: Addison-Wesley, p. 108.

Of course, this kind of daydreaming is *not* an advantage during competition or during training in weight-lifting or in team sports, when the mind must stay focused. However, on other occasions it can provide a kind of mental refreshment. Indeed, studies suggest that exercise can sharpen mental skills and enhance creativity. For instance, physical education professor Joan C. Gondola tested 60 young women on creative problem-solving before and after 20 minutes of aerobic dance. She found that creativity increased even after a single session of exercise.[34]

Keep Weight Down Reduce food portions, reduce fat intake, reduce alcohol you consume, and reduce Calories you eat—these are frequent tips one hears for reducing weight. Unfortunately, for many people, these measures aren't entirely successful, for once they stop, the pounds go right back on. What all respectable weight-loss plans recommend, in addition to "reduction," is an *increase* in physical activity. This is the principal way to keep your weight at its desirable limits. What's interesting is that although you may burn only a relatively few Calories during a workout, your body burns a great deal more throughout the day *following* the exercise. As one writer puts it, "Exercise helps you lose weight by turning your body into a calorie-guzzling machine."[35]

Two kinds of exercise are especially desirable for weight loss:

- *Aerobic conditioning: Aerobic exercise*—regular high-intensity workouts such as running, vigorous swimming, or bicycling—boost the body's consumption of oxygen. People who are in good shape aerobically are able to turn fat into energy in their muscle cells faster than people who are not as fit. (*See* ● *Figure 17.3.*)

- *Resistance training:* Doing sit-ups, lifting free weights, working out on weight machines—the kind of exercise called *resistance training*—builds muscle. Muscle burns more Calories a day (30–50 Calories per pound) than does fat (2 Calories per pound). The more muscle you have, then, the more Calories you will expend, even when you are just sitting around. Thus, resistance training may help you *add* pounds in muscle but *lose* even more pounds in fat.

Reduce Heart Disease Risk For couch potatoes thinking of taking up exercise, there is good news: it takes very little physical activity to achieve health benefits. As Ornstein and Sobel write, "Even the most dedicated sloth can make great gains in health and well-being merely by increasing activity from none to some."[36]

This conclusion was supported by findings from a long-term study involving nearly 17,000 Harvard alumni, which analyzed the relationship between heart-disease deaths and exer-

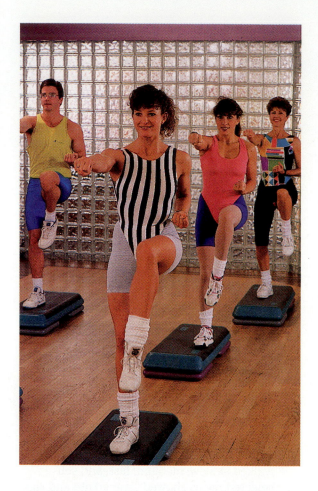

● **Figure 17.3 Workouts and weight loss**

❝*Studies show that aerobically fit people have more mitochondria, the tiny 'boiler rooms' inside muscle cells where fat is turned into energy, than do people who are out of shape. That means they can work harder and longer without huffing and puffing and feeling exhausted. It also means that, if they continue eating about the same amount, they're likely to burn more calories than they take in. So it's easier for them to lose fat.*❞

—Kathleen McCleary (1992, December/January). The no-gimmick weight-loss plan. *In Health*, p. 83.

cise.[37] Most of the benefits were found to occur in those who expended 500–2000 Calories a week, with some added benefits for those expending up to 3500 Calories. The loss of 500 Calories a week, which produced a decline in death rates of 20%, can be achieved by just a 15-minute walk a day.

More physical exercise may be even more helpful—but only up to a point. For instance, a study of 12,000 middle-aged men found that those who burned 1600 Calories a week had 40% fewer deaths from heart attacks than those who expended under 500 Calories a week. However, the expenditure of 4500 Calories a week did not result in any further lessening of fatal heart attacks.[38]

There is even some evidence that physical activity—along with a low-fat diet, no smoking, and stress-reduction techniques—can reverse coronary heart disease.[39] An anecdote is told of Eula Weaver, who at age 67 developed heart disease with angina and at age 75 was hospitalized with a severe heart attack. By age 81 she had such difficulty with congestive heart failure and poor circulation that she had to wear gloves on her hands in summer (because of cold fingers) and could not walk more than 100 feet. After adopting a high-carbohydrate diet and exercise program, her symptoms disappeared, and at age 85 she became a phenomenal success story: she trained for and won gold medals in the 800 and 1500 meters at the Senior Olympics![40]

We need to raise a warning here, however. The exercise-and-heart-disease issue is an example of how you should not base your opinion on just one study. For instance, several studies show that exercise seems to work directly in lowering blood pressure, one of the strongest risk factors in heart disease.[41–44] But other studies have found that aerobic exercise alone does not appear to be effective treatment for high blood pressure.[45,46] Even so, the director of one of the latter studies, James Blumenthal, says, "I still think there is something to exercise. Now it's a question of finding out exactly what it is."[47] Perhaps what's required is exercise *in conjunction with* other things, such as a regular, continuing, ongoing, exercise program along with smoking cessation and dietary changes.

Reduce Risk of Cancer and Diabetes Does exercise help diminish the risk of cancer and diabetes? Women who were involved in varsity sports in college were found to be less likely to develop breast cancer or cancers of the reproductive system in later life. A study of nearly 5400 college alumnae also found such women experienced lower risk of bone fractures and diabetes.[48]

A long-term study of over 17,000 Harvard alumni, men ages 30–79, found that regular vigorous exercise during the middle and later years of life reduced rates of colon and rectal cancer. Those who were moderately or highly active exercisers had half the risk of colon cancer compared to men who were inactive. The protection against cancer appeared to diminish or disappear if the subjects stopped exercising.[49] It has been speculated that exercise may help prevent colon cancer by speeding the final digestive process. Increasing intestinal speed means that potential cancer-causing substances in food have less exposure to the lining of the colon because food passes through the digestive and elimination system faster.[50]

At least 20% of the adult population is at risk for adult-onset diabetes, says Edward Horton, past president of the American Diabetes Association.[51] In **adult-onset diabetes,** also known as **noninsulin-dependent diabetes,** which affects 12 million Americans, the body does not effectively process **insulin,** a hormone produced by the body to regulate blood sugar levels. A study of nearly 6000 male graduates of the University of Pennsylvania, however, found that exercise reduces the chances of acquiring this disease—especially among those who are overweight, have high blood pressure, or have a family history of the disease. Exercising 4 or more hours a week could reduce the risk by more than 40%.[52]

Protect Against Bone Loss in Women The bone-crumbling disorder of **osteoporosis** is one that should be of concern to every woman. Indeed, osteoporosis occurs in one out of four women above 65 years of age.[53] This condition, which occurs following menopause and seems to be related to decreased estrogen levels, consists of bone loss—demineralization, during which bones become soft and porous and more apt to break easily. When bone density falls below the norm, a woman is said to reach the "fracture threshold." Her bones become weak enough so that even a simple fall can break them. As a result, women in later life frequently experience hip fractures. In some cases, even the weight of one vertebra pressing on another can collapse the spine, causing a deformity of the upper back known as "dowager's hump."

To prevent these painful problems in later life, women need to take steps early in their lives. The three components of osteoporosis prevention are (1) exercise, which stimulates new bone formation; (2) adequate daily intake of calcium, which helps to mineralize new bone being formed; and—for menopausal women (but not for most young women)—(3) hormone replacement therapy consisting of estrogen and progesterone. (We discuss these matters in more detail in the chapter on aging.)

Two forms of physical activity that all women can use to strengthen their bones are:

- *Weight-bearing, moderate-impact, aerobic exercises:* Jumping or running activities, in which the legs and feet must bear the body's full weight, can produce impact that stimulates bone development. Examples are walking, hiking, jogging, dancing, tennis, volleyball, basketball, low- or high-impact aerobics, and downhill and cross-country skiing.

- *Weight-bearing, nonaerobic, strength-training exercises:* This type of activity stimulates bone development by pulling on the muscles attached to the bone. Examples are weight training with free weights or weight (Nautilus-type) machines.

The least beneficial for bone development are such nonimpact activities as swimming or bicycling.

Make You Sexier Moderate exercise can dramatically improve a person's love life, although excessive exercise can diminish sexual motivation. Research suggests that although interest in sex continues into late adulthood, sexual activity tends to decrease with age. However, an investigation of men and women swimmers aged 40 and over found that the frequency of sexual activity was similar to that reported by many people in their 20s and 30s—about 7 times a month.[54] The study also found that

there was a threshold—about 3 days a week of exercise, 45 minutes a day—beyond which additional training failed to enhance sexuality. Athletes who swam 18 hours or more a week were found to have too little energy or time for lovemaking.

Why does moderate exercise make people sexier? The study authors speculate that the reasons lie less in some kind of hormonal link, if any, between exercise and sexual desire and more in the kinds of social and personal reinforcement they get about looking attractive and fit—and forestalling the normal aging process.

Slow Aging Says physician Walter Bortz II, author of *We Live Too Short and Die Too Long,* "We now know that a very fit body of 70 can be the same as a moderately fit body of 30."[55] In other words, as we said at the outset, the lesson seems to be: "Use it or lose it" (or "Move it or lose it"). Chronological age may be different from "functional age," so that some athletes over 40 can compete effectively against 28-year-olds.

Among the things that a lifelong program of physical activity can do to slow the aging process are the following:

- *Retain muscle mass:* As they age, most people lose their body muscle, primarily through nonuse. Exercise sometimes takes second place to the demands of work and family, but even minimal exercise such as walking 20 minutes a day or lifting weights twice a week can allow one to hang on to most of one's muscle mass well into old age.

- *Strengthen immune system:* Health science professor David Nieman studied 2300 applicants for the 1987 Los Angeles Marathon, looking at the incidence of colds and flus immediately preceding and following the race. He found that overexertion, as seen in those who ran more than 60 miles a week, seemed to depress the immune system, whereas moderate exercise, as shown in those who ran less than 20 miles a week, seemed to result in a reduced incidence of colds and flu. Nieman found in another study that moderate exercise also provided better immunity than lack of exercise.[56]

- *Foster independence:* Exercise does not necessarily help people live longer. But it can help people *stay independent longer* —that is, to live alone into their 80s and 90s, rather than have to submit to custodial care. (See ● *Figure 17.4.*)

Fitness for Fun and Feeling Good

Motivation is important, so exercise should be fun. Physical fitness consists of flexibility, aerobic endurance, and muscular strength and endurance. Guidelines exist for achieving fitness.

"No pain, no gain." If you hear people say this, pay no attention.

The notion that physical fitness cannot be achieved without sacrifice was promoted vigorously for a period of time, and certainly it's still true that competitive athletes may sometimes have to push themselves through pain in order to win. But if you're not in strenuous competition, this idea simply adds stress to an activity that is, among other things, supposed to be fun and *reduce* the stress in your life. Exercise may cause your body to protest somewhat, but you should *stop* doing what you're doing when you experience discomfort or pain. (See ● *Figure 17.5.*)

The Important Question of Motivation The belief that exercise involves discomfort, inconvenience, and great effort is one that puts a lot of people off. Indeed, this may be one reason why half of those who enroll in a supervised exercise program quit within 6 months.[57,58] It's important to note, however, that this 50% dropoff rate is found for *supervised, structured* exercise; it is likely that the decline is not so great for more moderate forms of physical activity.

Personal fitness is not about punishment; it's about *fun* and *feeling good*. The idea is not to think of exercise as training for "how far, how fast." Rather, it is to build in a strong component of fun and to remind yourself that exercise not only improves your health but also makes you feel better.

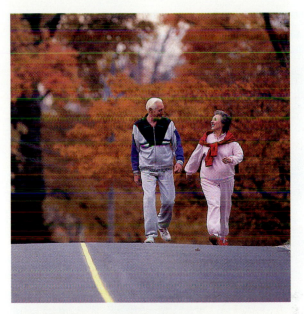

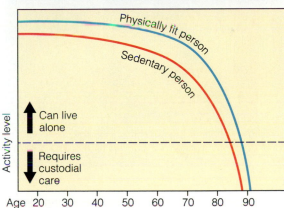

● **Figure 17.4 Staying independent.** Physically fit people are able to live alone longer than sedentary people.

The phases of physical activity where motivation plays a role are getting started or resuming exercise, continuing participation, and not dropping out.[59]

- *Getting started:* At the outset these factors are important:

  (1) Your *attitudes* toward the activity you're thinking of taking up—not exercise in general but specific activities, such as running or lifting weights. Your attitude will determine whether you

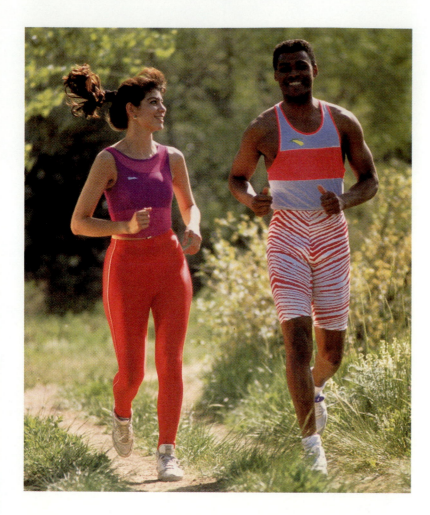

● **Figure 17.5 Pain versus challenge.** How hard should you exercise?

❝*My simple rule of thumb is as follows. If I am exercising so vigorously that I cannot talk easily (without gasping and panting), then I am probably exercising too vigorously. On the other hand, if my body does not feel some stimulation or challenge (an 'alive feeling'), then I probably am not exercising vigorously enough.*❞

—Howard S. Friedman, Ph.D. (1991). *The self-healing personality: Why some people achieve health and others succumb to illness.* New York: Henry Holt, p. 193.

think the activity is too uncomfortable or is worth doing. (Doing a more moderate activity, such as walking instead of running, may make a difference here.) Basically, you must find an activity that's right for you.

(2) *Social support* by friends or family.

(3) *Feeling of being in control,* resulting from making exercise a priority activity, managing time to fit it into your daily schedule, and setting achievable goals.

- *Maintaining participation:* Three motivators are important in helping people continue exercising.

(1) A positive and effective *exercise leader,* if the activity involves a structured class.

(2) *Good feelings* while exercising, helped by warm-up and cool-down sessions and by appropriate music.

(3) *Goal-setting and self-reinforcement* to accomplish specific goals—to lose so many pounds, to jog so far in so many minutes, to walk at least 30 minutes or 3 miles.

- *Preventing the "I quit" mentality:* Two ways to resist dropping out are:

(1) *Prepare for it.*

(2) *Identify it* as quickly as possible when it happens. When you stop exercising, determine what caused the change and use friends and goal-setting techniques to get started again. (See "Getting started" above.)

With it all, one overriding rule applies: *try to make it fun.* Sometimes it *will* be fun, sometimes it won't, but in any case the point is to enjoy it most of the time and to feel better afterward.

The Types of Physical Fitness The purpose of fitness is to enhance your body, mind, and spirit. *Total fitness* has mental, emotional, social, medical, nutritional, and physical elements. **Physical fitness** is defined as having above-average flexibility, aerobic endurance, and muscle strength and endurance:

- *Flexibility:* **Flexibility** is the suppleness of movement, your ability to move through the full range of motion allowed by your joints. This describes, for instance, your ability to touch your toes or twist your body without discomfort or injury.

- *Aerobic endurance:* **Aerobic endurance** describes how efficiently your body uses oxygen. An indicator is how out of breath you become while climbing stairs, riding a bicycle for a couple of miles, or any other **aerobic** activity in which the oxygen taken in is equal to or slightly more than the oxygen used by the body. You need aerobic endurance to achieve **cardiovascular fitness**—the ability to pump blood through your heart and blood vessels efficiently.

- *Muscle strength and muscular endurance:* The fitness of your muscles is measured in two ways:

  (1) **Muscle strength** is the ability to exert force against resistance, whether standing up from a chair or lifting a free weight.

  (2) **Muscular endurance** is the ability to keep repeating those muscle exertions, so that you can scoop not just one but several shovels full of snow.

As we suggested earlier, physical fitness may be achieved in two ways:

- *Physical activity:* **Physical activity** refers to *any* behavior that involves moving your muscles, from house cleaning and gardening to running and weight-lifting.

- *Exercise:* **Exercise** is a particular kind of physical activity, which involves consciously participating in activities that promote physical fitness. Such activity can range from walking to competitive sports.

Although any activity is better than no activity, and regular movement better than infrequent movement, the point of exercise is that it builds physical fitness in specific areas that are challenged during your workouts. Ideally, your exercise program will address the major areas of flexibility, aerobic endurance, and muscular strength and endurance.

Guidelines for Improving Fitness In 1990, the American College of Sports Medicine, the nation's principal sports and exercise research organization, presented its revised physical fit-

ness recommendations for adults. The 1990 guidelines for staying in shape are intended not just to keep people *healthy* (which even moderate levels of activity will do), but to achieve *fitness*. The guidelines are as follows:[60-62]

- *How often:* Exercise 3–5 days a week. Resistance training, such as weight lifting, should be at least two of those days.

- *How long:* Exercise at least 20–60 minutes per session at your recommended heart-rate level. To avoid injury, nonathletes should exercise at lower intensities for a longer period.

- *How much:* Exercise at an intensity level of 60–90% of maximum heart rate. A general idea about your maximum heart rate is found by subtracting your age from the number 220.

- *Aerobic training:* Exercise should be rhythmical and aerobic, using large muscle groups. Examples are walking, jogging, stair-climbing, bicycling, and rowing.

- *Resistance training:* Exercise should consist of 8–12 repetitions of 8–10 specific exercises that condition the major muscle groups. Weight machines, free weights, or calisthenics can be used for resistance training.

- *Flexibility:* No official guidelines exist— apparently, the jury is still out on how much stretching is enough. Nevertheless, flexibility exercises that involve stretching should be performed regularly, at least twice a week.

The American College of Sports Medicine points out that lower-intensity, longer-duration workouts offer less chance of injury. Moreover, it has been shown that people maintain these programs longer than those that involve higher-intensity, shorter-duration workouts. Finally, exercising beyond these limits doesn't really improve fitness.

In the next three sections we discuss the three important elements of physical fitness:

- Flexibility

- Aerobic endurance

- Muscular strength and endurance

Flexibility Test: Sit-and-Stretch

You will need a yardstick for this activity.

Directions

1. Sit on the floor with a yardstick between your outstretched legs. Slide the stick forward so that the 15-inch mark is even with your heels. Tape it to the floor, if you like.
2. Slowly lean and reach with both hands, touching the yardstick as far forward as possible with your fingertips.
3. Don't bounce or lunge. Hold for 3 seconds. Repeat three times, and record your best mark.

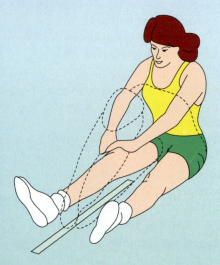

How you shape up for flexibility

The following are general guidelines indicating how flexible you are for your age.

Women

Age	Inches stretched				
	Excellent	High	Average	Low	Very Low
Under 30	24+	20–23	18–19	14–17	0–13
30–39	24+	20–23	18–19	14–17	0–13
40–49	23+	19–22	17–18	12–16	0–11
50–59	23+	19–22	17–18	11–16	0–10
60 and older	23+	19–22	17–18	10–16	0–9

Men

Age	Inches stretched				
	Excellent	High	Average	Low	Very Low
Under 30	23+	19–22	12–18	9–11	0–8
30–39	23+	19–22	12–18	9–11	0–8
40–49	22+	18–21	12–17	8–11	0–7
50–59	22+	18–21	11–17	8–9	0–7
60 and older	22+	18–21	11–17	8–9	0–7

Source: The President's Council on Fitness and Sports, YMCA.

Flexibility

Staying flexible prevents soreness and injuries and reduces stress. Stretching should be slow and relaxed. Flexibility activities should be done twice weekly.

Flexibility is suppleness of movement, your ability to move through the full range of motion allowed by your joints. How flexible you are depends in great part on the joint in question; even so, a test in one area can be indicative of your general flexibility. How supple you are depends on your sex, age, body fat/muscle mass, and the exercises you do to enhance flexibility. In general, women tend to be more flexible than men because of their builds and body composition. Children up to adolescence are quite flexible; as people age, joint mobility and flexibility decrease.

You may wish to test your flexibility before reading on. (*See Self Discovery 17.3.*)

The Benefits of Flexibility In general, flexibility exercises consist of *stretching*. The benefits of stretching are:

- *Decreased muscle stiffness and soreness:* When a joint is used infrequently, the muscles surrounding it become shorter, causing stiffness. If the joint remains unused, it leads to **contracture,** or a permanent shortening of the muscles.

- *Reduced risk of injury and improved coordination:* If you jump right into vigorous exercise without stretching, it can cause injuries. Stretching lengthens the muscles and helps prevent pulls or tears. Extending the muscles also helps your coordination by extending your range of motion.

- *Reduced stress:* Stretching can loosen up tight muscles and help you relax.

Activities for Flexibility The most important areas in which to maintain suppleness are your hips, chest, hamstring muscles, shoulders, and neck. (*See* ● *Figure 17.6.*)

Procedures for enhancing flexibility are as follows:

- *Warm up for 5–10 minutes before stretching.* The warm-up will help you increase your temperature and circulation, which will in turn increase the pliability of your muscles and help you to avoid the injuries that come with using cold muscles. The warm-up may consist of jogging in place, a brisk walk, or calisthenics.

- *Do slow, "static" (no-bounce) stretching.* Stretch gradually, while breathing deeply. Stretch until you feel slight resistance—a pulling sensation, not a pain. Hold the position for 30–60 seconds, then let go slowly. Relax for 20–30 seconds. This gradual, no-bounce stretching and holding is called **static stretching.**

- *Don't do bouncing, "ballistic" stretching.* Never bounce as you stretch. **Ballistic stretching,** such as bouncing on the balls of your feet or repeatedly forcing yourself to touch your toes, can tear muscle fibers and cause injuries.

- *Do at least 5 minutes of flexibility exercises twice a week.* Do stretching or range-of-motion exercises for 5–60 minutes at least twice a week, or after every aerobic endurance or muscular strength/endurance workout. (For optimal flexibility, add a third session, 30–60 minutes, of flexibility exercises, whether stretching or other activity.)

Besides stretching exercises, certain kinds of sports or activities are particularly useful for enhancing flexibility, ranging from such pastimes as gardening, golf, and swimming to yoga, martial arts, and rock climbing. (*See* ● *Table 17.1.*)

Aerobic Endurance

Aerobic activity, unlike anaerobic and nonaerobic activity, is effort without breathlessness. It reduces body fat, heart disease, and some cancers. Aerobic exercises, such as running or rowing, or cross-training for variety, should be done three times weekly or more. You should monitor your efforts by watching your target heart rate or rate of perceived exertion.

Aerobic endurance describes how efficiently your body uses oxygen. To appreciate how aerobic activities differ from other kinds of activities, consider these three distinctions:

● **Table 17.1 Customize your own exercise program.** You can get multiple benefits from each activity.

Physical activity	Flexibility (Do twice weekly)	Aerobic endurance (Do 3–5 times weekly)	Muscular strength and endurance (Do 2–3 times weekly)	
			Lower body	Upper body
Aerobics class*	●	●	●	●
Bench-stepping		●	●	
Bicycling		●	●	
Board-sailing			●	●
Bowling			●	●
Calisthenics			●	●
Canoeing	●	●		●
Dance, aerobic*	●	●	●	●
Gardening	●		●	●
Golf	●		●	●
Gymnastics	●	●	●	●
Hiking		●	●	
Ice-skating		●	●	
Kayaking	●	●		●
Martial arts	●	●	●	●
Racquetball		●	●	●
Rock-climbing	●	●	●	●
Roller-skating, in-line		●	●	
Rope-skipping		●	●	
Rowing		●	●	●
Running		●	●	
Sailing	●			●
Skiing, cross-country	●	●	●	●
Skiing, downhill	●	●	●	
Stair-climbing		●	●	
Swimming	●	●		●
Tennis		●	●	●
Volleyball		●	●	
Walking, fitness	●	●	●	
Weight training	●		●	●
Yoga	●		●	●

*Includes warm-up, cool-down, and strength activities.

Upper calves

Stand about 18 inches from a wall with your feet apart and your hands on the wall for balance. With your legs straight and your toes pointed ahead, lean toward the wall as you would in a pushup. Keep your body straight during the stretch. Good for: *any activity requiring walking or running.*

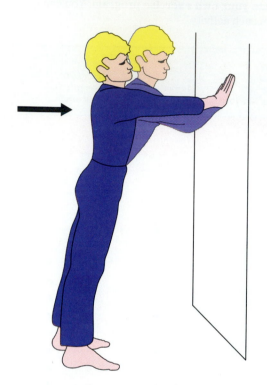

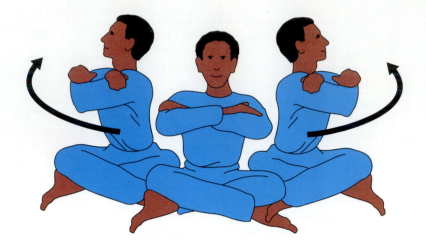

Spine rotation

Sit on the floor with your legs stretched out flat in front of you. (If you can't straighten your legs, bend them cross-legged.) With your arms folded across your chest, slowly turn your entire upper torso to the right, then to the left, keeping your legs and hips in place. Good for: *any activity requiring turning, twisting, or reaching.*

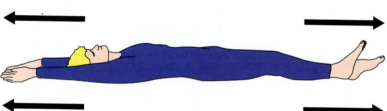

Overall stretch

Lie on the floor with your back flat, arms and hands on the floor above your head. Keeping your arms and legs as flat against the mat or carpet as possible, stretch your body in opposite directions by reaching up with your arms and down with your legs. Good for: *overall flexibility.*

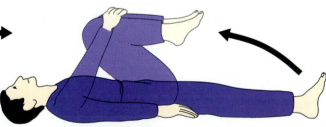

Hips

Lie flat on the floor. Pull one knee up toward your chest, keeping the opposite leg flat on the floor. Slowly return the bent leg to the start position. Repeat with the other leg. Good for: *walking, tennis, golf, or any activity requiring hip flexibility.*

● **Figure 17.6 Stretches for flexibility**

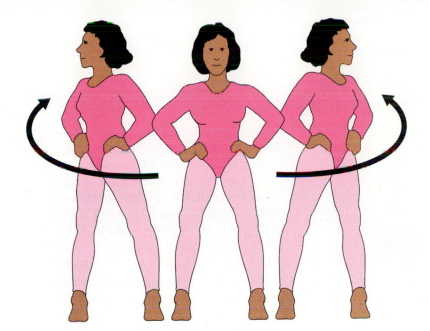

Spine and hip rotation
Stand with your hands on your hips. Do the same twisting motion as in the spine rotation exercise, but include the hips as you rotate. Keep your knees in place and your feet pointing straight ahead approximately your shoulders' width apart. Good for: *walking, golf, tennis, or any activity requiring reaching or hip rotation.*

Achilles tendons
Do the same exercise as for upper calves, but bend your knees. Good for: *any activity requiring walking or running.*

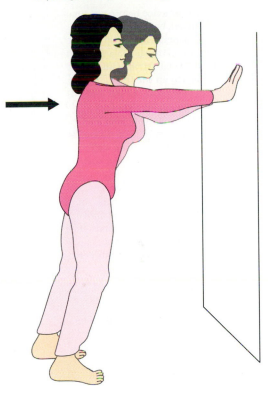

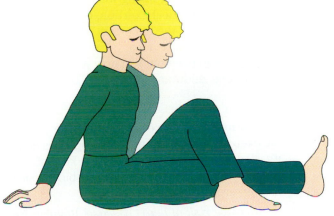

Hamstrings
Sit on the floor with one leg stretched out in front of you. Bend the other leg and cross it above the stretched leg's knee. Planting your hands on the mat next to your hips for support, bend forward from the hips, keeping your arms straight. Make sure you bend from the hips and not the upper back. Focusing attention on an object directly in front of you may help you do this properly. Good for: *most activities that require walking or running.*

Shoulders
Lie flat on the floor with your arms straight down at your sides, palms down. Bend your knees and slide your feet up close to your buttocks. Keep your lower back flat and elbows straight as you raise your arms in the air, then slowly lower them until the backs of your hands touch the mat above your head. Good for: *tennis, golf, or any activity that uses the shoulders.*

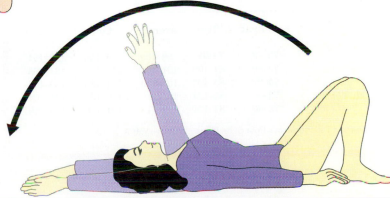

Aerobic-Endurance Test: 3-Minute Step Test

For this activity you will need a watch and a 12-inch-high step.

Directions

1. Don't practice before you time yourself, but do stretch.
2. For 3 minutes, step up and down on the step in a four-part movement: (a) up with the left foot, (b) up with the right foot, (c) down with the left foot, (d) down with the right foot.
3. You can alternate your lead foot, but try to keep pace at 24 steps a minute. (One step is a complete, four-part, up-and-down movement.)
4. Immediately after the 3 minutes, sit down and check your pulse. Count the number of heartbeats for 10 seconds, then multiply by 6 to get your exercising heart rate in beats per minute.

How You Shape Up for Aerobic Endurance

The following are general guidelines indicating how much aerobic endurance you have for your age.

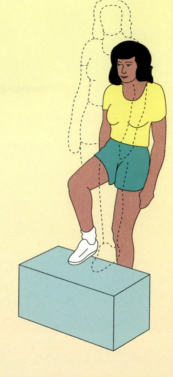

Women

Age	Step test—heart rate				
	Excellent	**High**	**Average**	**Low**	**Very Low**
Under 30	72–84	85–108	109–116	117–135	136–155
30–39	74–86	87–107	108–117	118–136	137–154
40–49	74–90	91–112	113–118	119–131	132–152
50–59	76–92	93–112	113–120	121–134	135–152
60 and older	74–90	91–109	110–119	120–133	134–151

Men

Age	Step test—heart rate				
	Excellent	**High**	**Average**	**Low**	**Very Low**
Under 30	70–78	79–97	98–105	106–126	127–164
30–39	72–80	81–100	101–109	110–126	127–168
40–49	74–82	83–103	104–113	114–128	129–168
50–59	72–84	85–104	105–115	116–130	131–154
60 and older	72–86	87–101	102–110	111–128	129–150

Source: The President's Council on Physical Fitness, YMCA.

- *Aerobic activity—effort without breathlessness:* Brisk walking, jogging, or long-distance bicycling or swimming are examples of aerobic exercise. The workout is strenuous, but you never become breathless to the point that you can't talk while engaging in the activity. In these activities the oxygen taken in is equal to or slightly more than the oxygen used by the body.

- *Anaerobic activity—effort that leaves you gasping:* Sprinting, as in track, football, or speed skating, is an example of **anaerobic** exercise. You expend tremendous effort for a short period of time, then are left gasping for air. The oxygen taken in is not enough to meet the oxygen required, leaving what experts call an "oxygen deficit" that must be made up later.

- *Nonaerobic activity—some effort with frequent rest:* Bowling, golf, tennis, and softball are examples of **nonaerobic** exercise. In these sports, the body gets frequent rests. The oxygen taken in is always sufficient to meet the need, to the point where the lungs and heart do not need to put out much effort.

There is nothing wrong with the second and third kinds of physical exertion, except that they don't deliver the important health benefits that aerobic exercise does.

Before proceeding, you may wish to test your aerobic endurance. (*See Self Discovery 17.4.*)

The Benefits of Aerobic Endurance Aerobic exercises consist of nonstop, vigorous activity. How vigorous depends on what kind of shape you're in. The payoffs of aerobic physical activity are of utmost importance:

- *Reduce risk of heart disease.* Regular, frequent exercise—along with a reduced-fat diet and quitting smoking—seems to be the best thing you can do to reduce the risk of heart disease, the No. 1 killer disease in the United States. Aerobic exercise can lower blood pressure and raise the "good" (HDL) cholesterol, thus decreasing two risk factors in heart disease. It can also strengthen the heart muscle.

- *Reduce body fat and increase lean muscle mass.* As we've suggested, the only kind of weight-loss program that makes any sense involves exercise and diet. This will build muscles while shedding fat; reductions in obesity lessen another heart-disease risk factor.

- *Reduce risk factors for some cancers.* Aerobic exercise may help reduce the risk of breast and reproductive cancers in women and colon and rectal cancers in men.

- *Improve mood.* Aerobic activity can reduce stress, relieve depression, and perhaps stimulate creativity.

Activities for Aerobic Endurance Unlike stretching, aerobic activities usually build physical fitness in more than one area at the same time—for instance, bicycling benefits your leg muscles, canoeing your arm muscles, and both benefit your heart and lungs. First and foremost, benefiting heart and lungs is what aerobics are really all about. The trick is to go about it in the right way. Here's how:

- *Before: do warm-up exercises.* It may be tempting to simply lace up your shoes and bolt out the door, but doing 5 minutes of calisthenics or jogging in place followed by 5 minutes of stretching before your walk, run, or whatever will help you avoid injury and will smooth out your form. For example, before running, do some calisthenics followed by stretching the Achilles tendon and heel. (*See* • *Figure 17.7.*)

- *After: do cool-down exercises.* The purpose of the cool-down is to return the blood to the heart from the body's extremities. Five to 10 minutes of walking and/or stretching is sufficient. Two good cool-down exercises are stretching for the front of your legs and behind-the-back or hands-over-head stretching to prevent shoulders from slumping. (*Refer to Figure 17.7.*)

- *Exercise from 20 minutes 3 times a week up to 60 minutes 4–5 times a week.* For people starting out, 20 minutes three times a week of brisk walking, dancing, bicycling, stair-climbing, swimming, and the like will be sufficient. An optimal exercise level might be 35–45 minutes of moderate exer-

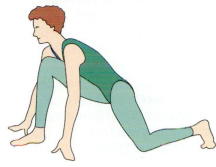

1 **Before your run:** Stand leaning against a solid support with one foot forward and knee bent to stretch the Achilles tendon. Now bend the back knee slightly, keeping the foot flat, until you feel a gentle stretching in the heel. Repeat on the opposite leg.

2 **After your run:** Get down on one knee, so that the other knee is aligned directly above the ankle. Lower your hips until you feel a stretching sensation in the front of your rear leg.

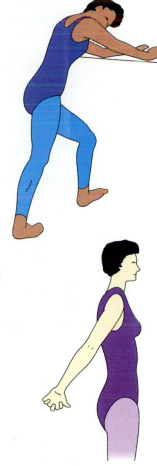

3 **After your run:** To stop your shoulders from slumping, lace your fingers together behind your back, palms in. Slowly turn your elbows inward while straightening your arms to stretch in your shoulders and chest.

• **Figure 17.7 Warm-up and cool-down stretches.** Several minutes of daily stretching will smooth out your form and help you avoid injury. Stretch slowly, without bouncing, to the point where you feel an easy stretching sensation. Hold this position for 5–30 seconds, until the tension diminishes, then stretch slightly farther and hold again.

cise 3–5 times a week, such as jogging, bicycling, or swimming. A peak level would be 45–60 minutes 4–5 times a week of strenuous exercise, such as running, rowing, or cross-country skiing.

During your workouts you should always monitor how hard you are pushing yourself. One way is to stop your workout and place your finger on your pulse to measure your heart rate. Another way is to visualize how hard you're working, using the Rate of Perceived Exertion (RPE) scale. We explain both methods next.

Monitoring Your Efforts: Target Heart Rate The heart rate is the best indicator of how much exercise you can tolerate and the level at which you are currently exercising. Here's how it works.

- *Step 1—Determine your maximum heart rate.* The **maximum heart rate** is the rate beyond which you do not want to push yourself during aerobic training, because of the danger of putting too great a strain on your heart. One general formula for finding your maximum heart rate is simple: *subtract your current age from 220.* Thus, if you are 20 years old, your maximum heart rate is 200. If you are 60 years old, your maximum heart rate is 160.

- *Step 2—Determine your target heart rate.* The **target heart rate** is the rate at which you derive maximum benefit from aerobic exercise. One formula for determining your target heart rate is as follows: *find 60% and 80% of your maximum heart rate.* Twenty-year-olds, for example, have a maximum heart rate of 200. Thus, when they train, they need to push their heart rates to between 120 (60% of 200) and 160 (80% of 200). The lower target rate is sufficient for those just starting out, who may then work toward achieving the higher rate over a period of 6 months or more of training.

- *Step 3—Learn how to determine your pulse rate.* To monitor your heart rate, you simply take your pulse. You can do this by placing two or three fingers (your forefinger and middle finger, not your thumb) as follows: (a) on your *radial artery,* located just below the base of your thumb on the inner side of your opposite wrist, or (b) on your *carotid artery* on the side of the neck below the angle of the jaw bone. (*See* ● *Figure 17.8.*)

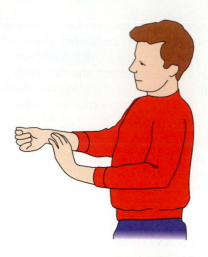

Wrist pulse
Two or three fingers on the radial artery, just below the base of the thumb, on the inner side of the wrist.

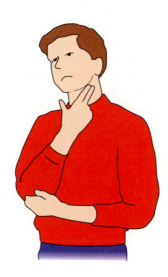

Neck pulse
The tips of two or three fingers on the carotid artery on the side of the neck below the angle of the jawbone.

● **Figure 17.8 Pulse-taking**

To determine your heart rate per minute, count the number of beats in 10 seconds, then multiply by 6. (Or count the number in 30 seconds, and multiply by 2.)

Try taking your pulse now. When you are sitting or lying down, your heart rate is called your **resting heart rate.** When you are doing aerobic exercise, you use the same pulse-taking method to determine your target rate.

Serious runners or athletes sometimes train with a *heart-rate monitor,* an electronic wrist unit that alerts them with a chirp when they are falling below or exceeding their target heart rate. The point of this gadget, of course, is that it provides more accurate feedback, so that you know when you are slacking off or going too hard.

Monitoring Your Efforts: Rate of Perceived Exertion Pulse-taking is now often supplemented with or replaced by the **Rate of Perceived Exertion (RPE) scale.** Even the American College of Sports Medicine, in its 1990 guidelines, suggests that the RPE is preferable to pulse-taking, unless one has a history of heart disease. The Rate of Perceived Exertion scale is based on the assumption that you can subjectively *feel* how strenuous your workout is and that the feeling can be expressed as a number corresponding to your heart rate.[63,64] The RPE provides a means of quantifying subjective exercise intensity. (*See* ● *Figure 17.9.*)

Aerobic Cross-Training for Variety Exercise can and should be pleasant, even fun. One way to do this is to add *variety.* Athletes and trainers speak of **cross-training,** combining a package of activities that will (1) provide variety to keep you from getting bored, (2) help you avoid injuries stemming from overuse, and (3) provide benefits to more than one part of your body.

Cross-training was born in the form of Hawaii's Ironman Triathlon, which begins with a 2.4-mile swim in the ocean, moves on to a 112-mile bicycle ride, and ends with a 26.2-mile run—all in one day.[65] Of course, a mix-and-match program is not intended to be anywhere near as strenuous as this, but at least you can subscribe to the same principles in order to use all your muscles and keep your interest level up. For instance, you can mix running, bicycling, and swimming on alternate days, depending on your mood, the weather, and the facilities

6		
7 Very, very light	How you should feel when warming up or cooling down — but not when aerobically exercising	
8		
9 Very light		
10	Between 10 and 15 is your aerobic workout zone.	
11 Fairly light		
12		
13 Somewhat hard	13 is your ideal. You should be sweating but still able to talk without effort.	
14		
15 Hard	Here you have trouble talking.	
16	Here you're beyond aerobic and into anaerobic. You can't talk.	
17 Very hard		
18	Muscles are aching!	
19 Very, very hard	This is like sprinting as hard as you can!	
20		

● **Figure 17.9 Rate of perceived exertion.** The Rate of Perceived Exertion (RPE) scale is an attempt to quantify how you *visualize* or *feel* about how strenuous your workout is. Assuming you're in good health, if you judge you're around "Somewhat hard" (13) while doing an aerobic task, you're probably at the right level of effort.

available. Many health clubs have set aside rooms for aerobic **circuit training,** whereby you begin with, say, a treadmill, then climb on an exercise bike, then a few minutes later get on a rowing machine, and so on.[66]

There are many ways to customize your program. (*Refer back to Table 17.1.*) Some popular categories of aerobic activities are as follows:

- *Walking:* This category may include anything from a brisk stroll to hiking to backpacking to race-walking. The same activity can also be done indoors on a stair-climbing machine at a gym or health club. Walking should be done 3–4 times a week 20–30 minutes at a time, at a fast enough pace to achieve target heart rate. **Race-walking** is a competitive form of walking, in which the stride is shorter than that of running. The walker stretches the hips forward and backward and also keeps the forward foot on the ground while the rear foot is pushing off.

- *Jogging and running:* In **jogging,** one moves at a pace slower than 9 minutes per mile; in **running,** one goes faster than that. Both jogging and running can be done on the same outing (or on a stair-climbing machine). Another variation is **interval training,** in which you typically alternate several minutes of aerobic running (at a 70–85% target rate) with 30–60 seconds of anaerobic *sprinting,* during which you push beyond the 85% target rate, so that you feel breathless.[67]

    Jogging or running should be done 25–30 minutes 3 times a week, with the aim of achieving and sustaining your target heart rate for 20 minutes. If you have had a long period of inactivity, begin by walking, then speed up the pace to slow jogging, and so on, until you can do 2½ miles in 25–30 minutes.

    For some, running goes beyond fitness to a kind of spiritual experience. Some of the Native Americans of New Mexico, for instance, still run as their ancestors did. "The sound is faint," said one writer, summing up the tradition. "It is a lone, lonely sound. It is the sound of ancient Indians running. It is one of the oldest echoes New Mexico knows."[68] (*See* ● *Figure 17.10.*)

- *Bicycling:* "For many of us," observes one writer, "learning to ride a bicycle was the magic spell that broke the earthly bonds holding us to our childhood homes. . . . Millions of us have recaptured that childhood sense of flight by discovering the sport of bicycling."[69]

    Whether done on a 10- or 12-speed touring bike riding to work or to class, an 18- or 21-gear mountain bike out in the hills on weekends (but good for on- and off-road use), or a variable-speed stationary bike set up in front of your television set or at a health club, pedaling is a great way to build aerobic endurance. It can also burn off 450–800 Calories per hour. The main thing is not to spend too much time coasting or changing gears to reduce effort, or the cardiovascular benefits will be lost.

- *Swimming:* At least once a year, 70 million Americans take a dip, making swimming the nation's No. 1 sports activity.[70] Of these, some 30 million are fitness swimmers.

Swimming is one of the best aerobic fitness activities, because it uses many of the body's muscles. An hour of vigorous swimming can burn 660 Calories. It also produces gentle stretching.

If you are using a pool, you have to swim laps to achieve aerobic conditioning, using the crawl, breaststroke, backstroke, or butterfly stroke. For beginners, a class such as that given at the local YMCA or YWCA is best. You need to improve your technique so that you can swim for 10 minutes at a time, then extend that to 20 minutes.

Regular swimmers find the activity supremely restorative. "For urban dwellers like me," says one writer, "the pool is a rare refuge of quiet and privacy, an oversized flotation tank. There are no intrusions. The telephone doesn't ring underwater. Horns don't honk. People don't shout. There is only the sound of water, the flutter kicking of the other swimmers, the bubbles of my own breathing."[71]

- *Skating, "blading," and skiing:* Both skating and skiing have made some advances over the last few years. For one thing, they can now be done year round.

    Ice-skating and roller-skating, which have been around for a century or more, are not only great fun for many people but also can be a terrific aerobic conditioner. Not long ago, the conventional roller skate, which had sets of wheels side by side, began to be superseded by **in-line skating,** better known as **rollerblading** or simply "blading," after the company, Rollerblade, Inc. Rollerblade revived an 18th-century Dutch design, patterned after ice skates, which put the wheels in a row.[72] "Blading" has turned out to be a popular activity for people looking for ways to have low-impact aerobics that are fun and fairly safe (if they aren't reckless and use protective gear). A half hour of blading can burn up 285–450 Calories, compared to 300–350 Calories for runners and bicyclists.[73] Blading also strengthens hip, thigh, and lower back muscles that are not well developed by running or bicycling.

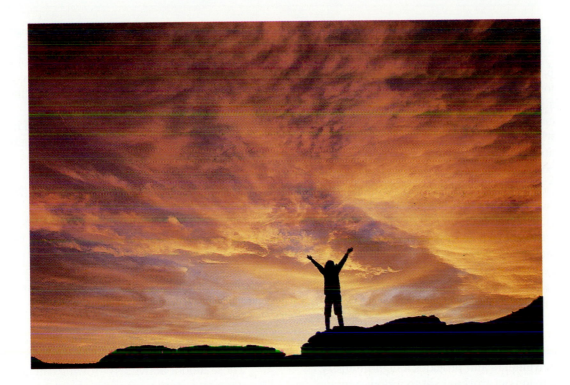

● **Figure 17.10 Running and the spirit.** Native Americans at Jemez Pueblo, New Mexico, still run as did their ancestors, who, for hundreds of years before horses arrived with the Europeans, ran to deliver messages, to hunt, for recreation, and for meditation and reflection.

❝*Out here, where North America's civilization was born, where rattlesnakes lurk in the rope cactus and hawks patrol the sun-scorched sky, there are no joggers—only runners keeping an ancient tradition alive.*

'Sometimes, when things are really bad, I will go out there and cry as I run,' said David Simone, a Navajo whose grandfather taught him the tradition.

'Running is as much a religion as a therapy,' Simone said. 'With the sky as my roof, the sun to give me energy, I do not think about the alcoholism, the young girls with babies, the lack of jobs.' . . .

Bart Humphrey, part Navajo and part Tewa, runs at dawn.

'My grandfather told me to run every morning, before sunrise, toward the sun,' Humphrey said. 'If you run in the morning, you absorb all the freshness of the day.' ❞

—Mike Clancey, Reuter news service (1991, July 21). Pueblo Indians sprinting toward sun, face new day. *San Francisco Examiner,* p. B-8.

Downhill skiing is a reasonably good aerobic sport, but cross-country skiing is an exceptionally good cardiovascular exercise, particularly when done correctly, with a long diagonal stride. Nowadays, in the absence of snowy fields, cross-country skiers can train by **roller-skiing** on pavement, which allows the same range of motion and exercises the same muscles as cross-country skis. (*See* • *Figure 17.11.*)

• *Dancing:* Aerobic dancing, made famous by Jazzercise classes, Jane Fonda Workout videotapes, and the like, began as a combination of upbeat music and calisthenics, kicks, and jumps. Now it has branched out into all sorts of variations, from reggae and Latin beats to low-impact step aerobics and inner-city street dances.

Step aerobics, for example, involve stepping on and off a 4- or 12-inch-high platform while making coinciding arm movements and provides a high-intensity, low-impact workout set to a slower tempo of music than regular aerobic dancing.[74]

"Street jam" is the name for a high-energy activity blending inner-city street dances (hip-hop) and low-impact aerobics. The activity is popular because it is easy to learn and is fun for people who don't like traditional forms of exercise.[75]

Nonimpact aerobics, developed in response to high-impact, jump-around aerobics that resulted in injuries, combines "the fluidity of tai chi and tae kwon do with the grace of modern dance, ballet, and yoga," according to one description.[76]

Even ballroom dancing, with steps such as the cha-cha, polka, samba, and the like, is recommended for people who have trouble sticking to a workout schedule. They find it is a lot of fun, yet it still increases the average person's heart rate enough to achieve some cardiovascular benefits.

• *Rowing, stair-climbing, running on a treadmill, jumping rope, and others:* These indoor activities—rowing can be done on a stationary rowing machine—are great fat-burning routines if you have ac-

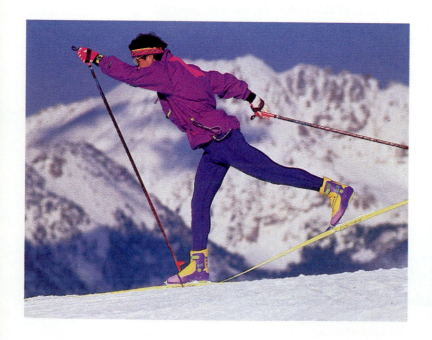

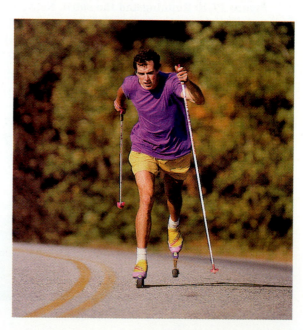

• **Figure 17.11 Cross-country skiing—winter and summer.** Traditional cross-country skiing (*left*) is one of the best exercises for building aerobic endurance. Roller skiing on wheels (*right*) duplicates most of the same motions when snowy fields are absent.

cess to a health club or gym. Clearly, having the opportunity to do these kinds of activities gives you an important option for cross-training during bad weather.

Muscular Strength and Endurance

Muscle strength is the measure of the force you are able to exert against resistance; muscle endurance is the ability to keep repeating those exertions. Such muscular activity makes you feel and look good, reduces heart disease and cancer risk, and strengthens bones. Resistance-training exercises, which should be done twice weekly or more, are specialized, involving use of free weights, weight machines, or calisthenics. Circuit training can be helpful.

People who get lots of aerobic exercise often have strong legs, but they may lack upper-body strength. When muscles are not used, they waste away, a condition called **atrophy.** Conversely, when they are used regularly, they increase in size, a state called **hypertrophy.**

As we stated, the fitness of your muscles is measured in two ways:

1. *Muscle strength* is the ability to exert force against resistance, as when you lift a box of books. To increase strength, you need to do a few repetitions with heavy loads.

2. *Muscle endurance* is the ability to keep repeating those muscle exertions, so that you can move not just a box of books into your house but all your fully loaded suitcases and other things besides. To increase endurance, you do many repetitions with light loads.

You may wish to test your muscular strength and endurance before reading on. (*See Self Discovery 17.5.*)

The Benefits of Muscular Strength and Endurance The benefits of strength training are that it not only makes you look good and feel good but gives you a body that can resist disease and survive the aging process a lot better. Specifically:

- *Look and feel good:* Whether you're male or female, overweight or not, strength training can tone up muscles and diminish the inevitable effects of gravity on body parts that tend to sag. When strength improves, posture improves, and so does breathing.[77] As you look better, your self-confidence also increases.

- *Reduce fat and lower heart disease and cancer risk:* Developing your muscles will decrease body fat and increase lean body mass, open up the tiny blood vessels called **capillaries** to increase the flow of blood and nutrients to the muscles, and increase efficient metabolism. The result is a lower risk of heart disease, some cancers, and adult diabetes.

- *Strengthen bones, reduce injury, and prolong independence:* Aging and less physical activity produce a decline in muscle strength—perhaps a 30% decrease in muscle mass between ages 30 and 70.[78] Strengthening the bones along with strengthening the muscles will improve your posture, prevent back pain, and enable you to remain active and independent as you grow older.[79]

Activities for Muscular Strength and Endurance The important muscle groups that need to be strengthened are your chest, back, legs, buttocks, arms, shoulders, and stomach. The key to fitness is to avoid emphasizing one group over another. For instance, some exercisers, often male, will do chest and arm repetitions but ignore back exercises, which can lead to back problems.

There are several principles to keep in mind for developing muscular strength and endurance:

- *General versus specialized exercises:* Certain activities such as swimming, cross-country skiing, rock-climbing, and even gardening can help you develop flexibility and aerobic fitness as well as muscular strength and endurance. (*Refer back to Table 17.1.*) However, development of the muscle groups we mentioned requires physical exercises aimed directly at strength training —namely, exercises with weight machines, free weights, or calisthenics.

Muscular Strength and Endurance Test: Push-Ups for Upper Body Strength and Sit-Ups and Curl-Ups for Abdominal Strength

Directions: Push-Ups/Upper Body Strength

1. Lie face down on the floor with your hands directly beneath your shoulders. Then, keeping your back rigid, push your body off the floor until your arms are straight.
2. If full push-ups are too difficult, lower your knees to the floor for support, but keep your back straight.
3. Stop 2 inches above the floor in the down position in standard push-ups. Touch your chest in the modified, knees-down version.
4. Down and up is one push-up. Do as many as you can without breaking form or resting.

Push-ups

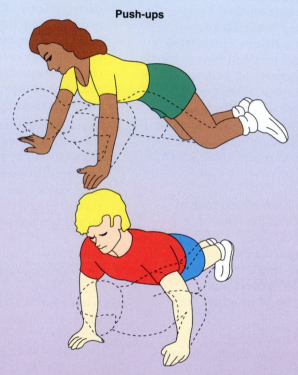

Directions: Sit-Ups and Curl-Ups—Abdominal Strength

1. Lie flat on your back, legs bent, with heels 6 inches from your buttocks. Cross your arms over your chest for sit-ups or extend them along your sides for curl-ups.
2. Keeping your feet on the floor, curl your upper torso upward. Touch your crossed arms to your knees for sit-ups. For curl-ups, make sure your hands slide 3 inches forward.
3. Do as many as you can in 1½ minutes.

Sit-ups and curl-ups

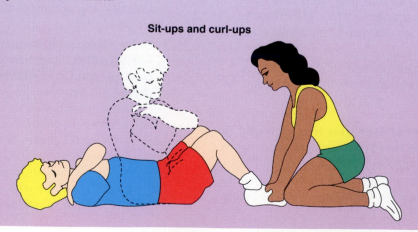

Push-Ups: How You Shape Up for Upper Body Strength

The following are general guidelines indicating how much upper-body muscular strength you have for your age based on number of push-ups.

Women

Age	Push-ups—number completed				
	Excellent	**High**	**Average**	**Low**	**Very Low**
Under 30	49+	34–48	17–33	6–16	0–5
30–39	40+	25–39	12–24	4–11	0–3
40–49	35+	20–34	8–19	3–7	0–2
50–59	30+	15–29	6–14	2–5	0–1
60 and older	20+	5–19	3–4	1–2	0

Men

Age	Push-ups—number completed				
	Excellent	**High**	**Average**	**Low**	**Very Low**
Under 30	55+	45–64	35–44	20–34	0–19
30–39	45+	35–44	25–34	15–24	0–14
40–49	40+	30–39	20–29	12–19	0–11
50–59	35+	25–34	15–24	8–14	0–7
60 and older	30+	20–29	10–19	5–9	0–4

Sit-Ups and Curl-Ups: How You Shape Up for Abdominal Strength

The following are general guidelines indicating how much abdominal strength you have for your age based on number of sit-ups and curl-ups.

Women

Age	Sit-ups—number completed				
	Excellent	**High**	**Average**	**Low**	**Very Low**
Under 30	45+	35–44	25–34	15–24	0–14
30–39	45+	35–44	25–34	15–24	0–14
40–49	40+	30–39	20–29	14–19	0–13
50–59	35+	25–34	15–24	10–14	0–9
60 and older	35+	25–34	15–24	8–14	0–7

Men

Age	Sit-ups—number completed				
	Excellent	**High**	**Average**	**Low**	**Very Low**
Under 30	50+	40–49	30–39	20–29	0–19
30–39	50+	40–49	30–39	20–29	0–19
40–49	45+	34–44	25–43	19–24	0–18
50–59	40+	30–39	20–29	15–19	0–14
60 and older	40+	28–39	19–27	14–18	0–13

Source: The President's Council on Physical Fitness, YMCA.

- *Resistance training for strength versus endurance:* All muscle-development training is based on the principle of resistance. During training you need to demand more of the muscles than usual; in short, you must overload them. Building *strength* requires *few* repetitions with *heavy* loads; building *endurance* requires *more* repetitions with *light* loads. In the beginning, you should strive to build strength, then as the muscles become developed, strive for endurance.

- *Isometric, isotonic, and isokinetic exercises:* Resistance training takes various forms, some of which work better than others.

  Isometric exercises—which are *not* recommended because they can raise blood pressure in some people—consist of pushing against a wall or other immovable object, holding each muscle contraction for a few seconds, and repeating 5–10 times.

  Isotonic exercises use free weights, weight machines, or calisthenics. The point is to strengthen muscles by creating muscular tension through shortening or lengthening the muscle, as in combining heavy weights with a low number of repetitions.

  Isokinetic exercises require specialized weight machines such as those found in gyms and health clubs. The principle is that the machines put tension on a particular set of muscles through an entire range of motion. For instance, Nautilus machines are built with cams that vary the load to match muscle strength in different joint positions.

  Whichever type of exercise is used, the idea is to apply the principle of overload to the muscles by increasing the resistance or load, increasing the number of repetitions, or increasing the number of sets (consecutive repetitions).

- *Free weights versus weight machines versus calisthenics:* The three principal means of developing muscular strength and endurance are through use of free weights, weight machines, or calisthenics. (*See • Figure 17.12.*)

  Free weights are a form of weight training mostly involving the use of dumbbells and barbells. A **dumbbell** consists of two weighted spheres (or sometimes adjustable weighted disks) joined by a short bar. A **barbell** consists of a long bar with adjustable weighted disks attached to each end. Beginners should get instruction by a trainer in how to use them because of the risks to safety they pose if dropped or lifted incorrectly.

  Weight machines duplicate many of the lifting exercises of free weights, but they are easier and safer to use because they control the range of motion and can't be dropped. Some of these machines can also offer variety for beginners. People often call these machines "Nautilus machines," but Nautilus is only one brand. (Some others are Universal, Paramount, Keiser, Hydrafitness, and Cybex Eagle.) Some weight machines are single-purpose, others can be adjusted for different exercises.

  Calisthenics are systematic rhythmic exercises, such as push-ups and pull-ups. These activities are usually performed without any apparatus, except perhaps for stretch bands or surgical tubing for light resistance exercises. Calisthenics are useful especially when one cannot get to a gym and does not wish to miss a training session.

- *Warm up:* Before lifting weights, be sure to warm up with a few minutes of walking, stretching, and light calisthenics.

- *Exercise from 20 minutes 2 times a week up to 90 minutes 5 times a week—or 1–3 sets of 8–12 exercises:* These recommendations should be thought of in terms of *sets of repetitions*. A **repetition** (or "rep") is the single execution of a movement—for example, lifting a barbell once. According to the American College of Sports Medicine, a **set** consists of 8–12 repetitions. Each exercise is for each of the important muscle groups: back, chest (pectorals), backs of legs, front thigh (quadriceps), buttocks (gluteus maximus), fronts and backs of upper arms (biceps and triceps), shoulders (deltoids), and stomach (abdomen).

For developing chest and triceps
Bench press using free weights: Keep hands 6–10 inches apart, push away

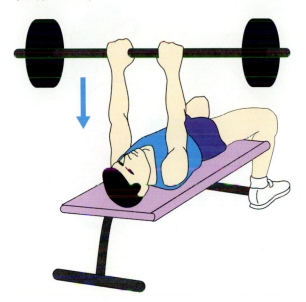

Bench press using weight machine: Back flat on bench, feet on floor, push away

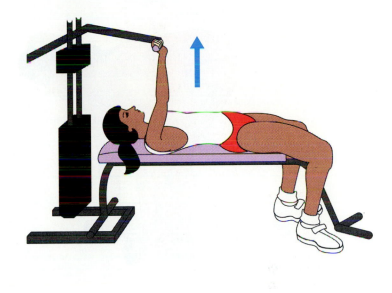

For developing biceps
Concentration curl using free weights: Sit with knees apart, bring weight toward chin

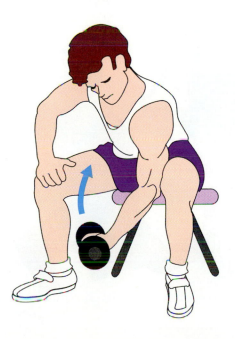

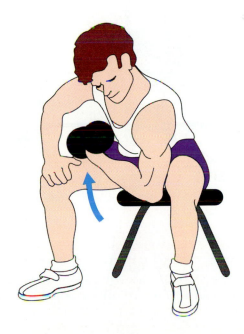

● **Figure 17.12 Exercises with free weights, weight machines, and calisthenics**

(continued)

For developing back muscles Bent-over row, using free weights: Pull weights straight up to the sides of the chest

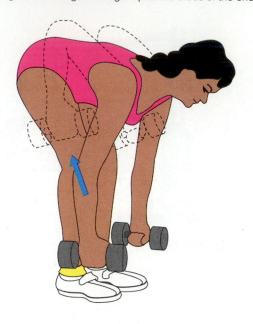

Bent arm curl Using weight machine: Shoulders should be slightly raised between lifts

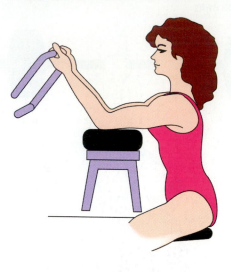

For developing leg muscles Lunge using free weights: Take a large step forward, then reverse

Lateral pulldown using weight machine: Pull bar down behind the neck

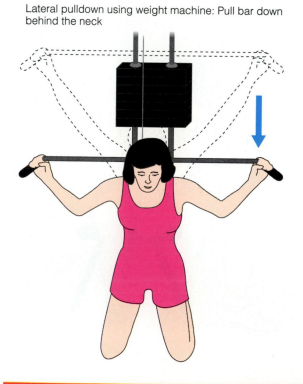

● **Figure 17.12** *(continued)*

Knee extension (top) and leg curls, using weight machine

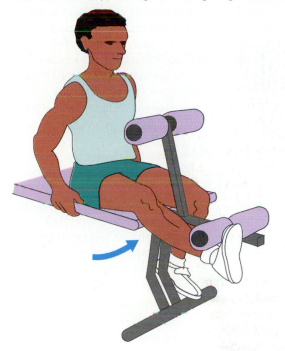

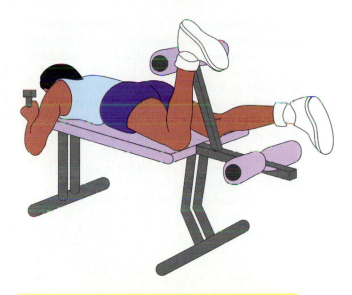

Calisthenic Alternatives to Equipment Exercises	
Equipment exercise	Calisthenic alternatives
Bench press	Push-ups (full)
	Push-ups (modified)
Overhead press	Lateral raise (with jugs)
	Arm stretch (with bands)
Lateral pulldown	Pull-ups (with spotter)
	Arm pulls (with bands)
Seated leg press	Standing squats
	Standing squats (with jugs)

As a beginner, you should start out with a set of 8 repetitions for each of 8–10 resistance exercises, which should be done within a 20- to 30-minute period of time twice a week. As you build your strength and endurance, you can increase to 2 sets of 10–12 repetitions for 12 exercises, each requiring 45–60 minutes 3 times a week. People pursuing maximum fitness may do 3 sets of 12 repetitions for 15 exercises, for 90 minutes 5 days a week.

- *Concentrate on form and technique:* When starting out on a weight-training program, you should work hard enough to feel some muscle fatigue. You should not, however, try to "go for the burn"—the experience of pain in the muscles—which may signal that you are overdoing it. Use enough weight to tax your muscles on the last few repetitions of each set.

If you're using weight machines, make sure they're adjusted to fit your body's dimensions. Don't squeeze the handgrips as you lift, just hold them. Move through the full range of motion for each exercise, concentrating on the specific muscles used in the exercise.[80] If you're using free weights (dumbbells and barbells), do each exercise in a slow, controlled manner, concentrating on feeling each contraction.[81] Don't let the weight drop between lifts.

Breathing and timing are important. Breathe *out* when you are doing the hardest part of the lifting, counting "one, two." Breathe *in* during recovery, counting "one, two, three, four."

Be sure to rest a few seconds between machines or sets. Allow your breath to return to normal.

- *Give your muscles time to rest:* It's important to avoid overtraining. In general, it's best to allow 48 hours for your muscles to recover from a workout. Thus, a good idea is to schedule your training sessions for aerobic endurance on alternate days from those you devote to training for muscle strength and endurance.

Circuit Training and Fitness Trails (Parcours) In many health clubs, you can take advantage of **circuit training,** a logical sequence of exercises that you perform at different stations of free weights or weight machines. The idea is to perform the exercises in sequential order so that no one muscle group is overworked and fatigue does not limit lifting ability.[82] For example, the first exercise might be for arm muscles, the second for stomach, the third for thighs, and so on.

Some community park departments and colleges offer **fitness trails,** also known as **parcours,** as they are called in Switzerland, where they were first invented. Fitness trails consist of a marked path—the ideal distance is 1 mile, but they can be much shorter or longer—comprising separate stations set at various distances. Each station has equipment (such as a bar for chin-ups) and posted instructions for self-paced exercises. The trails are designed for anyone from beginners to advanced athletes and provide self-tailored programs for walking or running between stations, then opportunities for stretching movements and endurance training.

Fitness trails provide ways of developing all three kinds of fitness—flexibility, aerobic endurance, and muscular strength and endurance—provided you do them on a regular basis, such as two or three times a week, not sporadically as an adjunct to other training. One problem can be the "impossible station," the one you find you can't perform. "Figure out which muscles are being worked," advises sports medicine physician James Garrick, "and look up modifications or alternative exercises in a fitness book."[83] It's important not to skip any stations or you won't be getting a well-rounded workout.

Exercise Dependency: How Much Is Too Much?

Overtraining, or "exercise dependency," can lead to injuries and mood disorders.

Too much exercise can have negative effects in that some people exercise compulsively regardless of illness or injury. A compulsion to overexercise, which lay people call *exercise addiction,* is known as **exercise dependency.** It

is characterized by a compulsion to exercise at the expense of physical and emotional health and to the point that exercise displaces other important areas of life, such as family, friends, sex, hobbies, and job.[84] Some who become dependent on exercise seem to show some of the same traits as substance abusers, such as aggressive or erratic behavior. Others also suffer from eating disorders (such as anorexia, or self-starvation).[85]

A study of New York City Marathon runners found that among the characteristics especially predictive of exercise dependency were the following: avoiding people after missing a workout, obsessing over skipping exercise, worrying about injuries disrupting his or her program, or feeling depressed after a workout.[86] (*See Self Discovery 17.6.*)

Even if you are not exercise dependent, overtraining can lead to a variety of problems:[87]

- *Bone and muscle injuries:* Of people who run under 9 miles a week, only about 20% suffer bone and muscle injuries. However, for those who run 30 miles, the injury rate jumps to 50%. Continuing to work out despite injuries can lead to arthritis and other problems.

- *Mood disturbances:* Although moderate exercise can relieve depression, too much exercise can *cause* depression, according to William P. Morgan of the University of Wisconsin–Madison Sports Psychology Laboratory.[88]

- *Amenorrhea in women:* Some women who overtrain, particularly runners, may lower their estrogen levels, which disrupts their menstrual cycles. The absence or suppression of menstrual cycles, called **amenorrhea,** can reduce fertility in the short run and perhaps produce osteoporosis in the long run.

- *"Sports anemia" and lower sexuality in men:* Men who overtrain show fatigue, weakness, and irritability, a condition known as *"sports anemia."* Overexercise can also lower sperm count, testosterone levels, and sex drive.

How much exercise is too much? Probably going beyond the guidelines set forth by the American College on Sports Medicine is excessive. A study of women who gradually increased

Exercise Involvement: What's Your Exercise IQ?

Answer the 40 questions below according to how accurately they reflect your actions, thoughts, and emotions:

A   Extremely accurate
B   Fairly accurate
C   Only slightly accurate
D   Not accurate

_____   1. I have often exercised in risk conditions (such as electrical storms) to avoid missing a workout.

_____   2. Family members or friends comment on or complain about the negative effect my exercise routine has on them.

_____   3. I get anxious when upcoming social events conflict with my exercise regimen.

_____   4. My physical appearance depends on my exercise.

_____   5. I exercise at least 4 days every week.

_____   6. I handle life's frustrations and make decisions more easily after exercise.

_____   7. I feel better if I stick to certain types of exercise (running, for example).

_____   8. Few things in life give me the satisfying sense of accomplishment I get from a good workout.

_____   9. I feel I need to work out more than others to maintain my level of fitness.

_____ 10. I get edgy and frustrated if work interferes with my exercise.

_____ 11. I would end a relationship if it prevented me from exercising.

_____ 12. If I have a bad workout I feel lethargic or depressed.

_____ 13. I often exercise despite injury, fatigue, or mild illness.

_____ 14. It's hard for me to work out with others because I have my own exercise preferences and my own routines.

_____ 15. I get upset when I hear about bad weather conditions (such as extreme heat) that could jeopardize my exercise plans.

_____ 16. I feel I have an advantage in my career over those people who don't exercise.

_____ 17. I am more concerned about aging than my peers are.

_____ 18. I need to exercise to get my digestive tract and metabolism to function effectively.

_____ 19. I am aware of my size and shape and gaze at my reflection in mirrors and windows more frequently than most people do.

_____ 20. I feel like punishing myself if I intentionally skip a workout.

_____ 21. I fear that I won't be motivated to exercise again if I take more than a day or so off.

_____ 22. I would choose exercise over social activities with family or friends.

_____ 23. To recover more quickly from an injury, I would take medication even if it caused side effects such as stomach irritation or bad breath.

_____ 24. I feel more self-conscious if I fail to exercise.

_____ 25. I feel that I have to keep increasing my exercise to maintain my desired level of fitness.

_____ 26. On days when I don't work out, I feel disoriented and sluggish.

_____ 27. I can't stop thinking about exercise if I miss a workout.

_____ 28. I would seriously consider refusing a new job, raise, or promotion if it meant the end of my exercise routine.

_____ 29. I feel that having a fit and attractive body is a better predictor of social success than loyalty or a sense of humor.

_____ 30. I think more about my problems and worries when I cannot work out.

_____ 31. I feel fat and bloated if I miss 2 days of exercise.

(continued)

SELF DISCOVERY 17.6

(continued)

_____ 32. There is a significant difference in my mood before and after I exercise.

_____ 33. I would continue to exercise with an injury even against the advice of a medical specialist.

_____ 34. When things are going badly in my life, I devote more time and thought to my workouts.

_____ 35. I avoid people if I miss my workouts.

_____ 36. If I miss a day of exercise, I feel as if my muscles have atrophied.

_____ 37. Since increasing my workout intensity has a beneficial effect on me, I try to exercise extra hard on special occasions such as my birthday so I'll be in a good mood.

_____ 38. Exercise is frequently on my mind.

_____ 39. I would consider using a potentially dangerous medication such as steroids if I knew it would enhance my physique or athletic ability.

_____ 40. If I sense an injury developing, I worry about not being able to exercise.

To Calculate Your Score

Give yourself 3 points for each A answer, 2 points for each B answer, and 1 point for each C answer. Then add to find your total score.

Below 20:   Low involvement.
20–40 points: Moderate involvement.
40–60 points: High involvement (the profile of the typical competitive athlete).
60–80 points: Very high involvement. (Exercise is important—maybe too important. You might want to reevaluate your workout program, and consider scaling it back.)
80 plus: Extremely high involvement. (This indicates you may be working out to the exclusion of other essential areas in your life. In extreme cases, counseling may be appropriate.)

Source: Morrow, J., & Harvey, P. (1990, November). What's your exercise IQ? *American Health, 9,* p. 32. [Information: J. Morrow, Dept. of Physical Education and Athletics, John Jay College, CUNY, 899 10th Ave., New York, NY 10019.]

their running mileage from 1 to 30 miles a week during a 6-month period, following these guidelines, found that none of the women experienced psychological or physiological problems.[89]

Because major variations exist, what would be exercise dependence or overtraining for one person would not be for another. The main thing is to listen to your body's signals. Remember that rest and restoration are necessary and that persistent soreness or fatigue means you're overextending yourself.

Injuries and Pain: Prevention and Management

Avoiding injuries means getting medical clearance; dressing right; knowing the hazards of hot weather, such as dehydration, and cold weather, such as hypothermia; making adjustments for smog or dim light or high altitude; avoiding anabolic steroids; and treating soreness and mishaps appropriately.

There are a lot of ways to put yourself *out of* action when performing any physical activity: not dressing right, not warming up or cooling down, doing high-impact activity, working out in smog or extremes of hot and cold, not giving your body enough recovery time from training, and taking drugs such as anabolic steroids in a misguided attempt to increase performance. Let's consider some of these.

Getting Medical Clearance Nearly every article or book on exercise suggests you get a physician's approval before starting an activity program. This is particularly true if you are overweight, over 40, have not exercised in many months, are taking any prescription medicines, are a smoker, or have any congenital or chronic condition—heart murmur, asthma, sickle cell anemia, high blood pressure, extreme tiredness—that could be a cause for concern.

Dressing Right Clearly, for some activities having the right clothes and gear is a must—rock climbing, for instance, or skiing. For most workouts and sports, however, the things that count are correct, properly fitting shoes, warm or light clothing to match the weather, and athletic supporters (jockstraps) for men and sports bras for women. The clothes should be comfortable and loose-fitting to allow freedom of movement.

Here are a few specifics:

- *Shoes:* There are now activity-specific shoes for nearly every sport, including some hundred-dollar-plus footwear featuring pillows, pumps, and bubbles. Runners need extra cushioning, tennis players need extra support, and aerobic dancers need both cushioning and all-over support.

  Unless you engage in three different sports more than once a week, however, you probably need *only two pairs of athletic shoes,* says Lloyd Smith, president of the American Academy of Podiatric Sports Medicine.[90] If you participate in any activity more than once a week, he says, your *first* sports shoe should be sport-specific. Your *second* shoe may be a **cross-trainer shoe,** a multipurpose shoe that covers the remaining activities—either principally for lateral movement (such as racquet sports) or for forward movement (such as running).

  When you shop for any sports shoe, you should always buy your shoes at the *end of the day,* when your feet are most swollen, and you should wear the kind of sock you wear for your particular activity. Try on both shoes, allowing a quarter inch of room between the end of the shoe and your longest toe and making sure the shoe does not slip in the heel or gap in the arch. Buy for the larger foot, since you can always accommodate the smaller foot with an inner-sole. Walk or jog around the store to see if they fit.[91,92]

- *Dressing for hot weather:* Loose-fitting, light-colored T-shirts and shorts—preferably cotton rather than nylon because cotton absorbs water quickly and is non-irritating—are the best clothing for many summer activities, such as running. A light-weight warm-up suit may be helpful in areas where the weather can turn cool.[93]

- *Dressing for cold weather:* The main point of dressing warmly in cold weather is that you want to retain your body heat while still allowing perspiration to evaporate. Thus, you should wear two or three loose-fitting layers of dark clothing (dark colors help retain heat), which can be removed. The outer garment should probably not be waterproof, since you want to avoid trapping body heat. A better choice is a wool garment, which wicks sweat away from the body, allowing it to evaporate.

  Besides keeping your hands and feet warm with mittens (preferred to gloves, which separate the fingers and thus don't conserve body heat as efficiently) and wool socks, you should be sure to wear a hat such as a wool stocking cap, since 50% of the body's heat can escape through the surface of your head. A face mask, scarf, and goggles may also be desirable.[94]

Hot Weather Hazards A hot day or heavy exercise leads to increased body heat, making the blood circulate nearer the cooler air of the surface of your skin and releasing excess body heat to the outside. The heat is dissipated by the evaporation of sweat, in which water vaporizes from the skin, causing a cooling effect. But problems can occur when both temperature and humidity are high, because the water-laden air prevents the water on your skin from evaporating. (See ● *Figure 17.13.*)

Heat and humidity chart

Numbers within the chart show equivalent temperatures. Shaded areas indicate when exertion may be dangerous.

Air temperature (F°)

Relative humidity	70°	75°	80°	85°	90°	95°	100°	105°	110°	115°	120°
30%	67	73	78	84	90	96	104	113	123	135	148
40%	68	74	79	86	93	101	110	123	137	151	
50%	69	75	81	88	96	107	120	135	150		
60%	70	76	82	90	100	114	132	149			
70%	70	77	85	93	106	124	144				
80%	71	78	86	97	113	136					
90%	71	79	88	102	122						
100%	72	80	91	108							

☐ Risk of heat exhaustion ☐ Risk of heat stroke ☐ High risk of heat stroke

Wind chill chart

Temperatures assume dry conditions. The greater the moisture, the higher the temperature at which your skin may be in danger.

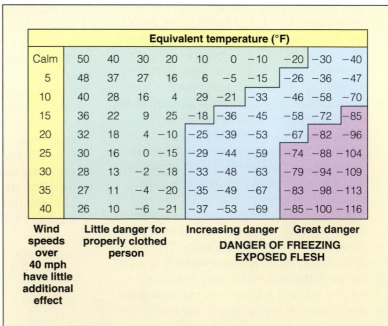

Estimated wind speed (mph)	Air temperature (°F)									
	50	40	30	20	10	0	−10	−20	−30	−40

Equivalent temperature (°F)										
Calm	50	40	30	20	10	0	−10	−20	−30	−40
5	48	37	27	16	6	−5	−15	−26	−36	−47
10	40	28	16	4	29	−21	−33	−46	−58	−70
15	36	22	9	25	−18	−36	−45	−58	−72	−85
20	32	18	4	−10	−25	−39	−53	−67	−82	−96
25	30	16	0	−15	−29	−44	−59	−74	−88	−104
30	28	13	−2	−18	−33	−48	−63	−79	−94	−109
35	27	11	−4	−20	−35	−49	−67	−83	−98	−113
40	26	10	−6	−21	−37	−53	−69	−85	−100	−116

Wind speeds over 40 mph have little additional effect

Little danger for properly clothed person

Increasing danger

Great danger

DANGER OF FREEZING EXPOSED FLESH

● **Figure 17.13 Weather warnings.** The dangers of too much heat (and humidity) and too much cold.

If you're not careful about shielding your-self from the hot weather or about drinking enough water to replace the fluids lost through perspiration, a number of things can happen:

- *Dehydration:* **Dehydration**—abnormal depletion of body fluids—occurs when not enough water is taken in to compensate for the amount lost. A loss of only 10% of the body's usual water content can cause se-vere problems; a loss of 20% may cause death.

- *Heat cramps and heat stress:* **Heat cramps,** caused by heavy sweating, are painful muscle spasms in the arms, legs, and abdomen. Heat cramps are frequently accompanied by **heat stress,** with a drop in blood pressure, dizziness, and blurred vision.

- *Heat exhaustion:* **Heat exhaustion** is de-fined as prostration caused by excessive fluid loss. It is characterized by increased sweating, higher body temperature, cool wet skin, and lack of coordination.

- *Heat stroke:* By far the most serious heat problem is **heat stroke,** with body temper-atures in excess of 107° Fahrenheit (42° Celsius), which may be fatal. Symptoms of heat stroke include *lack* of perspiration, hot and dry skin, rapid breathing, seizures— and coma. This requires *immediate* med-ical attention; the outcome is considered poor if diagnosis and treatment are delayed as little as 2 hours.

For heat cramps and heat stress, you should stop the physical activity, sit down in a cool place, drink lots of water, and not move un-til you've recovered. For heat exhaustion, you should do the same but also get medical treat-ment. Heat stroke is a medical emergency; until help comes, try to cool the victim's body down by applying ice to the back of the neck and armpits and by sponging him or her continu-ously with cool water. Don't try putting the vic-tim in the bathtub or pool of cold water as this may cause shock.

Strategy for Living: Exercising in Hot Weather Exercising safely in the heat is mostly a matter of drinking lots of fluids and following common sense. Some rules:

- *Take it easy:* Avoid strenuous exercise. Give yourself a chance to become acclima-tized or adjusted (10–14 days) if you are getting used to a new, hot climate.[95]

- *Avoid the hottest times of day:* Exercise early in the morning or in the evening or in-doors in air-conditioned health clubs or gyms.

- *Drink more water:* The thirst mechanism is somewhat faulty in that it doesn't always lead a person to replenish the water need-ed, particularly during strenuous physical activity. Indeed, it may cause only 60–70% of the needed water to be replaced.[96] Thus, it's important to drink *beyond* the point of quenching thirst, and 6–8 glasses a day in any event.

  You should drink fluids not only during and after workouts and competitions but also before. To prevent heat disorders, you should drink 2 or more cups of water 2 hours before an event and another 2 cups 15 minutes before. During the activity, you should drink ½–1 cup of water about every 15 minutes.

Water is considered better than commer-cially available sports beverages, such as Gatorade, because sports beverages often have a high sugar content, which tends to keep the fluid in the stomach rather than speeding it to the areas of the body needing replenishment. If sports drinks are used, they should be diluted by adding equal parts water. Fruit juices diluted with water (1 part juice to 2 parts water) are better because they replace minerals such as potassium.

Cold Weather Hazards You can look at an outdoor thermometer through your bedroom window in wintertime and decide that it's safe to go out and exercise. Indeed, it has been found that you can exercise at temperatures as low as −22°F (−30°C) without heavy cloth-ing.[97] However, what your thermometer proba-bly does not show is that the **wind-chill factor** —a measurement that expresses temperature as the equivalent of the absolute temperature combined with the wind velocity—results in environmental temperatures considerably lower than they appear. (*Refer back to Figure 17.13.*)

The dangers of overexposure to cold weather range from frost nip to frostbite to hypothermia:

- *Frost nip and frostbite:* If you go out without warm enough socks, mittens, or head covering, you may not even be aware that you have **frost nip** in your toes and fingers or about your head and face, because the condition is painless. You may only know it by a lightening of the skin.

  The real danger is that frost nip may go on to become **frostbite,** in which part of the body, such as fingers, toes, or nose, actually becomes frozen, a condition that may destroy the underlying tissue. One of the first signs of frostbite is a white, grayish yellow, or in the case of severe involvement grayish blue discoloration of the skin. Sometimes pain is present, sometimes not. In any event, as frostbite progresses, the body parts become numb, and the skin becomes glossy and pale. The bad news becomes apparent during thawing, when pain is really felt. One of the dangers of frostbite is tissue death and subsequent loss of the affected part.

- *Hypothermia:* In **hypothermia,** core body temperature drops to a dangerously low level—below 95°F (35°C)—the result not only of prolonged exposure to cold owing to inappropriate clothing or inadequate protection from the weather but also to immersion in cold water. Symptoms and signs of hypothermia include shivering, fatigue, slurring of speech, poor coordination, and blueness of skin. Vital signs are affected, including low body temperature, very slow pulse, and slowed respiratory rate.

  Hypothermia is a life-threatening condition, especially if one is exposed to the cold weather in damp clothes, is sweating in the presence of cold winds, or is in freezing water. In extreme cases, the victim may be disoriented, in shock, perhaps unconscious; breathing may stop and the person may die.

You may have heard that massaging or rubbing snow on frostbitten fingers or giving the victim a few stiff brandies will help to ease these problems. Don't do this. For frostbite, the affected area must be handled gently and very carefully. For both frostbite and hypothermia, you should get the victim indoors, give him or her a warm nonalcoholic drink, and get medical attention as quickly as possible; otherwise, the two conditions are treated differently.[98]

For frostbite, protect the frozen part and get medical attention. If no professional help will be available, place the part in lukewarm (not hot) water to rewarm it. Don't apply heat to the area. Avoid heat lamps, hot water bottles, or hot stoves. If the feet are affected, don't allow the victim to walk. Don't apply bandages. The rewarming process takes about 30 minutes and is very painful, especially during the last 10 minutes. (If the part is susceptible to refreezing after rewarming, as when a person must be moved through cold, it's best to delay rewarming until permanent shelter can be reached.)

For hypothermia, the victim should be wrapped in warm blankets. In mild cases, passive rewarming may be all that is needed. In serious cases, however, the person may be confused or comatose and no longer shivering. In such instances, heat must be applied, but *gradually* and *gently*. Warmed rocks or hot water bottles should be placed at the person's head, neck, underarms, trunk, and groin. Don't rub the extremities, don't put the person in a warm bath or shower, and don't allow the person to smoke or drink alcohol.

If the person has stopped breathing, he or she should be given cardiopulmonary resuscitation (CPR). People who appear dead after cold exposure should not be considered dead until their body temperature has returned to normal and they still have not responded to CPR.

Strategy for Living: Exercising in Cold Weather Exercising safely in cold weather is mostly a matter of common sense:

- *Consider the wind as well as the cold:* The wind-chill factor can make all the difference: a 20-mile-per-hour wind can transform 10°F air temperature into an equivalent temperature of −25°F—within the zone of increasing danger.

- *Wear appropriate clothing:* Always cover your head. Wear several layers of clothing and make sure the garments are loose-fitting. Remove wet clothing right away. To decrease heat loss from lips, cheeks, and nose, apply an oil-based ointment.

- *Don't stay out too long:* Don't spend long periods of time outdoors; intersperse your activity with time-outs indoors to warm up and drink warm liquids. Give yourself time to become acclimated to cold climates and reduce your intensity when starting out.

- *Work out with a friend:* A friend who is knowledgeable about hypothermia is more apt to notice your problems than you are.

- *Avoid alcohol and cigarettes:* Alcohol makes you *feel* warmer, because it expands (dilates) the blood vessels in the hands and feet, but it actually increases the escape of heat from the body, making you colder. Smoking (nicotine) constricts these same blood vessels, thereby reducing the body temperature and blood supply in these areas.

Strategy for Living: Exercising with Environmental Hazards If you jog alongside a busy roadway, you're most certainly breathing in some carbon monoxide from car exhaust. Carbon monoxide, sulfur dioxide, ozone, and **particulates**—chemical particles from industries, power plants, and cars—are considered dangerous air pollutants. Carbon monoxide can cause headaches, nausea, and respiratory failure. Sulfur dioxide can cause chronic bronchitis. Deep inhalation of these and other substances while exercising can be hazardous.[99]

Thus, besides weather, you need to know how to deal with such environmental conditions as air pollution, poor visibility, and high altitude:

- *Minimizing effects of air pollution:* In polluted areas, do your outdoor physical activity away from sources of air pollution (for example, in parks, not near four-lane highways), or early or late in the day, or indoors or not at all during smog alerts. If necessary, reduce the intensity of your exercise, and don't exercise if you have respiratory infections, such as a cold or bronchitis.[100]

- *Exercising outdoors at night:* Have you ever driven a car at night and found yourself abruptly swerving to avoid hitting a dark-clothed pedestrian, jogger, or bicyclist? This is the kind of experience that sets the heart pounding and the blood pressure sky-high for any driver.

If you must jog close to the roadway, be sure you wear highly visible, light-colored clothing. Add strips of reflector tape (available at sporting goods stores) to the back of your workout clothes and to the backs of your shoes or bicycle pedals. A flashlight will not only help you see where you're going but also warn approaching cars. Exercise in well-lighted areas and go accompanied with someone else.

- *Exercising at high altitudes:* The higher you are above sea level, the less oxygen is available, a situation that can put great stress on your heart and respiratory systems. A disorder known as **acute mountain sickness** can occur at altitudes of 9000–10,000 feet (3000–3300 meters). It is characterized by headache, nausea, vomiting, and insomnia. Other disorders are possible at extremely lofty elevations, such as altitude sickness, but are a problem mainly for high-altitude mountain climbers and the like.

If you move from sea level to a higher elevation, it's recommended you allow 1 week for every 3000 feet (1000 meters) as time to acclimatize yourself. During this adjustment period, you should reduce the intensity of your activity to about 25% of what you're used to at sea level.[101]

Strategy for Living: Avoiding Anabolic Steroids A former National Football League offensive lineman at age 36 needs a heart transplant and is given 2–3 years to live.[102] An 18-year-old male, a muscular high school senior, has breast enlargement, increased acne, and intermittent periods of depression and outbursts of anger.[103]

What both have in common is their use of **anabolic steroids** (slang names " 'roids," "juice"; taken orally or injected). Although other types of steroids are useful in the medical treatment of asthma and arthritis, anabolic steroids—mostly synthesized chemicals mimicking the male hormone testosterone—have been used in recent years by people interested in boosting their muscle size and strength and supposedly improving their appearance.

News about steroid use by top-level athletes brought this drug to public attention. In 1988 a Canadian sprinter was stripped of his

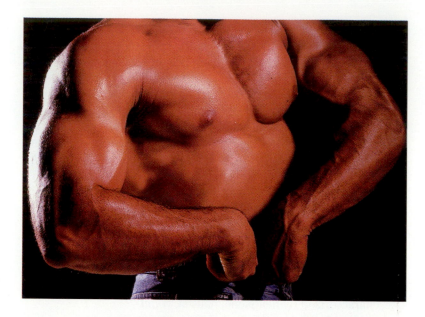

● **Figure 17.14 " 'Roid rage."** If people are predisposed to violence, steroids can push them over the edge.

“*He was an unlikely addict. Well-dressed and well-fed, he had the strong, sleek build of a man who regularly bench-pressed twice his weight. He was 24 years old, didn't smoke, drink, or eat junk food and sneered at psychoactive drugs as polluters of the mind. But when he drove himself to an emergency room in Ann Arbor, Michigan, one winter night in 1987, he was in trouble and he knew it.*

The anabolic steroids that fed the young weight lifter's muscles had also triggered alternating bouts of elation and rage. Two weeks before, his 5-year marriage had broken apart; his wife could no longer stand his angry outbursts. Once easygoing and content, he now found himself increasingly suicidal; the night before, he had struggled to keep from steering his speeding car into oncoming traffic. But over the last 9 months every time he had tried to quit using steroids, or even to cut the dose, he'd been thwarted by headaches, deadening fatigue, and bottomless depression.”

—Deborah Franklin. (1990, July 1). Stuck on steroids. *This World, San Francisco Chronicle*, p. 16. Reprinted from *In Health.*

Olympic gold medal for using anabolic steroids. Two American Olympic silver medalists, a 400-meter runner and a shotputter, tested positive for steroids in 1990 and were banned for 2 years from athletic competition.[104] However, steroid abuse is not limited to Olympic and professional athletes. It is also found among police officers, bouncers, gang members, and others who want to increase their body size and strength.[105] In addition, the U.S. Department of Health and Human Services estimates that 260,000 adolescents abuse steroids.[106] Two thirds of steroid-using 12th-grade boys said they started using the substances by age 16 to improve sports performance, but one out of four said they took them mainly to "improve appearance."[107]

Although they provide no more competitive edge than regular forms of rigorous athletic training, steroids *do* work as performance enhancers in the short run. When combined with heavy exercise, they promote gains in stamina, muscle, and weight, dramatically altering a person's physique in just a few months (for example, an increase of 15–20 pounds in 6–12 weeks). On the negative side, however, they also can alter temperament, and if people are predisposed to violent behavior, steroids can push them over the edge into increased aggressiveness and belligerence. This has given rise to the term " 'roid rage."[108] (See ● *Figure 17.14.*)

Mood swings, however, may be the least of the negative side effects. Indeed, the Food and Drug Administration has compiled a list of nearly *70* adverse effects, some of which are not reversible.[109] They include the following:[110–113]

- *Adverse psychological and physical side effects for both sexes:* Psychological symptoms include hostility, irritability, euphoria, and lessened fatigue, but when the drug is withdrawn it produces depression, suicidal tendencies, anorexia (self-starvation), and paranoia. Early on, the sex drive may increase, but with continued use it may decrease. Physical effects range from an increase in acne to higher blood pressure and blood cholesterol levels to increased risk of heart disease and liver and kidney cancer.

- *Adverse side effects for females:* Anabolic steroids produce **masculinizing** effects in women—the taking on of male characteristics—including deepened voice, facial hair growth, and male pattern baldness, all apparently irreversible. In addition, the clitoris may enlarge (also irreversible), breast size decrease, and menstrual cycles become irregular or cease.

- *Adverse side effects for males:* Men who use steroids may experience breast enlargement, shrunken testicles (an apparently irreversible change), decreased sperm production, impotence, and male pattern baldness.[114]

In January 1991, Congress reclassified anabolic steroids as a controlled schedule III substance, which means these drugs have medical uses but are subject to abuse. Although steroids are banned from college and professional sports, former National Football League lineman Lyle Alzado attributed the inoperable brain cancer from which he died in 1992 to his steroid abuse. He believed many players still use them—or use steroid-type drugs that aren't banned or can't be detected in drug tests. Other observers believe that as long as the emphasis in athletics is on winning—and, in professional sports, on big money—players will have incentives to cheat despite the ruinous effects of steroids on their health.[115,116]

What to Do About Strains and Sprains Different sports have different common injuries, which require different strategies for prevention and treatment. (*See* ● *Table 17.2.*) Strains and sprains are two of the most common injuries in athletics. A **strain,** also called a "muscle pull," is a stretch or tear in a muscle or in a tendon, the tissue connecting muscles with bones. A **sprain** is a stretch or tear of a ligament, the connective tissue attaching bones together at the joints.[117]

The treatment for strains and sprains, as well as for most other unexposed injuries affecting tissue, is with *R-I-C-E,* or *R*est, *I*ce, *C*ompression, *E*levation:

- *Rest:* Rest the injured area; 48 hours is a reasonable length of time.
- *Ice:* Ice wrapped in a towel should be applied for 20 minutes to the injured area to reduce swelling and pain, then removed for

20 minutes, then more ice applied for the next 20 minutes, and so on, up to several hours.

- *Compression:* Compress the injury by wrapping the area in an elastic bandage; this will help to reduce pain and buildup of fluid around the affected area.
- *Elevation:* Elevate the injury above the level of your heart to prevent swelling.

800-HELP

American Running and Fitness Association. 800-776-2732. Furnishes information on aerobic sports. Offers referrals to orthopedists, coaches, trainers, sports-medicine clinics, podiatrists, and chiropractors.

Nutrition for Athletes. 800-231-3438. Registered dietitians at the University of Alabama at Birmingham offer advice on high-performance nutrition.

Running Injuries. 800-843-8664. The American Running and Fitness Association offers free pamphlets on runners' injuries and tips on treatment.

Suggestions for Further Reading

American College of Sports Medicine. (1992). *ACSM fitness book.* Champaign, IL: Leisure Press. Comprehensive, easy-to-understand guide to physical fitness for people of all levels.

Stamford, Bryant A., & Shimer, Porter. (1990). *Fitness without exercise.* New York: Warner Books. Shows how to use small, nonstructured bouts of activity to develop and maintain fitness.

● **Table 17.2 Common sports injuries: treatment and prevention.** *R-I-C-E* stands for *Rest, Ice, Compression, Elevation.*

Type of sport	Common injury	Possible causes	Treatment	Prevention
Bicycling	Knee problems	Seat improperly adjusted	R-I-C-E, aspirin	Adjust seat position
		Using too high a gear		Learn to "spin" in lower gears
	Numb hands	Seat position causes weight to fall on hands	Massage	Ask expert to set correct seat position
		Wind chill		Wear gloves to keep hands from getting numb and to cushion palms
Dance, aerobic	Shin splints	Jumping, landing on toes	R-I-C-E, aspirin	Switch to low-impact aerobics
		Improper shoes		Wear appropriate shoes
	Back strain	Improper techniques or position (e.g., arching back)	R-I-C-E; rest with knee higher than hips	Ask instructor if you're performing correctly and ask for alternate exercises
Racquet sports: tennis, racquet-ball, squash	Tendonitis (tennis elbow)	Wrong size racquet	R-I-C-E, aspirin	Use equipment matching your body proportions and skills
		Improper technique		Get instruction to improve form
		Weak forearms		Exercise to strengthen wrist and forearm muscles
	Sprained ankle	Improper shoes	R-I-C-E, aspirin	Wear court shoes to control foot motion
Running	Runner's knee	Unstable heel	R-I-C-E, aspirin	Wear shoe with heel support
		Weak quadriceps		Gradually build up quadriceps
		Adding mileage too quickly	Cut down on mileage	Establish fitness base before increasing mileage

Table 17.2 (*continued*)

Type of sport	Common injury	Possible causes	Treatment	Prevention
Running	Achilles tendonitis	Insufficient stretching	R-I-C-E, aspirin	Thoroughly stretch hamstings, calf muscles, and Achilles tendons before and after running
		Uncushioned heel	Use heel lifts	Wear running shoes with adequate support and cushioning
		Increased mileage	Reduce mileage or stop running	Stretch thoroughly
Softball	Abrasions and bruises	Sliding into base, contact with ball, other players	Clean wound, use antiseptic, cover lightly; use aspirin and ice packs for bruises; for black eyes, see a health professional	Wear long pants and don't forget to duck
Swimming	Shoulder problems	Inadequate warm-up	R-I-C-E, aspirin, massage	Thoroughly stretch neck, back, chest, arm muscles
		Improper technique		Get instruction to improve form
Volleyball	Sprained fingers, thumb	Inattention	R-I-C-E; if pain continues, see health professional	Stay alert
		Improper technique		Get instruction to improve form
Walking	Sore feet or legs	Improper shoes	Elevate feet, take aspirin	Wear sturdy, comfortable walking shoes
		Rocky terrain		Walk on smooth, level paths
		Going too far too soon		Gradually increase distance

Source: Adapted from Chapman, V. (1988, January/February). Prevent fitness fallout. *View* [Group Health Cooperative], p. 22.

SELF DISCOVERY 18.1

How Good Are You in Bed?

	True	False
1. Some people sleep better in a strange environment.	___	___
2. The older you get, the more noise you need to fall asleep.	___	___
3. Spending more time in bed will help you sleep.	___	___
4. It's easier to sleep near an airport than a noisy refrigerator.	___	___
5. The kind of mattress you sleep on can make a big difference in how well you sleep.	___	___
6. Sleeping with a partner probably won't help you sleep.	___	___
7. Sleeping in a warm room won't help you get to sleep.	___	___
8. Overweight people have fewer serious sleep problems.	___	___
9. Alcohol is probably better than milk at bedtime.	___	___
10. Older people have more sleep problems.	___	___
11. Stopping smoking can help you sleep better.	___	___
12. Counting sheep actually helps you get to sleep.	___	___
13. Getting out of bed and engaging in some other activity may help you get to sleep sooner.	___	___
14. Not getting any REM sleep can lead to hallucinations.	___	___
15. If you are sick, your illness will get worse if you don't sleep.	___	___

Answers

1. *True.* Some insomniacs may actually improve in a new setting.
2. *False.* Some people fall asleep best when listening to music or watching television, but sensitivity to noise increases with age and is more prevalent in women.
3. *False.* Curtailing time in bed seems to help.
4. *False.* Occasional loud noises are more disruptive to sleep than constant noises. People living near airports had 45 minutes less sleep and less deep sleep than those living in quieter neighborhoods, according to one Los Angeles study.
5. *False.* Europeans seem to have a preference for soft mattresses with elevated heads. Americans prefer hard, flat mattresses. There is no evidence that either improves sleep.
6. *True.* Sleeping with a partner probably helps sex but may actually disturb sleep . . .
7. *True.* A moderate to cool room is probably better. A study of people in Chicago showed more sleep interruptions in the miserable Chicago summer than the miserable Chicago winter.
8. *False.* Although overweight people seem to be sleepier, they have a higher incidence of sleep apnea, a serious condition in which breathing can stop. On the other hand, dieting is associated with short and fragmented sleep.
9. *False.* Drinking has a rebound effect—you are initially sleepy and then wake up agitated. Milk seems to improve sleep, but this has not been proven.
10. *True.* The entire sleep/wake system becomes more disturbed as we grow older.
11. *True.* Nicotine is a nervous system stimulant and the sleep of smokers tends to improve after they stop.
12. *False.* Maybe if you've been working as hard as a shepherd. While an overactive mind can keep you up, counting sheep may encourage sleep worry.
13. *True.* Reading seems to be especially good.
14. *False.* Depriving people of REM sleep may actually be useful in treating depression.
15. *False.* No proof that lack of sleep slows healing.

Source: Adapted from: How good are you in bed? A quiz. In: Kahn, A. (1991, August 29). A nation of insomnoids. *San Francisco Chronicle*, p. D-3.

18   Sleep and Rest

▶ Discuss the principal sleep problems, the stages of sleep, the importance of sleep/wake cycles, and strategies for maximizing sleep.

▶ Why is leisure time important?

▶ What is "active rest"?

Sleep and rest are the opposite side of the coin from activity, and are equally important, since they are restorative. Although we may spend 8 hours or so sleeping (and many people another couple of hours reclining, as in front of a television set), we may actually know very little about the subject of rest. Indeed, people nowadays have a great many misconceptions about sleep and often worry about whether they get enough. But there is also rest beyond sleep, what sports psychologists call "active rest." Let us consider both kinds.

Sleep

Many people have sleep problems, from insomnia to narcolepsy. Understanding sleep stages and daily circadian, or sleep/wake, cycles can help fitness. Strategies are available to optimize sleep habits.

Most animals follow natural sleep cycles, and don't vary from them. But millions of humans—the 7 million Americans who have night jobs, for instance—routinely ignore their natural rhythms, staying awake at night and sleeping during the day. This and other variations cause a great number of problems in getting enough sleep. Indeed, you may find you have some sleep problems yourself. (*See Self Discovery 18.1.*)

The American Sleep Disorders Association now lists more than 140 accredited centers for treating sleep disorders—up from 25 a decade ago. The association has identified 84 varieties of sleep disorders, ranging from insomnia to sleepwalking.[118] Two important disorders are:

- *Insomnia:* **Insomnia** is defined as an inability to achieve adequate or restful sleep. Inadequate sleep is considered a major cause of the errors that people make. One leading sleep researcher, Stanford University's William Dement, says that sleep is such an important factor in accidents that perhaps someday "driving or going to work while sleepy may be as reprehensible and even as criminally negligent as driving or going to work while drunk."[119]

  Insomnia may be of three types:

  (1) **Transient insomnia** is occasional troubled sleep, such as that brought on by jet lag or worry about a test the next day.

  (2) **Short-term insomnia** is 3–6 weeks of disturbed sleep, generally linked to stress in one's life, such as relationship troubles or financial worries. Beyond 3 weeks it's time to see a doctor.

  (3) **Chronic insomnia** is a long-term sleep disturbance, which may stem from one of four causes: (a) medical causes such as a breathing problem; (b) psychological causes such as depression or anxiety; (c) lifestyle problems such as those associated with drug use, including coffee, nicotine, or alcohol, or insufficient exercise to promote sleepiness; (d) faulty bedtime or sleep habits, such as using the bed for activities other than sleep or sex (such as doing homework or paperwork or lolling late on Sundays).

- *Narcolepsy:* The opposite of insomnia, **narcolepsy** is an ongoing condition characterized by an irresistible urge to fall asleep. It differs from normal sleepiness in that it cannot be fully relieved by any amount of sleep. A second symptom of narcolepsy is **cataplexy,** a sudden muscle weakness usually brought about by excitement or high emotions such as laughter, anger, or fear, which causes one to collapse and be unable to move.[120] Narcoleptics number between 1 in 1000 and 1 in 10,000 people in the United States.[121,122]

The biggest problem in North America seems to be "sleep deficit." Sleep experts have

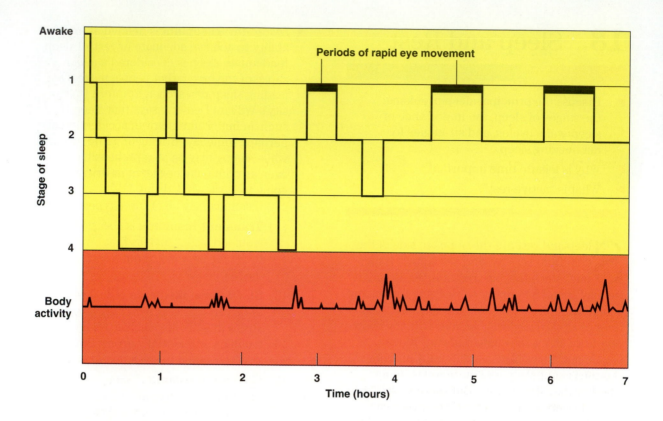

Figure 18.1 Sleep stages. The graph maps out one subject's sleep cycle during the course of one night. REM stages are shown as very thick bars. This cycle is very typical: there were four REM periods, and they tended to get longer as the night progressed.

found that most people get 60–90 minutes less sleep each night than they should. Whereas diaries and other personal accounts show that people in the 18th and 19th centuries used to sleep an average of 9½ hours a night, the invention of the electric light bulb a century ago seems to have been the beginning of a national sleep deficit, since people were able to rise before dawn's early light and retire long after sunset.[123]

The Cycles and Uses of Sleep In an 8-hour (or whatever) night's rest, your body may go through four or five sleep cycles, each cycle containing different stages of brain-wave activity. Sleep scientists distinguish between REM and non-REM sleep. **REM** stands for **rapid eye movement** and refers to times during the night

when the eyes shift rapidly back and forth beneath the closed lids. It is during REM sleep that most vivid dreaming occurs. Non-REM sleep is quieter, mainly nondreaming sleep, although it takes up about 6 hours of an 8-hour night's sleep. During the course of a cycle, as you fall deeper into unconsciousness, the brain waves become slower and larger, finally forming a jagged pattern. (*See ● Figure 18.1.*) After an hour-long descent into unconsciousness, you move into the stage of REM sleep—the stage of dreaming—in which the brain waves resemble those of ordinary wakefulness, with short, rapid strokes. During this time, your breathing, pulse, and blood flow increase; your eyes move rapidly back and forth beneath the lids; and you experience the bizarre, alluring, all-things-possible world of dreams.

The purpose of dreams remains a mystery, but it is possible they help us learn new mental strategies for dealing with difficulties and for coming to grips with traumatic events in our lives—for instance, the violence and despair of abused women or children.[124] Most dreams seem real to us as we are having them. However, psychologists have developed a technique called **lucid dreaming** that enables dreamers to become *aware* that what they are experiencing is unreal, which allows dreamers to work therapeutically with dream material to seek self-understanding.[125]

Whatever the importance of dreams, there seems to be no doubt about the importance of sleep. It used to be thought that mild sleep deprivation did not affect performance, but newer research seems to challenge that. Going without sleep even one night seems to diminish people's ability to think creatively the following day, according to British psychologist James Home.[126] And after 5–6 nights of shortened sleep, the way we work and feel is definitely affected. Researchers also have indications that sleep boosts the immune response against disease.

Strategy for Living: Understanding Your Circadian Rhythms An important physiological cycle to be aware of is your **circadian rhythm,** the built-in daily, or circadian, clock in everyone's body that determines individual blood pressure, body temperature, hormone output, cell division—and sleep/wake cycle. Circadian rhythms can be the reason you get sleepy after lunch, why you get those Sunday afternoon blues, and why your performance declines when you switch from day-shift work to night shift.

Consider some of these instances:

- *Afternoon sluggishness:* In general, the point at which you get sleepy after lunch is halfway between your usual wake-up and bedtime hours, although the timing will be affected by your genetically inherited circadian rhythm. Some countries, the so-called siesta cultures, such as those in Latin America, recognize this phenomenon by closing businesses for a long lunch hour, during which people go home and not only eat but nap. For most working people in North America, this may be difficult, although college students, many of whom have time between classes, may be able to take midday naps.

  Note: What you eat for lunch can also make a difference. A meal high in carbohydrates will make you sleepier than one high in protein, because the carbohydrates will release sleep-related chemicals in your brain. Exercising during your lunch hour can also lessen the likelihood of your wanting to take an afternoon snooze.[127]

- *The Sunday afternoon blues:* Many people experience a downward mood swing along about 3 o'clock Sunday afternoon, an attack of the blahs as one contemplates Monday morning's return to work or school. Part of this mild depression—which may extend to Monday morning—may not only derive from the end of the weekend's bright promise but also from, as one writer describes it, "the imbalance between weekend sleep/wake cycles and the internal biological clock set by evolution to the cycle of day and night."[128] Because people often stay up late and rise later on weekends, this disruption of the circadian rhythms may affect people's moods.

- *Night-shift work:* There are 7 million Americans who work at night but have difficulty adjusting to a night schedule. Not only does sleepiness lead to accidents, but the upset in body rhythms also produces insomnia, gastrointestinal disorders, and even increased incidences of heart disease and, in women, infertility. Many people who work at night apparently never adjust to their schedule, no matter how many years they work the night shift.[129] A new kind of therapy developed recently, however, provides a relatively easy way to shift rhythms quickly and efficiently. Researchers have discovered that night-shift workers can reset their internal clocks by exposure to very bright light (50–100 times brighter than ordinary indoor light) at work, with total darkness during the day. In the study, eight men took only 4 days to adapt to a night-shift schedule.[130]

Circadian rhythms also manifest themselves in other ways, such as the "jet lag" or tiredness that we associate with flying across several time zones. In addition, many people feel they are "night people," who do their best work at night. These are usually people who are under 40, are in general good health, and can catnap easily. As people grow older, however, most turn into "morning people." Many couples find themselves on mismatched sleep/wake cycles, which can mean troubles in a relationship unless the partners resolve to work at accommodating each other.[131] These ideas suggest it's worth paying attention to your inner body rhythms so that you can make maximum use of your high-energy time for work and study.

Strategy for Living: How to Pull an All-Nighter This is not advice we would recommend on a routine basis, but next time you find that you've let studying slide and have roughly 24 hours to prepare for a test or write a paper, give some thought to how best to pull an all-nighter. Should you plug in the coffeemaker, hit the books, and then catch a 4 A.M. snooze before going to class?

Actually, a better strategy for optimizing your performance is to take a nap *before* you light the midnight oil. "Prophylactic napping," as it has been called, will prevent sleepiness. In fact, according to a study led by biological psychologist David F. Dinges, a short nap before staying awake all night will enhance your performance even though the sleep will probably be lighter than it would during a nap later.[132]

Strategy for Living: How to Sleep Better Many people take pride in going without sleep. Some men in particular may see sleep loss as macho, taking pride in saying, "I get by on 4 hours," although in fact they are probably making up much of it on Saturdays and Sundays.[133]

Do you, in fact, *need* to sleep the 8 hours that everyone seems to consider standard? Sleep researchers say that people's sleep needs may range from 2–3 hours a night to 10 or more, although most adults seem to do their best work by sleeping 7–8 hours. Some people, who describe themselves as workaholics (including "Today" show host Bryant Gumbel and cookbook author Martha Stewart), apparently cut down on sleep in an effort to get more done, although Albert Einstein, for example, slept 11 hours a night.[134] If you are strongly motivated to sleep less, you can cut back slowly each night, going to bed 15–30 minutes later but al-

ways waking up at the same time. Still, you should expect to feel slightly under the weather while your body adjusts, and you should probably not try to sleep less than 6 hours a night.

Most people, however, have the opposite problem: they want more sleep, not less. Indeed, sleep scientists say there is virtually an epidemic of sleepiness in the nation: more than 100 million Americans get by with insufficient sleep—nearly every other adult and teenager.[135] Most short themselves 1–2 hours of sleep a night. This has important consequences, according to sleep researcher James Maas, because even one night's loss of 2 hours' sleep is not made up during the following 5–6 days of normal sleep. "There are some people who are literally walking zombies," Maas says. "If you need an alarm clock to get up in the morning, or if you feel more than a minor sag in the middle of the day, you need more sleep."[136]

Teenagers are particularly susceptible to sleep deprivation. Maas said studies show high-school seniors get an average of 6.1 hours of sleep a day but need about 10 hours to function effectively. A study of 150 Baltimore-area adolescents found the teenagers slept an average of 6½ hours a night.[137] Students whose schools had earlier starting times tended to have more problems in school, such as falling asleep in class, than those with later starting times. Even among college and graduate students ages 18–30 who got an average of 7–8 hours sleep a night, sleep researchers discovered that 20% of these apparently normal students could fall asleep almost immediately throughout the day if allowed to lie down in a darkened room. And students who did not fall asleep were found to improve their performance markedly on psychological tests if they spent 1 week getting to bed 90 minutes earlier than usual.[138]

Assuming you don't have chronic insomnia, in which case you should see a doctor (or contact the National Sleep Disorders Foundation), here are some tips on how to sleep better:

- *Follow a regular sleep schedule—7 days a week:* You don't have to go to bed at the same time every night, but you should get up at the same time every morning. Indeed, most experts recommend getting up at the usual time even on Saturdays and Sundays, in order to stick with your natural sleep/wake rhythms.

- *Save your bed for sleeping and sex:* The idea is to make sure bed is associated in your mind with these activities and not with such activities as studying or afternoon snacks. Incidentally, hormones triggered during sex can enhance sleep in some people.[139]

- *Develop a bedtime routine:* Develop bed-time rituals to allow yourself to wind down before sleep. Soak in a bath. Pick out the next day's clothes. Watch TV or read a book. After turning out the light, give your-self 15 minutes to drift off to sleep. If you don't become drowsy, don't stay in bed; get up and go into another room and read for a while until you feel sleepy.[140]

- *Watch what and when you drink and smoke:* Caffeine is a stimulant, so drinking coffee or caffeinated soft drinks after mid-day may affect your sleep. Nicotine is also a stimulant and won't help you sleep. In addition, there is the danger of fire if you fall asleep with a lit cigarette. Alcohol, even in small amounts, can make you sleep less soundly. A glass of warm milk before bed-time may help you relax.

- *Deal with worries before you go to bed:* If you find yourself lying awake worrying about a problem, write down what you can do about it in the morning, along with a list of reasons why it's not worth being upset about now. Earlier in the day you can take time for a "worry session," writing down how you will handle any upcoming events. Talk over your problems with someone else. (See ● *Figure 18.2*.)

- *Exercise at regular times:* Try to get at least some exercise every day. Although vigorous exercise is not recommended just before bedtime, a short evening walk may be helpful. Older people are apt to have more sleeping problems than younger, but a study by psychologist Michael Vitiello found that 12 men in their 70s, who exercised an hour a day 5 days a week for 6 months, all reported improved sleep quality and were more refreshed in the morning.[141]

- *Minimize distractions:* Try to eliminate distracting bedtime noises, or mask them with a soothing noise, such as music or the hum of a fan. Use heavy shades to darken

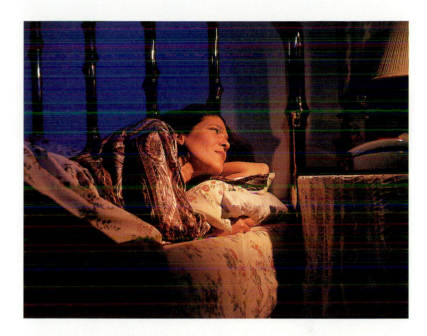

● **Figure 18.2 Worry time**

Some people report their minds start to race as soon as they flip off the lights. 'It's not that you worry too much,' [sleep psychologist Peter] Hauri tells them, 'but that you do it at the wrong time.'

His advice: Schedule 30 minutes earlier in the day as worry time. Sit in a quiet place. Write each worry on a separate 3-in. × 5-in. card. Sort the cards into categories. Take each in turn and think about it until you decide what to do. Write that plan of action down.

If no solution comes to mind, consider seeking advice from someone else. Write that down, too. The written word is a first step toward taking action. Often, writing things down literally puts your mind to rest.

—Lynne Lamberg. (1990, November). The boy who ate his bed . . . and other mysteries of sleep. *American Health*, p. 58.

your bedroom so you won't be awakened prematurely by the morning's first light.

- *Eliminate the use of sleeping pills:* The effects achieved by most sleeping pills usu-ally last only 2–4 weeks. Moreover, they only help you fall asleep faster, but do not help you achieve deep sleep. They also leave a hangover effect in the morning and decrease your alertness. Thus, if you must take a sleeping pill, try to limit yourself to one per week.[142]

Strategy for Living: Help for Snoring Snoring is caused by the vibration of tissues of the throat and soft palate that become relaxed during sleep. Maybe your own snoring doesn't bother you, but it may bother your bed partner or roommate. On the other hand, your snoring may indeed bother you (although you don't know it) because it may be a signal of **apnea.** In this sleep disorder, one stops breathing for brief periods each night (usually owing to the closure of throat tissues), and the lack of oxygen causes the sleeper to wake up. As though one were awakened by the phone ringing every 15 minutes throughout the night, the resulting sleep deprivation can cause daytime sleepiness.

Serious cases of snoring should be treated by a physician. However, there are several changes in lifestyle and sleeping habits that may help.[143] Some of these are simply the adoption of health habits that will benefit you in other ways as well.

- *Alter drug use.* Not smoking, avoiding or reducing alcohol consumption, and being careful with over-the-counter medications such as cold remedies have all been found to reduce snoring.

- *Lose weight.* Weight loss may reduce the tissue bulk in the neck and throat and diminish the size of a large abdomen pressing on the diaphragm when you lie on your back.

- *Change sleep habits.* Sleeping on a firm mattress with a low pillow can help reduce airway obstruction. If you snore only while sleeping on your back, try changing sleeping positions or sleeping without a pillow.

Leisure: More Than Rest from Work

Whether because of employer pressures, economic necessity, or a "work-and-spend" cycle, many people do not get enough or high-quality-enough leisure time, which can be harmful to health.

How you feel about work and leisure is an important value that has a profound effect on your health and your life.

Consider: Perhaps 108 million Americans drive to work each day; we spend more time than ever behind the wheel. Only a very few commuters (5%) use public transit; the dominant form of commuter transportation is the single-occupant vehicle in a suburb-to-suburb trip. Is all this car time good for us? In studies by psychology professor Raymond Novaco, a direct correlation was found between distance of a commute and rise in blood pressure. In addition, he found such commuting produced lowered ability to concentrate and to tolerate frustration, short-term memory loss, and family and relationship problems.[144]

In addition to spending more time commuting, we are also spending more time at work and having less leisure time as a result. During each of the last 20 years, Americans gradually added an additional day of work, so that, as economist Juliet Schor writes, today's work year (consisting of 1949 hours) is 163 hours longer—almost a month of 8-hour workdays—than in 1969.[145] Although many people are working more—the average is 43 hours a week—they also like it less. Nearly 1 in 6 employed adults works a second job and more than 1 in 3 regularly works evenings or weekends, but a 1991 Gallup poll found that two-thirds of workers say they prefer their off-hours to those on the job.[146]

Although for many people these extra hours at work are a matter of economic necessity, Schor, who authored *The Unexpected Decline of Leisure,* believes there is another important factor operating here—what she calls the insidious cycle of "work-and-spend." This occurs partly because "people get the income and then they automatically spend it," she says. "Once people have the income, it is very difficult to convince them that they'd be better off with less."[147] (*See ● Figure 18.3.*)

From an employer's standpoint, although many bosses use hours as the standard for judging their employees, too many hours at work actually impairs performance and productivity, as studies of army officers and oil-rig workers, among others, have shown. One researcher who interviewed over 1000 executives in the U.S.

and Britain about their work habits said: "Any manager who works over 50 hours a week in my view is turning in less than his [or her] best performance."[148] Work schedules with shorter hours, by contrast, can actually improve productivity, as different studies have shown. When hours are shorter, there is less fatigue, workers can sustain more intense effort, the time spent on less productive activity (breaks around the water cooler, for example) decreases, and morale is higher, so that workers spend less time at work on their personal business.[149]

American businesspeople who insist on longer hours often like to place the discussion in the context of competition with Japan. Compared to many European countries, for example, where by law or by contract workers put in shorter hours and receive vacations of at least a month each year. U.S. workers average 2 weeks' paid vacation a year, while the Japanese take only a week and a half. The Japanese experience a disturbing phenomenon known as *karoshi*. Defined as death from overwork, karoshi often appears in the form of fatal heart attacks. It is a serious problem among white-collar men, who adhere to grueling work days and commuter schedules, as well as obligatory after-hours socializing with coworkers.[150]

The effect of Americans' overwork on children is profound, particularly in one-parent families or two-parent families in which both mother and father work to meet the family's financial needs. One study found that as family incomes have gone up things have become worse for children, as represented by increased homicide and suicide rates among American teenagers and declines in standardized test scores. Adults seem to be spending more dollars and fewer hours on children.[151] According to a University of Maryland study, in 1985 American parents spent just 17 hours a week with their children.[152]

There are many signs that Americans actually *want* more leisure. For instance, most adults would rather work 10-hour shifts 4 days a week than 8-hour shifts 5 days a week, according to a fall 1990 Gallup poll.[153] Asked how they would spend another free day if they had it, the largest share (15%) said they would spend it with their families; 11% would relax; 9% would travel; and 6% would spend time on

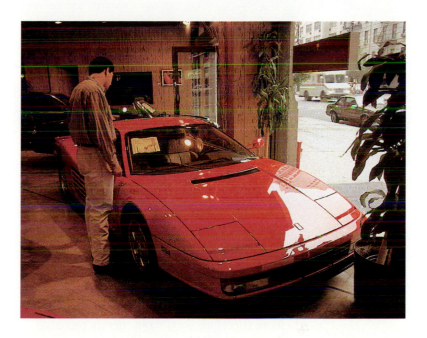

● **Figure 18.3 What keeps us from leisure?** How you feel about work and leisure are important values that relate to health. The dynamics of the "work-and-spend" cycle keep us working harder and away from relaxation, this economist asserts.

❝*In its starkest terms, the [work-and-spend] cycle operates like this: Employers ask for long hours from employees. They do so in part because long-hour jobs pay more and thus are more desirable to workers, who will labor more productively to keep them. Also, the fewer workers a firm needs to hire, the less it has to spend on fringe benefits. The high pay, in turn, creates a high level of consumption. People buy houses and go into debt; luxuries become necessities; Smiths keep up with Joneses— and workers accept, or even ask for, longer hours so they can go on spending. Work-and-spend has become a powerful dynamic keeping us from a more relaxed and leisured way of life.*❞

—Juliet B. Schor, Ph.D. (1991). Workers of the world, unwind. *Technology Review, 94*(8), 25–26.

crafts and hobbies, working around the house, or going back to school. Interestingly, 5% would spend their free time by working more.

There are, as Schor points out, two factors affecting the use of leisure time that seem important:

- *Overworked people choose low-energy leisure activities:* According to a 1986 Gallup poll cited by Schor, the most popular ways to spend an evening are television, resting, and reading—"all low-energy choices." Other potentially satisfying activities such as taking up a sport or musical instrument or voluntarism take more time.

- *People are encouraged to associate free time with spending money:* Many forms of leisure encouraged by the "leisure industry" cost money: vacations, hobbies, popular entertainment, eating out, and shopping, to name a few. Clearly, to escape the "work-and-spend" cycle, people must find more cost-free alternatives.

Perhaps the moral is this: the purpose of both working and leisure is to have a good life. Leisure therefore should not merely recharge us for more work; nor should it be so money-draining that it requires us to work more.

Active Rest

Active rest combines meditation and activity to lessen fatigue and enhance performance.

In recent times, athletes and others have found benefits in a form of personal self-renewal known as **active rest.** This state combines the benefits of meditation and physical activity to help us reduce stress, turn off disturbing "mind chatter," build energy and endurance, and enhance physical performance. Many athletes, for example, find that going into a workout while mentally uptight causes muscular tension that causes early fatigue and inhibits performance. Starting exercise while in a state of active rest lessens fatigue and helps one use the physical activity to sharpen concentration.

Some components of active rest are as follows:[154]

- *Meditative breathing exercises:* Prior to physical activity, 10 minutes of breathing exercises can help clear away the mental "noise" and focus your concentration. By counting each exhalation from 1 to 10 and then starting over, you learn to focus on the sensations of your body and induce relaxation. Breathing exercises may also be done following physical activity in order to calm the mind.

- *Visualization for mental relaxation:* Visualization can take the form of imagining a quiet, pleasurable experience, such as lying on a raft in the middle of a lake or walking on a beach, in order to induce a sense of peace. It also can take the form of making positive statements about the physical activity you are about to undertake—such as "I can bicycle 15 miles without fatigue"—in order to ensure greater probability of success.

- *Music:* During physical activity, music or other repetition can help to sustain the rhythm. For instance, many swimmers sing a song in their heads while doing laps. Researchers have learned that exercisers listening to slow, soft popular music (found to be better than rock 'n' roll, though rock was still better than silent exercise) felt better and could work out longer than those who exercised in silence.[155]

Suggestion for Further Reading

Hales, Dianne (1987). *How to sleep like a baby*. New York: Ballantine. Lists 101 suggestions for combatting insomnia.

High Performance: Energy Boosters

Successful people seem to be high-energy people. They seem able to put everything they've got into what they're doing. What are their secrets? Before we discuss these, answer the following with yes or no.

To be a high-energy person, you have to . . .

___ **1.** Eat like a top-performing athlete.

___ **2.** Be able to manage stress.

___ **3.** Find a way to get along with less sleep.

___ **4.** Be able to ignore your body's rhythms.

___ **5.** Fit exercise into your life.

The correct answers for the questions above are: (1) yes, (2) yes, (3) no, (4) no, and (5) yes. We describe these five components of a high-energy life below.

1. Food: Eat Like a Top-Performing Athlete

You don't have to eat the same *amounts* that high-performing athletes do—some of whom may well consume 7000 Calories a day—because their high levels of physical activity may require large amounts of food. But even desk workers can learn something from winning athletes about the kinds of foods to eat. The basic rules are:

- Eat a diet high in complex carbohydrates, such as vegetables, fruits, grains, and pasta, and low in fats and sugar. There's no need to increase protein consumption, since most people in North America get plenty. A balance athletes often strive for is to get 65% of their Calories from carbohydrates, 20% from fats, and 15% from proteins.

- Consume a variety of foods in order to ensure you get all the vitamins and minerals. This means fresh foods in particular.

- Drink lots of water, and avoid alcohol and caffeine.

Women should take supplements of iron and calcium but otherwise, with a balanced diet, vitamin supplements usually are not needed.

We described techniques for power eating in the Unit 6 Life Skill.

2. Mental Outlook: Be Able to Shut Out Stress

Sports psychologist Jim Loehr has coined the phrase *Ideal Performance State* (*IPF*), or *mental toughness,* to describe an athlete's ability to shut out stress, negative thoughts, doubts, and fears so that he or she can concentrate on the game at hand.[156] The Ideal Performance State is an internal feeling of high arousal, as expressed in the athlete's words of "being psyched," combined with a profound sense of calmness, clarity, and control.[157] The key seems to be to lose oneself in the moment, not worrying about the outcome, the competition, or what others think. These are moments of peak performance that psychologist Mihaly Csikszentmihalyi has described as "flow," the state in which people are so involved in activity that nothing else seems to matter.[158]

Recreational athletes—and people in stressful but nonathletic situations, such as public speaking—use the word "choking" to describe feelings of tension and nervousness and an adverse reaction to pressure. "Choking" means they are choking for air, with their inhalations much longer and deeper than their exhalations. Good players accept that choking is a normal response to pressure, but then reframe their outlook to eliminate the expectations that caused the stress in the first place. Among the techniques used are those for controlling breathing, relaxing muscles, using positive self-talk to replace negative internal messages, projecting a winning image, visualizing winning points before the play, and developing rituals between plays to maintain concentration.

We described some of these stress-reducing techniques in Unit 2.

3. Sleep: Find a Way to Get All the Sleep You Need

Although everybody's sleep needs are different, it is probably safe to say that most high-performance people *do not* short themselves on sleep. Moreover, it's highly likely that one principal cause of low energy is sleep loss. Studies have found that when young adults were deprived of sleep for 7 consecutive nights, allowing them just 5 hours of sleep per night, their daytime alertness progressively worsened.[159] Other research has also shown that sleep deprivation can lead to difficulty in concentration, fatigue, and poor performance on a variety of tasks.[160]

In general, most people need 7½ to 8½ hours of sleep per night, although a small percentage can get by on 5 or 6 hours and another small percentage need 9 or 10. Most people seem to benefit from sustained sleep (for example, 7 hours straight), although some people can profit from sleeping plus a nap (for example, 5 hours of sleeping and 2 hours of napping at a different time of day).[161]

4. Body Rhythms: Be Attentive to Your Energy Cycles

Timing can play a noticeable role in energy. Some researchers have discovered that athletes doing all-out workouts, such as sprinting, swimming, broad-jumping, or bicycling, can go longer and have more strength if they perform in the early evening. In other words, they may have a peak performance "window" that's available between 5 and 7 P.M.[162] Conversely, many people feel a gradual rise in energy through the morning, with a peak around noon, and a drop in energy in midafternoon. After an early-evening increase, their energy declines until sleep.[163]

Biopsychologist Robert E. Thayer suggests the existence of two bodywide energy systems of physical and emotional rhythms, a "physical energy cycle" and an "emotional tension cycle."[164] How the two come together determines whether you feel calm energy or tense

energy. *Calm energy,* the kind most of us would probably want, is when physical vigor is high and emotional tension is low. Calm energy is associated with enhanced thinking and learning. *Tense energy,* which is more difficult to sustain and more draining, is when both physical vigor and emotional tension are high. Although many people don't distinguish tense energy from calm energy, the former makes you anxious and leaves you in a state of "tense tiredness." Learning to become familiar with your own body rhythms can help you learn to manage your energy levels. Oftentimes all that's needed during the less-energetic times is to take a break—for socializing or for exercise. People who are slow risers may benefit from exercising first thing in the morning, others at noontime (followed by a light lunch) to fight midafternoon sluggishness, and others right before dinner.

We discussed body rhythms (circadian rhythms) in Chapter 18.

5. Fit Physical Fitness Into Your Life

Here is the paradox: to build energy, you have to use it. Exercise induces energy. Why this is so is not clear, but the anti-anxiety and antidepressant effects may result from the release into the bloodstream, and possibly brain, of the body's natural opiates known as endorphins, as well as the chemical norepinephrine, which is linked to feelings of alertness. In addition, exercise increases your blood flow, lowers your resting heart rate, and strengthens your heart, all of which enable you to accomplish your work with less physical effort.

Although these effects can be achieved in regular aerobic sessions of 15–20 minutes, Thayer suggests that even a 10-minute walk is a highly effective way of raising energy and reducing tension, as well as offering the break from routine that keeps you going. (And a workout of this duration means you won't work up a sweat, so you won't have to shower.) Aerobic exercise may offer the most energizing benefits, but even mind-body exercises such as yoga and t'ai chi ch'uan can lift energy levels.

Probably the two biggest objections raised to physical exercise are (a) finding time, and (b) getting bored. Finding time is indeed a problem for many people, as the work week (including commuting) has gone from an average of 41 hours in 1973 to 47 hours in 1987, according to a 1987 Harris survey.[165] The trick, then, is to squeeze exercise into any small chunks of time during the day. For example, you can walk, run, or bicycle to work or school. You can even plan to get off the bus at a distant stop or park your car in a far corner of the lot and walk the rest of the way. You can work out for a half hour or hour early in the morning, at noon, or early evening—by walking or running or by lifting weights at a college gym or health club. If you can afford it, you can buy an exercise bicycle and set it up at home in front of your TV set. Finally, you can mix work and play, moving briskly through errands, housework, and gardening in order to make these chores more active.[166]

Boredom is another matter. If you are to build exercise into your life, there must be a strong fun component or you won't do it. People have developed all kinds of tricks. The best way to forestall boredom is to change your exercise routine. You can change your route, your time, even the type of exercise itself. You can listen to music or motivational audiotapes on headphones. You can let your mind do dissociative thinking, focusing on job or school problems, on your love relationship, or on a song going through your head. Many people switch into cross-training, a mix-and-match approach, to keep exercise interesting. Switching between weight-lifting, roller-skating, and swimming, for instance, can provide a variety of challenges, as well as working out different muscle groups. Indeed, many competitors in the triathlon, the combination of three sports—usually swimming, bicycling, and running—said they started training for this grueling competition because they had become bored or dissatisfied with some other sport.[167]

Intimacy and Sexuality

In These Chapters:

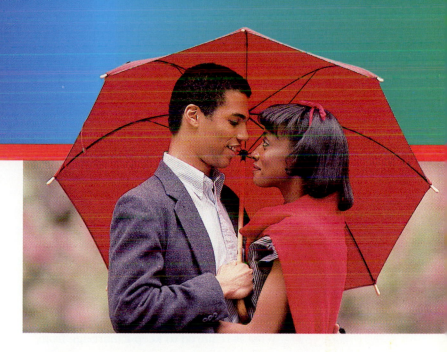

Life is short, and human attachments should be cherished.

One of the authors of this book came across that statement, was struck by it, and copied it for future reference: it seems like one of the best statements of a reason for living that I've seen. Throughout my life I've marveled at the number of people who chase money or position or possessions or "success" who seemed to have few friends and difficulties staying in a loving relationship—who seemed, in other words, to have scant human attachments.[1] On the other hand, there are those whose principal assets are friends and lovers and family members, people who like and love people and are liked and loved in return.

Loneliness is a common problem. That certainly was the case for one of the authors, who, throughout high school and college suffered from nearly crippling shyness, choked with anxiety about speaking up in class, telephoning a girl for a date, or getting out on a dance floor. My first girl friend was in 7th grade, when I was 13. After that, I didn't have another until I was 24.

I used to wonder why I was attracted to girls but they weren't attracted to me. Was it because I wasn't athletic? Although I was tall, I was awkward and gangly and couldn't seem to throw a ball straight. I also had a life-long hearing problem that interfered with my participation in sports.

To be sure, I wasn't a complete loss. Although my love life wasn't much, while I was both a high school and college student I had a great circle of friends of both sexes—many of whom remain friends a few decades later.

A great many people feel unattached, lonely, unlovable. Even some of those who for all appearances are handsome, poised, and outgoing are actually in great despair. They mistakenly believe that only a loving partner will deliver them from depression and boredom and make them feel happy and secure. In fact, however, one's feelings of loneliness and inadequacy may actually drive others away: potential partners are looking not for needy people but for people who are self-confident enough that they bring excitement and contentment to others' lives. Love, then, begins with self-love—a matter you can probably do something about.

19   Relationships

▶ Why is self-love important?

▶ Describe the various kinds of intimate relationships.

▶ Discuss five types of love.

▶ What is the "triangle of love"?

▶ Discuss what factors shape your "emotional availability."

▶ Describe some principal aspects of single-hood and dating and courtship.

▶ What are three types of committed relationships?

▶ What is required to keep a marriage from ending in divorce?

"Learning to like and love yourself is the key to intimacy," writes psychiatrist David Burns.[2] Self-love does not mean being selfish or conceited. It means appreciating who you are and your potential. To stop feeling inferior and rejected and project the self-confidence that will attract other people, Burns suggests taking four steps: Stop abusing yourself and get involved in life. Stop putting yourself down and think about yourself in a compassionate manner. Drop self-defeating attitudes and develop a more positive value system. Confront and conquer your fear of being alone.

When you include yourself in your positive feelings, you can then include others, and they will include you.

Intimate Relationships: From Being Alone to Being in Love

The capacity for love starts with self-love and the rewards of being alone. Intimate relationships include friendship but also various kinds of intimacy—recreational, social, intellectual, emotional, and physical—with another. Love may be of five types: passionate or romantic, erotic or sexual, dependent or addictive, friendship or companionate, and altruistic or unselfish. The "triangle of love" is interaction among intimacy, passion, and commitment. Loss of love means dealing with rejection and building self-esteem.

Many psychologists seem to measure mental well-being by the success of our relationships with others. Being able to be alone, however, may actually be a sign of strength, according to some. On the other end of the spectrum is love that is actually not love but neediness. Let us examine the range of relationship possibilities.

Being Alone   Twenty million Americans live alone. Some people are alone by choice, others by circumstance—new in town, separated, divorced, or widowed. Some people who don't live alone by choice may be angry and frustrated. Others, however, feel they have found true happiness by finding peace with themselves. (*See* ● *Figure 19.1.*)

Indeed, Oxford University lecturer in psychiatry Anthony Storr suggests that the solitary state plays an essential role in the life of thinking, creative people. For the artist, writer, composer, or philosopher, in fact, the flame of creativity burns most brightly in a mind working in solitude.[3] Because all of us are alone at some time in our lives, it is important to discover what the rewards of this state can be.

Friendship   Does every Butch Cassidy need a Sundance Kid? Does every Thelma need a Louise? How good a friend are you to *your* friends? **Friendship** is a relationship between two people that involves a high degree of trust and mutual support.

In the past an ignored topic in behavioral research, friendship has turned out to be important. Numerous studies find that people who have friends they can turn to for advice, empathy, assistance, and affirmation as well as affection have better odds of surviving serious life challenges such as heart attacks and major surgery. They are also less likely to develop cancer, respiratory infections, and other diseases.[4] Friends can help reaffirm your self-worth when you lose a job, suffer the breakup of an important love relationship or marriage, or have something else challenge your competence and good opinion of yourself.

Friendships may be hard to sustain for people who are taking classes and studying on weekends, who are upwardly mobile in a demanding job or otherwise on the move, or who are trying to find time for a two-career family with young children. A survey of 600 San Francisco residents found that only half regarded friendships as "very important" in their lives.[5]

Women seem to value friendships more than men do (58% of women found friendship "very important" versus only 46% of men), although men tend to retain their friendships longer than women do. The reason, suggests psychology professor Martin Fielbert, is that male friendships may involve less challenge but also less conflict. Women tend to have "face-to-face" friendships, in which they share their feelings and struggles; men have "side-by-side" friendships, in which they do things together but do not take risks by disclosing or talking about intimate life areas.[6]

Other psychologists who have explored friendship, such as Lillian Rubin, also find that women are more apt than men to share their hopes and fears with their same-sex friends.[7] As for men-women friendships, men feel they get more nurturing from these relationships than women feel they do. Women find they get more nurturing from their female friends.[8] Still, research shows that boys who aren't pushed to act tough and self-reliant—who are able to trust and feel close to their friends—seem just as likely as girls to forge close friendships with members of their own sex.[9]

In any event, friendship is important, both while growing up and later on.[10] The well-being of adults in all age groups seems to be related to the quality of social interaction they have with friends as well as with family.[11] (*See Self Discovery 19.1.*)

Intimacy Friendships can be close and can, though need not, involve intimacy. To some people, the word *intimate* means having sex. However, **intimacy** is defined as a close, familiar, affectionate, and loving relationship with another person.[12] Actually, intimacy can take any of five forms:[13]

- *Recreational intimacy:* **Recreational intimacy** is the sharing of interests, hobbies, and recreational activities, as, for example, if you and your partner spend a lot of time

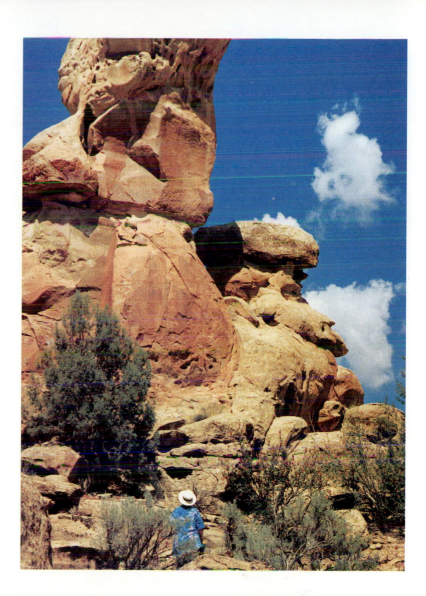

● **Figure 19.1 The joy of being alone**

❝*Living alone can be a positive experience at any age.*

It needn't be equated with loneliness.

Many people who live alone are lonely. And statistics indicate that loneliness leads to an increased risk of physical and psychological illness, including depression so severe that it can result in suicide. But what these statistics fail to point out is that there are thousands and thousands of people who are alone, alive, and well.

For every miserable, pathetic, and lonely individual who lives alone, there are many others who are healthy, involved in interesting, productive activities, and enjoying life.❞

—Barbara Powell. (1985). *Alone, alive, and well.* Emmaus, PA: Rodale, p. 2.

SELF DISCOVERY 19.1

How Good a Friend Are You?

Answer yes or no to each of the following statements.

	Yes	No
1. Do you promise to do things and then forget?	____	____
2. Do you try to "top" stories told by friends?	____	____
3. Do you exclude others from your clique?	____	____
4. Do you tell friends what's wrong with them?	____	____
5. Must you always be the center of attention?	____	____
6. Do you tell people about your loan to a friend?	____	____
7. Can you keep a secret?	____	____
8. Do you ask people to do trivial tasks for you?	____	____
9. Would you drop everything to help a friend?	____	____
10. Are you generally in good humor?	____	____
11. Is it easy for you to find good in others?	____	____
12. Do you drop in unannounced and then stay?	____	____

Scoring

Using the answer key below, determine how many questions you got right.

1. No	4. No	7. Yes	10. Yes
2. No	5. No	8. No	11. Yes
3. No	6. No	9. Yes	12. No

Interpretation

11–12	You have friends because you're a good friend—reliable, gracious, and giving.
7–10	You have friends, but some "put up" with you.
4–6	You're seeking friends, but can't find any.

Source: Klein, M. M. (1983, May 28). You can learn the fine art of friendship. *USA Today*, p. 4D.

playing tennis or being involved in environmental politics.

- *Social intimacy:* The experience of having common friends and similar social networks is called **social intimacy.** An example is when you and your partner enjoy spending time with other couples, or your partner's closest friends are also your closest friends.

- *Intellectual intimacy:* **Intellectual intimacy** is the closeness developed through the sharing of ideas, as when you find that you and your partner have an endless number of things to talk about. This form of intimacy is important because communication through words and **body language**—nonverbal communication through body posture, gestures, and so on—is important in being able to express feelings and desires. Communication has a great deal to do with sustaining a couple's satisfaction with their relationship.[14]

- *Emotional intimacy:* **Emotional intimacy** is closeness of feeling. This is when you feel your partner can understand your joys and your pains or when you feel you can describe your feelings without the other person becoming defensive.

- *Physical intimacy:* Closeness developed through physical contact, ranging from touching to hugging to caressing to kissing, is **physical intimacy.** This kind of intimacy may also, of course, include all forms of sexual contact. An expression of your level of comfort in physical intimacy might be measured by how much sexual expression is part of your relationship or your ability to tell your partner your sexual desires.

Our desire for touching and physical closeness—"contact comfort"—may be inborn, but it is also affected by cultural norms: American friends talking in a coffee shop will touch each other only 2 times in an hour, compared to 0 times for English friends, 110 times for French friends, and 180 times for Puerto Rican friends.[15] The American cultural prohibition (particularly for men) about adults touching each other, except in sexual situations, seems rooted in the tactile deprivation so many men experience in childhood. As a result, they may feel embarrassed and clumsy not only about expressing emotions but also about touching and expressing affection.[16] Both men and women, however, can learn to express their affection through touch. (*See ● Figure 19.2.*)

Love What is love? It is difficult to analyze this emotion, one of the grandest feelings a person can experience. If you look in the glossary of a textbook on human sexuality or marriage and the family, you probably won't find a definition of love. Look under *love* in the index, however, and you might find several listings. That is because love has several meanings or associations (parental love, brotherly love, "true" love, and so on). Indeed, the reason there is so much confusion about love is that this one lofty word is used to cover a multitude of feelings.

Professor F. Philip Rice describes five types of love—romantic, erotic, dependent, friendship, and altruistic loves—which together make up what he calls *complete love:*[17]

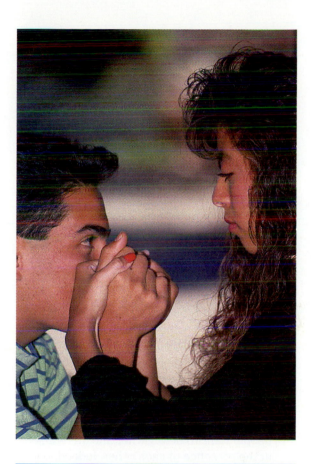

- *Infatuation, passionate, or romantic love:* When we experience that dizzying ecstasy and joy known as "falling in love"— the kind of wild exhilaration celebrated in so many songs, movies, and romance novels—we are actually in a state known as **infatuation, passionate love,** or **romantic love:** passionate, strong feelings of affection for another person. This kind of love is real enough in its physiological manifestations: pounding heart, breathlessness, sometimes the inability to eat or sleep.[18]

  The reasons people fall in love are probably proximity, commonality, and perceived attractiveness. People become attracted to those they see frequently and who share similar attributes.[19] Physical attractiveness is also often important at first, although sometimes a person's attractiveness is heightened by the perception of dangerous circumstances (which is why secret love may be so intense).[20,21]

  In the end, romantic love cannot be sustained. It becomes less wildly romantic and more rational, although love may continue to grow. In other words, the wildly emotional state of romantic or passionate love is replaced by the more low-keyed emotion of companionate love or friendship love (described below), with feelings of friendly affection and deep attachment.[22] But, assuming romantic love is not the *only* connection between a couple, infatuation has served its purpose: as psychiatrist Aaron Beck states, it forges the kind of powerful bond between a couple that spurs them to commit to a relationship.[23]

- *Erotic love:* **Erotic love** is sexual love. Many people can have sex without romantic love; indeed, they may be unable to handle emotional involvement. Others have found that having sex actually diminishes the

● **Figure 19.2 Touching**

❝*Touching is important because it develops bonding and affection between people. Touching is more than foreplay, more than a means of sexually stimulating another person. It is the basis of love and affection. To be able to touch and be touched is to discover new meanings of sex and love.*❞

—F. Philip Rice. (1989). *Human sexuality.* Dubuque, IA: Wm. C. Brown, p. 257.

power of romantic love previously felt for a person. Yet others find that tensions and resentments that diminish their loving feelings for each other also adversely affect the sexual aspect of their relationship. Finally, many couples find their sexual and loving feelings are not distinct from each other.

- *Dependent love:* **Dependent love** is love that develops for someone who fulfills one's psychological needs. For instance, someone who has not had much praise as a child may have his or her intense psychological needs for appreciation met by the beloved. Or a studious person may welcome appreciation for his or her playfulness.[24]

  At its extreme, this kind of love can become an addiction, when another person serves purely as the object of a need for security. At this point, love becomes a kind of "mutual protection racket," with two people hanging on because of a fear of loneliness or an extreme need for approval. This phenomenon has given rise to a number of popular books such as *Women Who Love Too Much* and *Love and Addiction.*[25,26]

- *Friendship love:* As mentioned, **friendship** or **companionate love** is more low key than romantic love is. It is love based upon companionship, with common respect and interest in the personality or character of the beloved. In a word, friendship love is *liking* for the other person, so that two people want to be together and are relaxed in the presence of each other. Indeed, one researcher believes that, despite the mass media's emphasis on romance and sexuality, companionate love is probably the most common and frequently experienced aspect of love.[27]

- *Altruistic love:* **Altruistic love** is unselfish concern for the welfare of another, finding meaning in making the other person happy. An example is a parent willingly and happily assuming care for a child. In a relationship such as marriage, altruistic love means accepting the beloved without insisting that he or she change. Altruism is also a feature, of course, of romantic love, as in stories about the great efforts a lover will make on behalf of the beloved.

The "complete love" of which Rice writes serves the point of showing that love consists of several elements. This idea is borne out by research by psychology professor Robert Sternberg, who asked subjects to describe their relationships with lovers, parents, siblings, and friends. The results showed close relationships have three necessary, interacting components —*intimacy, passion,* and *commitment*— which Sternberg calls the "triangle of love."[28] (*See* ●*Figure 19.3.*) In this triangle, *intimacy* refers to feelings in a relationship that promote emotional closeness and bonding. *Passion* includes the expression of one's needs and desires. *Commitment* consists first of the short-term decision to love the other person, then the long-term decision to maintain that love, although one phase may occur without the other. For most people, commitment results from intimate involvement combined with passionate attraction.

The End of Love The source of great joy can also be the source of great pain, but the process of falling out of love is equally as natural as falling in love—though it is not, of course, inevitable. The greatest difficulty is dealing with *rejection,* whether it is unrequited (unreciprocated) love at the beginning of an attempted relationship or love that "grows old and waxes cold," as the song goes.

For some people, the painful breakup of a love relationship can lead to what has been called "love addiction," when a person obsessively seeks to regain the pleasurable state that existed within a former love relationship. The distrust, feelings of rejection, loss of self-worth, and feelings of failure, loss, and anger in the emotionally hurt person are all feelings that must be dealt with, and counseling may help the person resume normal life and move into new relationships.[29,30]

In *How to Fall Out of Love,* Debora Phillips suggests some steps for recovering from the loss of love, using methods of behavioral therapy:[31]

- *Stop thoughts of the person:* You can learn to spend less and less time thinking about the loved one, mostly by making a list of positive scenes and pleasures that do not involve the former beloved. When a thought about the person enters your mind, say "Stop," then think about one of the best scenes on your list.

- *Build self-esteem:* Just as a love relationship builds self-esteem, being rejected lowers it. To raise your self-esteem, Phillips suggests you use index cards on which you write two good things about yourself every day, positive things you have done recently

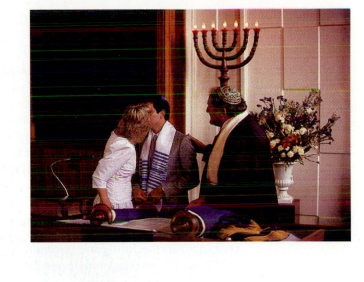

Intimacy

Includes
10 elements:
1. Desiring to promote the welfare of the loved one.
2. Experiencing happiness with the loved one.
3. Holding the loved one in high regard.
4. Being able to count on the loved one in times of need.
5. Having mutual understanding with the loved one.
6. Sharing oneself and one's possessions with the loved one.
7. Receiving emotional support from the loved one.
8. Giving emotional support to the loved one.
9. Communicating intimately with the loved one.
10. Valuing the loved one.

Intimacy

Passion

Commitment

Commitment

Includes two phases:
Short-term phase:
decision to love the other person.
Long-term phase:
commitment to maintain that love.

Passion

Includes the expression of one's needs and desires: sexual fulfillment, self-esteem, nurturance, belonging, dominance or submission.

● **Figure 19.3 The triangle of love.** Psychology professor Robert Sternberg's research shows that love is the interaction between intimacy, passion, and commitment.

or further in the past. When negative thoughts creep in, say "Stop," and think of one of these good things about yourself.

If you are the one being let down, don't spend a lot of time speculating *why:* the other person may not even know why he or she is not in love, and it doesn't help to torture yourself trying to figure it out. The best thing is to simply put some distance between yourself and the other person.

If you are the one trying to disengage from the relationship, remember how it feels to be rejected and try to be honest but gentle: "I no longer feel the way I once did about you." Don't promise to try to "work things out," and don't try to take care of or "rescue" the other person.

You and Your Committed Relationships

How well you were treated by others early in life—whether your family was loving or dysfunctional (withholding love)—affects your emotional availability, or ability to give yourself to others. Some people are happy with singlehood, others get involved with dating and courtship. Among the types of committed, or monogamous, relationships people have are living together or cohabitation, whether heterosexual or homosexual, and marriage. Without positive interaction and good problem-solving skills, many marriages will end in divorce.

When you were a newborn, everything from baby toys to mother seemed simply a part of you. This is why if people treated you well, you felt good about yourself, but if they ignored you or caused you pain, you felt badly about yourself—in other words, they affected your self-love. Later you began to learn that your self had boundaries and everything else was apart from the self. Still, perceived self-love or self-loathing established during childhood formed the basis for how you relate to others. As we mentioned, positive feelings of self-love mean you are capable of loving others.

Family Relationships and Emotional Availability Your emotional training began, most likely, with your **family of origin.** Those who directly influenced you might have been the adults who were parents to you and your brothers and sisters. You may also have been emotionally affected by people in your **extended family**—grandparents, aunts and uncles, cousins, and so on—especially if you lived in a multigenerational household, as is typical of families in Asia and Latin America.

The best that could be hoped for any child is to be raised in an atmosphere of openness, trust, and sharing, but far too often this is not the case. Too many people grow up in a **dysfunctional family,** in which the interaction between members holds back rather than fosters emotional expression, individual growth, and self-love. Sometimes a family is dysfunctional because someone in it has a dependency prob-

lem (alcohol, drugs, gambling, workaholism, religion, violence). Members of dysfunctional families are dishonest and distrustful of one another because one or more individuals try compulsively to control others, have unrealistic expectations about how they and others ought to be, and constantly seek self-gratification. The result is that family members suffer social isolation (for example, in keeping outsiders away from an alcoholic family). They also suffer a continuing cycle of pain (such as when the most dysfunctional member periodically rages at other members).[32]

Another damaging kind of upbringing is sexual abuse in childhood. This may consist of molestation—ranging from sexually suggestive remarks to fondling of breasts and genitals to intercourse and oral sex—by people inside the immediate family or others such as relatives, neighbors, or babysitters. One form of sexual abuse is **incest,** sexual relations between two people so closely related that the state would not permit them to marry, such as father and daughter. Some survivors of sexual abuse are so traumatized that they may actually not remember the abusive incidents, but it leaves them supremely wary and uncomfortable about opening themselves emotionally to prospective lovers.

How you were treated by others, then, is the basis for your **emotional availability.** This is your ability to give and receive emotionally from another person without the fear of being hurt or taken advantage of. Clearly, it has much to do with how you handle relationships and intimacy, now and in the future.

The Single Life Most of us pass through some period of singlehood, living by ourselves for a time (although some people may be involved in a relationship or marry just to get away from the dysfunctional family they were raised in). Being single is actually fairly common, with 66 million (37% of all adults) not involved in an intimate relationship, never-married, or "newly single"—the divorced and widowed.[33] The reasons for the large number of single people seem to be simply that more people are choosing to live alone, people are marrying for the first time later in life, and divorce rates are high. (*See Figure 19.4.*) Although adult men are more likely than women to live alone, women live longer than men, which is why they outnumber men in their later years.

Do people *like* being single? Many find it as appealing as being married, and indeed there are many committed relationships that do not involve marriage. Many people, both men and women, remain single because they are unable to find the right person, although they report they would like to get married some day. Psychologist Florence Kaslow, reporting on a survey of several states, said that, in addition, men say they don't want to marry because they are putting their independence and the resolution of personal issues first. Women, especially those over 30, often put their careers and quests for financial independence first.[34]

An interesting sidelight: many single people are also parents. Because half of all marriages now end in divorce and out-of-wedlock births have rocketed, the percentage of white children living with one parent has almost tripled (to 19.2%) during the past three decades, and it has doubled among blacks (to 54.8%). Thus, a majority of children born today will spend at least some of their youth in a single-parent household.[35]

Dating and Mating The 20s are an age when most people are seriously on the lookout for prospective mates—a time described by that old-fashioned word **courtship,** which includes the ritual known as *dating.* Courtship also takes the form of actively pursuing possibilities, such as going to dances, getting friends to "fix you up," and running personal ads.

The dating experience itself can be extremely difficult for people. Indeed, one study found that problems in dating relationships were the most frequent complaints voiced by undergraduates using a college counseling center.[36] In fact, says one writer, "Interaction with the opposite sex is a major factor in our development, and scars acquired during dating encounters may have long-lasting effects on later adjustment."[37] Feeling awkward about what to say and do on a date, being ill at ease about encounters of a potentially sexual nature, and being overcritical of one's own abilities may all lead to high anxiety. Anyone experiencing these kinds of worries about dating is well advised to go to a college counseling center or get similar assistance.

More people are living alone:

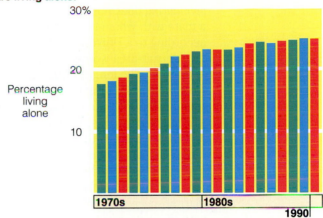

People are marrying for the first time later in life:

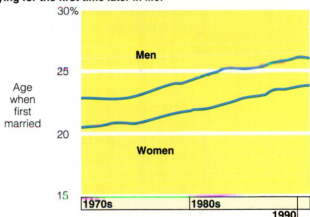

Divorce rates are high:

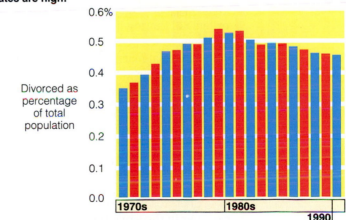

● **Figure 19.4 Single minded**

Contrary to popular belief, however, extensive dating does not have a bearing on selecting a mate with whom to live "happily ever after," according to a University of Michigan study of 459 Detroit-area women married between 1925 and 1984. "The length of the dating experience, the number of dating partners, the length of the relationship with the eventual first husband, and the degree of sexual intimacy with that husband—none of these predictors had any significant independent influence on the fate of the marriage," said Martin Whyte, a sociology professor who was involved in the study.[38] Rather, marital success seemed to be more associated with the degree of romantic love the woman felt at the moment of marriage, along with shared family values, leisure activities, and control of family finances.

Committed Relationships: Living Together

Once upon a time, the phrase "committed relationship" meant a long betrothal or courtship or being married. It still means those things, of course, but today it also can describe other kinds of mutually **monogamous** relationships—relationships in which two people are sexually faithful to each other. That is, there may be a committed relationship between an *unmarried heterosexual couple* living together as "domestic partners"—the Census Bureau recorded 2.7 million of these couples in 1990—or between a *homosexual couple,* male or female, sharing living quarters.

Sometimes people describe their relationship as a "trial marriage" rather than living together. Sometimes they may not even live together under the same roof, maintaining separate residences and "overnighting" with each other, but their intent is to maintain a union of permanence. The growth of such nontraditional households is happening not just in the United States but throughout other countries in the developed world.[39]

A heterosexual couple living intimately together in the same household outside of marriage is said to be **cohabiting.** The average length of cohabitation is only about 12 months.[40] However, if the relationship continues longer than 7 years, the law in some states considers it a **common-law marriage** for real estate or financial purposes. Cohabiting is most common among high-school dropouts, those on

welfare, and those raised in single-parent families, but more than 25% of college graduates have cohabited before marriage.[41,42]

Is living together in a "trial marriage" a good way to practice for the real thing? Some see cohabitation as simply a new development in the American courtship process. According to sociology professor Ronald Rindfuss, "In an earlier time, [a couple] would have gotten married or simply continued dating."[43] Yet some studies show that people who live together and then get married are actually *more* likely to divorce than people who did not live together first.[44,45] There may be several reasons for this: Long-term cohabitors who are unsure about or ideologically opposed to marriage may be pressured by friends or relatives to tie the knot. Cohabitors may also be less likely to pool incomes, to own joint property, and to share leisure activities, values, and interests that are essential to maintaining a healthy marriage.[46]

One psychotherapist who herself lived in an unmarried but committed relationship for many years points out that unmarried couples need legal contracts to cover many situations that they are bound to confront and that are automatically covered in marital law.[47] Buying a house or having children are two obvious concerns. So is the case where one unmarried partner works at a menial job to put the other through professional training such as medical school, so that later if the successful doctor abandons the relationship he or she is obligated to help the former partner progress professionally also. In the end, then, marriage may help to provide legal protection that otherwise must be consciously, even elaborately, arranged between a couple living together.

Committed Relationships: Homosexual Couples

Same-sex relationships are every bit as strong as opposite-sex relationships. In fact, people sexually and emotionally attracted to members of the same sex—that is, people with a **homosexual** orientation—have recently been focusing more and more on couples' rights and family issues. Indeed, many **lesbians,** or female homosexuals, are in long-term relationships and in fact are more likely than **gays,** or male homosexuals, to settle down with one partner. About one-third of lesbians are mothers through heterosexual relationships, artificial insemination, or adoption.[48,49] There are also many gay men who have long-term relationships, some of whom raise children.

As with unmarried heterosexual people living together, one of the greatest difficulties in a homosexual union is the absence of straightforward and automatic laws covering the relationship. Thus, when a gay or lesbian couple splits up, the recourses available in the dissolution of a heterosexual marriage—temporary spousal support, child support, equitable division of property—aren't in place unless the partners had the foresight to have lawyers write agreements for them beforehand.[50] Recently, however, there have been various efforts to legalize gay marriages—where legal, the law certifies them as "domestic couples"—which would extend gay couples societal recognition and legal protection.[51–53]

Children growing up in a gay home clearly are being raised in somewhat unconventional circumstances, and some may suffer insults from their peers in early adolescence, especially if their same-sex parents are open about their relationship—if they are active, say, in gay-rights political movements. However, studies suggest that most children of gay parents are well-adjusted.[54] Indeed, some experts find their experiences comparable to those of children of interracial marriages, where confronting prejudice in early adolescence builds character and enriches later life.[55]

Committed Relationships: Marriage The traditional committed relationship in North America and Western society is **marriage,** the legal, and often religious, union of two people of the opposite sex. Most people get married—70% of Americans at least once, although not necessarily "so long as ye both shall live," as the marriage oath suggests.[56]

In general, marriage is beneficial: married people are happier and healthier than people who are divorced, widowed, or never married.[57] Married people also live longer: the average mortality rate for unmarried men is twice as high as for married men, and 1½ times higher for unmarried women. Divorced people, especially men, generally have the highest death rates.[58,59]

In some countries, such as Japan and India, marriages are often arranged, usually by the parents for economic and social reasons. In North America, people marry for love, companionship, and security but also for reasons that have less to do with the partner than with fulfilling other needs: to get away from home, to legitimate a pregnancy, to prove to parents one is "grown up." Recently, however, Americans have been waiting longer to marry the first time and also longer to remarry: in 1991, the median age for the first marriage was 26 for men (up from 23 in 1970) and 24 for women (up from 21).[60] In the recession year of 1991, marriage rates hit a 16-year low, just as they dropped during the 1930s Great Depression and possibly for similar reasons: because of economic bad times, many young adults continued to live with their parents.[61]

Interestingly, although members of both sexes benefit psychologically from marriage, men seem to benefit more than women.[62] The reason may have to do with gender roles: whether working outside the home or not, being married is probably harder on women, who generally find themselves carrying a larger share of housework and childcare, making them feel stressed or unappreciated. The longer couples stay married, the more likely they are to become like each other, eventually sharing many of the same thoughts and perceptions, but even here women are more likely to change than their husbands are.[63]

Even though we live in a supposedly cynical age, there are many marriages in which partners can express the sort of love and devotion to each other that we now may associate with an earlier time. (*See ● Figure 19.5.*) Presumably such couples would be those whose marriages, in the 12-year study of 8000 couples by researcher David Olson, could be described as "vitalized" (9% of cases), "harmonious" (8%), or "balanced" (8%). Unfortunately, they are almost overshadowed by the 40% that fall into the lowest category—"devitalized," characterized by "dissatisfaction with all nine dimensions of the marital relationship."[64] The study is an assessment of nine dimensions of relationships, including communication, conflict resolution, leisure, parenthood, family and friends, religion, finances, and sexuality.

Perhaps, suggests Olson, the preponderance of unhappy marriages is partly because society does little to help the institution of marriage. "We assume that if people are going to do

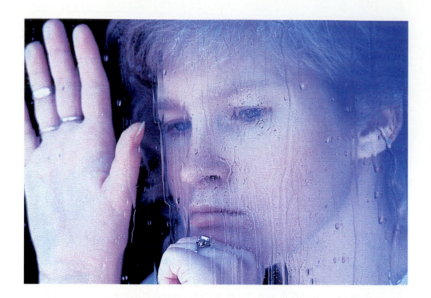

● **Figure 19.5 Devotion**

❝*Sarah, my love for you is deathless, it seems to bind me with mighty cables that nothing but Omnipotence can break, and yet my love of country comes over me like a strong wind and bears me irresistibly with all those chains to the battle field. The memories of all the blissful moments I have enjoyed with you come crowding over me, and I feel most deeply grateful to God and you that I have enjoyed them so long. And how hard it is for me to give them up and burn to ashes the hopes of future years when God willing we might still have lived and loved together and see our boys grow up to honourable manhood around us. I know I have but few claims upon Divine Providence but something whispers to me . . . that I shall return to my loved ones unharmed. If I do not my dear Sarah never forget how much I loved you nor that when my last breath escapes me on the battle field it will whisper your name.*❞

—Excerpt from a letter written during the Civil War by Sullivan Ballou, a Union Army major from Rhode Island, to his wife a week before he was killed at the first battle of Bull Run, July 21, 1861.

well in a career, they're going to have to invest time and money in education," says Olson. "But we don't assume that with marriage . . .. We shouldn't be surprised—if you don't invest anything, what can you expect?"[65]

Can science predict which marriages will survive and which will fall apart? One psychological study has found that the husband's disappointment with the marriage is the single most potent predictor of divorce, contrary to marital lore that the wife's feelings are the best indicator of the health of a marriage.[66] Frequent arguing is not a liability—provided it is outweighed by praise. *In couples that stay together, about five times more positive things are said to and about one another than negative ones.* In couples that divorce, there are about 1½ times more negative things said than positive ones. In addition, the couple's approach to problem solving—specifically whether or not the husband tended to withdraw from arguments—were more predictive of divorce. This corresponds with findings from another study which found that communication difficulties were the leading cause of divorce.[67]

Divorce When film star Elizabeth Taylor married construction worker Larry Fortensky in 1991, it was her eighth marriage and his third. Taylor had long since joined the club of 2 million American women ages 15–65 who have been married three or more times and 10 million who have been married twice (and 50 million once).[68] One divorce occurs for every two marriages in the United States, and—since some people don't remarry—at present 8% of Americans age 15 or over are divorced. (This compares with 7% who are widowed, 26% who haven't been married, and 59% who are married.)[69] Almost 80% of people who divorce will take a chance and marry again, usually within 3 years. Indeed, divorced people are more likely than singles to take the plunge, according to the National Center for Health Statistics.[70,71]

The mechanics of divorce have changed in recent years. No longer is it necessary to stage and photograph an act of "adultery," as used to be the case in New York, to prove grounds for divorce. Many states now have *no-fault divorce* laws, in which, instead of one party having to prove the other "at fault," it is assumed that no blame exists (or the blame is shared) and any alimony, spousal support, and child support are supposedly tailored by the court or by mutual agreement according to the particular circumstances.

Despite these attempts to bring some civility to the end of a marriage, for many people divorce is comparable to the loss one feels when a spouse dies. (*See ● Figure 19.6.*) "In both cases the person undergoes a grieving process," write sexuality authors Robert Crooks and Karla Baur. "There are important differences, however. When the grief is caused by death, there are rituals and social support available, which may be helpful to the survivor. In contrast, there are no recognized grief rituals to help the divorced person."[72]

Strategy for Living: The Importance of Communication Becoming one-half of a committed couple may be the end of a personal search of one kind, but it is the beginning of another kind. It has been said that no married couple alive has not thought about divorce. Probably no other kind of committed couple has never considered splitting up, for that matter. The number of subjects over which two people can disagree is limitless, but some principal ones that committed couples must adjust to are the following:[73]

- *Unrealistic expectations:* Dating and courtship involve pleasurable activities, but many people enter a committed relationship unprepared to deal with jobs, bills, housework, and so on. Confusion about domestic roles—who should do what chores, for example—may strain marital expectations.

- *Work and career issues:* Especially if both individuals work outside the home, there can be a great deal of work/family conflict, and adjustments may be necessary in spousal, parental, or domestic partnership roles.

- *Financial difficulties:* Having money does not ensure a couple's stability, but not having it can produce serious problems. Even when money is plentiful, however, there can be quarrels over how to spend it.

- *Problems with relatives:* Mobility may have made involvement with in-laws (or their equivalents in unmarried households) less of a problem, but they can still be a source of "interference."

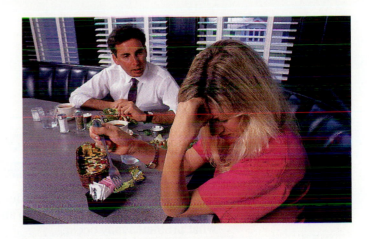

● **Figure 19.6 The pain of divorce**

“*Initially, a person may experience shock: 'This cannot be happening to me.' Disorganization may follow, a sense that one's entire world has turned upside down. Volatile emotions may unexpectedly surface. Feelings of guilt may become strong. Loneliness is common. Finally (usually not for several months or a year), a sense of relief and acceptance may come. . . . If after several months of separation a person is not developing a sense of acceptance, she or he may need professional help. Although many of the feelings triggered by divorce are uncomfortable, even painful, they can be steps toward resolving the loss so that a person can reestablish intimate relationships. Grieving can lead to healing.*”

—Robert Crooks & Karla Baur. (1990). *Our sexuality* (4th ed.). Redwood City, CA: Benjamin/Cummings, p. 522.

- *Sexual problems:* Sexual problems are often entwined with other cohabitation problems, but it's difficult to know which causes which. Inhibited sexual communication can be a source of great distress.

- *Jealousy:* It may be acceptable to imagine having a passionate love affair outside the committed relationship, but it is difficult to have an affair and have the at-home partnership remain the same. For many, infidelities are best left inside the mind—just as it is better to covet your neighbor's car than it is to steal it.

Most of the foregoing problems can be overcome with effective communication. Indeed, good communication—handling conflict, expressing wants and needs—is critical to a successful partnership. We discuss communication as a Life Skill at the end of the next chapter.

20 Your Sexuality

▶ Name the parts of the male reproductive system and describe what they do and what problems may occur.

▶ Name the parts of the female reproductive system and describe their function. Discuss the three phases of the fertility cycle and the role of relevant hormones. Discuss what problems can arise.

▶ Describe the difference between sex and gender and discuss the determinants of each.

▶ Discuss the types of sexual orientation.

▶ Describe the stages of human sexual response and different variations.

▶ Consider the different varieties of sexual expression and the concept of "normality."

▶ Name different types of sexual problems.

D o men and women have different feelings and fears? It might seem so: Men report fears of physical weakness, discomfort with any strong emotion except anger, powerful women, intellectual inferiority, and failure. Women report fears of being unattractive, victimized, and inadequate; of mismanaging a relationship; and of being estranged from close personal connections. At least these are the his-and-her concerns unearthed in research by Richard Eisler and others.[74,75]

Do these fears really only reflect **stereotypes,** oversimplified ideas and opinions about how men and women ought to be? Today the entire North American society is struggling to transcend the snips 'n' snails and sugar 'n' spice notions of masculinity and femininity—not only in childhood but also in the adult venues of workplace, bedroom, and nursery. Indeed, for many people the ideal of manhood or womanhood is not based on old notions of maleness and femaleness but on **androgyny,** a word meaning "having characteristics of both sexes." The ability of either sex to express both masculine and feminine traits can represent a profound liberation for both.

Because sexuality is such a private matter on the one hand and accorded such vast importance by the mass media (and the general public) on the other, it's sometimes difficult to sort out the facts from the myths about sex. Learning about basic reproductive anatomy, human sexual response, various sexual behaviors, and sexual problems helps you understand your own sexuality. It will also help you appreciate the complexity and influences of human sexuality in relationships with others. With this knowledge, we hope you will recognize sexuality as not only part of your own personality and basic to your well-being, but also learn to have a sense of caring and respect for the sexuality of others.

How much do you know about sex? Before proceeding you might wish to take the Self Discovery test about sex. (*See Self Discovery 20.1.*)

The Male Reproductive System

The visible, external parts of the male reproductive anatomy include the penis, which contains the urethra for carrying sperm and semen, and the scrotum, which covers the testes. Reproductive organs inside the body are the prostate gland, seminal vesicles, and Cowper's glands. In middle age, men may experience prostate enlargement and decline in production of the male sex hormone, testosterone.

Many notions about gender start with anatomy, most particularly sexual anatomy. We consider the reproductive systems for males first.

Male Reproductive Anatomy The male reproductive organs include two parts visible outside the body, the *penis* and the *scrotum*. The rest of the male reproductive system is inside the body. (*See* ● *Figure 20.1.*) Although many people think the word *genitalia* refers to the external organs, the term actually encompasses both internal and external reproductive structures. Let us consider these.

● *Outside and inside the penis:* The **penis,** the organ used for urinating and sex, aver-

SELF DISCOVERY 20.1

How Much Do You Know About Sex?

The Kinsey Institute/Roper Organization National Sex Knowledge Text

Circle one answer after reading each question carefully.

1. Nowadays, what do you think is the age at which the *average* or *typical* American *first* has sexual intercourse?

   a. 11 or younger   c. 13   e. 15   g. 17   i. 19   k. 21 or older
   b. 12   d. 14   f. 16   h. 18   j. 20   l. Don't know

2. Out of every 10 married American men, how many would you estimate have had an extramarital affair—that is, have been sexually unfaithful to their wives?

   a. Less than 1 out of 10   d. 3 out of 10 (30%)   g. 6 out of 10 (60%)   j. 9 out of 10 (90%)
   b. 1 out of 10 (10%)   e. 4 out of 10 (40%)   h. 7 out of 10 (70%)   k. More than 9 out of 10
   c. 2 out of 10 (20%)   f. 5 out of 10 (50%)   i. 8 out of 10 (80%)   l. Don't know

3. Out of every 10 American women, how many would you estimate have had anal (rectal) intercourse?

   a. Less than 1 out of 10   d. 3 out of 10 (30%)   g. 6 out of 10 (60%)   j. 9 out of 10 (90%)
   b. 1 out of 10 (10%)   e. 4 out of 10 (40%)   h. 7 out of 10 (70%)   k. More than 9 out of 10
   c. 2 out of 10 (20%)   f. 5 out of 10 (50%)   i. 8 out of 10 (80%)   l. Don't know

4. A person can get AIDS by having anal (rectal) intercourse even if neither partner is infected with the virus that causes AIDS.
   True   False   Don't know

5. There are over-the-counter spermicides people can buy at the drugstore that will kill the virus that causes AIDS.
   True   False   Don't know

6. Petroleum jelly, Vaseline Intensive Care, baby oil, and Nivea are *not* good lubricants to use with a condom or a diaphragm.
   True   False   Don't know

7. More than 1 out of 4 (25 percent) of American men have had a sexual experience with another male during either their teens or adult years.
   True   False   Don't know

8. It is usually difficult to tell whether people *are* or *are not* homosexual just by their appearance or gestures.
   True   False   Don't know

9. A woman or teenage girl can get pregnant during her menstrual flow (her period).
   True   False   Don't know

10. A woman or teenage girl can get pregnant even if the man withdraws his penis before he ejaculates.
    True   False   Don't know

11. Unless they are having sex, women do not need to have regular gynecological examinations.
    True   False   Don't know

12. Teenage boys should examine their testicles regularly just as women self-examine their breasts for lumps.
    True   False   Don't know

13. Problems with erection are most often started by a physical problem.
    True   False   Don't know

14. Almost all erection problems can be successfully treated.
    True   False   Don't know

15. Menopause, or change of life as it is often called, does *not* cause most women to lose interest in having sex.
    True   False   Don't know

16. Out of every 10 American women, how many would you estimate have masturbated either as children or after they were grown up?

    a. Less than 1 out of 10   d. 3 out of 10 (30%)   g. 6 out of 10 (60%)   j. 9 out of 10 (90%)
    b. 1 out of 10 (10%)   e. 4 out of 10 (40%)   h. 7 out of 10 (70%)   k. More than 9 out of 10
    c. 2 out of 10 (20%)   f. 5 out of 10 (50%)   i. 8 out of 10 (80%)   l. Don't know

17. What do you think is the length of the average man's *erect* penis?

    a. 2 inches   d. 5 inches   g. 8 inches   j. 11 inches
    b. 3 inches   e. 6 inches   h. 9 inches   k. 12 inches
    c. 4 inches   f. 7 inches   i. 10 inches   l. Don't know

18. Most women prefer a sexual partner with a larger-than-average penis.
    True   False   Don't know

(continued)

SELF DISCOVERY 20.1
(*continued*)

Scoring the Test

Each question is worth 1 point, so the total possible number of points you can get is 18. Using this chart, score each item and then add up your total number of points. When a range of possible answers is correct, according to currently available research data, all respondents choosing one of the answers in the correct range are given a point.

Question Number	Give yourself a point if you circled any of the following answers	Circle the number of points you received
1	f,g	0 1
2	d,e	0 1
3	d,e	0 1
4	False	0 1
5	(any answer; everyone gets a point)	1
6	True	0 1
7	True	0 1
8	True	0 1
9	True	0 1
10	True	0 1
11	False	0 1
12	True	0 1
13	True	0 1
14	True	0 1
15	True	0 1
16	g,h,l	0 1
17	d,e,f	0 1
18	False	0 1

Total Number of Points: _____

Now look up the grade you received:

If you got this number of points	You receive this grade
16–18	A
14–15	B
12–13	C
10–11	D
1–9	F

Compare yourself to other Americans: America's report card

Grade	Number of correct answers required to receive this grade	Number of participants receiving this grade	Percent of participants receiving this grade
A	16–18	5	<1
B	14–15	68	4
C	12–13	239	14
D	10–11	463	27
F	1–9	936	55

Note: Of the 1974 survey participants, 263 (13%) completed 10 or fewer of the 18 test items and were not included in the computation of these overall test scores. However, all those answering a question were included in the item-by-item analyses.

Source: Adapted from Reinisch, J., & Beasley, B. (1990). *The Kinsey Institute new report on sex.* New York: St. Martin's Press.

ages about 3¾ inches long when nonerect (a state described as *flaccid*) and *averages* 6¼ inches when erect (5–7 inches for 90% of men). An erection occurs when the penis becomes engorged with blood during sexual arousal. Penis length is a serious concern and sometimes an obsession with many men, but there is no relationship between the size of a man's penis and women's sexual satisfaction.

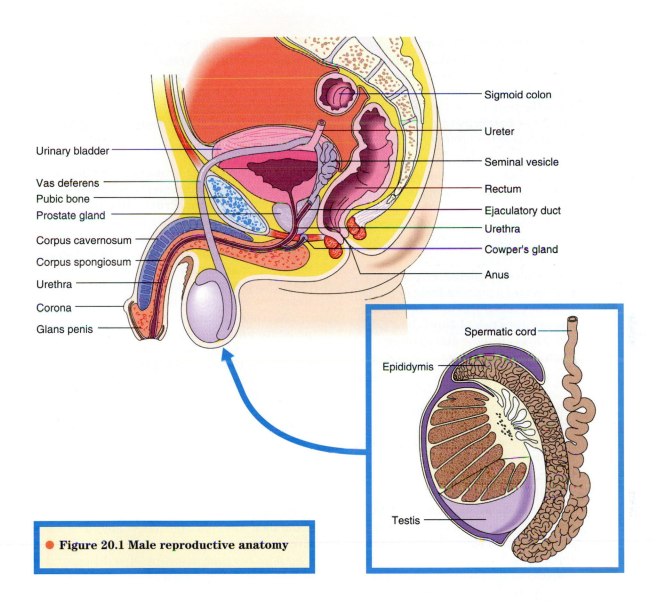

Urinary bladder

Vas deferens
Pubic bone
Prostate gland

Corpus cavernosum
Corpus spongiosum
Urethra
Corona
Glans penis

Sigmoid colon

Ureter

Seminal vesicle

Rectum
Ejaculatory duct
Urethra
Cowper's gland

Anus

Spermatic cord

Epididymis

Testis

● **Figure 20.1 Male reproductive anatomy**

At the head of the penis is the **glans,** a particularly sensitive part. (*Refer back to Figure 20.1.*) On newborns, the skin of the shaft of the penis extends past the glans, forming the **foreskin. In** the United States, about three out of five infant boys currently undergo **circumcision,** the surgical removal of the foreskin, either for religious or perceived health reasons. Scientists still debate whether circumcision truly yields health benefits (as we describe in a later chapter).

Inside the penis is the **urethra,** the main canal through which urine and semen

pass, although not at the same time. **Semen** is the whitish ejaculatory fluid that carries **sperm,** the male reproductive cells.

• *Inside the scrotum:* The **scrotum,** which contains the testicles, is the external pouch that hangs behind and below the penis. (*Refer back to Figure 20.1.*) The pair of **testicles,** also called **testes,** have two functions: (1) to produce sperm and (2) to produce about 95% of **testosterone,** the male sex hormone that stimulates male secondary sex characteristics such as facial hair. (The adrenal glands on top of the kidneys produce 5% of testosterone.)

Also within the scrotum are coiled tubes called the **epididymis,** in which sperm mature and are stored. The epididymis is a comma-shaped structure attached to the testicle. Two 18-inch tubes called the **vas deferens** carry sperm from the epididymis to the urethra.

- *Inside the body: Sperm* are produced by the testicles, but *semen*—the whitish fluid that carries sperm and that appears during ejaculation—is produced by three glands: the seminal vesicles, the prostate gland, and the Cowper's glands. (*Refer back to Figure 20.1.*)

  (1) The **seminal vesicles** are two glands that secrete a nutrient for sperm. The seminal vesicles join with the vas deferens to form a pair of 1-inch-long passageways called the **ejaculatory ducts,** which empty into the urethra.

  (2) The **prostate gland** is a gland located beneath the bladder and surrounding the urethra. Secretions from the prostate gland increase sperm motility and make the semen more alkaline and thus more life-sustaining for sperm.

  (3) The **Cowper's glands** secrete a fluid that alkalinizes the normally acid environment of the urethra prior to ejaculation and is sometimes called pre-ejaculatory fluid. This fluid often appears during sexual arousal as clear droplets on the tip of the penis. Since fluid from Cowper's glands may contain sperm, people who rely on the withdrawal method of contraception—in which the erect penis is withdrawn from the vagina immediately before ejaculation—may find themselves sorely disappointed in terms of pregnancy prevention. Withdrawal is not a reliable means of contraception.

The male reproductive system coexists with the system of elimination (bladder, rectum, anus) but does not intermingle with it. For instance, during sexual arousal, a sphincter (muscle) at the base of the bladder closes and thus prevents semen from getting into the bladder and urine from getting into the urethra.

Ejaculation is the emission of semen through the urethra to the outside. The experience of **orgasm** that usually accompanies ejaculation is the highly pleasurable feeling experienced at the height of sexual arousal, accompanied by a series of contractions of the pelvic muscles.

Prostate and Other Problems Like anything that is complex, the male reproductive system can develop problems. **Prostatitis,** which can occur in men of all ages, is an inflammation of the prostate, usually resulting from a bacterial or viral infection. Its symptoms include pain in the pelvic area, urinary complications, and backache. Depending on the cause, medical treatment using antibiotics is often required.

Another important prostate problem is **prostate enlargement** (also called *benign prostatic hypertrophy,* or *BPH*), which happens to most men at some point after age 40. Ever wonder why many older men often need to get up in the night to go to the bathroom? The reason is that the prostate enlarges and presses on the urethra. Symptoms of benign prostatic hypertrophy include a change in size and force of the urinary stream and a sensation of incomplete emptying. The problem may require surgery.[76,77] Indeed, the average 40-year-old American male has a 30–40% chance of undergoing such surgery (a prostatectomy) if he survives to age 80.[78]

Older men may also develop tumors, benign or malignant, of the prostate, one reason why all men over 40 should have yearly prostate evaluations. Surgical removal of the prostate or hormone treatment may be required.

The production of the male sex hormone declines after age 40, but this need not mean diminishing of sexual pleasure. However, older men may take longer to become sexually aroused, to achieve an erection, to have an ejaculation, and to resume intercourse.

The Female Reproductive System

Much of the female reproductive anatomy is inside the body. Externally, the vulva includes the labia, clitoris, and vaginal and urethral openings. Inside organs include

the vagina, cervix, uterus or womb, fallopian tubes, and ovaries. A woman's menstrual cycle has three phases. Menstrual problems may include menstrual cramps, premenstrual syndrome, and amenorrhea. In midlife, a woman's fertility cycle ends, an event called menopause.

Human males produce sperm continuously from puberty on. The reproductive capacity of human females, however, is cyclical and intermittent.

Female Reproductive Anatomy In the following paragraphs, we describe first those parts of the female reproductive anatomy that are on the outside, then those on the inside. (*See* ● *Figure 20.2.*)

- *The outside anatomy—from mons pubis to perineum:* The external organs of the female reproductive system are called the **vulva.** The vulva includes the *mons pubis,* the *labia majora,* the *labia minora,* the *clitoris,* the *urethral opening,* and the *vaginal opening.* We will also describe the *perineum.* (*Refer back to Figure 20.2.*)

(1) The **mons pubis** is the mound of fatty tissue over the pubic bone. In puberty it becomes covered with pubic hair.

(2) Beneath the mons pubis and covering the opening to the vagina and urethra are the vulva's outer and inner lips. The outer lips, the fleshy outer folds bordering the genital area, are called the **labia majora.** (The word *labia* means "lips.")

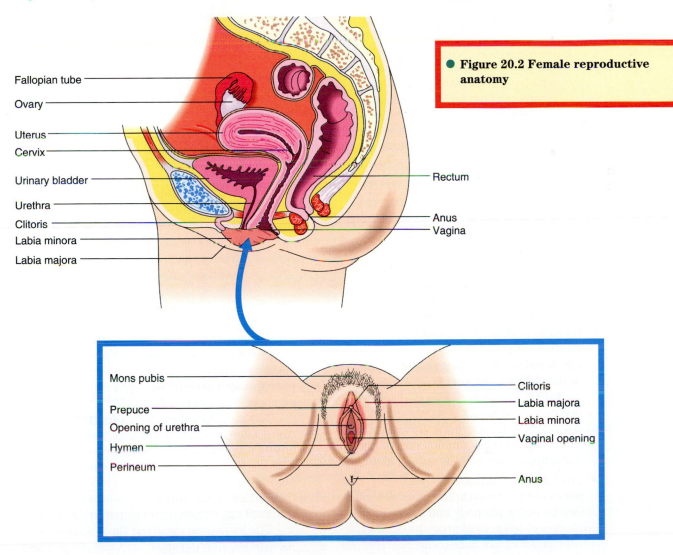

● **Figure 20.2 Female reproductive anatomy**

Fallopian tube
Ovary
Uterus
Cervix
Urinary bladder
Urethra
Clitoris
Labia minora
Labia majora

Rectum
Anus
Vagina

Mons pubis
Prepuce
Opening of urethra
Hymen
Perineum

Clitoris
Labia majora
Labia minora
Vaginal opening
Anus

(3) The **labia minora** come together to form the hood that covers the clitoris. These labia surround and protect the urethral and vaginal openings, and they surround and protect the clitoris and vaginal opening.

(4) The **clitoris,** protected at the top by a hood formed by the joining of the inner lips, is the most sexually sensitive portion of the external female genitals. For some women, it is extremely tender to the direct touch and is the source of much of a woman's sexual excitement.

(5) The tube through which urine is expelled from the bladder, the **urethra,** also has an opening in the vulva. Women's urinary and reproductive organs are separate systems.

(6) Beneath the urethra is a larger opening, the vaginal opening. The vaginal opening *may* be protected by a thin fold of mucous membrane called the **hymen,** which partly or (rarely) completely covers the opening. It was once thought that a broken hymen indicated a woman was no longer a **virgin** —had not had sex—but this is a myth. An intact hymen usually has openings through which vaginal secretions are discharged.

(7) The **perineum** is the name given to the area of skin between the vagina and the anus, the opening of the rectum.

- *The inside, accessible anatomy—from vagina to cervix:* Beyond the vaginal opening is the **vagina.** The vagina is an elastic muscular tube through which sperm must travel to fertilize an egg and through which a baby passes into the world (unless the infant is delivered by surgery). At the far end of the vagina is the **cervix,** the opening to the uterus. (*Refer to Figure 20.2.*) The opening of the cervix is tightly closed, but when a baby is being born, the cervix must dilate (open) considerably—a process that accounts for much of the pain of childbirth.

- *The inside, inaccessible anatomy—from uterus to ovaries:* On the other side of the cervix, inside the body and inaccessible to all except by medical procedures, are the *uterus, fallopian tubes,* and *ovaries.* (*Refer back to Figure 20.2.*)

(1) The **uterus,** or **womb,** is the pear-shaped and pear-sized muscle whose primary purpose is to contain and nurture a fetus until it is born. The internal lining of the uterus is called the **endometrium.** It is the endometrium in which the human embryo implants itself and develops. In adult women, the endometrium changes during the menstrual cycle and is shed during menstruation.

(2) Extending from the upper uterus is a pair of 4-inch-long **fallopian tubes.** These are the canals through which the eggs (ova) pass from the ovaries to the uterus. It is in the fallopian tubes that fertilization takes place.

(3) Near the end of each fallopian tube is an **ovary.** The **ovaries,** analogous to the testes in the male, are the pair of female reproductive glands that contain the eggs, called **ova.** Women do not produce eggs; they are born with all the eggs they will ever have. Generally, one ovary releases one egg, or **ovum,** one month, and the other ovary releases the other egg the following month. The egg moves down the fallopian tube into the uterus.

The ovaries also produce female sex hormones, estrogen and progesterone, which are important in the development of secondary sex characteristics (such as breasts) and in the menstrual cycle.

The Menstrual Cycle Understanding the menstrual cycle provides insight into conception, pregnancy, menopause, contraception, and other vital aspects of a woman's health. The cycle begins about age 12–14—the first menstruation is called **menarche**—and continues until menopause, around ages 45–55.

The **menstrual cycle** is a **fertility cycle.** About once a month, a woman's body matures an egg (ovum) to be available for fertilization by a male's sperm and also prepares the lining of her uterus for implantation, or embedding, of that fertilized egg. It is in the uterus that the fertilized egg begins to develop into the fetus.

The menstrual cycle has three phases— *menstrual, proliferative,* and *secretory.* These take place over *approximately* a 28-day period.

We say "approximately" because, although the *average* menstrual cycle is 28 days (from day 1 of one menstrual period to day 1 of the next menstrual period), normal cycles vary from 21 days to 34 days. Let us consider these three phases:

• *The menstrual phase:* The **menstrual phase** is the phase of **menstruation** or menstrual bleeding. (*See* ● *Figure 20.3, top.*) If a pregnancy does not occur, the endometrium—the lining of the uterus, composed of blood and tissue—is shed.

This shedding is what produces the bloody fluid, usually caught and disposed of using sanitary napkins, tampons, or other means. Because the muscle of the uterus contracts in order to expel this tissue, it

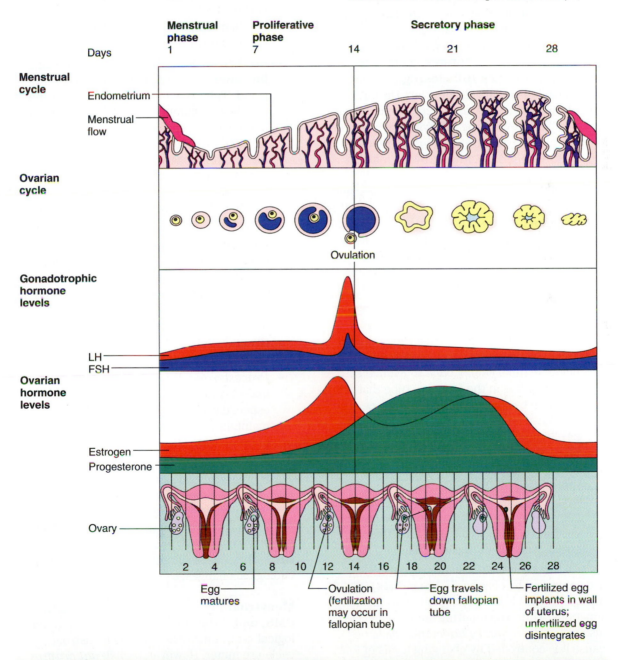

● **Figure 20.3 The menstrual cycle**

often produces the cramps that can cause women discomfort during this time.

- *The proliferative phase:* After menstruation and during the **proliferative phase,** a new endometrium develops into a thick spongy lining composed of blood and mucus. The purpose of the endometrium is to establish an environment conducive to the implantation and development of a fertilized egg. (*Refer back to Figure 20.3, top.*)

  During this time, an egg cell begins to mature in the ovary. (*Refer back to Figure 20.3, middle.*) The ovaries contain thousands of **ovarian follicles,** egg sacs in which individual eggs develop. During this phase of the cycle, about 20 ovarian follicles begin to grow. In the following days, *one* of the follicles, called the *graafian follicle,* matures fully; the other growing follicles degenerate.

  When the graafian follicle ruptures and releases a mature egg, the one-time event is called **ovulation.** The ruptured follicle left behind is called the *corpus luteum;* its purpose is to secrete progesterone, which helps maintain the endometrial lining for possible implantation of a fertilized egg.

- *The secretory phase:* During the **secretory phase,** which covers roughly the second half of the menstrual cycle, the released ovum enters and moves down the fallopian tube. (*Refer back to Figure 20.3, middle.*) It is in the fallopian tube that fertilization by the sperm may take place. The ovum can be fertilized during a period of 24–36 hours. If fertilization does not take place, the egg begins to disintegrate.

  Simultaneously, the endometrium continues its buildup, ready to receive a fertilized egg. At the end of the cycle, if the egg has not been fertilized, the uterine lining is shed during menstruation—and the menstrual cycle begins again at day 1.

All three phases of the menstrual cycle are controlled by changes in **hormones,** substances in the blood that regulate specific body functions. Thus, the monthly menstrual cycle is also called the *monthly hormonal cycle* because it is controlled by changing levels of four hormones throughout the 28 days: *FSH, LH, estrogen,* and *progesterone.*

- *FSH:* **FSH,** an abbreviation for **follicle-stimulating hormone,** is produced by the **pituitary gland,** a gland located within the brain which controls reproductive functions. In females, FSH stimulates the growth of ovarian follicles. Thus, FSH levels are elevated in the bloodstream during the second (proliferative) phase of the menstrual cycle. (*Refer back to Figure 20.3, bottom.*)

  In males, FSH stimulates the production of sperm.

- *LH:* **LH,** an abbreviation for **luteinizing hormone,** is also produced by the pituitary gland. The principal function of LH in the female is to stimulate ovulation, the maturing of ovarian egg cells. Thus, there is a surge of LH level in the bloodstream toward the end of the second (proliferative) phase of the menstrual cycle. (*Refer to Figure 20.3, bottom.*)

  In males, LH stimulates the production of testosterone.

- *Estrogen:* **Estrogen** is a female sex hormone secreted by the ovaries. Estrogen has many functions, including control of the menstrual cycle. An estrogen surge occurs toward the end of the second phase of the fertility cycle in order to start building up the endometrium. (*Refer back to Figure 20.3, bottom.*)

- *Progesterone:* **Progesterone** is another female sex hormone secreted by the ovaries, especially after ovulation. Its purpose is to maintain the endometrium in the event of pregnancy. (*Refer to Figure 20.3, bottom.*)

If pregnancy does not occur, blood levels of estrogen and progesterone drop, and the menstruation phase of the cycle begins.

Do these hormonal ups and downs affect how a woman feels? Indeed they do. In some cases, they cause significant physical and psychological changes, as we describe next.

Menstrual Problems: Menstrual Cramps, PMS, and Others Most physical and psychological symptoms related to the menstrual cycle are minor. However, *menstrual cramps premenstrual syndrome,* and *amenorrhea* are not.

- *Menstrual cramps:* **Dysmenorrhea,** or painful cramps during menstruation, is caused by excessive levels of *prostaglandins*. These hormones cause uterine muscles to contract. Dysmenorrhea affects about half of menstruating women and may entirely incapacitate 10–20% more for 1 or 2 days.[79]

  The condition may be relieved with over-the-counter medication and exercise.[80] Oral contraceptive use may reduce dysmenorrhea in some women.

- *Premenstrual syndrome:* **Premenstrual syndrome,** or **PMS,** occurs usually 7 or more days before the onset of the menstrual period and causes very severe physical and psychological distress in up to 15% of women.[81] The cause of PMS is not currently known. Some women experience extreme discomfort, including mood swings, irritability, hostility, muscle aches, pelvic cramps, breast tenderness, dizziness, bloating, and diarrhea. Other women are not so seriously affected.

  PMS relief may be obtained with medication, relaxation techniques, exercise, and eating a wholesome diet (one limited in salt, sugar, alcohol, and caffeine). However, no single remedy seems to work for all women.

- *Amenorrhea:* **Amenorrhea** is the absence of menstruation and, if continued for a long time, is associated with a bone-weakening disorder known as osteoporosis. The condition may be brought about as a result of strenuous exercise, extreme weight loss such as that occurring in the eating disorder anorexia nervosa, and changes in one's environment, but it may also be caused by hormonal changes or other problems.

Menopause: The End of Female Fertility

At some time usually between the ages of 45 and 55, a woman's cycles of ovulation and menstruation come to an end, an event called **menopause,** aptly described as "the change of life." The event is actually a process, foreshadowed by increasingly irregular periods, decreasing amounts of estrogen and progesterone, and the cessation of ovulation.

Some women experience problems linked to their declining hormones, especially estrogen: vaginal dryness that makes intercourse painful, surges of heat and perspiration that causes the physical reddening or flushes called "hot flashes," headaches, irritability, and depression. Many women, however, experience menopause as uneventful and view the years following menopause as among the best of their lives.

Sex and Gender: Your Sexuality and Sexual Orientation

The male or female sex is determined by biology—genetic instructions and sex hormones. Male and female gender identity and gender role are largely determined by social learning. Sexual orientation includes heterosexuality (attraction to other sex), homosexuality (to same sex), bisexuality (to both), and transsexuality (gender identity opposite of biological sex). Homosexual and bisexual orientations may have both social-learning and genetic bases.

Your maleness or femaleness begins with your biology and is shaped by your experience. That is, your **sex,** male or female, is determined by genetic and other biological factors. Your **gender** refers to how you perceive yourself as male or female and is determined by physiological, psychological, and sociological factors.

The Biological Bases of Sexuality Becoming a male or female depends on many factors, especially your chromosomes and hormones. We mentioned a number of hormones earlier, but the important ones that determine your sexual identity are three: *estrogen, progesterone,* and *testosterone*. Both sexes have these hormones, but what is important is that the *differences in their relative amounts significantly influence whether one grows up to be male or female*. Men have more testosterone than estrogen and progesterone, women more estrogen and progesterone than testosterone.

Immediately after conception, human embryos do not have **gonads**—testes or ovaries that indicate they are male or female. However, the embryos contain genetic instructions (in the form of X and Y chromosomes, as we describe in Chapter 24) that by the 7th week cause an embryo to begin to develop testes, if male, or by the 8th week ovaries, if female. The testes produce testosterone in males, creating the other male genitals. The absence of a Y chromosome or of testosterone leads to the formation of female genitals.

Years later, at **puberty,** the beginning of sexual maturity, the action of the sex hormones starts to be dramatized in the development of **secondary sex characteristics,** physical changes related to maleness and femaleness. Both boys and girls show rapid skeletal growth (as much as 6 inches in a year), produce pubic hair and underarm hair, and may experience hormonally influenced skin changes such as acne. Boys develop hair on their faces and bodies, their voices deepen, their muscles become stronger, their penises become longer. Girls develop wider hips, nipples enlarge and breasts fill out, external genitals become larger, and they begin to menstruate and later ovulate. Although humans are sexual beings throughout their lifespan, the sex hormones spur the **sex drive,** the desire to engage in sexual behavior, although the extent of the desire varies with individuals. Finally, at about age 18–21, as the bones stop growing, puberty comes to an end.

The Social-Learning Bases of Sexuality

Whatever the biological basis of your sexuality, the psychological and social influences on your sexuality are incredibly strong, perhaps beginning in the hospital bassinette with the pink card ("I'M A GIRL!") or blue card ("I'M A BOY!") on it.

Your **gender identity** refers to how you psychologically perceive yourself as either male or female. Children develop a strong sense of gender identity by 18 months.[82] **Gender role,** or sex role, is the collection of attitudes and behaviors considered appropriate within a given culture for people of a particular sex. Thus, for example, children in many parts of North America are raised to believe that it is not "masculine" for males to kiss each other on the cheek, although this is not the case in European cultures.[83] Similar social learning applies to the expression of aggression, which is not innately masculine behavior, and nurturing, which is not innately feminine behavior.

Once we become adolescents, gender roles are further reinforced as we worry about what others around us believe is acceptable or "normal" behavior. We then have to face pressures about looks, dating behavior, and how little or how much sexual activity we desire and are comfortable with.

People can and do express their sexuality in a variety of ways, many of which do not involve sexual intercourse. Perhaps the principal form of early sexual exploration is self-stimulation (masturbation), engaged in by two-thirds of females and nearly all males.[84]

Some people express themselves sexually by kissing, hand-holding, and touching genitals and other erotically sensitive areas but not sexual intercourse. Others, sometimes as a consequence of peer-group pressure, engage in sexual intercourse. According to the federal Centers for Disease Control and Prevention, 54% of teenagers surveyed in 1991 said they had had sexual intercourse, down from 59% in 1989. Thirty-five percent said they had had two or more sexual partners (versus 40% in 1989) and 19% reported four or more partners (down from 24% earlier).[85]

Even by young adulthood we may not be fully formed sexually, still trying to clarify the forms that sexual expression should take. Indeed, our sexuality and means of sexual expression may change throughout our lives and many people remain sexual beings in old age.

Sexual Orientation: Heterosexual, Homosexual, Bisexual, Transsexual

As we stated, your gender identity results from a combination of biological, social, and psychological factors. What is it, then, that draws us to one sex or the other—or maybe both? That is, what determines our **sexual orientation,** our attraction to a particular sex or both sexes?

Four sexual orientations have been described:

- *Heterosexual:* A person with a **heterosexual** orientation is sexually and emotionally attracted to members of the other sex. This is the orientation of the majority: 75% of men and 85% of women in the United States.[86]

- *Homosexual:* People with a **homosexual** orientation are sexually and emotionally attracted to members of the same sex. Many male homosexuals prefer the term **gay,** and many female homosexuals use the term **lesbian** to describe themselves (the term *gay* is sometimes used to refer to homosexual people of both sexes). About 2% of American men and 1% of American women have an exclusively homosexual orientation.[87]

- *Bisexual:* People who are sexually attracted to members of both sexes have a **bisexual** orientation. An estimated 23% of men and 14% of women in the United States have had bisexual experiences.[88]

  However, isolated sexual experiences —a few same-sex sexual experiences in adolescence, for example—are not a good indicator of true sexual orientation. What seems to count is *repeated* sexual and emotional attraction to members of either or both sexes during one's life.

- *Transsexual:* A small percentage of people are **transsexual.** That is, their gender identity, or feelings about whether they are male or female, is the opposite of their biological sex.[89] It is not clear what causes transsexualism.[90,91]

  Because psychotherapy has been generally unsuccessful in helping transsexuals adjust to their biological sex, sex-change operations that alter genitals and hormone injections that alter breasts and body hair are often performed after careful psychological assessment and preparation.[92,93]

Many of us are tempted to view our sexual orientation as solely heterosexual or homosexual. However, pioneer sex researcher Alfred Kinsey contended that sexual orientation is not an either/or phenomenon. Instead, he suggested, an individual's sexual orientation falls somewhere along a continuum. Kinsey developed a scale, or continuum, of sexual behavior, with 0 representing no homosexual desire or behavior and 6 representing no heterosexual desire or behavior.[94] Many people, he found, would find themselves somewhere in between. (*See* ● *Figure 20.4.*)

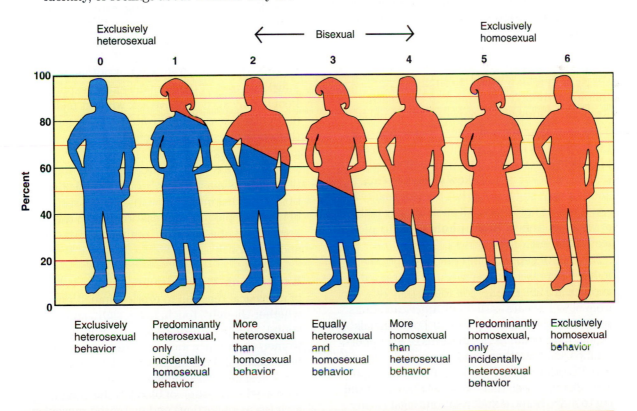

● **Figure 20.4 The continuum of sexual orientation**

Bisexuality, Homosexuality, and Homophobia Are homosexual and bisexual people "born that way" or is the behavior learned? There are numerous debates about this. In the animal kingdom, bisexual behavior is commonplace (for instance, among pygmy chimpanzees and dolphins), but the behavior may have less to do with sexual orientation than with animal power relationships and rituals. Among humans, bisexuality occurs among many male and female adolescents in many cultures. In some Latin and Muslim societies, it is reportedly a common but unspoken practice among men.[95] This seems to suggest a strong social-learning component.

Yet scientists have also discovered physiological differences between those who are homosexual and heterosexual, suggesting that homosexuality may be genetic.[96] For instance, one study of identical-twin brothers of homosexual men (the two have identical genes) found that a high percentage, 52%, were also homosexual, compared to only 22% among fraternal-twin brothers (who do not have identical genes).[97] Other studies have found anatomical differences between the brains of homosexual and heterosexual men, suggesting that homosexuality is at least partly inborn.[98,99]

Some psychiatrists still argue that homosexuality can be "cured" through psychotherapy, although the American Psychiatric Association long ago dropped homosexuality as a category of mental illness. Some religious groups have argued that homosexuality is simply a perverse choice. The "gay brains" research, however, could skew prejudices in another way, suggesting that homosexuality is some sort of deformity. All such antigay points of view may reflect **homophobia,** the irrational fear of homosexuality.

Public acceptance of homosexuality seems to have increased in one way and decreased in another. A 1992 Gallup poll found that 74% (up from 56% 15 years earlier) of American adults supported the general idea that homosexuals should have equal rights in terms of job opportunities. On the other hand, the poll also found that 57% think homosexuality is an unacceptable lifestyle. Less than half (48%) seemed willing to make homosexual relations legal (many states continue to carry laws making it a crime).[100] Still, the poll does suggest that the backlash toward gays seen in earlier polls seems to be subsiding.

The Human Sexual Response

The human sexual response may begin with desire and then proceed through four stages—excitement, plateau, orgasm, and resolution—with marked similarities and some differences between the sexes and among individuals, including the frequency of orgasm.

People have been having sex for thousands of years, but the *study* of sex was considered off-limits until the famous William Masters and Virginia Johnson began researching sex in their St. Louis laboratory in the 1950s. As a result of their investigations, they developed a four-phase model of how both men and women respond to sex physiologically: *excitement, plateau, orgasm, resolution.*[101]

This model is mainly concerned with genital or physiological changes. One thing missing from the Masters and Johnson model, as pointed out by sexuality writers Robert Crooks and Karla Baur, is a first phase suggested by sex therapist Helen Kaplan—*desire.*[102] We shall therefore add this to our discussion.

Desire Desire is a frequent but not necessarily inevitable part of the human sexual response. People may agree to have sex without feeling particularly sexually motivated at the time, although the desire may come about as they engage in the sexual activity.

Regardless of the source of erotic stimulation, such as masturbation, oral-genital stimulation, or sexual intercourse, the sexual response of most people more or less adheres to the following four-phase pattern outlined by Masters and Johnson.

Excitement The **excitement phase** consists of a physical reaction to erotic stimulation, whether thought, touch, taste, sight, and/or sound. (*See ● Figure 20.5, top.*) Both men and women experience increased respiration and heart rates and the nipples may become erect. Their responses are similar as they experience increased congestion of blood in the genital area (vasocongestion) and increased muscular tension (myotonia).

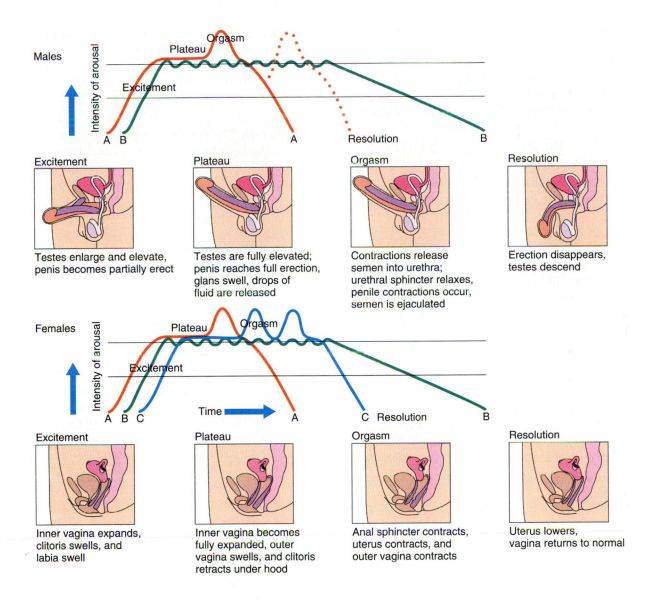

Males

Intensity of arousal

Orgasm
Plateau
Excitement
A B
A
Resolution
B

Excitement
Testes enlarge and elevate, penis becomes partially erect

Plateau
Testes are fully elevated; penis reaches full erection, glans swell, drops of fluid are released

Orgasm
Contractions release semen into urethra; urethral sphincter relaxes, penile contractions occur, semen is ejaculated

Resolution
Erection disappears, testes descend

Females

Intensity of arousal

Plateau
Orgasm
Excitement
A B C
Time
A
C Resolution
B

Excitement
Inner vagina expands, clitoris swells, and labia swell

Plateau
Inner vagina becomes fully expanded, outer vagina swells, and clitoris retracts under hood

Orgasm
Anal sphincter contracts, uterus contracts, and outer vagina contracts

Resolution
Uterus lowers, vagina returns to normal

● **Figure 20.5 Human sexual response.** The four phases as described by sex researchers Masters and Johnson. The letters indicate different basic patterns of sexual response.

- *Men:* The penis becomes erect, although the erection may subside and return several times. The testes lift and increase in size. A man's initial physical response to sexual arousal is erection.

- *Women:* The clitoris swells, as do the labia minor; the labia majora flatten and separate away from the vaginal opening. The vaginal walls begin to lubricate. The uterus enlarges. A woman's initial physical response to sexual arousal is believed to be vaginal lubrication.

Plateau During the **plateau phase,** sexual excitement and muscle tension continue to build, blood pressure and heart rate continue to rise, and breathing becomes faster. (*Refer back to Figure 20.5, middle.*) (The word *plateau* does not mean it is an unchanging state, only that no *new* behaviors can be observed.)

- *Men:* The penis becomes fully erect and testes continue to swell and elevate.
- *Women:* The clitoris retracts under its hood. The inner two-thirds of the vagina enlarges and the muscles in the outer third of the vagina tighten.

Orgasm The third phase observed by Masters and Johnson, the **orgasmic phase,** is the most ecstatic for those who experience it. (*Refer back to Figure 20.5, bottom.*) Here, rhythmic contractions cause the release of neuromuscular tension and feelings of intense pleasure—that is, an orgasm (also known as a "climax" or "coming"). Blood pressure, heart rate, and breathing reach their highest levels and there are involuntary muscle spasms throughout the body. All this lasts only a few seconds. The intensity of the orgasm seems to vary with experience, setting, partner, expectations, and level of anxiety.

- *Men:* Males ejaculate in two stages. First, the prostate, the seminal vesicles, and the vas deferens release semen into the urethra. It is during this time they may feel a sense of orgasmic inevitability. A few seconds later, the semen is ejaculated out of the urethra and out of the penis, accompanied by contractions of the urethra and anus. The first two or three contractions are most intense.
- *Women:* Contractions occur in the uterus, the vaginal opening, and anal areas. Masters and Johnson identified three patterns: (1) one or more orgasms without dropping below the plateau level; (2) extended plateau with no orgasms; and (3) a rapid rise to orgasm with no plateau.[103]

Some research suggests the presence of a G-spot (Grafenberg spot) that, when stimulated, results in orgasm. It is possible that some females ejaculate fluid (not urine) from their urethras during orgasm. This orgasm, which is very intense, follows stimulation of an area, the G-spot, located in the ceiling and toward the front of their vaginas. The G-spot is not noticeable until it is stimulated, when it may swell to the size of a dime or quarter.

Resolution The **resolution phase** is the return of the body to its unaroused state. Heart rate, blood pressure, breathing, muscle tension, and nipple erection all subside.

- *Men:* The penis returns to its nonerect or nonaroused state. The testes return to normal. Most men are unable to resume erection and ejaculation for a period of time that may range from seconds to hours. With age, the recovery period is considerably longer, up to several hours.
- *Women:* The clitoris, uterus, vagina, and vaginal lips return to their normal unaroused positions.

The Varieties of Orgasm We owe much to Masters and Johnson in getting beyond many of the mysteries of sex. For example, they found that most men, except for some in late adolescence, are not able to be **multiorgasmic**—that is, able to have multiple orgasms within a single period of sexual arousal. However, 10–30% of adult females are routinely able to have multiple orgasms. On the other hand, they found, some 10% of females are **anorgasmic,** unable to have an orgasm. Or they can experience orgasms during masturbation but not during conventional sexual intercourse.[104]

The Varieties of Sexual Expression: "Am I Normal?"

Sexual expression takes many forms and covers a wide range: sexual fantasies and dreams, masturbation, caressing and genital play, oral-genital stimulation, anal stimulation, and sexual intercourse or coitus in different positions. Some people are celibate—they don't have sex. Others indulge in pornography and prostitution, aspects of "commercial sex." Some forms of sexuality, ranging from voyeurism to sadomasochism to bestiality, are considered inappropriate.

Sexual intercourse occurs more than 100 million times around the world *every day,* according to the World Health Organization.[105] For all its frequency, however, sex remains basically a private matter. As one sex therapist notes, "We don't observe others having sex, don't hear anyone discussing sexual experiences seriously, and don't have access to reliable information about what other people feel and do."[106] The result, he says, is that many people have *normality anxiety:* they wonder if what they are thinking or feeling or doing about sex is normal. Basically what is "normal" is what any adult finds pleasurable as long as the experience is engaged in willingly, under noncoercive, nonmanipulated circumstances and places neither oneself nor one's partner (if a partner is involved) at risk for negative physical, emotional, or social consequences.

Sexual Fantasies and Dreams Many questions about normality have to do with fantasies. Sex is not just genitals and glands; a great part of it is the mind. For instance, a 24-year-old woman who had never had intercourse, interviewed by Nancy Friday, stated, "I am an extremely sexual person. I think about sex a lot and can become horny if just the right word, sound, or suggestion is made."[107]

A **sexual fantasy** is any mental representation of any kind of sexual activity.[108] It may be a single act, such as oral sex, or it may be like a movie, telling a story from beginning to end (for example, starting with a kiss and ending with orgasm). The fantasy may be stimulated by experience, imagination, through words or pictures, whether an underwear ad or an erotic video. A *sexual dream* occurs without a person's conscious control during sleep and may produce a **nocturnal orgasm,** an involuntary orgasm during sleep. In males, this is also called a "wet dream," because ejaculation occurs.

Perhaps the principal purpose of sexual fantasies, when they occur during masturbation or sexual intercourse, is to facilitate sexual arousal. Both men and women report that it is common to fantasize about one person—a former or an imaginary lover—while making love to another.[109] Sexual fantasies also allow one to overcome anxiety or boredom, rehearse new sexual experiences, and express forbidden wishes (such as forced or same-sex encounters).[110]

How "normal" is sexual fantasizing? Research by Alfred Kinsey and his associates found that nearly all the males and two-thirds of the females studied reported having sexual dreams and 84% of males and 67% of females reported having sexual fantasies.[111,112] People who feel more guilt about sex are less apt to be aroused by sexual fantasies than are people who feel less guilt about sex.[113]

Masturbation **Masturbation** is self-stimulation of the genitals for sexual pleasure, as with one's hand or with a vibrator, resulting in orgasm. Men often masturbate by gripping the penis and using an up-and-down movement to stimulate the shaft and the glans, speeding up the movement as orgasm nears. Women generally stimulate the clitoris or the area around it, caressing up and down beside the clitoral shaft or using a circular movement around or over it.

Do people in committed relationships or those with regular sexual partners masturbate? The answer seems to be yes. One study found that, among husbands and wives in their 20s and 30s, 72% of the males reported masturbating twice a month and 68% of the females once a month.[114] The practice is not considered abnormal unless it somehow interferes with one's life or with enjoyable sexual sharing in a relationship.[115] As might be expected, single and divorced people masturbate more often than people who are married or living together.[116]

There are a variety of reasons for masturbating: pleasure, relief from sexual tension, self-exploration, relaxation, even to induce sleep.[117] Crooks and Baur state that many people who masturbate "view the behavior with a mix of pleasure and a socialized sense of uneasiness or guilt." Indeed, they point out, a common concern of some writings is about "masturbating to excess," although "excess" is seldom defined. In general, they suggest, such self-pleasuring should not be viewed as a problem.[118]

Is masturbation normal? One study of young people ages 15–18 found that 80% of males and 59% of females masturbated.[119] The Kinsey studies in the 1950s found that males ages 16–20 masturbated an average of 57 times a year, males 21–25 an average of 42 times a year, and females ages 18–24 an average of 21 times a year.[120] However, men masturbate less as they approach age 30, whereas women masturbate more in their 20s and 30s.

Kissing, Caressing, Genital Play—and the Importance of Setting Kissing and touching need not, of course, be preliminary steps toward sexual arousal or intercourse. When they are, however, they are considered part of **foreplay,** or sex play, the kind of stimulating activity (sometimes including oral-genital sex) that leads to sexual intercourse. Touching sexually sensitive, or **erogenous,** areas—genitals, breasts, the anal areas in some people (but not others)—can build sexual excitement and even orgasm.

Kissing may be the tongue-thrusting, deep-in-the-mouth sort known as "French kissing," or it may be kissing of any other part of the body, from earlobes to the soles of the feet and everywhere in between. Caressing may begin with gentle, slow stroking anywhere on the body, then become more specific and excited. Likewise, genital play may begin with gentle stroking or kissing near the genitals, proceed to light, slow caressing of the penis and scrotum or of the clitoris or vaginal opening, then move on to more intensified stroking or kissing.

Setting is important for lovemaking. The mood for sex may be expressed to the prospective partner through clothing, music, a candlelit dinner, or by taking an evening bath or shower. Being clean and pleasant-smelling, in fact, may be vital, though heavy doses of cologne, perfume, and douches—cosmetics-industry advertising to the contrary—may actually work against sexual arousal.

Oral-Genital Stimulation **Oral-genital stimulation** consists of mouth-to-genital contact for the purpose of stimulating sexual pleasure. The three forms are:

- *Fellatio:* **Fellatio** is oral stimulation of the penis (and perhaps the scrotum) by the partner, usually by licking or sucking the glans and shaft of the penis. Most men find fellatio highly pleasurable. Partners differ in whether they want to stimulate the male to ejaculation or allow the male to ejaculate in the mouth, so this should not be done if it causes the partner discomfort.

  In addition, because fellatio risks the exchange of bodily fluids, and hence the passage of sexually transmitted diseases (including HIV) through small openings in the skin of the mouth or genitals, couples

not in a long-term mutually monogamous relationship should either avoid this practice or always use a condom.

- *Cunnilingus:* **Cunnilingus** is oral stimulation of the clitoris, labia, and vaginal opening by licking or penetration by the partner's tongue. Many women find the sensation highly pleasurable because the tongue is moist and gentle. Also, cunnilingus offers less roughness or discomfort than is sometimes experienced when the clitoris is stimulated by hand.[121]

  To avoid the risk of sexually transmitted diseases, couples not in mutually monogamous relationships should avoid practicing cunnilingus, or the woman receiving oral sex should cover her vulva with a latex square known as a *dental dam,* available in pharmacies and some dentists' offices.

- *Mutual oral-genital stimulation:* Couples sometimes practice simultaneous oral-genital stimulation by facing each other while lying in opposite directions (one atop the other or the two side by side), an arrangement known as the "69 position" because the numerals somewhat resemble the position of the two heads and bodies.

Couples sometimes begin their sex play with oral-genital stimulation and then when aroused proceed to sexual intercourse. Some people have reservations about this practice, considering it immoral, illegal (and it is in some states), or unsanitary because it is associated with organs that are close to the anus. Certainly washing the genital area would seem to be a basic prerequisite.

How commonplace is oral-genital sex? One 1974 study found that 90% of married couples under 25 years old had experienced it within the year.[122] A 1983 study of 203 Canadian college women found that 61% had performed fellatio and 68% had experienced cunnilingus.[123]

Anal Stimulation Some people don't care to do anything sexual with the anus, associating it with matters of excretion or "unnatural" acts. Others find touching of the anus to be highly erotic sex play. **Anal intercourse** consists of inserting the penis into the anus and is a sexual behavior engaged in by people regardless of sexual orientation.

Anal sex is one of the riskiest activities for transmission of sexual diseases, including HIV, the AIDS virus, because the lining of the rectum tears easily during penetration. Although use of a condom would seem to be mandatory for all but the most monogamous of sexual partners, whether homosexual or heterosexual, one should be aware that condoms have a higher breakage rate (1 in 105) for anal sex than for vaginal sex (1 in 165).[124]

Anal intercourse can be uncomfortable or painful for the recipient. Thus, the anus and penis (or other object) should first be well lubricated before insertion, and penetration should be done slowly and gently. Under no circumstances should anything inserted into the anus then be inserted into the vagina without thorough washing, or infection is apt to occur.

How frequently does anal intercourse occur among heterosexual partners? One survey found that 25% of married couples under age 35 said they performed it occasionally.[125]

Sexual Intercourse or Coitus The terms **sexual intercourse** and **coitus** usually mean penetration of the vagina by the penis. (*See* ● *Figure 20.6.*) This is the only sexual act designed for **procreation** or reproduction. It may or may not produce orgasm in one or both partners. Indeed, many females have difficulty experiencing a vaginal orgasm in coital positions

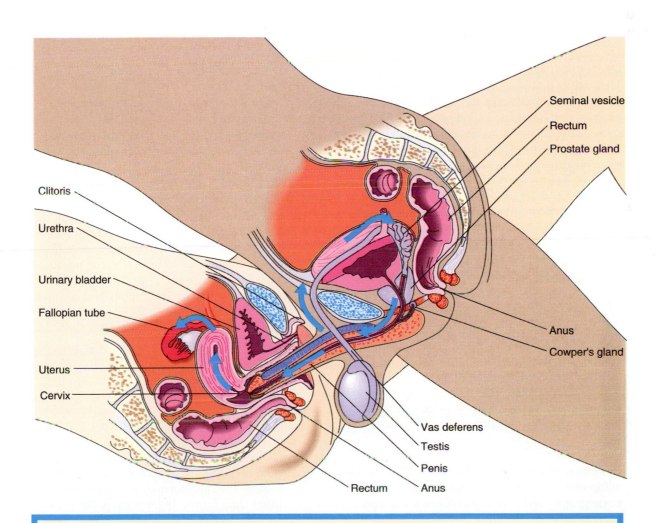

Clitoris
Urethra
Urinary bladder
Fallopian tube
Uterus
Cervix
Rectum
Vas deferens
Testis
Penis
Anus
Seminal vesicle
Rectum
Prostate gland
Anus
Cowper's gland

● **Figure 20.6 Sexual intercourse**

in which the clitoris is not readily stimulated. In coitus, men often appreciate the woman's using her hand or body to help guide the penis into the vagina (or to reinsert it).

What is the normal frequency of sexual intercourse? The answer is: there is no normal frequency, and this is not an area you need to feel concerned about (unless you're having problems with a partner). Kinsey found in the 1940s that 20-year-old husbands averaged 4 acts of sexual intercourse a week and 60-year-old husbands once a week—but some 20-year-olds had intercourse less than once a week and some 60-year-olds 10 or more times a week.[126] A 1974 study found that couples in their 20s and 30s have sex an *average* of 2–3 times a week.[127] However, the frequency among married couples tends to decrease as the relationship goes on, owing to the fatiguing demands of work and child-rearing as well as declining interest due to a familiar sexual routine.[128,129] A 1990 study by the National Opinion Research Center at the University of Chicago found that married and unmarried adults reported 57.4 instances of sexual intercourse in the preceding year—just a little more than once a week.[130] In sum: a wide range of frequency of intercourse is considered normal.

Celibacy **Celibacy** may either be complete— a person has no sex at all—or partial, meaning that he or she masturbates but has no sexual relations with others. Being celibate is not always a matter of religion or lack of sexual partners. Some people choose to "renew their virginity" because of concern about sexually transmitted diseases, because they want to avoid emotional upset while recovering from a broken relationship, or because of a health problem, including chemical dependency. How common is celibacy? A 1990 survey found that 22% of people—including 9% of married people—said they had no sex partners at all during the previous year.[131]

Pornography and Prostitution Is there a developed country in the world that *does not* have pornography and prostitution? Are these two aspects of "commercial sex"—which includes everything from phone sex (dial-a-porn) to child prostitution—simply part of the human condition? Paying for sex—or for sexual fantasies—seems to be as old as history. In the late 20th century, however, sex has also been exploited commercially in advertising to sell products and in movies to sell theater seats. In other words, sex has shifted from the private world to the public world: it has become popularized.[132] (*See ● Figure 20.7.*)

Here, however, let us consider just two aspects of commercialized sex—pornography and prostitution:

- *Pornography:* **Pornography** is depiction through words or pictures of sexual conduct involving same-sex or opposite-sex partners designed to cause sexual excitement. Most purchasers of pornography use it as a stimulus for masturbation. By identifying with the people in pornographic fantasies, it is suggested, some people may be able to deny their fears about sexual inadequacy, sexual fatigue, or failing sexual interest.[133]

Some pornography is simply explicit portrayal of sexual acts such as we have described so far, and some couples use it as an adjunct or stimulus for lovemaking. Some, however, is more violent, involving acts of rape, humiliation, degradation, and pain against women and men. Should pornography be allowed as free speech or censored as "an act of violence against women"? Censorship campaigns always blame unwanted speech for unwanted behavior; the intent of some recent antipornography movements has been to remove the "behavioral conditioner" (pornography) that supposedly stimulates men to perpetuate violence against women, as well as to rescue women abused in the making of pornography.

Even in countries in which pornography is prohibited (such as Saudi Arabia), women are not immune from violence against them by men.[134] Although there *may* be some link between violence in the media and violence in real life, it is complicated and difficult to prove. Moreover, it is possible that antipornography legislation, rather than protecting women in the porn industry, would drive pornography so far underground that it would be even more difficult to police.

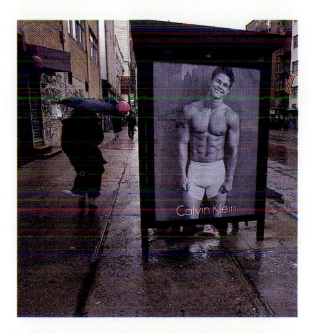

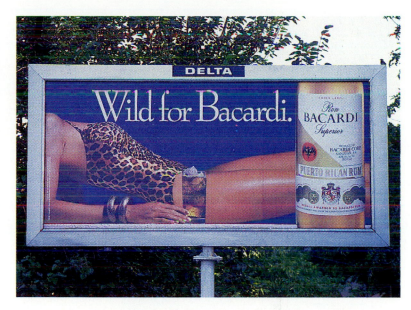

● **Figure 20.7 The popularization of sex**

● *Prostitution:* **Prostitution** is the exchange of sexual services for money. The reality of prostitution is not as depicted in glamorous fashion in the movie *Pretty Woman,* for example. The reality, as one writer puts it, is "about drugs and bad mistakes, and it's sometimes about violence."[135]

Some men sentimentally believe that prostitutes enjoy their work. However, there seems to be no such thing as a "happy hooker," say ex-prostitutes and psychological experts; the business kills body and soul. "Prostitution eats you alive," says one San Francisco female prostitute. "You have to numb out; you can't think about what you're doing—it's too disturbing, too weird, too creepy. You have to realize that the reason the man has come to you is that he wants you to do things that would have his girlfriend or wife running screaming out of the room."[136]

A prostitute may be female or male, adult or child, free agent or slave—in India and Thailand, for example, prostitution is often outright slavery, in which village girls are sold to brothel keepers.[137,138] Even in enlightened countries such as Holland, Norway, and Sweden, where prostitution is often legal, most prostitutes express a wish to quit. Life after prostitution is often equally sad, however: the emotional damage of having one's body used as a sex object does not always go away. Self-esteem and sexual pleasure may be replaced by self-hatred and depression.[139]

People are split over legalizing pornography and prostitution. Some feminists, for instance, believe the practices degrade not just the participants but all women. Others say that outlawing them may reduce them but never stop them, that if they have to exist, it's better that they take place safely and hygienically.[140] However, in an era of HIV infection and other sexually transmitted diseases, is it possible to have "safe sex" as a prostitute?

Atypical Sexuality The foregoing varieties of sexual expression may be considered within the realm of normality. There are, however, a host of sexual behaviors considered abnormal or atypical, although we may recognize glimpses of them within ourselves.

Most of these behaviors are principally practiced by males rather than females. Some behaviors are harmful to others. However, we are *not* concerned here with the very damaging sexual aberrations having to do with issues of power and violence—sexual harassment, rape, incest, and child molestation, which we describe in Chapter 29.

Forms of atypical sexual expression include, but are not limited to, the following, ranging from passive behavior (not involving contact with others) to more aggressive behavior:

- *Voyeurism:* **Voyeurism** is behavior in which one becomes sexually aroused by looking at people, often strangers, undressing or having sex without their being aware that they are being watched. Most, but not all, voyeurs are content just to look.

- *Fetishism:* **Fetishism** is behavior in which a person receives sexual arousal or pleasure from focusing on a nonsexual object, such as a shoe, or a nonsexual part of the body, such as the foot.

- *Transvestism:* People who practice **transvestism,** usually heterosexual males, achieve sexual excitement by putting on clothes of the opposite sex. Transvestism resembles fetishism, except that the object (often one garment, such as stockings or panties) is worn.

- *Exhibitionism:* **Exhibitionism** consists of exposing ("flashing") one's genitals in public to an involuntary observer, usually a female. The exhibitionistic male (who is often shy and unassertive) usually masturbates afterward, sexually excited by the victim's shocked reactions.

- *Obscene phone calls:* Men who make obscene phone calls experience sexual arousal in much the same way as the exhibitionist, and many masturbate during or immediately after the call. Often victims are called at random from the phone book. The best way to deal with such a call is not to show emotional upset (the kind of stimulation the caller is seeking), but just to calmly hang up.

In describing these (and not some of the more bizarre sexual behaviors, such as necrophilia—sexual contact with the dead), we do not mean to imply that these kinds of behavior are somehow all acceptable. If you express your sexual needs by engaging in any of these sexual behaviors, you may need professional assistance and support. Society regards these behaviors as being far off limits and some are illegal.

Strategy for Living: Don't Worry So Much About Normality The range of sexual activity is tremendous, as we have seen, from touching, to kissing, to sexual intercourse, to all kinds of variations. It is probably not useful to try to constantly compare ourselves with others. *Assuming one's sexual behavior is not exploitative, coercive, violent, or self-destructive and occurs between consenting adults,* what does it matter how "normal" or "not normal" it is? In sexuality as in many other aspects of life, perhaps the point is this: we should celebrate individual differences.

Sexual Difficulties and What to Do About Them

For both men and women, sexual problems include inhibited sexual desire or lack of interest, or compulsive sexual behavior. Men may experience erection difficulties and premature ejaculation. Women may be unable to have an orgasm or experience pain during intercourse or spasms of the vaginal muscles.

Our society raises all kinds of sexual expectations—about performance, about size, about having multiple orgasms. A lot of these ideas, which we get from our friends or from the mass media, promote an unrealistic view of sex. Even so, when real life gets in the way of our expectations, we may feel it as a personal failure, because these are matters that many of us are uncomfortable talking about.

Inhibited Sexual Desire Perhaps the greatest complaint most couples have about their sex lives is that one or both individuals experience

inhibited sexual desire (ISD)—lack of interest in sex, or an inability to feel sexual or get sexually aroused.[141] ISD has many causes. Perhaps the relationship has become too close for comfort and one partner is feeling suffocated, hence ISD is a way of getting some space. Or one person is feeling pushed around by a domineering partner, and ISD is a means of retaining some power in the relationship. Or there may be a lack of trust, fear of intimacy or rejection, or a continuing problem with unresolved issues, anger, or resentment. Or ISD may result from frustration over lack of sexual arousal and orgasm. Or there may be stress outside the relationship—a high-pressure job, two careers, children, the consumption of drugs, including alcohol—that turns a couple into roommates more than lovers. Indeed, many couples in long-term relationships have asexual partnerships—they haven't had sex in years.[142] A variation on ISD is dissatisfaction with the frequency or kind of sexual activity: one partner may want more or less sex than the other or want different varieties of sex.

How do you maintain a vital sexual relationship within a committed partnership or how do you rekindle the flame? Assuming there is no physical problem, therapists suggest a variety of techniques: break the cycle of routine sex, perhaps by having sex in a different place (the living room instead of the bedroom), setting aside time when you're not stressed out, trying different sexual positions, increasing daily physical contact with each other (more touching and hugging), having getaway weekends, buying sexy lingerie, watching erotic videotapes, and voicing the desires you may have been afraid to bring up.[143]

Sex Addiction: Compulsive Sexual Behavior The obsessive-compulsive may wash his or her hands 100 times a day. The sexual compulsive, on the other hand, may take sex to the extreme: compulsive masturbation, insatiable sexual demands within a relationship, feverish interest in pornography or phone sex, frenzied anonymous sex, or multiple affairs. **Sexual addiction,** or **compulsive sexual behavior (CSB),** is an intense preoccupation with sex that makes it difficult to have a normal sexual relationship.

Often such people were emotionally or physically abused as children and thus come to believe that sex is not a nurturing, natural experience. So they alternate between profound anxiety and self-loathing and, like alcoholics, are mainly intent on using sex to divert their pain.[144] Psychologists and other health professionals still are uncertain how to describe and treat the condition, but psychotherapy seems to be the best treatment. In addition, sexual compulsives may find support by joining such organizations as Sexaholics Anonymous or Sexual Addicts Anonymous.

Sexual Dysfunctions in Men Common sexual problems in men include *erection difficulties* and *premature ejaculation:*

- *Erection difficulties:* Because sexual adequacy is such an important matter for men, they can be devastated when they have **erection dysfunction,** also known as *impotence*—failure to achieve or maintain an erection. Actually, the problem affects almost every man at one time or another, but only when an erection cannot be maintained in 1 out of 4 sexual encounters is the problem considered serious. Problems can be caused by "performance anxiety" (self-consciousness about having an erection), tension, too much to eat or drink, some prescription or "street" drugs, tiredness, lack of privacy, or having a new partner. Sometimes there are physical causes, such as diabetes or blood-vessel disorders when the body cannot deliver enough blood to engorge the penis, or side effects from medication.

  A man cannot simply *will* an erection to happen; it develops involuntarily. Thus, therapists recommend that couples try nondemanding techniques, such as massage or simply lying together 10–20 minutes, in order to reduce anxiety so that sexual arousal may occur naturally.

- *Premature ejaculation:* After a long period of abstinence, almost any man will ejaculate rapidly. However, **premature ejaculation** is the inability of a man to *reasonably* control his ejaculatory reflex on a regular basis. That is, he reaches orgasm so quickly that his partner may consistently have trouble achieving orgasm. This is usually a psychological rather than physical problem.

Sometimes a condom will dull sensation and boost staying power. Sometimes masturbating before sex will make the second ejaculation occur less rapidly. Finally, there is a squeeze-and-release technique put forth by Masters and Johnson: when the man is about to ejaculate, the penis is withdrawn, the partner squeezes the neck of the penis between the thumb and the first and second fingers for 4 seconds, and 15–30 seconds later stimulation of the penis is resumed.

Sometimes men experience the inability to ejaculate, a temporary condition usually caused by fatigue, stress, alcohol, illness, or lack of emotional involvement with the partner.

Sexual Dysfunctions in Women Sexual enjoyment is now expected of women in a way that once it was not—which means that women too encounter sexual expectations that sometimes can't be met, as in the pressure to achieve multiple or simultaneous orgasms. Chief among the female dysfunctions are *inability to have an orgasm, painful intercourse,* and *spasms of the vaginal muscles:*

- *Inability to have orgasm:* **Anorgasmia** or **inhibited female orgasm** are terms now used instead of "frigidity" to describe an inability to reach orgasm. Perhaps 7% of women have never experienced orgasm.[145] Others have orgasms infrequently.

  There are a couple of reasons why a woman may not achieve orgasm. One is that her partner experiences premature ejaculation. Another is that orgasm is difficult to accomplish through sexual intercourse: what is required is additional, direct stimulation of the clitoris.

  Therapists may tell a woman to give herself permission to express her sexual feelings and eliminate inhibitions, instruct her how to explore her body, how to masturbate, and how to tell her partner to touch and stimulate her in a way that is pleasurable.

- *Painful intercourse:* Painful or difficult sexual intercourse is called **dyspareunia.**

Some women occasionally experience a burning or sharp pain when the penis is inserted into the vagina. There are a great many causes, ranging from inadequate lubrication or infection of the vagina to a tight hymen in young women, irritation by contraceptive creams, the penis touching the cervix, and a host of others. If the condition persists, the woman should see a physician.

- *Vaginismus:* **Vaginismus** consists of involuntary spasms of the muscles surrounding the lower third of the vagina so that the penis cannot enter. Sometimes it is a normal response when a woman is expecting pain (as on first intercourse) or does not want sex, perhaps as a reaction to sexual trauma, such as rape. When the problem is chronic, a woman needs to seek assistance from her health care provider. After exploring the underlying problem, some therapists may teach a woman to explore her genital area and learn to relax her vaginal muscles.

800-HELP

GETCHA—Group Energized to Terminate Caller Harassment and Abuse. 800-343-8242. A hot line for people who have been harassed by obscene phone calls.

Suggestions for Further Reading

Barbach, Lonnie. (1975). *For yourself: The fulfillment of female sexuality.* Garden City, NY: Doubleday. A classic self-help book for women by the innovator of a sex therapy treatment program for women.

Comfort, Alex. (1991). *The new joy of sex: A gourmet guide to lovemaking for the '90s.* New York: Crown. An update of the phenomenal bestseller on "advanced lovemaking" first published in 1972, which reflected the spirit of the era that sex is fun.

Zilbergeld, Bernie. (1978). *Male sexuality.* Boston: Little, Brown. A classic-self help book for men.

Conflict and Communication: Learning How to Disagree

Why can't couples get along better? Must there always be conflict in intimate relationships? Check which *one* of the following statements best describes your feelings when you approach a conflict with someone close to you.

___ **1.** I hate conflict. If I can find a way to avoid it, I will.

___ **2.** Conflict is such a hassle. I'd as soon let the other person have his or her way just to keep the peace.

___ **3.** You can't just let people walk over you. You've got to fight to establish your point of view.

___ **4.** I'm willing to negotiate to see if the other person and I can meet halfway.

___ **5.** Let's take time to explore our similarities and differences to see if we can solve the problem to the satisfaction of both of us.

Whichever one you checked corresponds to a particular style of dealing with conflict: (1) avoidance, (2) accommodation, (3) domination, (4) compromise, (5) integration. For an explanation, read on.

Conflict: Most People Adopt One of Five Styles of Dealing With Conflict

Researchers have identified five styles of dealing with conflict, one of which is probably closest to yours.[146,147]

1. Avoidance: "Maybe It Will Go Away." People who adopt this style find dealing with conflict unpleasant and uncomfortable. They hope that by ignoring the conflict or by avoiding confrontation the circumstances will change and the problem will magically disappear. Unfortunately, avoiding or delaying conflict usually means the situation will have to be dealt with later, at which point it may have worsened.

2. Accommodation: "Oh, Have It Your Way!" Accommodation does not mean compromise; it means simply giving in, although it does not really resolve the matter under dispute. People who adopt a style of easy surrender are, like avoiders, uncomfortable with conflict and hate disagreements. They are also inclined to be "people pleasers," worried about the approval of others. However, giving in does not really solve the conflict. If anything it may aggravate the situation over the long term because accommodators may be deeply resentful that the other person did not listen to their point of view. Indeed, the resentment may even develop into a role of martyrdom, irritating the partner.

3. Domination: "Only Winning Matters." The person with a winning-is-everything, dominating style should not be surprised if he or she some day finds an "I've moved out" note from the partner. The dominator will go to any lengths to emerge triumphant in a disagreement, even if it means being aggressive and manipulative. However, winning isn't what intimate human relationships are about; that approach to conflict only produces hostility.

4. Compromise: "I'll Meet You Halfway." Compromise seems like a civilized way of dealing with conflict, and it is definitely an improvement over the preceding styles. People striving for compromise recognize that partners have different needs and try to negotiate to reach agreement. Even so, they may still employ some gamesmanship, such as manipulation and misrepresentation, in an attempt to further their own ends. Thus, the compromise style is not as effective in resolving conflict as the integration style.

5. Integration: "Let's Honestly Try to Satisfy Both of Us." Compromisers view solutions to conflict as a matter of each party meeting the other half way. The integration style, on the other hand, attempts to find a solution that will achieve satisfaction for both partners. Integration has several parts to it:

- *Openness for mutual problem solving:* The conflict is seen not as a game to be won or negotiated but as a problem to be solved for mutual benefit. Consequently, manipulation and misrepresentation have no place; honesty and openness are a necessary part of reaching the solution. This also has the benefit of building trust that will carry over to the resolution of other conflicts.

- *Disagreement with the ideas, not the person:* An important part of integration, which we expand on below, is that partners criticize each other's ideas or specific acts rather than each other as persons. It is one thing, for instance, to say "You drink too much" and another to say "I feel you drank too much last evening." The first disparages character, the second states unhappiness with a particular incident.

- *Emphasis on similarities, not differences:* Integration requires more work than other styles of dealing with conflict (although the payoffs are better) because partners must put a good deal of effort into stating and clarifying their positions. To maintain the spirit of trust and problem solving, the two should also emphasize the similarities in their positions as they work toward a mutually satisfactory solution.

Communication: There Are Ways to Learn How to Disagree

Conflict is practically always present in an ongoing relationship between two people. That does not mean it is bad or that it should be suppressed. When handled constructively, researchers point out, conflict may "(1) bring problems out into the open, where they can be solved, (2) put an end to chronic sources of discontent in a relationship, and (3) lead to new insights through the clashing of divergent views."[148] The key to intimacy is the ability to handle conflict well, which means the ability to communicate well.

Bad Communication. Most of us *think* communication is easy, points out psychiatrist David Burns, because we've been talking since childhood.[149] However, it's when we have a conflict that we find out if we communicate well.

Bad communication, says Burns, author of *The Feeling Good Handbook,* has two characteristics:

- *You become argumentative and defensive:* The natural tendency of most of us when we are upset is to argue. The habit of contradicting others, however, is self-defeating, for it creates distance between you and them and prevents intimacy. Moreover, in this stance you show you are not interested in listening to the other person or understanding his or her feelings.

- *You deny your own feelings and act them out indirectly:* You may become sarcastic, or pout, or storm out of the room slamming doors. This kind of reaction, known as *passive aggression,* can sometimes be as destructive as *active aggression,* in which you make threats or tell the other person off.

Good Communication. "Most people want to be understood and accepted more than anything else in the world," says Burns.[150] Knowing that is a first step toward good communication.

Good communication, according to Burns, has two attributes:

- *You listen to and acknowledge the other person's feelings:* Instead of showing that you are only interested in broadcasting your feelings and insisting that the other agree with you, you encourage the other to express his or her feelings. You try to listen to and understand what the other person is thinking and feeling.

- *You express your own feelings openly and directly:* If you only listen to the other person's feelings and don't express your own, you will end up feeling shortchanged, angry, and resentful. When you deny your feelings, you end up acting them out indirectly. The trick, then, is to express your feelings in a way that will not alienate the other person.

Becoming Expert at Listening. Besides the Burns book, perhaps one of the best books on communication is *Love Is Never Enough* by Aaron Beck.[151]

Some listening guidelines Beck suggests:

- *Tune in to your partner's channel:* Imagining how the other person might be feeling—putting yourself in the other's shoes—is known as *empathy,* trying to experience the other's thoughts and feelings.

- *Give listening signals:* Use facial expressions, subtle gestures, and sounds such as "uh-huh" and "yeah" to show your partner you are really listening. Beck particularly urges this advice on men, since studies find that women are more inclined to send responsive signals.

- *Don't interrupt:* Although interruptions may seem natural to you, they can make the other person feel cut off. Men, says Beck, tend to interrupt more than women do, although they interrupt other men as often as they do women.

- *Ask questions skillfully:* Asking questions can help you determine what the other person is thinking and keep the discussion going—provided the question is not a *conversation stopper.* "Why" questions can be conversation stoppers ("Why were you home late?"). So can questions that can have only a yes-or-no answer. Questions that ask the other's opinion can be *conversation starters* ("What do you think about always having dinner at the same time?"). Questions that reflect the other's statements ("Can you tell me more about why you feel that way?") help convey your empathy. The important thing is to ask questions *gently,* never accusingly.

- *Use diplomacy and tact:* Everyone has sensitive areas—about their appearance or how they speak, for example. This is true of people in intimate relationships as much as people in other relationships. *Problems in relationships invariably involve feelings.* Using diplomacy in your responses will help build trust to talk about difficulties.

An especially wise piece of advice about listening comes from David Burns: find *some* truth in what the other person is saying and agree with it, even if you feel convinced that what he or she is saying is totally wrong, unreasonable, irrational, or unfair. This technique, known as *disarming,* works especially well if you're feeling criticized and attacked. If you resist the urge to argue or defend yourself and instead agree with the other person, it takes the wind out of the other person's sails and has a calming effect. That person will then be more open to your point of view. Adds Burns: "When you use the disarming technique, you must be genuine in what you say or it will backfire. You can always find some valid way to agree, no matter how illogical the person's accusations might seem to you. If you agree with them in a sincere way, they will generally soften and will be far more willing to listen to you."[152]

Becoming Expert at Expressing Yourself. In expressing yourself, there are two principal points to keep in mind:

- *Use "I feel" language:* It's always tempting to use accusatory language during the heat of conflict ("You make me so mad!" or "You never listen to what I say!"), but this is sure to send the other person stomping out of the room. By using the simple method of saying "I feel" followed by the word expressing your feelings ("frustrated," "ignored," "attacked," "nervous," "unloved"), you don't sound blaming and critical, as you would by saying "You make me . . ." or "You never . . ." By telling your partner how you feel, rather than defending the "truth" of your position, you are able to express your feelings without attacking the other person.

- *Express praise and keep criticism specific:* In any conflict, we may disagree with a person's *specific act or behavior,* but we need not reject the other as a person. For example, to express criticism alone, you might say, "When we make love you seem so inhibited." Better to combine criticism with praise by saying, "I appreciate the way you respond to me when we make love, and I think it could be even better if you would take the initiative sometimes. Does this seem like a reasonable request?"[153]

Safer Sex, Birth Control, and Abortion

Love and passion are among the most powerful human forces.

Love, or the belief in love, sometimes leads people to take chances. Even if her boyfriend was also seeing other women, the San Francisco 17-year-old reports, "nothing would happen because he says he'll never do anything that would mess me up, and I believe him." They don't need a condom, she states, "because he says he loves me."[1]

Sexual passion also leads people to sometimes take chances or to make decisions they might not otherwise make. A survey of Stanford University students found that nearly three-quarters of those who engaged in heterosexual intercourse did not always use a condom. Two-thirds of homosexuals did not use a condom during anal sex. Students who did not use a condom often reported they had gotten carried away, "out of control," or had not planned ahead when they became sexually involved.[2]

Love or sexual passion has often steam-rolled over rationality in the past, as people have risked their marriages, jobs, social standing, or concerns about morality or ethics to have sex with someone they really liked. That, however, was before the Age of AIDS. Has the knowledge that sex can be associated with a potentially fatal disease changed human behavior? It doesn't seem so.

We are surrounded by words and images about sex. However, a great many people, including many college-educated people, are surprisingly uninformed about the subject. For instance, the *majority* of women and men in the United States do not know the most likely time in the monthly menstrual cycle when a woman can become pregnant.[3] However, in sexual matters, ignorance can no longer be considered bliss, if it ever could.

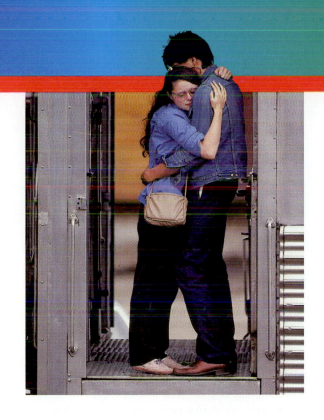

As we have stated elsewhere, our sexuality encompasses more than just biology and the physiology of sexual response. It includes how we see ourselves as men and women and how our behavior and attitudes are influenced by cultural and social norms and legal restraints. To these we must add our feelings about passion and risk. In the following three chapters, we provide you with information you can use to understand your risks and make informed choices that will enhance your well-being—how to reduce your vulnerability to potentially life-threatening illness such as HIV infection, how to avoid an unplanned pregnancy, and what to do if an undesired pregnancy occurs.

21 Safer Sex

▶ Discuss all the considerations in avoiding exposure to sexually transmitted diseases.

Know your sexual partner, medical authorities advise.

Many college students have taken the advice to heart. Unfortunately, says psychologist Jeffrey D. Fisher, they may go about it the wrong way. Rather than try to determine directly whether a prospective partner has been infected with the AIDS virus—**HIV,** the **human immunodeficiency virus**—or another sexually transmitted disease, they ask about home town, family, and major. Using those useless and irrelevant facts, says Fisher, they draw a conclusion about how safe it is to have sex with that person.[4]

Other young adults make similar kinds of decisions. They decide whether to use condoms on the basis of the other person's perceived *social class,* judging a person who seems "lower class" to be more promiscuous or more risky. Or they base their risk assessment on *appearance,* considering a person who is attractive and well educated to be less risky.[5] Do such external clues work? No, says Fisher. To use them as guides to safe sex, he says, is to believe in superstition.

How can you be *sure* that sex is really safe? The answer is: you can't. However, there are things that you can do to reduce your risks. That is the subject of this chapter.

Unsafe Sex and Knowing Your Partner

To reduce your risk of exposure to sexually transmitted organisms such as HIV, you need to ask the right kinds of questions of prospective sexual partners, although the answers are no guarantees. The law may also require partner notification about sexual disease.

AIDS, or **acquired immunodeficiency syndrome,** the final and fatal stages of infection from HIV, has been in North America since at least 1975. In the years following, it has become more and more apparent that it is not a disease limited to male homosexuals and intravenous drug users. Indeed, the fastest-growing group of HIV-infected people worldwide is heterosexual women. Women account for half of new AIDS cases, and an official for the World Health Organization (WHO) says that by the year 2000 most new AIDS infections worldwide will be among women.[6] "To put it simply, AIDS is becoming a heterosexual disease," says Michael Merson, director of WHO's Global Program on AIDS. Even in the United States, "the greatest rate of increase is among heterosexuals," he says.[7]

The Concerns About Unsafe Sex The message about the dangers of unprotected sex seems to have gotten through to many people, but clearly more must be done.[8-10] For instance, even some students in a Stanford survey who used condoms said they tended to rely on them more to prevent pregnancy than to avoid sexually transmitted diseases.[11] Other studies show that teenagers who use condoms are swayed less by health concerns than by the popularity of condoms among peers and by their ease of use.[12] A 1992 survey of 10,000 heterosexual Americans ages 18–75 found that the vast majority of those with multiple partners were engaging in sexual intercourse without condoms.[13] One author of the study, Joseph Catania, said the situation might reflect "a denial of personal risk" by a segment of the population that "still believes [AIDS] is a gay disease."

It's time to "Get real!", as the expression goes. AIDS is only one of several sexually transmitted diseases (STDs) that have shown an alarming rise. The rates are up for syphilis, chlamydia, genital warts, genital herpes, and other STDs. Gonorrhea, pelvic inflammatory disease, genital warts, and hepatitis B continue to pose serious problems. Indeed, according to a 1993 report by the Alan Guttmacher Institute, *more than one in five of all Americans is infected by a sexually caused viral disease.*[14] About 12 million new sexually transmitted infections occur every year, two-thirds of them to people under 25, one-quarter in teenagers.[15]

The sexually transmitted diseases caused by viruses—such as hepatitis B, genital herpes, genital warts, and HIV infection—cannot be cured, although they can in many cases be controlled. Some, such as genital warts, have been linked with an increased risk of cervical cancer in women. STDs caused by bacteria (such as gonorrhea, chlamydia, and syphilis) can be cured, but unfortunately many have no obvious symptoms and so they can continue to develop. Thus, they pose special threats to women of childbearing age as well as to men because, if not treated, they can lead to serious complications (infertility, tubal pregnancies, and chronic pain).

Asking Partners About Their Sexual History However embarrassing the conversation, it can be helpful for people to explore their prospective partners' sexual histories before getting involved. Here are some questions to ask:[16]

- *STD tests:* "Have you ever been tested for HIV or for other STDs? Would you be willing to have an HIV test done?"

- *Previous partners:* "How many sexual partners have you had?" (The more partners, the higher the STD risk.)

- *Prostitution:* "Have you ever had sex with a prostitute?" (If so, was protection used?)

- *Bisexuality:* For a woman to ask a man: "Have you ever had a male sexual partner?" For a man to ask a woman: "Have you ever had a sexual partner who was bisexual?"

- *IV drug use:* "Have you—*or your sexual partners*—ever injected drugs?" (A previous sexual partner can transmit AIDS or hepatitis by sharing needles.)

- *Blood transfusion:* "Have you ever had a transfusion of blood or blood products?" (This fact is particularly important if it occurred before 1985, when blood wasn't screened for HIV.)

Even if you ask all the right questions, however, you still can't be sure of the answers. Someone may look at you and state with absolute honesty and sincerity that he or she is "clean," yet may have an infection and not know

it. Even people who flash a card showing they visited a county health department for an HIV test can't actually offer proof of lack of infection. The test measures the presence of antibodies (which fight the HIV infection) that can take up to 6 months to develop, and there's no guarantee the person hasn't been infected since the test. Indeed, a person can have HIV and be able to infect others during the 2 weeks to 6 months necessary to show antibodies.

Blood-donor cards are equally suspect: though the cards show the bearer has given blood that was subsequently screened for HIV infection, they do not prove that one hasn't been infected after the donation and is a safe partner.

Dating and Sexual Honesty Truth is the first casualty in war, it is said. Some think it is also the first casualty in sexual behavior.[17]

A survey by psychologists Susan Cochran and Vickie Mays of 422 sexually active college students found that 60% of the women and 47% of the men said that someone had lied to them in order to have sex. In turn, 10% of the women and 30% of the men said that they had told a lie to obtain sex. And 42% of the women and 47% of the men said that, if asked, they would understate the number of previous sexual partners they had had. Finally, asked hypothetically if they would lie about having tested positive for HIV, 4% of the women and 20% of the men said they would not reveal they were HIV positive.[18]

Although male respondents were more willing to lie than women, Cochran says it would be a mistake to say that men are more dishonest about sex. Rather, "women will lie in order to achieve a relationship, while men will lie for both sex and relationships," she says. Clearly, the bottom line, as Cochran points out, is that simply "asking one's partner about AIDS is a risky technique" and does not by itself guarantee safer sex.[19]

Partner Notification of Sexually Transmitted Diseases In recent years, *partner notification* has become a major issue.[20–24] There are two kinds of partner notification:

1. *Notification in advance by one partner to another:* Some persons have been sued or prosecuted for failing to inform a sexual

partner before having sex that they had an STD, or for not wearing a condom when they presumably knew they were infected and could transmit the disease. Some people being sued have claimed they were not even aware themselves that they were infected at the time, but the courts have still made them pay damages (up to $150,000 in one case) to the person they infected. Most of the court cases were brought by victims of herpes (a nonfatal STD that is treatable but not curable).

2. *Partner notification afterward by health authorities:* The question of partner notification may also arise later, after people have been tested to see if they have been infected with an STD, particularly HIV. An important concern is whether states should allow anonymous testing for the AIDS virus. Such policies enable people to find out whether they have become infected but maintain their privacy, since the results of their tests are not reported to any health agencies. Or, should states require all people whose tests show they are HIV infected

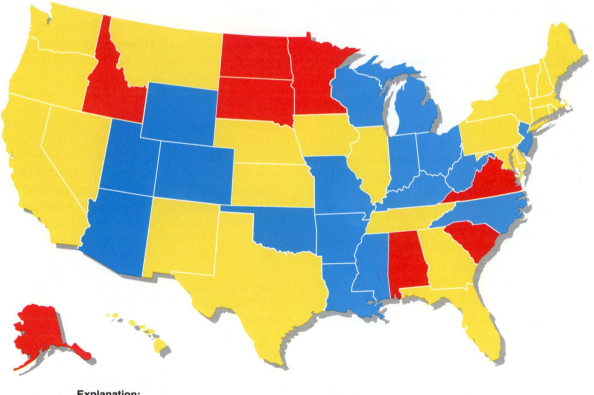

Explanation:

■ States with mandatory name reporting of people who test positive for the AIDS virus.

■ States with "mixed" name reporting that allows some anonymous testing.

■ Most of the other states rely on anonymous testing entirely or require name reporting only in special cases.

● **Figure 21.1 States with mandatory reporting of people testing positive for HIV.** These states are required to contact infected persons and ask for their cooperation in providing the names of sexual partners, who are then notified of their possible infection (without identifying who may have infected them).

to be identified so that their sexual partners, past and present, can be warned?[25]

Several states have various forms of "mandatory name reporting." (*See ● Figure 21.1.*) This means that when people test positive for the AIDS virus, their names are reported to the state health department. They are then contacted and asked to *voluntarily* provide the names of their sexual partners, so that the partners can be notified by health officials. It's important to note that no state so far forces people to divulge partners' names. In addition, stringent precautions are taken by health officials to prevent partners from finding out the identity of the person who may have infected them.

Reducing Risks of Acquiring Sexually Transmitted Diseases

The safest form of sex for preventing transmission of STDs is abstinence and other behavior in which body fluids are not exchanged. The next least risky is protected sex, such as that using condoms and dental dams. High-risk behavior involves sexual exchange of body fluids or use of intravenous needles. Long-term mutually monogamous relationships are an especially important consideration.

So how *should* one pursue sexual relationships? There are two principal pieces of advice:

1. *Use precautions universally:* If you choose to have sex, then CONSISTENTLY use safer-sex measures (such as a condom) with ALL partners. This means *all* sexual partners, not just those you don't know well or those you think may be higher risk.

2. *Keep your head clear:* Be careful about using alcohol and other drugs with a prospective sexual partner. They may cloud your judgment, placing you in a position of increased vulnerability.

No doubt you have heard the phrase "safe sex." However, only abstinence is considered safe—that is, no sexual contact at all, or no contact with a partner's body fluids, including semen, vaginal secretions, saliva, or blood. Ac-

tually, even if no body fluids are exchanged, some STDs, such as genital herpes or pubic lice, can still be transmitted under certain conditions by skin-to-skin contact.

In general, then, there are three levels of risk in sexual behavior: "saved sex," "safer sex," and high-risk sex. (*See ● Table 21.1.*)

● **Table 21.1 Relative risks of various sexual behaviors**

Level of risk	Behavior
Lower risk	Abstinence Massage Hugging Rubbing bodies Dry kissing (not exchanging saliva) Masturbation Mutual manual stimulation of genitals (avoiding contact with body fluids)
Somewhat risky	Deep (French) kissing Vaginal intercourse, using latex condoms with the spermicide nonoxynol-9 Fellatio, with the male wearing a condom Cunnilingus, with a nonmenstruating female using a latex dental dam
Very risky	Vaginal or anal intercourse without a condom Fellatio without a condom Cunnilingus without a dental dam Oral-anal contact Semen in the mouth Contact with a partner's blood, including menstrual blood Sexual behavior leading to bleeding or tissue damage Behavior involving shared IV needles Sexual contact with an IV user Sexual contact with someone whose previous partner was an IV user Sexual contact with someone who sells or buys sex

Lower Risk: "Saved" Sex, Including Absti-nence The safest kind of sex avoids the ex-change of semen, vaginal secretions, saliva, or blood. The principal kind of "saved sex" is **ab-stinence,** defined as the voluntary avoidance of sexual intercourse. Saved sex also includes massage, hugging, rubbing of bodies, dry kissing (not exchanging saliva), masturbation, and mu-tual manual stimulation of the genitals (if con-tact with body fluids is avoided).

Thus, abstinence can be taken to mean any-thing from avoiding all forms of sexual activity to avoiding only those, such as intercourse or oral sex, in which fluids are exchanged in a way that can transmit disease. Of course, if you *do* want to practice only safe sexual behaviors, the trick is not to get swept away and end up prac-ticing unsafe sex in spite of yourself.

Some people are more comfortable being with dates, potential mates, and just plain friends who do nothing more than kiss and cud-dle. In other words, practicing abstinence is becoming increasingly acceptable.[26] (*See* ● *Fig-ure 21.2.*)

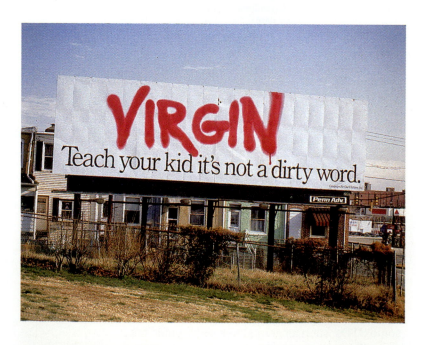

● **Figure 21.2 The acceptability of abstinence.** A Maryland sex education program has helped make abstinence acceptable.

Somewhat Risky: "Safer" Sex, Including Use of Condoms Abstinence may be unrealis-tic for some people. The next best step to en-suring safe sex—actually, only saf*er* sex—is to use *latex:* condoms and dental dams. "Safer" sex is still somewhat risky, but at least it mini-mizes the exchange of body fluids (semen, vagi-nal secretions, saliva, or blood). Examples of safer-sex behavior include dry kissing, vaginal intercourse using latex condoms with the sper-micide nonoxynol-9 (which kills STD organ-isms), fellatio with the male wearing a condom, and cunnilingus with a nonmenstruating female using a latex dental dam. Let us consider the two principal means of protection, condoms and dental dams:

- *Condoms:* A **condom** ("prophylactic," "rubber," "safe," "French letter") is a thin sheath made of latex rubber or lamb intes-tine (called "natural skin," but only latex is recommended for HIV protection). Pack-aged in rolled-up form, the condom is un-rolled over a male's erect penis, leaving a little room at the top to catch the semen. Some condoms are marketed with a "reser-voir" at the end for this purpose. (*See* ● *Figure 21.3.*)

  The purpose of a condom is to provide protection for both partners during vaginal, oral, or anal intercourse. On the one hand, it keeps semen from being transmitted to a man's sexual partner and shields against contact with any infectious problem on his penis. On the other hand, the condom also protects the male's penis and urethra from contact with his partner's secretions, blood, and saliva.

- *Dental dams:* Every major sexually trans-mitted disease can be acquired during oral sex, although not as easily as during inter-course. Males receiving oral sex should wear a condom. If a female is the recipient, she should use a **dental dam.** Sold in med-ical supply stores and pharmacies, a dental dam (designed for use in dental surgery) is a flat 5-inch-square piece of latex that may be placed over the vaginal opening and sur-rounding area. (*See* ● *Figure 21.4.*) Some people use plastic wrap (for example, Saran Wrap) for the same purpose, although this has not been tested to see how well it pro-tects.

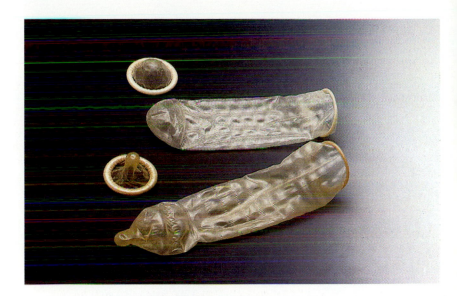

● **Figure 21.3 Condoms.** (*Right*) Two kinds of condoms, one with a "reservoir" tip. (*Below*) How to put on a condom.

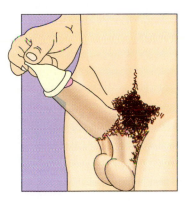

Pinch or twist the tip of the condom, leaving one-half inch at the tip to catch the semen.

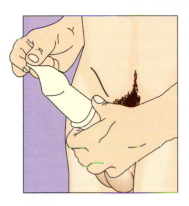

Holding the tip, unroll the condom.

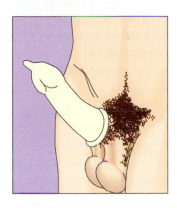

Unroll the condom until it reaches the pubic hairs.

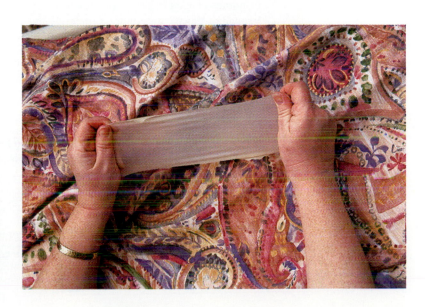

● **Figure 21.4 A dental dam.** Sold in medical supply stores and pharmacies, the dental dam is a thin latex square that can be used to cover the vagina when the couple is engaging in cunnilingus (a woman is the recipient of oral sex).

Unfortunately, *condoms are not perfect protection.* They only *reduce* the risk of acquiring HIV infections and other STDs. Note that *reducing the risk is not the same as eliminating the risk.* If the condom slips off or breaks during intercourse or is flawed to begin with, there is, obviously, 100% exposure—possibly to a disease that is 100% fatal.

How often do condoms come off or tear during intercourse? One way to judge is that there are typically 12 pregnancies per 100 women using condoms during the first year of use.[27] A nonprofit family-planning research agency in North Carolina, Family Health International, conducted a 2-year study in nine countries and found that married or cohabiting couples broke only 1–2% of the condoms they used. However, among other couples, such as those having casual sex or extramarital affairs or lovers not living together—people who actually need the highest protection—there was a higher breakage rate: 3–5%. About 1 couple in 20 broke condoms 20% of the time, according to the study.[28] Condoms break most frequently when couples use oil-based lubricants, attempt their own "quality testing" (such as blowing up condoms to test for leaks), or engage in prolonged sex. There are several precautions people can take to ensure that condoms are used properly. (See ● *Figure 21.5.*)

Condoms, whether made by U.S. or overseas manufacturers, are tested for leakage by the Food and Drug Administration. As of February 1988, 12% of the samples of domestically produced condoms and 21% of foreign-made condoms failed the FDA tests.[29] In March 1989, Consumers Union tested condoms and listed 43 brands and models in terms of their features and performance in resisting breakage. Your physician, health department, or campus student health service can provide additional information. Planned Parenthood will also answer questions about condoms.

● **Figure 21.5 How to buy and use condoms**

How to Buy

Materials: Buy latex, not natural membrane or lambskin. Latex is less apt to leak and better able to protect against HIV transmission. Inexpensive foreign brands are suspect.

Sizes: The Food and Drug Administration (FDA) says condoms must be between 6 and 8 inches in length when unrolled. (The average erect penis is 6½ inches.)
　　Condoms labeled *Regular* are 7 ½ inches.
　　Instead of "Small" for condoms under 7½ inches, manufacturers use labels such as *Snug Fit.*
　　Instead of "Large" for condoms over 7½ inches, manufacturers use labels such as *Max* or *Magnum.*

Shapes: Most condoms are *straight-walled.* Some are labeled *contoured,* which means they are anatomically shaped to fit the penis and thus are more comfortable.

Tips: Some condoms have a *reservoir* at the end to catch semen upon ejaculation. Others do not have a reservoir, in which case they should be twisted at the tip after being put on.

Plain or Lubricated: Condoms can be purchased *plain* (unlubricated) or *lubricated,* which means they feel more slippery to the touch. There are four options:

1. Buy a plain condom and don't use a lubricant.

2. Buy a plain condom and use your own lubricant, preferably water-based (such as K-Y Jelly or Astroglide).

3. Buy a lubricated condom pregreased with silicone-, jelly-, or water-based lubricants.

4. Buy a *spermicidally lubricated* condom, which contains *nonoxynol-9,* a chemical that kills sperm and HIV. This is probably the best option.

Strength: A standard condom will do for vaginal and oral sex. Some people believe an *"extra-strength"* condom is less apt to break during anal sex, although this is debatable.

Gimmicks: In addition, condoms come with all kinds of other features:

1. *Colors:* Red, blue, green, and yellow are safe. Avoid black and "glow in the dark," says the FDA, since dyes may rub off.

2. *Smell and taste:* Latex smells and tastes rubbery, but some fragranced condoms mask this odor.

3. *Adhesive:* Condoms are available with adhesive to hold them in place so they won't slip off during withdrawal.

4. *Marketing gimmicks:* Condoms are sold with ribs, nubs, bumps, and so on, but unless the additions are at the tip and can reach the clitoris they do no good whatsoever.

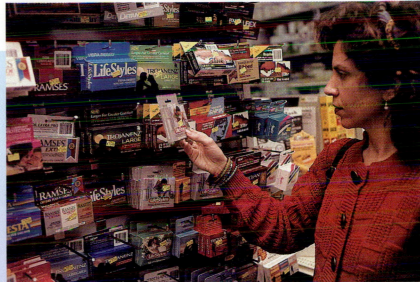

How to Use

Storage: Condoms should be stored in a cool, dry place. Keeping them in a hot glove compartment or wallet in the back pocket for weeks can cause the latex to fail.

Opening package: Look to see that the foil or plastic packaging is not broken; if it is, don't use the condom. Open the package carefully. Fingernails can easily damage a condom.

Inspection: Make sure a condom is soft and pliable. Don't use it if it's brittle, sticky, or discolored. Don't try to test it for leaks by unrolling, stretching, or blowing it up, which will only weaken it.

Putting on: Put the condom on before any genital contact to prevent exposure to fluids. Hold the tip of the condom and unroll it directly onto the erect penis. (If the man is not circumcised, pull back the foreskin before rolling on the condom.) Gently pinch the tip to remove air bubbles, which can cause the condom to break. Condoms without a reservoir tip need a half-inch free at the tip.

Lubricants: *Important!* If you're using a lubricant of your own, *don't use an oil-based lubricant.* Oil-based lubricants—examples are hand lotion, baby oil, mineral oil, and Vaseline—can reduce a latex condom's strength by 90% in as little as 60 seconds. Saliva is not recommended either.

Use a water-based or silicone-based product designed for such use, such as K-Y Jelly or spermicidal compounds containing nonoxynol-9.

Add lubricant to the outside of the condom before entry. If not enough lubricant is used, the condom can tear or pull off.

Slippage and breakage: If the condom begins to slip, hold your fingers around the base to make it stay on. If a condom breaks, it should be replaced immediately.

If ejaculation occurs after a condom breaks, apply a foam spermicide to the vagina at once.

After ejaculation: After sex, hold the base of the condom to prevent it from slipping off and to avoid spillage during withdrawal. Withdraw while the penis is still erect. Throw the used condom away. (Never reuse condoms.) Wash the genitals.

Very Risky: Unprotected Sex and Other Behavior Behavior that is high-risk for the transmission of STDs includes unprotected sex plus any behavior that involves sharing intravenous needles. This includes vaginal or anal intercourse without a condom, fellatio without a condom, cunnilingus without a dental dam, and unprotected oral-anal contact. It includes all forms of sex in which body fluids may be exchanged: semen in the mouth, contact with a partner's blood (including menstrual blood), and any sexual behavior that leads to bleeding or tissue damage.

Finally, the category of high risk has to be extended to people or behavior that involves the exchange of blood, especially by means of injectable drugs or any other situation in which blood-contaminated needles or other objects may be shared (tatooing, ear-piercing, shaving, and so on). Thus, you should not only not share IV needles yourself but should avoid sexual contact with someone who is an IV drug user or whose previous partner was an IV drug user. And you should avoid having sexual contact with people who sell or buy sex, who are often IV drug users.

Mutual Monogamy Most men and women in the United States have more than one sexual partner during their lifetime. Indeed, two-thirds of all American women who have ever had intercourse have had more than one partner, and some young women have more than one partner within a short time.[30]

Having multiple sexual partners is one of the leading risk factors for the transmission of STDs. Clearly, mutual monogamy is one way to avoid infection. However, in "this day and age" (as the euphemism goes for the Age of AIDS), even apparent monogamy *may* have its risks:

- *"Cheating hearts":* If one partner is having sexual contacts (whether heterosexual, bisexual, or homosexual) outside the supposedly monogamous relationship and is not using condoms—and is not telling his or her principal partner about such activities—it does not just breach a trust. It endangers the other's life. AIDS makes this old problem much more agonizing than, say, 15 years ago, when there was a possibility of passing along herpes, syphilis, or gonor-

rhea, diseases that are serious but, in North America today, not usually fatal.

- *The AIDS time bomb:* The AIDS virus can be present in a person for perhaps 10 years before AIDS itself begins to appear. *And there may be no outward signs or symptoms at all during that time*. This poses a real dilemma, for you could be in a monogamous relationship with someone but have no idea if he or she was previously infected with HIV. Only by waiting 6 months while remaining faithful to each other and then taking a test to see if AIDS virus antibodies are present can one be reasonably sure that the partner is free of HIV infections.

Having extramarital affairs or otherwise "cheating" outside the relationship means, of course, that the commitment is not truly monogamous. The world has changed, but many of our cultural images have not: movies and magazines still celebrate the glories of passion, of losing oneself in sexual ecstasy, of having relationships with exciting strangers. Still, the best strategy for living includes acknowledging the risks associated with sexual behavior, making rational, informed choices that enhance your well-being, and using universal precautions during sexual activity.

800-HELP

AIDS Hotline. 800-533-AIDS (in Canada, 800-668-AIDS)

AIDS Information Hotline. 800-342-AIDS

STD National Hotline. 800-634-3662 (in California, 800-982-5883)

Suggestion for Further Reading

Consumers Union. (1989, March). Can you rely on condoms? *Consumer Reports,* pp. 135–141. Consumers Union tested condoms in 1989 and listed 43 brands and models in terms of their features and their performance in resisting breakage.

22 Birth Control

▶ Describe how conception occurs.

▶ Discuss the various types of contraception and rate them for effectiveness.

▶ Describe the new contraceptive directions for men and women.

The biological purpose of sex, of course, is not to put life at risk but to begin it. The reproduction-related motivation for sex has evolved over 500 million years and shows no sign of abating. If anything, human fertility seems to be escalating out of control, with 1.7 million new infants born worldwide *each week*. An understanding of conception and contraception can be helpful in reducing your pregnancy-related risks.

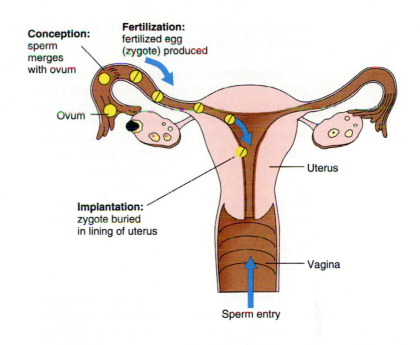

Conception: sperm merges with ovum

Fertilization: fertilized egg (zygote) produced

Ovum

Implantation: zygote buried in lining of uterus

Uterus

Vagina

Sperm entry

● **Figure 22.1 Conception**

Conception: The Merging of Sperm and Ovum

Contraception, or birth control, begins with understanding conception—how sperm and ovum merge to form a fertilized egg or zygote, which implants itself in the lining of the uterus, where it grows into an embryo and then a fetus.

When during sexual intercourse (or artificial insemination) the male reproductive cell, the **sperm,** meets the female reproductive cell, the egg or **ovum,** and the two merge, that is known as the moment of **conception** or **fertilization.** (*See* ● *Figure 22.1.*) Let us explore the process by which sperm and ovum proceed to produce a human being.

The Ovum The eggs are stored in the two **ovaries,** the female reproductive glands, or gonads, near the ends of the **fallopian tubes,** channels whose opposite ends connect with the uterus. (*Refer back to Figure 22.1.*) As a consequence of the hormonal changes associated with the menstrual cycle, one egg matures every month. The release of a mature ovum from an ovary (approximately 14 days before

the onset of menstruation) is called **ovulation.** In most cases, once a month one egg becomes available for fertilization, but sometimes multiple eggs are released, and the subsequent fertilization produces multiple births.

Women do not produce these eggs; they are born with all the eggs they will ever have. In most women, only 300–400 eggs become mature during their lifetimes.

The Sperm A single ejaculation contains as many as 500 million sperm. Each sperm resembles a tiny tadpole that moves by means of whip-like motions of its tail. The life span of a sperm is 1–3 days, though some experts suggest that sperm can live as long as a week once they enter the fallopian tubes.

Each sperm released into the vagina attempts to move through the cervix, into and through the uterus, and up into the fallopian tubes. (*Refer back to Figure 22.1.*) Most never make it. Of the 1% that do, most find themselves in the wrong tube or their timing is wrong. An egg can be fertilized only within 24–48 hours of ovulation. If conception fails to occur, the unfertilized egg is reabsorbed or passes out of the vagina unnoticed, sometimes during menstruation.

Fertilization and Implantation In the event that a sperm and an ovum meet, they will probably meet in the fallopian tube, in the part closest to the ovary. (*Refer back to Figure 22.1.*) By this time, the sperm probably number less than 250 and have already undergone changes that make fertilization possible. They cluster around the egg, each contributing an enzyme that works to dissolve the outer layer of the ovum. When one sperm finally penetrates the ovum, the lining of the ovum immediately changes, preventing additional sperm from entering. Thus, only one sperm combines its genetic material with the egg.

The initial fertilized egg is called a **zygote.** Within about 36 hours of fertilization, cell division begins. This division continues as the egg is moved by the action of hairlike structures (called cilia) through the fallopian tube toward the **uterus,** the site where the baby grows and is nourished until birth. The trip is a relatively slow one, taking about 3–5 days.

Once in the uterus, the fertilized egg (now called a *blastocyst*) floats around for a day or two before it burrows itself into the **endometrium,** the lining of the uterus; this burrowing is called **implantation.** (*Refer back to Figure 22.1.*)

For 8 weeks after fertilization, the product of conception is called an **embryo.** From the beginning of the ninth week on, it is called a **fetus.** In most cases, a fetus cannot sustain life outside the uterus before the 24th week.

The Gambling Casino of Reproduction As we have described it, conception might seem to be a fairly unusual occurrence, a hit-or-miss proposition. In fact, this may seem to be the case for the many couples who want to have a child and discover they cannot conceive. In general, however, the chances of pregnancy for a couple having unprotected intercourse over a 1-year period is 85–90%. As the number of unplanned pregnancies in the United States indicates—about 1 million unplanned adolescent pregnancies occur every year and 1.5 million abortions are performed annually—the gambling casino of reproduction all too frequently works in nature's favor. Still, almost all U.S.

women—95% of those who have ever had sex—use contraceptives at some time.[31]

Avoidance of unwanted pregnancies requires the practice of **contraception** or **birth control,** the prevention of ovulation, fertilization, and/or implantation.

Choosing a Contraceptive Method

Methods of contraception vary greatly in effectiveness, side effects, cost, and other matters. Here we consider abstinence, douching, withdrawal, vaginal spermicides, vaginal sponges, condoms, diaphragms, cervical caps, IUDs, oral contraceptives, implants, injectable contraceptives, tubal sterilization, and vasectomy.

There are many different contraceptive methods. Today, however, concerns about preventing pregnancy often have to be linked with concerns about protection from sexually transmitted diseases. In general, for anyone who is sexually active and not involved in a long-term, mutually monogamous heterosexual relationship, these two concerns come down to a single method of contraception and protection that can be used with other methods: condoms combined with **nonoxynol-9,** an antiviral, antibacterial spermicidal agent. Heterosexual couples who need not worry about STDs, however, have a great many choices in contraception.

Choices Available: Five Categories of Birth Control There are many criteria for choosing a method of contraception, ranging from availability, to effectiveness, to cost, to considerations of personal comfort, health, and religious beliefs. (*See Self Discovery 22.1.*) Since no method of contraception is 100% effective, a combination of methods is recommended.

The five categories of birth control are:

1. *Natural family planning methods:* Various methods that include a period of abstinence, such as fertility awareness, the rhythm method, or withdrawal are examples of natural family planning methods of preventing conception.

2. *Barrier methods:* Condoms, diaphragms, and the vaginal contraceptive sponges are examples of contraceptive devices that put physical barriers between egg and sperm.

3. *Chemical methods:* Vaginal spermicides are examples of chemical contraceptives that destroy sperm. The contraceptive sponge is both a barrier and a chemical contraceptive. Oral contraceptives—The Pill—are chemical or hormonal contraceptives that prevent ovulation or implantation.

4. *Invasive methods:* Intrauterine devices (IUDs), male sterilization (vasectomy), and female sterilization (tubal sterilization) are methods that require that the body be entered ("invaded") in order to insert a device or perform surgery for the purpose of contraception.

5. *After-intercourse methods:* The morning-after pill (RU 486) is an example of an after-intercourse contraceptive option.

We describe contraceptive methods from these five categories, proceeding from contraceptive methods that are *least effective* to those that are *most effective.* (See ● *Figure 22.2.*)

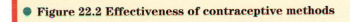

● **Figure 22.2 Effectiveness of contraceptive methods**

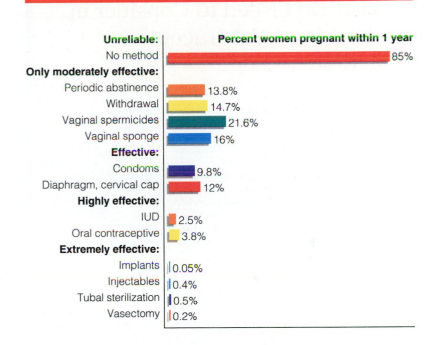

	Percent women pregnant within 1 year
Unreliable:	
No method	85%
Only moderately effective:	
Periodic abstinence	13.8%
Withdrawal	14.7%
Vaginal spermicides	21.6%
Vaginal sponge	16%
Effective:	
Condoms	9.8%
Diaphragm, cervical cap	12%
Highly effective:	
IUD	2.5%
Oral contraceptive	3.8%
Extremely effective:	
Implants	0.05%
Injectables	0.4%
Tubal sterilization	0.5%
Vasectomy	0.2%

No Method At All Using no method of contraception at all has the highest failure rate for birth control: in one study, 85% of women ages 15–44 who didn't think they were infertile were estimated to have become pregnant within 1 year.[32] This was at least four times as high as the rate among those using *any* method of birth control.

Breast-Feeding Nursing delays fertility in many women after childbirth. However, it is an unreliable form of birth control, since no one can predict in whom ovulation is suppressed and for how long. About 80% of women ovulate before their menstrual periods return after childbirth. Nursing mothers should therefore use other methods of contraception.

Douching The practice of rinsing out the vagina with a chemical right after sexual intercourse is called **douching.** From the standpoint of birth control, it is almost worthless. Douching is an attempt to "wash out" the ejaculate. Instead, however, it often brings the sperm into contact with the cervix. Moreover, some sperm are able to enter the uterus within seconds of ejaculation, before a woman has a chance to begin douching.[33]

Periodic Abstinence The voluntary avoidance of sexual intercourse is called **abstinence.** Periodic abstinence goes under the names of **fertility awareness, natural family planning,** and the **rhythm method.** All three terms refer to the avoidance of sexual intercourse during perceived fertile periods of the woman's menstrual cycle.

This method cannot be used by women who have irregular menstrual cycles or who are at risk for STD exposure owing to unprotected intercourse. Using this method to prevent pregnancy requires a motivated, knowledgeable couple who has undergone training. The couple must be able to abstain or use another contraceptive method during those times the woman is estimated to be at risk for fertility. Actually, the method has been successfully used by some couples who are not trying to *prevent* conception but are attempting to become pregnant.

SELF DISCOVERY 22.1

What Do I Need to Consider in Choosing a Contraceptive Method?

If you are considering choosing a method of contraception, apply the following criteria to see if that method seems right for you. Answer the following yes or no:

	Yes	No
1. *Effectiveness:* Am I satisfied this method is effective enough in preventing pregnancy?	____	____
2. *Comfort:* Will I find this method personally acceptable and comfortable? (For example, women uncomfortable with touching themselves may find a diaphragm difficult to use.)	____	____
3. *Safety:* Do I consider this method safe enough for me? (For example, although oral contraceptives are relatively safe for non-smokers under age 35, they do have the potential for serious side effects.)	____	____
4. *Cost:* Is this method affordable on an annual basis?	____	____
5. *STDs:* Are my sexual relationships such that I should be concerned that the contraceptive method be effective against sexually transmitted diseases?	____	____
6. *Protection:* Does the method I am considering offer protection against STDs?	____	____
7. *Access:* Do I have access to the kind of health care that will make this method available to me? (For example, oral contraceptives, the IUD, and Norplant require a prescription.)	____	____
8. *Health:* Do I have existing health problems that would prohibit use of this method?	____	____
9. *Religion:* Is this method compatible with my religious beliefs?	____	____
10. *Partner:* Are there concerns about this method I must consult about my sexual partner? (Examples are cost, personal preference, issues of shared responsibility.)	____	____

The time in a woman's cycle when she is at increased risk of ovulation is assessed in four ways: by the *calendar method,* the *basal-body-temperature method,* the *cervical mucus method,* and the *sympto-thermal method:*

- *Calendar method:* The **calendar method** involves counting days. Each month for 6–12 months the first day of the menstrual period is charted on a calendar. At the end of this time, the shortest and longest cycles are determined. (See • *Figure 22.3.*) A cycle ranges from day 1 of one menstrual period to day 1 of the next menstrual period. A formula then is used to estimate the days of the month a woman is most likely to be fertile. Needless to say, this method alone is not particularly reliable, given that women can ovulate at unpredictable times.

- *Basal-body-temperature (BBT) method:* In the **basal-body-temperature (BBT) method,** a woman uses a special thermometer to record her body temperature daily *immediately* upon waking (before going to the bathroom or any physical activity). Records are kept for 6–12 months. The pattern that many women experience is a slight drop in *basal body temperature* 1–3 days before ovulation, then a sharp rise marks the beginning of ovulation. (See • *Figure 22.4.*) Ovulation is confirmed if the rise is sustained at least 3 days. It is unsafe to have intercourse from the day the temperature drops until 3 days after it rises.

- *Cervical mucus method:* The **cervical mucus method** (Billings method, or fertility awareness method) requires that a woman evaluate the appearance, amount, and consistency of the daily mucus discharge from her cervix. Unsafe days for intercourse are indicated by a discharge that is clear, thin, and elastic rather than cloudy and thick. With this method, which must be learned from a family-planning professional or physician, a woman has to abstain from intercourse 9–15 days out of each cycle.

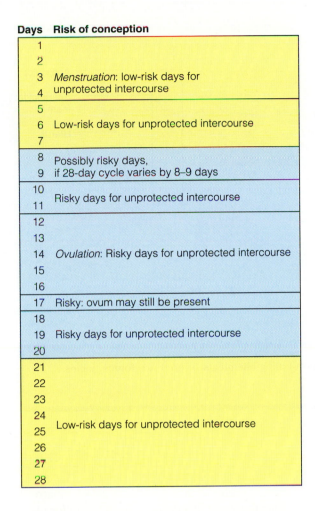

Days	Risk of conception
1	
2	
3	*Menstruation*: low-risk days for
4	unprotected intercourse
5	
6	Low-risk days for unprotected intercourse
7	
8	Possibly risky days,
9	if 28-day cycle varies by 8–9 days
10	
11	Risky days for unprotected intercourse
12	
13	
14	*Ovulation*: Risky days for unprotected intercourse
15	
16	
17	Risky: ovum may still be present
18	
19	Risky days for unprotected intercourse
20	
21	
22	
23	
24	
25	Low-risk days for unprotected intercourse
26	
27	
28	

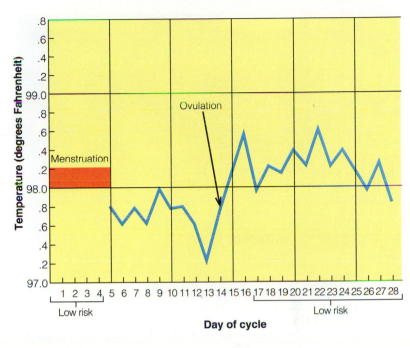

● **Figure 22.4 The BBT method**

● **Figure 22.3 The calendar method.** Most women's cycles are not a consistent 28 days but may vary up to 9 days (21–35 days). This method is *not* reliable.

• *Sympto-thermal method:* The **sympto-thermal method** combines all three previous methods—calendar, BBT, and the cervical mucus—and provides the most reliable means of determining high- and low-risk times for sexual intercourse.

One of the problems with the methods described above is that ovulation is difficult to accurately and consistently predict. The only relatively accurate way to determine ovulation is by hindsight: one can look *back* on day 1 of the menstrual period and say that 2 weeks *ago* ovulation probably occurred. The problem, however, is in trying to predict ovulation *ahead* of time.

Withdrawal The birth-control technique known as **withdrawal,** or **coitus interruptus,** which dates back to biblical times, consists of removing the penis from the vagina before ejaculation, so that no sperm are deposited in or around the vagina. This is an unreliable contraceptive method with a failure rate of 15% to 18%. Probably one reason is that withdrawal requires unusual willpower, but in any case all it takes is the small amount of pre-ejaculatory fluid from Cowper's glands that appears at the end of the penis during sexual arousal to cause a pregnancy—the fluid contains some sperm.

Vaginal Spermicides Alone Vaginal spermicides are sperm-killing chemicals, such as

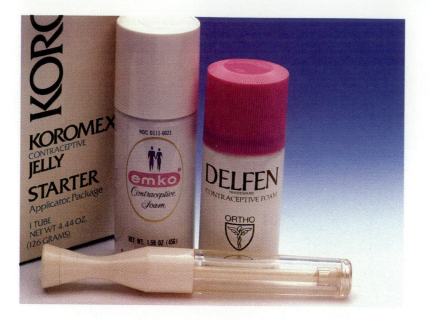

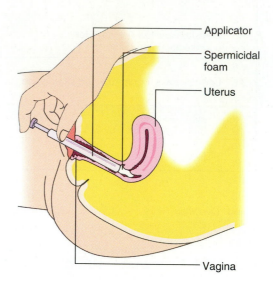

Applicator

Spermicidal
foam

Uterus

Vagina

● **Figure 22.5 Vaginal spermicides.** Among the sperm-killing chemicals offered are foams, jellies, creams, suppositories, and films.

spermicidal foam, cream, jelly, film, or suppositories, which are placed in the vagina within 30 minutes or so before intercourse, depending on product instuctions. (*See* ● *Figure 22.5.*) Some require the use of an applicator. Others, such as the suppositories, require a waiting time of 10–15 minutes after insertion before intercourse can take place.

Spermicides can be effectively used as lubricants during sexual intercourse. Those that contain nonoxynol-9 also kill bacteria and viruses in addition to sperm. It is recommended that these agents be used with other methods such as condoms and diaphragms. Spermicides can be purchased without a physician's prescription in many drugstores and supermarkets. Some people are sensitive to these agents. If burning or itching occurs, switching to another brand may alleviate the problem.

One of the newer spermicide contraceptives is the **vaginal contraceptive film (VCF),** which consists of a thin, small (2-inch × 2-inch) film impregnated with nonoxynol-9. The VCF can be inserted into the vagina from 5 to 90 minutes before intercourse. Body heat causes the film to dissolve into a gel-like material that covers the cervix. It is effective for up to 2 hours. One of the chief benefits is that it can be used by people who are allergic to foams and jellies.

Vaginal Sponge The **vaginal contraceptive sponge** is a soft, mushroom-shaped spongy disk saturated with spermicide (nonoxynol-9). (*See* ● *Figure 22.6.*) Moistened and inserted into the vagina over the cervix up to 24 hours before intercourse, the device blocks sperm from entering the uterus and kills them. The sponge is left in place for 6–8 hours after intercourse.

The vaginal sponge is a one-size-fits-all method that is available in pharmacies without prescription and does not require individual fitting. It does require that users be able to feel that the sponge is properly placed so that it covers the cervix.

Condoms Condoms present a physical barrier between sperm and egg. These thin, tight-fitting sheaths of latex rubber or animal skin are available in all kinds of colors, shapes, and textures, with or without a reservoir tip, dry or lubricated. Spermicide-coated condoms, including those with nonoxynol-9, have been shown to be effective in killing sperm.[34] When buying condoms, always check the expiration date, and don't store them in places where they might be exposed to heat (wallets, glove compartments), which causes latex to deteriorate.

The condom should be put on before any genital contact in order to prevent exposure to fluids. The condom should be held at the tip and unrolled directly onto the erect penis. Condoms without a reservoir tip need to have a half-inch left free at the tip. Gently pinch the tip to remove air bubbles, which can cause the condom to break. Petroleum-based lubricants such as Vaseline should never be used with condoms since they cause the rubber to deteriorate.

After ejaculation, the condom should be held at the base of the penis, and the penis should be immediately withdrawn from the vagina in order to avoid letting the condom slip off or semen leak out. If the condom does slip off, it should be removed from the vagina immediately, with the open end held tightly closed. If a condom appears to have torn during use or if semen has escaped into the vagina, a spermicidal agent should be inserted into the vagina immediately to help avoid conception.[35]

Note: Natural skin condoms provide effective contraception and increased sensitivity during intercourse but do not effectively prevent the transmission of some STDs, in particular HIV.[36] (*For further information on condoms, refer to Figure 21.5 in Chapter 21.*)

Diaphragm and Cervical Cap Diaphragms and cervical caps are barrier contraceptives that are always used with spermicidal creams or jellies. They are available only by prescription. Both come in various sizes and require a fitting by a health care professional to determine correct size and style.

Diaphragms and cervical caps can be inserted up to 6 hours before intercourse (although a shorter time between insertion and intercourse may afford better protection) and must remain in place for 6–8 hours afterward. Both should be checked for holes after every use (just hold them up to the light). Both increase the woman's risk of *toxic shock syn-*

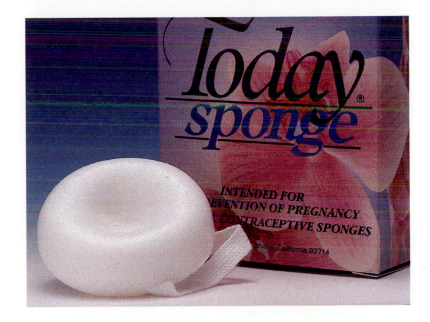

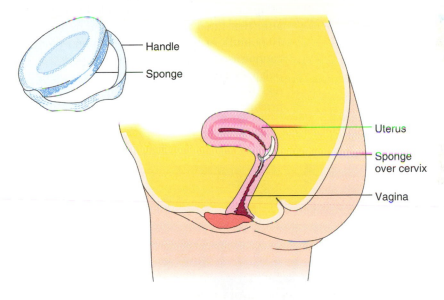

● **Figure 22.6 The vaginal sponge**

drome—a severe, potentially life-threatening bacterial infection—if they remain in the vagina for prolonged periods of time.

When used with spermicides containing nonoxynol-9, diaphragms and cervical caps may be helpful in reducing the risk of exposure to some STDs. Because they lower the risk of gonorrhea and chlamydia infection, they may help protect women against future infertility.

Let us now distinguish between the two devices:

- *Diaphragms:* A **diaphragm** is made of a soft latex rubber dome stretched over a flexible metal spring or ring. The size varies from 2 inches to 4 inches, depending on the length of the vagina. When in place, the diaphragm covers the ceiling of the vagina, including the cervix. (See ● *Figure 22.7.*) It works primarily by holding spermicide in contact with the cervix and by blocking sperm from entering the cervix. If possible, diaphragms should be removed before 24 hours has elapsed from the time of insertion. They should not, however, be removed within 6 hours of the last act of intercourse.

  Diaphragms can be reused for a period of up to 1 year. A refitting should be done after that time, after a weight gain or loss of 10 pounds, or after childbirth. Some women cannot use a diaphragm, owing to poor pelvic muscle tone. Some diaphragm users may be more prone to urethral irritation or urinary tract infections.

- *Cervical caps:* The **cervical cap** operates in much the same way as the diaphragm. This is a much smaller, thimble-shaped rubber or plastic cap that fits directly onto the cervix. (See ● *Figure 22.8.*) Insertion of the cervical cap tends to present more of a challenge to first-time users than does the diaphragm.

  Unlike diaphragm users, cervical cap users do not need to reapply spermicide with each subsequent intercourse after insertion. In addition, they can leave the cap in place for up to 48 hours. Not all women can use the cap, owing to fitting problems or problems with cervical damage.

The IUD The **IUD,** the abbreviation for the **intrauterine device,** is a small plastic device that is placed inside the uterus. (See ● *Figure 22.9.*) The IUD, which must be inserted by a

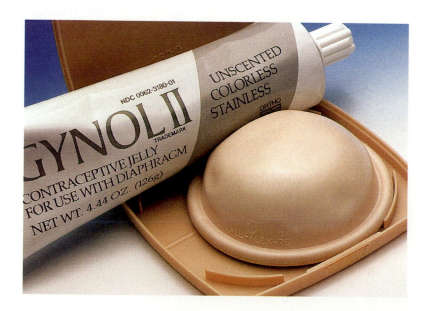

● **Figure 22.7 The diaphragm**

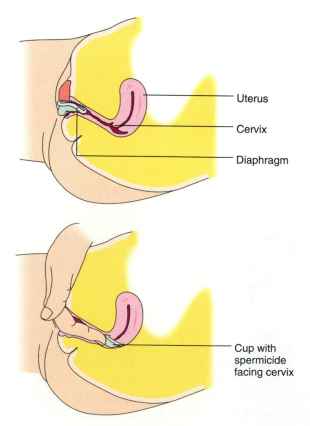

Uterus

Cervix

Diaphragm

Cup with spermicide facing cervix

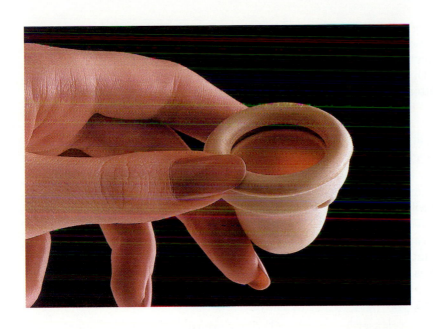

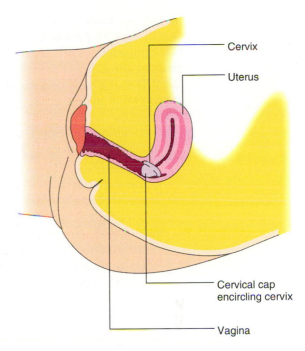

Cervix

Uterus

Cervical cap
encircling cervix

Vagina

● **Figure 22.8 The cervical cap**

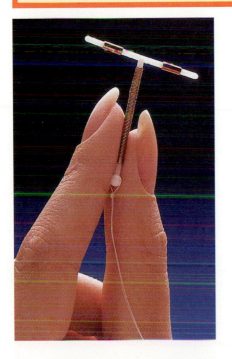

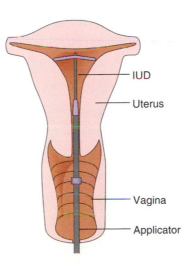

IUD

Uterus

Vagina

Applicator

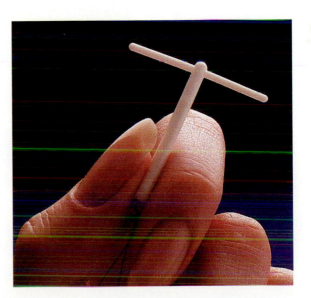

● **Figure 22.9 The IUD.** Two types of intrauterine devices are shown, copper (Paragard T 380A) (*left*) and medicated (Progestasert) (*right*).

health care professional, may prevent fertilization in some women or, if fertilization takes place, interferes with implantation because it changes the lining of the uterus. Once inserted, the IUD string must be located after every menstrual period to be sure the device remains in place.

Depending on the type used, an IUD may remain in the uterus for 1–6 years. Presently two principal types are:

- *Copper-T:* The *copper* (Paragard) IUD is made of plastic and covered with fine copper wire. The copper seems to cause biochemical reactions in the uterine lining, which interferes with implantation. The IUD may be worn for as long as 6 years, after which it must be replaced because the copper is completely dissolved.

- *Medicated:* The *medicated* (Progestasert) IUD contains the hormone progesterone, which inhibits implantation and also reduces cramping. The device must be replaced after 1 year, when the hormone has run out.

Because IUDs increase users' risk of pelvic infection and infertility, women planning to use the device should try to meet certain criteria: be over 25, have at least one child, not have a history of menstrual cramps or other reproductive-system problems, be certain they are free of STDs, be in mutually monogamous long-term relationships, and have access to health care.

Oral Contraceptives The **oral contraceptive** or **birth-control pill,** famously known as simply The Pill, consists of synthetic female hormones that prevent ovulation or implantation. (*See* ● *Figure 22.10.*) It is one of the most effective *reversible* birth control method available (surgery, for instance, may not be reversible). Nearly 14 million women use the pill in the United States, and it appears to be the contraceptive of choice among women ages 15–24.[37]

There are three basic types of pills—the combination, the multiphasic, and the minipill:

- *Combination pill:* The **combination pill** contains two hormones, *estrogen* and *progesterone*. These hormones, independently or together, prevent pregnancy in three ways:

 (1) They primarily prevent ovulation.

 (2) They change the mucus in the cervix, making it difficult for the sperm to enter the cervix.

 (3) They change the lining of the uterus, preventing implantation.

 The combination pill provides a steady dosage of the two hormones, estrogen and progesterone. The pill is taken for 21 days, with 7 days off.

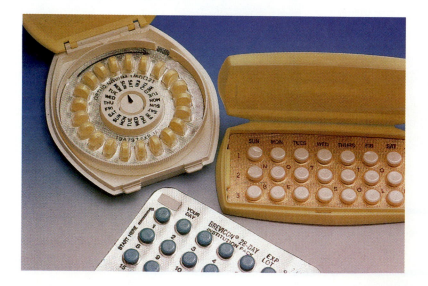

● **Figure 22.10 Oral contraceptives.** Pills are taken daily for 3 weeks, then stopped during the fourth week to allow menstruation to occur.

- *Multiphasic pill:* The **multiphasic pill** is a variation on the combination pill. Whereas the combination pill provides a steady dosage of the two hormones, the multiphasic pill provides a changing dosage of estrogen and progesterone that more nearly mimics the body's natural cycle of hormones.

  Like the combination pill, the multiphasic pill is taken for 21 days, with 7 days off.

- *Minipill:* The **minipill** contains progesterone only. It thus has fewer side effects than the other two, but it is also less effective in preventing pregnancy. Because it contains no estrogen, the minipill does not consistently prevent ovulation. It does, however, change cervical mucus and change the lining of the uterus.

  Unlike the combination and multiphasic pills, the minipill is taken every day.

Users should check with their health care practitioner regarding the pill-taking schedule and find out what to do in the event a pill is missed.

Oral contraceptives have several advantages and disadvantages that any prospective user must weigh:

- *Advantages:* Besides their effectiveness in preventing pregnancy, oral contraceptives have the following benefits:[38]

  (1) They tend to reduce menstrual cramps and the amount of menstrual flow.

  (2) They regulate the menstrual period— that is, help women with irregular cycles have regular periods.

  (3) They decrease the incidence of non-cancerous (benign) breast disease, ovarian cysts, and *endometriosis* (the growth of endometrial tissue outside the uterus, such as the ovaries and fallopian tubes).

  (4) They reduce the incidence of ovarian and endometrial (uterine lining) cancer.

  (5) They may even help reduce the incidence of rheumatoid arthritis.

- *Disadvantages:* Unfortunately, oral contraceptives also have significant disadvantages:

  (1) One of the biggest is that they do not protect the user against STDs, including HIV.

  (2) They increase the risk of blood clots (especially in the legs), stroke, migraine headaches, gallbladder disease, and benign liver tumors.

  (3) They cause 1 in 20 pill users to develop hypertension, a risk factor in heart disease.[39]

  (4) For smokers, they cause increased cardiovascular risks. For users of combination pills in particular, there is increased risk of heart attacks, especially for women over the age of 35 who are smokers.

  (5) They may cause swollen, tender breasts, nausea, and weight gain, especially among new users. However, these symptoms often subside after 1–3 months of use.

  (6) Users may also experience acne, a change in their sex drive, mood swings or depression, spotting between menstrual periods, and vaginal yeast infections.

  (7) Women are often concerned about the risk of breast cancer with use of The Pill. The association between the two is inconclusive. It may be that users of oral contraceptives simply are screened for breast cancer more frequently than nonusers are, so that their breast cancers are detected earlier.[40]

Women who are not good candidates for oral contraceptive use are those with a history of blood clots, stroke, heart disease, impaired liver function, or cancer. Those with diabetes, migraine headaches, hypertension, mononucleosis, or other problems should discuss the risks with a health care practitioner.

Despite the side effects, use of oral contraceptives is relatively safe if the user is knowledgeable about the risks and is monitored by a health care professional. It may help to realize that *any* method of contraception, including use of The Pill, is safer than pregnancy. For pregnancy, the risk of death is 1 in 10,000; for a pill user who is a smoker the risk is 1 in 16,000, and for a nonsmoker it is 1 in 63,000.[41]

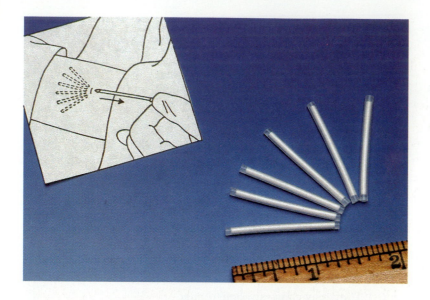

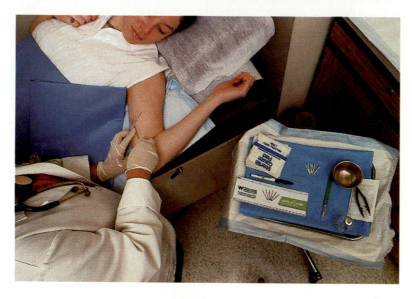

● **Figure 22.11 Implants.** Norplant silicone rods surgically implanted in a woman's arm release progestin over a 5-year period.

Implant Contraceptive (Norplant) In 1990, the FDA approved for use in the United States contraceptives called *implants,* marketed under the brand name *Norplant.* Norplant consists of small, removable silicone-rubber rods or capsules filled with synthetic progestin, which are embedded in a woman's arm or leg. (*See* ● *Figure 22.11.*) The capsules, which can be implanted surgically by a physician in 15 minutes using a local anesthetic, release low levels of synthetic progestin, preventing ovulation and thickening the cervical mucus, to prevent sperm from entering the uterus. The implants may stay in place for 5 years and can be removed surgically if a woman wants to become pregnant.

Some women experience irregular patterns of menstrual bleeding, but otherwise side effects appear minimal. Implants are considered extremely effective, with only an estimated 0.05% of women becoming pregnant in the first year.

Injectable Contraceptive (Depo-Provera) An *injectable contraceptive* known as *Depo-Provera,* finally approved for use in the United States in 1992 by the FDA, consists of a long-lasting progestin that is administered once every 3 months. (*See* ● *Figure 22.12.*) During the time between injections, a woman has no menstrual periods or irregular ones. Fertility returns after the use of injectables is discontinued.

The risk of pregnancy from injectable contraceptives is extremely low—only 0.4% of women are estimated to become pregnant within the first year.

Tubal Sterilization—Female Sterilization
Sterilization is the surgical—and generally permanent—interruption of a person's reproductive capacity, whether male or female, preventing the normal passage of sperm or ova. Sterilization is the most popular contraceptive method among American couples. In females, the procedure is called **tubal sterilization** and is accomplished by blocking or cutting the fallopian tubes, thus preventing the passage of the egg through the fallopian tube to the uterus. (*See* ● *Figure 22.13.*) Tubal sterilization may take the form of either **tubal ligation,** the cutting and tying of the fallopian tubes, or **tubal**

occlusion, the blocking of the tubes by cauterizing (burning) or by use of a clamp, clip, or band of silicone. Either way, tubal sterilization is extremely effective: only an estimated 0.5% of women become pregnant within the first year after the procedure, probably because of improperly performed operations.

There are three procedures for accomplishing tubal sterilization: *laparotomy, laparoscopy,* and *colpotomy.* The choice of method often has to do with the surgeon's skill, the potential for reversibility (in case a woman decides she later wants to have children), the place and extent of the incision, and the anticipated anesthesia and length of hospitalization needed.

- *Laparotomy:* In a **laparotomy,** a surgeon makes a 2-inch-long incision in the woman's abdomen and cuts the fallopian tubes. The procedure is performed with anesthesia in a hospital and requires up to 5 days' stay in the hospital, as well as several weeks of recovery at home.

  A laparotomy leaves a 2-inch scar. A **minilaparotomy** attempts to make the scar less visible by making a 1-inch-long incision just above the pubic hairline. Often the minilaparotomy can be done under local anesthesia in just 30 minutes, and the patient can go home the same day.

- *Laparoscopy:* In a **laparoscopy,** the most common means of female sterilization, a tube-like instrument called a laparoscope is inserted through a half-inch incision in the area of the navel. After the abdomen is filled with carbon dioxide, the procedure of closing the fallopian tubes is accomplished with instruments inserted through the laparoscope. Called "Band-Aid" surgery, because the incision can be closed with a single stitch, the operation may be performed in 30 minutes and the patient discharged in a few hours.

- *Colpotomy:* In a **colpotomy** (sometimes spelled *culpotomy),* an incision is made through the back of the vagina (the *cul de sac*). Though the operation leaves no outside scar, it is somewhat more difficult and hazardous.

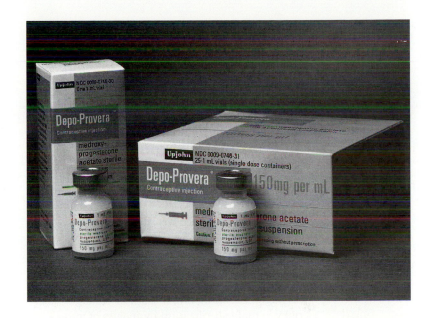

● **Figure 22.12 Injectable contraceptive.** Depo-Provera is injected once every 3 months.

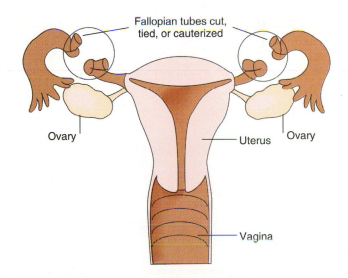

● **Figure 22.13 Female sterilization: tubal sterilization.** The fallopian tubes are interrupted surgically—cut and tied or blocked—to prevent passage of the eggs from the ovaries to the uterus.

About 3% of women who have tubal sterilizations later seek to have the procedure reversed, but in only about half the cases of restoration surgery (an expensive operation) is the woman actually able to have children.[42,43] Clearly, then, a woman should be sure that she does not want to have children before having tubal sterilization.

Sterilization may also be a consequence of operations intended for other purposes. For example, a **hysterectomy,** removal of the uterus because of cancer or other disorders, will result in sterilization. So will an **ovariectomy** (also called an *oopherectomy*), removal of the ovaries, for similar reasons.

The risks associated with female sterilization are low but include such problems as hemorrhage, infection, and intestinal damage. Less risky is male sterilization by means of vasectomy, as we discuss next.

Vasectomy—Male Sterilization Male sterilization is accomplished by means of a **vasectomy,** a surgical procedure that involves making a pair of incisions in the scrotum and cutting and tying the two sperm-carrying tubes called

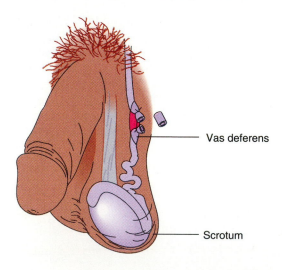

Vas deferens

Scrotum

● **Figure 22.14 Male sterilization: vasectomy.** A pair of incisions is made in the scrotum, and the vas deferens—the tubes connecting the testes and the urethra—are cut and tied off to prevent the passage of sperm to the urethra.

the *vas deferens*. (See ● *Figure 22.14*.) The vas deferens connect the testes, which produce the sperm, with the urethra, through which semen is ejaculated. After vasectomy, sperm continue to form, but are absorbed by the body. The man continues to be able to have erections, enjoy orgasms, and produce semen, but the ejaculate contains no sperm cells.

Vasectomies, which can be performed as a 20-minute procedure in a doctor's office with local anesthetic, are considered extremely effective: only 0.2% of women whose mates have had vasectomies are estimated to become pregnant in the first year. Failures may result because the vasectomy was improperly performed or because the couple engaged in unprotected sex before all sperm had disappeared from the ejaculate (normally about 8 weeks or 5–15 ejaculations after the operation). Although vasectomy is a relatively safe procedure, there may be complications owing to swelling, infection, or hemorrhage.

A man contemplating a vasectomy should proceed as though the procedure were irreversible. Although 90% of the operations to reopen the tubes are successful, only 40–70% result in the ability to father children.[44]

New Directions

Methods of birth control that are relatively recent or still under development include the female condom, vaginal ring, RU 486 pill, and male contraceptive pill.

Numerous new contraceptives and barrier devices against STDs are in development, but the approval process by the Food and Drug Administration puts the United States behind Europe in releasing these for use.[45,46] As you read this, some of the following may have become recently available.

Female Condom One of the more promising contraceptive devices is the female condom. Already sold in Europe, the *female condom* or *vaginal pouch* (brand name: Reality) is a soft, loose-fitting polyurethane sheath, about 6½ inches long, that lines the vagina.[47] It is held in place by two flexible plastic rings, a 2-inch-diameter ring outside the body and a 1½-inch-diameter ring at the cervix. (*See ● Figure 22.15.*) This one-time-use-only device is inserted much like a diaphragm.

Alternative women's condoms under development are the Women's Choice Female Condomme, which is inserted with an applicator (like a tampon), and the Unisex Condom Garment, a polyurethane "bikini condom" with attached sheath, which becomes a penis cover or a vaginal liner, depending on which sex wears it.

Vaginal Ring The *vaginal ring* is something like a diaphragm, but is worn for 3 months before being replaced. Each ring slowly releases estrogen and progestin (or progestin alone), and the hormones are slowly absorbed into the blood through the vagina. The vaginal ring has been found to be comparable in safety to other low-dose, progestogen-only contraceptives.[48]

RU 486 Pill Developed in France, **RU 486** is a hormonal compound available in pill form that can be used to terminate a pregnancy within 5 weeks of conception. The pill works by blocking the action of progesterone, a hormone that enables the endometrial lining to be retained during pregnancy and prevents uterine contractions. By blocking progesterone, RU 486 induces menstrual bleeding and uterine contractions, thus expelling the fertilized egg. Women experience some discomfort, which has been compared to menstrual cramps. One study found that RU 486 was effective 96% of the time when the drug was taken within 49 days of a missed period.[49] Researchers have also found that it can enable women to avoid abortions by serving as an effective morning-after pill, when taken within 72 hours of unprotected intercourse.[50]

Over 100,00 women have used RU 486 in Europe, but as of this writing it is not generally available in the United States. It may also not be imported into the United States for personal use, a government ban upheld by the U.S. Supreme Court in 1992.[51] As far as seeking to obtain the drug abroad, both France and Britain restrict the drug to residents.[52]

Male Contraceptive Pill For several years there have been attempts to develop a contraceptive pill for males, particularly since, according to one study by the World Health Organiza-

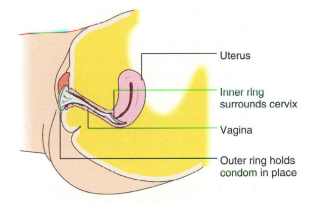

Uterus

Inner ring surrounds cervix

Vagina

Outer ring holds condom in place

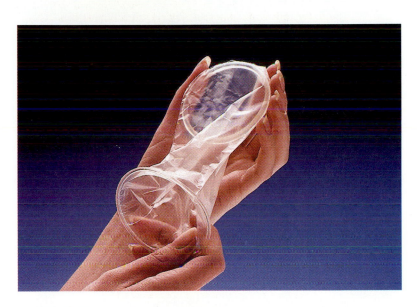

● **Figure 22.15 The female condom.** The 6½-inch-long sheath lines the vagina, held in place by two plastic rings.

tion, 75% of men would welcome a reliable non-surgical form of male contraception.[53]

Among the possibilities are the following:

● *The gossypol pill, the Chinese solution:* Derived from cottonseed, **gossypol** has been used in China in pill form for over a decade to reduce sperm counts. Fertility generally returns after the pill is discontinued, although it is reported that in up to 20% of cases fertility has not come back within a year's time.[54] Recently, however, U.S. expectations for the "Chinese wonder drug" have dissipated.

- *TE shots, synthetic male hormone:* Injecting males once a week with *TE* (for testosterone enanthate), a synthetic version of the male sex hormone, has been under study by the World Health Organization. TE has been found to suppress sperm production and to be as effective a form of contraception as female injectable contraceptives and better than the IUD, pill, or condom.[55]

800-HELP

Planned Parenthood Federation of America. 800-829-7732. Information on contraception and abortion

Suggestion for Further Reading

Consumers Union. (1989, March). Can you rely on condoms? *Consumer Reports,* pp. 135–141. Consumers Union tested condoms in 1989 and listed 43 brands and models in terms of their features and their performance in resisting breaking.

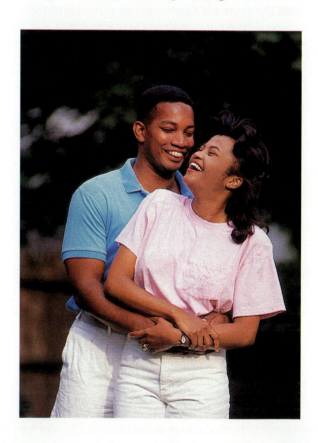

23   Abortion

▶ Name five principal types of induced abortion.

▶ Describe the emotional effects of abortion on women with unintended pregnancies.

Abortion is the removal or expulsion of an embryo or fetus from the uterus of a pregnant woman before it can survive on its own. An abortion can happen spontaneously, owing to medical, hormonal, genetic, or other problems, in which case it is called a **spontaneous abortion** or **miscarriage.** A spontaneous abortion is a miscarriage that occurs within the first 20 weeks of pregnancy. About 20% of all pregnancies end in a spontaneous abortion, most of which happen during the first 3 months (trimester) of pregnancy. A miscarriage often represents a significant loss to the woman and her partner that must be grieved for.

In contrast with spontaneous abortions, **induced** or **elective abortions** are those in which a decision has been made to purposefully terminate a pregnancy. Every year over a million women terminate their pregnancies by means of abortion.

Types of Induced Abortion

Five principal methods of induced abortion, ranging from those appropriate earlier in pregnancy to those late in pregnancy, are suction curettage, D and C, D and E, saline induction or use of prostaglandins, and hysterotomy.

Five principal methods of induced abortion that we will describe (there are others as well) are as follows:

- Suction curettage
- D and C
- D and E
- Saline induction/use of prostaglandins
- Hysterotomy

Each method is appropriate for a different stage or stages of pregnancy. From a medical standpoint, abortions are least risky during the first 3 months of pregnancy. During the second 3 months, the woman is more apt to suffer complications. Abortions are generally not performed after the 24th week of pregnancy.

Suction Curettage: Performed in First 12 Weeks The most common method of abortion—96% of all abortions are induced with this method—is **suction curettage,** which is usually performed during weeks 6–12.[56] The procedure itself usually takes about 10–15 minutes. After the cervix is numbed with a local anesthetic, the cervix is dilated. A small, plastic tube called a curette is then inserted into the woman's cervix into the uterus. The curette is attached to a suction pump, and the contents of the uterus are then drawn out into the vacuum system. (See ● *Figure 23.1.*)

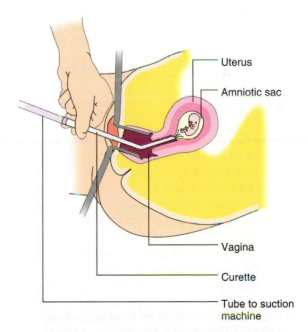

Uterus

Amniotic sac

Vagina

Curette

Tube to suction machine

● **Figure 23.1 Suction curettage.** The contents of the uterus are sucked out with a suction machine. This method is most often used during the first 3 months of pregnancy.

When performed during the first trimester, this kind of abortion usually takes place in a clinic or physician's office. Although suction curettage is one of the safest surgical procedures when performed by a trained, experienced health care professional, like any other surgical procedure there can be side effects. Such side effects include perforation of the uterus, bleeding, uterine cramping, or incomplete evacuation of the uterine contents.

D and C, Dilation and Curettage: Performed in Weeks 9–14 A benefit of suction curettage is that it reduces the risk of the physician accidentally perforating the uterus. From the 9th to 14th weeks, however, a physician will often use the **D and C** technique, which stands for **dilation and curettage.** In this surgical procedure, after general anesthesia has been administered, the cervical canal is **dilated**— that is, gradually expanded. The physician then uses a small, spoon-shaped instrument called a **curette** to scrape the uterine wall of fetal tissue. Hospitalization is usually required for a D and C because of the risk of perforation of the uterus and bleeding and infection. A D and C is rarely used to perform abortions today because it requires general anesthesia and wider cervical dilation, and it results in more blood loss than suction curettage.

D and E, Dilation and Evacuation: Performed in Weeks 13–20 Similar to the D and C method, **D and E** techniques stand for **dilation and evacuation.** Performed with general anesthesia in a hospital, because of the risk of perforation, the D and E first involves dilation of the cervix. Then the physician uses a combination of suction curettage and forceps (an instrument for grasping) to extract fetal tissue the suction machine has been unable to remove.

Saline Induction/Use of Protaglandins: Performed in Weeks 16–20 The **saline-induction method,** or **instillation,** uses what is known as a hypertonic saline (salt) solution, which is injected (instilled) through a needle by a physician through the abdominal wall and into the amniotic sac surrounding the fetus. This induces the uterus to simulate labor, which results in the expulsion of the fetus within 24 hours.

Instead of using salt solutions, physicians may also use **prostaglandins,** naturally occurring hormone-like substances, which produce labor contractions faster but may also cause vomiting and diarrhea.

Hysterotomy: Performed in Weeks 16–24 A **hysterotomy,** which should not be confused with a hysterectomy (removal of the uterus), is a surgical procedure performed late in a woman's pregnancy, in weeks 16–24, mainly when the woman's life is in danger and when saline-induction or other abortion methods are considered too risky. Called a "small cesarean section," this procedure, which requires that the woman be in a hospital and under general anesthesia, consists of the physician's making a surgical incision in the abdomen and uterus and removing the fetus.

After the 24th Week After week 24, abortion by any method is not considered advisable, or at least will not be performed by very many doctors. This can create a great deal of anxiety and hardship for women and their partners who discover late in a pregnancy (via sonogram or other technology) that the fetus is severely deformed or brain-damaged and want to exercise the option of a legal abortion.[57]

Abortion, Psychological Health, and Moral Issues

Abortion is only one alternative; bringing the baby to term is another. Abortion may be emotionally difficult for the woman if the child is wanted but is often not if the child is not wanted. Some women denied abortions experience difficulties in later life. Abortion is an issue about which there is much disagreement in the United States.

It needs to be mentioned that there are alternatives to abortion, of course. Assuming absence of a serious threat to a woman's life or health, the pregnancy can be carried to term. The child can then be kept, placed for adoption, or placed in a foster home. Abortion is therefore one of several available options regarding pregnancy.

Women who have planned or wanted pregnancies and then lose their babies, as in a spontaneous abortion (miscarriage), may become quite distraught, although some seem not to be affected at all.[58] How, then, might women be expected to react psychologically to an *induced* abortion?

In some ways, the reactions are predictable: The more a pregnancy is wanted and is personally meaningful to the woman, the more difficult emotionally abortion may be for her and her partner. On the other hand, if a pregnancy is unintended and holds little personal meaning, women seem not to experience negative psychological responses—provided the idea of abortion does not violate their deeply held values or beliefs or have a perceived social stigma. In point of fact, emotional distress is usually greatest *before* an abortion rather than afterward, when women frequently report relief and other positive emotions.[59,60]

Equally important, at least one study reports that women who are denied abortions only rarely give up their unwanted babies for adoption, and many harbor resentment and anger toward their children for years. In addition, the study found, children born to women whose requests for abortion were denied are much likelier to be troubled and depressed, to have drug and alcohol problems, to drop out of school, to commit crimes, to suffer from serious illnesses, and to express dissatisfaction with life than are the offspring of parents who wanted their children.[61]

Abortion is an issue about which many Americans profoundly disagree, which is why laws about it vary from state to state. Strictly from a public-health standpoint, however, it seems clear that when abortions are illegal there are many maternal deaths owing to botched illegal abortions by unqualified practitioners. In 1972, there were probably thousands of deaths from illegal abortions in the United States. The next year the U.S. Supreme Court upheld the case of *Roe v. Wade,* which stated that an abortion in the first 3 months of pregnancy is a matter to be determined by a woman and her physician (and can be performed in later months on the basis of health risks and the danger to the mother's health). By 1985, there were only six deaths from abortion—making it safer than pregnancy or childbirth.

One writer points out that in all of human history, no culture has been able to satisfactorily answer three questions: When is a fetus a person? What circumstances justify abortion? Who decides? And in our time abortion continues to polarize the political dialogue.[62]

800-HELP

National Abortion Federation. 800-772-9100. Consumer hotline

Planned Parenthood Federation of America. 800-829-7732. Information on contraception and abortion

Suggestions for Further Reading

Baird, Robert M., & Rosenbaum, Stuart E. (Eds.). (1989). *The ethics of abortion: Pro-life vs. pro-choice*. Buffalo, NY: Prometheus. Twelve essays on both sides of the complex issue of abortion.

Lunneborg, Patricia. (1992). *Abortion: A positive decision*. South Hadley, MA: Bergin & Garvey. A counselor and former professor at the University of Washington presents results of interviews with over 100 people who experienced abortion or work as abortion providers. Their experiences support the author's conviction that abortion is rarely a negative experience and can actually be empowering.

Developing Assertiveness: Speaking Out for Safe Sex

Safe sex is important not only for preventing AIDS but also for preventing other STDs. However, few people feel comfortable discussing the use of condoms with prospective sexual partners. How would you react, for instance, if someone said, "Hey, what's the problem? People like us don't get AIDS!" Or, "I don't like to use condoms; it's like taking a bath with your boots on." Or, "All this talk about protection spoils the mood."

Answer yes or no to the following:

I am embarrassed or would be embarrassed . . .

____ **1.** To ask a pharmacist or drug store clerk where condoms are located in the store

____ **2.** If a new partner insists or insisted that we use a condom

____ **3.** To tell my partner during foreplay that I am not willing to have sexual intercourse unless we use a condom

____ **4.** If my partner watched me dispose of a condom after we had used it

These are based on 4 of 18 questions used on a questionnaire called the Condom Embarrassment Scale.[63] (*See the Self Discovery opposite.*) If you answered "Yes" to a number of these statements, it may mean you have difficulty asserting yourself.

Embarrassment is a very frightening and powerful emotion. So is shyness. The fear of being put down, of looking like a fool, of being held in contempt, can be trivial or it can be traumatic. Being slavish in trying to avoid this fear, however, means always feeling angry, guilty, put down, self-denying. The cure for these feelings of powerlessness is *assertiveness,* a form of behavior essential to the art of living.

Assertiveness doesn't mean being pushy or selfish but rather being forthright enough to communicate your needs while respecting the needs of others. Being assertive is important not only in sexual relationships but in many other kinds of social interactions in which speaking out, standing up for yourself, or talking back is necessary.

Aggressive, Nonassertive, and Assertive Behavior

Let us see what is meant by these three types of behavior: aggressiveness, nonassertiveness, and assertiveness. Distinctions among these behaviors have been put forth by two psychologists, Robert Alberti and Michael Emmons, in two interesting, readable books, *Your Perfect Right* and *Stand Up, Speak Out, Talk Back!*[64,65]

- *Aggressiveness—expressing yourself and hurting others:* **Aggressive behavior** means you vehemently expound your opinions, accuse or blame others, and hurt others before hurting yourself.

- *Nonassertiveness—giving in to others and hurting yourself:* **Nonassertive behavior**—also called *submissive* or *passive behavior*—means consistently giving in to others on points of differences, agreeing with others regardless of your own feelings, not expressing your opinions, and hurting yourself to avoid the chance of hurting others. Nonassertive people have difficulty making requests for themselves or expressing their differences with others. In a word, they are *timid.*

- *Assertiveness—expressing yourself without hurting others or yourself:* **Assertiveness** is defined as acting in your own best interests by expressing your thoughts and feelings directly and honestly. It means standing up for yourself and openly expressing your personal feelings and opinions but at the same time not hurting either yourself or others. Assertiveness is important in enabling you to express or defend your rights.

How Embarrassed Are You About Using a Condom?

Answer each of the following by circling one of the numbers 1 through 5. The numbers represent the following reactions to the statement:

1 = strongly disagree (very low embarrassment)
2 = somewhat disagree (somewhat low embarrassment)
3 = in between

4 = somewhat agree (somewhat high embarrassment)
5 = strongly agree (very high embarrassment)

I am embarrassed or would be embarrassed . . .

1. About buying a condom from a drug store near campus.	1 2 3 4 5
2. About buying a condom from a drug store close to where my parents live.	1 2 3 4 5
3. About buying a condom from a place where I could be certain no one I know would see me.	1 2 3 4 5
4. About obtaining condoms from Student Health Services (infirmary).	1 2 3 4 5
5. About obtaining condoms from a local health department.	1 2 3 4 5
6. About asking a pharmacist or drug store clerk where condoms are located in the store.	1 2 3 4 5
7. About asking a doctor or other health care professional questions about condom use.	1 2 3 4 5
8. About stopping during foreplay and asking my partner to use a condom.	1 2 3 4 5
9. If a new partner insists/insisted that we use a condom.	1 2 3 4 5
10. To tell my partner during foreplay that I am not willing to have sexual intercourse unless we use a condom.	1 2 3 4 5
11. About being prepared and providing a condom during lovemaking if my partner didn't have one.	1 2 3 4 5
12. About carrying a condom around in my wallet/purse.	1 2 3 4 5
13. About talking to my partner about my thoughts and feelings about condom use.	1 2 3 4 5
14. If my partner watched me dispose of a condom after we had used it.	1 2 3 4 5
15. (*Female:*) About watching my partner put on a condom.	1 2 3 4 5
(*Male:*) If my partner watched me put on a condom.	1 2 3 4 5
16. (*Female:*) About helping my partner put on a condom.	1 2 3 4 5
(*Male:*) If my partner helped me put on a condom.	1 2 3 4 5
17. (*Female:*) About watching my partner remove a condom.	1 2 3 4 5
(*Male:*) If my partner watched me remove a condom.	1 2 3 4 5
18. (*Female:*) About helping my partner remove a condom.	1 2 3 4 5
(*Male:*) If my partner helped me remove a condom.	1 2 3 4 5

Score

This Condom Embarrassment Scale was developed to assess the level of embarrassment associated with condom use. The possible range of scores is 18–90, with 90 indicating the highest embarrassment and 18 indicating the lowest.

In one study at a public university in the Southeast of 163 women and 93 men, it was found that the mean score was just under 45. Women scored significantly higher than men (women about 47, compared to men about 42). This would suggest that women experience more embarrassment around condom use than men do. Scores were also higher among people who had not purchased condoms (about 50) than those who had (about 40).

Finally, scores were higher among people who were not sexually active (about 54) as opposed to those who were sexually active (about 44).

Source: Adapted from: Vail-Smith, K., Durham, T. W., & Howard, H. A. (1992). A scale to measure embarrassment associated with condom use. *Journal of Health Education, 23,* 209–214.

It's important to learn to *ask for what you want in a civilized way, without bruising the feelings of the other person*. This is what assertive behavior is all about. Consider what happens if you try aggressive or nonassertive behavior: Aggressive behavior probably won't help you get what you want because your pushiness or anger creates disharmony and alienates other people; it may also make you feel guilty about how you treated others. Nonassertive behavior also may not help you get what you want because, though it may be an attempt to please others by not offending them, it may actually make them contemptuous of you.[66] In addition, nonassertive behavior leads you to suppress your feelings, leading to self-denial and poor self-esteem.

Note that assertive behavior will *not* always get you what you want; probably no one form of behavior will. Still, it may improve your chances because, if performed correctly, the behavior is not offensive to other people, making them more willing to listen to your point of view.

Assertiveness and Gender Stereotypes

It has been suggested that behaving assertively may be more difficult for women than men, because many females have been socialized to be more passive and submissive than men.[67] For example, some women are concerned that if they act boldly in the pursuit of success they will appear unfeminine.[68] Indeed, by the college years, women are inclined to view a given kind of assertive behavior as more aggressive when engaged in by females than by males.[69]

However, many men have assertiveness problems, too. Some males have been raised to be nonassertive, others to be aggressive rather than assertive. Some researchers suggest that actually more males than females need to be trained in assertiveness in order to modify their typically more aggressive behavior.[70]

Examples of Different Behaviors

The best way to see how the different behaviors work is to show three different scenarios. Here we use an example in which a woman who is attracted to a man tells him that, for them to have sex, she wants him to wear a condom, an idea he resists:

HE: *For sex to be good for me, it has to be spontaneous and passionate. All this talk about protection, it gets in the way and turns me off.*

The aggressive response:

SHE: *Okay, so buzz off, then! You obviously don't give a damn about me!*

HE: *Hey, it's not that! I took the AIDS test two months ago, and I got a clean bill of health!*

SHE: *Yes, but you could've picked up another kind of STD that the AIDS test can't detect. How're you going to prove to me you're clean on that?*

The problem with her aggressive response is that it's apt just to infuriate him and make him even more resistant. Thus, even though she may want to have sex, she has now created a locked-horns situation where one of them must give in to the other for it to happen.

The nonassertive response:

SHE: *Well, I don't know . . .*

HE: *Look, you're just using AIDS as an excuse not to have sex with me.*

SHE: *Um . . . Oh, all right.*

If she goes ahead and has sex with him without a condom, she will not only have to worry afterward whether she has contracted an STD but will also feel she has sacrificed her self-respect. She will probably feel guilty for having had unsafe sex, guilty for having given in against her better judgment, and angry at herself (and probably him) for not having stood up for her rights. He, on the other hand, may feel contemptuous of her for having been such a pushover.

The assertive response:

SHE: *[when he says talking about protection is a "turnoff"] I've never found that talking about sex or protection gets in the way for me. It's really the opposite — once I know I don't have to worry about the consequences, I'll feel free to enjoy myself and get passionate.*

HE: *You don't have to worry about me. I took the AIDS test two months ago, and I got a clean bill of health.*

SHE: *I'm glad you're concerned enough to take the test, but it takes a while for it to turn positive, and you could have picked up the AIDS virus since then, or have something else the AIDS virus can't detect.*

HE: *You're just using AIDS as an excuse not to have sex with me.*

SHE: *No way. I like you and I want to make love with you, but I can't feel sexy unless I know I'm protected. I'm sorry, but it's a rubber or nothing.*

In this last scenario, her responses are not threatening to him. Her responses are designed not to hurt him but at the same time to express her true thoughts so that she won't get hurt herself.

We have taken most of the dialogue above from the transcript of an audio tape, "How to Talk with a Partner About Smart Sex."[71] (*See the resources at the end of this essay.*) The tape was developed by sex therapist Bernie Zilbergeld, author of the classic self-help book for men, *Male Sexuality,* and Lonnie Barbach, author of the classic self-help book for women, *For Yourself.*

Barbach and Zilbergeld also recommend that discussions of safe sex happen early in the relationship, before the clothing hits the floor. Some examples:

So, what do you think about all this AIDS business?

I don't know what to think. Sometimes I think the only answer is celibacy.

Well, I haven't gone that far yet, but I don't have sex with anyone anymore until I've gotten to know them, and then I always use condoms. How about you?

Do you think it's true what the media have been saying about AIDS? Do you think everyone is at risk?

I don't know what to think. The media have a way of blowing things out of proportion. But on the other hand, sex today can involve real risks. So I play it safe.

Yeah, how?

I'm more cautious than I used to be. I make sure I get to know people before I go to bed with them. And I always use condoms.

If some of this dialogue almost seems like a radio or television commercial for condoms, it still makes a point: the embarrassing subject of safe sex, or sex in general, *can* be talked about. What you need to do is select or make up lines you feel most at ease with and then rehearse them so you feel comfortable delivering them.

To get an idea of your assertiveness outside the realm of sex and condoms, try the other questionnaire presented here. (*See the Self Discovery on the next page.*)

Developing Assertiveness

There are different programs for developing assertiveness, but most consist of four steps:[72]

- *Learn what assertive behavior is:* First you need to learn what assertive behavior is, so that you know what it is supposed to be like. You need to learn how to consider both yours *and* others' rights.

- *Observe your own behavior in conflict situations:* You then need to monitor your own assertive (or unassertive) behavior, seeing what circumstances, people, situations, or topics make you behave aggressively or nonassertively. You may find you are able to take care of yourself (behave assertively) in some situations, but not in others.

- *Visualize a model for assertiveness:* If possible, you should try to find a model for assertiveness in the specific situations that trouble you and observe that person's behavior. Role models are important in other

How Assertive Are You?

Answer yes or no to each of the following statements.

	Yes	No
1. When a person is blatantly unfair, do you usually fail to say something about it to him or her?	___	___
2. Are you always very careful to avoid all trouble with other people?	___	___
3. Do you often avoid social contacts for fear of doing or saying the wrong thing?	___	___
4. If a friend betrays your confidence, do you tell him or her how you really feel?	___	___
5. Would you insist that a roommate do his or her fair share of cleaning?	___	___
6. When a clerk in a store waits on someone who has come in after you, do you call his or her attention to the matter?	___	___
7. Do you find that there are very few people with whom you can be relaxed and have a good time?	___	___
8. Would you be hesitant about asking a good friend to lend you a few dollars?	___	___
9. If someone who has borrowed $5 from you seems to have forgotten about it, would you remind this person?	___	___
10. If a person keeps on teasing you, do you have difficulty expressing your annoyance or displeasure?	___	___
11. Would you remain standing at the rear of a crowded auditorium rather than look for a seat up front?	___	___
12. If someone kept kicking the back of your chair in a movie, would you ask him or her to stop?	___	___
13. If a friend keeps calling you very late each evening, would you ask him or her not to call after a certain time?	___	___
14. If someone starts talking to someone else right in the middle of your conversation, do you express your irritation?	___	___
15. In a plush restaurant, if you order a medium steak and find it too rare, would you ask the waiter to have it recooked?	___	___
16. If a landlord of your apartment fails to make certain necessary repairs after promising to do so, would you insist on it?	___	___
17. Would you return a faulty garment you purchased a few days ago?	___	___
18. If someone you respect expresses opinions you strongly disagree with, would you venture to state your own point of view?	___	___
19. Are you usually able to say no when people make unreasonable requests?	___	___
20. Do you think that people should stand up for their rights?	___	___

Answers

There is no scoring system. You can figure out what the answers *should* be. Now it becomes a matter of rehearsing or role-playing the responses so that you will be able to act assertively next time the landlord fails to make repairs, your roommate fails to do his or her fair share of cleaning, or you need to ask the waiter to have your steak recooked.

Source: Lazarus, A. A. (1971). Assertive questionnaire, in *Behavior theory and beyond.* New York: McGraw-Hill.

parts of life, and this area is no exception. If possible, note how rewarding such behavior is, which will reinforce the assertive tendencies.

- *Practice assertive behavior:* Of course the only way to consistently behave assertively is to practice the behavior. You can do this as a rehearsal, carrying on an imaginary dialogue in private with yourself. Or you can actually role-play the behavior, practicing the assertive behavior with someone you're comfortable with, such as a counselor, therapist, or good friend.

Sharon and Gordon Bower, authors of *Asserting Yourself: A Practical Guide for Positive Change,* provide examples of verbal scripts that provide models of assertiveness. One technique they suggest, useful in handling most interpersonal conflicts, is that called *DESC scripts.* DESC stands for Describe, Express, Specify, and Consequences. The following examples were reproduced in Philip Zimbardo's famous book *Shyness: What It Is, What to Do About It,* which also contains many techniques helpful to nonassertive and aggressive persons.[73,74] The first example involves a dialogue with an auto mechanic who is overcharging you, the second a wife's discussion with her husband who criticizes her in front of other people.

- *Describe:* Begin your script by describing as specifically and objectively as possible the behavior that is bothersome to you:

    "You said these car repairs would cost $35 and now you're charging me $110."

    "The last three times we have been with other people you have criticized me in front of them."

- *Express:* Say what you feel and think about this behavior:

    [To the auto mechanic:] "This makes me angry because I feel I'm being ripped off."

    [To the husband:] "This makes me feel humiliated and hurt."

- *Specify:* Ask for a different, specific behavior:

    "I would like you to readjust my bill back to the original estimate unless you can clearly justify these extra charges."

    "I would like you to quit criticizing me, and I will signal you every time that you start to do it."

- *Consequences:* Spell out concretely and simply what your reward will be for changing the behavior. Sometimes you have to specify the negative consequences of not following the changes:

    "If you do this, I will tell all of my friends that I have gotten good service at Bob's repair shop."

    "If you quit criticizing me, I'll feel a lot better and bake you your favorite apple pie."

The best way to make these scripts effective is to write them out ahead of time. Can you think of situations that are continually troubling to you? Perhaps you can begin to change them by writing out some scenarios for changing them.

Suggestions for Further Reading

Alberti, Robert E., & Emmons, Michael, L. (1970). *Your perfect right: A guide to assertive behavior.* San Luis Obispo, CA: Impact. One of the early books on self-assertive behavior.

Alberti, Robert E., & Emmons, Michael L. (1975). *Stand up, speak out, talk back!* New York: Pocket Books. Includes a 13-step self-training course.

Bower, Sharon Anthony, & Bower, Gordon H. (1976). *Asserting yourself: A practical guide for positive change.* Reading, MA: Addison-Wesley. One of the most specific, systematic books for recognizing unassertive behavior and changing it.

Zilbergeld, Bernie, & Barbach, Lonnie (1989). *How to talk with a partner about smart sex.* 60-minute audiotape available for $11.95 from Focus International, 14 Oregon Dr., Huntington Station, NY 11746. 800-843-0305.

Zimbardo, Philip G. (1977). *Shyness: What it is, what to do about it.* Reading, MA: Addison-Wesley. The classic book on the study of shyness and techniques for overcoming it, by a psychologist who is head of the Stanford University Shyness Clinic.

Family Matters: Decisions About Parenting, Pregnancy and Childbirth

In These Chapters:

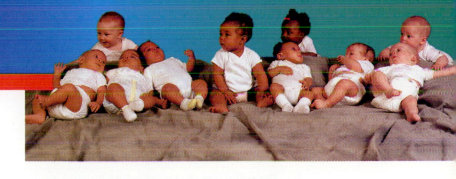

Some things are hard to imagine until an important life event happens.

Such a life event gives you cause to think more deeply about the meaning of your life and your relationship with others. This could be the beginning or end of a relationship, a moment of terrible violence, a spiritual revelation, getting or losing an important job, a death in the family—or a birth.

Becoming a parent is one of those notable life changes: suddenly one has the major responsibility of having to protect and care for a fragile human being. When this happens, people may abruptly feel themselves become more "grown up" and begin to think about themselves and their obligations differently.[1,2]

Parenting has been described as a "chronic emergency" by Northwestern University psychologist David Guttman.[3] As he explains, "After children come, dedicated parents can never completely relax into self-absorption or self-indulgence. From then on, even rest becomes a nurse's sleep, the parent waiting for the child's cry or the alarm in the night." Although there are exceptions, parenting forces one to move toward a less self-centered view of the world.[4]

One of the authors of this book recalls the torrent of emotion as he went to work bleary-eyed and over-coffeed the morning after his first child was born. The months leading up to the birth had been filled with expectations, trepidation, and excitement. The future mother and I had attended birthing classes, rehearsed breathing exercises, stockpiled baby food, furniture, and diapers. Then one night the baby had sent unmistakable signals that it was ready to be born, and we dressed hurriedly and rushed to the hospital.

"It's a girl!!", I shouted as I entered the office, ecstatic over the memory of the squished, mouse-colored thing that had emerged in the delivery room as I excitedly clicked away with a camera. But, like most new parents, as I passed around the proud father's box of candy I had little idea how dramatically the experience of parenting would change me.

10.2

Unit 10
Family Matters:
Decisions About
Parenting,
Pregnancy, and
Childbirth

24 The Job of Being a Parent

▶ What are the status and rights of children, and what are the different kinds of parenthood and options?

▶ What are some considerations to think about before becoming a parent?

▶ Describe the causes of infertility and explain the options of infertility treatments and adoption.

▶ Why are genetics important in considering whether to be a parent?

▶ What kinds of preconception care should mothers and fathers be concerned about?

With parenting, there is just not one of you or two of you. Even if you and your spouse or partner have been together for some time, the arrival of a baby makes you realize you don't just come from a **family**, a group in the same household united by marriage, blood, adoption, or other commitment; now you are *making* a family yourself.

Parenthood: The Varieties of Experience

Ideally, children should be born because parents want them and can afford them. But many children suffer from ill health, poverty, and worse. Many such problems result from unwanted pregnancies, especially among teenagers. The varieties of parents include single mothers, older people, single fathers, relatives, and gays. The increase in numbers of two working parents raises the issues of career-parenting conflicts, parental leave, and child-care services. Most people say they want two children but may need to consider the cost. Choosing to be childless can mean happiness. A clue to your future parenting abilities may be found in whether you were raised in a functional or dysfunctional family.

A family can take many forms. In a 1950s television sitcom, a family consisted of a father who worked and a mother who stayed at home. Today 61% of children live with both biological parents, both of whom often work at paying jobs. Eleven percent live with a formerly married mother and no father, 9% live with a mother and stepfather, 8% live with a never-married mother and no father. The rest live in other types of family arrangements.[5]

What is the purpose of a family? Historically, perhaps even biologically, we might say it is to nurture and protect the young. Here, then, is an important consideration: *if people are not ready to protect and nurture children, should they become parents?* All children *should* be wanted children, and parenting is one of the most important responsibilities anyone can ever have. Is this a responsibility you want to undertake? Let us consider what this means and what some of the various parental arrangements are.

The Status and Rights of Children Children are not doing well in the United States, let alone the world. A great many of the 64 million American children and adolescents are suffering:

- *High mortality rate for babies:* Many children do not even live to see their first birthday. The United States ranks 22nd in the world in the number of babies who survive their first year of life, according to a March 1992 report of the National Commission to Prevent Infant Mortality.[6] This occurs despite the fact that the United States spends more on health care than any other country in the world. Black infants were more than twice as likely as whites to die within their first year. By contrast, Japan's rate, the best in the world, is less than half that of the United States. Canada and the United Kingdom are tied for 11th place.

- *Low birth weight:* U.S. infants born with low birth weights—under 5.5 pounds, a condition foreshadowing many problems—were 7% of all births, the highest level since 1978. Infants weighing less than 3.5 pounds at birth are 40 times more likely to die within the first month of life.[7–9]

- *Epidemic of childhood diseases:* Preventable childhood diseases—mumps, whooping cough, rubella (German measles) —have reached epidemic levels. Indeed, in the United States, rubella was well on the way to being wiped out in 1987, but has since returned. The epidemic of these diseases is especially deplorable because vaccines are available (most were developed in the United States) to prevent them.

- *Childhood poverty—and other ills:* The gap between rich and poor grew wider for children over the past 30 years, according to a study by two Stanford University economists.[10] At the same time, American children and adolescents are less physically fit and have higher suicide and murder rates than in the past.[11]

Why are children in this terrible situation? Economics is the biggest reason. An increasingly selective health care system in the United States has left a rising percentage of children without health insurance.[12] In addition, from 1980 to 1989, more than 1 million children slipped into poverty, according to the U.S. Census Bureau. (By contrast, only 175,000 people over 65, who have the social safety nets of Social Security and Medicaid, fell below the poverty line.)[13]

Economic factors have also meant that two-parent families have become more dependent than ever on the mother's income to meet the family's financial needs. As a result, adults in households with children had 10–12 fewer hours available per week to provide children with things like home-cooked meals and help with homework. In addition, the growing incidence of divorce and single motherhood has led to an increase in the number of children living in single-parent families (14% in 1988 versus 5.5% in 1960) and a consequent decline in the money available to spend on children.[14]

Elsewhere in the world, the status of children is even more tragic. Millions are starved, undernourished, sick, uneducated, homeless, enslaved; are brutally exploited sexually and for their labor; are both victims and killers in war; are even hunted down and murdered by sadistic police or death squads. It was with a sense of urgency, therefore, that the leaders from 70 nations met in 1990 in New York for the first-ever World Summit for Children.[15–17] Earlier, in 1989, the Bill of Rights for Children was adopted by the United Nations General Assembly after a decade of discussion. It has been signed by 109 countries and ratified by 40—but the United States has done neither. (*See* ● *Figure 24.1.*)

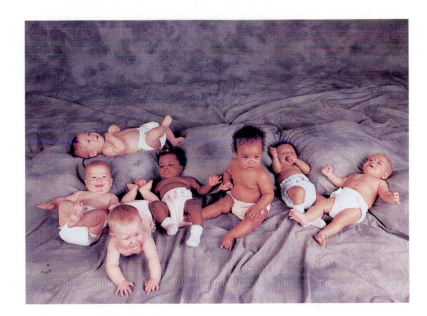

● **Figure 24.1 Children's rights.** The United Nations Bill of Rights for Children states that every human being below the age of 18 should have these rights.

- The right to affection, love, and understanding.
- The right to adequate nutrition and medical care.
- The right to free education.
- The right to full opportunity for play and recreation.
- The right to a name and nationality.
- The right to be among the first to receive relief in times of disaster.
- The right to learn to be a useful member of society and to develop individual abilities.
- The right to be brought up in a spirit of universal peace and brother/sisterhood.
- The right to enjoy these rights, regardless of race, color, sex, religion, national, or social origin.

10.4

Unit 10
Family Matters:
Decisions About
Parenting,
Pregnancy, and
Childbirth

Young Parents: Teen Pregnancies Although the teen pregnancy rate seems to be declining, about 1 out of 10 girls ages 15–19 becomes pregnant each year; one-fifth of all U.S. births are to teenagers; 32% of unintended pregnancies to all women occur in adolescents; 55% of the teen pregnancies will result in birth.[18]

The problems with children having children are twofold:

- *Difficulties for the parent:* Studies show that girls who have babies end up poorer and less educated than other women. For many young women already in poverty, having babies may follow from their sense that they have nothing better to look forward to.[19] Yet having babies makes it even more difficult to break out of poverty. Managing schoolwork and childcare is difficult when social support systems such as counseling and day-care are absent. On top of that, many teenagers are single parents: over half the children of teenage mothers never live with their biological fathers.[20]

  Women who bear only one child during adolescence seem to have a better chance of educational and economic achievement. Teenage women who bear a second child are less able to achieve an education, independence, and financial security.[21]

- *Difficulties for the child:* Some good news: only about a third of the daughters of poor teenage mothers became teenage mothers themselves, according to one study, indicating that a cycle of adolescent parents repeating from generation to generation is not inevitable.[22] The bad news: those offspring that *do* become teenage mothers, the study found, may have less chance of breaking out of poverty than their mothers did.

  Children of adolescent parents are more apt to fail a grade in school, suggests the study, with up to half repeating at least one grade. Incidents of substance abuse, fighting, and problems with the law are also higher among offspring of teenage parents.

Single Parents: Unmarried and Divorced
Single-parent families are definitely on the upswing. In 1989, 17% of white children, 29% of Hispanic children, and 61% of black children were in single-parent families, nearly double the percentages of 20 years earlier.[23] Indeed, a 1992 report by the Population Reference Bureau predicts that about *half* of all children today will spend some part of their childhood in a single-parent home.[24] Another report, from the National Center for Health Statistics, predicts that about one-third of today's children will experience the divorce of their biological parents, and one-fourth will live with a stepparent by age 16.[25]

Who are today's single parents? Probably the two largest groups are the *unmarried* and the *divorced*. (Other single parents include the widowed, grandparents and other guardians, and gay families.)

- *Unmarried parents:* According to the U.S. Census Bureau, increasing numbers of new mothers of all ages are unmarried. In the early 1960s, about half the unmarried women who became pregnant got married before the child was born; by the late 1980s, only a quarter did so.[26] Among teenage women, 92% of first births were conceived out of wedlock in 1985–89.

  This does not mean that children of unwed mothers are necessarily born into single-parent families. About one-quarter of the children born to unmarried parents are born into two-parent families because the parents live together.[27] Often a child lives in a single-parent situation for only a year or two, until the parent marries.

- *Divorced parents:* Married adults now divorce 2½ times as often as adults did 20 years ago and 4 times as often as 50 years ago. In fact, for every two American marriages that occurred in 1985 there was about one divorce. More than 90% of the time, the mother winds up having custody of the children.[28]

  Divorced women with children often don't do as well as their ex-husbands financially. Many experience a marked decline in their standard of living.[29] The primary reason is that ex-husbands contribute far less to child care than they did before the divorce. (By 1994, employers must make all child-support payments for workers, whether the absent parent is delinquent or not. A lack of child-support is a major cause of poverty among American children.[30])

  Divorced fathers, on the other hand, tend to become less and less involved with their children's lives.[31] One survey of children from divorced families found that only 17% had at least weekly visits with the noncustodial parent in the previous year and over half had no direct contact.[32]

Older Parents At one time, physicians routinely advised women not to wait until they were older to have children. However, more effective birth control and the increased opportunities for women for education and careers have allowed many women to delay childbearing until their later years, bringing about a profound shift in childbearing patterns. First births to women aged 30 and older have been increasing (it was 10 per 1000 women among 30- to 44-year-olds in 1986).[33] Although women who postpone childbirth until their 30s may have more pregnancy complications, older parents often speak enthusiastically about having children and say they are more prepared emotionally to be parents than when they were younger.[34,35]

Nontraditional Parents: Single Fathers, Relatives, Gays Today parents don't consist of just the traditional biological mom 'n' dad. Among American households with working parents and children, those headed by single fathers are increasing fastest and now account for more than 1 million families.[36] In addition, grandparents or other relatives increasingly end up raising children because the biological parents are incapable of doing so themselves (perhaps because of chemical dependency) or a court determines that the biological parent is not the best nurturer for a child. Finally, children become part of gay and lesbian families through custody in the dissolution of heterosexual marriages (in which one parent may also be homosexual), through adoption, and through alternative means of conception, such as artificial insemination or surrogate birth mothers.[37]

Working Parents Mom's role has undergone a serious change in the last decade—and this has affected Dad's role. The change: Mom has gone to work, either because she wants to or because she has to help meet the family budget. Indeed, 61% of women with children under age 18 are employed outside the home (compared with 19% in 1947).[38] Even more significant, the greatest increase in employment over the past 20 years has been among mothers with the youngest children.[39]

The fact of both parents working has amounted to a social revolution. Among the consequences:

- *Career-parenting conflict:* Mothers (and fathers) who don't work outside the home —who choose to stay home, particularly when the children are old enough to go to school—may find their role devalued by their own family members, other parents, and society in general.[40] Alternatively, parents who want to pursue a career may worry about the effect of their absence on their child's upbringing.

- *Parental and maternal leave:* Until recently, the United States has not required employers to allow workers to take unpaid leaves of absence from their jobs for pregnancy, maternity or paternity, or care of sick children or family emergencies. Family leave has been a reality for some time in countries such as Germany and Japan, with government and/or employers supporting a certain number of paid weeks. Only in 1993 did Congress finally pass legislation allowing unpaid family leave.[41,42]

  At present, some parents who take time off either for pregnancy or childbirth experience employer discrimination and often suffer career setbacks.[43–46] Men seem reluctant to use unpaid leaves, even in the 28 states that require large employers to provide them. According to a 1990 survey, only about 1% of eligible men actually use the leaves, perhaps in part because of a social and cultural stigma associated with men taking care of children.[47]

- *Child-care services:* Single working parents find worries about child care and flexible scheduling one of their major concerns.[48] Indeed, the youngest children of working women are now more likely to be cared for by a nonrelative than by a family member.[49,50] (See ● *Figure 24.2.*)

  Child care is also a preoccupation of married working parents, particularly those who are poor. Although the average family pays about 10% of its family income for child care, the costs are 23% for low-income parents, about the same proportion as housing.[51]

10.6

Unit 10
Family Matters:
Decisions About
Parenting,
Pregnancy, and
Childbirth

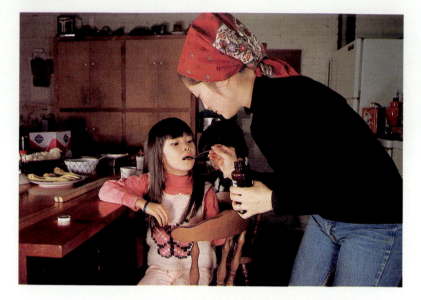

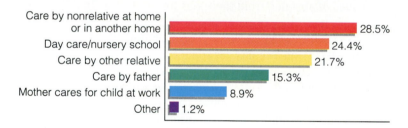

Care by nonrelative at home or in another home	28.5%
Day care/nursery school	24.4%
Care by other relative	21.7%
Care by father	15.3%
Mother cares for child at work	8.9%
Other	1.2%

● **Figure 24.2 Who's watching America's children?** Primary care arrangements for children under age 5 used by employed mothers, 1987. (Total number of children: 9,124,000.)

Child care is such a major dilemma for many two-paycheck couples with children that they try to avoid child care and its costs by asking their employers for split shifts. Others borrow money to pay for high-quality care. Because child care is expensive, some parents are forced to leave their children alone at home; indeed, nearly *half* of school-age children are "latchkey children."[52] Preteens and teenagers left unsupervised after school may be far more prone than other kids to get involved with alcohol and illegal drugs.[53]

Although some day-care centers offer children excellent age-appropriate care and

educational opportunities, some resort to "child packing"—rows of children in cribs and high chairs with an adult sitting nearby reading a magazine.[54] Whether or not child-care facilities have a negative or positive impact on the children depends, of course, on the level of care, which depends in turn on such matters as pay and training of staffers. (*See ● Table 24.1.*) Overall, some studies have found that children whose mothers worked outside the home when their children were less than 1 year old, children who had been put in full-time day-care, did less well on tests predicting school performance than those whose mothers stayed at home.[55]

Even working parents who have satisfactory child-care arrangements come to dread the phone call from the sitter or child-care center saying, "I'm sorry to bother you at work, but your child is running a high temperature and needs to go home." Work and sick children are one of the top conflicts in a working parent's life. Despite all the talk about changing gender roles, it is mothers rather than fathers who bear most of the burden for child care. Among parents with preschoolers, more women than men missed work in an average week, usually owing to sick children or problems in child-care scheduling arrangements.[56]

● *Making time for children:* Jobs, school, and financial responsibilities can be terribly demanding of adults. Sooner or later, many find they've reached a decision point: Should they continue a single-minded devotion to career at the expense of attention to their family? Or should they scale back their career ambitions in order to devote more time to their families? Certainly the stress of overwork does not make for good parenting or a good relationship with one's partner. Yet the transition from a socially and intellectually involving job to a renewed emphasis on family is not always easy. Some people who cut back on work to focus on family may initially feel a sense of loss. Still, on balance, the news is encouraging: a Canadian study found that professional women who take time out to marry and have children are far more content than those who put their career above all.[57] Unfortunately, we know little about the effect on men of scaling back on or taking a hiatus from their careers for the sake of their children.

Family Size and Cost In 1957, at the height of the postwar Baby Boom (generally considered to be from 1945 to 1964, when American families produced children in record numbers), the average number of children for American families was 3.7. That figure then sank like a stone (to about 1.8 in 1970) but has since climbed back—to an average of 2.1 in 1990.[58]

If you were contemplating having children, how many would you want? According to a Gallup poll, these percentages of Americans think these numbers of children would be ideal:[59]

- One child—3%
- Two children—57%
- Three children—18%
- Four or more children—11%

Only a minority of Americans—about 4%—say they never want or are glad they don't have kids. For Americans under 40, 58% have already had children and 84% of those who have not say they want to someday.[60]

Before you decide how many, if any, children sound right to you, you might want to consider: *what are the important things to think about before having a child?* Children should be thought about in terms of love, but they also have to have to be thought about in terms of *cost*. For a child born in 1990, the *minimum* cost of raising him or her during the first 17 years of life will exceed $150,000. Affluent families will spend nearly twice that much.[61] (*See* ● *Figure 24.3.*)

Choosing to Be Childless The fastest-growing household type in the 1990s will be married couples with no children at home and the second fastest will be women who live alone.[62] Many of these households will be childless by choice.

People who choose not to have children may actually be *happier* than those with children.[63] This may be because they have avoided the tremendous amount of work associated with parenting, beginning with feedings, diaperings,

● **Table 24.1 Child-care quality checklist**

Basics

- Is the program licensed or registered?
- Is the group's size OK for my child's age?
- Is the care giver trained and experienced?

The Place:

- Is there enough space?
- Are there different places for different activities?
- Is the outdoor play area fenced, hazard-free, and completely visible to the care giver?
- Is the space bright and pleasant?
- Is there an acceptable child-to-staff ratio?

Parents' Role:

- Are unannounced visits OK?
- Are there ways for you to get involved?

Do the Care Givers . . .

- Genuinely like children?
- Talk to children at their eye level?
- Share your beliefs about discipline?
- Greet your child when you arrive?
- Comfort children when needed?
- Keep you up to date on your child's activities?
- Make themselves available to answer your questions?

Activities:

- Are active and quiet experiences balanced?
- Are activities correct for the child's age?
- Are toys safe for each age, clean, and available?

Source: Child Care Aware, Dayton Hudson Corp.; coordinated by Bonneville Communications, Salt Lake City, UT.

and night wakings. It may also be because they realize that the presence of a baby would make them lose some of their own intimacy and closeness. Many voluntarily childless women, says psychologist Mardy Ireland, who studies childless women, "often express their nurturing capacity through relationships, community involvement, or creative pursuits."[64]

Those who choose to be childless often face disapproval, even scorn, from friends and family.[65] This pressure is especially difficult for voluntarily childless women, who may be viewed as not "whole" or "normal," according to Ireland.[66] Choosing not to be a parent, then, means being clear in your own mind that you are bucking the views of a "pro-natal" society.

10.8

Unit 10
Family Matters:
Decisions About
Parenting,
Pregnancy, and
Childbirth

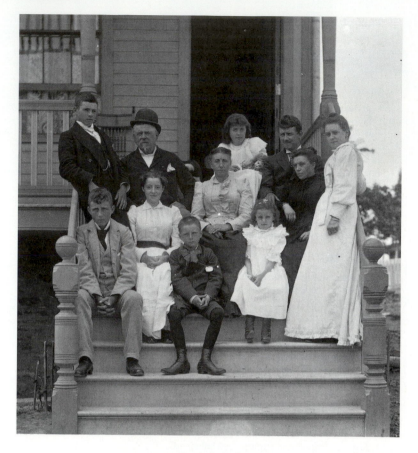

| Year | Age of child | Income group* | | |
		Low	Middle	High
1990	under1	$4,330	$6,140	$8,770
1991	1	4,590	6,510	9,300
1992	2	4,870	6,900	9,850
1993	3	5,510	7,790	11,030
1994	4	5,850	8,260	11,690
1995	5	6,200	8,750	12,390
1996	6	6,550	9,220	12,950
1997	7	6,950	9,770	13,730
1998	8	7,360	10,360	14,550
1999	9	7,570	10,690	15,120
2000	10	8,020	11,340	16,030
2001	11	8,500	12,020	16,990
2002	12	10,360	14,190	19,680
2003	13	10,980	15,040	20,860
2004	14	11,640	15,940	22,110
2005	15	13,160	17,950	24,610
2006	16	13,950	19,030	26,090
2007	17	14,780	20,170	27,650
Total		$151,170	$210,070	$293,400

* Low income is under $29,900 in 1990; middle is
$29,900 to $48,299; high is $48,300 or more. Projection
assumes 6 percent for annual inflation.

● **Figure 24.3 The costs of growing up.** The projected annual expenditures in current dollars on a child born in 1990, by income group for married-couple families.

A Key to Choosing Children: Was Your Own Family Functional or Dysfunctional?

Are you willing to devote 18 years of your life to being responsible for a child? How would having a child affect your career, your interests, your intimate relationship with your partner? Do you *like* children—and will you like them if and when they turn out to have different ideas and goals from yours? (*See Self Discovery 24.1.*)

Many people say that becoming a parent gives them self-esteem, a sense of accomplishment, and the sense of exploring new frontiers within themselves. The presence of a child is not a substitute for happiness they may feel is missing in their lives. Rather, they feel a child brings them *additional* happiness. Others say that children don't make life better, they make it different.

The best place to start in deciding whether you want to be a parent and whether you would be a good one is to look at how you were brought up. If you were raised in a *functional family*, you were raised (generally) with love and respect, then this positive picture of parenthood is probably one you would bring to your own parenting.

Unfortunately, many people are raised in dysfunctional families, such as those in which a parent is impaired by alcohol or other drugs, bringing many of the woes to his or her children. A **dysfunctional family** is one in which the parents demonstrate negative or destructive behavior toward each other or toward their children. Children may be physically or sexually abused, emotionally or verbally abused, neglected, isolated, overcontrolled, overburdened, or otherwise maltreated. As a result, they usually have a low sense of self-esteem, feeling unworthy, unvalued, unloved. Unfortunately, the children of abusive or neglectful parents may themselves become abusive or neglectful with their own children, perpetuating a cycle that may well extend back several generations. (*See the Life Skill essay at the end of this chapter.*)

Being raised in a dysfunctional family should not negate the possibility of becoming a parent. Rather it should serve as an invitation to prospective parents to actively participate in their own recovery from the impact of their dysfunctional families. In addition, parenting programs can be helpful in developing the knowledge, skills, and perspectives needed to be a nurturing, effective parent.

Infertility: Medical Solutions and Adoption

Infertility is when a sexually active couple is unable to conceive after trying for a year. Most causes are physiological, although some are psychological. Treatment is with artificial insemination, ovulation-stimulating hormones, in vitro fertilization, embryo transfer, or use of surrogate mothers. Another option is adoption.

Baby-making would seem to just happen naturally. One researcher found that the average (median) time for a sexually active couple using no contraception to conceive was 2½ months. (The majority was within 6 months, but some couples took 2 years or more.)[67]

For about a third of all couples in the United States, however, having a child is difficult—either because they cannot conceive or because the woman is physiologically unable to carry the child to term. About 1 couple in 10 cannot ever have children.[68]

The Causes of Infertility Although definitions vary, by **infertility** we mean the failure to conceive after 1 year of regular sexual intercourse without contraception. It is differentiated from **sterility,** which is total inability to conceive.[69,70] Infertility is a couple's problem that requires an evaluation of both partners. One of the most important causes of infertility

---

SELF DISCOVERY 24.1

Are You Ready to Be a Parent?

Check the following. There are no right answers—the responses only show what surveys by the Gallup poll have found in questioning a sample of American adults on the subject of child raising.

1. What do you think would be the greatest plus or the thing that you would gain most from having children? (Check one.)
   _____ a. The love and affection children bring
   _____ b. Having the pleasure of watching them grow
   _____ c. The joy, happiness, and fun they would bring
   _____ d. The sense of family they create
   _____ e. The fulfillment and satisfaction they bring
2. What do you think would be the minus or the greatest problem you would encounter in raising children? (Check one.)
   _____ a. The cost
   _____ b. Worries about their using drugs
   _____ c. Worries about the world and society they have to be brought up into
   _____ d. Trying to teach children right from wrong
   _____ e. Worries about peer pressure and its effects
   _____ f. The teenage years
3. Which of the following would you consider to be the ideal family situation for children? (Check one.)
   _____ a. A family in which the father has a job and the mother stays home and cares for the children
   _____ b. A family in which both parents have jobs and both take care of the children when they are home
   _____ c. A family in which the mother has a job and the father stays home and cares for the children
4. Do you think parents today are too strict with their children, not strict enough, or just about right? (Check one.)
   _____ a. Too strict
   _____ b. Not strict enough
   _____ c. About right
   _____ d. Don't know

Answers

The percentage of adults answering each possibility, according to Gallup, were as follows:
1. a—12%; b—11%; c—10%; d—7%; e—6%.
2. a—22%; b—13%; c—5%; d—3%; e—3%; f—3%.
3. a—63%; b—33%; c—1%.
4. a—2%; b—81%; c—14%; d—3%.

Source: Based on: Gallup, G. H., Jr., & Newport, F. (1990, June 4). Parenthood—a (nearly) universal desire. *San Francisco Chronicle,* pp. B3–B4.

---

today is infection and tubal scarring that results from untreated STDs—STDs cause about 20% of female infertility problems. Other causes are:

- *Causes of infertility in couples:* A couple's inability to conceive can have any number of causes; here are five:[71] (1) not enough

10.10

*Unit 10
Family Matters:
Decisions About
Parenting,
Pregnancy, and
Childbirth*

intercourse (once or less per week); (2) too much intercourse (several times a day or over the course of several days, which prohibits sperm from building up); (3) intercourse during times of the month when the woman is less apt to conceive; (4) use of vaginal lubricants such as Vaseline, which may prevent sperm from entering the cervix; and (5) anemia, fatigue, emotional stress, poor nutrition, or general poor health in either one of the couple.

• *Causes of infertility in males:* Principal causes of infertility in men are the following:[72] (1) reduced number of sperm or defective sperm, owing to untreated sexually transmitted diseases and environmental toxins; (2) blockage somewhere between testicle and end of the penis; and (3) inability to ejaculate or to sustain an erection.

• *Causes of infertility in females:* The causes of infertility in women are as follows:[73] (1) age of the mother, since fertility decreases slightly as women become older; (2) failure to ovulate, owing to such factors as hormonal deficiencies, defective ovaries, metabolic imbalances, genetic factors, various medical conditions, cigarettes or other drugs; (3) blockage of fallopian tubes; (4) abnormalities of the uterus, such as **endometriosis,** in which some cells of the inner lining of the uterus grow in the pelvic and abdominal cavities; and (5) an immune response or acidic chemical climate in the vagina, which may immobilize sperm.

If none of these events take place, and the sperm and egg are united in conception, there is still no guarantee of full-term pregnancy. About 20–30% of pregnancies end in **miscarriages,** or spontaneous abortions.[74]

Treating Infertility: High-Tech Baby Making After a couple has tried to conceive for a year or more, they may seek alternative methods of conception. Medical breakthroughs have provided a variety of techniques for overcoming infertility. In 1990, more than a million new patients sought treatment for infertility (six times as many people as were treated for lung cancer and 10 times the number of reported cases of AIDS).[75] Physicians cannot manipulate every aspect of the reproductive cycle, but here are some techniques they do try:

• *Artificial insemination:* Sometimes sperm don't have the strength, the mobility, the necessary enzymes, or the ability to bypass hostile vaginal secretions and pierce the outer shell of the egg (ovum). Or a man may be unable to produce sperm at all. **Artificial insemination** consists of collecting sperm from the man—or an anonymous male donor—by masturbation and, with the help of a powerful microscope, injecting the sperm cells by syringe directly into the woman's vagina or uterus in order to induce pregnancy.

One result of the success of artificial insemination has been an increase in the establishment of *sperm banks* to meet demand. From 1980 to 1987, the births of children conceived by this method more than doubled.[76] In 1988, a study by the Congressional Office of Technology Assessment revealed a lack of testing of semen donors by sperm banks, so that women inseminated artificially were unknowingly putting themselves at risk of contracting infectious diseases (including AIDS and hepatitis).[77] Thus, couples should select sperm banks and physicians with care, reviewing testing and record-keeping procedures and choosing banks that have provided sperm for many cases of artificial insemination.

• *Ovulation-stimulating hormones:* Some women have difficulty ovulating naturally. Others produce eggs that cannot be fertilized. When large doses of ovulation-stimulating hormones (clomiphene or Pergonal) are administered, an ovary may produce dozens of eggs. One common result of this treatment is multiple births—twins, triplets, even quadruplets. Unfortunately, many multiple births are premature and low-birth-weight babies, which puts them at risk for many problems.[78,79] (*See* ● *Figure 24.4.*)

• *In vitro fertilization:* The term *in vitro* means "in glass"; thus the origin of the term "test-tube babies." During an **in vitro fertilization (IVF)** procedure, the egg and sperm are taken from the parents and kept in a laboratory setting until the mother's uterus is hormonally ready; the fertilized egg is then implanted in the wall of the uterus. This procedure is particularly use-

Rate per 1000 live births	Singleton	Twins	Triplets
Very low birth weight (3.3 pounds or less)	10.3	98.7	336.3
Low birth weight (5.5 pounds or less)	59.2	502.0	911.8
Mortality	8.6	56.6	166.7

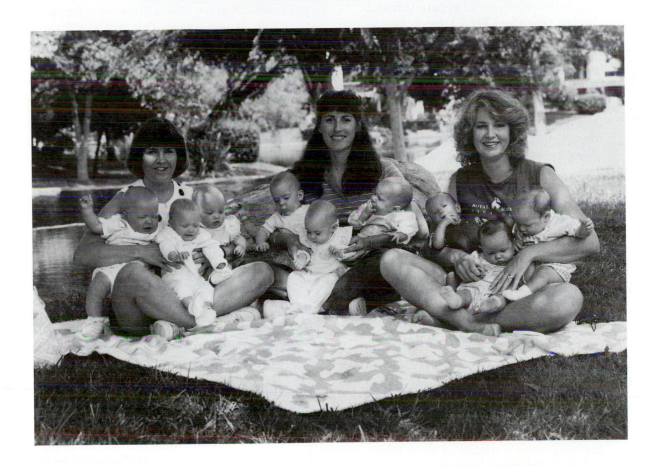

● **Figure 24.4 The risks of being a twin or triplet.** Babies born in multiple births have higher risks of low birth weight and infant mortality.

ful when the woman's fallopian tubes are blocked or otherwise unable to transport an ovum.

Sometimes the donor of the egg is not the woman who bears the child. A women who is infertile because of premature menopause or who wants to become pregnant after menopause may be implanted with her husband's sperm and another, often anonymous, woman's egg. One concern is that the donor of the egg may at some point try to insist on the rights to the child.[80] Even so, women older than 40 are just as successful at bearing healthy babies with donated eggs as younger women, as long as the eggs come from a younger donor.[81,82] About 22% of embryo transfers following IVF of donated eggs resulted in live births.

10.12

*Unit 10
Family Matters:
Decisions About
Parenting,
Pregnancy, and
Childbirth*

- *GIFT and ZIFT:* The technique of **gamete intrafallopian transfer (GIFT)** involves collecting the woman's egg and the man's sperm and uniting them inside the woman's fallopian tubes. The procedure, which has a 50–60% success rate, is often tried when the cause of the infertility is unclear.

  In the technique of **zygote intrafallopian transfer (ZIFT),** the mother's egg and father's sperm are collected and placed in a laboratory dish. Then, one day after fertilization takes place, the zygote, or single-celled fertilized egg, is placed in the woman's fallopian tubes.

- *Embryo transfer:* In an *embryo transfer,* the sperm of a male partner of an infertile woman is placed in another woman's uterus during ovulation. Five days later, the embryo is transferred to the uterus of the infertile woman, who carries the embryo and delivers the baby. Sometimes, in a technique known as *frozen embryo transfer,* the embryo is frozen and later implanted in an infertile woman's uterus.

- *A surrogate mother:* A surrogate mother is a consenting woman who is artificially inseminated with the sperm of the male partner of an infertile woman. For a fee, the surrogate mother carries the child through pregnancy and upon delivery turns the child over to the couple with whom she contracted.

  Important issues must be clarified before a surrogate can be considered. For instance, some surrogate mothers have changed their minds and refused to surrender the baby upon delivery. Some states require that the contracting couple legally adopt the child.

High-tech baby making can be quite expensive and usually is not covered by health insurance. IVF, for instance, may cost about $10,000 a try, and several tries may be necessary to achieve a single pregnancy.[83]

Adoption Adults who cannot become biological parents may still become parents by adopting children who have been relinquished by their birth parents or who have been orphaned. Traditionally, people wanting to adopt have been infertile couples, but in recent years single parents and gay and lesbian couples have also adopted children. In addition, some couples who are biological parents have widened their families by adopting disabled and older children.

Most adoptions are arranged through public or nonprofit agencies or private counselors. In recent years, however, adoptions have become more difficult in the United States as relinquishment rates have declined. This may be a consequence of more single parents keeping their babies. For instance, over one-quarter of all children are born to unmarried mothers today, four times the percentage of just 25 years ago.[84] Because there is an imbalance between prospective parents and adoptable children, some Americans seek to arrange adoptions of babies from other countries, principally South Korea, Romania, Latin America, and India.[85]

Deciding to Be a Parent: What Is Your Genetic Legacy?

Through sperm and egg, the biological information from each parent is passed along to the offspring as chromosomes. These structures which contain the body's genetic life plan and which are composed of DNA, carrying the organism's hereditary information in the form of units of heredity called genes. Traits such as eye color are determined by dominant or recessive genes. Sex is determined by X and Y chromosomes. Inherited birth defects include Down syndrome, sickle-cell disease, cystic fibrosis, and PKU, some of which can be detected by genetic testing. Some inherited disorders can be treated with gene therapy and genetic engineering techniques.

Are you left-handed? Is left-handedness an inherited trait? If you're a lefty, you're constantly having to adjust to the tools (from scissors to power saws) and prejudices of a right-handed world. Unlike animals such as gorillas and chimpanzees, which show no hand preference, humans are unique in that they generally favor the right hand.[86]

The consequences of being left-handed are startling. According to psychology professor Stanley Coren, left-handers statistically are more accident-prone (perhaps because so many tools are designed for right-handers). They are also more apt to suffer from such problems as bed-wetting, dyslexia, speech defects, deafness, epilepsy, and alcoholism.[87] (Previous assumptions that lefties die up to 14 years sooner have been disproved.[88]) On the other hand, left-handed children tend to have better mathematical and verbal skills and be superior in musical and visual abilities.

Is left-handedness a genetically fixed trait? Perhaps sometimes it is: before birth, according to one study, only 5% of 212 fetuses sucked their left thumb in the womb, which suggests that heredity determines handedness.[89] On the other hand, a greater percentage, 10–15%, of the American adult population is left-handed. This suggests, then, that handedness is also affected by the environment. Indeed, it turns out that there is a higher percentage of left-handers among people who suffered some sort of stress at birth: they were premature, endured prolonged labor, had breathing difficulties, and the like. The theory, then, is that the left side of the brain, which is more sensitive to lack of oxygen, was affected, shifting dominance to the right brain (which directs parts of the left side of the body).[90]

This example shows how heredity and environment mix to influence who you are. Your heredity may only partly determine handedness, but it may determine other, equally important things about you. And *your* heredity may determine some important characteristics of your children.

The Master Plan for Your Body: Chromosomes, DNA, Genes When the male reproductive cell, the **sperm,** from your father and the female reproductive cell, the **ovum,** from your mother met at the moment of conception, they fused to create a new cell, the **zygote,** the beginning of life for you. (See ● *Figure 24.5.*) Amazingly, that one cell—which, of course, later diversified into many others—contained all the biologically inherited information from each of your parents that determined most of your principal characteristics: hair color, foot size, heart shape, blood type, and so on.

The biological information from each parent was passed along as *chromosomes, DNA,* and *genes.* Let's explain how these work:

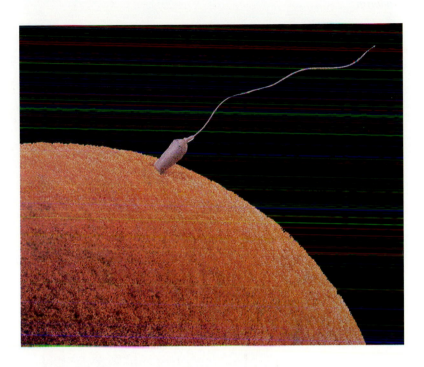

● **Figure 24.5 The moment of conception: when a sperm unites with an egg**

"*Like space voyagers approaching a huge planet, the sperm approach a cell 85,000 times bigger than themselves. The relatively few sperm that make it to the egg release digestive enzymes that eat away the egg's protective coating, allowing one sperm to penetrate. . . . As it does so, an electrical charge shoots across the ovum's surface, blocking out other sperm during the minute or so that it takes the egg to form a barrier. Meanwhile, fingerlike projections sprout around the successful sperm and pull it inward. The egg nucleus and the sperm nucleus move toward each other and, before half a day has elapsed, they fuse. The two have become one.*

But even at that moment, when one lucky sperm has won the 1 in 300 million lottery, an individual's destiny is not assured. Fewer than half of fertilized eggs, called zygotes, survive beyond the first week . . . and only a fourth survive to birth. . . . If human life begins at conception, then most people die without being born."

—David G. Myers (1989). *Psychology* (2nd ed.). New York: Worth, pp. 59–60.

10.14

*Unit 10
Family Matters:
Decisions About
Parenting,
Pregnancy, and
Childbirth*

• *Chromosomes:* Within the nucleus of each of the trillions of cells in your body are **chromosomes,** which contain the master life plan for your body. (*See* • *Figure 24.6.*) When egg and sperm unite at the time of conception and new life is created, the 23 chromosomes carried in the egg are paired with the 23 chromosomes in the sperm. Every human cell (including the first one, the zygote), except the sperm and

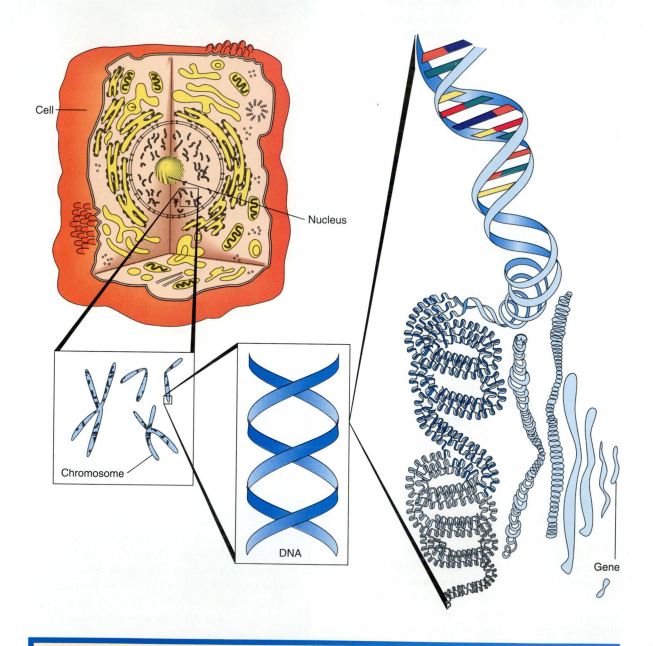

Cell

Nucleus

Chromosome

DNA

Gene

• **Figure 24.6 Your genetic heritage.** Within the nucleus of each of your cells are chromosomes, which contain the master plan for your body. Each chromosome is composed of long threads of the molecule DNA. Genes, which are segments of DNA, direct the production of proteins that determine specific biological characteristics or traits.

the ova, contains 46 chromosomes in the form of 23 chromosome pairs, one pair member coming from each parent. Each chromosome is composed of long threads containing *DNA*, which transmit genetic information from generation to generation.

- *DNA:* **DNA,** which stands for **deoxyribonucleic acid,** is considered the basic unit of control of human life, the carrier of an organism's hereditary information. (*Refer back to Figure 24.6.*) DNA is made up of thousands of molecules or segments called *genes*.

- *Genes:* **Genes** are the units of heredity, the transmitters of hereditary information—your sex, your eye color, and so on. Genes direct the manufacture of proteins that determine biological traits. Genes "specialize" to carry specific biochemical instructions appropriate to a particular physical characteristic or trait.

Dominant and Recessive Genes A particular pair of genes, one from each parent, may determine a specific inherited characteristic. When the actions of the two genes are alike, they are said to be **homozygous genes.** However, sometimes the actions of the two genes are different, in which case they are said to be **heterozygous genes.** That is, one gene is a **dominant gene,** having greater influence in determining a particular characteristic. Such a gene is more powerful than a **recessive gene,** whose influence is not as great.

Many physical characteristics follow the rule of dominant-recessive genes, but one in particular is that of eye color. Brown is dominant over blue. Thus, if one parent has two genes for brown eyes, and the other has two genes for blue eyes, they will produce brown-eyed children, because brown is the dominant color. However, if both parents are brown-eyed but both carry the recessive blue gene, odds are they will have one blue-eyed child for every three brown-eyed children. (*See ● Figure 24.7.*)

Sex Chromosomes: Is It a Boy or a Girl?
Of the 23 pairs of chromosomes you inherited from your parents, 22 (called *autosomes*) control the development and functioning of most of the body. The remaining pair determine a person's sex and are called the *sex chromosomes.*

Brown is dominant over blue. Thus, if a parent with 2 genes for brown eyes joins with a parent who has 2 genes for blue eyes, all possible combinations are for brown eyes; no matter how many children they have, all will have brown eyes.

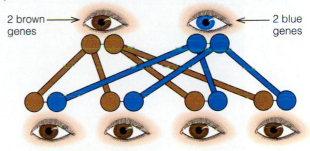

2 brown genes   2 blue genes

If a brown-eyed parent with a recessive blue gene joins with another brown-eyed parent with a recessive blue gene, and they have 4 children, one possible combination is for blue eyes and three are for brown eyes; on average 3 of their children will have brown eyes and 1 child will have blue eyes.

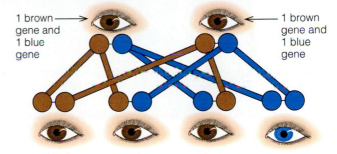

1 brown gene and 1 blue gene   1 brown gene and 1 blue gene

● **Figure 24.7 Eye color**

The sex chromosomes are of two types, X and Y, and their particular combination determines whether a particular offspring of two parents will be female or male. (*See ● Figure 25.8.*)

- *X sex chromosome:* The **X chromosome** is found in both males and females. Men have one X chromosome; women have two X chromosomes. When an X chromosome is paired from each parent, a *female* offspring is produced.

- *Y sex chromosome:* The **Y chromosome** is found only in males. When a Y chromosome is paired with an X chromosome from the mother, a *male* offspring is produced.

10.16

Unit 10
Family Matters:
Decisions About
Parenting,
Pregnancy, and
Childbirth

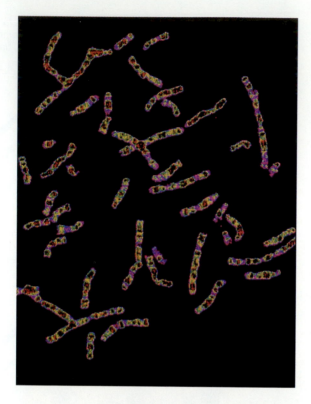
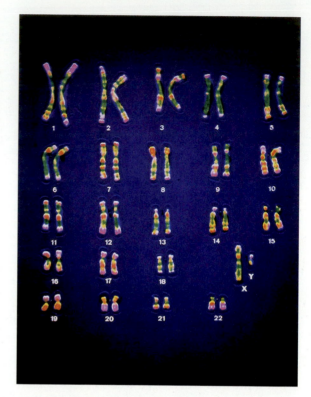

● **Figure 24.8 Forty-six chromosomes—including the sex chromosomes, X and Y.** *(Left)* The 46 chromosomes as they appear under a microscope. *(Right)* The 46 chromosomes arranged in pairs. Note the X and Y sex chromosomes.

What causes the differences in development? To greatly oversimplify, it seems that if a Y chromosome is present in the unborn child during the first 8 weeks after conception, the baby develops testes; if the Y chromosome is absent, the infant develops ovaries. Thus, the X chromosome seems to have no effect on initial sexual determination; it is the presence or absence of the Y chromosome that determines sex.

Inherited Birth Defects Most babies are born healthy and normal, but perhaps 1 in 16 is born with a serious physical birth defect.[91] Birth defects may be the result of environmental factors—for example, a prenatal problem (such as the mother's drinking) or birth injuries—but some are the result of hereditary factors. Each of us has perhaps 50,000–100,000 genes in every cell in our body, of which perhaps 5–7 could pose serious problems to an offspring who inherited the identically defective gene from each parent.[92] Most of the time, of course, one parent's defective genes are different from the other parent's. A missing gene, or a malfunction in one, can cause aberrations in the proteins and chemicals essential to life.

Several diseases and disorders have been linked to, or have a suspected link with, hereditary causes or defective genes. *(See ● Table 24.2.)* Some of the most common are the following:

● *Down syndrome:* **Down (or Down's) syndrome** occurs in 1 out of every 650 births. The most common condition caused by a chromosomal abnormality, Down syndrome leads to various degrees of mental retardation and physical deformity.

● **Table 24.2 Some genetic disorders**

Disease	Description
Alcoholism	In April 1990, researchers announced a suspected link. The connection is still not confirmed as a genetic disorder.
"Bubble boy" disease	ADA deficiency is rare disorder called "bubble boy" disease, because child lacks a working immune system and must live in a bubble-like enclosure to protect against infection.
Colon cancer	Researchers have discovered one major gene that contributes to it.
Coronary atherosclerosis, premature	Hardening of the arteries.
Cystic fibrosis	Mucus in the lungs is so thick it cannot be cleared, killing most victims by age 27.
Down syndrome	Physical and mental retardation; occurs in 1 of 650 births.
Duchenne muscular dystrophy	Wasting muscle disease, affecting 1 in 5000 males.
Emphysema, premature	A breathing disorder usually associated with smoking, emphysema can also strike early in life. Found in people with genetic defect known as alpha 1-antitrypsin deficiency.
Fragile-X syndrome	Common genetic form of mental retardation, striking more than 1 in 1000 males.
Hemophilia	Disorder in which blood fails to clot.
Huntington's chorea	A lethal degenerative brain disease that strikes between ages 15 and 80.
Lesch Nyhan syndrome	Disorder causing spasticity and self-mutilation, affecting 1 in 100,000 babies.
Neurofibromatosis	A hereditary disease of the nervous system that produces birthmarks, tumors of the skin and nerve cells, and learning disabilities in about 100,000 Americans.
Phenylketonuria (PKU)	Genetic disorder in which crucial liver enzyme, phenylalanine, is absent. Produces severe mental retardation if not treated.
Polycystic kidney disease	Genetic disease causing kidney cysts, leading to kidney failure; it affects 1 in 1000.
Retinoblastoma	Eye cancer.
Sickle-cell anemia	Severe anemia brought about by abnormal form of hemoglobin, the molecule that carries oxygen to the blood. It affects 8–10% of African-Americans.
Tay-Sachs disease	Fatal enzyme deficiency, affecting 1 in 3600 Ashkenazi Jews.
Thalassemia	Forms of blood disease (anemias) found in people of Mediterranean, African, and Southeast Asian descent.

Source: Adapted from Gladstone Foundation Laboratories, San Francisco General Hospital, San Francisco, CA.

- *Sickle-cell disease:* **Sickle-cell disease** is a genetic disorder of the blood characterized by sickle-shaped red blood cells. About 10% of African-Americans in the United States carry sickle-cell trait, and 1 in 500 has sickle-cell disease.[93,94] Because the sickled cells are unable to transport enough oxygen to important organs, the disorder causes tiredness, weakness, irritability, shortness of breath, and severe pain. Half of those born with the disorder die before the age of 20.

- *Cystic fibrosis:* At least 30,000 Americans have **cystic fibrosis,** a severe abnormality of the respiratory system and sweat and mucous glands. It is one of the most common genetic diseases, with 12 million people thought to be carriers.[95] The symptoms of cystic fibrosis are serious digestive and respiratory problems, caused by a sticky

10.18

*Unit 10
Family Matters:
Decisions About
Parenting,
Pregnancy, and
Childbirth*

mucus that clogs the lungs and leads to chronic infections. The average life span of victims is 26, and few live beyond 40.

- *Phenylketonuria (PKU):* **Phenylketonuria,** or **PKU,** is a condition that leads to severe retardation unless preventive steps are taken soon after birth. The condition is caused by the absence of a crucial liver enzyme (phenylalanine). Most newborns are routinely screened for PKU, and those found to have it are put on a strict diet that prevents brain damage.

The chances of having a baby with chromosome abnormalities, such as Down syndrome, increase as the mother gets older. More than one in four women who gave birth in 1988 were over 30, according to the National Center for Health Statistics.[96] (*See* ● *Figure 24.9.*)

Controversy: How Desirable Is Genetic Testing? Genetic testing or screening, the science of scrutinizing human genes for abnormalities, has come a long way in recent years, raising profound implications for the future. Consider a few ethical issues:

- *Should the sex of babies be determined in advance?* The technology already exists, as we discuss later in the chapter, for determining the sex of a baby before it is born. Medical procedures (amniocentesis, chorionic villus sampling, ultrasound) must be conducted on the fetus in the uterus. Now researchers can determine the sex of a test-tube baby before it is implanted in the mother's womb.[97]

The good news is that this pre-implantation testing helps couples carrying genetic defects to make decisions about children, such as whether to continue the pregnancy despite evidence of a problem. Ensuring that a baby is a girl is especially important to parents in which the woman is a carrier for Duchenne muscular dystrophy or hemophilia, for example, which primarily affect males. The bad news is that this kind of screening to determine sex could be used to *prevent* the birth of a child of an unwanted sex. In many societies, there is a strong social preference for male children. In India, for instance, a pregnant woman

When the mother's age is . . .	20	25	30	35	40	45	49
Her chances of having a baby born with Down syndrome is 1 out of . . .	1667	1250	952	378	106	30	11
And her chances of having a baby born with some chromosomal abnormality is 1 out of . . .	526	476	385	192	66	21	8

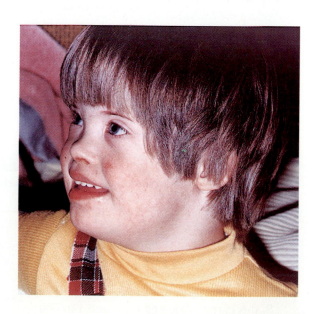

● **Figure 24.9 The older mother and risk of genetic abnormalities.** The chances of having a baby with chromosomal abnormalities, such as Down syndrome, increase with age, as this risk table shows.

who has access to medical technology to ascertain the sex of the infant she is carrying often chooses to abort the fetus if tests show it is a girl. As a result, census data is showing a dramatic skewing of sex ratios in favor of males in India.[98]

- *Should genetic testing be done even if it is expensive and uncertain?* Because cystic fibrosis is so common, should everyone be screened for it—even though the test is expensive and not all carriers can be identified unless doctors know exactly what to search for? Screening the general population might give thousands of people a false sense of security.[99,100]

- *Should genetic screening be done if it affects insurance risk and employment?* What if testing *might* reveal a genetic problem with your child that could cause the health insurer to limit or deny coverage or charge a higher premium?[101] What if employers used the results of genetic tests taken for health purposes to discriminate against people who have indicators for heart disease, cancer, or certain personality traits?[102]

- *Should genetic testing be done if results might have a negative effect on the person's mental well-being?* Suppose you knew that you or your children carried the gene for a serious health problem. For example, symptoms of the genetic disease of Huntington's chorea (which don't show up until middle age) include personality changes, dementia, jerking and writhing movements, and a progressively failing mind and body for many years until death.

Genetic testing can predict with great accuracy whether someone with a family history of Huntington's chorea will be affected. Would you want to know about it—or your child to know about it—when nothing can be done to prevent it? This is truly a terrible dilemma.[103,104]

Strategy for Living: Genetic Counseling and Gene Therapy The concerns just discussed are all legitimate ones. Fortunately, however, one of the greatest stories of our time is the unfolding discovery of not only how genes cause problems but also how defective ones can

be repaired or replaced or how genetic engineering may reverse the effects of illness. A genetically engineered drug called DNase, for example, has been found to help break up the infected mucus in the lungs of patients suffering from cystic fibrosis.[105] Biomedical researchers have also done laboratory experiments that replace the defective gene that causes cystic fibrosis with normal copies that correct the crucial defect that cripples the lung cells.[106] Genetic scientists are also doing experiments in the treatment of sickle-cell anemia, diabetes, cardiovascular disease, and cancer.

Because of these and other rapid advances in medicine and biotechnology, it makes sense to make an analysis of your family's "health tree." The **family health tree** resembles the kind of family tree that genealogists put together, except that, in addition to your parents', grandparents', and other relatives' birth and death dates, it includes diseases they may have died of and (if possible) the age at which the diseases were diagnosed. This kind of family tree can be of value as a tipoff not only for possible genetic disorders but also for various cancers, heart disease, diabetes, and other conditions considered "familial." (*See Self Discovery 24.2.*) Whether or not you are contemplating having children, if you have any suspicion a disorder runs in your family, you would probably benefit from talking to a genetic counselor. If you and your partner are considering having a baby, and you suspect some history of genetic disorders, genetic counseling is a must.

Strategy for Living: Preconception Care for Parenthood

Preconception care is care prospective parents take before even conceiving a child: not smoking, not consuming alcohol or other drugs, eating right, and being careful about pollution and radiation.

Aside from being aware of their genetic heritage, there are various kinds of preconception care that prospective parents can take to improve the chances that their child will be born

10.20

*Unit 10
Family Matters:
Decisions About
Parenting,
Pregnancy, and
Childbirth*

SELF DISCOVERY 24.2

Your Family Health Tree

The purpose of the family health tree is to help you establish any genetic disorders or familial diseases for which you or your children may be at risk. Besides genetic diseases such as sickle-cell anemia, PKU, Down syndrome, and cystic fibrosis, you should try to establish any patterns for various types of cancers, heart disease, diabetes, addictions, and mental disorders (depression, schizophrenia, "senility"). You can get information by interviewing parents and close relatives.

Once your information is as complete as you can get it, look for similar diseases (such as cancers or heart disease) among your parents and brothers and sisters (your *primary relatives*), then among your grandparents and aunts and uncles (your *secondary relatives*), then among your great-grandparents and your cousins (your *tertiary relatives*). If similar disorders or diseases exist in your primary and secondary relatives particularly, that may be a warning sign.

In each area below, include *name, date of birth, age at death, cause of death, incidence and type of disease*, and *age of diagnosis of disease*. Of course, not all this information may be available to you.

Explanation

Squares = male relatives
Circles = female relatives

Red = primary relatives
Blue = secondary relatives
Yellow = tertiary relatives

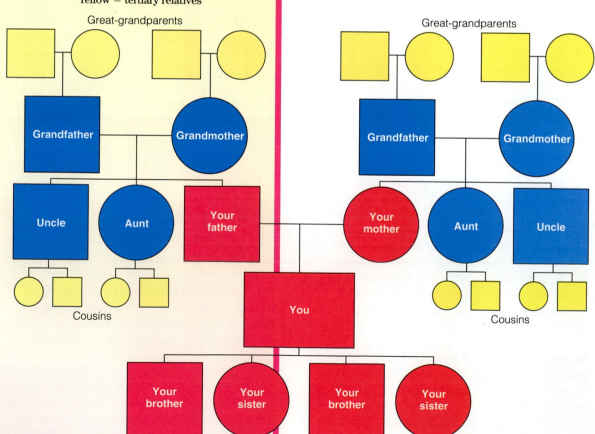

healthy. **Preconception care** is the care you take before conceiving a child in order to ensure its health. Preconception care can be valuable for both women and men. Indeed, the lifestyles and occupations that fathers follow can be every bit as important as those of mothers in affecting the health of the future offspring.

The Mother's Self-Care If you are a woman who has thought it was time "to get in shape," plans to become pregnant should give you all the reasons you need. Smoking, alcohol, drugs, and a nonnutritious diet are not only bad *during* pregnancy but also *before* the baby is even conceived. So are being overweight or underweight and being exposed to radiation and various fumes and solvents.[107–109]

Some diseases contracted by the mother are particularly risky for the baby. All women of childbearing age should be vaccinated against rubella (German measles), which can cause birth defects ranging from deafness to congenital heart disease. Women should also be tested for genital herpes. One study found that 32% of 277 pregnant women had herpes, although two-thirds reported no history of blistering or other symptoms.[110]

The U.S. Public Health Service has also recommended that all women of childbearing age take folic acid supplementation (a B vitamin) to prevent such birth defects as spina bifida (in which a piece of the spinal cord protrudes from the spinal column) and anencephaly (in which most of the brain is missing). The government recommends that *all* women of childbearing age take 400 micrograms (0.4 milligrams) of folic acid a day.[111,112]

The Father's Self-Care The man who really wants healthy children has two pieces of business to take care of—making sure he does nothing to reduce the potency of his sperm and avoiding environmental and lifestyle hazards that could lead to birth defects.

- *Healthy sperm:* Men may already have a problem. According to one study, the past 50 years may have seen a significant reduction in men's average sperm count, possibly because of environmental pollution.[113] Starting with this possible disadvantage, they must then try to avoid worsening the situation.

  Men who have an unbalanced diet or who smoke may have low levels of vitamin C, which may increase the likelihood of producing children with birth defects and certain types of cancer (leukemia and lymphoma).[114] It is recommended that they include more fruit and vegetables in their diet or take a vitamin C supplement every day.

  Men who are heavy drinkers are known to have comparatively low sperm counts. Alcohol, particularly binge drinking, also suppresses the body's ability to produce sperm, as research on rats shows.[115] Indeed, drinking a six-pack of beer in less than 2 hours blocks the genetic messenger that orders the testicles to produce sperm.

(But don't rely on this phenomenon for contraception!)

- *Habits and working conditions:* The male reproductive tract is extremely vulnerable to poisons and gene-damaging substances, some of which men may be exposed to in the course of their work. (*See* ● *Figure 24.10.*)

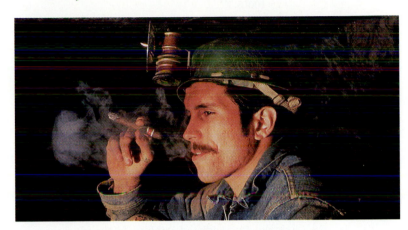

● **Figure 24.10 Fathers' jobs and habits and babies' health**

66. *Men who work in the glass, clay, stone, textile, and mining industries have twice the average risk of fathering premature infants.*

- *Fathers who smoke have above-average rates of low-birth-weight babies and children with brain cancer and leukemia.*

- *The wives of men exposed to vinyl chloride, an ingredient in plastic, and water treatment materials have elevated miscarriage rates.*

- *Men exposed to low levels of radiation in a British nuclear power plant fathered children with increased rates of leukemia.*

- *Fireman exposed to the wide variety of poisons in smoke have an increased risk of having children with heart defects.*

- *Children of men who work with hydrocarbons, solvents, spray paints, and toxic metal fumes have increased rates of cancer and birth defects.*

- *Children of male aerospace workers have higher rates of brain tumors.* 99

—Sandra Blakeslee (1991, April). Father figures: The male link to birth defects. *American Health*, pp. 54–57.

10.22

Unit 10
Family Matters:
Decisions About
Parenting,
Pregnancy, and
Childbirth

Among the sperm-damaging substances are lead, paint thinners and other industrial solvents, pesticides, and ionizing radiation. Alcohol and marijuana smoke are also dangerous.[116] One study suggests that men in certain jobs—janitors and certain mill workers, for instance—have a higher risk of becoming parents of children with birth defects.[117]

Perhaps, as one writer suggests, the day will come when businesses and governments establish policies for a workplace that is safe for everyone—mother, father, and fetus. That would mean establishing policies to protect the unborn even before conception occurs.[118]

800-HELP

AASK-America (Aid to Adoption of Special Kids). 800-232-2751. Nonprofit adoption program that places so-called unadoptable children—for example, drug-addicted children, fetal alcohol syndrome infants, those with AIDS, and older, abused, abandoned children.

Alliance of Genetic Support Groups. 800-336-GENE. An umbrella organization of support groups for people or parents of children with genetic disorders.

American Adoption Congress. 800-274-6736. Support group for adoptees seeking their birth parents.

Childhelp USA/IOF Foresters National Child Abuse Hotline. 800-4-A-CHILD. Provides crisis counseling and referrals for child abusers and their victims.

Childwatch. 800-222-1464 (in Canada 800-248-1464). Hotline of National Child Safety Council.

Cystic Fibrosis Foundation. 800-FIGHT-CF. Information about this inherited disease and its treatment.

National Center for Missing and Exploited Children. 800-843-5678

Parents Anonymous. 800-421-0353. A California-based organization set up to fight child abuse. It has steered troubled parents into more than 1100 inexpensive group-therapy sessions where abusive parents can vent feelings, find out they are not alone, and learn better ways of parenting.

RESOLVE. 800-662-1016. Nonprofit, nationwide information network serving needs of infertile couples; gives support-group referrals for people coping with infertility.

Suggestions for Further Reading

Anton, Linda Hunt (1992). *Never to be a mother: A guide for all women who didn't—or couldn't—have children.* New York: HarperCollins. A clinical social worker directs this comforting guide to women who are not childless by choice.

Berman, Claire (1991). *Adult children of divorce speak out: About growing up with—and moving beyond—parental divorce.* New York: Simon & Schuster. A journalist who served as national president of the Stepfamily Association of America reports interviews with grown children of divorce and offers ways to mitigate the ongoing effect of divorce on a child's life.

Cowan, Carolyn Pape, & Cowan, Philip A. (1992). *When partners become parents: The big life change for couples.* New York: Basic Books. Two University of California at Berkeley professors, married to each other, report on a 10-year project tracking parent and nonparent couples. They conclude parenthood is more difficult now than in the past and that it is easy to fall into traditional mom-and-dad roles, however egalitarian one's ideals.

Hewlett, Sylvia Ann (1991). *When the bough breaks: The cost of neglecting our children.* New York: Basic Books. An economist's examination of why America is so far behind in the care of its children.

25 Pregnancy, Childbirth, and Homecoming

▶ Explain the experience of pregnancy from the baby's, mother's, and father's points of view.

▶ What kind of prenatal care should a mother-to-be concern herself with?

▶ Explain the kinds of possible birth-related complications parents should be aware of.

▶ Describe the process of labor and delivery.

▶ What kinds of decisions about childbirth are available to prospective parents?

▶ Explain what kinds of things could happen after the baby is born.

At what time of year are obstetricians least likely to take their vacations? Late summer, especially September, says one report.[119] That's when the largest group of babies is born—at least in the United States. Although most people would prefer to have their babies in the spring, it can take 3–4 months or more to conceive—which is why most birth dates can't be preplanned.[120]

In other parts of the world, peak months for births vary according to latitude and climate when conception occurred, according to one study.[121] Air conditioning and heating in industrialized nations change this somewhat.[122]

Pregnancy: The Inside Story

The 9 months of pregnancy are divided into three parts called *trimesters*. The first trimester consists of conception, implantation, and early growth of the embryo and fetus. At the end of the second trimester the infant has a small chance of surviving outside the womb. In the third trimester the infant develops surfactant, which enables it to breathe on its own.

If your mother's pregnancy met the average and went full term, your stay inside her body lasted 266 days from conception to birth, or about 9 calendar months. These 9 months are divided into thirds called **trimesters.** (*See ●Figure 25.1.*) Actually, the first trimester is dated from the beginning of the last menstrual period, about 2 weeks before conception.

The First Trimester: Conception, Implantation, and Early Growth You began life with conception. **Conception,** or **fertilization,** was the uniting of the ovum or egg from your mother with a sperm cell from your father in one of the two **fallopian tubes,** attached to the uterus. The **ovum** is the female reproductive cell, the **sperm** the male reproductive cell, and the fertilized ovum is called a **zygote.**

Moved along by hairlike projections called **cilia,** which line the fallopian tube, the zygote was propelled into the **uterus,** or **womb,** where it grew and was nourished until birth. (*See ●Figure 25.2.*) As it moved along, the zygote underwent cell division—one cell divided into two cells, two into four, four into eight, and so on. The subdivided cells were smaller, so the total zygote remained the same size as the fertilized ovum. Three to four days after conception, the zygote entered the uterus, and in another three or four days buried itself within the uterine lining, called the **endometrium,** a process called **implantation.** At this point, from the second through the eighth week, the growing baby is called an **embryo.** After implantation, a

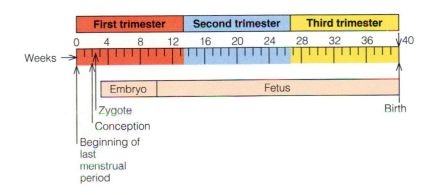

● **Figure 25.1 The three trimesters of pregnancy**

10.24

*Unit 10
Family Matters:
Decisions About
Parenting,
Pregnancy, and
Childbirth*

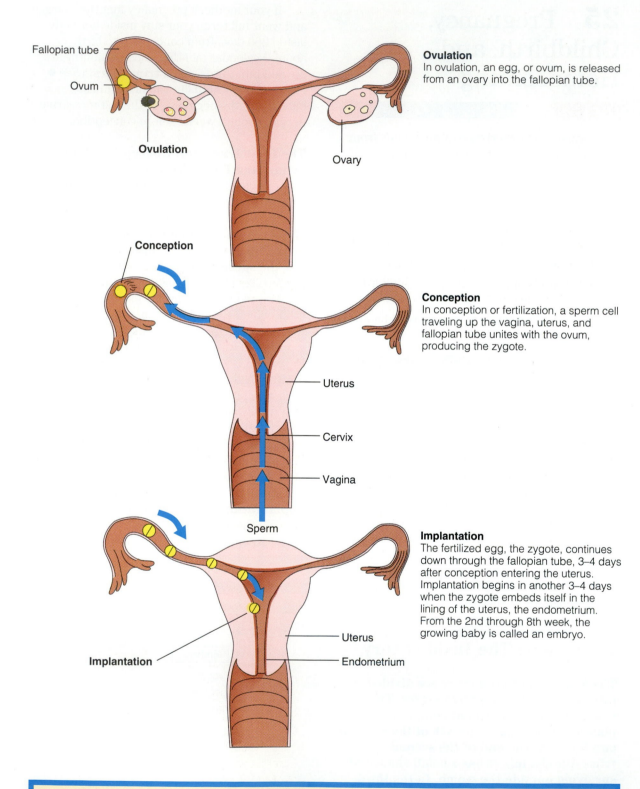

Ovulation
In ovulation, an egg, or ovum, is released from an ovary into the fallopian tube.

Conception
In conception or fertilization, a sperm cell traveling up the vagina, uterus, and fallopian tube unites with the ovum, producing the zygote.

Implantation
The fertilized egg, the zygote, continues down through the fallopian tube, 3–4 days after conception entering the uterus. Implantation begins in another 3–4 days when the zygote embeds itself in the lining of the uterus, the endometrium. From the 2nd through 8th week, the growing baby is called an embryo.

● **Figure 25.2 Conception and implantation**

hormone called **human chorionic gonadotropin (HCG)** was secreted first by special cells of the developing embryo and later by cells that make up the placenta. HCG is the substance measured in most pregnancy tests.

From the embryo, **chorionic villi,** small fingerlike growths, began to burrow into the endometrium, the uterine blood supply. From these villi and the uterine wall, a **placenta** began to form. (See ● *Figure 25.3.*) Beginning about 4 weeks after conception, the placenta supplied you, the growing infant, with nourishment and oxygen from your mother's blood and returned wastes back to your mother's body for disposal. This was accomplished through the **umbilical cord,** which contained two arteries and a vein and which carried blood from the placenta to you and vice versa. Your blood never directly mixed with that of your mother. Even so, the placenta was not sufficient to prevent any drugs or some diseases that were in your mother's bloodstream from entering your blood. Inside the uterus, you floated in a sac of liquid called **amniotic fluid,** also called the "bag of waters."

By the end of your first month, you had multiplied to 10,000 times your original size, though you were still only about a quarter inch long and weighed only one-seventh of an ounce. (See ● *Figure 25.4.*) Did you look like a person? Barely. Your head was disproportionately large, because of brain development. The forerunners of your throat, jaw, and mouth had developed, but they looked like gills. You had only the rudiments of eyes, ears, and nose. A fold called the neural groove had appeared, which later became your nervous system. (See ● *Figure 25.5.*)

By the end of the second month, you were a **fetus.** (The *embryo* describes the fertilized egg from conception to week 8, the *fetus* from week 9 to delivery.) At that point you were 1.2 inches long, had fingers and toes in human form, and had developed a circulatory system.

By the end of the third month—the end of the first trimester—you were about 3 inches long, most major organs were present, a heartbeat could be detected (with a stethoscope), and your face and head were formed. Your sex was also apparent. You probably also were moving a bit within your watery environment, although your mother could not feel it yet.

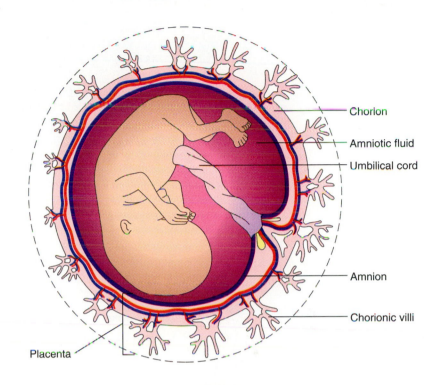

Chorion
Amniotic fluid
Umbilical cord
Amnion
Chorionic villi
Placenta

● **Figure 25.3 The protected infant.** Formed by the embryo's chorionic villi and the mother's uterine wall, the placenta provides the growing infant, through the umbilical cord, with nutrients from the mother's bloodstream and removes wastes. The infant floats in a liquid environment called amniotic fluid.

The Second Trimester By the end of the fourth month, you had become more than 6 inches long and weighed perhaps 5 ounces. Your skeleton developed and your skin was covered with a fine hair, called **lanugo,** which you probably shed before birth.

At the end of the fifth month, you could have been as much as 12 inches long and weighed about a pound. You had developed nails on your fingers and toes, and your ears were able to hear sounds. You were capable of grasping and sucking, and you slept and woke by turns. Your mother could feel you kicking and moving about in her womb. Your skin was covered by a cheeselike coating called the **vernix caseosa,** which remained until it was absorbed into your skin within the first 24 hours after you were born.

10.26

Unit 10
Family Matters:
Decisions About
Parenting,
Pregnancy, and
Childbirth

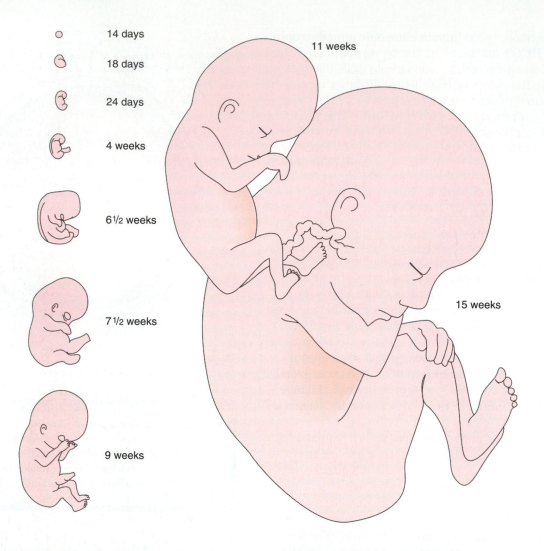

14 days

18 days

24 days

4 weeks

6½ weeks

7½ weeks

9 weeks

11 weeks

15 weeks

● **Figure 25.4 Actual size.** Growth of the embryo and fetus from 2 to 15 weeks after conception.

By the end of the sixth month, you were perhaps 13 inches long and your eyes had become light sensitive. Eyebrows and eyelashes were formed. You were sucking your thumb and perhaps even had hiccups. If you were born at this age, you appeared thin and scrawny. Your organs, including your lungs, remained immature. If you were born at this age, you had a 10% chance of surviving.

A critical matter during the second trimester was your brain development, which is essential to your attaining the **age of viability,** the point somewhere between the 20th and 26th weeks after conception when you would have some chance of survival outside the womb, if expert care were provided.

The Third Trimester At the end of the seventh month inside your mother, you had reached 14 or 15 inches in length and you had gained weight, mainly as fat layers under your skin, so that you weighed perhaps 3 pounds. Your head had abundant hair, your eyelids were open, and—particularly critical—you probably had developed **surfactant,** a substance produced in your lungs that enabled you to breathe on your own.

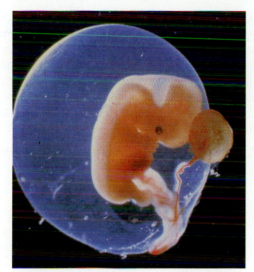

5–6 weeks

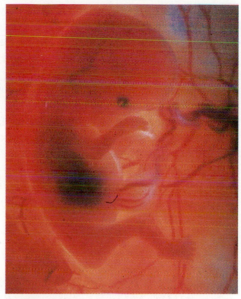

8–12 weeks

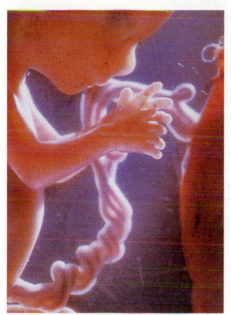

16 weeks

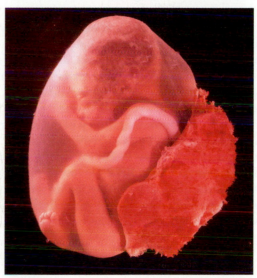

36 weeks

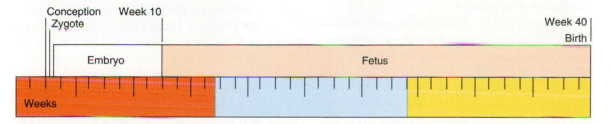

● **Figure 25.5 Development of the embryo and fetus**

10.28

Unit 10
Family Matters:
Decisions About
Parenting,
Pregnancy, and
Childbirth

By the end of the eighth month, you may have reached 18 inches long and weighed about 5 pounds. Your skin had a wrinkled appearance. By this time, you had also probably assumed a head-down position in your mother's uterus.

By the end of your third trimester, you had reached about 19 inches and weighed 6 or 7 pounds. Your limbs were proportional, your face had features, your skin was smooth, the bones of your skull had hardened but had not completely connected, since some flexiblity was needed to enable you to pass through your mother's pelvis.

Ready or not, here you came—into the world.

Pregnancy: The Mother's Story

Pregnancy detecting begins in the first trimester with presumptive signs that lead a woman to guess she's pregnant, such as missed menstrual period. A physician looks for probable signs, such as laboratory tests to detect the placental hormone HCG, and then positive signs, such as hearing a fetal heartbeat. In the second trimester, the woman gains weight, experiences changes in body secretions, and feels the baby move inside of her. The third trimester may be a period of increasing discomfort as the infant gains weight, putting pressure on her organs, until at last the baby is ready to be born.

Perhaps your mother had what is known as an "easy" pregnancy, perhaps not. First pregnancies are usually more "difficult," it is said, than subsequent ones.

The terms "easy" and "difficult" are relative. The fact is, nearly any pregnancy can be an uncomfortable experience, characterized by such complaints as fatigue, nausea, indigestion, constipation, breathlessness, and trouble sleeping. On the other hand, there are few thrills to compare with those of feeling the stirrings of a new life within.[123]

The First Trimester: Detecting Pregnancy
The stirrings don't happen right away, of course. At first, a woman may have just the vaguest suspicion she may be pregnant, which she may then voice to a physician, who in turn may order some tests. Pregnancy detection is based on a variety of signs and symptoms, some of which are more reliable indicators of pregnancy than others. Depending on their reliability, these signs are categorized as *presumptive, probable,* and *positive.*[124]

- *Presumptive signs:* **Presumptive signs** are the subjective signs by which the woman herself guesses she may be pregnant. The classic presumptive sign is a missed menstrual period. Actually, pregnancy has been known to occur in women who have never menstruated, in menstruating women (though often they notice a change in their normal periods), and in nursing mothers not currently menstruating.

  Other symptoms of pregnancy are **morning sickness**—nausea and vomiting that occur on rising in the morning or during other times of the day—and frequent need to urinate, primarily owing to the pressure of the fetus on the bladder, and fatigue. There are also changes in the body itself: the breasts become enlarged and more tender as milk glands develop, and the areolae (the ring around the nipples) become darkened.

- *Probable signs:* **Probable signs** are those by which a physician determines that pregnancy is probable. Probable signs include positive pregnancy tests, slight increase in body temperature, softening and enlargement of the uterus, and bluish discoloration of the cervix.

  Pregnancy tests are based on detecting the presence of *human chorionic gonadotropin (HCG),* which is secreted by the placenta. Blood pregnancy tests are the most accurate pregnancy tests and can be used as early as 10 days after conception. Home pregnancy tests, which test urine for HCG, are generally used after the first day of a missed period. They are inexpensive and easy to use, although not always accurate (they are in error 20% of the time), especially in the early weeks of pregnancy. Laboratory pregnancy tests, by contrast, have only a 1% error rate.[125] Thus, a woman worrying about an unwanted pregnancy who finds herself testing "not pregnant" on a home pregnancy test should not breathe a sigh of relief just yet; rather she should wait a week and take the test again, or have a professionally administered laboratory test.

- *Positive signs:* **Positive signs** are those detected by the physician that definitely indicate pregnancy. Many of these signs are present only later in pregnancy. There are five positive signs: The examiner (1) feels the fetus move, (2) hears the fetal heartbeat, (3) detects the fetal skeleton through an X ray, (4) obtains an electronic tracing of the fetal heart rate, and (5) sees an outline of the fetus by means of ultrasonic equipment.[126]

Of course, one of the first things people want to know is, When is the baby due? Since 266 is the *average* number of days from conception to birth, some babies will be early, some late. (However, only about 4% of pregnancies continue 2 weeks beyond 266 days.)[127] A rule for calculating the expected date of childbirth, called **Naegele's formula,** is to add 1 week to the first day of the last menstrual period, subtract 3 months, and add 1 year. This works out to 9 months and 7 days from the beginning of a woman's last menstrual period.[128]

How the woman reacts to the news of her pregnancy depends in great part on whether the pregnancy is planned or not, on whether she is in love with the father, whether financial hard times mean the baby is merely another mouth to feed, and all kinds of other matters. Women having second or subsequent pregnancies view them more negatively than first ones, perhaps because of their awareness of the costs and responsibilities.[129] Pregnancy seems more desirable if the man is employed.[130] In addition, the woman's reactions can vary depending on the extent of the father's support.[131]

The Second Trimester During the second 3 months of pregnancy, the mother will definitely begin to notice the transformations within her body. Her waistline begins to expand, and she will find herself having to think about getting maternity clothes.

Many women experience the second trimester as an enjoyable time, as the morning sickness and fatigue recede. Still, there are many adjustments. She may find herself craving certain foods—not just the classic pickles and peppermint ice cream, but foods she may not even have liked before. She may experience indigestion, constipation, and hemorrhoids. The pigment around her nipples will darken further, and a dark line will appear down the center of her abdomen. Body secretions increase: perspiration, saliva, vaginal fluids, and perhaps **colostrum** in her breasts, a yellowish milk that will exist until a few days following childbirth. As her heart works harder to supply blood to both herself and the fetus, it enlarges somewhat and shifts position. By the fourth or fifth month, she will experience "quickening"—the baby moving and kicking inside her.

The Third Trimester During months 7–9, the mother-to-be may experience increasing discomfort. The growing infant puts pressure on her internal organs, including her bladder, causing frequent urination; her lungs and diaphragm, causing breathlessness; and her stomach, causing heartburn. She may have difficulty sleeping, because of the baby's constant movements or because she needs to get up and urinate. She may have backaches. She has swollen legs if she stands too long. She may find it awkward to move, sit down, stand up. About 2–4 weeks before birth, the baby "drops"—its head settles low in her pelvis. As she nears the end of the ninth month, her moods may swing from anxiety and apprehension to excitement and anticipation of the impending arrival.

Then one day—or, often, one night—the time she thought would never come finally does. The baby signals it is ready to be born.

Pregnancy: The Father's Story

If fathers-to-be often get less attention than prospective mothers, many are still excited participants. Some even experience "couvade," completely identifying with the woman's physical symptoms.

The father's story is mainly an emotional one. Even the most involved father, however, is less apt to get attention than the prospective mother. (See ● *Figure 25.6.*)

10.30

*Unit 10
Family Matters:
Decisions About
Parenting,
Pregnancy, and
Childbirth*

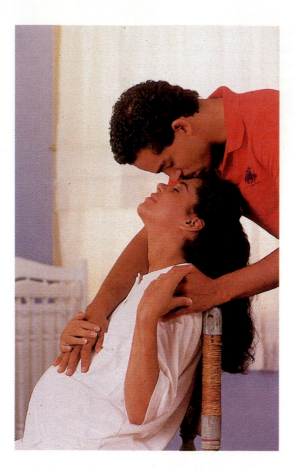

● **Figure 25.6 The overlooked father**

❝ . . . Although fathers-to-be may need as much social support as mothers-to-be, they are less likely to get it. For one thing, their imminent parenthood is not visible, so their friends, family, and co-workers are less likely to express interest in the pregnancy. For another, men at all points of the life span are less likely to reveal their need for help. Especially as fatherhood approaches, many men make a special effort to appear strong and protective, frequently camouflaging their understandable feelings of panic by springing into action. Some build a crib, a room, or even a house; others become intensely involved in physical fitness or sports; others eat too much or develop physical symptoms of their own.❞

—Kathleen Stassen Berger (1988). *The developing person through the life span* (2nd ed.). New York: Worth, p. 94.

Some fathers are excited participants, identifying with all the stages of pregnancy.[132] Indeed, there are men who so completely identify with the woman's pregnancy that they even experience some of the same physical symptoms.[133] This psychosomatic behavior, called *couvade*, from a French word meaning "to sit on or to hatch," may affect a great many fathers.[134,135] Some fathers-to-be become preoccupied with themselves, overexercising or overeating.[136] Others become so resentful that they actually harm their partners; in fact, the incidence of wife-beating actually increases during pregnancy.[137] Many couples, however, find that the event brings them closer together than they have ever been before.[138]

One study found that whether or not men felt *ready* to be receptive to a pregnancy depended on the stability of the relationship, their sense of financial security, whether or not they intended to be parents at some point, and the sense of coming to an end of the childless part

of their life.[139] Their readiness, then, depended on the goals they had set earlier in their lives.

Pennsylvania dairy farmer Jeff Kennedy, 22, was ready. He had even gone to classes at the hospital so he could be present during the delivery. "I want to be right there the whole time," he said. "They even told us at the last class that we get to cut the baby's navel cord, and I'm looking forward to that one. A lot of people wouldn't do such a thing, but I guess, being farm oriented, I'm used to that kind of stuff and I'm just excited to see. It's my first baby to see born."[140]

Mother Care: Prenatal Care for Mother and Infant

Prenatal care is care the expectant mother takes of herself and her infant during pregnancy. This includes medical care, a

well-balanced diet, exercise and rest, and stress reduction. Pregnant women who smoke risk having premature or low-birth-weight babies. Those who drink alcohol risk producing babies with fetal alcohol syndrome, a form of retardation, or fetal alcohol effects, which cause other problems. Marijuana, cocaine, and other drugs also cause trouble. Pregnant women should also avoid radiation and environmental pollution.

If you are a new mother-to-be, with a child growing within, you may be suddenly struck by the awesome pending responsibility of having to take care of a new life. Actually, that responsibility begins now. **Prenatal care** means taking care of yourself and the baby before birth.

Poor health care for expectant mothers leads to many problems. Of the 3.8 million infants born in the United States in 1987, 38,408 died before their first birthday, with black infants perishing at twice the rate of white infants.[141,142] In addition, more than 250,000 low-birth-weight infants are born each year. Low birth weight is associated with increased risk of death and a wide range of disorders, including nervous system disorders, cerebral palsy, low IQ, learning disorders, behavior problems, and lower respiratory tract infections.[143] Children with these kinds of problems can place a tremendous emotional and financial burden on their parents. One study found that for every 100 babies born in American hospitals, women are hospitalized 22 times for pregnancy complications.[144] In addition, although the number of maternal deaths each year is small, many are preventable good prenatal care.

Among the things an expectant mother must think about are:

- Medical care
- Nutrition
- Exercise and rest
- Stress
- Caffeine, tobacco, alcohol, and other drug use
- Environmental hazards

Of course, all these factors affect her own health, but now she has the added responsibility of thinking about her baby's health as well.

Prenatal Medical Care As soon as a woman suspects she may be pregnant, she should see a health care professional and have a complete physical examination. This is important because the first trimester of pregnancy is critical to the fetus's health and well-being. Because both parents are (or should be) participants in this event, it is beneficial if both come to the examination.

The health care professional may be a physician assistant nurse, nurse practitioner, or nurse-midwife. Or it may be a physician such as a general practitioner or family practitioner. Most often it is an **obstetrician/gynecologist (OB/GYN),** a doctor who specializes in the female reproductive system and pregnancy. A pregnant woman will usually see her health care professional once a month through the first 2 trimesters, then every 2 weeks and finally every week during the last trimester.

Nutrition: Eating for Two If indeed "You are what you eat," as the saying goes, so is your baby, if you're pregnant. Some physicians will prescribe special vitamin supplements during pregnancy, but the expectant mother also needs to make sure she gets *increased* amounts of vitamins and minerals from a well-balanced diet, as well as increased protein. A serious protein deficiency can lead to low birth weight, premature birth, and mental retardation.[145] Increased calcium may also help prevent one of the most common complications of pregnancy, hypertension (high blood pressure).[146]

An important part of prenatal nutrition is *weight gain*—25–35 pounds is normal, according to recent guidelines by the National Academy of Sciences' Food and Nutrition Board.[147] (Overweight women should gain 15–25 pounds, underweight women 28–40 pounds.) The exact amount of extra weight should be worked out between the mother-to-be and her doctor, but even a 30-pound weight gain should be considered normal. The new guidelines are higher than was recommended in the 1970s, the reasoning being that the mother's weight gain helps to lower the risk of low-birth-weight babies. It is particularly important that pregnant women gain enough weight in the first and second trimesters, if the risk of low-birth-weight babies is to be avoided.[148]

10.32

Unit 10
Family Matters:
Decisions About
Parenting,
Pregnancy, and
Childbirth

Why, you might wonder, if the average baby weighs 7½ pounds at birth, should a woman put on more than three times that amount in extra weight? The fetus is only part of it. The rest goes to increased body fluid, blood, breasts, the placenta, the uterus, and maternal stores of various nutrients. (*See ● Figure 25.7.*)

Exercise and Rest "Pregnancy is like an athletic event," says obstetrician Douglas Hall. "A woman should prepare for it the way an athlete would."[149] Expectant women can continue doing the kinds of activities they're used to—although they shouldn't *take up* strenuous new activities while pregnant.

Rest is important, and women who find the baby's exertions and the pressure on the bladder keeps them awake at night are advised to nap during the day, if possible. Sleeping pills or any other drugs, however, should be avoided.

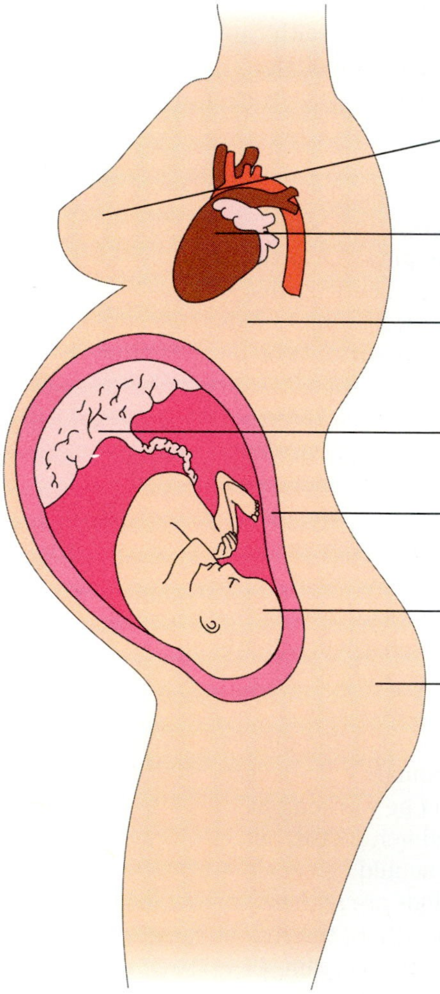

Stress Here are the results of one study: Pregnant women who took adversity hard and fretted for extended periods were far likelier to have premature or low-birth-weight babies than pregnant women who reacted to stressful situations with equanimity.[150] And here are the results of another: long hours and hard, stressful work do not increase early deliveries, low-birth-weight babies, miscarriage, and the like.[151]

So, should you try to avoid stress or not (as if avoiding stress were possible)? The first study compared two groups of low-income women. The second compared higher-income female physicians, who became pregnant during their residencies, with wives of medical residents. Perhaps, then, the matter comes down to other factors: being in good health during pregnancy, eating well, avoiding cigarettes and alcohol, and reacting well to stress. Even so, although many pregnant women have stressful lives and must work right up to the day of their delivery, if you as a pregnant woman have a choice it's probably advisable to try to lower your stress levels.

Incidentally, women who wind down in the high temperatures of hot tubs and saunas should stay away from them during pregnancy. One study found that women who continued to use them during the first 6 weeks of pregnancy faced up to triple the risk of bearing babies with spina bifida or brain defects.[152]

Caffeine, Tobacco, Alcohol, and Other Drugs The benefits and risks of using any drug during pregnancy must be carefully weighed. Some drugs have both positive and negative effects. Aspirin is a good example. Some studies indicate that low doses of aspirin may prevent pregnant women from developing pregnancy-induced high blood pressure and reduce their risk of having low-birth-weight infants by 44%.[153] Aspirin is also a potent antiprostaglandin agent that may interfere with uterine contractions during labor, thus prolonging childbirth.

1–2 pounds—Breast enlargement

3–4 pounds—Increased blood volume

2–3 pounds—Increased volume of fluids other than blood

1½ pounds—Placenta

2 pounds—Uterus

6–8 pounds—Fetus

4–6 pounds—Stores of fat, protein, and other nutrients to nourish fetus

● **Figure 25.7 Where the extra pounds go**

However, all drugs, whether available in a pharmacy, liquor store, or on the street, should be avoided unless prescribed by a doctor. The reason, of course, is that any drug taken by the mother readily crosses the placenta and enters into the baby's bloodsteam. This means that if the mother is dependent on or addicted to some drug, the baby will be too.

Some of the most common drugs to think about are the following.

- *Caffeine:* Is a cup of coffee or tea or a glass of Coke harmful? In moderation, probably not. However, research suggests that mothers who usually consume caffeine fairly heavily (300 milligrams or more a day—3 restaurant-size cups of coffee or 6 cans of cola) may produce low-birth-weight babies.[154,155]

- *Tobacco:* A pregnant woman who smokes— and 1 in 5 pregnant women do smoke—is in a real dilemma: you're not just smoking for yourself but for the both of you, and the effects on infants are serious.[156] Experts estimate that the elimination of smoking during pregnancy would reduce infant mortality by 10%, or 2500–3000 deaths per year.[157]

  Smoking reduces the flow of blood to the infant and reduces the amount of oxygen carried by the blood.[158] As a result, smoking mothers have increased rates of miscarriage, stillbirths, and premature babies; often produce smaller, low-weight babies; and have babies with higher infant death rates.[159–161] Lower birth weight does not mean merely a smaller baby. Cigarette smoking deprives the fetus of essential growth of *all* its body organs, including the brain, which can lead to developmental delays in children.[162]

  In sum: The more cigarettes a woman smokes during pregnancy, the more the baby's weight is reduced. Conversely, the earlier a woman quits smoking during her pregnancy, the more positive the impact on her baby's birth weight.[163] Because pregnancy is difficult enough in itself, women trying to have children are well advised to try to quit smoking *before* they become pregnant. A final reason for quitting is this: the more a mother smokes *after* giving

birth, the more behavioral problems her children are likely to have and the higher the likelihood of childhood asthma.[164]

- *Alcohol:* Pregnancy and alcohol are always a dangerous combination. The leading known cause of preventable mental retardation and birth defects in the United States is **fetal alcohol syndrome (FAS).** FAS is characterized by a common pattern of mental retardation and other central nervous system problems; delayed language development and low IQ; malformations of various organ systems (heart, urinary, genital, and skeletal); and growth deficiency and facial abnormalities (small heads, small eyes, and abnormal facial features, including an underdeveloped midface).[165]

  About 1 in every 750 babies born has FAS, and many more have a condition known as **fetal alcohol effects (FAE).** The symptoms of FAE include low birth weight, abnormalities of the mouth and the genital and urinary systems, and altered behavioral patterns.[166]

  Perhaps 30–40% of the children of chronic alcoholic mothers who were drinking during pregnancy will have FAS, but even more children whose mothers were abusing alcohol during pregnancy are at risk for various learning problems even without FAS.[167] As the FAS child grows into adolescence and adulthood, he or she will experience major psychosocial problems and lifelong adjustment problems.[168] Even moderate drinking during pregnancy can produce newborns who are more excitable and irritable than the average newborn, perhaps because alcohol in the mother's bloodstream temporarily reduces oxygen to the fetus, causing slight brain damage.[169,170]

  Signs in restaurants now carry the U.S. Surgeon General's advisory: WARNING: DRINKING ALCOHOLIC BEVERAGES DURING PREGNANCY CAN CAUSE BIRTH DEFECTS. So, how much alcohol is safe? None? One glass a day? One glass a week? All the childbirth books seems to hedge on the issue, and for good reason: the experts aren't sure. Scientists can't experiment on pregnant women, and pregnant women who drink may underreport the amount they consume in alcohol surveys.

10.34

Unit 10
Family Matters:
Decisions About
Parenting,
Pregnancy, and
Childbirth

One thing researchers do seem to agree on is that the worst damage seems to occur in the first trimester, when the fetus's basic growth takes place.[171] Thus, some women may decide, for instance, that a glass of wine with dinner a couple of times a week *after* the first trimester is a conservative risk (if they don't drink caffeine, smoke, or do other drugs). Others may feel more comfortable by playing it totally safe and having no alcohol at all. (*See ● Figure 25.8.*) At this time, until more is known about the effects of alcohol on fetal development, no amount of alcohol can be considered safe during pregnancy.

- *Street drugs:* If street drugs (illegal drugs) are trouble for adults, they are trouble for babies, too. Babies whose mothers are addicted to heroin and methadone, for instance, are born addicted and may die of withdrawal symptoms if they do not receive the drug shortly after birth. Those who survive are apt have a low birth weight and suffer a variety of problems.[172]

    Moderate consumption of marijuana has also led to complications, some of them resembling those produced by alcohol.[173–175] Cocaine can lead to spontaneous abortions, stillbirths, and premature births.[176–178]

- *Prescription drugs:* Several physician-prescribed drugs have been shown to be harmful to the fetus: examples are streptomycin, tetracycline, anticoagulants, and bromides. Tranquilizers and barbiturates such as Valium, chlorpromazine, and phenobarbital are also dangerous.[179,180] Tell all health care professionals and pharmacists that you are pregnant to ensure the safety of any drugs you may be prescribed.

Environmental Hazards: Radiation and Pollution A pregnant woman can control many important aspects of her life that affect her developing fetus—alcohol, drugs, nutrition, exercise. What about certain environmental hazards? Two that she should be aware of are *radiation* and *pollution*.

- *Radiation:* The largest dosage of radiation a pregnant woman is apt to receive is during a pelvic X ray in conjunction with a medical emergency or radiation therapy (as

for cancer). In most cases, the dosages are low enough that the fetus will not be harmed.[181] However, especially during the first trimester, X rays slightly increase the risk of leukemia during childhood.[182] An expectant mother thus should consult with her doctor about the benefits of any X rays (including dental X rays) and risks to her baby.

- *Pollution:* PCBs are a manufacturing chemical and have also become an environmental pollutant. In recent years, PCBs have found their way into the human body through polluted fish. It is not clear whether small amounts of PCBs by themselves will cause birth abnormalities, but women who ate more PCB-polluted fish from Lake Michigan were discovered to have infants who were premature, smaller, and slower to react to stimuli.[183]

    A more likely source of environmental pollution harmful to the fetus is automobile emissions—such as carbon monoxide and lead—as might happen if a woman lives near a heavily traveled street with lots of stop-and-go traffic. Such circumstances have been associated with low birth weight and slow neurological development.[184]

With all the possible hazards, it's easy for pregnant women to worry that they run the risk of doing *something* wrong. However, we need to point out that *most* women are exposed to some of these risks, yet have healthy babies anyway. What is important is the interaction among hazards: the more the hazards and the longer the mother's exposure to them, the more the possibility of some sort of harm to the infant.

Coping with Complications: "Will My Baby and I Be All Right?"

Expectant women need to be aware of possible complications. These include premature labor and preterm births, miscarriage or stillbirth, and ectopic pregnancy, improper implantation that endangers both mother and fetus. Other possible complications are placenta praevia, premature

separation of the placenta, and high blood pressure and toxemia. Diseases that might endanger the unborn baby are rubella, cytomegalovirus, toxoplasmosis, and sexually transmitted diseases. Rh disease may occur in second and later pregnancies. Prenatal tests—ultrasound, amniocentesis, the AFP plus test, chorionic villus sampling, and percutaneous umbilical blood sampling—may help to detect birth defects and other problems.

Most pregnant women give birth to babies with little risk to themselves or to their infants. Even so, in 1987, for every 100 deliveries there were 22 hospitalizations for pregnancy-related complications—*prior* to delivery.[185] Expectant women need to be aware of what some of these common complications are. Here we describe:

- Premature labor and preterm births
- Miscarriages and stillbirths
- Ectopic pregnancy
- Placentia praevia
- High blood pressure and toxemia
- Exposure to infections, such as rubella, cytomegalovirus, toxoplasmosis, and STDs, which can result in birth defects
- Rh disease

Premature Labor and Preterm Births
About 27% of the hospitalizations for pregnancy complications are for premature labor.[186] **Premature** (or "preterm") **labor** is defined as labor occurring before 36 weeks' gestation. Whereas a *mature infant* at birth or near full term (40 weeks) weighs 5.5 pounds or more, an *immature infant* is born before the 28th week and weighs less than 2.2 pounds and a *premature infant* is born after the 27th week and before full term and weighs 2.2–5.5 pounds. Depending on the weight, the chances of a premature infant's surviving range from poor to good.

The earlier a baby is born during pregnancy and the less it weighs, the lower its chances for survival. About 5000 of the babies born between the 24th and 32nd weeks weighing less than 2 pounds die every year, although intensive-care nurseries and a new drug called Exosurf promise to greatly reduce that figure.[187] It is not known why some babies arrive prematurely, but pregnant women who experience such

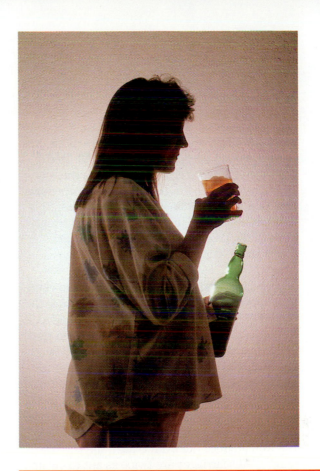

● **Figure 25.8 Pregnancy and drinking.** How much alcohol is too much?

"*Even though 'How much is too much?' is what women really want to know, many experts now believe that the very question may be a bit of a red herring. 'People can argue forever about how much alcohol is safe,' says University of Washington's [pediatrics professor Sterling] Clarren, 'but it's not just how much a woman drinks that's important. It's the specific blood alcohol level that is reached, and that's going to depend on a whole host of variables.'*

A woman's size is one important factor. Clarren explains that a woman who weighs 120 pounds would have to drink only about two-thirds of the amount that a 180-pound woman would need to reach the same blood alcohol level. How and when a woman drinks also figures prominently in the equation. Wine consumed on an empty stomach, for instance, will be absorbed more quickly than wine drunk during dinner. And binge drinking, which can mean something as simple as getting drunk on just one occasion, can be more dangerous than the regular consumption of smaller amounts. Since the fetus is constantly undergoing some kind of change, Clarren theorizes, a high dose all at once can cause damage to whatever part of the body happens to be developing that day."

—Nan Wiener (1992, March 22). Unfair warning? *This World, San Francisco Chronicle*, p. 7. A version of this article appeared earlier in *Parenting* magazine.

10.36

*Unit 10
Family Matters:
Decisions About
Parenting,
Pregnancy, and
Childbirth*

early-warning signs as uterine contractions, low backache, and intestinal cramps should see a physician immediately.[188] Sometimes these contractions will turn out to be **false labor,** which usually stops spontaneously. In false labor, the contractions of the uterus are brief and irregular, and the pain is limited to the groin and lower abdomen.

Miscarriages and Stillbirths A **miscarriage,** also known as a **spontaneous abortion,** is the expulsion of the fetus when it is too young to live outside the womb, especially between the 12th and 28th weeks. A **stillbirth** is the delivery of a dead fetus. Most miscarriages and stillbirths result from chromosomal abnormalities, bacterial or viral infections, and rejection by the immune system.[189] About 1 in 6 pregnancies is miscarried, most early in the pregnancy; often the woman does not even realize she is pregnant.[190] Miscarriages are twice as apt to occur in women over age 35 as in women under age 24, because of the increase in chromosomal abnormalities with age. This is why the older the woman trying to conceive, the greater her anxiety about miscarriage may be. Miscarriages do not result from physical exercise, sexual activity, or any psychological matters.

A miscarriage can be a heavy psychological blow for a woman or couple who have been strongly desirous of having a child, and indeed the loss may be experienced as deeply as the death of a child, with consequent depression.[191] The pain may be particularly acute if the couple has been trying to conceive for some time or if the woman has had a miscarriage before. Friends and family who are aware of the loss can offer support and understanding.

Ectopic Pregnancy The potentially fatal (to the mother, as well as fetus) pregnancy complication known as **ectopic pregnancy** occurs when a fertilized egg becomes implanted somewhere other than the lining of the uterus. A growing embryo that is implanted in the fallopian tubes (through which eggs move from the ovaries to the uterus) may rupture the surrounding tube and blood vessels, putting the woman at risk of bleeding to death. Ninety percent of ectopic pregnancies take place in the fallopian tubes and are called *tubal pregnancies.*[192] Other ectopic pregnancies take place in the abdomen, cervix, or ovary.

Ectopic pregnancies have tripled in recent years.[193] One cause may be that many women have delayed childbearing until they were older, when the fallopian tubes too are older. Another reason is the increased prevalence of sexually transmitted diseases, such as chlamydia, and subsequent pelvic inflammatory disease. According to one study, women who have been smoking at the time of conception have been found to have twice the risk of nonsmokers for developing ectopic pregnancy.[194]

The diagnosis of ectopic pregnancy continues to be challenging. Signs and symptoms include a blood pregnancy test, missed period, abnormal vaginal bleeding, pelvic pain, and sometimes dizziness and nausea. Earlier diagnosis, including the use of ultrasound, has helped physicians to treat the problem before it becomes life-threatening.

Placenta Praevia This disorder, which usually occurs in the third trimester, affects 1 in 200 pregnant women. **Placenta praevia** is the premature separation of the placenta from the wall of the uterus. This usually occurs because the placenta has grown over all or part of the cervical opening. About 80–85% of the infants survive, if treated properly.

High Blood Pressure and Toxemia Because of the extra weight gain of pregnancy and the strains on the circulatory system, women are more apt to develop high blood pressure—hypertension—in pregnancy than at any other time. In the early stage of a health problem called **toxemia,** the mother experiences high blood pressure, sudden weight gain, swollen fingers and ankles (owing to increased water retention), protein in the urine, blurring vision, and headaches. If it is not treated, it can produce convulsions, which can be fatal to the mother and child.

Exposure to Infectious Diseases: Rubella, Cytomegalovirus, Toxoplasmosis, and STDs It's difficult enough having a disease oneself; it's even worse when the disease affects the unborn. Some that severely affect the unborn child are the following:

- *Rubella (German measles):* **Rubella,** or **German measles,** is a virus that is reasonably mild outside of pregnancy. However, if contracted during pregnancy, it can cause the fetus to develop serious handicaps, including blindness and deafness.

Fortunately, this is one disease that can be prevented. Immunity to the organism that causes rubella is conferred by previous exposure to rubella or by a vaccine. A rubella vaccination is one of the standard immunizations that one receives in childhood and its protection is usually lifelong. A woman wanting to become pregnant should be sure she has had this vaccine. (It should not be given during pregnancy, however, because of the possible risk to the fetus.)[195] A blood test can also assess a woman's prior exposure to this infection.

- *Toxoplasmosis:* **Toxoplasmosis** is a disease caused by a parasite found in uncooked or undercooked meat and in dust or water contaminated by cat feces. Although healthy adults rarely experience symptoms, the disease can cause blindness and serious brain damage to the infant.

  A blood test early in pregnancy may determine whether the mother is vulnerable to toxoplasmosis. If she is, she should avoid eating rare meat and should avoid any contact with a cat's litter box.[196]

- *Cytomegaloviral (CMV) infection:* Like rubella, **cytomegaloviral (CMV) infection** has only mild effect on healthy adults, but may have severe consequences for the fetus. Some infants experience brain damage, mental retardation, blindness, deafness, cerebral palsy, seizures, and liver damage.

  Adults usually get CMV by such intimate contact as kissing, sexual contact, or handling infected children's diapers. A transmission to the newborn can occur during childbirth if CMV is present in cervical secretions and during breast feeding. Pregnant women who are around children should wash their hands frequently.

- *Sexually transmitted diseases (STDs):* **Sexually transmitted diseases (STDs)** cover all those diseases spread by sexual contact: HIV, chlamydia, gonorrhea, genital herpes, human papilloma viruses, syphilis. These can lead to a great many unpleasant consequences for fetuses and infants.

For instance, in an infected woman, the virus that causes AIDS—human immunodeficiency virus (HIV)—can cross the placenta into the blood of the fetus. A pregnant woman with genital herpes virus may pass it to her infant during the birth process, causing brain infection in the baby. Gonorrhea and chlamydia may be passed from an infected woman to her infant at birth, infecting the baby's eyes and possibly causing blindness unless treated.[197] Syphilis cannot cross the placenta in the early part of pregnancy but can later, rendering the fetus susceptible to bone, liver, and brain damage.[198]

Rh Disease **Rh disease,** or **erythroblastosis,** is a condition that occurs when antibodies produced by the mother's blood damage the fetal blood supply, causing the fetus to be stillborn or suffer severe brain damage. Rh disease can occur when a woman whose blood type is Rh negative conceives a child with a man whose blood is Rh positive—a combination that exists in about 12% of all couples.[199] Most such children inherit the father's positive blood, but during childbirth that blood, which has been in the placenta, may come in contact with the mother's negative blood, causing her to develop antibodies to the positive blood. This first Rh-positive baby born to an Rh-negative mother usually will have no problem. However, in future pregnancies, antibodies cross the placenta from the Rh-negative mother and destroy the red blood cells in the Rh-positive fetus, causing Rh disease and its complications.

Fortunately, this problem is now easily prevented by giving such mothers RhoGAM or RhoImmune, which stop the mother from making anti-RH antibodies. The antibodies disappear, so that when the woman becomes pregnant the second time she has no antibodies to attack the blood of the Rh-negative baby.

Prenatal Tests "Will my baby and I be all right?", a pregnant woman may ask. The odds are generally good, if she has followed the kind of prenatal program we described above. If she seems at risk for any of the conditions we've just described, she should be closely monitored by her physician. There are a number of prenatal tests that can be used to identify more than

10.38

*Unit 10
Family Matters:
Decisions About
Parenting,
Pregnancy, and
Childbirth*

250 diseases and disorders. The most common are the following:

- *Ultrasound:* In **ultrasound,** also known as *ultrasonography* or *prenatal sonography,* a physician passes a hand-held instrument over the pregnant woman's abdomen. Sound waves beam into the body, make contact with the fetus, and send back echoes, which are translated into an image on a television monitor.[200] (*See* ● *Figure 25.9.*) There is no danger from radiation (ultrasound is not an X ray), and ultrasound can be used to count the number of fetuses during pregnancy, check for fetal anomalies, and monitor the growth of the infant. Ultrasound is called a "noninvasive" technique, because there is no surgical incision or insertion of an instrument.

- *The AFP Plus Test:* A combination of three blood tests, called the **AFP Plus Test** (AFP stands for alpha-fetoprotein), offers an improvement over past tests (such as amniocentesis) in detecting Down syndrome. The tests look for three substances (alfa-fetoprotein, unconjugated estriol, and

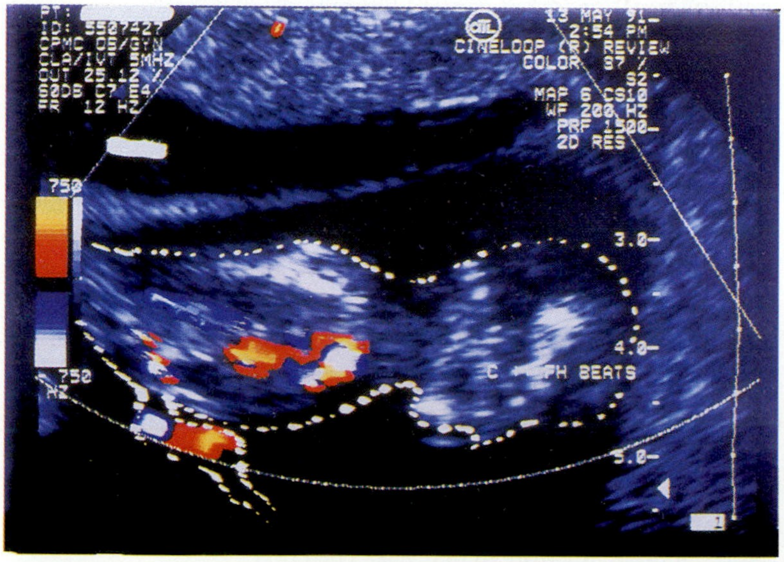

Figure 25.9 Ultrasound. An ultrasound image showing head and torso of a human fetus at 26 weeks.

chorionic gonadotropin) that can determine which women are at risk for bearing afflicted children. The test predicts Down syndrome correctly 60% of the time.[201] A similar test developed in England is called Bart's Triple Test.[202]

- *Amniocentesis:* If fetal abnormalities are suspected, amniocentesis may be used to discover if they are present. **Amniocentesis** is performed during the 14th through 16th week of pregnancy. Using ultrasound for guidance, the physician inserts a needle through the woman's abdominal wall into the amniotic sac surrounding the fetus and removes a small amount of amniotic fluid. (*See* ● *Figure 25.10.*) The fluid contains fetal skin cells, which are grown as a culture in a laboratory and analyzed for genetic defects. Results take up to 4 weeks.

  Because it is an invasive procedure, amniocentesis poses some risk to the fetus, so it is not recommended for every pregnancy.

- *Chorionic villus sampling* (*CVS*): In **chorionic villus sampling (CVS),** the physician, guided by an ultrasound device, inserts a tube into the cervix (or, alternatively, a needle through the abdomen, as in amniocentesis), and a sample of the developing placenta is suctioned out. (*Refer back to Figure 25.10.*) Genetic tests can be performed on the tissue sample, and results of the analysis can be available within 5 days.

  CVS can be performed as early as 9 weeks into pregnancy, earlier than amniocentesis. Thus, if a birth defect is detected and the woman chooses to end her pregnancy, she can do so during the first 3 months of pregnancy, when abortion is safest. At one point there was some debate within the medical community as to whether CVS might actually be associated with an *increase* in a small number of serious congenital deformities; however, later research seems to have alleviated this concern.[203–205]

- *Percutaneous umbilical blood sampling* (*PUBS*): The procedure called **percutaneous umbilical blood sampling** is a technique for getting a blood sample from a

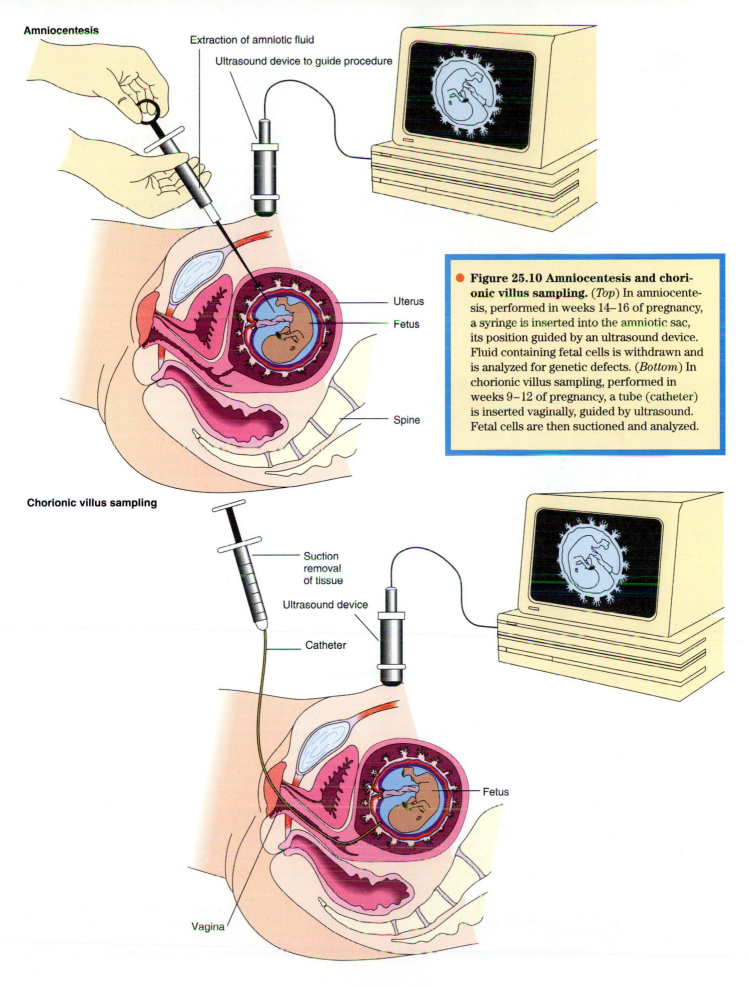

Amniocentesis

Extraction of amniotic fluid

Ultrasound device to guide procedure

Uterus

Fetus

Spine

Chorionic villus sampling

Suction removal of tissue

Ultrasound device

Catheter

Fetus

Vagina

● **Figure 25.10 Amniocentesis and chorionic villus sampling.** (*Top*) In amniocentesis, performed in weeks 14–16 of pregnancy, a syringe is inserted into the amniotic sac, its position guided by an ultrasound device. Fluid containing fetal cells is withdrawn and is analyzed for genetic defects. (*Bottom*) In chorionic villus sampling, performed in weeks 9–12 of pregnancy, a tube (catheter) is inserted vaginally, guided by ultrasound. Fetal cells are then suctioned and analyzed.

10.40

Unit 10
Family Matters:
Decisions About
Parenting,
Pregnancy, and
Childbirth

fetus. Guided by ultrasound, the physician inserts a needle into a blood vessel in the umbilical cord of a fetus, drawing a blood sample out that may be analyzed for diseases and disorders. Because the cells are taken directly from the fetus's bloodstream, they need not be cultured in a laboratory and so can produce results within a couple of days. However, there is a greater risk to the fetus than from either amniocentesis or chorionic villus sampling.

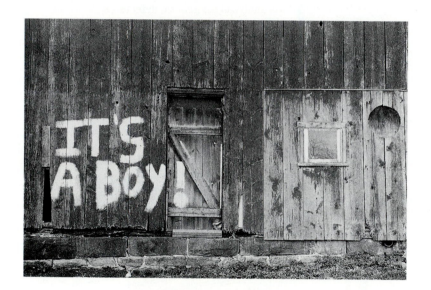

Childbirth: Labor and Delivery

Labor consists of regular muscular contractions to propel the baby through the birth canal. Labor takes place in three stages: (1) dilation of the cervix; (2) passage of the baby through the birth canal; (3) expulsion of the placenta, or afterbirth.

The baby was born a week early. Janice Kennedy, 22, the pregnant wife of Pennsylvania dairy farmer Jeff Kennedy, explained the first sign: "[In the] morning when I got up, I could tell my water had broke. So I came down and told Jeff that I thought today was the day. And he was like, no!"[206] Thus began baby Justin's passage into the world. (*See* ● *Figure 25.11.*)

When Labor Begins Labor begins when a woman experiences regular contractions and expels the mucous plug from her cervix (called "bloody show"). The "breaking of the waters," which Janice referred to, is the rupturing of the amniotic sac ("bag of water"), which is followed by the rushing or leaking of fluid from the vagina. In one-eighth of all pregnancies, especially first pregnancies, the breaking of the amniotic sac happens before labor begins and is usually followed by the beginning of labor within 6–24 hours. However, the sac often does not break until the last hours of labor.

● **Figure 25.11 The birth of Justin**

"*I called the doctor, and I packed, and we got to the hospital about ten-thirty. They hooked me up to the monitor to hear the baby's heart beating and find out how long the contractions were. They were about six minutes apart. They got me ready and told me I could walk around, so we walked around a little bit and then came back to the room and watched TV.*

I just kept working through the contractions till about four, and they were getting too much for me, so the doctor came in and said I could have a painkiller. So then I was more or less in and out of it. Then about six, I guess, it started getting too much for me again, and I asked for another painkiller. The nurse told me no. She came in one time and caught me pushing, and she said, 'Do you have to push?' I said yes, and she went and called the doctor. And they had everything ready to go, and when they told me I could push, it was maybe five or six contractions, and I had him."

—Janice Kennedy, 22, about the birth of her son Justin, quoted in: John Kotre & Elizabeth Hall (1990). *Seasons of life: Our dramatic journey from birth to death.* Boston: Little, Brown, p. 18.

Labor is defined as the rhythmic muscular contractions of the uterus that propel the baby through the birth canal. At the beginning of labor, the time between contractions may be 15–20 minutes and irregular. As labor progresses, the contractions become regular, more frequent, and longer lasting. The contractions themselves may progress from half a minute to a minute.

The Three Stages of Labor Labor takes place in three stages. The first stage begins with the appearance of the first contraction and the third stage ends with the delivery of the placenta (afterbirth). (*See* ● *Figure 25.12.*) For women experiencing their first labor, the average (median) number of hours is 10.6, though 1 in 9 takes more than 24 hours and 1 in 100 requires less than 3 hours. For women giving birth to their second or subsequent child, the average number of hours is 6.2.[207]

- *First stage—dilation of cervix:* The first stage of labor is the longest. The *early* first stage begins with the **dilation,** or opening up, and thinning (effacement) of the **cervix,** the opening between the vagina and the uterus. (*Refer back to Figure 25.12.*) The mother is not supposed to bear down at this point, only to try to relax and let the contractions do their work and use breathing exercises to help control discomfort.

    The dilation continues until the opening is the equivalent of five fingers (4 inches or 10 centimeters), at which point the baby is ready to come down the birth canal. The *transition* phase occurs during the *late* first stage of labor. At this point the contractions become more frequent and more painful, and the woman must concentrate on each contraction. Fortunately, this stage averages only 30–60 minutes. Dilation is complete when the baby's head can start to pass through the cervix.

- *Second stage—passage of baby through birth canal:* The second stage of labor begins when the cervix is fully open and the baby moves through the cervix into the birth canal, or vagina. (*Refer back to Figure 25.12.*) In this stage, which may last an hour or more, the contractions will occur every 2–3 minutes and will be quite strong.

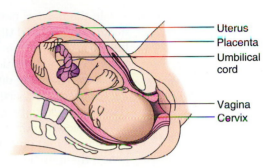

First stage
Dilation of cervix, followed by transition phase, when baby's head can start to pass through the cervix

— Uterus
— Placenta
— Umbilical cord
— Vagina
— Cervix

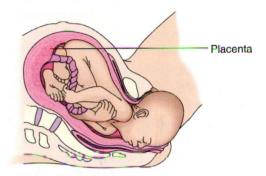

Second stage
Passage of the baby through the birth canal, or vagina, and delivery into the world

— Placenta

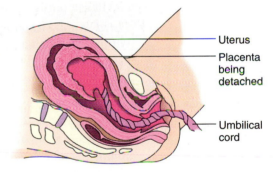

Third stage
Expulsion of the placenta, blood, and fluid ("afterbirth")

— Uterus
— Placenta being detached
— Umbilical cord

● **Figure 25.12 The three stages of labor**

At this point, the woman needs to alternately push and relax to help the baby move through the birth canal.

Each contraction moves the baby further down the birth canal. First the head emerges, then the neck and shoulders, then the body is quickly expelled. At this point, an attendant clamps the baby's umbilical cord a few inches from the navel. Mucus covering the baby's nose and mouth, which came from the birth canal and amniotic fluid, is suctioned off with a rubber syringe.

10.42

Unit 10
Family Matters:
Decisions About
Parenting,
Pregnancy, and
Childbirth

In the movies, newborns are spanked to make them cry and thus begin breathing, but this is not done in real life. Most babies begin crying automatically after their oxygen stops when the umbilical cord connecting the placenta is clamped. Sometimes they may need to be gently rubbed or have oxygen blown in their faces to stimulate breathing. Now, unless there is an emergency, the umbilical cord is cut and the baby is usually given to its mother to hold.

Some parents are surprised, even disappointed, when they get their first look at their newborn. Expecting to see the round head of a 3- or 4-month old, they may be dismayed to see the baby's head molded like a long melon—the molding is necessary to fit the infant's skull through the mother's pelvis. Some newborns will be bald, some will have hair, some will have flattened ears and squashed noses, some will be bowlegged. The face may be puffy and bluish until the circulation improves.[208]

- *Third stage—expulsion of placenta:* Within about half an hour of the birth of the baby, the contractions of the uterus begin again until the placenta or *afterbirth* is separated and expelled, a process that may take about 10 minutes. (*Refer back to Figure 25.12.*)

Putting the baby to the mother's breast stimulates breast-feeding and contraction of the uterus, beginning to return the uterus to its normal size and the control of uterine bleeding.

After the delivery, mother and child may be together in the hospital or the mother may have help in taking care of the baby. If there are difficulties, as when the baby is born prematurely or with low birth weight, the infant may be kept for a time in a separate nursery. At one point newborns were principally isolated in nurseries, but research has shown that they do better when they are allowed to stay with their parents immediately after birth.[209]

Decisions About Childbirth

Prospective parents have several decisions they can make. Should the baby be delivered by obstetrician, midwife, or a trained woman companion called a *doula*? Should the baby be born in a hospital, a birthing center inside or outside a hospital, or at home? Should an episiotomy be done? Should a woman opt for anesthesia (general or regional) or try natural childbirth (no medication) or prepared childbirth (using Lamaze or Leboyer methods)? Under what circumstances should cesarean sections be performed?

There is more than one way to deliver a baby, more than one kind of "birth style." Thus, expectant parents, both fathers and mothers, should be aware of the options available to them.

Choice of Birth Attendants: Obstetrician, Midwife, Doula? Expectant parents should anticipate being part of a team in terms of preparing for childbirth. One of the most important decisions they make is who will be the primary health care provider both during the pregnancy and at the time of labor and delivery. Who should deliver the baby, where, and how much will it cost?

Let's start with the costs: According to the Health Insurance Association of America, a normal pregnancy and delivery cost an average of $4334, about two-thirds of which goes to the hospital and one-third for physician's fees.[210] Complications, such as a cesarean birth, will increase the cost. The services of a midwife average just under $1000, compared to $1492 for those of a physician.

The choices of birth attendants are:

- *Obstetrician/gynecologist:* An obstetrician/gynecologist (OB/GYN) is a physician who specializes in female reproductive health and pregnancy. Some physicians limit their practice to **gynecology,** which deals with the reproductive health and diseases of women. A physician will be required if the pregnancy seems to be a high-risk one to either mother or child, as when a physical examination shows poor nutrition, inadequate prenatal care, unwanted pregnancy, genetic abnormalities, multiple pregnancy, maternal age over 35, and similar problems.[211]

Interestingly, in the United States, a sizable number of obstetrician/gynecologists no longer deliver babies in order to avoid lawsuits and the high cost of malpractice insurance.[212]

- *Midwives:* **Midwives** are specialists who are not medical doctors who assist in uncomplicated pregnancies and deliveries. Midwives may be of two types, *certified nurse-midwives* and *lay midwives.*[213,214]

    Certified nurse-midwives (CNMs) are registered nurses who have completed graduate programs in normal pregnancy and birth, are state-licensed, and practice primarily in hospitals.

    Lay midwives lack nursing education, are often trained by other lay midwives, and primarily do home deliveries. Lay midwives shun the use of medications and technology and are not able to practice (or simply practice illegally) in many states.

    In recent times, nurse-midwives have filled a void left by the withdrawal of physicians from the obstetrics field. More than that, they provide family- and women-centered care that many patients find satisfying. In addition, because they specialize in normal births, midwives free physicians to work on more complicated deliveries.

- *Doulas:* Recently, a birthing practice used in developing countries has been found to offer important lessons for North America. A **doula** is simply a trained woman companion, a person who has given birth herself, who provides constant support, such as hugging and hand-holding, during labor and delivery.

    Interestingly, one study of mainly indigent mothers in Houston found that the presence of such a supportive companion in hospitals reduced the need for cesarean sections, forceps delivery, labor-inducing drugs, and other high-tech measures.[215] "Remarkably, human support is more powerful than the modern obstetric techniques we have at the present time," said John Kennell, lead author of the study.[216] The study's authors believe the doula's presence has a calming effect on the laboring woman and the hospital staff.

    In the five European countries with the lowest infant mortality rates, midwives preside at more than 70% of all births.[217] For many reasons, midwifery has been slow to catch on in

the United States, many of them having to do with liability and malpractice coverage. For lay midwives, especially if they practice illegally, there may be the difficulty of finding a physician or hospital to provide backup support when there are birth complications. Nurse-midwives do not have this problem: because so many work in hospitals with lots of backup, and many are part of a nurse-physician team, they are about as safe as doctors.[218] In addition, there is some evidence that midwifery significantly reduces the number of cesareans, episiotomies, and necessity for pain medication compared to the usual obstetrician-attended delivery.[219]

The Birthplace About 99% of births occurred in hospitals in 1988.[220] More than 96% of these hospital deliveries were attended by physicians. If the expectant mother chooses the services of a physician, she will no doubt have her baby in a hospital. A hospital delivery will be necessary if the woman or child seem to be high-risk. However, for uncomplicated pregnancies, there are a number of alternatives:

- *Hospital-based birthing centers:* The main difference between a traditional hospital delivery room and a birthing center within the hospital is that birthing centers have a more home-like atmosphere. The advantage of an in-hospital birthing center is the immediate access to emergency care.

- *Free-standing birth centers:* These facilities, which are not in a hospital but may be near one, provide a comfortable environment in which family and friends can participate in uncomplicated deliveries. Childbirths are generally supervised by certified nurse-midwives. These centers are cheaper than hospitals, more family-centered, less likely to use high-tech procedures such as episiotomies, and emphasize the mother's and her partner's control over how her labor is handled.

    Although infant mortality in birth centers appears to be no higher than that in hospitals, further studies are needed to evaluate the safety of this alternative.[221] The problem is that it is currently impossible to predict which women will have rare complications for which hospital-based assistance is needed.

10.44

Unit 10
Family Matters:
Decisions About
Parenting,
Pregnancy, and
Childbirth

Most states now license birthing centers, and about 135 such centers have opened in the United States since 1975.[222]

- *Home births:* Although three generations ago nearly all births took place at home, today this is a somewhat uncommon event. Still, some studies show that under certain circumstances home births attended by lay midwives can be accomplished as safely as, and with less intervention than, physician-attended hospital deliveries.[223–225]

Controversy: Should Episiotomies Be Performed? At some point in a physician-assisted delivery in a hospital setting, the physician *may* do an **episiotomy,** a small, straight surgical incision in the **perineum,** the area of skin between the anus and the vagina. The theory here is that the episiotomy allows more room so that the baby's head can pass through the birth canal without tearing the mother's vaginal tissue.[226,227]

Although in North America episiotomies are done on 50–90% of first-time mothers and 25–30% of women who have given birth before, not everyone in the birthing field believes they are necessary. Indeed, one Swedish study found a significantly higher infection rate and a longer healing period in the episiotomy group than those not receiving an episiotomy. In fact, the results indicated that many women suffer unnecessarily after an episiotomy.[228]

The American College of Obstetrics and Gynecology does not recommend episiotomy in normal deliveries, and the organization's standards state that the procedure should not be considered routine. Thus, an expectant mother should be sure to let the delivering physician or midwife know if she does not wish to have this surgical procedure except in emergencies.

Pain Management Some birth practitioners believe that for many women pain during childbirth can be alleviated without medication, particularly if prepared childbirth techniques can be used for pain management. However, the expectant mother should know what painkilling drugs are available. She should also know that, because every drug may cross the placenta, the medication will affect her baby, too. Indeed, with some drugs (such as the tranquilizer Valium), the concentration of the drug may be higher in the blood of the fetus than it is in the mother and may last for days after delivery.

Drugs used for pain control are generally administered in two ways:

- *General anesthesia:* **General anesthesia** affects the whole body, rendering the mother unconscious. The problem is that general anesthesia can actually slow or stop labor and may decrease the responsiveness of the newborn.[229] Today general anesthesia during childbirth is used only in emergencies or when there is not enough time to administer a regional anesthetic.

- *Regional or local anesthesia:* **Regional anesthesia** or **local anesthesia** involves injecting of a drug into a localized area or region to alleviate pain confined to that area. This kind of anesthesia rarely affects the baby. Among the kinds of regional anesthesia available are:

  (1) The *pudendal block,* in which an anesthetic is injected into the pudendal nerves inside the vagina

  (2) The *paracervical block,* in which anesthesia is injected into the cervical area

  (3) The *epidural block,* in which an anesthetic is injected slowly into the lower back, numbing the lower half of the body and easing the pain of contractions

  (4) The *spinal block,* a short-acting anesthetic that is also injected into the lower back

Natural Childbirth and Prepared Childbirth The term **natural childbirth** means a normal vaginal delivery during which the mother uses no medication. The term **prepared childbirth,** or **participatory childbirth,** refers to childbirth that follows a series of classes intended to prepare the expectant mother to actively participate in the delivery of her baby and to avoid painkilling drugs. Sometimes "natural childbirth" and "prepared childbirth" are used interchangeably. The difference, however, is that in prepared childbirth the mother *may* use medication if she wishes.

In general, prepared childbirth stresses the preparation of the woman and the partner who will accompany her during the delivery (father or friend, referred to as the "coach") in special classes. These classes teach not only about nutrition and exercise during pregnancy but also about the birth process. The woman and her partner are also taught how breathing and pushing (coached by the partner) can help in the delivery and reduce the pain.

Two variations on prepared childbirth are the *Lamaze* and the *Leboyer* methods:[230,231]

- *The Lamaze method:* The **Lamaze method** involves teaching women breathing, massage, and pushing techniques so they learn not to focus on the pain during labor. The partner offers emotional support and helps the woman to focus on her breathing and to release muscular tension that causes pain. Lamaze classes, which may begin as early as the first trimester or as late as the seventh month, attempt to teach the expectant mother that she can be in control during labor and delivery.[232,233]

- *The Leboyer method:* The **Leboyer method** attempts to make the birth as nontraumatic as possible for the infant.[234] A Leboyer delivery includes dim lights, lowered voices, caressing of the infant and delay in cutting the umbilical cord while the newborn rests on the mother's abdomen, followed by bathing in soothing water.

The Lamaze method in particular has won a great deal of acceptance among obstetricians in North America.

Father Participation In the Lamaze method, the "coach" is often the father, though it need not be, provided the partner is allowed to participate in the birthing process. Men may have mixed feelings about being in the delivery room or birthing center, although one estimate is that 60–80% of American fathers are present at their childrens' births.[235] Certainly a father should not be forced to be there just because it is currently popular to do so (as once the reverse was true).

Still, as part of the parents' "birth plan," there should be discussion about the father's role in the delivery. His participation may be extremely important to the mother's comfort as well as his own.[236,237] Moreover, it has been found that fathers who participated in the prenatal classes and were present at the delivery showed more interest in their babies than fathers who did not.[238]

Controversy: Are Cesarean Sections Done Too Often? A **cesarean section** is a procedure in which the obstetrician makes a surgical incision in the abdominal and uterine walls to remove the baby. The cesarean (or Cesarean—the name comes from Caesar, who was said to have been plucked from the womb) section has become the most common operation in the United States. Nearly 1 million babies a year are born by "C-section" rather than by normal vaginal delivery—18–25% of all U.S. births, the highest rate in the world.[239,240]

The four most common reasons given for cesareans are these: the woman has had a prior cesarean delivery (35.6%); labor is not progressing normally (28.9%); the baby is positioned buttocks or feet first rather than head down, called a **breech birth** (12.3%); or there is fetal distress (9.9%).[241] But are these the real reasons? For instance, according to one article, the most frequently cited reason for the mounting cesarean rate is physicians' fear of malpractice suits.[242] Another report states that a hospital's profit motive may be nearly as important as concerns for medical safety. Women who give birth at private, for-profit hospitals are more likely to have repeated cesareans than those who go to public or teaching hospitals.[243] Finally, it appears that many women who have had cesareans for their first child opt to have it again for their next delivery, even though physicians encourage them to try vaginal births. The main reason is that women want to avoid the pain and unpredictability of labor.[244]

Maternal deaths from cesareans are rare, less than 2%.[245] Even so, the risk is two to four times higher than that for vaginal delivery. Moreover, there are a great many medical complications, such as infection (of the uterus, urinary tract, or surgical wound), which occur in perhaps 40% of cesarean mothers.[246] Other factors are that cesarean mothers have to remain in the hospital twice as long as women delivering vaginally, have more pain and fatigue, and suffer unanticipated emotional reactions—many to the extent of joining cesarean self-help groups. Finally, cesareans may also harm the baby—breathing problems may result from delivery before labor begins.

10.46

Unit 10
Family Matters:
Decisions About
Parenting,
Pregnancy, and
Childbirth

We do not mean that cesareans should be avoided should an emergency arise, only that the expectant mother should understand that it is major abdominal surgery, with all the complications such surgery entails.

After the Baby Is Born

After the baby is delivered, it may be placed with the mother in a rooming-in arrangement at the hospital or taken home. New parents need to think about diapers (cloth or disposable) and safety matters. They need to be aware of the phenomenon of sudden infant death syndrome. They may wish to become knowledgeable about the pros and cons of circumcision and of breast-feeding versus bottle-feeding. New mothers need to be aware of the difference between postpartum blues and postpartum depression.

Sometimes separation between mother and child immediately after birth cannot be avoided, although if it is prolonged it can have important negative effects. In general, however, the more time the family can spend together after the baby's arrival, the better the emotional attachment or **bonding** between them.[247,248] Indeed, frequent contact between both parents and the baby is important in developing future attachments.[249]

Rooming-In and Homecoming Many hospitals now offer **rooming-in** arrangements, a room or place where the mother can stay and take care of her baby and be visited by the father and other members of the family. Besides enabling the new family to get to know each other, rooming-in also gives the mother the opportunity to learn from the hospital staff some fundamentals of baby care.

It is to be hoped that the parents will have made some preparations for homecoming before the baby actually arrived. That is, they will have prepared a place for the infant to sleep, bought necessary clothes and supplies, and perhaps enlisted the help of a friend or a (new) grandparent to assist with household chores and taking care of the baby's siblings, if any.

Among the concerns that new parents need to address are the following:

- *Diapers:* An often appreciated gift to new parents is a few months' subscription to a commercial diaper service. These firms will deliver a supply of freshly laundered cloth diapers and will pick up dirty ones for cleaning. The diapers are usually washed with soft detergents to avoid giving infants diaper rash. (Incidentally, baby powder with talc should be avoided because infants can develop life-threatening respiratory problems if they accidentally inhale powdered talc.)[250]

  Disposable diapers are also a convenient alternative. Indeed, some day care centers will not accept youngsters in cloth diapers. In recent years, there have been environmental concerns that disposable diapers add to the world's trash and will last 500 years in a landfill. However, it turns out they account for only 2% of the contents of landfills in the United States, and if everyone switched to cloth tomorrow, there would not be enough cloth diapers in the United States to accommodate them.[251] Even so, disposable diapers are still an environmental concern.

- *Safety matters:* New parents need to plan for everything from obtaining car safety seats for their infant to safety covers on electrical outlets to gates at the head of indoor stairways. The vertical bars in cribs should not be more than 2⅜ inches apart, so that the baby will not get its head stuck between them. Parents should not leave infants alone on a regular bed, even for a brief nap, because they may get caught between the mattress and the bed frame or wall and may suffocate.[252]

In addition, parents need to stay in close touch with their pediatricians to make sure their children get the immunizations and other treatments they need (as we describe in Unit 11). For example, in the first 6 months, infants should be immunized against diphtheria, tetanus, pertussis, and polio, and in the second year of life against measles, mumps, and rubella.[253]

Sudden Infant Death Syndrome Commonly known as "crib death," **sudden infant death syndrome (SIDS)** is the unexpected death of an apparently healthy baby, usually between the ages of 1 week and 1 year (most likely between 2 and 4 months). It is the second leading cause of infant death in the United States.[254] The cause remains unexplained, even after an autopsy. SIDS is not a diagnosis; it is simply medicine's way of saying "We don't know what the cause is." It is not caused by suffocation, aspiration, regurgitation, immunization, or child abuse, and it cannot be predicted. A few babies may show signs of a slight cold before death. One study suggests that the supine position (lying on the back) is the safest sleeping position for babies.[255]

Controversy: Is Circumcision Beneficial?

Circumcision is the removal of the foreskin from a male infant's penis for religious, cultural, or health reasons. Beginning in the 1940s, circumcision was a standard procedure for newborns in the United States. Then in the 1970s, the American Academy of Pediatrics declared there was no medical indication for routine circumcision, and during the 1980s circumcision rates dropped dramatically, from 85% to 58%.[256,257] Lately, there have been arguments that there may be some benefits associated with circumcision.

Today there seem to be two points of view:

- *Arguments for circumcision:* Recent research suggests that circumcision helps prevent urinary tract infections, which are experienced 9–20 times more often in uncircumcised infants as in circumcised babies in their first year of life, although such infections occur infrequently.[258,259] If the urinary tract infection affects the kidney, it can predispose the baby to kidney infections later in life.[260]

  In addition, uncircumcised males also face a 5000 times higher risk of cancer of the penis—although the condition is rare (only 1000 cases reported a year in the United States).[261]

- *Arguments against circumcision:* The counterargument is that the risks to the uncircumcised are too small to cause concern—that, in effect, 100 babies will be circumcised just to prevent one baby having a urinary tract infection that could be treated with antibiotics anyway. On the other hand, as many as four of those cir-

cumcised babies will experience complications (such as operations that have to be redone) as a result of the procedure.[262,263]

The American Academy of Pediatrics states that newborn circumcision has potential benefits as well as risks and emphasizes that these issues need to be explained to parents. Compared with circumcised males, uncircumcised males are at greater risk for urinary tract infection, sexually transmitted disease, and other problems. On the other hand, complications of circumcision include infection and hemorrhage, and the academy recommends that painkillers should be prescribed for the substantial pain during the procedure.[264,265]

Breast-Feeding or Bottle-Feeding? Most authorities agree that breast-feeding is better than bottle-feeding, at least for the first 6

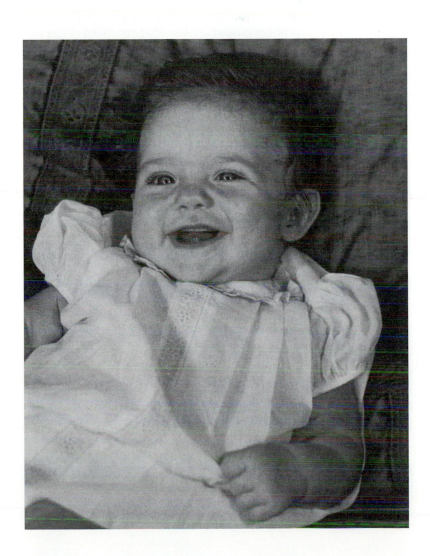

10.48

*Unit 10
Family Matters:
Decisions About
Parenting,
Pregnancy, and
Childbirth*

months. Antibodies present in *colostrum*, the fluid secreted from the mother's breast for 2–3 days after birth, help protect infants from a number of infectious diseases for which the mother has developed immunity. In recent years, there was an increase for a while in mothers breast-feeding their young, then in the early 1980s there was a steep decline, raising concerns about a possible public-health crisis from lowered protection against infection. The decline apparently occurred because breast-feeding is no longer considered fashionable, the popular media has promoted breast-feeding less, and infant formula is marketed aggressively.[266]

Babies who are breast-fed get better nutrition, develop fewer allergies, and have fewer intestinal infections.[267] Indeed, some physicians are of the opinion that the benefits of breast-feeding extend even into adulthood: people breast-fed as infants have a lower incidence of allergies and are less likely to develop the painful intestinal disorder called inflammatory bowel disease.[268] They are also less apt to develop a bad bite compared to bottle-fed babies.[269] Children fed breast milk as premature infants scored significantly higher (an IQ advantage of 8.3 points) on intelligence tests than children also born prematurely who had not received their mothers' milk, a British study found.[270] Nursing also helps the mother shrink the uterus back to normal and return to her pre-pregnancy shape. Recently, research suggests that drinking cow's milk during infancy may trigger juvenile diabetes in some people later in life.[271]

Needless to say, nursing a baby creates some disadvantages for any woman who takes her infant anywhere in public. (See ● *Figure 25.13.*) Even so, the woman-made substance is superior to the infant formula because it has all the essential nutrients.

What influences a woman to decide to breast-feed her baby? According to one study, a supportive partner makes a difference.[272] Partners of women who favored infant formula didn't know that breast-feeding was good for babies and had misguided ideas that breast-feeding was bad for the breasts. Partners of the breast-feeding women, on the other hand, believed nursing would encourage bonding and protect infants against disease. In addition, some women believed that breast-feeding was better for a baby but chose to bottle-feed because of negative attitudes toward breast-feeding, conflicting schedules, and convenience.[273]

Postpartum Adjustment After 9 months of pregnancy, several hours of fatiguing and stressful labor, hormonal changes after delivery, and the incredible emotional high of seeing the baby born, many women (perhaps 25–50%) experience a period of sadness and anxiety, the *postpartum blues*. A woman may cry easily, be alternately ecstatic and lethargic, feel helpless and out of control, even crazy.[274] Because these fluctuating moods may persist for weeks or even months, it helps to know that they are normal, universal, and temporary.

However, we need to distinguish *postpartum blues* from **postpartum depression,** severe, persistent symptoms of a major depression, which warrant the assistance of a health care professional. The consequences of postpartum depression for those who have limited or no emotional support or who have a history of depression can be serious.[275]

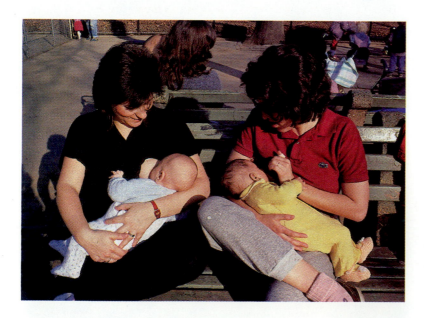

● **Figure 25.13 The public difficulties of breast-feeding**

Of course the emotions of both parents are strained by the sudden responsibilities of caring for a new infant and the continuing fatigue because the baby does not sleep through the night and often fusses during the day. As one expert put it, "One of the frustrating things is the lack of control, especially during the first 3 months. The baby is constantly demanding things of you, but is giving very little back."[276] In addition, there are all the other responsibilities that must be attended to, whether taking care of other children, doing housework, or going off to a job. One way to reduce this stress is for the mother to mobilize her social support network, including her partner, close relatives, or friends to help her.

Strategy for Living: Treating a Baby as Human The headlines say it all: BABIES' SOCIAL INSTINCTS ARE REMARKABLY SOPHISTICATED.[277] BABIES' SENSES SHARPER.[278] BABIES AT 5 MONTHS GRASP SIMPLE MATHEMATICS.[279] BABIES LEARN SOUNDS OF LANGUAGE BY 6 MONTHS.[280] In other words, babies are not just passive blobs waiting to be molded into human beings. They are remarkably responsive and aware from the day of delivery, able to distinguish bright from dim light, moving objects from still ones, patterns from solids. Even in the seventh month in the womb they can be startled by outside sounds. Four-day-olds can discriminate among odors. And newborns prefer human faces to dangling mobiles.[281] For the mother and father, the exciting adventure of relating to a new intelligence begins with the first day of the baby's presence in the world.

Some parents learn only belatedly that learning how to manage children involves learning how to manage themselves first. Children are often frustrating, and disciplining them is often fraught with emotional conflicts. Before you can learn to be an effective disciplinarian of a child, you must learn how to manage your own anger, learn how to solve problem situations, and how to get support from others.[282]

800-HELP

Childwatch. 800-222-1464 (in Canada, 800-248-1464). National Child Safety Council

National Pregnancy Hotline. 800-852-5683 (in Oklahoma, 800-493-6425)

National SIDS Foundation. 800-221-SIDS (in Maryland, 301-459-3388). Hotline for Sudden Infant Death Syndrome (crib death)

Pregnancy Crisis Center. 800-368-3336

Suggestions for Further Reading

Lamaze, Fernand (1970). *Painless childbirth*. Chicago: Regency. French obstetrician's techniques for controlled breathing and concentration to release muscular tension during childbirth.

Leboyer, Frederick (1975). *Birth without violence*. New York: Alfred Knopf. French obstetrician emphasizes gentle, loving treatment for newborns to introduce them to the world gradually.

Shapiro, Jerrold (1987). *When men are pregnant: Needs and concerns of expectant fathers*. San Luis Obispo, CA: Impact Publishers. A Santa Clara, California, clinical psychologist writes on how men can handle their partner's pregnancy.

Simkin, Penny (1989). *The birth partner: Everything you need to know to help a woman through childbirth*. Boston: Harvard Commons Press. A Seattle childbirth educator's help book for prospective fathers.

Spock, Benjamin, & Rothenberg, Michael (1992). *Dr. Spock's baby and child care* (6th ed.). New York: Pocket Books. The famous guidebook of baby and child care that has served parents for five decades. The latest edition breaks new ground with discussion of medical updates on injuries, AIDS, immunizations, headaches, choking, as well as treatment of stepfamily dynamics, homosexuality, and open adoptions.

Taffel, Ron, & Blau, Melina (1991). *Parenting by heart: How to connect with your kids in the face of too much advice, too many pressures, and never enough time*. Reading, MA: Addison-Wesley. A psychotherapist and his co-author's down-to-earth guide for child raising.

"Toxic Parents" and Child Abuse

Even if you're not immediately engaged in raising children yourself, you may be interested in how you were affected by the way you were raised yourself. You might also wonder about how your own abilities as a parent are affected by how you were parented. Answer true or false to the following questions.

___ **1.** Child abuse is any violence to a child beyond spanking.

___ **2.** The problem of child abuse has really been exaggerated.

___ **3.** Even abused and neglected children can still recover from their early childhood experiences.

___ **4.** Parents tend to raise their children the way they were raised themselves.

The answers for the questions above are: (1) true-but, (2) false, (3) true-but, (4) true. (We explain what we mean by the "buts" below.)

1. "Toxic Parents": There Is a Difference Between Discipline and Abuse

Even the best of parents are only human. They lose their tempers with their children, aren't always emotionally available, and are occasionally domineering or controlling. And in the United States, at least, physical force, ranging from slaps to batterings, is a common form of punishment.[283] Indeed, a 1992 survey in Ohio found that more than two-thirds of family physicians and pediatricians supported the use of spanking—even though the U.S. Surgeon General in 1985 said corporal punishment should be discouraged.[284]

If your parents acted this way from time to time, does it mean they were abusive? Probably not. Parents are subject to many stresses and strains, and we might argue that they may be excused if *occasionally* they have such lapses, especially if the rest of the time they treat their children with warmth and affection. However, there are some parents (including stepparents and guardians) who *consistently* act in negative ways toward their children, inflicting ongoing trauma, abuse, and denigration. Sometimes the trauma is not ongoing but happens only once, as in the case of sexual abuse. Quite often the maltreatment may take the form of emotional abuse, such as excessive criticism or withholding of affection. Dr. Susan Forward has dubbed such harmful parents "toxic parents." The emotional damage inflicted by such parents, she says, spreads throughout a child's being like a chemical toxin, and as the child grows, so does the pain.[285]

Are such parents *legally* considered abusive and hence subject to criminal prosecution? It depends. The short answer is that, as far as the law is concerned, if a parent hits a child and leaves a mark, that parent has crossed the line from discipline into abuse.[286] Actually, neglect —whether inattentiveness to the child's safety, withholding of food, or withholding of affection —is the most common form of maltreatment, causing more deaths, injuries, and eventual problems than outright physical abuse.[287,288]

Under the Child Abuse Prevention and Treatment Act, *child abuse and neglect* is defined as physical or mental injury, sexual abuse or exploitation, negligent treatment, or maltreatment of a child under age 18. Four types of child abuse and neglect are as follows:[289]

- *Physical abuse:* Inflicting physical injury by punching, beating, kicking, biting, burning, and so on, whether the injury is intended or not, is abuse.

- *Child neglect:* Neglect, or failure to provide for the child's basic needs, may be physical, educational, or emotional. An example of physical neglect is causing a child to run away or not allowing a runaway to return home. An example of educational neglect is failure to pay attention to a special educational need. An example of emotional neglect is spouse abuse in the child's presence or permission of alcohol use by the child or just plain ignoring the child.

- *Sexual abuse:* Sexual abuse includes fondling a child's genitals, intercourse, incest, rape, sodomy, exhibitionism, and sexual exploitation. Many experts believe that sexual abuse is the most underreported form of child maltreatment.

- *Mental injury:* Mental injury is psychological or emotional abuse, such as belittling or scapegoating a child, or withholding affection. This may not *legally* be considered child abuse and negligence—that is, the kind in which authorities would intervene—but it may have had a damaging effect.

If you were sexually abused, beaten, left alone a lot, repeatedly humiliated, made to feel guilty, or overprotected, you probably suffer what most abused children feel: feelings that you are worthless, unlovable, and inadequate. These feelings come about, Susan Forward points out, because children of "toxic parents" largely blame themselves for their parents' abuse. As she writes, "It is easier for a defenseless, dependent child to feel guilty for having done something 'bad' to deserve Daddy's rage than it is for that child to accept the frightening fact that Daddy, the protector, can't be trusted."

A final thought: *Is* spanking abusive to children? Consider: If you spanked a grown-up, such an act could be treated by the law as assault and battery. Some experts believe that, far from making children behave better, continuing physical punishment only makes them angry, hostile, anxious, fearful, apathetic, depressed, and aggressive. In Sweden people apparently *do* think such corporal punishment to children is harmful.[290] There spanking is outlawed.

2. Child Abuse Is a "National Emergency"

Fallon calls itself "the Oasis of Nevada," but it is an ordinary small town like many others, with the county courthouse in the old part and the McDonald's, Pizza Hut, and AM-PM Mini Market in the newer part. The town is choked with dust from construction fueled by newcomers fleeing other Western cities and from unplanted nearby fields because of a 6-year drought. Fallon is also suffering from a phenomenal rise in child abuse and neglect cases—157% from 1987 to 1991.[291]

Why so high? According to the Nevada Division of Child and Family Services, the leading factor behind the state's child abuse and neglect problem is that "the parent can't cope," which translates mainly into neglect: physical neglect, lack of supervision, educational neglect, medical neglect, abandonment, emotional abuse/ neglect. Other family stress factors, which contribute to the parent's inability to cope, are: insufficient income, alcohol/drug dependency, marital problems, inadequate housing, and job-related problems.[292] In Fallon, for instance, many people are struggling economically: the unemployment is the highest in the state, unskilled jobs are hard to find, housing is scarce, rents are high, and nearly three-quarters of the single mothers with children under 5 in the county are below the poverty line. Finally, it is suggested, because of a "John Wayne" I-will-take-care-of-myself mentality, adults don't seek help when they are stressed and end up striking their children.

Alcohol plays a major role in child abuse, in Nevada and elsewhere. Indeed, children of mothers who are problem drinkers have more than twice the risk of serious injury (resulting in hospitalization, surgical treatment, missed school, or a half day or more in bed) compared with nondrinking mothers. Children of female problem drinkers married to moderate or heavy drinkers had a relative risk of abuse that was 2.7 times those of children of nondrinkers. Because 7 million American children live with an alcoholic parent and 18% of American adults lived with an alcoholic or problem drinker when they were children, it's clear that alcohol and child abuse affect a tremendous number of people.[293]

A recent report declares child abuse and negligence a "national emergency." Hundreds of thousands of children, it states, are "being starved and abandoned, burned and severely beaten, raped and sodomized, berated and belittled."[294] According to a 1988 study, 63% of child maltreatment cases involved neglect (over a million children, or nearly 16 out of 1000 children); 43% involved physical, emotional, or sexual abuse (675,000 children, or nearly 11 out of every 1000 children).[295]

What children are more apt to be abused or neglected?[296] Race and ethnicity make no difference: maltreated children come from all racial and ethnic groups. Geographic location also makes no difference: child abuse can occur in any community—urban, suburban, or rural. In addition to parental chemical dependency, there are some higher risk situations, however:

- *Family income—being poor is a risk:* As usual, being poor never helps. Children from families whose income is less than $15,000 a year experience maltreatment *five* times higher than do children from higher income families. Very poor parents, those earning under $5000 a year, are especially apt to abuse their children.[297] (But even upper- and middle-income families produce abused and neglected children.)

- *Family size—large families are a risk:* Families with four or more children show higher rates of both physical abuse and physical neglect.

- *Gender—females are at increased risk:* Boys and girls suffer equal amounts of neglect. However, girls experience more sexual abuse than boys do—four times the rate for females as for males.

- *Stress—stressed parents are a risk:* Parental stress plays an important role in abusive families. Physically abusive families are not only more often low-income but also have younger mothers with less education, more frequently report a family history of child abuse, are more likely to be abusing alcohol, and report more depression and anxiety, all of which add up to more stress.[298]

3. Transcenders: Even Abused Children Can Turn Out All Right

Some people from abusive childhoods have managed to overcome problems or disabilities that would seem to sink most others. Called "transcenders," they offer lessons for those who have trouble rising above the circumstances of their lives. *Transcenders,* writes psychologist Donna LaMar, author of *Transcending Turmoil: Survivors of Dysfunctional Families,* are "individuals who grow up in difficult, painful, destructive families and emerge with a meaningful, productive way of life."[299]

Several famous people were abused as children. Television talk-show hostess Oprah Winfrey was sexually molested by male relatives and family friends when she was 9. British actor Michael Caine was physically abused by his foster mother and kept on a starvation diet until rescued by his natural mother. U.S. Senator Paula Hawkins was molested at age 5 by an elderly man. Poet Rod McKuen was battered by his stepfather, to the extent of having both arms broken, and was raped by a male family member at age 7.

Other transcenders are "ordinary heroes." A young West Virginian named Elizabeth was abandoned by her mother, subjected to bone-breaking beatings by her aunt, and sexually molested by her uncle from the age of 8. The turning point came in fourth grade, when her aunt shaved her head of her long, blond curls, her secret pride. "After that," reports Karen Northcraft, a psychiatric social worker who wrote her doctoral dissertation on transcenders, "she was able to reject what her aunt was saying and start making her life better."[300] Even when Elizabeth was admitted to college and told she was dyslexic and should drop out, she persevered, working her way through school, earning a graduate degree, and becoming a therapist.

What is it that transcenders have that others don't? Why do they not succumb to the pressures of the psychological and social problems of their surroundings? "They have self-confidence, and early on they think for themselves," says Northcraft. "They emotionally distance themselves from their parents, and they choose their actions rather than do what would be expected in their environment." When things are at their worst, they are able to imagine themselves somewhere else, envisioning that they can do great things despite their present circumstances.

But many other children never rise above their abusive backgrounds. Some develop health problems that require more than usual medical care as adults.[301,302] Some who experienced harsh punishment at home become accustomed to expressing violence against other children, teachers, and society.[303] Some become the homicidal teenagers who make headlines for killing their parents.[304] Others continue to have problems accepting and valuing themselves and forming intimate relationships with others.

4. Like Father (or Mother), Like Son (or Daughter): Parents Copy Their Own Parents' Child-Raising Styles

There are no skills tests to earn the right to parenthood, of course. Should there be? A volunteer counselor in the war against child abuse describes a scenario that is repeated over and over: "You're told you're stupid by your parents," says Norma Lemily, "so you're attracted to a man who says the same thing. It's perversely comfortable. Then your child regularly spills his juice. And out comes all that anger."[305] And another child is abused, and the cycle continues for another generation.

A theme repeated over and over is that abused children come from parents who were themselves abused.[306–308] For instance, youngsters who have been abused were found to be more apt to respond to provocative social situations aggressively.[309] When hit on the head by a ball on the playground, a child with no history of abuse was found to be more apt to assume it was an accident; a child who had been abused would be more apt to assume he or she had been attacked and would respond aggressively.

Somehow, the cycle of abused children growing up to be abusive parents has to be broken. If you come from an abusive or neglected background yourself, you need to be aware that not only does this kind of "discipline" not work but that there are far better alternatives. (*See accompanying figure.*) Parenting programs, support groups, *and* individual counseling can be immeasurably helpful to these parents who were raised in abusive homes.

How, in fact, *do* you help children grow up to be happy—to enjoy their work, to have close friends, to have a satisfying marriage? One important study shows that having warm, loving parents in early childhood—parents (both mothers and fathers) who cuddled, hugged, and spent time with their children—can make all the difference.[310] Indeed, the fact of having warm and affectionate parents turned out to be more important than such other factors as being from rich or poor families or having parents who were divorced or alcoholic.

Interestingly, in 1951, at the time the children in the study were 5, the conventional wisdom of experts was that children should be raised with a firm parental hand and strong discipline. Going against the grain of this advice was Dr. Benjamin Spock, author of the famed *Baby and Child Care*, first published in 1945, which became the major child-care guidebook for parents of the last five decades.[311] "I'd agree that the most significant thing is parents' warmth," said Spock, feeling vindicated by the study. "I've always said so, and I'm glad it's turned out to be true."[312]

UNIT

11 Infectious and Sexually Transmitted Deseases

In These Chapters:

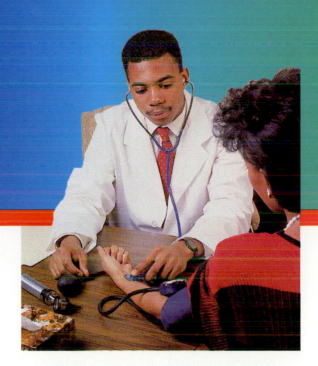

Where do those new diseases come from?

A mere decade or so ago, we might have thought medical science was well on its way to wrapping up some of the dread diseases of the past. Bubonic plague, which had swept medieval Europe, was no longer considered a problem. Syphilis, which had afflicted the Spanish colonizers of the New World, seemed to be behind us. Yellow fever, once a killer in American port cities, had disappeared. Tuberculosis and smallpox seemed to have been overcome.

Then, almost as punishment for our complacency, *new* diseases began to appear. One of the authors owns a 1975 medical dictionary. Here are three now-familiar diseases that I found that were *not* listed in it: *Lyme disease,* a disease transmitted by ticks, first recognized in 1975; *AIDS,* the famous sexual disease of acquired immunological deficiency named in 1982; and *chronic fatigue syndrome (CFS),* another immune system disease, characterized by extreme tiredness, first detected in 1984.

Then, as if the development of new diseases were not enough, there has been a comeback among old diseases: tuberculosis, measles, influenza, gonorrhea, and others. Some of these resurgences are the results of the inadequacy of existing public health surveillance and prevention systems. Some of them represent the appearance of antibiotic-resistant strains.

This unit provides important information to help you understand what the disease enemies are, how to boost your body's defenses, and what treatment to seek if you need it.

11.2

*Unit 11
Infectious and
Sexually
Transmitted
Diseases*

26 The Immune System and Infectious Diseases

▶ Explain the causes of infection, the pathogens, and discuss each of the six types of pathogens.

▶ Describe the process of infection—the transmission and four stages of infection.

▶ Discuss the defenses against infection—physical, chemical, and cellular, including the immune system and response.

▶ Compare and contrast the following types of infections: the common cold, the flu, mononucleosis, chronic fatigue syndrome, hepatitis, staph infections, strep infections, pneumonia, tuberculosis, and Lyme disease.

▶ Explain the principal types of immunizations for children and for adults.

Everyone who is born holds dual citizenship, in the kingdom of the well and in the kingdom of the sick," states philosopher and critic Susan Sontag in *Illness as Metaphor*.[1] When we are well, it is difficult to understand what it is like to be unwell. When we are sick, it is difficult to avoid self-pity, but it is important to go beyond it. Illness has lessons for us. As Arthur Frank writes, "Illness takes away parts of your life, but in doing so it gives you the opportunity to choose the life you will lead, as opposed to living out the one you have simply accumulated over the years."[2]

Many factors contribute to illness, or disease. Some of them you can do nothing about, such as heredity, aging, or certain environmental pollutants outside your control. Some of them you probably can do something about, such as drug use and lifestyle. A third area is both: **microorganisms** or **microbes**—organisms, such as germs, that are microscopic in size and thus escape easy detection. Avoiding some of the diseases transmitted as microorganisms may take a bit of luck. On the other hand, consider the observation of baseball

mogul Branch Rickey: *"Luck is the residue of design."* This represents a strategy for living: Good luck is not always just a fortuitous bolt from the blue. Good luck is frequently brought about by design—by thoughtful planning.

The forms of illness transmitted by microbes may be thought of as a battle between invaders and defenders of your body. There are three important factors that influence one's vulnerability and ability to cope with communicable diseases:

1. *The causes of infection:* The invaders are called **pathogens,** microorganisms that have gained entry to the body and that cause disease. The ability of a particular pathogen to cause disease is affected by its type, number, and **virulence**—the capability of a pathogen to overcome the body's defenses.

2. *The process of infection:* Disease caused by a pathogen is called an **infection.** The infection proceeds through four steps, as we will describe.

3. *The protection against infection:* The body protects itself against infection using physical, chemical, and cellular forms of defenses. One important part of the body's protection is the **immune system,** a system of cellular elements that protect the body from invading pathogens and foreign materials.

Causes of Infection: Pathogens

Six kinds of harmful microorganisms, or pathogens, are viruses, bacteria, rickettsia, fungi, protozoa, and parasitic worms. Viruses are the smallest yet toughest, are commonplace (as in the common cold), and vary in seriousness, means of transmission, and incubation periods; drug treatment is limited. Bacteria are single-celled organisms that cause a variety of diseases such as pneumonia and tuberculosis and may be treated with antibiotics. Rickettsia grow inside living cells. Fungi consist of yeasts and molds. Protozoa are responsible for many tropical diseases, such as malaria. Parasitic worms may attack the intestines.

11.3

*Chapter 26
The Immune
System and
Infectious
Diseases*

Many of the microorganisms that surround us are beneficial, such as the bacteria in our intestines, which help in digestion. Here, however, we consider the types of microorganisms that are harmful—namely, pathogens. There are six kinds of pathogens, ranging in size from smallest to largest: *viruses, bacteria, rickettsia, fungi, protozoa,* and *parasitic worms.* (See ● *Figure 26.1.*)

Viruses: The Smallest and Toughest

Viruses may be the smallest of the pathogens, being visible only under an electron microscope. However, they are also the toughest to fight because it is difficult to find drugs that will kill a virus without also killing the cell it has taken over. In addition, viruses withstand heat, formaldehyde, and radiation.

A virus is such a primitive form of life that it cannot exist on its own. Indeed, a virus is simply a protein structure containing the nucleic acids DNA or RNA. To survive and reproduce, it must attach itself to a cell and inject its own DNA or RNA, which tricks the cell's reproductive functions into producing new viruses. These new viruses expand the cell until it bursts, setting the viruses free to seek other cells to take over.

Common characteristics of viruses that are important to know are the following:

● *Viruses are common:* There are many viruses—200 for the common cold alone—making them the most prevalent form of contagious disease. **Contagious** means a disease is "catching"—it is easily transmitted from one person (carrier) to another. Viruses include the common cold, influenza (flu), mononucleosis (mono), hepatitis, mumps, chicken pox, measles, rubella, polio, and **HIV,** the human immunodeficiency virus that causes AIDS.

● *Viruses vary in seriousness:* Some viruses cause relatively mild, short-lived illnesses, such as a 24-hour flu that produces gastrointestinal upset. Other viruses have far

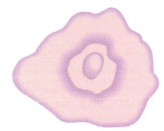

Viruses: Smallest pathogens
Typical diseases: Colds, influenza, herpes, rubella, mononucleosis, hepatitis, mumps, chicken pox, HIV

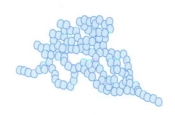

Bacteria: One-celled pathogens
Typical diseases: Strep throat, tetanus, bacterial pneumonia, Lyme disease, tuberculosis, scarlet fever, gonorrhea

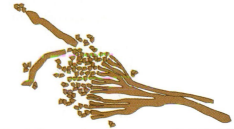

Fungi: Plant-like pathogens
Typical diseases: Athlete's foot, candidiasis, ringworm

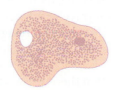

Protozoa: Simplest animal form
Typical diseases: amebic dysentery, giardia, malaria

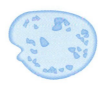

Rickettsia: Virus-like microbes
Typical diseases: Typhus fever, Rocky Mountain spotted fever

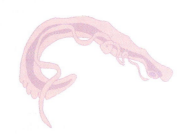

Parasitic worms: Many-celled
Typical diseases: Pinworm, elephantiasis

● **Figure 26.1 Pathogens.** Examples of each of the six types of pathogens are shown.

11.4

*Unit 11
Infectious and
Sexually
Transmitted
Diseases*

more serious consequences, such as mononucleosis, hepatitis, polio, or AIDS. The key is which cells the viruses attack. For example, cold viruses attack respiratory cells, which can be replaced. However, the polio virus attacks nerve cells, which cannot be replaced, resulting in paralysis.

- *Viruses are transmitted in different ways:* Some highly contagious viruses are transmitted in the air. When cold sufferers sneeze or cough, they spray extremely fine droplets of virus-bearing mucus and saliva into the environment. Hepatitis A is transmitted by water contaminated by sewage or by another fecal-oral route, as when infected food handlers don't wash their hands. HIV is transmitted by means of infected body fluids through anal, vaginal, or oral sex with an infected partner, through sharing drug needles with a person who has the virus, or by an infected pregnant woman to her fetus.

- *Viruses have varying incubation periods:* An **incubation period** is the time lapse between exposure to an organism and the development of symptoms. Cold viruses have short incubation periods, taking perhaps only 24 hours and lasting only 4–5 days. The flu, on the other hand, may develop after 4 days and last about 2 weeks. AIDS may not appear for 10–11 years after infection by HIV and may last 2 or more years.

- *Drug treatment for viruses is limited:* Viruses are hard to reproduce in laboratories, which makes antiviral drug development difficult. Drugs may block viral reproduction for some viruses. For other viruses, drugs may control symptoms but not cure the problem.

  A natural protection against some viruses is **interferon,** a protein substance produced by our bodies, which helps protect healthy cells in their battle with invaders.

Unfortunately, in recent years some old viruses (such as polio) have been causing what seem to be "new" diseases and what seem to be "new" viruses (such as influenza A and B) are causing old diseases.[3] New viruses and diseases emerge because of such factors as urban-

ization and travel, which help disease travel faster and further afield; agriculture, which exposes humans to animal-borne diseases; and organ transplants and blood transfusions, which can spread undetectable viruses.[4]

Bacteria: The Most Plentiful Next larger in size to viruses are **bacteria.** These single-celled organisms, visible through a standard microscope, are the most plentiful of the pathogens. Unlike viruses, many bacteria do not enter cells but thrive on and around the cells. Some bacteria are actually helpful, such as those (*Escherichia coli*) in the digestive tract. However, when people are ill, these bacteria can become harmful. About 100 of the several thousand species of bacteria actually cause disease in people.

The characteristics of bacteria include the following:

- *Bacteria cause a variety of diseases:* Three types of bacteria are spirilla, cocci, and bacilli. Among the types of bacterial infections they cause are strep infections (such as strep throat), staph infections, pneumonia, tuberculosis, scarlet fever, and gonorrhea.

- *Bacteria are transmitted in various ways:* Some bacteria are transmitted through consumption of contaminated water or food. A type of bacteria called chlamydia (discussed in Chapter 27) is largely transmitted by sexual intercourse.

- *Bacteria can harm the body in several ways:* Many bacteria release **toxins,** poisonous substances, that can lead to diseases such as tetanus, diphtheria, or even that unpleasant traveler's diarrhea sometimes called "Montezuma's revenge."

  Within the body, some bacteria work locally, killing cells near the source of infection; the infection then spreads to other tissue, producing boils, abscesses, and soreness. Other bacteria spread via the bloodstream, causing fever or attacking organs. Some bacteria simply grow until they obstruct vital organs, as in pneumonia.

- *Antibiotics may fight specific bacteria:* **Antibiotics** are bacteria-killing drugs in pill, cream, liquid, or injectable form. One of the most well known antibiotics is **peni-**

11.5

Chapter 26
The Immune
System and
Infectious
Diseases

cillin, a substance produced from a fungus. (Other antibiotics you may recognize are such drugs as erythromycin, tetracycline, streptomycin, gentamicin, and the cephalosporins.)

Specific antibiotics work on specific bacteria. No antibiotic, therefore, can be used to treat all bacterial infections. Nor are antibiotics appropriate for treating viral infections. In addition, antibiotics have to be taken properly in order to be effective. (*See* ● *Figure 26.2.*)

- *Some bacteria are drug-resistant:* Because of inappropriate use and overuse of antibiotics, some antibiotic-resistant strains of bacteria have developed. In addition, some strains of bacteria—for instance, some forms of tuberculosis—are transforming themselves into "superbugs" highly resistant or even invulnerable to some or all antibiotics.[5-7]

Rickettsia Resembling bacteria but more complex than viruses, **rickettsia** are disease-causing microorganisms that grow inside living cells. These organisms are generally transmitted by insects such as mites, ticks, and fleas. Rickettsia may cause rashes and fever, such as **typhoid fever (typhus),** a disease characterized by high, disabling fever. Infected ticks transmit **Rocky Mountain spotted fever,** a disease marked by chills, fever, prostration, and pain in muscles in joints.

Fungi: Yeasts, Molds, and the Like Fungi are single-celled organisms (like yeasts) or multicelled organisms (like molds), some of which cause diseases on the skin, mucous membranes, and lungs. The itching, burning, and scaling disorders of the feet and of the scrotal skin known as **athlete's foot** and **jock itch** are caused by a fungus that thrives in moist environments, such as locker-room shower floors. Another kind of fungal disorder is **candidiasis,** a yeast infection of the vagina. Treatment is with antifungal medications.

Protozoa: The Smallest Animals The smallest animals in existence are **protozoa,** single-celled organisms responsible for many tropical diseases. One example is **malaria,** the severe, recurrent disease borne by mosquitos. It re-

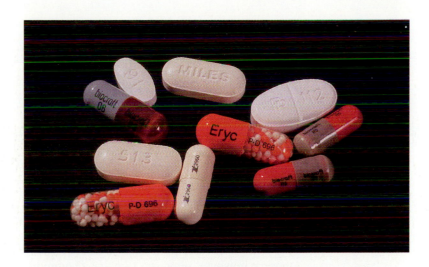

● **Figure 26.2 Using antibiotics right.** The safest way to use antibiotics is to take them only when you need them and to make sure you use them properly.

Some advice on using antibiotics:

1. **Take the drug *exactly* as prescribed.** Many antibiotics are prescribed for 7 days or more, and you should not stop taking them sooner even if you feel better sooner. Bacteria may be launching another attack, and if you're not taking the antibiotic, you may have a relapse. This not only means that you'll have to start over again but that you're increasing the chances the bacteria will become drug-resistant.

2. **Watch for a decline in symptoms.** You will probably know an antibiotic is working within a day or two by experiencing fewer symptoms. If they aren't disappearing, you may need to contact your health professional about changing medication. You could be fighting a resistant strain of bacteria.

3. **Never use someone else's prescription.** That person's antibiotic may not be the appropriate treatment for your problem. Moreover, some people have strong allergic reactions to some antibiotics.

4. **Throw out year-old prescriptions.** Old antibiotics have probably lost strength and are no longer effective.

mains one of the most serious and widespread tropical diseases, killing up to 2 million people a year.[8,9] Others are **African sleeping sickness,** a recurring disease whose chief characteristic is weariness and listlessness, and **amoebic dysentery,** an infection of the intestines.

11.6

Unit 11
Infectious and
Sexually
Transmitted
Diseases

If you spend time hiking or camping in North America, you need to be particularly aware that drinking unpurified water—even that from mountain streams—may produce a protozoan infection called **giardia,** characterized by diarrhea, abdominal cramps, and fatigue.

Parasitic Worms **Parasitic worms** may be microscopic in size or may range up to 10 feet long. Intestinal parasites, such as the tapeworm or pinworm, which cause anal itching in children, may be contracted by eating undercooked beef or pork. Some of these parasites are more a problem in developing countries than in North America; however, pinworm remains a common problem among school-aged children.

The Process of Infection

Infectious diseases are transmitted in three ways: from person-to-person contact, via contaminated food- and water-borne organisms (such as salmonella, botulism, trichinosis, cholera), or via animal- and insect-borne diseases (such as encephalitis). Infection occurs in four phases: incubation, prodromal, peak, and recovery.

We move among trillions of exotic viruses, bacteria, fungal spores, and other unseen microorganisms. How shall we avoid the harmful microbes and ignore the others?

Transmission Infectious diseases are transmitted in three ways—by people, by food or water, and by animals and insects.

- *People-to people-diseases:* Most of us need human contact of some sort, but not the sort that gives disease, which is transmitted by coughing, sneezing, touching, kissing, and sexual contact. You can't always avoid people coughing or sneezing in your presence and it's considered unfriendly if you don't shake hands. Still, you can wash your hands after going to the bathroom and before handling food, avoid sharing toothbrushes or other personal items, and make sure eating utensils are clean.

You can also use judgment about kissing someone who seems to have cold symptoms or cold sores. And you can ask a prospective sexual partner about any problems they may be having in the genital area—any blister or lesion, for example—and try to get a sense of his or her sexual history. Finally, as we shall describe, you can take steps to avoid getting infected blood, as happens with shared needles or blood transfusions with improperly screened blood donations.

- *Food- and water-borne organisms:* Spoiled or incorrectly prepared or processed food can transmit diseases, especially bacteria. Three in particular are worth mentioning—salmonella infections, botulism, and trichinosis. Two examples of water-borne diseases include cholera and typhoid fever.

  (1) **Salmonella** is a leading agent in bacterial food-borne diseases and is found throughout the environment. Salmonella bacteria are found in about a third of the poultry in the United States and appear in some eggs as well. If food is not properly handled, cooked, or refrigerated—as when eggs are consumed raw or undercooked—the salmonella can produce **gastroenteritis (food poisoning):** nausea, vomiting, diarrhea, fever, and abdominal cramps lasting 1–3 days.

  (2) **Botulism** is a food-related disease produced by a bacterium (*Clostridium*) that grows in improperly canned foods, as may happen in home canning, especially home-canned vegetables and fruits. Without treatment, botulism can produce paralysis and even death.

  (3) **Trichinosis,** a disease caused by an intestinal worm, is transmitted as a result of eating raw or undercooked meat, especially pork (a rarity in commercially processed meats), produces diarrhea, nausea, fever, and later stiffness, pain, sweating, and insomnia.

  (4) **Cholera** is an example of a water-borne disease transmitted by contaminated drinking water or in food washed with such water. The disease causes se-

11.7

Chapter 26
The Immune
System and
Infectious
Diseases

vere diarrhea and vomiting, draining the body of vital fluids and often causing rapid death if treatment is not available. Cholera is considered a footnote to history for many Americans, although it has shown up among many impoverished Texans living along the Mexican border. Cholera is a threat when natural disasters cause contamination of community water supplies. With the increase in international travel, as to Latin America, where the disease is widespread, travelers must be alert to its presence.[10,11]

- *Animal- and insect-borne diseases:* You can't catch warts from a frog (warts are a virus that you can get from another person, particularly if you have a cut or scratch and your resistance is low). However, you can catch other diseases from animals. Dogs and cats, for example, may carry rabies. Houseflies may spread dysentery, which is why food should be kept covered. Some types of mosquitos may carry **encephalitis,** such as *eastern equine encephalitis,* a relatively rare but usually fatal virus that attacks the brain, causing it to swell.[12]

The Four Periods of Infection After a disease is transmitted, whether by people, water, food, animals, or insects, it then goes through four periods of infection—incubation, prodromal, peak, and recovery:

- *Incubation period—the beginning of the battle:* The period between the time a pathogen is transmitted to you and the time you actually notice its symptoms is called the *incubation period.* For some diseases (the common cold, for example) this may be mere hours, for others (HIV) it may be years. For most illnesses, this is not a particularly contagious stage, although infection of others is possible.

- *Prodromal period—the invaders build their strength:* In the short second stage, or *prodromal period,* you begin to show vague, nonspecific signs and symptoms of a problem. With a cold, for instance, you may experience coughing, sneezing, and watery eyes. During this time, you are apt to be most contagious, capable of infecting other people.

- *Peak period—the battle is at its height:* Also called the *acute period,* the *peak period* is when the illness is full-blown, reaching its highest point of development—and unpleasantness. All the symptoms of the disease are now in full force. You may continue to be infectious, likely to transmit the illness to others. At this point, your body is using all its available defense mechanisms.

- *Recovery period—the invaders are beaten back:* In the *recovery* or *convalescence period,* your body (and any disease-fighting drugs) has triumphed over the invader, the pathogen is killed or reduced in power, and the signs and symptoms of the disease disappear. Until the time when all signs and symptoms have vanished, you are still somewhat contagious, but transmission is not as likely. With some infections (such as syphilis), the symptoms may disappear by themselves, but the pathogen has not gone away.

During the recovery period, you may be somewhat vulnerable to illness, perhaps from another pathogen. However, after recovery, in some cases you may be better able to resist the same invading agent because of the buildup in your immunity.

Defenses Against Infection

The body's three lines of defense against disease are physical, chemical, and cellular, the cellular defenses being the immune system that protects against pathogens and foreign materials. Two systems of immunity are cell-mediated (T-cells) and humoral (B-cells). Humoral immunity provides antibodies against specific invaders. Immunity is acquired naturally, artificially (vaccinations), and passively. Repelling the invasion of disease is known as the *immune response,* which is carried out by phagocytes, helper T-cells and killer T-cells, B-cells and antibodies, memory cells and suppressor T-cells. When the body overreacts to disease, the result is known as an *allergy.* When the body attacks itself, it produces autoimmune disorders, such as rheumatoid arthritis and multiple sclerosis.

11.8

Unit 11
Infectious and
Sexually
Transmitted
Diseases

Consider hair in the nose: Is it just some relic of our furry ancestors or is it truly useful?

Actually, it is quite useful, it turns out. Nose hairs trap inhaled dust and other debris, preventing some of it from moving on into the nasal passages. Inside the nose and respiratory passages, other tiny hair-like *cilia* sweep the foreign matter you breathe in, trapping them in *mucus* (thick secretions). When the debris is moved to the back of the throat, it is then coughed out or swallowed and eliminated or destroyed by the digestive system.

The Body's Defenses The body has three lines of defense—physical, chemical, and cellular (the immune system) against disease. (*See* ● Figure 26.3.)

- *The first line—physical barriers:* The first line of deterrence consists of *physical defenses,* both *external* and *internal.*

  Examples of external defenses are nasal hairs and cilia that filter the air. Another is the skin, which (when not broken) keeps out pathogens. Sweat, tears, and saliva wash away bacteria. The mucous membranes of the respiratory and gastrointestinal tracts trap invaders, as does the wax in the ears.

  Internal defenses include the spleen and the liver, organs that filter and purify the blood and eliminate dangerous substances. The **lymph nodes** are small pea-sized glands in the neck, underarms, and groin that filter out and destroy harmful debris. (*See* ● *Figure 26.4.*)

- *The second line—chemical barriers:* The second line of defense consists of *chemical barriers.* These include digestive enzymes and acids in the stomach and upper gastrointestinal tract. Sweat, tears, and saliva contain substances that repel or destroy bacteria. Vaginal enzymes also make life inhospitable for some microorganisms.

- *The third line—cellular barriers, the immune system:* The third line of defense consists of *cellular barriers.* This is called the **immune system,** the internal system of cellular elements that protects the body from pathogens and foreign materials.

Two Systems of Immunity: Cell-Mediated and Humoral When invaders slip by the physical and chemical barriers, the immune system—the cellular defense system—goes to work. The immune system actually consists of two groups of white blood cells (called lymphocytes), which work with each other to provide two kinds of immunity against invaders:

- *T-cells—cell-mediated immunity:* One group of cells are called *T-cells* because they originate in the thymus gland. (*Refer back to Figure 26.4.*) These kind of cells provide T-cell-mediated immunity, or simply **cell-mediated immunity.** The thousands of T-cells in cell-mediated immunity

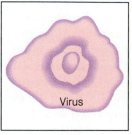

Virus

Invading
pathogen

**First line
of defense:
physical
barriers**

Skin
Hair and cilia
Sweat, tears, and saliva
Mucous membranes
Ear wax
Spleen and liver
Lymph nodes

**Second line
of defense:
chemical
barriers**

Stomach acids and enzymes
GI tract acids and enzymes
Sweat, tears, and saliva
Mucous membranes
Vaginal enzymes

**Third line
of defense:
cellular
barriers**

Cell-mediated immunity
Humoral immunity

● **Figure 26.3 The body's three lines of defense against disease**

11.9

Chapter 26
The Immune
System and
Infectious
Diseases

mainly protect the body against cancer cells, fungi, parasites, and foreign cells.

- *B-cells—humoral immunity:* The other group of cells are called *B-cells,* because they originate in the bone marrow, and they provide what is known as **humoral immunity.** Humoral immunity is mainly effective in protecting against infections caused by viruses and bacteria.

  In particular, humoral immunity provides **antibodies,** specific chemical compounds derived from the B-cells that destroy specific kinds of invaders. These invaders—toxins, foreign substances, and microorganisms—are called **antigens.** An antigen is any foreign matter that enters the body and causes it to form antibodies. Moreover, *once your body produces antibodies, you're protected against that particular antigen for life.* This is important to understand because it is the principle on which vaccines (for example, against polio) operate.

An example of how antigens and antibodies work is seen in a case of German measles, or rubella. Many colleges are requiring students to show proof that they have had rubella or been inoculated against it before they are allowed to enroll. What they want to know is whether students have built up or acquired *antibodies* against the *antigen* of rubella, so they are protected from the infection.

Let us see how the body acquires an immunity to an infectious disease such as rubella.

Three Ways of Obtaining Acquired Immunity The two cellular systems of immunity—cell-mediated and humoral—are in place when we are born. However, they will not actually work against specific disease threats until they encounter antigens representing that disease. Once this encounter has happened, then the immune system is "armed and ready," able to fight if that antigen appears again. That is, the body has now developed **acquired immunity;** it has formed antibodies and specialized blood cells that can destroy the specific pathogen.

This protection of acquired immunity can come about in three ways:

- *By exposure to the disease:* **Naturally acquired immunity** means that you were ex-

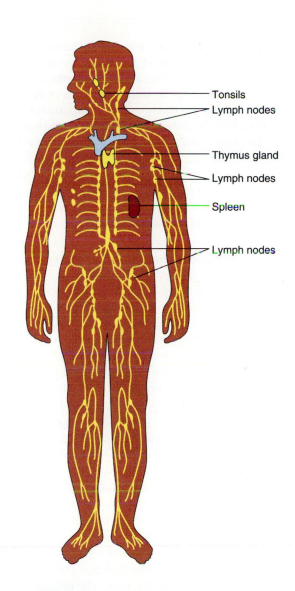

Tonsils
Lymph nodes

Thymus gland

Lymph nodes

Spleen

Lymph nodes

● **Figure 26.4 The defense effort.** Location of lymph nodes, the thymus gland, tonsils, and spleen, which are important in resisting disease organisms.

posed to the disease naturally. For example, a family member had rubella and transmitted the rubella virus to you. Your body fought the infection, thereby developing antibodies that will protect you against ever being reinfected.

- *By receiving a vaccination:* **Artificially acquired immunity** means that you

11.10

*Unit 11
Infectious and
Sexually
Transmitted
Diseases*

developed antibodies as a result of having pathogens introduced artificially into your body through a vaccination. A **vaccination** —also known as an **immunization** or **inoculation**—is the injection of organisms, prepared in a laboratory, into the body for the purpose of building antibodies against a particular disease. The injected organisms may be killed or they may be weakened but live. In any case, they constitute only a mild case of the disease against which they are supposed to build antibodies.

- *By receiving antibodies from outside the body:* **Passively acquired immunity** means that you acquired antibodies from outside your body—for example, microorganisms from animal sources or other people who have recovered from the disease. In other words, you didn't develop the antibodies within your own body; you got them from somewhere else. Gamma globulin is administered as a preventative for hepatitis.

Note that an antibody is specific: any one antibody can deactivate only one type of antigen. A polio antibody, for example, won't work against a measles antigen.

The Immune Response: Repelling the Invasion Assuming your immune system is armed and ready, what happens when the invaders invade? Once the antigens—whether microorganisms, foreign substances, or abnormal cells—have penetrated physical and chemical defenses and are inside the body, the cellular defense goes into operation, as follows:[13]

- *"Eating cells" first:* Frontline defenders consist of specialized white blood cells called **phagocytes,** from the Greek for "eating cells." Phagocytes confront the enemy and attempt to engulf and digest them. These eating cells are of two types—**granulocytes,** which roam the bloodstream, and **macrophages,** large white blood cells that line the blood vessels.

- *Helper T-cells and killer T-cells:* On encountering the foreign organism, the macrophages summon helper T-cells to the scene. **Helper T-cells** (components of cell-mediated immunity) identify the intruders, then call in **killer T-cells** (also a component of cell-mediated immunity) to destroy the antigen.

- *B-cells and antibodies:* In addition, the helper T-cells notify the *B-cells* (components of humoral immunity). The B-cells are transformed into producers of *antibodies* capable of destroying the specific intruder.

- *Memory cells and suppressor T-cells:* Finally, two other cells also become activated. **Memory cells** "remember" the specific attacking microbes and enable the body to respond more quickly against the antigen in subsequent infections. In other words, they give your body acquired immunity. **Suppressor T-cells** reduce or suppress the production of antibodies by B-cells once it is apparent that the battle against infection is being won.

How can you tell these great struggles are going on inside you? Sometimes you may develop signs and symptoms such as a slight fever. Sometimes you develop an **inflammation** in a specific place. That is, there will be a buildup of cells and fluid, causing blood vessels to expand, making a site red and swollen. Sometimes, as the body struggles with the invader in a specific location, it will form an **abscess,** a cavity filled with pus—battling cells, fluid, and dead white blood cells.

Sometimes our body's defense systems don't work the way they should to combat invading substances. When the immune system underreacts, the result is *infection:* the invaders win, as when pelvic inflammatory disease results from gonorrhea. At other times, in what are called **immune disorders,** the immune system overreacts or the body even attacks itself. We consider these next.

Allergies: When the Body Overreacts Lots of people have allergies—hay fever alone afflicts 41 million Americans, according to the American College of Allergy and Immunology.[14] An **allergy** is defined as a hypersensitivity to a particular substance or environmental condition. What happens is that the immune system overreacts to the stimulus, producing antibodies that attack it. The results are runny nose, watery eyes, itching, swelling, redness, rashes, and wheezing—or even worse.

11.11

*Chapter 26
The Immune
System and
Infectious
Diseases*

The sources of allergies, called **allergens,** can be almost anything: dust, molds, plants, animals, insects, foods, medicines, chemicals, perfumes, and cigarette smoke. Some people are allergic to things most of us would not suspect, such as tap water or paper money.

The outdoors can be particularly hazardous. **Pollen,** a natural, powdery substance produced by trees and grass, is a common allergen. Most people who come into contact with *poison ivy* or, on the West Coast, *poison oak* get itchy, blistered skin on the affected part. Poison sumac, a native of the Southeast, also sometimes shows up in the West and Canada.[15]

Common allergic reactions take several forms, ranging from mild to life-threatening:

- *Hay fever:* **Hay fever** is an allergic reaction not just to hay but to pollens and other allergens; it produces runny nose and eyes, itching, sneezing, and loss of appetite.

- *Hives:* **Hives,** a reaction to insect bites, drugs, chemicals, and certain foods, is characterized by raised, itchy red blotches on the skin.

- *Asthma:* **Asthma,** a chronic affliction of the airways in the lungs marked by constriction in the chest, labored breathing, wheezing, gasping, and coughing, affects 15 million Americans.[16]

- *Anaphylaxis:* In the worst cases, people get near-fatal and even fatal allergic reactions called **anaphylaxis,** or **anaphylactic shock.** In these instances, the air passages become constricted, causing great difficulty breathing; the blood vessels expand, causing the blood pressure to drop; and the victim faints and feels like he or she is going to die. Indeed, without medical treatment, anaphylaxis can be fatal.[17]

Autoimmune Disorders: When the Body Attacks Itself Some of the most difficult disorders to treat, called **autoimmune disorders,** come about because the immune system fails to recognize its own tissue and attacks itself, causing progressive degeneration. Three examples are:

- *Rheumatoid arthritis:* **Rheumatoid arthritis** is a chronic, crippling form of arthritis (of which there are more than 100 varieties) that inflames small joints, such

as those in the fingers and wrists, but it can also attack the organs and connective tissues.[18]

- *Multiple sclerosis:* **Multiple sclerosis** is a condition in which cells in the immune system turn against the body and attack the brain and spinal cord, leading to progressive, irreversible paralysis and death.[19]

- *Myasthenia gravis:* **Myasthenia gravis,** an autoimmune disorder most common in women ages 20–40, consists of a weakening of the muscles, to the point where double vision may appear and even combing one's hair becomes difficult.[20]

These diseases, although they may progressively worsen, may be treated with drugs that suppress the immune system.

Let us now turn to some of the most common infectious diseases.

The Common Cold

The common cold, an infection of the lining of the upper respiratory tract, is caused by any of 200 viruses and is transmitted by people contact. Treatment is with time, decongestants, expectorants, and cough suppressants, depending on the symptoms.

The common cold can definitely be a pain in the head—or the chest—and most adults get at least two colds a year. That it is "common," however, does not mean that it is simple: a cold can be caused by not just one but any of 200 or so different viruses. Indeed, in 1990, the Common Cold Research Institute in London finally closed down after 44 years and the efforts of 18,000 sniffling volunteers, conceding defeat at any attempt to develop a vaccine against humanity's most infectious disease.[21] If such a defense is ever developed, it will probably be through genetic engineering techniques.[22]

Prevention The **common cold** is an infection of the membrane lining the upper respiratory tract: nose, sinuses, and throat. The symptoms, as all of us know, are runny nose, watery eyes, general aches and pains, and sometimes a slight fever. Later symptoms might include a stuffy nose, sore throat, and coughing.

11.12

*Unit 11
Infectious and
Sexually
Transmitted
Diseases*

Whatever people have told you about staying away from drafts or avoiding getting your hair wet, these are not ways you catch a cold. Frequent temperature changes also make no difference.[23] If college students are particularly apt to get colds, it is because they spend so much time in crowded classrooms and living spaces with other people who may have colds.

Colds are rarely spread through the air; most are hand-delivered. You could avoid shaking hands with people, but can you avoid touching doorknobs and telephones, some of which are apt to be virus-contaminated? Washing your hands often and keeping your unwashed fingers away from your eyes and nose may lessen your chances of infection by cold viruses. So will using tissues rather than handkerchiefs, since cold viruses don't survive as long on tissues.[24]

High levels of stress may double your chances of getting a cold.[25] This may be because stress impairs some of the body's defenses, such as the production of interferon, a natural antiviral agent.

Treatment Actually, you don't "treat" a cold so much as manage it, since there is no cure. Recommended cold management includes staying home, resting, eating moderately (your sense of taste will be diminished), and drinking plenty of fluids such as water and juices. Steam inhalation seems to have no beneficial effects.[26]

Since there are more than 800 over-the-counter cold remedies, which should you use? Here are some thoughts:

- *Avoid aspirin and acetaminophen:* The common painkillers aspirin and acetaminophen (Tylenol) may help your headache and muscle pain, if you have them, but they may also suppress the body's immune system, slowing down the production of antibodies against infection.[27] These drugs are just pain medications, but colds aren't usually painful, just uncomfortable. (Some cold medications include these painkillers.) Children and teenagers especially should avoid aspirin because of a possible link with a rare but potentially fatal illness called *Reye's syndrome.* This disorder is characterized by fever, vomiting, and swelling of the kidneys and brain.

- *Use decongestants with care:* **Decongestants** are drugs that suppress mucus production by constricting the blood vessels in the nose. Spray decongestants are considered the most effective for runny noses. Overuse sometimes leads to **rebound congestion**—excessive congestion that can worsen the problem. (Oral decongestants can constrict blood vessels throughout the body, causing mouth dryness and other side effects in some people.)

- *Expectorants:* **Expectorants** are supposed to stimulate coughing so that mucus in the chest will be loosened and can be coughed up.

- *Use cough suppressants for dry coughs:* **Cough suppressants** act on the brain's cough reflex to suppress the cough. Coughing is important for clearing phlegm from the throat and chest, and so cough suppressants should be used only when there is a dry cough. A *dry cough* is marked by the absence or scantiness of secretions.

In recent years, many of these products have been combined into multipurpose or "shotgun" cough remedies. These remedies often contain antihistamines—useful for hay fever and similar allergies but not for the common cold—and decongestants. Some also have pain relievers, such as aspirin or acetaminophen. Cold experts consider these combinations irrational because people differ greatly in their cold symptoms. Most effective are single-ingredient drugs because you can target just the symptoms you have. Why take more medication than is really needed? Whatever course you take—even if you do nothing—the symptoms will subside after a few days.

In 1970, Nobel Prize–winning chemist Linus Pauling suggested that high doses of vitamin C—up to 10 grams a day—would help prevent colds or diminish cold symptoms.[28] Studies have failed to support this, but the enormous sales of vitamin C supplements show that many people believe the idea anyway.[29]

11.13

*Chapter 26
The Immune
System and
Infectious
Diseases*

The Flu: More Serious Than It Seems

Influenza, or the flu, is caused by three contagious viruses. Influenza is quite serious and has caused worldwide epidemics (pandemics) killing millions of people. Flu viruses are airborne, transmitted by sneezing and coughing. Inoculation with flu shots may help prevent infection.

The "flu" is the name most people give to influenza. Influenza is different from a cold, although distinguishing the two isn't always easy. Like the common cold, **influenza** is caused by contagious viruses, although there are only three principal strains (strains A, B, and C, within which are several subtypes). However, people don't die directly from a cold, whereas flu and resulting complications kill an average of 10,000 Americans in a mild year, sometimes up to 70,000 in a severe one.[30] Indeed, the most common misconception about the flu is that it is not serious.[31] Yet it has caused some of the worst **pandemics**—the word experts use for an epidemic that rages across national boundaries. Pandemics occur every 10–12 years and minor regional epidemics every 2–3 years.[32] One of the worst epidemics was the 1918 influenza pandemic, which killed 20 million people worldwide—far more than the casualties from combat in World War I. (*See ● Figure 26.5.*)

Distinguishing Flu from Colds Whereas cold viruses are not thought to be airborne, flu viruses, which are transmitted by sneezing and coughing, can be airborne for up to 2 hours. This ability to be transmitted by air droplets makes them extraordinarily contagious. In general, influenza is much more uncomfortable

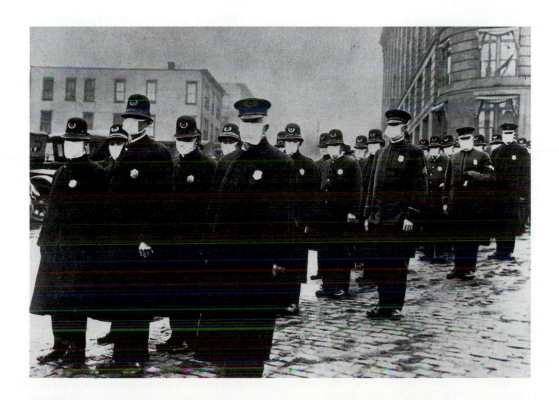

● **Figure 26.5 Influenza.** Chicago police officers wearing masks to protect themselves against influenza during the 1918–1919 epidemic.

11.14

Unit 11
Infectious and
Sexually
Transmitted
Diseases

than a cold. Most colds produce only slight aches and pains and do not often cause fevers or headaches. The flu, on the other hand, produces all of these. In addition, chest discomfort can be severe. If the condition advances to bronchitis or pneumonia, it can be life-threatening.

Influenza and its complications present a major cause of debilitating illness and premature death in the United States. The risks are especially high for people over 65 years of age and those with chronic medical conditions.

Prevention Most health officials recommend annual influenza immunization for older adults and anyone with a chronic medical problem. The vaccines used consist of viruses that have been grown in laboratories and then killed. When injected into the body, the vaccine stimulates the production of antibodies that will fight an invading flu virus, thus reducing the likelihood of infection and the severity of disease if an infection occurs.

In about a third of cases, people receiving the vaccine experience pain and redness at the vaccination site for 1–2 days. Some persons, especially children, may also suffer fever and malaise. People who are strongly allergic to eggs may develop immediate allergic reactions to the vaccine.[33]

The vaccine is effective in 70–90% of people under the age of 65 and about half the people over age 65.[34,35] Unfortunately, less than a third of the 50 million Americans in high-risk categories get immunized.[36]

Because the flu season is usually the winter months and because it takes the body a couple of weeks to develop the virus-fighting antibodies, people are advised to get their flu shots in the fall.[37] Mid-October through mid-November are best.[38] However, even an inoculation in February may lessen the severity of the flu, although it may not protect one from the virus.

Treatment If you already have the flu, a physician might prescribe the antiviral drug *amantadine*. This drug can be 70–90% effective in reducing flu symptoms—provided it is started within 48 hours after symptoms begin. Otherwise, treatment is similar to that used for a cold: bed rest and fluids. As with colds, children and teenagers should *not* take aspirin, which may cause Reye's syndrome.

Mononucleosis: The "Kissing Disease"

Mononucleosis is a common infectious disease that affects people ages 15–24 and can bring long periods of low energy. Treatment involves rest.

Mononucleosis, sometimes called the "kissing disease" and frequently called just "mono," is a common infectious viral disease among college students and other people 15–24 years old. Initially, mononucleosis is experienced as a fever, headache, sore throat, chills, nausea, and prolonged tiredness or weakness. Later the lymph nodes may become enlarged, body rashes and joint aches develop, and there may be kidney and liver complications. One of the most difficult aspects of the illness is the long period in which one feels devoid of energy, a real hardship for students attempting to keep up with school work.

Mono is usually caused by the *Epstein-Barr virus (EBV)*, which is present in over 90% of American adults, though usually in latent form. Mono is diagnosed by means of a blood test. Despite being known as "the kissing disease," mononucleosis is not thought to be highly contagious, although kissing is always a possible mode of transmission.

Treatment is much the same as for colds and the flu but principally involves extended rest. Alcohol should be avoided because it may increase the risk of liver complications.[39] A physician's advice should be sought. Returning to normal activity prematurely can bring about relapse.

Chronic Fatigue Syndrome: The Mysterious Disease of Exhaustion

Chronic fatigue syndrome is a disease of mysterious origins, perhaps a virus, whose principal effect is profound exhaustion, sometimes lasting for years. Various kinds of treatments are still being developed.

Chronic fatigue syndrome (CFS) starts out resembling mononucleosis (indeed, it was

11.15

*Chapter 26
The Immune
System and
Infectious
Diseases*

once called "chronic mono"), with patients reporting the same flu-like symptoms: sore throat, tender lymph nodes, fever, chills, headaches, joint pain, and prolonged, debilitating fatigue and depression. However, the symptoms linger from 6 months to several years.[40,41] For instance, months after the mysterious ailment was discovered among members of a Lake Tahoe high-school girls' basketball team, 200 people in the region were still feeling overwhelming fatigue plus, in many cases, disorientation, memory loss, and sleep disorders.[42]

Many early medical observers thought that CFS was little more than depression or psychological problems. Skeptics referred to the illness as the "yuppie flu" because many who were stricken came from affluent families. The cause of the problem has still not been identified. However, research suggests the debilitating disease could be linked to an immune system disorder that causes inflammation of the central nervous system.[43] Researchers also have found evidence of a virus among CFS sufferers, although it is not clear whether it is the cause of the syndrome. It is possible that each case may arise from a mix of causes—viruses, immune abnormalities, genetic predisposition, and psychological makeup.

Because no treatment has proven effective for all CFS patients, those affected may be vulnerable to schemes geared to profit from people's distress.[44] In general, doctors prescribe reducing stress, getting plenty of sleep, eating a balanced diet, and exercising lightly while avoiding overexertion. Antidepressants have been tried. An antiviral drug named Ampligen is also being studied. Having hope is crucial: CFS often gradually subsides, allowing full recovery.

Hepatitis: Five Diseases of the Liver

Hepatitis is a name given to five virally caused inflammations of the liver, all of which have similar symptoms. Hepatitis A is spread by fecal contamination of food and water and sometimes oral-anal sex. Hepatitis B—100 times more contagious than the AIDS virus—is transmitted by infected blood, as in sexual contact or sharing of drug needles; vaccination against it is recommended. Hepatitis C is bloodborne, spread by shared needles and other blood contacts.

The Centers for Disease Control (CDC) recorded about 57,000 cases of viral hepatitis in 1988 in the United States, although the number may actually be as high as 300,000.[45] **Hepatitis** is generally defined as a virally caused inflammation of the liver. Its symptoms include fever, chills, headache, nausea, diarrhea, loss of appetite, skin rashes, and sometimes the yellowing of skin and eyes called *jaundice*.

Actually, the term "hepatitis" includes at least *five* inflammatory diseases of the liver, covering 95% of viral hepatitis cases: hepatitis A, B, C, D, and E. These five diseases have similar symptoms but otherwise are different. We describe the first three, considered the principal health threats.

Hepatitis A—Transmitted by Hygiene Lapses Hepatitis A generally enters the body through the mouth. The virus is found in the feces of infected people and is spread by fecal contamination of food and water. Thus, it may be spread by restaurant workers or people working in day-care centers or homes with children in diapers. Another source of contamination is raw shellfish.

However, the virus may also be transmitted by oral-anal contact during sex, which would seem to explain the rise in hepatitis A among gay or bisexual men in 1991. This may reflect a return to unsafe sex practices or a misperception regarding the relative safety of such contact.[46]

The period of illness usually lasts 2–6 weeks. There is no treatment, although doctors can ease the symptoms of fever, lethargy, and pain. A vaccine called *immune globulin (IG)*, recommended for travelers in developing countries, is available to boost immunity.[47,48]

Hepatitis B—Transmitted by Infected Blood This hepatitis virus is transmitted through infected blood (or saliva, mucus, or semen), typically by sexual contact, sharing of drug needles, needle-stick accidents (a risk to health care workers, who may accidentally be stuck with used needles), or even sharing of

11.16

Unit 11
Infectious and
Sexually
Transmitted
Diseases

razors and toothbrushes. (*See ● Figure 26.6.*) It can also be transmitted by an infected mother to her baby at birth.

Although you might not think of it as a sexually transmitted disease (STD), today hepatitis B is second only to gonorrhea as the most common STD in America. In 1990, it was reported to be spreading almost nine times faster than HIV, the virus that causes AIDS, among gay men, mainly because of anal intercourse.[49]

Among those at risk are people who live with the 1.2 million Americans who are infected with the virus and 10 million heterosexuals who have multiple partners or whose partners have multiple partners.[50] Adolescents are particularly at risk because they tend to have sex more often with more partners and many do not use condoms.

Symptoms of hepatitis B include dark urine, muscle and joint aches, and fatigue. The disease lasts 2–6 months. People usually recover on their own, although in a small percentage of cases (1–3%) there are fatalities from liver failure. A drug called alpha interferon has shown promise of being effective in treatment.[51,52] A vaccine has been available for about a decade that has been found to be 80–95% effective, but health officials are concerned that many children and at-risk individuals have not been immunized.[53]

Hepatitis C—"Classic" Hepatitis, Also Blood-Borne It is not clear whether hepatitis C is spread by sexual contact, but as another blood-borne virus it has been found to be transmitted by IV drug use, needle-stick accidents, blood transfusions, and contact between infected women and their fetuses. Often the virus produces no symptoms, so that victims may infect others without knowing it. The disease is fatal in 2% of cases. No vaccine is available, but alpha interferon can manage the illness in some patients.

Protecting Against Hepatitis The hepatitis viruses, particularly hepatitis B, continue to spread principally because of ignorance. Hepatitis B is 100 times as contagious as HIV and may be spread not only through sexual contact but also through sharing toothbrushes or razors or even by kissing in which there is an exchange of saliva.[54] All sexually active people with a chance of being infected by it should use condoms. All babies should get the vaccine for hepatitis B as part of their standard immunization program, according to the CDC. Indeed, *anyone*—every person in America—would be wise to be vaccinated against this widespread disease.

Staph Infections: From Acne to Toxic Shock Syndrome

Staph infections are caused by *staphylococci* bacteria. Commonplace staph infections are acne, boils, and styes. A potentially fatal disease is toxic shock syndrome.

Staph (or staphylococcal) infections are caused by bacteria called *staphylococci*. These bacteria are usually present on the skin and don't create problems unless they enter through a wound or cut.

Acne, Boils, and Styes Three commonplace staph infections are the following:

- *Acne:* **Acne** is, of course, the disorder of the skin caused by inflammation of the oil glands in the skin and hair follicles, which produces pimples, cysts, and even scarring on the face and elsewhere. This is not just a teen-age problem; many adults are also plagued by breakouts. Moreover, contrary to widespread belief, acne is not caused by

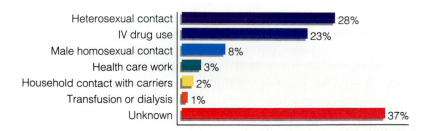

Heterosexual contact	28%
IV drug use	23%
Male homosexual contact	8%
Health care work	3%
Household contact with carriers	2%
Transfusion or dialysis	1%
Unknown	37%

● **Figure 26.6 Hepatitis B.** Risk of infection by source, 1989. Heterosexual sex is the most common means of transmitting the disease, followed by IV (intravenous—by needles) drug use.

11.17

*Chapter 26
The Immune
System and
Infectious
Diseases*

consuming chocolate, colas, or shellfish. Rather the fluctuation in hormones brought about by puberty cause the oil glands in the skin to become overactive, producing excess oil and plugging up the glands, leading staph bacteria to attack. In defense, the body's white blood cells move to the area, forming pus, creating a "white head." Later, pigment-producing cells cause the formation of a "black head."

- *Boils and styes:* **Boils,** that famous affliction of the biblical Job, are localized swellings and inflammations of the skin resulting from staphylococcal infection in a skin gland; the swellings have a central hard core and form pus. **Styes** are inflamed swellings of the oil glands at the margin of an eyelid.

Acne is quite often solved by simply getting older, when the adolescent hormones subside. Pharmacies carry many over-the-counter preparations containing so-called *peeling agents* (salicylic acid, benzoyl peroxide) to treat acne. Physicians may also prescribe *antibiotics* (tetracycline, erythromycin, minocycline), although there may be some side effects. A derivative of vitamin A called *Accutane,* which reduces acne by halting oil production of the oil glands, may be helpful for severe cases.

Toxic Shock Syndrome Acne and boils may be unsightly and bring about emotional pain, but at least they aren't fatal. However, **toxic shock syndrome (TSS)** can be. TSS is a rare infection in which the bacteria *Staphylococcus aureus* releases toxins into the bloodstream. The "shock" in toxic shock syndrome is associated with symptoms such as faintness, rapid pulse, and low blood pressure. TSS is also characterized by fever, headache, vomiting, sore throat, diarrhea, muscle aches, rash, peeling of skin on palms and soles of feet, reduced urination, and disorientation. Without prompt treatment, TSS can cause permanent damage and is potentially fatal.

Although sometimes occurring in people recovering from wounds or surgery and women within 6–8 weeks of giving birth, TSS has been most dramatically discovered in women using high-absorbency tampons. In the last 10 years, TSS has declined because manufacturers have changed the absorbency and composition of tampons.[55] Even so, besides avoiding superabsorbent tampons, women are advised to change tampons every 3–4 hours and to allow themselves some tampon-free time every day of their menstrual period.

Strep Infections: More Than "Strep Throat"

Strep infections include strep throat and the very serious disorders of rheumatic fever, which can lead to heart damage, and group A strep, linked to a fatal pneumonia.

Strep throat is familiar to most people. This is a severe sore throat caused by streptococci bacteria and characterized by white or yellow pustules at the back of the throat and fever. Indeed, strep throat is quite common, with as many as 20 million Americans developing it every year.[56]

Most strep infections are not serious, especially in children, but some forms, including rheumatic fever and group A strep, can be fatal to adults if not treated.

- *Rheumatic fever:* **Rheumatic fever** is a streptococcal infection that occurs principally in children ages 5–15 and young adults such as military recruits. The disorder is characterized by fever, inflammation and pain around the joints, jerky and involuntary movement, skin rashes, and in half the victims a condition called rheumatic heart disease, which damages heart valves.

  Rheumatic fever, like scarlet fever (an acute fever, sore throat, and rash), virtually disappeared in the United States in the mid-1900s, but in recent years it was observed to be making a return in parts of the United States. Because it is difficult to predict who will get rheumatic fever, everyone who might have strep should see a doctor.[57]

- *Group A strep:* **Group A strep** is a bacteria that was linked to the return of rheumatic fever in the U.S. and to a rare and fatal form of pneumonia, one that killed world-famous Muppet puppeteer Jim Henson in May 1990.[58] (See ● *Figure 26.7.*) The new disease, also known as *streptococcal toxic-shock-like syndrome,* progresses

11.18

Unit 11
Infectious and
Sexually
Transmitted
Diseases

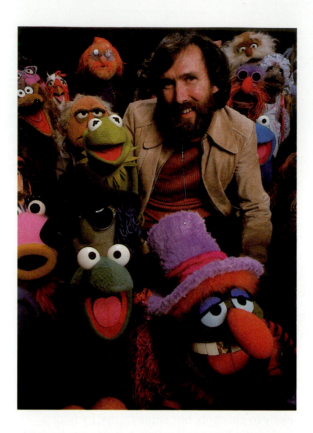

● **Figure 26.7 Mean strep.** Famous Muppet puppeteer Jim Henson (shown with some of his creations) died suddenly in May 1990 from a mysterious strain of Group A strep, or streptococcal toxic-shock-like syndrome.

quickly, causing a high fever, cough, chills, skin rash, dizziness, sudden drop in blood pressure, and an interruption in circulation. Henson, for instance, complained of flu-like symptoms the weekend before his death but did not get treatment until he checked into a hospital 2 days later. By then, however, the infection had spread from the lungs to other organs.

Penicillin and other antibiotics are still effective in treating strep infections, if they are caught early. Still, it is important to be aware of the dangers. Many people carry strep bacteria in their throats, where a cough can transmit them in airborne droplets—dangerously to

some susceptible people. No one knows why some people become ill and others don't. To guard against the toxic-shock-like syndrome, if you get a cut or burn you should wash the wound, keep it covered, and see a doctor if the site becomes red and swollen or if flu-like symptoms develop.

Pneumonia: Inflammation of the Lungs

Pneumonia is an infection with different causes in which fluid fills the lung's tiny air chambers. Pneumonia, the most frequently fatal infection in the United States, is distinguished from a cold by its length and severity.

Pneumonia is an infection in the lungs, in which fluid fills the tiny air chambers. It can be brought on by bacteria (such as Group A strep), viruses (such as a strain of influenza), or chemicals or other substances in the lungs (such as smoke). It can be a complication of childhood diseases such as measles, mumps, and rubella. Seventy-five years ago, pneumonia and influenza were the leading killers in the United States; today they are the fifth leading cause of death. Every year, of the 2 million Americans who catch pneumonia, at least 40,000 die.[59]

Pneumonia caused by a bacterial infection can be controlled with antibiotics. Antibiotics are not effective for those strains caused by viruses or environmental exposure. A vaccine is available for bacterial pneumonia and is recommended for everyone over age 65, those with weakened immune systems, and people with heart, lung, and kidney disease.[60]

How do you tell pneumonia from a cold? If cough, runny nose, fever, headache, muscle ache, and loss of appetite last more than a few days or if they are accompanied by shortness of breath and by difficulty breathing, you should seek the assistance of a health care professional to determine if you have something more complicated than a cold. Some strains produce a sharp, severe chest pain that worsens with deep breathing or coughing.[61]

11.19

*Chapter 26
The Immune
System and
Infectious
Diseases*

Tuberculosis: A 19th-Century Killer Returns

Tuberculosis is a contagious bacterial disease that lodges in the lung and then spreads to the rest of the body. TB is transmitted in airborne droplets via breathing, coughing, and the like, but the risk of acquiring it rises only with prolonged contact with a carrier. People most at risk are prisoners, the poor, immigrants, refugees, and people with HIV. People may be infected with TB, but it may not become active. The early form can nearly always be cured. People who drop out of treatment may develop drug-resistant TB strains.

The headlines began to appear in 1990 and multiplied through the early '90s—BIG RISE IN U.S. TUBERCULOSIS RATE; WEAKENED BY AIDS, PRISONERS ARE DYING OF NEW TB STRAINS; TB RETURNS TO HAUNT THE POOR—finally exploding in a cover story in *Newsweek* and a five-part series in the *New York Times*.[62–67] Tuberculosis is an important cause of disability and death in many parts of the world, but it was thought to be largely controlled in North America. However, in a stunning development, the scourge once called "consumption"—which killed more Americans in the 19th century than any other infectious disease—has come back.

Tuberculosis (TB) is a contagious bacterial disease (caused by a germ called *mycobacterium*) that mainly lodges in the lungs and slowly and painfully multiplies there. It can spread to and damage the brain, bone, eyes, liver and kidneys, spine, and skin. Common symptoms include coughing, chest pain, night sweats, and spitting up blood.[68] Serious outcomes of initial TB infections most frequently occur in infants, adolescents, and adults.[69]

Who Gets TB and How TB is an airborne disease: it travels from person to person in airborne droplets when someone with active TB exhales, coughs, or sneezes. Since it is airborne, it is far easier to transmit than blood-borne illnesses like hepatitis or AIDS. "Catching tuberculosis requires no consensual act: only breathing," says one physician specializing in communicable diseases.[70] (*See* • *Figure 26.8.*)

Even so, it is not as contagious as influenza, measles, or chicken pox, in which sick people can infect nearly anyone who has not already had the disease.[71] TB occurs only after close and prolonged contact with an infected person. On average, healthy people have a 50% chance of becoming infected if they spend 8 hours a day for 6 months or all day for 2 months working or living with someone who is sick with TB, according to an administrator with the American Lung Association.[72]

In general, the people most at risk in the resurgence are as follows:

- *People living in close contact and poorly nourished:* The homeless who sleep in public shelters or flophouse rooms are more at risk than those who sleep in cars, stay with relatives, or sleep outdoors, according to a preliminary study by University of California at San Francisco researcher Andrew Zolopa.[73] The reasons are overcrowded, inadequately ventilated shelters, combined with the poorly functioning immune systems of many homeless people brought on by malnutrition, drug use, or AIDS infection, according to a CDC report.[74]

  Researchers who studied poor migrant workers in South Carolina found that of the native-born African Americans they studied, 3.6% had active tuberculosis—more than 300 times the national average. Researchers found these cases were not an imported problem, brought in by foreign workers, but rather the result of poor living conditions and inadequate medical care.[75] Tuberculosis killed 12 inmates and a guard in the New York prison system in 1991, raising concern among officials.[76,77]

- *Immigrants and refugees:* About one-fourth of reported tuberculosis cases are in people who were born outside the United States. Thus, health officials are concerned about inadequate screening and prevention programs among immigrants and refugees from countries where TB rates are higher than in the United States.[78]

- *People with impaired immunity:* People with HIV, the virus that causes AIDS, are particularly at risk. As many as 40% of AIDS patients have active TB. They are apt to develop it faster because their immune systems are already ravaged.[79,80]

11.20

*Unit 11
Infectious and
Sexually
Transmitted
Diseases*

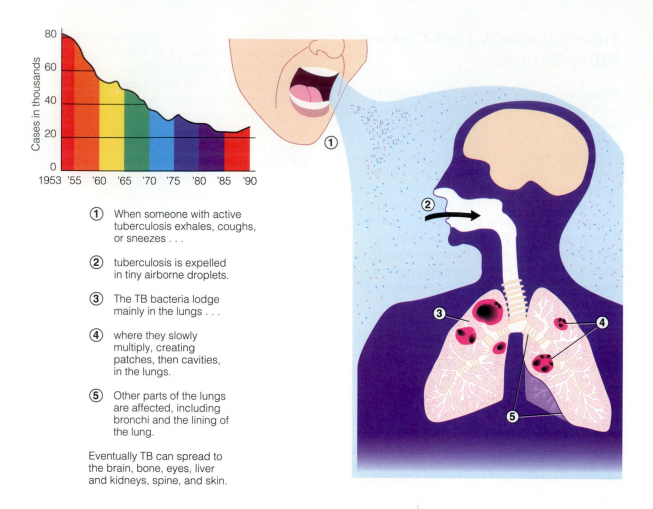

① When someone with active tuberculosis exhales, coughs, or sneezes . . .

② tuberculosis is expelled in tiny airborne droplets.

③ The TB bacteria lodge mainly in the lungs . . .

④ where they slowly multiply, creating patches, then cavities, in the lungs.

⑤ Other parts of the lungs are affected, including bronchi and the lining of the lung.

Eventually TB can spread to the brain, bone, eyes, liver and kidneys, spine, and skin.

● **Figure 26.8 The spread of tuberculosis**

Although TB mainly attacks the poor and the HIV-infected, there have been instances where low-risk people have been infected. In 1992, for instance, a Maine man unknowingly infected 417 fellow shipyard workers, as well as others with whom he socialized.[81]

People such as hospital workers, prison guards, and shelter workers who are around TB victims are insisting on the installation of ultraviolet lights, which kill the TB germ in the air; the upgrading of ventilation systems, especially in closed spaces; and the wearing of face masks.

Treatment Tuberculosis may exist in two forms—*latent,* in which no outward symptoms

and signs are present, and *active,* when people become ill with coughs, fevers, and night sweats. To determine whether a person has latent TB, doctors use skin tests, chest X rays, and cultures of sputum. Active TB is diagnosed with a chest X ray.

Millions of people in North America are infected with the latent form but have no sign of the disease. Their immune systems control the latent infection, so that they have only a 1 in 10 lifetime chance of developing active TB.[82] Physicians don't know what makes TB progress from the latent to active stage, but it may be changes in the immune system that come with age and existing diseases such as HIV.

11.21

Chapter 26
The Immune
System and
Infectious
Diseases

The good news is that the common, latent form of tuberculosis, if detected early, can nearly always be cured, unless the person has a drug-resistant strain of the disease. Drug therapy must continue for at least 6 months and may mean taking several drugs daily. A difficulty, however, is that patients must comply with the prescribed treatment *exactly* as ordered if they are to be cured.[83,84] The bad news is that many of those who do not comply with treatment may become sick again. Some have strains of TB that are *resistant* to most drugs—and they can transmit those strains to others. Some drug-resistant strains can be cured—at a cost of perhaps $250,000 versus $11,000 for a simple TB case—but the process may take much longer.[85-87] As is usually the case, every dollar spent on prevention saves several dollars later in treatment.

In the old days, tuberculosis patients were sent—often against their will—to special hospitals called sanitoriums. The advantage of such a **quarantine,** or state of enforced isolation, was that it prevented the spread of the TB organism to others and ensured that patients followed their prescribed treatment plans. Although most such facilities no longer exist, society may again face the question of whether to detain patients against their wishes in the interests of public health.

Lyme Disease: The Summer Nemesis

Lyme disease is spread by tick bites and can lead to difficulties such as heart problems. The most prominent symptom is a ring-like rash at the site of the bite and flu-like symptoms. Prevention means taking precautions when walking outdoors.

Lyme disease was identified only a few years ago, after a 1975 outbreak in Old Lyme, Connecticut, although the bacteria that causes it (the bacterium *Borrelia burgdorferi*) seems to have been around since 1940 in the United States.[88] **Lyme disease** is spread by deer ticks. (See ● *Figure 26.9.*)The bites may cause extremely serious complications, including joint inflammation, heart problems, severe headaches, and nervous system disorders.[89,90] Two-

thirds of those who have been bitten develop a ring-like rash at the site of the bite about 2 days to a few weeks later. Within 48 hours after infection, most people also experience flu-like symptoms such as fatigue, fever, headache, chills, a stiff neck, and muscle aches. Without treatment, the disease can spread to other organs, eventually leading to memory loss, poor coordination, and an irregular heartbeat. Weeks or even years after the bite, half of untreated patients develop arthritis.

Cases of Lyme disease have been reported in most states, but three parts of the country are hotbeds: the Northeast from Maryland to Massachusetts, especially New York; the Upper Midwest, especially Wisconsin and Minnesota; and Northern California and the Pacific Northwest.[91]

Prevention Fear of Lyme disease might make you want to stay indoors during the time of year when transmission is highest, especially May through July, but the real answer is simply to take precautions. Avoid tick-infested areas, if possible, and be vigilant about walking in tall grass or woods. Wear long-sleeved shirts and

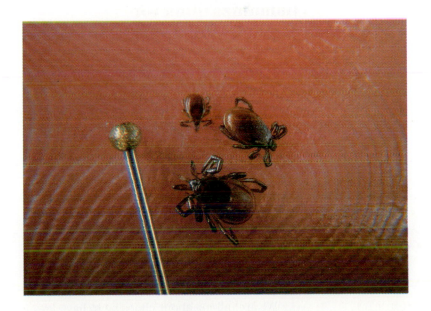

● **Figure 26.9 Lyme disease.** The deer tick that spreads Lyme disease is the size of a poppy seed.

11.22

*Unit 11
Infectious and
Sexually
Transmitted
Diseases*

long pants rather than shorts. Wear light colors, so you can see the ticks, and tuck trousers into socks or cinch them at the ankle. It is also helpful to spray your pant legs and shirt sleeves with tick or insect repellent (preferably containing DEET).[92] When outside during tick season, inspect your body every 3–4 hours. If you find a tick, remove it as soon as possible with tweezers, and save it if possible for professional identification. The greatest risk for infection is when a tick has been attached to the skin for more than 24 hours.[93] Children and furry pets should also be inspected for ticks.

Treatment If you suspect you have been bitten, you should see a health care professional at once. Treatment is with antibiotics, and it is safer and more cost-effective to begin treatment immediately rather than waiting for signs or symptoms.[94] When administered early, antibiotics can cure virtually all cases. Later, however, treatment is more difficult. Medical researchers have been working to come up with a vaccine that protects against Lyme disease.[95]

Strategy for Living: Immunizations for Staying Well

A vaccine is a preparation of organisms that helps increase one's immunity to a particular disease. All children ages 2 months to 16 years should have scheduled vaccinations: DPT combination, polio, MMR combination, meningitis, and hepatitis B. Adults, including college students, should also be immunized against specific diseases, depending on need: diphtheria-tetanus booster, MMR, hepatitis B, polio, and influenza and pneumococcal disease.

Our forebears had no choice, many people in developing countries have no choice, but we in North America do—or at least we should.

We are talking about choosing to have immunizations or vaccinations, the injection of laboratory-prepared organisms into the body to increase one's immunity to a particular disease. The first **vaccine**—the preparation of organisms—was the virus of cowpox, used to produce immunity to smallpox. So successful has

the immunization campaign been that *smallpox,* a once-dreaded disease that killed millions of people, was wiped out in 1977. Indeed, in 1990 the United States and what was then the Soviet Union agreed to discuss destroying stores containing the last live smallpox viruses, which for several years had been held under tight security.[96]

Both children and adults should receive immunizations. Vaccines needed during adulthood include "booster" shots or revaccinations for many common infectious diseases and vaccines for diseases specific to countries to which a person may be traveling.

Immunizations for Children All children from ages 2 months to 16 years should have vaccinations, on a scheduled basis, that include the following immunizations: *diphtheria-tetanus-pertussis (DPT) combination, polio, measles-mumps-rubella (MMR) combination, meningitis,* and *hepatitis B.* (*See* ● *Table 26.1.*)

Unfortunately, there is no legal mechanism in the U.S. to ensure that children under age 5 have had vaccinations. Children must be immunized before entering school, but that is the earliest it is required. As a result, there is better health protection for children under 5 in Algeria, El Salvador, and Uganda than for children in New York City (where only 40% have their recommended series of vaccinations by age 2).[97] A principal reason for immunization deficiencies in the American population is the 25% cut made in 1983 in public health programs. As a result of the failure to immunize children before age 2, there was a national measles epidemic in 1990, during which 27,672 people contracted measles and 89 died.[98,99]

The major kinds of vaccinations that should be given to children are as follows. The schedule of immunizations may vary slightly according to the recommendation of a child's pediatrician.

- *DPT—diphtheria-pertussis-tetanus:* This shot, which should be given six times in a child's life, protects against three diseases:

    (1) *Diphtheria,* an infection involving the membranes of the mouth and throat, is a rare but dangerous disease that can result in death from an obstructed windpipe or heart failure.

11.23

Chapter 26
The Immune
System and
Infectious
Diseases

● **Table 26.1 Childhood immunization schedule.** DPT is combined vaccination for diphtheria-pertussis-tetanus; MMR is combined vaccination for measles-mumps-rubella.

Immunization	2 mos.	4 mos.	6 mos.	12 mos.	15 mos.	15–18 mos.	4–6 yrs.	11–12 yrs.	14–16 yrs.
DPT	●	●	●			●	●		●
Polio	●	●				●	●		
MMR					●		●[1]	●[1]	
Meningitis or HIB influenza	●	●	●	●		●			
Hepatitis B	●								
Cholera, typhoid fever, yellow fever	If possibility of being exposed								

[1]Advisory groups differ on whether final MMR shot should be given at 4–6 years or 11–12 years; parents should consult their pediatrician.

Sources: Combined recommendations from the American Academy of Pediatrics and the Advisory Committee on Immunization Practices.

(2) *Pertussis* (whooping cough) is a bacterial infection that can develop into pneumonia, with possibly fatal results. Concern that the pertussis vaccination itself might lead to brain damage and death seems to have been allayed.[100–102]

(3) *Tetanus*, called "lockjaw" because one symptom is a painful stiffening of the jaw, can produce difficulty breathing and death. It is transmitted by puncture wounds, such as stepping on a nail, and by contamination with soil, dust, or feces that contain the causative organism.

● *Polio:* Immunizations and booster shots for *polio* (short for *poliomyelitis*) should be given at four separate intervals for infants and young children. Often they coincide with the schedule for DPT vaccinations, depending on the pediatrician.

After three decades of a program of vaccination, polio has almost disappeared in the United States. One complication is that some of today's adults who overcame the disease as children have found themselves weakened by a condition called *post-polio syndrome*, which has put them back on crutches.[103,104] Symptoms include fatigue, weakness, joint and back pain, and intolerance to cold.[105,106]

● *MMR—measles-mumps-rubella:* This immunization, given once at 15 months and again later in childhood, is intended to prevent three diseases:

(1) *Measles* produces a rash on the face and body, eye inflammation, high fever, runny nose, cough, and fatigue, and serious cases may produce ear infections and pneumonia. One in 1000 cases produces *encephalitis*, an inflammation of the brain that can produce neurological disorders, mental retardation, or even death. As mentioned, the reduction in MMR vaccinations produced an epidemic in the United States in 1990.

(2) *Mumps* is generally a mild though uncomfortable disease in childhood, although in some cases it can produce deafness in one ear and other complications.[107]

11.24

Unit 11
Infectious and
Sexually
Transmitted
Diseases

(3) *Rubella* is also known as German measles, because it is a measles-like disease. Rubella can be devastating for the unborn.[108]

- *Meningitis or HIB:* The vaccine to immunize infants against bacterial *meningitis* is so effective that the potentially lethal illness is being virtually eliminated, according to one study.[109] Meningitis is an acute and sometimes deadly infection of the lining of the brain and spinal cord. Before the vaccine, it struck up to 15,000 young children in the United States a year and killed 5–10% of its victims.

● Table 26.2 Adult vaccination schedule

Immunization	How often to get it
Diphtheria-tetanus	If received no DPT shots as a child, should have series of 3 shots (second one 4–6 weeks after first, third one 6–12 months after second)
Diphtheria-tetanus booster	If did receive DPT shots as a child, should have booster shot once every 10 years
MMR—measles-mumps-rubella	Recommended for college students, health care workers, and travelers born after 1956 or anyone born after that year and not diagnosed with having had those diseases. (People born before 1957 are considered immune.)
Hepatitis B	Recommended for all health care workers, sexual partners of homosexual and bisexual men, heterosexuals who have multiple partners or whose sex partner does, hemophiliacs, and IV drug users; series of 3 shots anytime (second one 4 weeks after first, third one 5 months after second).
Polio	Booster shot recommended for travelers to less-developed countries before traveling.
Influenza and pneumococcal disease	Recommended for people 65 and older, anyone with chronic illness (heart or lung problems), or in contact with high-risk individuals. Influenza shot once a year before the flu season. Pneumococcal disease shot once or twice (second one at least 6 years after first).
Tuberculosis	Recommended for those exposed to active tuberculosis

Sources: Adapted from: Anonymous. (1992). Immunization: Important for adults, too! *Patient Care, 26* (15), 124–129; Weinstock, C. (1992, January/February). Revaccinating adults. *American Health*, p. 15.

The bacterium that can cause meningitis in children (called *Haemophilus influenzae* type B) is abbreviated as HIB. *HIB* diseases include not only meningitis but also other invasive childhood diseases such as pneumonia, arthritis, inflammations of the bone marrow and the membrane around the heart, and infection of tissue in the throat that can end in suffocation. The vaccine used to resist these diseases is known as the HIB vaccine.

We described the effects of, and vaccines for, hepatitis B and influenza in the sections about those diseases.

Immunizations for Adults, Including College Students Maybe you think you had all the vaccinations you needed as a child, or maybe you've simply "outgrown" those childhood diseases. Even adults, however, need to be immunized for some things, particularly since many of your childhood immunizations cannot confer lifetime immunity. (*See* ● *Table 26.2.*) Unfortunately, some of those so-called childhood diseases can be serious, even fatal, to adults. If, for instance, you are a parent and your child catches measles, you can catch the disease yourself. Indeed, measles is a serious health threat to college students.[110,111]

Even if you were vaccinated as a child, you may need to be *revaccinated,* particularly if you are planning to travel to less-developed countries and if you were born after 1956, one study suggests.[112] Here are some recommendations to consider:

- *Diphtheria-tetanus booster:* All college students and adults should have one of these every 10 years. Diphtheria can produce death from an obstructed windpipe or heart failure. Tetanus produces difficulty breathing and death.

- *MMR—measles-mumps-rubella:* All college students and adults (especially health care workers and travelers to undeveloped countries) born after 1956 should talk to a health care professional about having one of these immunizations, which can be done any time. This is particularly recommended for anyone born after 1956 who has never had measles, mumps, or rubella (German measles) who has not been vaccinated with

11.25

Chapter 26
The Immune
System and
Infectious
Diseases

live measles vaccine. Measles and rubella are particularly dangerous to women of child-bearing age.[113,114]

(1) *Measles* in adults can cause severe pneumonia, ear infections, and encephalitis, and death occasionally occurs. Measles also can cause a pregnant woman to deliver a stillborn child.[115]

(2) *Mumps* in adults can cause inflammation in the testicles and sometimes may cause sterility or meningitis.[116]

(3) *Rubella* (German measles) during pregnancy can cause miscarriage, stillbirth, or birth defects ranging from deafness to congenital heart disease.[117] All women of childbearing age are particularly urged to be vaccinated against rubella, which is increasing steadily in the United States.

- *Hepatitis B:* All health care workers, people living with someone with the disease, sexual partners of homosexual and bisexual men, heterosexuals with multiple partners (or a partner with multiple partners), hemophiliacs, and intravenous drug users should take the three-shot series of vaccinations at any time.

- *Polio:* Travelers to less developed countries should get a polio booster shot.

- *Influenza and pneumococcal disease:* People 65 or older, anyone with chronic illness (especially heart or lung problems), or in contact with such high-risk individuals should be vaccinated each year before the flu season for influenza or vaccinated any time against bacterial pneumonia.

- *Tuberculosis:* The homeless, poor, drug-addicted, or HIV-infected should be vaccinated, as should anyone coming into contact with such individuals.

Rabies is passed along to humans bitten by (or exposed to the saliva of) infected raccoons, opossums, foxes, bats, or dogs and cats. Rabies is still rare among humans, with only 16 cases being reported in the United States in the years 1980–1991.[118] In 1990, there was a rise in animal cases in the New York–New Jersey area.[119] Several hundred people in those two states underwent the series of five inoculations necessary to halt the disease, which otherwise invariably leads to death from attacks on the brain and nervous system. Pet owners were urged to have their pets vaccinated.

In less developed countries, travelers may be exposed to cholera, yellow fever, and typhoid fever. Thus, vaccinations are recommended before travel to those regions.

800-HELP

Acne Helpline. 800-222-SKIN (in California, 800-221-SKIN)

Allergy Information Hot Line. 800-727-5400. Sponsored by Allerest, this hotline offers a free allergy calendar

Asthma and Allergy Foundation of America. 800-7-ASTHMA

Lungline. 800-222-LUNG (in Colorado, 303-355-LUNG). National Asthma Center

Myasthemia Gravia Foundation. 800-541-5454

Suggestions for Further Reading

Kunz, Jeffrey R. M., and Finkel, Asher J. (1987). *The American Medical Association family medical guide, revised and updated.* New York: Random House. Describes 650 illnesses, with flowcharts that lead the reader through self-diagnosis.

Mayo Clinic family health book. (1990). New York: William Morrow. In-depth descriptions of medical conditions, including symptoms and treatments.

11.26

*Unit 11
Infectious and
Sexually
Transmitted
Diseases*

27 Sexually Transmitted Diseases

▶ Discuss fully the causes, diagnosis, treatment, and prevention of HIV and AIDS.

▶ Explain the two types of herpes simplex virus.

▶ Describe the human papilloma virus.

▶ Discuss chlamydia, gonorrhea, and syphilis.

▶ Explain parasite infections and infections of the urinary and reproduction systems.

▶ Describe how to avoid acquiring sexually transmitted diseases.

It came seemingly out of nowhere, around 1981 in the United States, a baffling disease bringing sickness and death, at that time principally to male homosexuals and intravenous drug users. At first it had no name, then several names, and finally an international committee gave it an appellation that became famous worldwide: *AIDS*.[120]

More than any other sexual type of disease, AIDS changed human behavior, making people more cautious about sexual relations than they were in previous times. However, AIDS is only one of over 20 **sexually transmitted diseases (STDs),** infectious diseases formerly called *venereal diseases* that are usually transmitted by sexual contact. Although AIDS is the most lethal, STDs as a whole are growing rapidly and may double by the end of the century, bringing considerable suffering and anguish.

HIV and AIDS: The Modern Scourge

HIV (human immunodeficiency virus) may progress over about 10 years through

● **Figure 27.1 The age of AIDS**

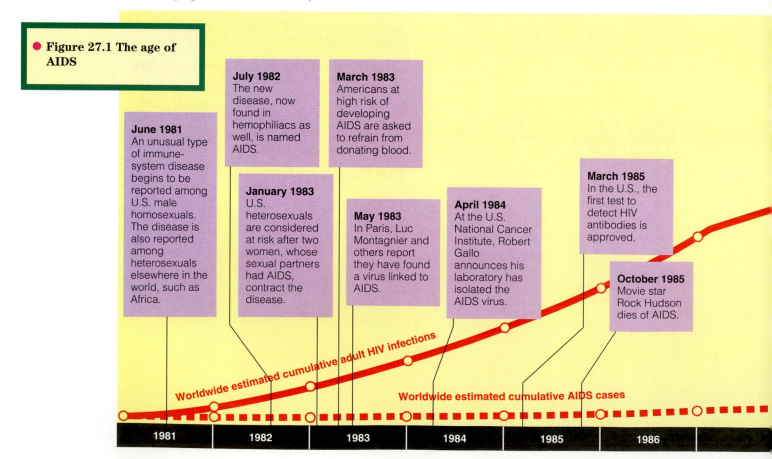

June 1981
An unusual type of immune-system disease begins to be reported among U.S. male homosexuals. The disease is also reported among heterosexuals elsewhere in the world, such as Africa.

July 1982
The new disease, now found in hemophiliacs as well, is named AIDS.

March 1983
Americans at high risk of developing AIDS are asked to refrain from donating blood.

January 1983
U.S. heterosexuals are considered at risk after two women, whose sexual partners had AIDS, contract the disease.

May 1983
In Paris, Luc Montagnier and others report they have found a virus linked to AIDS.

April 1984
At the U.S. National Cancer Institute, Robert Gallo announces his laboratory has isolated the AIDS virus.

March 1985
In the U.S., the first test to detect HIV antibodies is approved.

October 1985
Movie star Rock Hudson dies of AIDS.

Worldwide estimated cumulative adult HIV infections

Worldwide estimated cumulative AIDS cases

1981   1982   1983   1984   1985   1986

four stages into AIDS (acquired immune deficiency syndrome). HIV is diagnosed through an antibody test, but the test cannot predict if the virus will become AIDS. A few drugs are available to extend lives, but none kill the virus or cure the disease. HIV may infect both sexes and is principally transmitted by unprotected sex and by shared drug needles.

AIDS stands for **acquired immune deficiency syndrome,** a sexually transmitted disease that is caused by a virus, HIV. AIDS is characterized by irreversible damage to the body's immune system. **HIV,** or **human immunodeficiency virus,** the virus causing AIDS, brings about a variety of ills, including the breakdown of the immune system, which leads to the development of certain infections and cancers. Two variants of the virus are *HIV-1,* which causes most of the AIDS cases in the United States, and *HIV-2,* which is the dominant strain in Africa and cases of which are now

showing up in the U.S. Because AIDS is relatively new, there are all kinds of fears and misunderstandings about it. Since it is a life-and-death matter, however, it's important to have *accurate knowledge* about it. The accompanying Self Discovery will help you determine what you know. (*See Self Discovery 27.1.*)

In the years since 1981, when the first gay man walked into San Francisco General Hospital with a mysterious immune disorder, HIV has raged across the United States, now affecting about 1 million Americans, about a fifth of whom have developed AIDS.[121] (*See ● Figure 27.1.*) In the early years, the epidemic in the United States

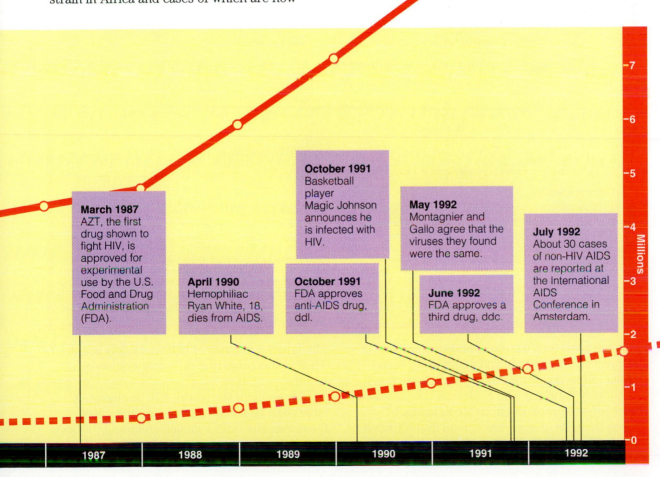

Year 2000 estimate: 30 million to 40 million worldwide

1992 12 million to 14 million worldwide

March 1987 AZT, the first drug shown to fight HIV, is approved for experimental use by the U.S. Food and Drug Administration (FDA).

April 1990 Hemophiliac Ryan White, 18, dies from AIDS.

October 1991 FDA approves anti-AIDS drug, ddI.

October 1991 Basketball player Magic Johnson announces he is infected with HIV.

May 1992 Montagnier and Gallo agree that the viruses they found were the same.

June 1992 FDA approves a third drug, ddc.

July 1992 About 30 cases of non-HIV AIDS are reported at the International AIDS Conference in Amsterdam.

Millions

7
6
5
4
3
2
1
0

1987 1988 1989 1990 1991 1992

11.28

*Unit 11
Infectious and
Sexually
Transmitted
Diseases*

SELF DISCOVERY 27.1

What Do You Know About HIV and AIDS?

Answer true or false to each of the following statements:

	True	False
1. There is no known cure for AIDS.	____	____
2. AIDS is caused by inheriting faulty genes.	____	____
3. AIDS is caused by bacteria.	____	____
4. A person can "carry" and transmit the organism that causes AIDS without showing symptoms of the disease or appearing ill.	____	____
5. The organism that causes AIDS can be transmitted through semen.	____	____
6. Urinating after sexual intercourse makes infection with AIDS less likely.	____	____
7. Washing your genitals after sex makes infection with AIDS less likely.	____	____
8. Sharing drug needles increases the chance of transmitting the organism that causes AIDS.	____	____
9. The organism that causes AIDS can be transmitted through blood or blood products.	____	____
10. Donating blood makes it more likely you will be exposed to HIV.	____	____
11. You can catch AIDS like you catch a cold because whatever causes AIDS can be carried in the air.	____	____
12. You can get AIDS by being in the same classroom as someone who has AIDS.	____	____
13. You can get AIDS by shaking hands with someone who has AIDS.	____	____
14. A pregnant woman who has HIV can give AIDS to her baby.	____	____
15. Having a steady relationship with just one sex partner decreases the risk of getting AIDS.	____	____
16. Using condoms reduces the risk of getting AIDS.	____	____
17. A test to determine whether a person who has been exposed to HIV is available.	____	____
18. A vaccine that protects people from getting AIDS is now available.	____	____

Correct Answers

1. True	4. True	7. False	10. False	13. False	16. True
2. False	5. True	8. True	11. False	14. True	17. True
3. False	6. False	9. True	12. False	15. True	18. False

Sources: Anderson, D. M., & Christenson, G. M. (1991). Ethnic breakdown of AIDS related knowledge and attitudes from the National Adolescent Student Health Survey. *Journal of Health Education, 22,* 30–34; Timoshok, L., Sweet, D. M., & Zich, J. (1987). A three city comparison of the public's knowledge and attitudes about AIDS. *Psychology & Health, 1*(1), 43–60; Weiten, W., Lloyd, M. A., & Lashley, R. L. (1991). *Psychology applied to modern life: Adjustment in the 90s* (3rd ed.). Pacific Grove, CA: Brooks/Cole, p. 408.

was primarily an affliction of homosexual men, intravenous drug users, and people with hemophilia (a blood clotting defect) and others (such as surgery patients) who contracted the disease from infected products from blood banks.[122] Since then, the disease has spread in the United States along with epidemics of drug use and of sexually transmitted diseases such as syphilis.

The number of cases of heterosexually acquired AIDS in this country is now doubling every 15 months.[123]

Throughout the world, HIV has infected more than 10 million adults—perhaps 40% of them women—and 1 million children.[124] (*See* ● *Figure 27.2.*) About 2.5 million are already dead of AIDS. An estimated 40 million people

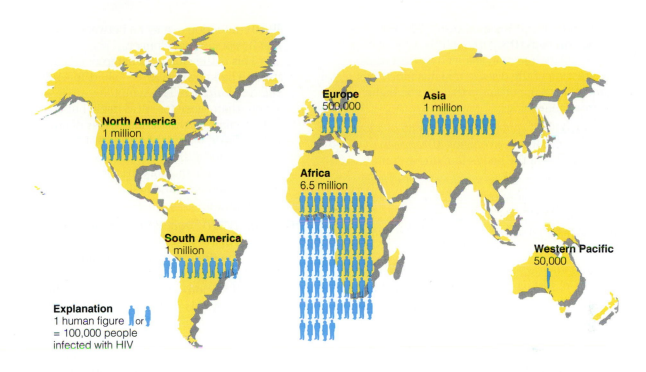

North America
1 million

Europe
500,000

Asia
1 million

Africa
6.5 million

South America
1 million

Western Pacific
50,000

Explanation
1 human figure ▌ or ▐
= 100,000 people
infected with HIV

● **Figure 27.2 HIV, the global epidemic.** Estimated number of people infected with HIV.

will be infected with HIV by the end of the century.[125] One reason for the spread of the disease, as one commentator pointed out, is that "Never before in history have so many people travelled to so many faraway places so frequently as today. . . . HIV may be the first virus to take advantage of this uniquely modern opportunity. . . ."[126]

Who Has AIDS: The Politics of Definition

Who has AIDS? For a long time, people weren't considered to have AIDS until they showed symptoms of any of 23 indicator diseases delineated by the federal Centers for Disease Control and Prevention (CDC); this list included a rare pneumonia, specific cancers, and other infections. However, the definition became a political as much as a medical question in part because in the United States and Europe, for instance, the definition influences a person's ability to get care. This previous AIDS definition was based on symptoms first found in homosexual men,

but women were found to have different symptoms throughout the course of the illness.

After hearing complaints that many ill people were being excluded from the count of AIDS casualties, in 1993 the CDC revised the definition. AIDS now includes HIV-infected people whose level of the body's master immune cells —called **T4 helper cells** or **CD4 cells** (or CD4 positive lymphocytes)—falls to 200 per cubic millimeter, or one-fifth that of a normal person. A T4-cell count is an important measure of immune-system strength, with the normal level being around 1000.[127]

In addition, the CDC's new definition of AIDS also includes pulmonary tuberculosis, recurrent bacterial pneumonia, and invasive cervical cancer—diseases that are fatal to women infected with HIV. Adding such disorders to the official definition of HIV, AIDs activists say, is a red flag to physicians that women with these symptoms—which are also found in other diseases—should be tested for AIDS.[128]

11.30

*Unit 11
Infectious and
Sexually
Transmitted
Diseases*

The Four-Stage Progression of HIV: From Infection to AIDS Although the official definition of HIV infection changed in 1993, the progression of the disease remains much the same. What's important is that you be highly aware of four things:

1. AIDS itself comes only at the end of a long, slow collapse—averaging 10 years in adults—of the body's immune system.[129]

2. Often there are *no symptoms of illness* during the development of the disease, which means for perhaps 7–9 years.

3. So far *no one has ever recovered from AIDS.*

4. *Not everyone who is exposed to HIV gets AIDS,* just as not everyone exposed to the polio virus develops paralysis.

There are four stages of development of HIV-related problems:

- *Group I HIV infection, starting in the first 1–8 weeks—short-term illness may develop:* The time from the virus entering the body until the occurrence of a short-term illness—known as group I HIV infection—ranges from 1 to 8 weeks. Many people show no symptoms, but some show signs similar to mononucleosis—fatigue, fever, swollen lymph nodes, and possibly a rash—signs that most people may simply ignore. These initial symptoms disappear in a few weeks, and most people continue to feel normal, although some may complain of chronically swollen lymph nodes.

- *Group II HIV infection, starting 6 weeks to a year or more after transmission— no symptoms, diagnosis requires antibody test:* The time from the virus entering the body until the person tests positive on an HIV antibody test—known as group II HIV infection—may occur within 6 weeks of transmission, but it can also be a year or more. During this period, people with HIV often show no symptoms and feel fine. The HIV antibody test is a standard blood test that tests for antibodies to HIV, not the virus itself.

- *Group III HIV infection, starting 1 week to 2 years or so after transmission—enlarged lymph nodes:* The time from the virus entering the body until the occurrence of new symptoms—known as group III HIV infection—may be between 1 week and 2 years or even longer.

This is the cluster of symptoms that used to be known as *ARC*—short for *AIDS-related complex.* The symptoms are less severe than those for AIDS itself, but consist of enlarged lymph nodes, loss of appetite, fever, lethargy, night sweats, diarrhea, and rashes. Later there may be slurred speech, memory loss, loss of feeling in hands and feet, and mental deterioration.[130]

- *Group IV HIV infection, starting 6 months to 10 years after transmission— AIDS:* The time from the virus entering the body until the AIDS disease occurs—group IV HIV infection—ranges from 6 months to 10 years. By this point, the T4-cell count has dropped from 1000 per cubic millimeter of blood (normal) to 200. The AIDS patient experiences rapid swelling of the lymph glands, weight loss, diarrhea, fatigue, headaches, fever, shortness of breath, dry cough, white coating on the tongue, and reddish-purplish bumps on the skin.

As the HIV gradually weakens the body's immune system, other infections— called "opportunistic infections," diseases the body would normally repel—and cancer may invade the body. The principal infectious disease is a type of pneumonia caused by the *Pneumocystis carinii* organism. The principal cancer is **Kaposi's sarcoma,** a cancer of the connective tissues that may occur on the skin or in the mouth.

As the immune system continues to deteriorate, other opportunistic infections may occur, attacking the brain, nervous system, liver, bones, and skin.

The estimated average time from the time of HIV infection to first symptom is approximately 5 years and to AIDS approximately 10 years. Very few patients are diagnosed with AIDS the first 2 years after infection, but after that the risk seems to be 5–10% per year, although the use of anti-HIV medication might alter that.[131]

Although there do seem to be survivors of HIV infection, no one has survived AIDS itself. It is not known why some people infected with the virus develop AIDS while others do not.

Is There a "Mystery Virus"? Journalists at a 1992 international AIDS conference in Amsterdam seized on medical reports about 30 patients from widely scattered geographic areas who showed unexplained T4-cell depletion without evidence of HIV infection. Over half the cases had no apparent risk factors for acquiring HIV. The medical consensus is that the virus is unlikely to be an infectious agent and poses no general threat to the public health, though it still remains a mystery. One reporter dubbed it MTV for "media transforming virus," after the alacrity with which journalists embraced it.[132]

Diagnosing HIV: The Antibody Test As mentioned, the *HIV antibody test* is a standard blood test for HIV. Actually, the test does not detect the virus itself but rather the antibodies that the body forms in response to the appearance of the virus. **Antibodies** are blood proteins that are secreted into the bloodstream, where they bind to the invading virus, incapacitating it.

Two principal blood tests are used in sequence to detect HIV infection. The first one is the *EIA* or *ELISA*—short for the *enzyme immunoassay* and the *enzyme-linked immunosorbant assay,* respectively. Because the ELISA may produce a positive result that is actually false—that is, the test may erroneously suggest HIV antibodies are present—it is followed by the more expensive but more accurate *Western blot* test. *Negative* test results *can* mean positive news: the HIV may not be present. *Positive* test results *can* mean negative news: the HIV may be present. Still, anyone taking these tests needs to be aware of certain cautions:

- *Antibodies to the virus may not develop immediately:* If the test results are negative, it may mean the body has not been exposed to HIV. But it may also mean that antibody formation has not yet taken place. The time it takes for most people to develop antibodies is about 2–12 weeks, though this can be quite variable. Some people do not develop antibodies until 6–12 months after exposure to the organism. (Meanwhile the person may be infected and continue to infect others.)

- *Be aware that testing labs can make errors:* If performed correctly, the tests themselves can be highly accurate, detecting antibodies in 99.6% of HIV-infected people. The problem is that some medical labs have problems with high error rates in their testing.[133]

- *Tests cannot predict AIDS:* Currently, tests can indicate HIV infection. They cannot predict whether that HIV will develop into AIDS.

Treating HIV and AIDS In the absence of treatment, the path from HIV infection to AIDS is usually about 8 years. If the HIV virus is detected, and the T4-cell count is found to have dropped to 500 per cubic millimeter of blood, half of normal, treatment with antiviral drugs is recommended, even if no signs or symptoms are apparent. Unfortunately, viruses in general are more difficult to treat with drugs than bacteria are, and HIV has turned out to be a very difficult virus to treat.

At present only three drugs are approved by the Food and Drug Administration (FDA) for treatment of HIV in the United States—AZT, ddI, and ddC:

- *AZT:* First approved in 1987, AZT (azidothymidine or zidovudine) extends life an average of 18 months by postponing some of the symptoms of AIDS. Eventually, however, HIV mutates into a form that is less vulnerable to AZT, and the drug's side effects of anemia and bone-marrow damage force patients to stop using it.[134]

- *ddI:* Approved by the FDA in October 1991, ddI (didanosine) works like AZT, but causes less viral resistance. The drug helps to protect uninfected cells, but does not destroy the virus in already-infected cells.[135]

- *ddC:* ddC (dideoxycytidine) is the same type of drug as AZT and ddI, but has less severe side effects. Before being approved by the FDA in June 1992, it was widely used in the AIDS underground, where buyers clubs smuggled the drug into the United States from other countries.

AZT, ddI, and ddC are similar drugs and are likely to work best in combination. Although they do not rid the body of the virus and have limited effectiveness, they are thought to

11.32

Unit 11
Infectious and
Sexually
Transmitted
Diseases

extend lives of some patients by 1–3 years. Another drug-treatment candidate is d4T, which may have fewer side effects than other AIDS drugs.

Drug researchers have developed a number of other compounds that were first thought to be promising, but all have been rejected as being ineffective or potentially toxic. Experimenters continue to push forward at top speed, but they warn that it may be years before any breakthrough is forthcoming and that nations must prepare to care for millions of sick people who cannot be saved by drugs.[136]

If the achievement of truly effective HIV or AIDS drugs seems elusive, what about preventive vaccines? Some laboratory research with monkeys and chimpanzees suggests that a vaccine is possible, and at least 13 vaccines are under study. Still, that could leave 5 years for development and another 5 years for testing and regulatory work—a decade in which many people would die.[137,138]

Interestingly, one nonpharmaceutical method that may lengthen the lives of people with HIV infection is something that anyone can do without a doctor's prescription: relaxation and aerobic exercise. One study found that such activities apparently enhanced the strength of the immune system and slowed the progress of HIV.[139,140]

Who Gets HIV/AIDS and How In the technological and pharmaceutical age in which people in North America live, we have come to expect that disease will be prevented or treated by means of drugs and high-tech medicine. In fact, however, most of the improvements in the last 40 years in physical health—in all aspects— have taken place because of *changes in lifestyle*. This particularly applies to preventing the spread of HIV and AIDS. Today an estimated 1 million living Americans carry HIV, a tragedy that will play itself out over the next 20 years or more, spreading to more and more people.

In the United States, AIDS was initially discovered among gays and intravenous drug users, although it was already well established in Africa as a heterosexually transmitted disease. However, if there is one thing this disease has taught us is that the past may not be a guide to the future. In 1992, the predominant number of reported U.S. AIDS cases were transmitted by male homosexual sex (58%), followed next by those transmitted by intravenous drug use (23%), with a small percentage of men (6%) falling into both categories. Heterosexual sex, as a means of transmission, was only 6%. (*See* ● *Figure 27.3.*)

However, the sources of transmission of the disease may well be changing. Let's consider the major sources of *heterosexual sex, male homosexual sex, intravenous drug use, blood transfusions and blood products, from mothers to infants,* and *accidental contacts:*

- *Heterosexual sex—HIV risk is rising:* Basketball player and sports hero Magic Johnson called attention to the dangers of unprotected heterosexual sex with multiple partners when in November 1991 he announced he was infected with HIV.[141] So did a lesser-known figure, Alison Gertz, a New Yorker who at 22 was beginning a career as an illustrator. In 1988 she began suffering puzzling symptoms that were diagnosed as AIDS. The source of the disease was traced to an old friend with whom she spent *one* romantic evening 6 years earlier, when she was 16. He, it turned out, was bisexual and had since died of AIDS. Ms. Gertz herself died in August 1992 at the age of 26, after becoming an AIDS crusader who publicized her story as a warning to heterosexuals, women, and teenagers.[142]

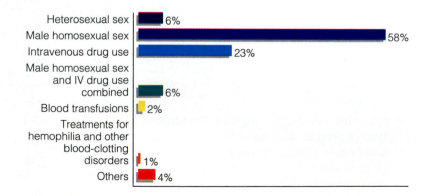

Heterosexual sex	6%
Male homosexual sex	58%
Intravenous drug use	23%
Male homosexual sex and IV drug use combined	6%
Blood transfusions	2%
Treatments for hemophilia and other blood-clotting disorders	1%
Others	4%

● **Figure 27.3 Where AIDS comes from.** Reported U.S. AIDS cases by type of transmission.

There is some evidence that *men are more efficient at infecting women than women are at infecting men.*[143] Studies seem to show that increasingly women are becoming HIV-infected through unprotected sex with bisexual men or male intravenous drug users.[144] Indeed, women are the fastest-growing category of people affected by the epidemic, particularly women of color.[145]

In contrast with the pattern in North America, HIV and AIDS in Africa are spreading mainly through heterosexual intercourse, striking men and women alike.[146] Indeed, heterosexual sex is thought to account for more than 80% of the adult cases of AIDS in Africa.[147]

- *Male homosexual sex:* By December 1991, according to the Centers for Disease Control, there were 206,392 men and women with AIDS in the United States. Most cases (59%) occurred among homosexual or bisexual men.[148] Although HIV is no longer spreading explosively among gay men as it was in the late 1970s and 1980s, infecting many before they knew it existed, AIDS is still the second leading cause of death for men ages 25–44 in the United States.[149] As we shall discuss, part of the reason for the epidemic among men is that men are more apt to engage in risk-taking behavior.[150]

- *Intravenous drug use:* HIV infection has dropped in Canada, where clean needles have been distributed free to drug addicts in large cities. For instance, in Toronto, which began a clean-needles program in 1989, a study found a 17% drop in the number of people testing HIV-positive, compared to a year earlier.[151,152]

In the United States, needle-swapping programs for intravenous drug users such as heroin users, in which clean needles are exchanged for used ones, were resisted for years on the grounds that free needles would increase drug use. The Canadian experience, however, found that there was no such increase in drug abuse: participants are almost always long-term abusers, not new recruits. A similar clean-needle program in New Haven, Connecticut, was found to reduce new HIV infections by 33%,

also with no increase in drug users.[153] As one female New Haven addict, 45, who works as an executive assistant, said, "Just because I shoot drugs doesn't mean I don't care about AIDS. I care a lot."[154]

Today there are numerous cities with needle-exchange programs, ranging from legal efforts in Seattle, Honolulu, and Boulder, Colorado, to underground (illegal) programs in San Francisco, Baltimore, Boston, Philadelphia, Chicago, and New York.[155]

- *Blood transfusions and blood products:* The Centers for Disease Control and Prevention in 1991 reported that 2.2% of the AIDS cases in the United States came from blood transfusions. Another 0.8% of the cases were found in the nation's 25,000 **hemophiliacs.** Hemophiliacs are people (nearly all males) with a blood defect characterized by delayed clotting of the blood, causing difficulty in controlling hemorrhage after even minor injuries. Hemophiliacs require the administration several times a week of a blood-clotting substance (Factor VIII) made from donated blood. HIV has infected almost every hemophiliac born before 1985, the year all blood donations and products were screened for HIV antibodies.[156]

Though not risk-free, the U.S. blood supply is now safer than ever, as a result of new HIV-screen policies by the Red Cross and other blood banks. The odds of getting infected from a transfusion are said to be extremely low—perhaps 1 in 60,000 units.[157,158]

Still, people who are heading into surgery and are worried about getting a transfusion from an unknown donor may arrange to donate their own blood prior to the operation or seek out a friend or family member whose health history and lifestyle are familiar to them. They may also have their own blood recycled during surgery, through the use of an **autotransfusion machine.**

Experts say the chances of getting HIV from an organ or tissue transplant are minimal because potential organ donors are screened for the virus.[159]

- *From mothers to infants:* Mothers who are HIV-infected may transmit the disease

11.34

*Unit 11
Infectious and
Sexually
Transmitted
Diseases*

to their young in several ways: during pregnancy, labor and delivery, and breast-feeding. Unfortunately, many women are unaware that they are infected with HIV until they give birth and their babies later develop AIDS.[160–162]

- *Accidental contacts:* HIV is not contracted by casual contact, as many people once believed.[163] You won't get it from being on a crowded bus or in a swimming pool, from a toilet seat, from mosquitos, or from sharing eating utensils, toothbrushes, razors, or toilets with AIDS patients, according to several studies. HIV survives poorly in saliva and is rarely recovered from the saliva of HIV-infected persons; of 31 persons bitten by AIDS patients, none have turned out to be HIV-positive. The risk of HIV infection from sticking oneself with a needle used on AIDS or HIV-infected persons is low, about 1% or less per stick.

  At one time, people were worried about getting HIV from health care workers, but there seems to be no cause for alarm. The risk of being infected by a doctor, for instance, is considered "so remote that it may never be measured," as former Surgeon General C. Everett Koop put it.[164]

  In addition, even though HIV is rarely transmitted in the workplace, the federal Occupational Safety and Health Administration has issued rules covering use of rubber gloves and protective clothing and housekeeping procedures, which are intended to prevent more than 200 deaths and 9200 blood-borne infections a year—most *not* related to AIDS. The rules are directed not only to health care workers but also to people employed by funeral homes, linen services, and law-enforcement agencies.[165]

The Abuse of Persons with HIV/AIDS You might think having a possibly fatal disease is the worst thing that could happen to you. Unfortunately, it's even harder than that. Those who are HIV-positive face job and housing discrimination, and illegal evictions, despite laws against such practices. They may face criminal charges if they don't inform their sex partners of their HIV status. And, often at an earlier age than most of their peers, they have to seek legal help with wills and similar matters.[166]

In addition, a third of Americans infected with HIV report being physically or verbally abused because of their disease, according to a 1992 survey by the National Association of People with AIDS.[167] Often the violence comes from members of their own families. They also have soaring medical bills that leave about half of them destitute, unable to pay the rent or buy groceries. Many formerly affluent people find themselves poverty-stricken, facing losses and dependencies they never imagined.[168]

Still, living with HIV need not be this grim. Taking aggressive medical action against the virus, sharing feelings with friends or members of an HIV support group, following health-promoting habits to delay the progression of the illness (exercising, avoiding drugs, practicing stress-reducing techniques), and living life to the fullest can make the remaining years more bearable. If you yourself know people with HIV, probably the best thing you can do is to offer them support, to let them know they are not alone.

Strategy for Living: The Relationship Between Gender Roles and HIV Most people become HIV-infected in two ways: (1) from unsafe sexual behavior or (2) from sharing drug needles.

One thing that is important is that both men and women need to think about how they feel about behaviors they consider masculine or feminine and how such behaviors increase their risk of contracting HIV.

- *Men's roles:* What, ask sociologists Michael Kimmel and Martin Levine, is the relationship between AIDS and masculinity? Perhaps, they suggest, many men act in a "real man" kind of role of engaging in high-risk behaviors that ignore health risks.[169] (*See* ● *Figure 27.4.*) Indeed, for a time, and even today, they suggest, many gay men tried to act more like "real men" than even most straight men, wearing leather and short haircuts, and engaging in exciting, quick, and often anonymous sex. Similarly, IV drug users found drug use provided both risk and adventure.

  Recently, the patterns seem to have changed. As we have seen, drug users have eagerly embraced needle-swapping programs. Both gay and straight men are apparently having fewer sexual partners than in previous years and reporting more condom use.[170–172] Even so, many gay men apparently see themselves as less vulnerable to AIDS—a kind of optimism also found among sexually active adolescents.[173]

- *Women's roles:* Women are at risk for HIV, as we have shown, and many may not even know they are at risk. At the end of 1990, half the women with AIDS were found to have contracted it from IV drug use and another 16% from blood transfusions and other categories. A third, however, contracted HIV through heterosexual contacts.[174] Presumably some HIV-positive women became infected from bisexual partners.

In North American culture, it used to be that women traditionally were given responsibility for birth control.[175] This is no longer tolerable. The HIV epidemic now means that *both* men and women must address resistance about the use of condoms and other latex barriers such as dental dams used during oral sex. Thus, it becomes an urgent matter that both women and men learn negotiation and communication skills, assertiveness and refusal skills, and otherwise improve their self-protection with regard to HIV.

Other Sexually Transmitted Diseases

Besides HIV/AIDS, other serious STDs include hepatitis B, herpes, human papilloma virus, chlamydia, gonorrhea, syphilis, and parasite infections.

HIV/AIDS is perhaps the most dangerous and recent of the sexually transmitted diseases, but it is not the only one.

As mentioned in the preceding chapter, **hepatitis B** is also a serious STD, second only to gonorrhea as the most common one in America. Symptoms of the disease, which lasts 2–6 months, include dark urine, muscle and joint aches, and fatigue. Although people often recover on their own, others are treated with a drug called alpha interferon. A vaccine is available that is 80–95% effective.

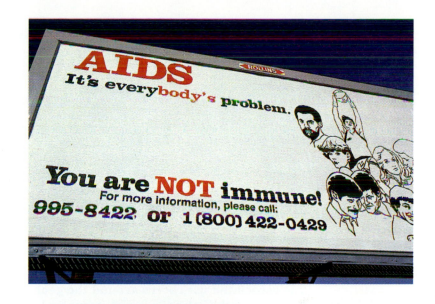

● **Figure 27.4 Is high-risk sex sexy?**

"*How does one get AIDS? Not by being a homosexual or IV drug user, but by engaging in high-risk behaviors that ignore health risks. These behaviors also can confirm masculinity since masculinity typically is associated with risk-taking. Indeed, those whose masculinity is least secure are precisely those most likely to enact hypermasculine behavioral codes. . . .*

To men, . . . that which is safe is not sexy. Sex is about danger, risk, excitement; safety is about comfort, softness, security. Seen this way, it isn't surprising that one-fourth of gay men report they haven't changed unsafe sexual behaviors. What's astonishing is three-fourths are practicing safer sex.

What heterosexual men can learn from the gay community's response to AIDS is how to eroticize responsibility—something women have been trying to teach men for decades."

—Michael Kimmel & Martin Levine. (1991, May 10). AIDS is a disease of men involved in risky behavior. *San Francisco Chronicle*, p. A25.

11.36

*Unit 11
Infectious and
Sexually
Transmitted
Diseases*

The STDs we will describe in the rest of this chapter include:

- Herpes
- Human papilloma virus
- Chlamydia
- Gonorrhea
- Syphilis
- Parasite infections: pubic lice and scabies

Herpes: The Secretive Virus

The STD known as the herpes simplex virus is of two types: type 1 typically causes cold sores around the mouth, type 2 is associated with sores around the genitals, although both types can be acquired through oral-genital sex. The virus never completely disappears and may recur with or without symptoms, often triggered by stress.

A decade ago, genital herpes sent a wave of panic through participants in the the so-called sexual revolution, reports health writer Jane Brody, but now, with all the publicity about AIDS, it is nearly forgotten.[176]

Forgotten, perhaps, but far from gone. Indeed, a great number of people—30 million, or perhaps 16% of all Americans ages 15–74—have been infected with the virus, and perhaps as many as 1 million more join their ranks every year.[177] This is unfortunate, for genital herpes can inflict a great deal of emotional as well as physical suffering.

Herpes is a viral infection that evades the body's immune defenses by hiding in the nervous system until reactivation of the virus occurs. There are six major types of herpes virus that affect humans (varicella-zoster virus, Epstein-Barr virus, cytomegalovirus, human herpes virus 6, and herpes simplex virus types 1 and 2). The *herpes simplex virus, types 1 and 2,* the most common strains of the herpes virus family, are sexually transmitted strains (as is the cytomegalovirus) that produce cold-sore-like blisters in the areas of the genitals and mouth.

Two Types of Herpes Simplex: 1 and 2 Herpes simplex 1 and 2, which are closely related to each other, are associated with STDs. (*See* ● *Figure 27.5.*)

- *Herpes simplex type 1:* **Herpes simplex virus type 1** is extremely common. It has been estimated that 90% of adults have been exposed to this virus. The type 1 virus, which lies dormant in a nerve in the face, typically causes cold sores around the mouth, but it can also cause genital herpes.

- *Herpes simplex type 2:* **Herpes simplex virus type 2,** which lies dormant in a nerve track at the base of the spine, is commonly associated with genital herpes. However, it too can be found in and around the mouth.[178] Generally, this strain recurs more frequently than the type 1—some people experience four or more recurrences a year.

Oral-genital sex makes these distinctions less relevant, however. The type 2 genital virus can be acquired through oral sex with a partner who has a type 1 herpes virus outbreak in or on the mouth.

How It Feels, How It Spreads Many occurrences of herpes of the genitals and lips are so mild they may not be noticed. For those who do have symptoms, two common patterns have been identified that depend on whether it is a primary (first) experience with the virus or a recurrence of the virus.

In both types, the individual may experience numbness, itching, or tingling where contact with the virus occurred, followed by an often painful eruption of water-filled blisters. Within 10 days of an initial exposure to the virus, one may feel flu-like symptoms: fever, chills, nausea, headaches, fatigue, and muscle aches. The eruption crusts and scabs over, and about 2 weeks later the skin appears normal.

After the first episode, the virus seems to disappear. Thereafter it emerges from time to time—sometimes as frequently as four or more times a year. Sometimes it will produce no symptoms. At other times it will produce outbreaks of blistering sores, although the flu-like symptoms do not reappear. As time goes on, many find that the symptoms become shorter-lived and less severe. When the infection is active—that is, any time between the initial itch

and tingle and the appearance of symptoms—
the virus may be spread by skin-to-skin contact.
However, in some men and many women, the
symptoms of infection are so slight that they
easily escape notice.[179] Such women are said to
have *asymptomatic virus shedding*. Thus,
even highly motivated people who avoid sex
during herpes flare-ups face the possibility of
transmitting the disease to their partners.[180] Indeed, even doctors' standard methods of diagnosing genital herpes in women—routine
physicals and patient histories—miss many
cases.[181] If you think you should be screened
for herpes, you should ask for a blood test, although no single lab test can detect all cases.

The Effects of Herpes Among adults, the
principal effects of herpes are sometimes feelings of desperation and social inhibition. At
first, many herpes victims feel isolated and depressed and fear rejection in social situations.
Although the negative effect of herpes on work
and school performance and on nonsexual social pleasures diminishes, it may continue to
cause distress in areas of sexual relations.[182]
One of the best coping mechanisms is to develop a social support system.

Much less well off is the baby born to a
woman who has a herpes infection at the time
of the birth, for the baby is apt to contract the
disease during the birth process.[183] Among the
babies born with the virus, as many as 60%
die. Half of the rest suffer blindness or brain
damage.[184]

Most women with recurrent genital herpes
deliver normal infants. Those who do pass the
herpes simplex virus to their babies usually
have had their first infection during the third
trimester. In addition, women who have asymptomatic herpes simplex shedding virus at the
time of delivery may need to take steps to avoid
passing the disease to the infant. If a pregnant
woman suspects she has herpes, her physician
will probably test for it during the last few
weeks of pregnancy. If the virus is active, the
physician will recommend a cesarean operation
to avoid infecting the baby.[185]

Prevention and Treatment As with AIDS,
the law in many states is clear: those who have
herpes are *legally* obliged to inform their partners about it.

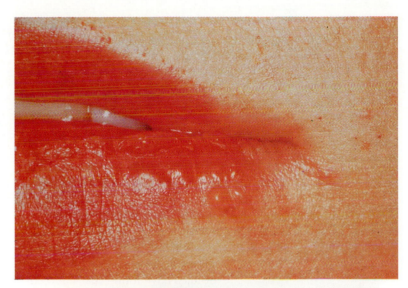

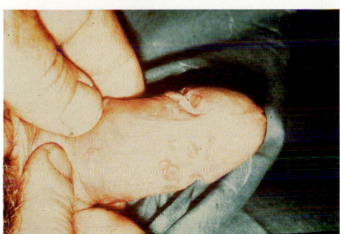

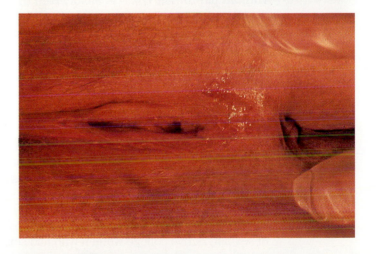

● **Figure 27.5 Herpes simplex.** (*Top*) Fever blister—sore on lower
lip. (*Middle and bottom*) Blisters on male and female genitals.

11.38

*Unit 11
Infectious and
Sexually
Transmitted
Diseases*

People who know they have herpes are advised to abstain from sex until all symptoms have disappeared. At other times, they should use latex condoms with a spermicidal jelly or cream containing nonoxynol-9. They should avoid touching infected areas and should wash their hands with soap and water if they do touch infected areas accidentally. Still, there are no guarantees. People who only have sex when they are free of symptoms and who use condoms may still have some potential to transmit the virus.[186]

There is no cure for herpes. Still, it has been noticed that stress, depression, conflict, and other psychological upsets seem to trigger recurrences among people infected with the virus.[187–189] Studies have found that infected people who have learned relaxation and other coping techniques suffer fewer herpes outbreaks.[190]

In addition, a prescription drug called *acyclovir*, if taken during the initial herpes outbreak, can ease the symptoms, even if it does not destroy the virus. The drug may also be taken regularly (with a break every 6 months) for those suffering frequent outbreaks.

Human Papilloma Virus: The Fastest-Growing STD

Human papilloma virus is associated principally with "genital warts," or fleshy growths in genital and other areas. Sometimes it has no symptoms at all. The disease is dangerous because it may lead to cancer.

What is perhaps the *fastest-growing* STD in the United States? It might be one you've never heard of: **HPV,** short for **human papilloma virus,** which causes genital warts. There are presently an estimated 12–24 million cases of HPV in the United States, with 750,000 new cases being added every year.[191] Indeed, some researchers found that nearly *half* of a sample of sexually active college women who had sexual relations with an average of four partners were HPV positive.[192]

HPV should not be taken lightly. At one time, it was thought that HPV caused only **genital warts**—unpleasant but supposedly harm-

less fleshy growths on a man's penis, scrotum, anus, or **urethra** (the tube from the bladder to the outside), and on a woman's vulva, perineum, cervix, and anus, and warts in areas of the mouth of both sexes.[193] However, some types of HPV have also been associated with cancer: of the anus, penis, vulva, and cervix.[194,195] Unfortunately, HPV may be painless and show no symptoms, both in males and females. Many people with genital warts also have other STDs.

HPV is very contagious, being readily transmitted by sexual contact (including oral-genital sex) and from afflicted women to their newborn babies during passage through the birth canal. On average the incubation period is 2–3 months after contact. Women who have had HPV should get an annual Pap smear, the standard test for cervical cancer. However, the Pap smear will not diagnose a *new* HPV infection; other tests (such as one called the Southern blot technique) are required for this.

Treatment is required not only for the patient but for his or her sexual partner as well, who may otherwise reinfect the patient.[196,197] Genital warts are treated by freezing (cryotherapy), heat (diathermy), cauterization, laser therapy, chemicals, or surgical removal.

Chlamydia: The Most Common STD

Chlamydial infections, perhaps the most common of STDs, often show no symptoms. Three serious complications in women are pelvic inflammatory disease, which can cause infertility; infections of the cervix, also possibly causing infertility; and infections of newborns during childbirth. Two complications in men are epididymitis, which can lead to sterility, and nongonococcal urethritis.

If HPV is the fastest-growing sexually transmitted disease in the United States, chlamydia is perhaps the most common STD, affecting 3–4 million Americans every year, according to the Centers for Disease Control and Prevention.[198] Indeed, a New Orleans study found that about 20% of sexually active adults had the infection, making it more common than gonorrhea or syphilis.[199] Yet, according to one study, most college students have no knowledge of the disease, have several misconceptions about it, don't understand the severity of untreated infection, and cannot distinguish between effective and ineffective means of prevention.[200] No wonder chlamydial infection has been called "the quiet epidemic."[201]

Chlamydia—or more accurately **chlamydial infections**—consists of a family of sexually transmitted diseases caused by a bacterium (*Chlamydia trachomatis*). The disease is usually transmitted by sexual contact, including anal-genital and oral-genital sex.[202] A major problem associated with this STD is that the organism *often does not cause any symptoms*—especially early in the disease and especially in women—yet if untreated it can cause lifelong damage. For example, one consequence is the eye infection trachoma, causing blindness.

Infections in Women and Newborns About 50–70% of infected females show no signs of early symptoms. Those that do show early signs may experience bleeding between menstrual periods, painful urination, abdominal pain, and vaginal discharge. Often women only become aware they have chlamydia when their sexual partners are diagnosed with it.

Untreated chlamydial infections in women can lead to some serious complications. Perhaps the three most important are *pelvic inflammatory disease, cervical infections,* and *infections of newborns:*

- *Pelvic inflammatory disease:* **Pelvic inflammatory disease (PID)** is an infection that is a consequence of the ascending spread of organisms from the vagina or cervix to the uterus, fallopian tubes, ovaries, and pelvis. The infection sometimes spreads to the liver and appendix. PID is characterized by lower abdominal pain, painful intercourse, irregular menstrual bleeding, abnormal vaginal discharge, painful urination, fever, and nausea and vomiting. On the other hand, sometimes there are no symptoms at all.

  About half of all PID cases result from chlamydia—perhaps half a million American women a year, most among women under age 25 who are sexually active.[203] (PID also results from gonorrhea.)

At least a fourth of the women who develop PID suffer long-term consequences: One is chronic lower abdominal pain. Another is scarring of the fallopian tubes, which is held accountable for up to 30% of cases of infertility a year. PID is also associated with half of all cases of **ectopic pregnancy** (tubal pregnancy), which occurs when a fertilized egg (ovum) implants itself outside the lining of the uterus in the fallopian tube or elsewhere.[204]

PID is treated with antibiotics (such as tetracycline). The earlier the treatment, the better in terms of preventing scarring of the fallopian tubes and other complications. The risk of acquiring PID is reduced by avoiding high-risk sexual behaviors and by using condoms and diaphragms with a spermicidal agent containing nonoxynol-9.[205] Oral contraceptives may also protect some women against PID who are already infected with chlamydia.[206]

- *Cervical infections:* Chlamydial infections of the cervix usually cause no symptoms or only symptoms such as a slight vaginal discharge, which are sometimes missed or ignored. An untreated cervical infection, however, can lead to PID and result in infertility and even death.

- *Infections of newborns:* About two out of three infants born to women with chlamydial genital infections will become infected, primarily by coming into contact with an infected cervix during childbirth. Such infants, who may also be born prematurely and with low birth weights, can develop eye infections (conjunctivitis) and pneumonia if not treated at birth.[207,208]

Infections in Men As in women, early chlamydial infection in men often goes unrecognized. About 30% of infected men show no symptoms.[209] Those who do have symptoms may have a watery, puslike discharge from the penis and may experience difficult, painful urination.

If untreated, two of the most common results of chlamydial infection in men are epididymitis and nongonococcal urethritis:[210]

- *Epididymitis:* **Epididymitis** is an inflammation of the comma-shaped structure

11.40

Unit 11
Infectious and
Sexually
Transmitted
Diseases

leading out of the testicle called the epididymis. Most commonly found in sexually active males under age 35, epididymitis is characterized by tenderness in the testicles, fever, and swelling. If untreated, it can produce sterility.

- *Nongonococcal urethritis:* Chlamydia causes perhaps half the cases of **nongonococcal urethritis (NGU),** an infection of the urethra in men. (The other half of NGU cases are caused by other organisms.) The symptoms include mild burning during urination and discharge from the penis.

The symptoms of rectal infection are rectal pain, soreness, and anal discharge; oral-genital sex may produce inflammation in the throat.[211] Diagnosis is through a lab test, and treatment is with repeated antibiotic therapy.

Treatment The standard treatment for chlamydia for both men and women is antibiotics, usually tetracycline. It is important to continue treatment as prescribed to prevent the continuation of the infection. Unfortunately, many people with the infection show no symptoms and thus aren't treated. A one-dose antibiotic (Zithromax) may help address this problem.[212]

Gonorrhea: An Old Enemy Comes Back

Gonorrhea is an easily transmitted STD presently on the increase after declining for some time. Infection is through sexual contact and during childbirth. Infected men may show inflammation called *urethritis;* infected women may show infections of cervix and pelvic inflammatory disease. Both sexes may show rectal and throat infections and severe systemic blood-borne infection. Gonorrhea is treated with penicillin, although a penicillin-resistant strain has emerged.

Once upon a time, when the phrase "venereal disease" was in use, when people thought of sexually transmitted diseases they thought principally of gonorrhea (called the "clap" or "drip") and syphilis. For a time, in the 1970s

and early 1980s, the incidence of these two diseases declined.[213] Unfortunately, both the old enemies—especially gonorrhea—had a resurgence. Unfortunately also, some strains are more resistant to treatment than before.

What It Is, How It Spreads Gonorrhea is caused by the sexual transmission of a bacterium (*Neisseria gonorrhoeae*). It is an organism that is easily transmitted. A man who has had sexual intercourse *once* with an infected woman has a 20–25% risk of getting the disease; a woman who has intercourse *once* with an infected man has a 50% chance of getting it.[214]

The disease may be spread from one person to another via genital, oral, or anal contact, both heterosexual and homosexual, and also to babies during childbirth. Specifically:

- *Infection from sexual contact:* Because the gonorrhea bacterium needs warmth and humidity to thrive, it is harbored principally in warm, moist areas of the human body. Thus, one may contract gonorrhea from an infected person through genital, anal, and oral contact—including kissing.[215]

- *Infection of newborn babies:* Babies born to mothers who have gonorrhea may become infected as they pass through the birth canal. If not treated, they risk becoming blind. Thus, it is standard for newborns to have antiseptic or antibiotic placed in their eyes at birth to prevent blindness.

- *Probably not from toilet seats:* Toilet seats may harbor the gonococcus bacterium for a few seconds. However, despite the theoretical possibility of—and the folklore about—contracting the disease from toilet seats, the evidence does not show this to be a means of transmission.[216]

Infections in Men Some infected men, perhaps 10–20%, show no signs of infection at all.[217] Otherwise, the main manifestation is urethritis. **Urethritis** is a painful inflammation of the urethra, which discharges urine from the bladder. Whether the form of urethritis is nongonococcal urethritis (NGU), as we discussed above under chlamydia, or gonococcal urethritis (GCU), the symptoms are unpleasant: burning pain during urination and discharge of pus—

often watery or milkish at first, then greenish yellow—from the tip of the penis.

Although the burning sensation may subside in 2–3 weeks, if the disease is not treated it spreads throughout the urinary and reproductive systems, causing scarring, obstructions, and sterility.

Infections in Women Early gonorrhea symptoms in women may be so slight that they are apt to be overlooked. Indeed, up to 80% of infected women show no symptoms at all, and women may only begin to suspect they have a problem when their partners are diagnosed.[218] When symptoms appear, they may take the following forms:

- *Infections of cervix:* Cervical infections can produce a yellowish or yellow-green pus-like vaginal discharge, which can cause irritation of the vagina and painful and frequent urination. Someone who has an infected cervix may experience pain during sexual intercourse.

- *Pelvic inflammatory disease:* If untreated, gonorrhea, like chlamydia, can lead to pelvic inflammatory disease (PID) as the disease moves through the urinary and reproductive system. Scar tissue in the fallopian tubes, the long-term consequence of PID, may lead to sterility or ectopic pregnancies.

Infections in Either Sex In addition to or instead of the gender-specific symptoms, gonorrhea may produce the following problems in either men or women:

- *Rectal infections:* Among men with a history of anal intercourse, there are almost as many rectal infections as there are instances of urethritis. Half such men, however, show no symptoms.[219] Women who practice anal sex may also experience gonorrhea infection.

- *Throat infections:* Men or women who practice oral-genital contact may experience throat infections, which feel much like a sore throat.

- *Severe systemic blood-borne infection:* Gonorrhea can develop into a serious blood-borne systemic infection, which may lead to a form of arthritis in the joints and attack

important organs in the body, from heart to brain to skin. At times, this systemic infection can even be fatal.

Diagnosis and Treatment Gonorrhea is primarily diagnosed through laboratory tests, principally microscopic analysis of cultures taken from sites of infection. One test that is now available can detect the organism within 3 hours.

The principal treatment is use of antibiotics, especially penicillin. A very great problem recently, however, is the appearance of **PPNG**—short for **penicillinase-producing *Neisseria gonorrhoeae***—penicillin-resistant (and tetracycline-resistant) strains of gonorrhea. The spread of PPNG went up 131% from 1988 to 1989.[220,221] In place of penicillin, doctors are using other antibiotics (such as ceftriaxone).

Syphilis: The "Great Imitator" Returns

The symptoms of syphilis mimic some other disorders and diseases. Transmitted by sexual and mouth contact and through infection of newborns during childbirth by infected mothers, syphilis has four stages: primary, secondary, latent, and tertiary. The disease is detected by means of blood tests.

Syphilis, another old enemy like gonorrhea, is known as the "great imitator" because its sores and other symptoms mimic other disorders and diseases, such as cancers, abscesses, hemorrhoids, and hernias.[222] Once thought to be under control in the United States, syphilis returned with a vengeance: in 1990 it reached its highest level since 1949, zooming 75% in just 5 years. One reason for this epidemic, experts say, was the surge in crack cocaine use, which promotes high-risk sexual behavior, such as trading anonymous sex in exchange for money or drugs.[223,224]

What It Is, How It Spreads **Syphilis** is a sexually transmitted disease that is characterized by four stages. Like gonorrhea, the disease is caused by a bacterium, in this case a long,

11.42

Unit 11
Infectious and
Sexually
Transmitted
Diseases

slender, spiral bacterium, or **spirochete,** called *Treponema pallidum.* Syphilis is a serious STD because it can become a systemic infection, leading to possible brain damage, heart failure, and death.

The syphilis bacterium is a frail organism that requires warm, moist skin or mucous-membrane surfaces for survival. These spirochetes are present in a dime-sized or smaller sore, called a **chancre,** which may originate where the spirochete enters the body and exist on the outside of the body—such as the lip, tongue, or finger—but also may be hidden within the vagina or rectum. (See ● *Figure 27.6.*) The disease can be transmitted to another person when these sores are present. Because the sores do not cause pain, they may not be noticed.

Specifically, syphilis is transmitted as follows:

- *Infection by sexual and mouth contact:* Syphilis is transmitted to a sexual partner through vaginal intercourse, anal inter-

course, or oral-genital contact—including kissing, if the sores are present in or around the mouth.

- *Infection of fetus during pregnancy:* A baby in the womb may acquire *congenital syphilis* because its mother is infected and the spirochetes cross the placental barrier. Syphilis can cause deafness, anemia, and damage to bones and teeth. In extreme cases, the infant may die before birth (stillbirth).

Accordingly, pregnant women are advised to have blood tests for syphilis. Because infection of the fetus apparently does not occur before the fourth month of pregnancy, treatment of a woman with syphilis prior to the fifth month can prevent damage to the baby.[225]

The Four Stages of Syphilis Syphilis appears in four stages—primary, secondary, latent, and tertiary—as follows:

1. *Primary syphilis—painless sores that go away:* The first stage is characterized by the appearance, within 10–90 days of infection, of one or more of the pink or red raised sores called chancres at the point of sexual contact: penis, vagina, cervix, anus, tongue, lips, breast, or wherever. The edges of the sore are hard, like cartilage. Because it is painless, it is often ignored or not noticed.

    The chancre disappears by itself in 3–6 weeks. This may give the impression that the disease itself also has disappeared, but it has not.

2. *Secondary syphilis—rash and sores:* About 6–8 weeks after the disappearance of the chancre, the spirochete spreads through the blood, leading to symptoms that signal the second stage. These symptoms may be mistaken for the flu: swollen lymph nodes, sore throat, headache, and fever. There may also be loss of hair. The disease also produces a rash, which may appear on the hands or feet or all over the body and which does not itch. (See ● *Figure 27.7.*)

    In addition, large, moist sores may appear around the mouth or genitals. Because they are swarming with spirochetes, the

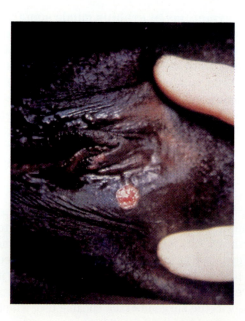

● **Figure 27.6 A chancre.** This dime-sized, painless sore, which may appear in the vagina (as shown), rectum, or on the outside of the body, contains the spirochetes that are the bearers of syphilis.

sores make this second stage especially contagious to sexual partners. If untreated, the second-stage sores disappear in 2–6 weeks. This only means the disease has entered the next stage.

3. *Latent syphilis—unnoticed invasion of the body:* In this stage, which may last from a few months to a lifetime, the disease goes underground and only a blood test can show whether a person has the disease. The spirochetes burrow unnoticed into the blood vessels, bones, spinal cord, brain, and other organs. Although 50–70% of those with untreated syphilis remain in this latent stage for the rest of their lives and experience no further problems, the rest develop late-stage syphilis.[226]

   During the first two years of the latent stage, the symptoms of secondary syphilis may reappear. On these occasions the person is highly contagious to sexual partners. After a year or two, the person is no longer contagious. An infected pregnant woman, however, can always transmit the disease to the fetus.

4. *Tertiary syphilis—destruction of nervous system and organs:* Years or even decades after the initial exposure, untreated syphilis may result in damage to the heart and major blood vessels or the central nervous system, causing impaired muscle control, paralysis, insanity, and death. This late-stage syphilis can also affect nearly all other organs: eyes (causing blindness), muscles, skin, lungs, liver, digestive organs, and endocrine glands.

Diagnosis and Treatment The re-emergence of syphilis forced physicians to become highly suspicious about a disease that once had become relatively rare in North America.[227,228] Health officials have also worried that the open sores of syphilis made it easier for the AIDS virus to enter the body.[229]

Syphilis is diagnosed by means of blood tests and the microscopic analysis of cultures of suspected spirochetes taken from sores. Blood tests are used as a standard screening device; indeed, blood tests for syphilis are usually required to obtain a marriage license.

Penicillin is the most common treatment for syphilis and can be highly effective if given during the primary stage. Syphilis is treated by antibiotics.

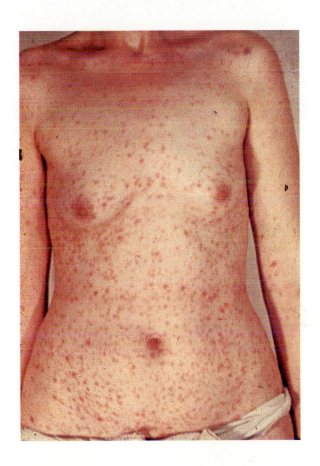

● **Figure 27.7 Rash of secondary syphilis.** A sign of the second stage of syphilis, this rash does not itch. It may appear all over the body or only part of it.

Parasite Infections: Pubic Lice and Scabies

The parasite infections of pubic lice and scabies are transmitted by sexual means. They are far easier to control than other STDs.

The STDs we have described are transmitted by organisms that are microscopic in size.

11.44

*Unit 11
Infectious and
Sexually
Transmitted
Diseases*

However, at least one of the class of parasitic insects transmitted by sexual contact, pubic lice, can actually be seen, at least with a magnifying glass. (*See ● Figure 27.8.*)

Pubic Lice: "Crabs" Called "crabs" because of their crab-like appearance, **pubic lice** are wingless, gray insects, about ¹⁄₁₆ inch long. They live in human hair, particularly pubic hair, although they may move to underarm hair, eyebrows, eyelashes, and beards. Pubic lice feed on blood, causing itching and skin discoloration. Female lice lay eggs, or *nits,* that are attached to the hair.

Pubic lice are mainly transmitted during sex but may also be picked up from bedding and infected clothing. Treatment is by washing with insecticide-containing shampoo available from health care professionals and as over-the-counter preparations available at pharmacies. In addition, the nits may be combed out with a fine-toothed comb, and contaminated clothing and linen should be washed.

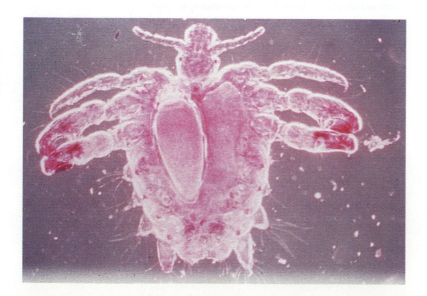

● **Figure 27.8 Pubic louse.** About one-sixteenth-inch long, the pubic louse is often transmitted by sexual contact. Pubic lice live in body hair, feed on human blood, and cause itching.

Scabies: Skin Mites Scabies is a parasitic infection that is spread the same way as pubic lice—that is, by sexual contact or by contact with contaminated clothing or bedding. **Scabies** are tiny mites (lice) that burrow under the skin and lay eggs, producing itching and discolored lines on the skin. Treatment consists of washing oneself and other members of the household with insecticide-containing soap. Bedding and clothing should also be thoroughly washed.

Infections of the Reproductive and Urinary Systems

Troublesome disorders of the urinary and reproductive systems include bacterial vaginosis, trichomoniasis, yeast infections, and cystitis. These infections happen in both sexes.

Some infections of the urinary and reproductive systems are not transmitted exclusively by sexual contact, although sexual contact represents one possible means of transmission. Still, that doesn't make them any less troublesome. We describe *bacterial vaginosis, trichomoniasis, yeast infections,* and *cystitis.*

Bacterial Vaginosis Bacterial vaginosis **(BV),** characterized by slightly increased quantities of malodorous vaginal discharge, is the most prevalent cause of vaginal symptoms among women of childbearing age.[230] BV may be a risk factor for pelvic inflammatory disease. The bacteria (*Gardnerella vaginalis*) leading to BV is probably transmitted by male partners during sexual intercourse, although BV may also be present in the absence of sexual activity. Although some women show no symptoms, others reveal a white vaginal discharge. Diagnosis is made by performing laboratory tests, and treatment is with Flagyl or antibiotics. Although males may have no symptoms, both partners should be treated at the same time.

Trichomoniasis The infection **trichomoniasis** ("trick"), found in both sexes, is caused by a parasitic protozoa (*Trichomonas vaginalis*). Some women show no symptoms at all, but 50–75% experience itching, burning, and vaginal discharge and find sexual intercourse painful. The infection generally remains in the genital and urethral area. Some women experience urinary symptoms. Many men show no symptoms. Those that do may experience a slight burning during urination. Trichomoniasis is highly contagious and is usually transmitted sexually, but it may also be transmitted in other ways, as from public toilet seats.[231] Treatment for both oneself and one's sexual partners is with oral or vaginal medications such as metronidazole (Flagyl).

Yeast Infections About 75% of women will at some point experience vaginal **yeast infections.**[232] These are caused by a fungus called *Candida albicans* and other candida species that normally inhabit the intestinal tract, mouth, and vagina but cause no problems or symptoms unless overgrowth of the organism occurs. In women, the symptoms of vaginal yeast infection can include severe itching, pain during intercourse, vaginal redness and soreness, and a white vaginal discharge. In men, the fungus may be present under the foreskin or scrotum, but most men have no symptoms.

Vaginal yeast infections can be precipitated by poor diet (excessive intake of sugar), use of antibiotics, diabetes, frequent douching, or pregnancy. Treatment of oneself and one's sexual partner is with antifungal vaginal suppositories or creams.

Urinary Tract Infections: Cystitis As with so many other disorders of the urinary system, women appear more vulnerable than men to **cystitis,** inflammation of the urinary bladder. The reason for this particular inequality of the sexes may be that the urethra in women is quite short (about 1½ inches long), compared to the urethra in men (6 inches), which means that bacteria have to travel a shorter distance to reach the bladder in females. One in five women have a urinary tract infection in their lives, and many of them are prone to recurrent infections. Sexual intercourse is a common way that bacteria gets introduced into the female urethra.

Cystitis can be caused by a variety of microorganisms and it may be associated with vigorous sexual activity. Symptoms include burning during urination, urgency and frequency of urination, blood in the urine, fever,

lower abdominal pain, and fatigue. Diagnosis is through a laboratory analysis of a urine culture. Early treatment, which usually consists of 7–10 days of antibiotics, is important to prevent the infection from migrating to the kidneys, where it may produce **pyelonephritis,** inflammation of the kidneys.

Strategy for Living: Preventing STDs

Avoiding STDs means taking such preventive measures as practicing abstinence or minimizing the number of sexual partners; trying to learn your partner's sexual history; being alert to your passions, especially when drinking alcohol; using condoms, spermicides, and dental dams; and using care after having sex.

It's clear that some STDs can be treated, but some cannot, and in any case they nearly all produce discomfort, ranging from unpleasantness to extreme anguish. So let us state the obvious: *Prevention matters.*

Here are some tips, possibly life-saving ones:

- *Practice abstinence or minimize the number of sexual partners:* Clearly, the best defense is to have no sex at all—to practice *abstinence* or *celibacy.* This kind of behavior might have been scoffed at in the free-wheeling 1970s and 1980s, but it makes a whole lot of sense now.

  Failing that, the next best defense is to minimize the number of sexual partners you have. A long-term, monogamous relationship is best. Next best is to have sexual relations with only a handful of partners, preferably spread out over a long period of time. The more partners, of course, the higher the probability of contracting an STD.

- *Try to learn your partner's sexual history:* This can be difficult, perhaps impossible. Clearly, a prospective sex partner who has had numerous previous relationships may not want to level with you. A woman who has had bisexual partners or IV drug-using partners may not want to own up to this. Sometimes she may not even be aware

11.46

*Unit 11
Infectious and
Sexually
Transmitted
Diseases*

of her previous partners' histories. A bisexual man may not wish to acknowledge his bisexuality to a woman. This is a reason for moving into a new relationship slowly and not having sex until you can get a sense of the person.

These days, to enter a new relationship is to enter uncharted waters, so you need to be especially alert. *During foreplay, for example, inspect your partner's body for any symptoms of a possible STD, such as urethral discharge or genital lesions.* Try to remember the bottom line: sex may be fun, but it also may be fatal.

- *Crucial to the art of living: Be alert to your passions—and drinking:* Being "swept away"—letting your passions overwhelm you—is an ongoing feature of novels, magazines, and movies, ranging from supermarket romances to *Penthouse* to the film *Fatal Attraction.* It is also a feature of real life. The breakdown of resistance and good intentions *is particularly apt to happen when alcohol is involved.*[233] In addition, for some people, romance, love, one moment of shattering pleasure, may be worth more than longevity.[234]

  One of the important arts of living is not to let your heart rule your head in these instances. That you had a momentary lapse in judgment and didn't use a condom can have extremely serious consequences.

  Incidentally, condoms are sold in many interesting and erotic styles and can actually become an intrinsic part of sexual pleasure.[235]

- *Use protection—condoms, spermicides, and dental dams:* Condoms help prevent the spread of HIV, herpes, chlamydia, gonorrhea, syphilis, and most other STDs. It's important *to put the condom on before the penis touches the other person's body.*

  Using a spermicide, such as vaginal creams, foams, and jellies, also helps. Men receiving oral sex (fellatio) should use a condom, women receiving oral sex (cunnilingus) should use a dental dam, a square piece of latex held over the genitals. Oral-anal stimulation (anilingus) should be avoided altogether.

- *Use care after sex:* There are two important things that both men and women should do *immediately* after sex to reduce the risk of STDs:

  (1) *Urinate,* which will help prevent urethral infection and bladder infection;

  (2) *Wash with soap and water,* which will kill STD pathogens that can enter the body through those parts of the skin not protected by a condom.

Of course, if in the following days or weeks you begin to experience discomfort or notice signs such as those described in this chapter, you should not simply shrug them off but should seek medical help. Antibiotics, for instance, can be very effective for some STDs if given early after exposure but will not be as effective later on.

800-HELP

AIDS Hotline. 800-533-AIDS (in Canada, 800-668-AIDS)

Centers for Disease Control and Prevention National AIDS Hotline. 800-342-2437 (800-344-7432 for Spanish-speaking). Provides confidential and anonymous information and referrals to local health organizations, counselors, and support groups

STD National Hotline. 800-634-3662 (in California, 800-982-5883)

Suggestions for Further Readings

Baker, Ronald A., Moulton, Jeffrey M., & Tighe, John Charles (1992). *Early care for HIV disease* (2nd ed.). San Francisco: San Francisco AIDS Foundation. Paperback book available at bookstores as well as from the foundation.

Stine, Gerald J. (1993). *Acquired immune deficiency syndrome: Biological, medical, social, and legal issues.* Englewood Cliffs, NJ: Prentice Hall. A well-written, up-to-date, and thorough discussion of all aspects of HIV/AIDS.

Your Image: Personal Care and Habits

Answer the following yes or no:

At least once a day, I . . .

___ **1.** Shower or bathe.

___ **2.** Use an underarm deodorant or antiperspirant.

___ **3.** Shampoo my hair.

___ **4.** Floss my teeth.

Is your answer that you don't do *any* of these things on a daily basis? Then clearly you prize your outsider or outlaw image, you lack access to a shower or tub, or you're simply indifferent to the people around you. But if this is indeed the case, ask yourself: How are such habits advancing my life?

Most readers, we assume, do most of these activities—if not daily then at least fairly often. Personal grooming and hygiene—seemingly old-fashioned terms mainly associated with habits of cleanliness that may have been drilled into you by your parents—are not just for beautification purposes. Of the five dimensions of health (physical, intellectual, emotional, social, and spiritual), they advance you not only in the physical but also on the social dimensions.

Skin and Hair Care

Aging of the skin is not something programmed to happen at a certain rate. Such aging occurs in part because of environmental and lifestyle factors such as exposure to the sun, wind, cold, indoor heat, stress, smoking, alcohol, poor diet, and lack of exercise.

Washing Going to bed with clean skin helps the nightly repair processes to the day's damage to take place. Washing your face—or, even better, washing and then applying a moisturizer—before turning in will keep the dirt and debris from clogging up the pores and will prevent the skin from drying out. If you wear makeup, you should first use a makeup remover, then a skin cleanser. Or, if you have normal skin, try a combination makeup remover and skin cleanser.

Most people begin the day with a shower or a bath, or at the very least splashing water on the face. Don't shower with extremely hot water, which can cause your skin to dry out. Use a cleanser, lotion, soap, or shower gel that is appropriate for your skin.

Skin Cleanser What kind of skin cleanser should you use? That depends on whether your skin is dry, oily, sensitive, or dull.[236]

- *Dry skin:* Dry skin needs protection against moisture loss. Look for cleansing creams with plant oils or sodium TEA/lauryl hydrolyzed protein, which mimic the skin's natural protective barrier.

- *Oily or acne-prone skin:* This kind of skin needs deep cleansing but also needs moisture because oily-skinned adults often experience dryness on the cheeks. Clean the skin with warm water twice a day, using a gentle, pH-balanced soap that does not contain chemicals or perfumes.

- *Sensitive skin:* Some people's skins are very sensitive to fragrances and preservatives. Many new cleansers use botanicals to reduce skin irritation.

Moisturizer Your skin is always losing moisture through evaporation and perspiration, and dryness is what causes the skin to age. Moisturizers help protect against dry skin, helping it stay moist for up to 24 hours.[237, 238]

Deodorizer A *deodorant* is intended to mask or absorb body odor, but it will not keep you from perspiring. An *antiperspirant* is intended to reduce sweating, but it will do nothing for your odor. To be both dry and free of odor, you need to use something that's a combination of both—a deodorant/antiperspirant. Whether it's a stick, roll-on, or spray makes no difference in effectiveness.

For Men: Shaving [239] Shower before you shave to soften up your beard. Moisturize the beard with shaving cream. Use a sharp razor (don't reuse a disposable blade or razor more than three or four times). "Stroke gently, drawing the razor slowly in the direction your beard grows," advises one writer. "Shave smooth areas first, and save the difficult parts of your face, such as under the chin, for last. This gives the shaving cream more time to take effect." [240]

Use of a medicated shaving cream or washing the face first with medicated soap can minimize rashes or acne-like pimples that develop on the faces of some men from shaving. If you have difficulty with ingrown hairs, a problem for African Americans and men with heavy beards, always use a sharp blade and be careful not to shave against the grain.

For Women: Cosmetics Makeup, such as lipstick, eye shadow, and blush, are not needed to keep your skin healthy. If you do wear them, consider the following: [241]

- *Effective use:* Are you using cosmetics in a way that really enhances your looks? Ask your friends for their reactions, giving them permission first to be honest in their opinions.

- *"Natural" versus synthetic cosmetics:* Many cosmetics are promoted as being "natural," which means they probably contain no petroleum-based substances, chemicals, additives, preservatives, artificial dyes, or animal products. Still, even "natural" products may contain substances created in a laboratory. Read the labels to be sure most of the ingredients are from plant, herbal, or other natural sources.

- *Allergic reactions:* If you suspect you may be sensitive to a new product, apply a small amount somewhere on the inside of your arm. If your skin remains clear after several hours, you are probably not allergic. Certain "hypo-allergenic" cosmetics have been developed for people with allergies.

Shampoos and Conditioners The hair should be washed regularly—every day or twice a week, depending on the type of hair—in order to remove dandruff, dirt, oil, and bacteria. If you have oily hair, you should shampoo every day. You can tell if your hair is oily if it has a sheen to it and tends to mat against the scalp. If you have dry hair, you need shampoo only every other day or a couple of times a week. If your hair is frizzy or has a straw-like feel to it, or if your scalp is itchy, these are signs of dry hair.

If you wash your hair every day, use one of the milder (pH-balanced) shampoos and don't repeat the wash-and-rinse cycle.

Conditioners The purpose of conditioners is to add moisture or to add protein to the hair (hair is 3% moisture, 97% protein). Conditioners add body to the hair, make it appear soft and smooth, get rid of snarls, and make it easier to comb and handle.

Dandruff Just as the rest of your skin sloughs off flakes of skin every 28 days, so does your scalp, causing dandruff, the small flakes of dead skin appearing in your hair. If the flakes are normal, you can use a rubber scalp brush when you shower. If the dandruff is severe—the kind called *seborrheic dermatitis,* which can be caused by stress, illness, or allergies—you can use medicated or dandruff shampoos containing zinc, selenium, sulfur, or coal-tar formulas. These should be used in moderation (such as once a week); otherwise, they can actually *cause* dandruff.

Hair dressings are of several types. *Lotions,* which give a light hold, are all that is necessary for thin hair. *Mousses,* which come in foam dispensers, and *gels,* which come in a jar or tube, will give a stronger hold; they should be put on while the hair is wet. *Sprays* will also give a strong hold, but they should be put on hair that is dried. [242]

Tooth and Gum Care

Watch your mouth—at least if you want to keep your teeth. Of course, people have probably been warning you about cavities since you were in grade school. Actually, for most people, tooth decay is less a problem than gum disease. The difficulty, however, is that only when the damage is severe—when the sticky film of bacteria called *plaque* has attacked the bones and ligaments that secure your teeth—and you have bleeding gums or wobbly teeth will you know that you have a gum problem. Since this can take a while, it is a surprise to many people when the dentist tells them their teeth are at risk.

Dental care consists of the following steps:

- *The twice-daily duty:* You should brush *and* floss your teeth at least twice a day—before you go to bed and in the morning. "Oral bacteria reach their highest count when you're asleep because the fluids in your mouth stagnate (that's why your mouth is ripest when you first wake up)," says one writer. "So the nighttime cleaning is tantamount to a strategic strike—cutting down the bacterial population before it can rally. The morning cleaning lets you mow down the bacteria again when their numbers have peaked."[243]

- *Toothbrush:* Use a *soft*-bristled brush, rather than a hard one. Soft bristles are not only gentler on the gums, they also yield when pressed against the tooth enamel and expand to surround the tooth.

- *Toothpaste:* Most toothpastes are similar in formula and price, and any variation in ingredients makes no difference, with one exception—fluoride. Fluoride toothpaste, combined with the fluoridation of water, is widely credited with helping to reduce cavities.

   The newer antiplaque and antitartar formulas act against plaque and tartar on the exposed tooth, which do not cause gum disease; however, making these deposits softer helps dentists penetrate to the disease-producing agents beyond the gum line.[244]

- *Brushing:* There is a very specific, correct way to go about manipulating the toothbrush:

  1. Place the brush so it is tilted at a 45-degree angle against the gum line.

  2. *Gently* move the brush in small circular motions.

  3. Start with your upper back teeth, on the outside, and move the brush

around to the other side of your mouth. Then move to the outside of your lower teeth. Finally, move to the inside of your upper and lower teeth.

  4. Brush your tongue, too. (It is a source of bacteria.)

- *Flossing:* It does not matter whether your floss is waxed or unwaxed, tape or thread, flavored or unflavored. Nor does it matter whether you floss before or after brushing.[245]

   Flossing has a set procedure:

  1. Take an 18-inch to 3-foot strand of floss.

  2. Wind it around the middle (or little) finger of one hand and the same finger on the other hand. Use your index fingers to guide the thread.

  3. Slip the thread behind an upper back tooth and below the gum line, but not so deeply that you cut into the gum. Wrap the thread part way around the tooth.

  4. Slide the floss up and down against the tooth two or three times.

  5. Slip the floss down and unwind a clean segment of thread. Slide it between the next pair of teeth, and continue until you've worked your way around the top and bottom of your mouth.

   If you're still unsure about how to floss, have a dental hygienist show you when you make your next visit to a dentist.

- *Mouthwashes:* Use of a mouthwash (Plax, Scope) might seem to be a nice alternative to the chore of brushing and flossing, but at best it is only a supplement, not a substitute, for your other bacteria-killing and breath-freshening efforts.

In These Chapters:

When bad luck happens, are we merely hapless victims?

Or are we the makers of our own luck, good and bad, and therefore responsible?

No doubt about it, bad things do happen to good people. But is it their fault or not? Being hit by a falling airplane part is bad luck. Or being in an old brick building when an earthquake happens. So is being born with some of the noninfectious illnesses described in this chapter, such as epilepsy. Bad things may happen randomly. Indeed, you may be genuinely unlucky and suffer a *run* of bad luck.

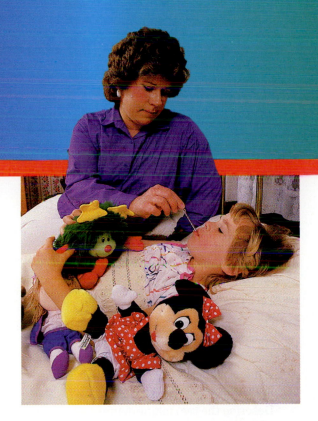

Once bad luck happens to you, your task is damage control. You need to take action to keep your fate from becoming worse, as patients do who have learned they have a serious illness. You also need to take the steps to recover psychologically. Psychologist Elise Labbe advises people to deal with their devastation as they would grief. "First, I urge them to get angry," she says. "Then, to get sad, to cry if they can. And finally to get on with their lives with a new, objective, even optimistic outlook."[1]

However, not all bad things that happen may be the result of bad luck. As psychologist William F. Vitulli says, "We are responsible for a good deal more of what happens to us than we realize."[2] This may be good news because it means that once you realize your own role in your misfortune, instead of shaking your fist at the wrathful gods, you are in a position to change your so-called bad-luck behavior.

If you think you are prone to bad luck, here are some things to think about:[3] Could it be that you are *more impulsive* than other people? Do you speak without thinking, buy things without checking them out, start things without reading instructions, fail to plan ahead, or confuse wishful thinking with intuition? Do you have blind spots in one area of life, such as personal rela-

tionships, where you seem to have difficulty judging life realistically? Do you unconsciously wish to have failures or accidents because you get some sort of emotional comfort from others when they happen?

The topics in this unit—noninfectious illnesses and matters of personal safety—exemplify both kinds of luck. Some are accidents of fate, disorders for which a person is not responsible but that must be dealt with nonetheless. Some, however, are instances of *self-induced* bad luck. These are illnesses and injuries that you can avoid.

28 Noninfectious Illnesses

▶ Explain the two types of diabetes.

▶ Describe three principal disorders of the nervous system: the different types of headaches, multiple sclerosis, and two types of seizure disorders or epilepsy.

▶ Discuss the two disorders of low-back pain and arthritis.

▶ Describe inflammatory bowel disease and gallbladder disease.

▶ Discuss two principal disorders of the kidneys—kidney failure and kidney stones.

▶ Explain asthma and chronic obstructive lung disease.

▶ Describe the two major dental diseases of cavities and gum disease.

Becoming ill because you caught some free-floating microorganism is easy to understand. All of us have been suddenly laid low by a cold virus or flu microbe—in other words, an infectious disease. Noninfectious illnesses may also seem to come from out of nowhere, but they may seem baffling because we can't point to them and say, "A germ did this to me." But such disorders, which range from diabetes to headaches to low-back pain to asthma to tooth decay, can be as inconvenient and impair health and well-being as can any infection. This chapter explains some of the principal noninfectious conditions.

Diabetes: Failure to Use Glucose

Diabetes is a disease in which the body cannot properly metabolize food, especially carbohydrates. In people with diabetes, the pancreas cannot produce any insulin (Type 1 diabetes) or insufficient insulin is produced or there is inability to effectively use the insulin produced (Type 2 diabetes).

As the seventh leading cause of death in the United States, diabetes is a serious disease.[4] Every year, 30,000 Americans die from it, and 300,000 more die from complications stemming from it. It doubles the risk of heart attack or stroke, is the leading cause of blindness in adults, and is associated with one-third of all cases of kidney failure.[5] Pregnant women with diabetes have higher risks of miscarriage or producing infants with developmental delays and birth defects.[6-8] Most disturbing, perhaps half of all Americans who have diabetes have not been diagnosed as having the disease. (*See Self Discovery 28.1.*)

Diabetes: What It Is, What It Does The disorder **diabetes**—more precisely known as **diabetes mellitus**—is a disease in which the body cannot properly metabolize food, especially carbohydrates. A one-sentence definition only begins to cover it, however. The details are as follows:

1. For the body to have energy and make replacement materials for itself, it must metabolize—that is, chemically break down—food. In the case of diabetes, the foods of particular concern consist of carbohydrates and simple sugars.

2. Carbohydrates—fruits, milk, sugar, pasta, bread, vegetables, and other foods that include sugars and starches—act as the body's immediate fuel.

3. The body breaks down carbohydrates into *glucose,* or blood sugar. Glucose is the primary form of sugar that provides the body with energy. Both nondiabetics and diabetics are capable of producing glucose. The difference is what happens after that.

4. A critical organ is the pancreas. In healthy people, the level of glucose rises in the blood after a meal. This automatically causes the pancreas to release a hormone called **insulin** into the blood. *The body needs insulin in order to move the sugar from the blood into the cells—to convert glucose and other foods into energy.*

5. In people with diabetes, unfortunately, the pancreas produces either no insulin or insufficient insulin. When *no* insulin is produced, the condition is called **Type 1 diabetes,** or **insulin-dependent diabetes**

mellitus (IDDM). When *insufficient* insulin is produced—or the body is unable to effectively use the insulin produced—the condition is called **Type 2 diabetes, or insulin-independent diabetes mellitus (IIDM).**

6. Without any insulin or not enough insulin, the glucose rising in the blood after a meal is unable to enter most body cells. This has two consequences: (a) The unused glucose has to go somewhere else, since it can't go into the cells. (b) The energy needs of the cells are not being met.

7. The unused glucose in the blood that is unable to go into the cells accumulates to such levels that the kidneys cannot process it, and this excess glucose spills over into the urine, which is expelled.

8. When the energy needs of the cells are not met, the body begins to look elsewhere within itself for some other source of energy. Specifically, the body burns stored fats and proteins, in the course of which it produces dangerous acids called *ketones*. Ketones can lead to nausea, vomiting, drowsiness, and even coma and death.[9]

Diagnosis, Onset, and Risk Factors Symptoms of diabetes include excessive thirst, frequent urination, fatigue and weakness, irritability, and a craving for sweets. Diagnosis is made on the basis of blood glucose tests.

The two types of diabetes have different patterns:

- *Type 1 diabetes:* The onset of Type 1 diabetes, in which the body does not produce insulin at all, usually strikes in childhood or adolescence, but can develop at any time up to 35 years of age. Type 1 diabetes often comes about suddenly, the result of the body's own immune system destroying the insulin-producing cells of the pancreas.[10] Although the cause is unknown, in some cases it may spring from virus-caused infection of the insulin-producing cells.[11]

- *Type 2 diabetes:* Type 2 diabetes, in which insulin production is insufficient rather than totally lacking, is the less severe of the two types although far more common. Type 2 generally occurs gradually, most often in adults who are over 35 and overweight.

SELF DISCOVERY 28.1

Are You at Risk for Diabetes?

Answer yes or no to each of the following statements:

	Yes	No
1. I have been experiencing one or more of the following symptoms regularly:		
a. Excessive thirst	___	___
b. Frequent urination	___	___
c. Extreme fatigue	___	___
d. Unexplained weight loss	___	___
e. Blurry vision from time to time	___	___
2. I am older than 30.	___	___
3. I am at least 20% over my ideal weight.	___	___
4. I am a woman who has had more than one baby weighing more than 9 pounds at birth.	___	___
5. I am of Native American descent.	___	___
6. I am of Hispanic or African American descent.	___	___
7. I have a parent with diabetes.	___	___
8. I have a brother or sister with diabetes.	___	___

Scoring

Score your yes answers as follows:

1a. 3	1c. 1	1e. 2	3. 2	5. 1	7. 1
1b. 3	1d. 3	2. 1	4. 2	6. 1	8. 2

Add your score: _____

Interpretation

3–5 points: You are at low risk for diabetes.

Over 5 points: You may be at high risk or even have diabetes. *See your doctor without delay.*

Preventive Steps

You can't change your heritage or your age, but you can change habits that may affect whether or not you get diabetes. Best are a low-calorie diet and a regular aerobic exercise program, which will keep your weight down.

Source: Adapted from The Diabetes Risk Test, American Diabetes Association, National Center, 1660 Duke Street, Alexandria, VA 22314.

Fully 90% of all diabetics have Type 2 diabetes. It can occur in people with no family history of diabetes, but people with relatives or parents who are diabetic are at high risk. Perhaps 75% of diabetics are overweight and don't exercise. Most are also over age 45. People of

Native American, African American, or Hispanic descent are also more at risk.[12,13]

Treatment Diabetes cannot be cured, but it can be managed. The course of treatment is similar in many ways for the two types but differs in terms of blood sugar management.

- *Type 1:* People with Type 1 diabetes cannot go much more than a day without insulin, usually self-administered either via injections (1–4 daily) or via an insulin pump.[14] (*See ● Figure 28.1.*) Too much or too little

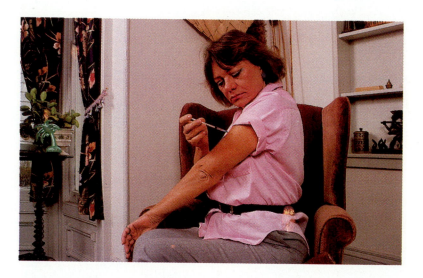

● **Figure 28.1 Insulin injection.** People with Type 1 diabetes require daily doses of insulin.

❝*Every moment of every day, the healthy human body performs an array of life-sustaining chores: The kidney filters toxins from the blood, the immune system battles foreign invaders, the lungs exchange carbon dioxide for precious oxygen. But for 14 million Americans stricken by diabetes mellitus—a chronic, incurable disease—one 'automatic' function, normally regulated by the pancreas, demands unrelenting attention: the conversion of sugar into fuel to power the body's cells.*

Diabetes robs its victims of the automatic pilot that regulates sugar processing. To compensate, diabetics must control their condition with an individually tailored regimen of diet, exercise and, when necessary, oral medication; many require daily insulin injections.❞

—Clare Collins. (1993, January/February). Diabolical diabetes. *American Health,* p. 68.

insulin can cause life-threatening complications. If a Type 1 diabetic shows such insulin-overdose signs as weakness, impaired vision, tingling in hands, and drowsiness, he or she should take a fast source of sugar, such as sugar cubes or orange juice, and seek medical help.

Type 1 diabetics also need to take many of the same dietary and exercise measures as Type 2 diabetics do.

- *Type 2:* People with Type 2 diabetes may not need daily insulin injections, but they do need to take steps to maintain their glucose and blood fat levels as closely to normal as possible. This means exercising, keeping their weight down, and watching their diet.

The American Diabetes Association guidelines state that Type 2 diabetics may include up to 60% complex carbohydrates (cereals, grains, breads, pasta, beans, fruits and vegetables) in their diet but should go easy on proteins (meat and milk) and fats and *very* easy on sugar and alcohol.

Neurological Disorders

Three neurological disorders, or disorders of the nervous system, are (1) headaches, such as tension headaches induced by stress, migraine headaches, or cluster headaches; (2) multiple sclerosis (MS), caused by a virus in which the immune system turns against the body; and (3) seizure disorders, or epilepsy, which includes convulsive seizures and nonconvulsive seizures.

There are a great many **neurological disorders,** disorders of the nervous system. Three that you may encounter are headaches, multiple sclerosis, and epilepsy.

Headaches Those mild or severe pounding pains in the head known as **headaches** can have all kinds of causes, sometimes psychological, sometimes organic. If they persist, they should always be taken seriously.

Among the kinds of headaches are:

- *Tension headaches:* The most common kinds of headaches are **tension headaches,** discomfort caused by involuntary contractions of muscles in the neck, head, and scalp, usually brought about by stress. They may be alleviated by stress-reduction techniques (as we described in Unit 2).

- *Migraine headaches:* **Migraine headaches** have different causes. Blood vessels expand (dilate) in the brain, and chemicals leaked through the blood vessel walls inflame nearby tissues, sending pain signals. Migraine attacks are often preceded by the sensation of glowing spots before the eyes, a condition known as an *aura*. Migraine headaches, which often run in families and can become increasingly severe over time, are treated with strong chemical painkillers and/or with relaxation.[15]

- *Other headaches:* One type of headache, most common in men, is the severely painful **cluster headache,** which strikes on one side (and always the same side) of the head and occurs 1–14 times a day for many weeks. Treatment is with prescription medications.

    Some headaches are *secondary headaches* caused by some other condition—hunger (low blood sugar), common colds, eyesight problems, badly fitting dentures, sexual activity, exposure to second-hand cigarette smoke, and so on. To treat the headache, one must first identify and treat the underlying cause.

    Toxic headaches are types of secondary headaches caused by poisonous chemicals, such as toxins from bacterial infections, engine fumes, or alcohol.

Multiple Sclerosis According to current theory, the neurological disorder **multiple sclerosis (MS)** occurs when an unidentified virus causes cells in the immune system to turn against the body and attack the brain and spinal cord, slowing the nerve impulses. In the beginning, symptoms include tremors, speech impediment, prickling and burning in the arms and legs, blurred vision, and changes in manner of walking. Often the disease goes into remission, in which one is free of symptoms for months or years. Ultimately, however, people suffer irreversible paralysis, and death occurs 20–25 years after onset.[16] The disease strikes as many as 350,000 Americans every year, primarily young adults around age 30.[17]

Treatment is with steroid, anti-inflammatory, and other drugs to relieve muscle spasms; physical therapy to reduce incapacitation; and psychotherapy and other forms of emotional support to alleviate depression.

Epilepsy and Seizure Disorders *Seizure disorders,* also called **epilepsy** or **epilepsies,** are a collection of neurological disorders caused by abnormal electrical activity in the brain. They are characterized by sudden attacks, or seizures, of involuntary, violent muscle contractions and loss of consciousness. About 1% of Americans suffer from some form of seizure-related disorder. The disorders are seldom fatal, although they can be dangerous if a seizure occurs while one is driving or swimming, or if a seizure episode is prolonged.

The Epilepsy Foundation of America has simplified the classification of epilepsy into *convulsive* and *nonconvulsive,* as follows:[18]

- *Convulsive:* An episode of **convulsive seizures** is often mistaken for a heart attack or a stroke. The person suffering a generalized major seizure (grand mal seizure) shows sudden rigidity and falls. This is followed by **convulsions**—muscle jerks or involuntary muscle contractions—shallow breathing or loss of breathing, perhaps loss of bladder or bowel control, frothy saliva on lips, and bluish skin. The seizures usually last 2–5 minutes, followed by normal breathing, some confusion, and return to consciousness.

    If you see a person having such seizures, the main thing is to make sure he or she is not injured during the attack. Loosen clothing and do not attempt to restrain his or her movements. After the seizure, turn the person on his or her side to keep the airway clear, check for medical identification, and take the person to an emergency room if the seizure lasts *longer* than 10 minutes. Do not try to restrain the person, put any implements in the mouth, or try to hold the tongue (which cannot be swallowed), and do not try to give liquids during or just after the seizure.

- *Nonconvulsive:* An attack of **nonconvulsive seizures** can be mistaken for daydreaming, intoxication, poor coordination, or mental illness. The category covers a range of seizures, from brief muscle jerks to loss of contact with surroundings (psychomotor seizures) to loss of consciousness for a few seconds (petit mal seizures).

If you are in the presence of a person in the midst of a nonconvulsive seizure, usually no first aid is required, although you should expect the person to show momentary confusion and not understand you. The main thing is to provide reassurance and emotional support.

People with seizures are usually able to control their disorder with medications (such as carbamazepine and phenytoin) and most are able to drive, participate in athletics, go to school, and work.

Disorders of the Bones and Joints

Important disorders of bones and joints are low-back pain and arthritis, especially osteoarthritis and rheumatoid arthritis.

Disorders of the bones and joints are commonplace in part because we use them so frequently that they are more likely to be injured. Among the most common problems are *low-back pain* and *arthritis*.

Low-Back Pain Your posture, as well as good nutrition and exercise, may well make some difference in avoiding problems with your back. Still, your chances of *not* experiencing back pain at some time are, unfortunately, not good. Sometime in their lives, 60–90% of people develop a chronic back condition.[19] Indeed, low-back pain is the second leading cause of missed work in the United States, right after the common cold.[20,21] Even highly active people have bad backs. (Examples: sports heroes Joe Montana, Larry Bird, Jack Nicklaus.) Chronic back conditions are the most frequent cause of activity limitation in people younger than age 45, and account for 23% of the activity limitation among people ages 18–44.[22]

Why is the back such a problem? One reason is that the disks, the gel-like pads separating each vertebra in the spine, wear out over time. Once they have deteriorated past a certain point, it may take only a small bit of

stress—a cough, bending to pat the dog—to send a person into a paroxysm of pain. The sufferer may discover that he or she has a **herniated disk,** the protrusion of the disk from its position between two vertebrae, which may require surgery to correct.

As you might expect, people whose jobs involve heavy lifting (garbage collectors, warehouse workers, mechanics, nursing aides) are apt to suffer more from low-back pain.[23] However, people who sit inactive all week at their desks and then jump into a weekend of sports activity are also prime candidates for problems.

To avoid a back problem, here are the factors that matter most:

- *Don't demand too much of your back muscles:* The familiar advice for lifting something heavy is to keep the object close to your body, keep your back straight, *bend your knees,* and *lift with your legs*. This advice is ignored with astonishing regularity, eventually to the sorrow of the lifter.[24]

  Any sport requiring lots of twisting, arching, and sudden starts and stops, such as racquet sports, golf, baseball, or basketball, can put you at risk for back problems. Thus, you should do warm-ups, stretches, and cool-downs before and after activity. Stretching helps lubricate the spinal joints.[25]

- *Build strong abdomen and back muscles:* Strong abdominal and back muscles help to support the spine and stabilize the lower back. Weak muscles allow your back to have an exaggerated curve that puts pressure on the nerves and disks.

  The best way to improve your abdominals is with exercise. The YMCA Healthy Back Program is devoted to strengthening the abdominal muscles. In one evaluation of the YMCA program, 82% of patients found their usual back pain stopped or decreased significantly.[26]

- *Move your body and don't smoke:* If you sit a lot, find ways to keep moving. It's all right to slump, fidget, cross and uncross your legs, stand up, sit down, and otherwise keep oxygenated blood circulating to the lower back muscles. If you smoke, you should be aware that it also restricts the flow of blood and oxygen.

If you suffer from periodic low-back pain, you can try to alleviate it with rest, aspirin, heat, hot tubs, and massage. Always sitting with good back support is also important. If it persists, however, you should consult a physician.

Arthritis **Arthritis** is an umbrella term covering over 100 different types of inflammation of the joints. The inflammation is frequently painful and often disabling and affects over 37 million Americans.[27] (See ● *Figure 28.2.*) Among the most common forms are *osteoarthritis* and *rheumatoid arthritis:*

- *Osteoarthritis:* **Osteoarthritis,** which usually develops in people over age 40, is progressive deterioration of the bones and joints caused largely by weight bearing and aging. Symptoms include swelling, pain, deformity, and restricted movement of joints.

- *Rheumatoid arthritis:* **Rheumatoid arthritis** is a deterioration of the joints that, for unknown reasons, results when the body's immune system attacks healthy cells in the joints. In about 2% of the population over age 15—more women than men—all the joints show symptoms of this disease: stiffness and joint pain in the beginning, followed by swelling, deformity, and limitations in mobility.

If you find yourself with early morning stiffness, swelling or recurring pain in a joint, or inability to move a joint normally, you should see a physician. Treatment often includes drugs to reduce inflammation and relieve pain and physical therapy to maintain mobility. Sometimes artificial joints are implanted surgically.

Digestive-Related Disorders

Some serious digestive-related disorders are inflammatory bowel disease, which include Crohn's disease and ulcerative colitis, and gallbladder disease.

Some digestion-related disorders are merely uncomfortable. Others, however, are quite serious, such as inflammatory bowel disease and gallbladder disease.

Inflammatory Bowel Disease: Crohn's and Colitis The term **inflammatory bowel disease** encompasses two entities, Crohn's disease and ulcerative colitis. Both are disorders of unknown origin characterized by chronic inflammations of sections of the digestive tract.

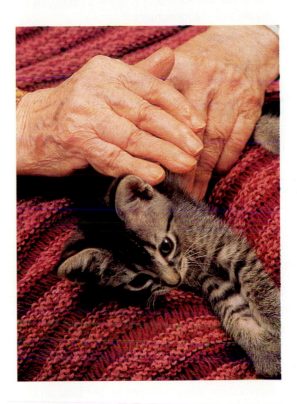

● **Figure 28.2 Arthritis.** Besides pain, arthritis often produces deformity of the joints.

"*Osteoarthritis is so common that nearly everyone over 40 shows some signs of it on X rays—a gradual loss of the soft, smooth cartilage at joint surfaces, and frequently a compensatory overgrowth of bone at the joints. It's estimated that 20 million Americans have symptoms of this joint disease at any given time. . . .*

Because of the pain and stiffness, the natural tendency is to minimize movement of arthritic joints. Unfortunately, this can simply to lead to stiffer joints—and thus more pain—since inactivity weakens the muscles that stabilize joints."

—Editors of the University of California *Wellness Letter.* (1991). *The wellness encyclopedia.* Boston: Houghton Mifflin, p. 383.

- *Crohn's disease:* The symptoms of **Crohn's disease** depend on the region of the bowel that is affected, but diarrhea, abdominal pain, cramps, and fever are most common. Diagnosis is made with an X ray and examination of the inside of the intestine with a flexible, lighted tube (the exam is a colonoscopy).

  Treatment is with drugs, including steroids and a drug called sulfasalazine. Surgery may be necessary to remove the diseased segment of the bowel.[28]

- *Ulcerative colitis:* **Ulcerative colitis** affects the colon and causes bouts of rectal bleeding and diarrhea. After about 20 years of the disease, a patient has a significant chance of developing cancer of the colon.[29]

  Treatment is with antidiarrhea medications, drug therapy such as steroids and sulfasalazine, and change in diet.

Gallbladder Disease Imagine having a hot poker thrust through your rib cage. That can be the feeling caused by a large gallstone. Roughly 20 million Americans have gallbladder disease, although only half seek treatment.[30] The disease typically affects middle-aged women who are overweight.

The gallbladder is a small, pear-shaped sac attached to the underside of the liver. Its purpose is to store bile produced by the liver and release it into the small intestine to aid digestion. **Gallbladder disease** occurs when the gallbladder has been irritated by infection or overuse, producing *gallstones*—formations of calcium, cholesterol, and minerals. Often these are as small as grains of sand and produce no symptoms. However, when they become enlarged, perhaps to the size of walnuts, they become stuck in the bile duct. They can cause several hours of intense pain, which may be mistaken for a heart attack. Diagnosis is made on the basis of X rays and other imaging techniques.

Treatment may be through the removal of the gallbladder, an operation performed on an estimated 500,000 Americans every year.[31] Nowadays many people have this done in a 45-minute "keyhole surgery" that uses imaging equipment. Called a *laparoscopic cholecystectomy,* the operation leaves only a tiny scar and usually allows the patient to go home in less than a day.[32,33]

Kidney Disorders

When kidneys fail, owing to infection or other causes, a person must have a kidney transplant or have waste fluids cleared by means of kidney dialysis. Kidney stones, which temporarily block the urinary system, are extremely painful.

In 1990, Steven Katona was a 30-year-old human development and family studies major at Pennsylvania State University, living in an unusual residence hall. Every Sunday, Tuesday, and Thursday he went one floor below his apartment and hooked himself up to a special piece of equipment that is not usually considered part of the undergraduate support system: a kidney dialysis machine. Penn State is, in fact, the only college that has a dialysis center in a students' residence building, and it is the reason, Katona said, he made it to college at all. Normally, patients requiring dialysis must make a trip to a hospital three times a week.[34]

Kidneys and Kidney Dialysis Your two kidneys are part of the excretory system, organs for removing excess water, toxic waste products, and surplus chemicals from the body. For some whose kidneys fail, the damage is permanent. Kidney damage can be produced by infection, diabetes, poisoning by mercury or lead, high blood pressure, or other problems.

Once permanent damage has occurred, the only alternatives are kidney dialysis or kidney transplants. Kidney transplants are an involved surgical procedure requiring a tissue-matched organ from a living relative or other donor. **Kidney dialysis** consists of a mechanical process for doing what the kidneys can no longer do themselves—clear waste fluids from the body. The patient is connected to a sophisticated filtering machine through which blood is circulated and impurities are removed.

Kidney Stones Having kidney stones, it is said, may be the closest men can come to knowing what women experience during the pain of childbirth.

The kidneys are located in the abdominal cavity, below the lowest rib. When difficulty with the kidneys occurs, it may at first be mistaken for a backache. However, the pain could indicate the presence of a **kidney "stone"** (technically called a *urinary calculus*). The stone usually consists of crystallized salts and minerals that stick together.[35] When it blocks the flow of urine from the kidney or bladder, the stone can cause excruciating agony. About 350,000 Americans every year have this frightening experience. Men, especially those ages 20–50, are more likely than women to have problems with kidney stones.[36]

Most of the time, the stones pass through on their own, bringing instant relief. However, if they do not, medical help must be sought to avoid kidney damage. The main procedure uses ultrasound to break up the stone.

To avoid kidney stones and other kidney disorders, you should drink lots of fluids, perhaps 8 ounces every waking hour. This is especially necessary when you're very active or during the summer months when your body loses fluids through perspiration.

Respiratory Disorders

One serious respiratory disorder is asthma, a chronic illness of the airways of the lungs. Another is chronic obstructive lung disease, which includes chronic bronchitis and pulmonary emphysema.

Take a deep breath, if you can. A couple of breaths not only momentarily relaxes you, it can remind you what a privilege it is to be able to perform this most elemental of life's activities. Some people, after all, have great difficulty doing this. Among the worst of the respiratory afflictions are asthma and chronic obstructive lung disease (COLD).

Asthma A chronic illness of the airways in the lungs, **asthma** leaves a person wheezing, coughing, and gasping for air, and afflicts 15 million Americans.[37] It is the most common cause of chronic illness for children and adolescents. Repeated attacks can damage the lungs and heart. Death rates from asthma have increased significantly in recent years.[38,39]

Asthma attacks may be mild or severe. In an asthmatic person, the attacks may be triggered by an allergic reaction, as to dust, pollen, or cigarette smoke; bacterial infections; weather changes; exercise; or stress or fatigue. During the attack, there is swelling of the mucous membrane lining the small tubes in the lungs called bronchioles. This causes the bronchioles to constrict, obstructing airflow and producing blockage and spasms.

Asthma is diagnosed using lung-function tests and by exposing the patient to whatever agent is suspected of triggering the attacks. Treatment, which should be under the direction of a physician, consists of identifying the triggering factors to avoid, increasing exercise endurance, alleviation of any emotional distress, and medications, often in the form of bronchodilators that, when inhaled, widen the airways in the lungs. (*See ● Figure 28.3.*)

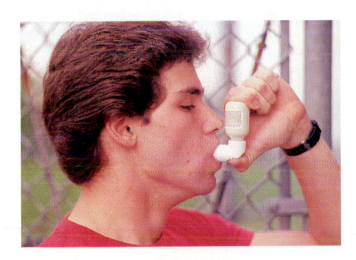

● **Figure 28.3 Asthma treatment.** Some asthma patients need a bronchodilator to relieve attacks.

“*Once asthma begins, it establishes a powerful feedback loop that may not even need an allergen to trigger an attack. General irritants such as cigarette smoke and urban smog can cause the already inflamed airways to constrict. 'It is my opinion that parents and caregivers who smoke in the presence of a child are guilty of child abuse,' says Dr. Allan Luskin of the Rush Medical Center in Illinois. 'Smoke not only increases the risk of a child getting asthma in the first place, it makes asthma worse when it is there.'*”

—Christine Gorman & Mary Cronin. (1992, June 22). Asthma: Deadly but treatable. *Time*, pp. 61–62.

Chronic Obstructive Lung Disease A slow, progressive interruption of air flow within the lungs characterizes **chronic obstructive lung disease (COLD).** People who have COLD may have *chronic bronchitis, pulmonary emphysema,* or both:

- *Chronic bronchitis:* **Chronic bronchitis** consists of inflamed airways to the lungs and the resultant increased production of mucus. These narrow air passages produce shortness of breath, labored breathing, and **sputum,** mucus coughed up from the throat.

- *Pulmonary emphysema:* **Pulmonary emphysema** is characterized by the loss of elasticity in the tiny air sacs (alveoli) of the lungs. The air sacs become less elastic and thus less able to expand and contract. In time, these air sacs are stretched to the point that they rupture. The chest cage becomes enlarged as it tries to accommodate the nonfunctional or overstretched air sacs, which makes the diaphragm work less efficiently.

  Ultimately, the impaired lung function interferes with the ability to exchange oxygen and carbon dioxide. This leads to continual shortness of breath and an overworked heart, which often leads to heart failure. Once the airways are destroyed, there is no way to reverse the process.

The biggest contributor to both chronic bronchitis and pulmonary emphysema is cigarette smoking.[40] Chronic bronchitis may also be brought about by the inhalation of sidestream (secondhand) smoke and environmental irritants such as chemicals. Both conditions are treated with drugs (such as antibiotics and epinephrine) and physical therapy.

Dental Disorders

Two major, and very preventable, dental diseases are cavities, caused principally by the teeth-coating film called *plaque,* and gum disease. The principal defense is brushing and flossing.

Do you go to the dentist? Do you floss? According to a one poll, 97% of Americans say regular dental checkups are important, but only 51% actually get a checkup at least twice a year. In addition, 80% say flossing is very important, but only 36% floss at least once a day.[41] In short, dental care is an area where people don't practice what they preach.

Cavities and Gum Disease Most of us are concerned about having great smiles and avoiding bad breath. However, dental checkups and flossing are subjects a number of us don't want to think about. Half of Americans hate going to the dentist, surveys show, and perhaps 12 million people show the sweaty-palms, heart-racing fear of dentists that constitutes a genuine phobia.[42] (*See ●Figure 28.4.*) Still, there are two major, and very preventable, dental diseases that can eventually affect your smile and your breath—cavities and gum disease:

- *Cavities:* About 95% of Americans have one or more cavities, or **dental caries,** the demineralization of tooth enamel often called "tooth decay."[43] Cavities are caused by **plaque,** a sticky, colorless film comprising bacteria that coats your teeth. When mixed with sugar and starches or allowed to reproduce, plaque bacteria produce toxic substances that lead to tooth decay and gum disease. Sometimes you can recognize a cavity as a hole or discoloration in the tooth, but more often it is discovered during a dental exam or because of a toothache.

- *Gum disease:* Cavities have actually been in decline, as a result of fluoridated water and toothpaste, and so today only 4% of Americans under age 65 are toothless, compared to 40% a generation ago.[44] The culprit that dentists now worry about is gum disease, or **periodontal disease.**

  In its early and still reversible form, periodontal disease is manifested as **gingivitis.** Signs of gingivitis include red and swollen gums that bleed easily, especially during brushing. Gingivitis is caused by the migration of plaque bacteria beneath the gum line.

  If not treated, gingivitis is followed by the more serious periodontal disease **periodontitis (pyorrhea),** characterized by permanent tooth, gum, and bone loss.

If you're concerned about bad breath (halitosis), you should know that it can be a tip-off to a form of periodontal disease. Gum disease now afflicts most children and adolescents, according to the American Academy of Periodontology.[45]

Strategy for Living: Brushing and Flossing
The weapons against bad breath and gum disease are well known—the toothbrush and dental floss:[46,47]

- *Brushing:* Soft-bristle brushes are better than hard. Hard bristles can cause gum abrasions, wear down the tooth enamel, and even cause a groove in the soft roots of your teeth if your gums recede. Because plaque is soft, it can be removed with a soft brush moved with a small, circular, vibrating motion. As one dentist advises, "You should brush your teeth as if you were waxing an antique Porsche, not scrubbing the kitchen sink."[48] Electric toothbrushes are also effective, and, if your dentist advises it, use an oral irrigator (such as Water Pik or Via-jet).[49]

- *Flossing:* "You don't have to floss all your teeth," says one writer, "only the ones you want to save."[50] People who say they don't have to time to floss should consider keeping the floss next to the TV set or carrying it in the car for use during traffic stoppages.

  Break off an 18-inch piece of floss (waxed or unwaxed, plain or flavored), wind one end around the middle finger of one hand, the other around the middle finger of the other. Insert the floss between your teeth and move it back and forth in a gentle sawing motion.

Even conscientious brushing and flossing won't eliminate all the plaque. Thus, you need to visit the dentist twice a year to have the dentist or dental hygienist remove this for you, as well as to check for signs of cavities and gum disease.

800-HELP

Crohn's and Colitis Foundation of America. 800-343-3637. For information on support groups for people coping with Crohn's disease and ulcerative colitis

Juvenile Diabetes Foundation. 800-223-1138 (in New York 212-889-7575)

National Asthma Center. 800-222-LUNG (in Denver 303-355-LUNG)

National Headache Foundation. 800-843-2256 (in Illinois 800-523-8858). Information on all types of headaches

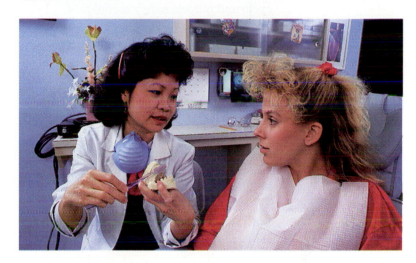

Figure 28.4 Fighting dental fear

❝*If you're among the millions who avoid the dentist because of a fear of pain, remember that you are not without recourse, as these steps suggest:*

- *Ask dental schools to help you find phobia and pain clinics in your area.*
- *Ask for referrals to dentists who treat phobic or anxious patients.*
- *Ask the dentist how he or she deals with a patient's fear or pain. If your dentist seems unsympathetic, go to another.*
- *Make sure you take control. You need not be a victim.*
- *If one dentist hurts you, find another who doesn't. You'll keep smiling that way—with your own teeth.*❞

—Carol Berczuk (1992, July 5). Are you afraid to go to the dentist? *Parade Magazine,* p. 13.

29 Personal Safety: Preventing Accidents and Violence

▶ Explain people's different reactions to involuntary and voluntary risks and what matters affect risk.

▶ Describe traffic safety techniques for avoiding hurting others and hurting yourself with a motor vehicle, including motorcycle and bicycle safety techniques.

▶ List the various types of home accidents and some rescue techniques.

▶ Describe the principal types of accidents that may happen in the outdoors.

▶ Discuss some important disorders that are work-related, including those involved with chemicals and computers.

▶ Explain the importance of murder, gunfire-related violence, and other forms of assault in the United States and some precautions to take.

▶ Discuss the dynamics of abusive relationships, and describe the abuse of children, including incest.

▶ Describe sexual harassment and rape, including date rape.

Who can forget the sight of a wrecked airliner on the television evening news? Such pictures make some people so afraid of flying they can hardly get on an airplane. However, if you go up in a commercial airliner, you'll be 10 times safer than if you made the same trip by car.[51] In fact, every time you fall down, you are six times more likely to be killed than when you travel in an airplane.[52]

Do these odds sound correct to you? The study of risks and odds is interesting because it often disproves our common perception as to what events are most threatening.

Chances Are: Risks and Accidents

We may worry more about involuntary risks, or those we can't control, than about voluntary risks, or those we can control. Risk assessment is determined by (1) how long one is exposed to a particular hazard, and (2) by legislation that decides what a risk is. Attitudes that affect personal safety include those relating to thrill seeking, drug taking, stress, aggression, inattention, denial, and failure to anticipate. Principal types of accidents are traffic, home-related, outdoor, and work-related.

If you're a white-knuckled flyer, you may be inclined to obsess about all that television news footage you've seen of crashed jetliners, whereas you almost never worry about driving in a car. Television and newspapers can have that effect. Because they often emphasize the sensational, the media can make us worry unduly about death from airplane crashes, shark attacks, lightning, tornados, or earthquakes. In fact, however, your risk of death is far, far greater from being in an auto accident. (*See ● Tables 29.1 and ● 29.2.*)

Voluntary Versus Involuntary Risks: The Question of Control "We worry much more about involuntary risks," observes one writer, "than those we choose of our own free will. Most of us seem to be willing to accept far greater risks—maybe 1000 times greater—in activities we choose than dangers that are imposed on us."[53] This is an extremely important point.

- *Involuntary risks:* Many people become upset at *involuntary* risks, risks over which they have no control, even if the odds are small. For example, in 1991, a notorious dentist, Dr. David Acer of Florida, who was believed to be criminally irresponsible in his sanitary practices, infected five patients with HIV—the only actual cases of HIV transmission in a health care setting. (Another Acer patient later also turned out to be HIV positive.)

12.13

*Chapter 29
Personal Safety:
Preventing
Accidents and
Violence*

No other cases of health care providers infecting patients with HIV are known. The Centers for Disease Control and Prevention (CDC) estimated that the risk of transmission of HIV from a surgeon to a patient was somewhere between 1 in 41,000 and 1 in 416,000. The risk of transmission from a dentist to a patient, the CDC estimated, was between 1 in 263,000 and 1 in 2.6 million.[54]

Despite these absurdly small risks, people were so upset about Dr. Acer that there were several attempts to pass laws regarding the transmission of AIDS by health care workers (for example, to allow sentencing HIV-positive surgeons to 10 years in jail for failing to reveal their health status). Similar levels of worry dominate discussions of nuclear safety, pollution control, food safety, pesticide contamination, airline security, and exposure to chemicals, all areas over which we often have no control.[55]

- *Voluntary risks:* By contrast, people take *voluntary* risks because they see some benefits associated with the behavior. (Indeed, there exists a whole field called *risk/benefit analysis.*) The "benefits" often are those of immediate pleasure or excitement or convenience. This is why people drink alcohol, smoke, do drugs, drive too fast, or take up risky hobbies such as scuba diving or hang gliding.

The acceptance of voluntary risks versus the reluctance to accept involuntary risks explains many ironies—for example, that of mountain climbers who protest the risk of nuclear power.[56]

Risk Analysis: The Effects of Time Duration, Legislation, and Politics Risk analysis (or risk assessment) is not an exact science. Still, the field is important because so many health regulations and lawsuits depend on its findings. Besides the voluntary and involuntary notion of risk, perhaps the two most important factors to understand are (1) the importance of the length of time you're exposed to a risk and (2) how legislation and politics affect the actions taken on risks.

- *Short-term versus long-term odds:* The risk of being killed in a quarry is 1 in 3100 if

Table 29.1 Threats: A comparison. Estimated risk for an American over a 50-year period

Type of risk: Risk of death from . . .	Odds over 50 years
Automobile accident	1 in 100
Homicide	1 in 300
Firearms accident	1 in 2000
Electrocution	1 in 5000
Airplane crash	1 in 20,000
Tornados	1 in 50,000
Fireworks	1 in 1,000,000
Botulism	1 in 2,000,000

Source: Adapted from: Chapman, C. R., & Morrison, D. (1991, June 18). Threats: A comparison. *New York Times*, p. B5.

you work there only a year. However, if you work there for 40 years, the risk of being killed is 1 in 80—significantly greater.[57] Thus, the duration of time and exposure to a risk is important data.

- *Legislative and political effects:* In the United States, food safety regulations are based on the Delaney Amendment of 1958, which requires chemicals be banned that are capable of causing cancer in animals or humans when used in processed food in *any* amount. However, does a chemical that causes cancer in laboratory rats in huge doses cause cancer in humans in small doses? Scientists don't think so, but the Delaney clause sets a limit of absolute zero. This was the reason that the pesticide Alar was banned from apples in 1989, although apple growers insisted a human would have to eat 28,000 pounds of apples a day before getting as much Alar as caused cancer in rats.[58]

Such political considerations also figure in implementing regulations on toxic-waste cleanup, automobile safety, and occupational hazards of all sorts.

The Importance of Attitude in Reducing Risks Every time you walk home in the dark, stand on a chair to change a light bulb, or get in

● **Table 29.2 Voluntary and involuntary risks**

Type of risk	Odds of death per person/year
Voluntary Risks	
Motorcycling	1 in 50
Smoking, 20 cigarettes per day	1 in 200
Horse racing	1 in 740[a]
Pregnancy (in United Kingdom)	1 in 4350[c]
Automobile driving (in United Kingdom)	1 in 5900[a]
Abortion, legal—after 14 weeks	1 in 5900[c]
Power boating	1 in 5900[a]
Rock climbing	1 in 7150[b]
Automobile racing	1 in 10,000
Drinking, 1 bottle of wine per day	1 in 13,300
Professional boxing	1 in 14,300
Soccer, football	1 in 25,000[a]
Taking contraceptive pills	1 in 50,000
Abortion, legal—under 12 weeks	1 in 50,000[c]
Canoeing	1 in 100,000[b]
Skiing	1 in 1,430,000[b]
Amateur boxing	1 in 2 million[a]
Involuntary Risks	
Influenza	1 in 5000
Leukemia	1 in 12,500
Struck by automobile	1 in 20,000
Floods	1 in 455,000
Tornados (Midwest)	1 in 455,000
Earthquake (California)	1 in 588,000
Bites of venomous creatures (in United Kingdom)	1 in 5 million
Falling aircraft	1 in 10 million
Lightning (in United Kingdom)	1 in 10 million
Release from atomic power station at site boundary	1 in 10 million
Flooding of dike (in the Netherlands)	1 in 10 million
Explosion, pressure vessel	1 in 20 million
Meteorite	1 in 100 billion

[a] Based on deaths per million participants per year.

[b] Based on deaths per million hours per year spent in sport.

[c] Based on deaths per million pregnancies per year.

Source: Adapted from: Dinman, B. D. (1980). The reality and acceptance of risk. *Journal of the American Medical Association, 244,* 1226–1228.

12.15

*Chapter 29
Personal Safety:
Preventing
Accidents and
Violence*

a car, you are consciously or unconsciously making an assessment of your risks. Indeed, your *attitude* about risks is the whole reason for having this chapter.

In the United States, your chances of being murdered are 1 in 170 in the course of your lifetime, odds that most of us think are unacceptable. Yet your lifetime chances of being killed in a home accident are even greater—about 1 in 130. And your lifetime chances of being killed in a road accident are greater still—about 1 in 60.[59] The latter two kinds of risks, however, are those most of us cheerfully assume.

You cannot control some risks inherent in voluntary situations: in a car, for example, you're at risk from the unpredictability of other drivers. However, you can improve your odds in other ways. This is where your attitude comes in. Do you or do you not drive fast, drive drunk, drive half asleep, drive with mechanical defects, drive without using a seat belt? All these are risks *you* can control.

Attitudes that affect your safety include thrill seeking, drug taking, stress, aggression, inattention, denial, and failure to anticipate:

- *Avoiding boredom and seeking thrills:* A lot of things we have to do in life are boring, but some people have trouble with that fact. Indeed, some people don't think they're alive unless they're living on the edge. Such sensation seekers clearly increase the risk of accidents to themselves. Are you one of them? (*See Life Skill, "Boredom and Risk-Taking: Understanding Your Need for Excitement," at the end of this chapter.*)

- *Alcohol and other drugs:* Excessive drinking is so widespread that you probably know of someone who has been arrested for drunken driving or drinking-related crimes. You may also know someone who has been injured (or injured someone else) as a result of alcohol-related behavior. Is there a lesson in this?

  The same observations apply with other drugs, such as cocaine. While one is on them, drugs *may* make a person feel almost larger than life, impervious to mistakes. But the statistics on accidents, as well as suicides and homicides, run almost entirely the other way.

- *Stress:* Stress can distort your thinking. If you're late for a job interview, for example, you may tend to take chances on crossing the street or race the light at intersections. Stress can also distract you, as when you're worrying about an important exam or breaking up with your lover. Stress, in a word, makes you *careless*. Thus, when you're feeling tense, you should do what you can to lower your stress level.

- *Aggression:* Nothing can cloud your judgment like getting mad at somebody. You see this happen with drivers all the time. Otherwise civilized people become enraged when another driver cuts them off or beats them out of a parking place and try to exact "revenge" ("That turkey needs a lesson!"). People become walking (or driving) accidents because they allow matters of supposed "honor" or "respect" or "payback" to overwhelm more rational ideas about personal safety.

- *Inattention:* Daydreaming or letting your mind wander can do you in. Many a driver has looked down to adjust the car radio and rear-ended the car ahead. Farmers, who work around dangerous equipment, have become injured when they looked away at a crucial moment. Boaters have gotten in trouble because they didn't look at tide tables and skiers because they didn't attend to weather reports. Pedestrians in crime-prone areas learn how to keep their wits about them and avoid trouble, as we shall discuss.

- *Denial:* Some of the biggest risks aren't flashy and so they are easy to ignore or explain away. For instance, terrorism fears caused thousands of Americans to cancel overseas travel plans during the 1991 Persian Gulf War, although the chance of dying by a terrorist's hand has been pegged at only 1 in 650,000.[60] Yet you can be sure that many of these same Americans refused to reconsider their smoking, drinking, and driving habits. Denial ("That will never happen to me") enables many people to disregard the threat of low-profile calamities such as car crashes and home accidents.

- *Failure to anticipate or prepare:* Although some accidents cannot be anticipated or prevented, many can. For example, some truck drivers with excellent safety records make a point of mentally practicing "what-if" possibilities so that they can react appropriately to avoid accidents. ("What if I rounded the bend and found a car stopped dead in the middle of the highway . . ." "What if a car pulled out of that side road . . .")

Besides mental preparation, there are also other kinds of preparation. If you're driving for a weekend of skiing, for example, you need to listen to weather reports; carry tire chains, flares, and food and water (in case you get stuck); wear appropriate clothing; and once you get to the ski slopes take lessons or otherwise become properly trained. The way to avoid bad luck, in other words, is to *anticipate the possibility* of bad luck.

Types of Accidents Accidents are defined as unexpected events that produce injury or death. In the United States, accidents are the fourth leading cause of death, after heart disease, cancer, and stroke.[61] For people between the ages of 1 and 37—which certainly includes a lot of readers of this book—accidents are *the* leading cause of death.

Some people have accidents more often than others, and some types of accidents are more common than others. As you might expect, children are at risk for many accidents, simply because they do not have the judgment to recognize dangerous situations. Older people also are at risk, because of impaired sight, hearing, agility, reflexes, and resilience. People ages 15–24 years are at particular risk for accidents, including motor vehicle, drowning, firearms, and poisoning by gases and vapors.[62] About 69% of all accidental deaths involve males.[63] Left-handed people have more accidents than right-handed people, perhaps because they are operating in a world not designed for lefties.[64]

As for types of accidents, they may be classified as follows:[65]

- *Traffic accidents:* Motor vehicle accidents (including motorcycle accidents) cause the greatest number of deaths, about 50,000 a year in the United States. In addition, 2 million people are seriously injured. We also consider bicycle accidents in this category.

- *Home-related accidents:* Because people spend so much of their time at home, that is where most accidents happen: falls, burns, poisonings, suffocations, electrical shock, and the like.

- *Outdoor accidents:* Outdoor accidents are often associated with recreation. The most common include drowning and near drowning, diving accidents, falls, overexposure to heat and cold, and athletic injuries.

- *Work-related accidents:* Deaths from work-related accidents are apt to be associated with farm machinery, construction, and heavy industry. However, severe injuries can happen in jobs you might not suspect, such as office work involving heavy computer use.

Let us consider some of these.

A Crash Course in Traffic Safety: Strategy for Living

Part of traffic safety is driving to avoid hurting others: surrounding yourself with a defensive "bubble" of space, not speeding, running red lights, drinking and driving, driving while fatigued, driving with distractions. The other part is driving to avoid hurting yourself: using seat belts, learning crash-avoidance techniques, being patient, being in a safe car. Riding on motorcycles and bicycles requires particular vigilance.

Not everyone knows how to drive, but probably most readers of this book, including bicyclists and pedestrians, are exposed to the dangers of driving. As the driver of a car, motorcycle, or bicycle, you have two concerns: to avoid injuring others and to avoid injuring yourself. Often the two concerns overlap.

12.17

*Chapter 29
Personal Safety:
Preventing
Accidents and
Violence*

Driving to Avoid Hurting Others The young driver looked down to change a music tape in her dashboard tape deck. When she looked up again, she had drifted slightly off the road and was too late to avoid hitting four bicyclists riding single file, all of whom were killed. This young college student was not only convicted of manslaughter but will have to bear the pain of her experience for the rest of her life.

About 95% of the automobile deaths and injuries are due to careless or reckless driving such as this. (The rest are caused by mechanical failure of the vehicle.)[66] To avoid having a similar tragic episode in your life, here are some tips:

- *Surround yourself with a "bubble" of space:* Don't tailgate cars in front, avoid traveling next to cars in other lanes, and try not to let cars behind you crowd you (let them go around). This "bubble" or "defensive space" keeps you away from other cars and gives you some room to maneuver. When you enter situations such as interchanges or heavy traffic, slow down to allow for a smaller bubble.[67]

- *Don't speed:* Speed is a leading cause of accidents in general. The reasons are simple: the faster you go, the less reaction time you have to stop and the heavier the force of impact when you hit something. Speeding on rain-slick or icy roads means you have no control over the vehicle. Speed-limit signs indicate the *maximum* speed allowed under *ideal* conditions. This means if you are driving at night or during bad weather, you should drive more slowly.

  We realize that so many people speed that it can almost make you feel uncomfortable to drive under the speed limit because people may crowd you from behind. But that's *their* problem. *Your* problem is to not let yourself feel harassed just because you're holding up someone who wants to go faster.

- *Don't be a red light bandit:* Not surprisingly, the rules-don't-apply-to-me drivers who try to beat the yellow light at an intersection and find themselves going through on the red are extremely dangerous. In San Francisco, for instance, up to 29% of the injury accidents are caused by drivers who run red lights.[68]

- *Don't drink and drive:* Alcohol is responsible for about *half* of all automobile accidents and is the leading cause of automobile fatalities. No stronger message can be sent about the reasons for the steady drumbeat of advertising begging you not to drink and drive.

- *Don't become fatigued:* After alcohol, the second cause of serious accidents is fatigue (which is worst from 3 P.M. to 2 A.M.). Drowsiness can be caused not only by lack of sleep but also by certain medications, such as tranquilizers, muscle relaxants, antidepressants, antihistamines, and some cold and flu remedies.[69]

- *Don't smoke and drive:* People who smoke while driving are 50% more likely to be involved in a mishap than those who don't smoke.[70] Fumbling with cigarettes, eye irritation, filmy windshields, and the interference of carbon monoxide with night vision are all reasons.

- *Don't try to do two things at once:* A nonscientific study of 500 traffic-school students in South Florida found that three-quarters of them drink a beverage, eat, or do both while driving. About half admitted applying makeup or writing notes. More than 40% said they sometimes kiss and drive at the same time.[71] You can't do these things and keep your mind on your driving.

  Incidentally, many people are convinced they can hold a cellular phone to one ear while maneuvering 1½ tons of metal through traffic. There are no statistics on traffic accidents related to these wireless phones, but clearly mobile callers don't have their full attention on the road.[72]

Driving to Avoid Hurting Yourself Young drivers, ages 15–24, have the highest death rates, owing to lack of experience and judgment. The second highest death rate is among drivers over the age of 75 (nearly tied with those ages 25–44), owing to slowing of reaction times and deterioration of the senses. (See ● *Figure 29.1.*) Regardless of the current age group in which you find yourself, you can reduce the chances of injuring or killing yourself by adopting the habits described above and then also doing the following:

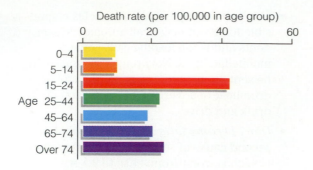

Death rate (per 100,000 in age group)

Age

Figure legend axis values: 0, 20, 40, 60

Age groups: 0–4, 5–14, 15–24, 25–44, 45–64, 65–74, Over 74

● **Figure 29.1 Deaths from motor vehicle accidents, by age.** People ages 15–24 have the highest rate of deaths in motor vehicle (car and motorcycle) accidents. Those over age 74 have the second highest rate.

- *Use seat belts:* The percentage of people admitting they don't use seat belts varies tremendously, from a low of 6% in Hawaii to a high of 62% in South Dakota.[73] However, there is no valid reason *not* to use seat belts.

  Whereas some health behaviors are somewhat complex, such as exercising or losing weight, there is nothing complicated about putting on a seat belt. Yet the 2 seconds it takes to buckle up can reduce the chances of accidental death by 50%—an incredible amount of protection in return for the tiny effort invested.[74]

  Some people think there's no need to buckle up when on short trips or when not driving fast. However, three-quarters of all crashes are within 25 miles of home and 80% of deaths and injuries occur under 40 mph.[75] Some people also think that in a crash they would be better off being "thrown clear," although actually they would be 25 times more likely to be killed. Finally, although you may be a good driver yourself, you may not be able to prevent someone else—a drunk driver, say—from hitting you.

  We repeat: *The single most effective thing you can do in a car to protect your life is to use a seat belt.*

- *Know crash-avoidance driving techniques:* Many people don't know how to handle themselves when driving in bad weather. They drive as fast on rain-slicked pavements as they do when it's dry, and wonder why they go into a skid when they hit the brakes. In fog they pull close to the car or truck in front and follow its lights, eliminating room to stop.[76] When someone veers into their lane, they choose a head-on accident rather than risk a less lethal crash to the side or off the road. Some crash survival techniques don't square with most people's driving habits but are well worth learning. (See ● *Figure 29.2.*)

- *Learn patience to avoid stress:* It has been found that the longer people commute, the higher their blood pressure afterward, the worse the stress they feel, and the more they carry over that stress into the office or home afterward.[77] How does one deal with this? You can practice patience, or what psychotherapist Todd Berger, co-author of *Zen Driving,* calls "moving meditation"—driving with full awareness and relaxed concentration.

  "In Zen driving," he says, "you let go. You drop what you were thinking about before, and you drop your destination. All that matters is what you are doing *right now.* Anything that gets in the way, like anger, fear, or tension, is calmly acknowledged. Then you let the emotion go, and return your attention to the pure experience, and awareness of the present moment. A guy in a pickup truck cuts you off. It makes you mad. You acknowledge the anger, and let it go. Then you go back to total awareness and feeling the car around you."[78]

- *Drive or ride in a safe car:* Big cars are usually safer than small cars in crashes. However, a large car is not necessarily a safer car.[79–81] The critical factor is design, which can compensate for small size and light weight. Cars of whatever size built with tough roofs and sides, a frame designed to absorb collision, interior padding, anti-lock brakes, and air bags are more apt to protect drivers and passengers than cars not so designed. Air bags in particular have proven to be a lifesaving feature.

12.19

*Chapter 29
Personal Safety:
Preventing
Accidents and
Violence*

Making sure the car you are in is mechanically sound or fully equipped can also make a big difference. For instance, nearly half of all taxicabs nationwide have no seat belts in the rear seat or the belts are broken or inaccessible behind the seat cushions, leading to serious head and neck injuries of passengers in the estimated 100,000 crashes cabs are involved in each year.[82]

Motorcycle Safety Mile for mile, motorcycles are more dangerous than cars, the chief reasons being that they are hard to see and other motorists often forget that motorcycles are there. Some motorcyclists add to their chances of injury by "lane splitting," riding between traffic lanes when cars are slowing or stopped. Despite the argument (not true) that a helmet decreases vision, helmet laws have been shown to reduce head injuries.[83–87]

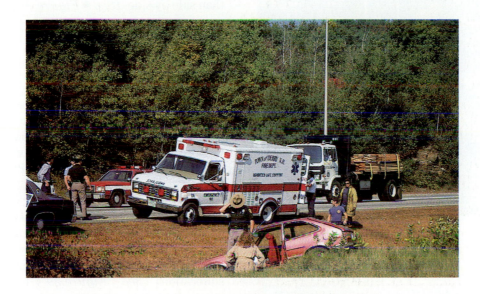

● **Figure 29.2 Crash-avoidance techniques**

1. **ALWAYS try to avoid a head-on crash.** Your chances of surviving almost any other crash are better than of surviving a head-on collision.
2. **Go off-road, if necessary.** Get rid of the idea that your car *always* belongs on the pavement. If you are close to having an on-road collision, and pedestrians, bicyclists, or motorcyclists are not in your way, *drive off the road*. Driving onto a sidewalk or lawn or into a field may save your life.
3. **Steer your way clear and brake gently off-road.** As you drive off the pavement, try to steer to avoid skidding. Also, don't brake too hard when you're off road, which may trip up the vehicle and cause it to roll over.
4. **Hit a car going your way.** If you are about to crash into a car stopped in front of you or approaching you, and have to hit another vehicle, *hit one going in the same direction you are*. Hitting one traveling beside you in the next lane will have less impact than hitting one in front.
5. **Hit objects that will yield somewhat, and hit with a glancing blow.** If you have to have a collision, don't hit a massive immovable object, such as a concrete abutment or a brick building. Try to pick something that has some "give," such as small trees, parked cars, or wood-frame buildings. Whatever object you run in to, try to give it a glancing blow, which will lessen the impact.

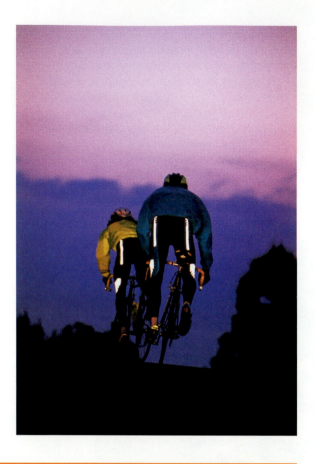

Bicycle Safety Bicyclists also benefit from having helmets.[88] Of the 1300 bicyclists killed each year, most die from head injuries, and the odds of injury are six times greater for the un-helmeted compared to the helmeted.[89] In addition, bicyclists need to be sure they are visible to motorists, using bright-colored clothing, reflectors, and headlights and taillights at night. Ride as though your life depended on it, because it does: stop at stop signs, signal for turns, use bike lanes when available, and when riding with others proceed single file rather than side by side. (*See* ● *Figure 29.3.*)

Home Safe: Strategy for Living

Common home accidents are from falls, burns and fires, poisonings, electrical shocks, choking, and eye and limb injuries. Good rescue techniques to know are cardiopulmonary resuscitation (CPR) and the Heimlich maneuver.

People tend to feel safest in their own homes, so it's ironic that that's where most accidents and injuries occur. Most of these are the result of falls, fires and burns, poisonings, and suffocations. (*See* ● *Figure 29.4.*)

Falls Falls are the leading cause of nonfatal injuries in the United States and the second leading cause of death from injury (after motor vehicle accidents).[90] In one survey of 70,000 Americans by Rand Corporation, it was found that almost 2 out of 5 nonfatal injuries were due to slips and falls.[91] Falls on stairs and falls on the floor are the two leading causes of emergency-room visits for injuries.

Falls are a particular affliction of older people. In older bones, falls often produce hip fractures—about 172,000 every year in the United States—and roughly half the survivors never recover normal function.[92,93]

Falls in the bathroom may be caused by the combination of slippery and hard surfaces. A nonskid rubber tub mat and handrails (not towel bars, which may break) in the tub or shower may help avoid them. Falls in the kitchen may occur because of spills, inadequate lighting, and attempts to reach items on high

● **Figure 29.3 Bicycle safety**

Bicycling is . . .

- *. . . Like driving a car in some respects:* Many of the same traffic laws apply, including those of stop signs and traffic signals. Signal (using hand signals) your intention to change directions. Go in a straight line and don't weave. Slow down on rainy days.

- *. . . But you're much less visible than a car:* Drivers don't see bicycles as readily as they do other cars. Thus, at night you should have a rear red reflector, a light emitting a bright beam forward and to the sides, and reflectors on the frame or wheels, or reflecting tape on your clothes. In the daytime, wear bright clothes.

- *. . . And much more vulnerable than a motorist:* You need to be especially alert to the hazards of the road. Check for cars before you make a turn. Watch for sewer grates, pot holes, gravel, and low-hanging branches. Keep at least one hand on the handlebars. Avoid clothing that might get caught in the chain or spokes (long scarves and coats or baggy trousers or dresses). Wear a helmet.

12.21

*Chapter 29
Personal Safety:
Preventing
Accidents and
Violence*

shelves. Spills should be wiped up immediately and you should not carry loads you can't see over. In other rooms, electrical and phone cords should be taped down.

Burns and Fires Fires are the third leading cause of unintentional injury death in the United States (following falls and drownings). Each year, residential fires—in which most injuries from fire occur—are responsible for about 5000 deaths.[94]

Interestingly, even though the United States has some of the fastest fire departments in the world, it has more fire deaths than nearly any other industrialized country. The United States has twice Japan's population and 40 times as many fires. It spends a great deal less on preventing fires than on fighting them.[95] Fire-safety lessons are aimed mostly at children, but they cause only 9% of all fire deaths.

It is adults who leave pans on the stove, overload house wiring, and buy unsafe heaters.

Adults also drink, and experts say alcohol plays nearly as important a role in fires as it does in auto accidents: alcohol is involved in 40% of all fatal fires and burns.[96] In addition, adults smoke, and cigarettes cause about 25% of residential fires, usually by setting fire to bedding or upholstery.[97] Smoking is responsible for 29% of deaths in home fires, and cooking causes 22% of injuries.[98]

Three factors can be significant in preventing fire injuries and fatalities:

- *Smoke detectors:* Fire deaths have dropped steadily in the United States during the last few decades in part because 85% of all homes now have smoke detectors.[99] Still, smoke detectors often fail to operate because of incorrect installation or inadequate testing. Moreover, some people (the elderly) may not hear them, and others (children) may not respond to them.

- *Responsibility:* Other industrialized countries, such as Japan and those in Western

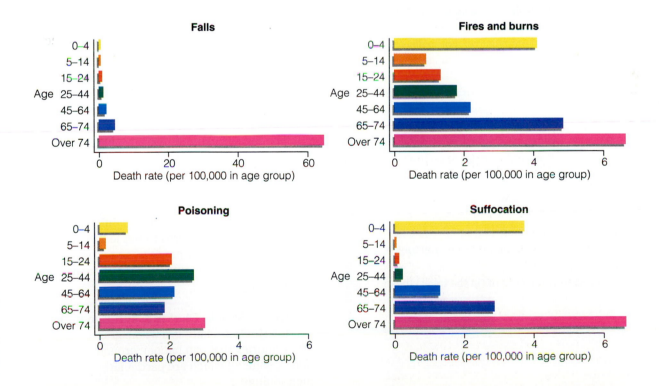

● **Figure 29.4 Common types of accidental deaths.** Many of these occur at home.

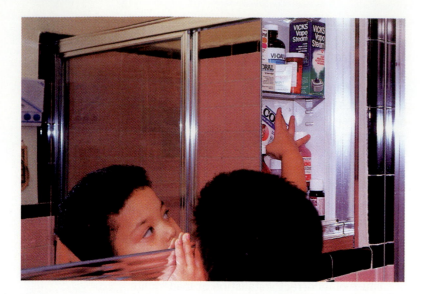

● **Figure 29.5 Sheer poison**

To prevent poisoning in children:

- Keep pills, drugs, vitamins, and cosmetics out of children's reach. Buy products in child-resistant packaging or containers.
- Store cleaning supplies, rat and ant poisons, mothballs, and aerosol cans in a locked place. Never store them under the sink.
- Be sure hazardous materials in the garage or intended for outdoor use—paint, gasoline, lighter fluid, antifreeze, certain toxic plants—are secure.
- Don't leave a child alone with a toxic product even for a minute; take it with you to answer the phone or doorbell.

To prevent poisoning in older adults:

- If you are over 65, read the label before taking a pill. (Don't take it at night with the light off or without glasses.)
- Post a sheet and regularly check it off every time you take medication so you'll never be uncertain whether you took a pill or not.
- Check the expiration date and get rid of (in the toilet) those that are outdated.

Europe, treat fires as either a personal failing or a crime, punished by social rejection and prison, just as the United States does with drunken drivers. In the United States, however, the attitude is that "fires are not really anyone's fault."[100] You're in a position to adopt a new attitude as a strategy for living: the view that no one is to blame for careless fires is simply incorrect.

- *Escape plan:* Many people grew up with fire drills at school. Do you have one for you (and your family or housemates) where you live? Safety experts urge residents to draw floor plans of their dwellings and mark not just one but *two* ways of escaping from each room. Then you should practice, with all other members of your household, getting out of the building and regrouping at a predesignated meeting place.[101]

Poisoning Unintentional poisonings account for 3300 deaths per year in the United States.[102] The largest group is of children under age 5, who think household chemicals and medications are food or candy. The next largest group is people older than age 65, who may take medications without checking the labels. (*See ● Figure 29.5.*) Reduction in childhood poisoning has been associated with federal legislation requiring child-resistant containers for aspirin, prescription drugs, household chemicals, and similar substances.

The biggest cause of gas poisoning is carbon monoxide, which is colorless and odorless. The way you know you've been affected is first when you feel headache, blurred vision, and shortness of breath, followed by dizziness and vomiting. Make sure wood stoves, furnaces, and gas and kerosene heaters are not leaking. Work on car engines, power mowers, and other gasoline-powered equipment outside rather than in closed garages.

Electrical Shock, Choking, and Eye and Limb Injuries There is a whole grab-bag of other injuries that can happen around the house, some of which are particularly worth mentioning:

- *Electrical shocks:* Any electrical equipment that causes a tingling sensation when you touch it can mean bad news—especially if

12.23

*Chapter 29
Personal Safety:
Preventing
Accidents and
Violence*

you have wet hands or are standing in water. People tend to shrug off electrical shocks, but the jolt can actually cause more damage to your heart or other organs than it first seems. Avoid using frayed extension cords, buy irons that turn themselves off when not in use and space heaters that shut down when tipped over, and above all don't use electrical appliances when you're wet or touching water.

If you are with someone who has suffered electrical shock that has knocked him or her unconscious, the first order of business is to remove or shut off the electrical current. Next quickly call (or have someone call) 911 or another emergency number to get medical assistance.[103] If you have been properly trained, you may then attempt life-saving measures such as **cardiopulmonary resuscitation (CPR).** This technique consists of two parts: (1) **rescue breathing,** in which you force air into the nonbreathing victim's lungs; and (2) heart massage, in which you do chest compressions to stimulate a stopped heart.

- *Choking:* Most choking is the result of haste. Food, such as a big piece of meat, that has not been chewed properly can block the windpipe. Often this happens with someone who has been drinking alcohol or using other drugs, but not necessarily. To avoid choking, it's best to eat in a relaxed fashion—cut your food into small pieces, chew thoroughly, and don't try to talk when swallowing.

  If you see someone choking, or if you are choking yourself, you should *quickly* act to dislodge the food in the windpipe. The procedure for doing this is the **Heimlich maneuver,** the manual application of sudden upward pressure on the abdomen to force the object from the windpipe. (*See* ● *Figure 29.6.*)

- *Eye and limb injuries:* Power tools and lawn mowers, as well as games such as racquetball and squash, can be hazardous to the unprotected eye. As one emergency-room physician writes, "Virtually all eye injuries can be avoided by remembering three words: goggles, goggles, goggles."[104] If you wear eye glasses, an eye doctor can prescribe prescription goggles.

When working around power tools, such as lawn mowers, chain saws, and snow blowers, you need to exercise extra care to avoid the involuntary removal of fingers and toes. Wear special gloves and steel-toed boots. Make sure long hair is tied back out of the way. Be certain to shut off the engine before unjamming equipment.

Survival in the Outdoors

Accidents in the outdoors result from lack of preparation for changes in weather, drowning, and animal bites.

You can get into as much trouble outdoors as indoors. Elsewhere in this book (Chapter 17) we described the dangers from not adjusting your clothing and physical activity to accommodate hot weather (heat exhaustion and heat stroke) and cold weather (frostnip, frostbite, and hypothermia). Even when weather is not a problem, however, there are at least two other hazards that bear your attention—drowning and animal bites.

Drowning About 7700 Americans die each year by drowning, including about 1200 in boating accidents.[105,106] The people at greatest risk are small children ages 1–3. Small children most often drown in backyard swimming pools, because adults are unaware they have wandered near the water; these accidents are preventable with fences and latchgates.

The next group at greatest risk is males ages 15–24. (*See* ● *Figure 29.7.*) Adolescents and adults most often drown in lakes, rivers, and ponds while swimming, wading, diving, boating, rafting, and fishing—in other words, at places that are not organized facilities with lifeguards.[107] Many drownings occur when people are exhausted or are swept into deep water.

It's important to know that alcohol and other drugs figure prominently in drowning and boating mishaps. About half of drowning victims have a high blood alcohol level, and about 10% show evidence of having taken other drugs.[108]

First aid for drowning victims consists of administering CPR for as long as possible. Some people have recovered who have been submerged for more than an hour.

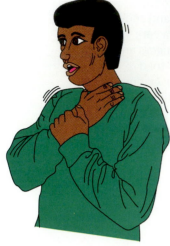

Step 1: Establish if the person is choking: Ask, "Are you choking?" or "Can you speak?" If the person nods and cannot speak, something is obstructing the windpipe. If the person can make some sounds, it may be better to let him or her clear the airway by coughing.

Step 2: Perform the Heimlich maneuver: If the person cannot speak, perform the following:
• Stand behind the person.
• Make a fist and put it slightly above the navel (higher on the chest in an obese or pregnant person). The thumb should be toward the choking person. Grasp the fist with your other hand (drawing).

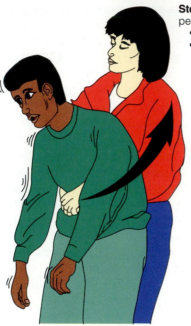

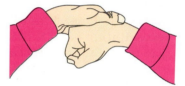

• Thrust **forcefully and quickly** inward and upward against the person's abdomen to dislodge the obstruction. Repeat if necessary.

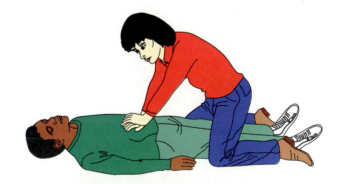

• If the person is unconscious, roll him or her on his back, straddle the person, place one hand above the navel with the second on top, and thrust both hands quickly upward into the abdomen.

● **Figure 29.6 The Heimlich maneuver**

"*If you're choking, you don't have to rely on someone else to come to your rescue. Stand up and make a fist with one hand and place the thumb side on the abdomen just above your navel. Now grab your fist and press inward and upward with a quick, sharp thrust. If that doesn't dislodge the stuck food, try again, this time throwing your weight forward over the back of a chair, so your fist is driven up hard into your abdomen.*"

—Emergency-room physician Arnold G. Robinson, M. D. (1991, April). Painful mistakes. *Men's Health*, p. 33.

12.25

Chapter 29
Personal Safety:
Preventing
Accidents and
Violence

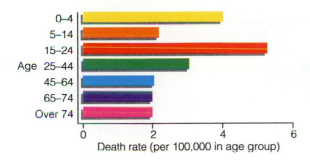

● **Figure 29.7 Drowning**

Animal Bites So you think meter readers, mail carriers, and dogcatchers are most apt to be bitten by animals? Actually, people in such lines of work are usually cautious and therefore rarely bitten. More likely victims are children. The great majority of the 2 million bite wounds reported annually in the United States, 80–85%, are inflicted by domestic dogs; cats account for about 10%. About 20 Americans die every year from dog attacks, half of them by pit bull terriers.[109] Treatment must first be for traumatic damage and then for bacterial infection. A health professional should always examine the wound. As a preventative, you should make sure that immunizations are up to date—tetanus and hepatitis B for people and rabies for pets.

Caution: Work May Be Hazardous to Your Health

Overexertion, being struck, and falls produce the most common work-related disabling injuries. Other injuries are caused by breathing tobacco smoke and exposure to industrial chemicals. Computer-related jobs may lead to serious repetitive strain injury (RSI), as well as eye strain, headache, and back and neck pains.

Work, says one writer, "kills more people each year than die from AIDS, drugs, or drunken driving and all other motor vehicle accidents."[110] Since the passage of the Occupa-

tional Safety and Health Act of 1970—legislation designed to enhance worker safety—some 200,000 workers have been killed on the job in the United States, 2 million more have died from diseases caused by the conditions in which they worked, and 1.4 million have been disabled in workplace accidents.[111]

Work-related fatalities actually dropped to 10,500 in 1991 from 12,500 a decade earlier; however, that is partly because steel, shipbuilding, logging, and other highly unsafe industries were in recession. Meanwhile, job-related illness and crippling injuries increased.[112–114] Much of the lack of safety in worker conditions has been attributed to the fact that the Occupational Safety and Health Administration (OSHA) is understaffed and enforcement is too limited: a mere 3% of American workplaces are inspected annually for safety.[115]

Restaurants and bars account for the largest number of occupational injuries, but meat packing and motor-vehicle manufacturing are by far the most dangerous industries.[116] The most common disabling work injuries are overexertion, followed by being struck by or against an object and falls.[117] (*See* ● *Figure 29.8.*) However, some other workplace hazards particularly deserve mention—chemicals and computers.

The Hazards of Smoke and Certain Chemicals Waiters and waitresses, although they might not smoke themselves, have as much as five times more exposure to cigarette smoke than people in other workplaces and have a significantly higher risk of lung cancer—perhaps 50–90% more, according to one study.[118] Indeed, the study found that waitresses die of lung cancer nearly four times more often than other women and twice as often of heart disease.

Tobacco smoke is not the only harmful chemical found in the workplace. Toxic solvents, dyes, lead dusts, plastics, metals, or other chemicals are part of the work environments of artists, art teachers, chemistry and biology teachers, operating room personnel, laboratory workers, machine operators, electrical or circuit board workers, launderers, dry cleaners, book binders, furniture refinishers, cosmetologists, health aides, telephone operators, automobile mechanics, and many other workers. If you are in such an environment, you

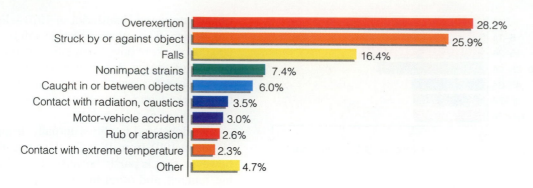

- **Figure 29.8 Accidents on the job**

should follow safety guidelines and use protective clothing and equipment. Women who are pregnant should try to ask for a temporary job transfer.[119]

The Hazards of Computers The computer is supposed to make us more efficient, but for some people—clerical workers, word processors, postal clerks, journalists—it has turned out to be quite uncomfortable and for some even to disable them so that they can no longer perform their jobs. The reasons are repetitive strain injury, eyestrain and headache, and back and neck pains.[120]

- *Avoiding repetitive strain injury:* **Repetitive strain injury (RSI)**—also called **repetitive motion injury** and **cumulative trauma disorders**—is the name given to a number of wrist, hand, arm, and neck pains resulting from fast, repetitive work. Whereas once RSI victims were mainly slaughterhouse, textile, and automobile workers, and musicians (because of long hours of practice), the increase in computer users during the last decade has made the disorder the fastest-growing work injury in recent years.[121–127]

  One kind of RSI called **carpal tunnel syndrome (CTS),** consisting of damage and pain to nerves and tendons in the hands, is virulent among heavy computer users, some of whom may make as many as 23,000 keystrokes a day. (*See* ● *Figure 29.9.*) Some CTS sufferers cannot type or

even open a door. As a result of this and similar computer-related injuries, there has been considerable interest in **ergonomics,** the study of human factors to consider in designing and arranging tools for safe and effective use. Ergonomics is concerned with fitting the job to the worker rather than the reverse.

- *Avoiding eyestrain and headache:* Human eyes were made for most efficient seeing at a distance. However, computer screens require that you use your eyes at reasonably close range for a long time. This can lead to eyestrain, headache, and double vision.

  To avoid these difficulties, you should take a 15-minute break every hour or so. Position the screen so it's not in direct sunlight and doesn't reflect glare from lights. Make sure the brightness of the screen and the surrounding area are about the same, so your eyes won't have to keep adjusting. Consider installing an antiglare filter.

- *Avoiding back and neck pains:* Many people work at computers in work situations that produce back and neck pain. Often the computers are simply installed on desks intended for typewriters, but the two kinds of equipment are not alike. To avoid problems, you should have a chair that is adjustable for height and back. The height of the keyboard, the computer screen, and the document holder should also all be adjustable.

12.27

*Chapter 29
Personal Safety:
Preventing
Accidents and
Violence*

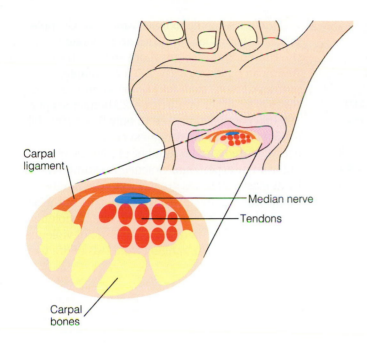

Carpal Tunnel Syndrome

The carpal ligament creates a tunnel across the bones of the wrist. When tendons passing through the carpal tunnel become swollen, they press against the median nerve, which runs to the thumb and first three fingers.

Carpal ligament

Median nerve

Tendons

Carpal bones

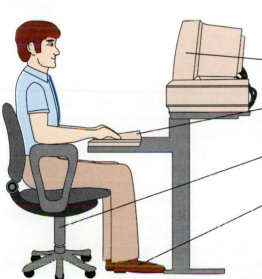

Ideal Setup for Working at Computer

The position of the computer and your posture are important.

Screen: At eye level or slightly lower. Your head should be about an arm's length from the screen. Avoid having light throw glare on the screen.

Keyboard: At or below elbow level. Elbows should be at about right angle. Hands and wrists should be straight and relaxed. Fingers should be gently curved. A wrist rest helps.

Chair: Chair should keep back upright or inclined slightly forward from the hips. Knees should be slightly lower than hips. Backrest should maintain the slight natural curve of the lower back.

Footrest: Feet should be planted firmly on floor; otherwise, use a footrest.

● **Figure 29.9 Computer injury, computer safety.** Prolonged computer use can lead to carpal tunnel syndrome (*top*), in which tendons passing through a tunnel created by the carpal ligament swell and painfully press on the median nerve, disabling wrist and forearm. To prevent such injuries, experts recommend an ideal setup (*bottom*) for using computers that avoids wrist, neck, back, and eye strain. Frequent breaks are also advised.

The Culture of Violence: From Murder to Sexual Harassment

Murder is the 11th leading cause of death in the United States and is highest among young males. Next to traffic accidents, gunfire is the most common cause of death for young Americans. Avoiding assault and other violence means learning precautions about when and where to walk and drive, protecting your residence, and knowing what to do if attacked.

Violence seems to be as American as apple pie. Not that other countries aren't violent, but the United States seems more so than most. American males ages 15–24, for example, are murdered more than four times as often as are those of 21 other countries—22 homicides per 100,000 people compared to only 5 per 100,000 for Scotland, the next highest country on the list.[128] Moreover, the number of injuries resulting from interpersonal violence is estimated to be at least 100 times greater than the number of homicides.[129] Obviously, a critical part of the art of living, then, is learning how to avoid violence in your life. We will discuss the issue of violence along a continuum, ranging from loss of life to sexual harassment.

Murder Homicide is the 11th leading cause of death in the United States.[130] The number of murders in the United States in 1991 was more than *twice* as many as the *combined* figures for Canada, France, Germany, Britain, and Japan for 1988, the latest year for which statistics are available. Although even Canada's reputation as a safe country has been tarnished by a rapidly rising murder rate (762 cases in 1991, up 14% from the previous year), that is a very long way from the 24,000 homicides in the United States that year, especially among young males.[131] (*See* ● *Figure 29.10.*) Among young African American men ages 15–24, the homicide rate was more than seven times that for white American males of similar age (87 per 100,000 people versus 11 per 100,000).[132] The majority of murders were perpetrated by members of the same race: 90% of black male victims were murdered by blacks, and 87% of white males were murdered by whites. Moreover, in the majority of cases victims were murdered by someone who was known to them.[133]

The chances of being murdered or otherwise a victim of violence vary according to who and where you are:

- *Gender and age:* Three-quarters of all homicide victims are males, perhaps because of gender differences in weapon-carrying behavior and social expectations for males and females.[134–135] Violent behavior is committed disproportionately by young males in their late teens through early 30s. Those are also the very people who are apt to be victims of violent acts.

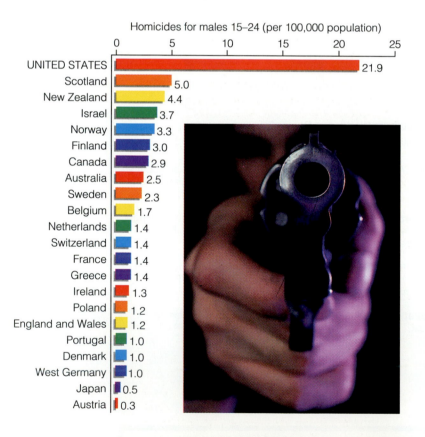

Homicides for males 15–24 (per 100,000 population)

UNITED STATES	21.9
Scotland	5.0
New Zealand	4.4
Israel	3.7
Norway	3.3
Finland	3.0
Canada	2.9
Australia	2.5
Sweden	2.3
Belgium	1.7
Netherlands	1.4
Switzerland	1.4
France	1.4
Greece	1.4
Ireland	1.3
Poland	1.2
England and Wales	1.2
Portugal	1.0
Denmark	1.0
West Germany	1.0
Japan	0.5
Austria	0.3

● **Figure 29.10 World murder rates, males 14–24.** The homicide rates for males ages 15–24 in 1986 or 1987 was 4 times higher in the United States than it was for Scotland, the next highest country.

12.29

*Chapter 29
Personal Safety:
Preventing
Accidents and
Violence*

- *Race and social class:* "Although there is an overrepresentation of blacks (44% of all homicide victims are black) and other non-whites in U.S. violence statistics," points out one group of scholars, "it is increasingly clear that socioeconomic status is a greater predictor of violence than racial status."[136] Both perpetrators and victims of violence are apt to be in the lowest socioeconomic levels.[137]

- *Urban and suburban areas:* Between 1980 and 1988, there was a 50% increase in mortality of children and adolescents living in cities as opposed to suburbs. Firearm-related homicides accounted for the majority of homicide deaths.[138]

- *Friends and murderers:* Most murders occur between people who have some sort of prior relationship with each other. In only 15% of murders are assailant and victim strangers to each other.[139]

- *Arguments, alcohol, and weapons:* Half of homicides are precipitated by an argument. Alcohol and other drugs seem to lead to violence by stimulating aggression and reducing inhibitions and impairing judgment. Indeed, nearly half of all convicted criminals, whatever the crime, were intoxicated at the time of their offense.[140] Having immediate access to a weapon or carrying a weapon also increases the possibility for violence.[141]

- *Homicide on the job:* Murder is the No. 3 cause of death on the job and is the leading cause of death of women at work.[142]

Guns and Harm There are about 200 million guns in the hands of American civilians. Four million more guns, including 2 million handguns, are being added each year.[143] Next to traffic accidents, gunfire is the most common cause of death for Americans ages 15–19.[144]

Every day, an average of 10 Americans who are 19 years of age or under are killed by guns, in homicides, suicides, or accidents. Only 5% of all firearms fatalities are unintentional.[145] The largest number of deaths from guns happen from nonaccidents. Thus, there are two areas of concern—the safe handling of guns to prevent accidents, and their safe handling to prevent their deliberate use.

- *Firearms safety:* Most inadvertent firearm injuries occur in or around the house. Too often the victims are children. To prevent such accidents, the Center to Prevent Handgun Violence recommends that guns should be stored in a locked container, unloaded and uncocked, and stored separately from their ammunition.

  A revolver may be child-proofed with a special padlock that goes around the cylinder and behind the trigger. A semiautomatic pistol may be child-proofed by locking the trigger with a special lock, by disconnecting the slide encasing the barrel, or at the least by pulling out the magazine or clip of bullets from the handle.[146]

- *The question of gun control:* The Justice Department estimates that over one-half million Americans are confronted each year by criminals carrying pistols, including 9200 people who are killed.[147] But what is the best solution—allowing more guns or fewer?

  In the U.S. national debate over crime control, declared one writer, "a gun, depending on one's view, is either an agent of evil that ought to be banned or restricted, or a constitutionally enshrined defense against evil."[148] Even a small decrease in firearms deaths would mean some progress, however: in 1989, there were 35,000 firearms-connected deaths, including 15,000 homicides, 18,000 suicides, 1500 accidents, and other unspecified.

  The dilemma is that, with so many guns in circulation, should new laws try to do a better job of keeping firearms away from criminals, or should they also restrict legal gun ownership in order to reduce the number of guns in the public's hands?[149] By contrast, consider that Canada passed a 1991 gun-control law that banned the import of military assault weapons, made it harder to obtain gun permits, and raised the minimum age for gun ownership from 16 to 18.[150] Few of these controls exist in the United States.

Dealing with Crime and Violence: Strategy for Living Just as crime has risen in American society at large, so it has also come to the college campus. Safety is a major issue on many campuses. At your college, you may see posters, brochures, and newspaper articles that address dormitory security, date rape, and use of night-time escorts to parked cars. The federal Campus Security Act requires that students and prospective students and their parents be provided with crime statistics for the previous 3 years, as well as a description of security procedures.[151]

Whether you are on campus or off, there are a number of precautions you can take to decrease your risk of becoming a victim of crime:

- *When walking or out in public:* At night or in early morning, don't walk or jog alone. Stay with groups. Take advantage of campus escort services. Stick to well-populated, well-lighted areas.

  Don't show money or valuables in public. Discreetly tuck away your cash after using an automatic teller machine.

  When on foot, walk rapidly and look as though you're going somewhere. If someone makes signs of wanting to talk to you, just keep on going. It's less important that you be polite than that you be safe.

- *When in a car:* When in a car, make sure all doors are locked. Don't open them for anyone you don't know. Keep windows rolled up so someone can't reach in and snatch your purse, wallet, or keys. Remain alert when stopped at intersections, day or night. If you stop for gas or to use a pay phone, choose well-lighted, busy facilities. Park in well-lighted areas, and get an escort to your car whenever possible.

  If your car is bumped from behind and you don't feel comfortable getting out, signal to the other person to follow you and drive to the nearest police station, service station, hospital, or fire station.[152,153]

  If you are the victim of a **carjacking**—a crime in which someone approaches you with a weapon and demands your car or money—turn it over to them.

- *When in your residence or campus buildings:* Lock your dorm-room or residence doors, even when you go to the shower. Theft is a big problem in some residence halls. Don't let strangers into your residence hall. Ask any stranger whom he or she wants to see. Don't leave backpacks,

purses, or briefcases unattended, even in your residence lounge.

- *If you sense you might be attacked:* If you are facing an armed criminal, the risk of injury may be minimized by cooperating with his or her demands. Avoid any sudden movements and give the criminal what he or she wants.

  If you sense your life is in immediate danger, *use any defense you can think of: screaming, kicking, running.* Your objective is to get away. In a violent crime, it is generally ineffective for the victim to cry or plead with the attacker. Such actions tend to reinforce the attacker's feeling of power over the victim.[154]

Intimate Violence: Abusive Relationships, Child Abuse, and Incest

Both men and women are involved in abusive relationships. It's important to understand why people abuse and why people stay in abusive relationships. Many children are also physically, mentally, and sexually abused, by their parents and others. Incest can be a difficult matter to detect and to deal with.

When Gregory Kottke opened his Milwaukee bodyguard agency in 1992, he figured his clients would be wealthy business executives and professional athletes and entertainers. Instead, he found most of his clients were low-income, physically abused women terrified of being beaten or worse by former husbands and boyfriends. Kottke found he had become a bodyguard for battered women, offering protection where the legal system could not.[155]

The epidemic of family violence is not limited to male perpetrators. In some cases, there are female perpetrators, and quite often it is adults of both sexes against children. Oftentimes the abuse is verbal or psychological rather than physical. Let us consider three types of intimate violence—abusive relationships, child abuse, and sexual assault and incest.

12.31

*Chapter 29
Personal Safety:
Preventing
Accidents and
Violence*

Abusive Relationships and Domestic Violence "American women have far more to fear from the men they know and once loved than from any stranger on the street," writes health reporter Jane Brody. "Domestic violence is the leading cause of injury and death to American women, causing more harm than vehicular accidents, rapes, and muggings combined."[156]

Domestic violence is found in all types of families, among all races, religions, economic groups, and educational levels.[157] Although some men are abused by women, siblings are abused by siblings, and some gays and lesbians by their partners, most abuse is experienced by women in what has been called "domestic captivity."[158] Sometimes the effects have been compared to the terror men feel in war, inflicting post-traumatic stress disorder.[159] Perhaps 6 million women—wives and girlfriends—every year are beaten by the men they live with. An estimated 30% of murdered women are killed by men with whom they have a "family" relationship.[160] Perhaps 30–40% of teenage girls, including women in college, have been hit in the course of dating.[161] (*See Self Discovery 29.1.*)

Some critical questions need to be answered: What kind of men are abusers, and why? Why do women stay in abusive relationships?

- *Men who are abusers and why:* Michigan psychologist Donald Saunders finds there are three types of men who abuse their partners:[162]

  (1) Men who are violent only in the home, who overcontrol their hostility, acting like doormats until they drink too much and then erupt. Half the time their violence is linked to alcohol.

  (2) Men who are violent inside and outside the home, whose violence is severe and tied to alcohol; they have rigid attitudes about sex roles and often have arrest records.

  (3) Less violent men who are psychologically abusive, who have rigid attitudes about sex roles and fear losing their partners.

  Why do men do it? The speculation is that many abusive men were abused themselves as children or observed their fathers

physically or verbally abusing their mothers.[163] Perhaps also men in general have been socialized by cultural stereotypes about masculinity—reinforced by violence in the media and toy manufacturing—in the varied acts of violence and destructiveness.[164] Finally, if men are domineering and aggressive, it may be because of raging hormones—specifically, the male sex hormone testosterone.[165]

- *Why women stay in abusive relationships:* If you had been assaulted, even seriously injured, why would you stay in the

---

SELF DISCOVERY 29.1

Are You Abused?

Answer the following yes or no:

Does your partner . . .   **Yes** **No**

1. Constantly criticize you and your abilities?
2. Become overprotective or extremely jealous?
3. Threaten to hurt you, children, pets, family, or friends?
4. Prevent you from seeing family or friends?
5. Have sudden bursts of anger?
6. Destroy personal property?
7. Deny you access to family assets or control all finances and force you to account for what you spend?
8. Use intimidation or manipulation to control you or your children?
9. Hit, punch, slap, kick, shove, or hit you?
10. Prevent you from going where you want when you want?
11. Force you to have sex when you don't want to?
12. Humiliate or embarrass you in front of others?

Interpretation
If you answer yes to *any* of these questions, you may be in an abusive relationship.

Source: Victim Services, New York City. (212-577-7777). Questionnaire appeared in: Brody, J. E. (1992, March 18). Each year, six million American women become victims of abuse without ever leaving home. *New York Times*, p. B6.

relationship? Often women first try to accommodate their abusers, and some may even believe their batterer's rationalization that the beating "is for your own good."[166] Indeed, some researchers think the behavior of battered women falls in the category of the so-called **Stockholm syndrome,** a condition named for a 1973 bank holdup in Sweden in which victims held hostage came to "bond" themselves to their captors out of fear that it was the only way to survive.[167]

Economics presents one major reason why women stay with those who batter them. Many do not have enough money to live by themselves (particularly if they have children requiring day-care). Many also have trouble finding places to live, since there are not enough shelters for battered women and the majority of shelters do not accept children.[168]

Perhaps fear is the biggest part. Women who leave are afraid their spouses will gain custody of their children. They are also afraid the law will not protect their safety and that their abusers will track them down. Indeed, there is some basis for this belief: Justice Department statistics show that 75% of assaults against lovers or wives occur *after* separation.[169]

Violence against women is not a cultural aberration. In fact, it has been found in almost every culture of the world.[170] However, the reverse is also true: men are battered, too. One 1985 study of 6000 couples found that women were slightly more likely than men to have slapped, kicked, bitten, or punched their partners or to have threatened them with a knife or a gun.[171,172] Still, a major difference between the sexes is that when battered men leave a relationship, the violence almost always stops. However, when battered women leave a relationship, the violence often escalates—sometimes leading to incidents of men stalking women and of women feeling they must kill or be killed.

Child Abuse In 1991, an estimated 2.7 million youngsters were physically, mentally, and sexually assaulted by their parents, according to the National Center for Child Abuse and Neglect.[173] According to the center, parents are more likely to maltreat their children if they are emotionally immature or needy and are isolated, with no family or friends to depend on. Many abusive parents have experienced abuse, deprivation, and neglect as children. As a result, they feel worthless and feel they have never been cared about. In addition, such parents are frequently alcohol or drug abusers.[174] Child abuse is more likely to occur in lower-income families (under $15,000 a year) than higher-income families, although abuse is found at all economic and educational levels.

Children are most likely to be at risk for abuse if they are unwanted, resemble someone the parent dislikes, or have physical or behavioral traits that make them somehow different or difficult to take care of—such as being retarded or very intelligent.[175] Parents may actually not intend to harm the children—indeed, they may feel remorseful for their behavior—but they are so concerned with their own problems they find it difficult to stop their abusive behavior. Abuse may be particularly aggravated when there is a financial condition or family structure that shakes the family's stability.[176]

Childhood Sexual Abuse, Including Incest
How hard is it to prosecute sexual abuse cases involving small children? Consider this: In Delaware in 1992, state prosecutors gave a man his freedom in return for his signed statement admitting that he had repeatedly raped his 3-year-old daughter. They did so because the child was too young to testify in court and there was not enough other evidence to persuade a jury to convict.[177]

Child sexual abuse is a crime—and a social taboo—that all involved, adult and child, frequently want to keep hidden. Yet the phenomenon may be widespread: perhaps as many as 500,000 children are sexually assaulted in the United States each year.[178] In one study in Los Angeles, 15% of 6th–12th graders, both boys and girls, reported having had at least one unwanted sexual experience; in a number of cases, the incident occurred with an adult authority figure, usually male family members and friends.[179] The sexual assault may include sexual contact, but it may also mean coercion to watch or perform sexual acts.

The most common form of child sexual abuse is incest. **Incest** is defined as sexual contact between a child or adolescent and a person who is closely related or perceived to be related

12.33

Chapter 29
Personal Safety:
Preventing
Accidents and
Violence

to the child.[180] The abusive person may be a parent, stepparent, sibling, uncle, or cousin. If the child is repeatedly abused by trusted non-family members, such as neighbors or child-care workers, the abuse may be experienced with the same emotional impact as incest. The abuse may range from fondling of genitals or breasts to vaginal, oral, or anal sex. Incest often involves some form of coercion and psychological manipulation.[181]

In recent years, incest has emerged from the dark as many Americans have become willing to talk about it, including celebrities such as talk-show host Oprah Winfrey and comedian Roseanne Arnold.[182,183] It has also spawned an incest-recovery movement. Incest may well cause women to be more depressed and have lower self-esteem as adults, although there are no studies to support this, points out social psychologist Carol Tavris. Nor does it follow, she says, "that all women who are depressed, [or who] are sexually conflicted, . . . were abused as children."[184] Still, at least this problem is at last coming into the open.

Unwanted Sex: From Sexual Harassment to Rape

Members of either sex may be victims of forced or unwanted sexual attentions or actions. Unwanted sex ranges from sexual harassment to sexual assault, including statutory, acquaintance, and date rape. It's important to learn techniques for preventing, resisting, or coping with acquaintance or stranger rape.

A grave problem for both sexes, but particularly for women, is that of dealing with unwanted sexual attention or demands. This may range from listening to sexual remarks to rape.

Sexual Harassment Your instructor or supervisor puts his or her hand on your shoulder, says "Can we discuss your coursework/possible promotion over dinner?", winks, and glides away. You don't want to do it, but you're worried about your grade or promotion. This really isn't about sex, it's about power. What do you do?

Sexual harassment is defined as unwelcome sexual attention, whether physical or ver-bal, that creates an intimidating, hostile, or offensive work or learning environment. Such harassment may include sexual remarks, suggestive looks, pressure for dates, letters and calls, deliberate touching, or pressure for sexual favors. From a legal standpoint, the U.S. Supreme Court has ruled that sexual harassment is a form of employment discrimination that is every bit as serious and as illegal as racial or religious discrimination.[185]

Men and women may see each of these matters differently. For instance, in one study, 95% of women felt that "deliberate touching" by a supervisor constituted sexual harassment, but only 89% of men said the same.[186] However, men, too, occasionally experience harassment by women (or men).

So what do you do if you are confronted with sexual harassment by someone who has power over your college or work career? Proving harassment in court is difficult, and other institutional arrangements are predisposed to protect the harasser.[187,188] Thus, one needs to proceed deliberately. First keep a log, recording dates, times, nature of incidents, and any witnesses. According to one survey, just asking or telling the person to stop worked for 61% of the women. Telling coworkers, or threatening to, worked 55% of the time. Pretending to ignore the offensive behavior usually didn't work at all.[189] If the harassment persists, stronger measures may be required. (*See ● Figure 29.11.*)

Rape: Date Rape and Other Sexual Assaults Sex may be pleasurable, but forced sex is in the same category as any other attack. Assault is assault, whether it is with a gun, a club, a fist—or a penis. **Rape** is defined as sexual penetration of a male or female by intimidation, fraud, or force. Most rape victims are women, but one study of 3000 randomly chosen Los Angeles residents found that one third of victims of attempted sexual assault were men.[190] In a 1988 survey done of Stanford University students, 1 in 3 women and 1 in 8 men reported having unwanted sexual activity.[191]

Rape victims can be of all ages, but the shocking fact is that 61% of female rape victims were younger than 18 at the time of their attack, according to the National Victim Center.[192] In almost 80% of cases, the victim knew her rapist. (*See ● Figure 29.12.*)

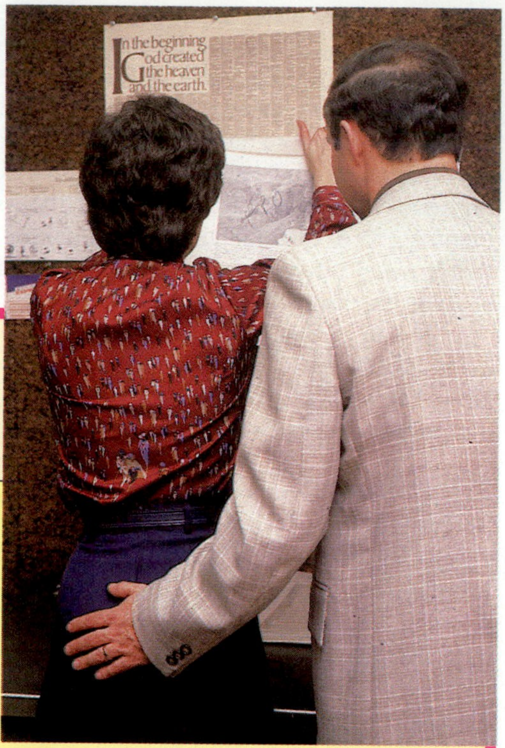

● **Figure 29.11
How to fight
sexual harass-
ment**

*If sexual harass-
ment persists, here
are some steps to
take:*

- *Document:*
  Keep a detailed
  written record
  of the incidents,
  with dates, times, places, names, and quotes. Keep any notes you
  receive.
- *Confide in co-workers or friends:* You may tell trusted co-
  workers, friends, family members, a minister, or others, saying you may have to file a grievance and that you want them
  to know what is happening.
- *Find witnesses or supporting evidence:* If there are witnesses, ask them to write a statement for you. If you are receiving harassing phone calls, have someone be an "ear
  witness" by listening in and taking notes. Look for other people in your same situation who may have been harassed by
  the same person.
- *Confront the harasser:* Say the behavior must stop immediately, and let him or her know you will file a complaint if it
  does not. If necessary, write a letter—or follow up your conversation with a memo summarizing your talk—and hand it
  to the harasser in the presence of a witness. Keep a copy.
- *Talk to the harasser's supervisor:* Talk to an appropriate third
  party such as the harasser's supervisor or someone in the human resources department or equal opportunity officer.
- *File a complaint:* If your company or institution does not
  take steps to stop the harassment, file a legal complaint based
  on state or federal antidiscrimination laws. Your state may
  have a department of fair employment or you may take your
  case to the U.S. Equal Employment Opportunity Commission
  (call 800-USA-EEOC).

Three kinds of rape are particularly worth
mentioning:

- *Statutory rape:* **Statutory rape** is unlaw-
  ful sexual intercourse between a male over
  age 16 and a female under age 12 or 21, depending on the state. As the National Victim Center report showed, 3 out of 10 rape
  victims had not reached their 11th birthday.

- *Acquaintance rape:* **Acquaintance rape**
  is rape by a person known by the victim,
  whether related or unrelated. The National
  Victim Center report found that 78% of
  rapists were known to their victims.

- *Date rape:* **Date rape** is a particular kind
  of acquaintance rape in which the rapist is
  someone with whom the victim has had a
  date. Whereas once nonconsensual sex between men and women on dates might have
  been thought to be a form of female error
  or lack of resistance, today sexual activity
  that is unwanted by females is considered
  assault by males.[193]

On some college campuses, there is still
some uncertainty as to when sex is considered
consensual and when sex is considered rape.
For instance, one male student, asked whether
a woman he had dated had consented to having
sex, replied, "No, but she didn't say no, so she
must have wanted it, too."[194] He added that
both had been drunk and the woman had struggled initially. Others pointed out that the young
man's behavior is reinforced by pressure from
other men to "score" and by many men's assumptions that when a woman enters their bedroom in a dorm or fraternity house, it is an
unspoken invitation to sex. Whatever one
party's assumptions about the other and whatever the state of intoxication of either person, it
is *always* rape if sex is not consensual.

**Strategy for Living: Avoiding and Coping
with Rape** Men and women interpret sexual
cues differently. For instance, according to one
study, when asked whether going back to a
date's room, kissing, French kissing, and taking
off one's shirt indicate an interest in and a willingness to have sex, men interpreted all these
behaviors as more indicative of consent than
women did.[195] These are the kinds of misunderstandings, resulting from misinterpretations of
nonverbal cues, that can hurt someone.

12.35

*Chapter 29
Personal Safety:
Preventing
Accidents and
Violence*

To cope with rape, here are some suggestions:

- *To avoid acquaintance or date rape:* Be aware of your surroundings and intentions. Stay out of ambiguous situations (such as bedrooms) and be clear in communicating what you want and don't want. Learn to listen carefully to your partner's messages about what he or she wants and doesn't want. Use a neutral tone and speak in "I" statements: "I want to be taken home."

- *Trust your instincts.* If you're uncomfortable with a situation, follow your intuition. Don't be afraid of hurting somebody's feelings.

- *To avoid stranger rape:* When on the street, be aware of your surroundings, anticipate how you would respond to an attack, look behind you, stay in the middle of the sidewalk, and walk with a confident stride. Use extra caution in parking garages. If you're alone on an elevator, get out if a stranger gets on and pushes the button for the basement. Have your keys in hand when you approach your car so you won't have to stand there fumbling.

- *To resist rape of any kind:* Don't be too polite to fight. Be loud, be rude, cause a scene. Attackers count on the fear of embarrassment. Research shows that women who fight back, especially against acquaintances, have a better chance of escaping rape than those who plead or cry.[196]

- *To cope with rape:* Call the police and a rape crisis center or rape treatment center. Don't bathe or wash yourself or your clothes or touch anything in the location of the rape. If a condom was used, try to remember where it was discarded. Try to remember everything about the rapist, his car, clothing, scars, haircut, and things he said and did. Report any weapons or restraints used, and if bruises show up later, have photographs taken by the police. Go to a hospital and be tested and/or treated for sexually transmitted diseases.

Afterward, expect emotional aftershocks, even if you weren't hurt physically. Tell your physician and try to institute a health strategy that includes psychological as well as physical factors. Confide your feelings to a friend.[197]

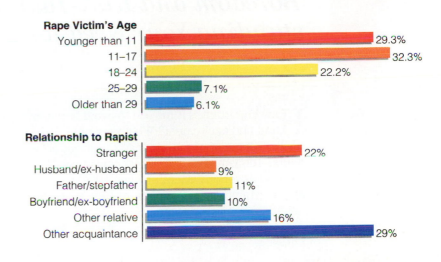

Figure 29.12 Age of rape victim and relationship to rapist

Many women tend to blame themselves when attacked, especially by men they trust, then only later—perhaps years later—decide that they have been sexually assaulted.[198]

800-HELP

Auto Safety Hotline. 800-494-9393 (in Washington, D.C., 202-366-0123)

Battered Women's Shelter. 800-333-SAFE

Child Help National Child Abuse Hot Line. 800-422-4453. For incest victims and others suffering sexual assault as children

9to5 Job Problem Hotline. 800-522-0925. For sexual harassment and other work-related problems. A service of the Cleveland-based 9to5 National Association of Working Women.

Suggestions for Further Reading

Evans, Patricia. (1992). *The verbally abusive relationship: How to recognize it and how to respond.* Holbrook, MA: Bob Adams. A valuable book in the literature of domestic violence.

Nisbet, Lee (Ed.) (1990). *The gun control debate: You decide.* Buffalo, NY: Prometheus. Essays by historians, criminologists, jurists, and public health officials pro and con on public access versus prohibition of handguns in the United States.

Boredom and Risk-Taking: Understanding Your Need for Excitement

How important is it for you to avoid boredom and find excitement? What kind of kicks or thrills—some of which can lead to serious accidents—do you seek out? These questions deserve your serious attention, since they have an important bearing on your attitude toward health.

Answer the following T for True or F for False:

I often . . .

___ **1.** Get fidgety and start yawning when I have to sit still.

___ **2.** Can't remember what people have said when they finish talking.

___ **3.** Flick through the TV channels even though I know there's nothing worth watching.

___ **4.** Think about someone other than the person I'm with.

These are 4 of 10 questions adapted from a questionnaire on boredom.[199] (*See Self Discovery.*) If you answered True to a number of these statements, it may mean you are bored a lot of the time.

Boredom and Its Discontents

"Somebody's boring me," wrote Welsh poet Dylan Thomas. "I think it's me."

Is boredom a part of life—or a part of you?

Bored people have differing characteristics, but researchers agree that people prone to boredom are often young—in their late teens or 20s.[200] Bored people also turn up frequently among younger people in management: "my generation . . . expects to be fascinated all the time on the job," said one 33-year-old vice president, who has since learned better.[201] Women executives may also be more bored than their male counterparts, not having expected to spend their lives in 9 to 5 jobs.

Boredom may come about because of forced attention: you are compelled to listen to Mr. Drone's tedious lecture or Aunt Chatty's unending stories or to yawn your way through weekly inventory reports. Or boredom may occur because skills and challenges are mismatched: you are exercising your high level of skill in a job with a low level of challenge, such as licking envelopes.

In the view of psychology professor Mihaly Csikszentmihalyi, author of *Beyond Boredom and Anxiety* and *Flow,* boredom is the opposite of anxiety. Anxiety arises when one has low levels of skills but a high level of challenge.[202,203] When skills and challenges are in balance, he says, the result is *flow.* "Flow," or moments of peak concentration, refers to those times when things seem to go just right, when you feel alive and fully attentive to what you are doing.

But feelings of boredom may be caused less by the lack of challenge than by having too few inner resources. For instance, research by Csikszentmihalyi found that one assembly-line worker had a job in which he simply tightened a set of screws all day long.[204] But after several years he was still experimenting with ways to increase his performance, a challenge that kept him interested in the job. Long-haul truck drivers with excellent safety records were also able to stave off tedium by playing mental games and otherwise finding ways to keep their minds active.[205]

What do people do when they are bored? If the problem is chronic, they may perform poorly in their jobs or at school, have difficulty relating to other people, and spend too much time sleeping. They may also have troubles with alcoholism, drug addiction, or sexually transmitted diseases—disorders that can be brought about by the need for excitement.

How Bored Are You?

To assess whether boredom is causing problems in your life, take the 10-step quiz below. Check off, honestly, how often each statement applies to you.

1. I get fidgety and start yawning when I have to sit still.

    a. _____ Rarely   b. _____ Sometimes   c. _____ Frequently

2. I can't believe how fast time goes.

    a. _____ Rarely   b. _____ Sometimes   c. _____ Frequently

3. I sigh and think, "I don't care."

    a. _____ Rarely   b. _____ Sometimes   c. _____ Frequently

4. I can't remember what people have said when they finish talking.

    a. _____ Rarely   b. _____ Sometimes   c. _____ Frequently

5. I eat when I'm not hungry.

    a. _____ Rarely   b. _____ Sometimes   c. _____ Frequently

6. I flick through the TV channels even though I know there's nothing I want to watch.

    a. _____ Rarely   b. _____ Sometimes   c. _____ Frequently

7. I think, "I'll never get to everything I want to do."

    a. _____ Rarely   b. _____ Sometimes   c. _____ Frequently

8. I take a nap when I'm not tired.

    a. _____ Rarely   b. _____ Sometimes   c. _____ Frequently

9. I think about someone other than the person I'm with.

    a. _____ Rarely   b. _____ Sometimes   c. _____ Frequently

10. I can't think of anything to do.

    a. _____ Rarely   b. _____ Sometimes   c. _____ Frequently

Scoring

For questions 1, 3, 4, 5, 6, 8, 9, 10: a = 0, b = 5, c = 10.
For questions 2 and 7: a = 0, b = subtract 5, c = subtract 10.

Interpretation

If your total score is:

Less than 20: You're enjoying life. Boredom's not a problem. You even want to take some time out for contemplation.

20–35: You're probably bored about as much as the average person. It is not a problem overall but does bother you in some situations. Think about what they are, and try to see what simple changes you can make.

40–55: You're bored a lot of the time. Think about the times when you *aren't* bored. See if you can figure out what *really* interests you, and make it more a part of your life.

60–80: Boredom is really a problem for you and may even be masking more serious depression. You might want to consider some changes in your life to give you more satisfaction. Consider involving family, friends, or even a professional counselor in helping you with these changes.

Source: Darden, D. (1990, May). How bored are you? *Self*, p. 237.

Excitement and Risk-Taking

Some people take up skydiving, rock climbing, motorcycle racing, or rodeo riding. Others go in for fast driving on city streets, unprotected sex in the age of AIDS, intravenous drug abuse—even violence and murder.

Perhaps one element that all such behavior has in common is risk-taking or thrill-seeking action that reflects a thirst for excitement. "Excitement is an important form of human satisfaction," writes economist Tibor Scitovsky. "Looking at newspapers, movies, and television screens, books of fiction, and advertisements, one gets the impression that the advanced economies of the West cater to a greatly increased public demand for excitement."[206] (*See table, opposite.*)

Does everybody seek excitement? Some people may be biologically predisposed "sensation seekers," according to psychologist Marvin Zuckerman of the University of Delaware.[207] Zuckerman has devised a four-part sensation-seeking scale, which measures a person's penchant for (1) thrill- and adventure-seeking—the desire to engage in activities with some physical risk; (2) experience seeking—the desire for new experiences through travel or nonconforming lifestyle; (3) disinhibition—the propensity for drinking, partying, and a variety of sexual partners; and (4) boredom susceptibility—the aversion to routine experience and predictable people.

Teenagers and Criminals

Risk-taking and recklessness are particularly common among teenagers and young people.[208] Violence is the leading cause of teenage mortality, with accidents, homicides, and suicides accounting for more than three-quarters of adolescent deaths. Such acts indicate a lethal propensity for risk-taking.[209] Accidents alone account for 60% of these deaths.[210] Substance use contributes to this carnage, as in the high number of young people who drink or use drugs and drive.[211] To this must now be added the number of young people who still engage in unprotected sex—despite the high level of awareness (74–98%) among college students of the potential dangers of having sexual intercourse without using a condom.[212]

Sensation-seeking, high-risk behavior is certainly not confined to adolescents, of course. UCLA sociologist Jack Katz has found that crime has an important psychological payoff for criminals.[213] Shoplifting and vandalism, for instance, are seductive to offenders because of the "sneaky thrills" they offer—including the thrill of being caught. Career criminals, such as armed robbers, are dedicated to their carefully constructed self-images as "bad" characters, so the prospect of jail time may not offer much of a deterrent.

The Qualities of Recklessness

Why are adolescents and young adults particularly susceptible to recklessness? There seem to be a number of reasons—some of which apply to people in general, not just teenagers:

- *Hormone-related thrill-seeking:* According to Zuckerman, people who score highest on a personality test for sensation-seeking have higher levels than others of the sex hormones that are released in puberty, particularly the principal male sex hormone (testosterone).[214]

- *Inability to perceive risks accurately:* Teenagers' ability to evaluate risk seems to be skewed, according to pediatrician Charles Irwin of the University of California at San Francisco.[215] He found that some adolescents, when asked to state what activities become more or less dangerous with repetition, stated that addiction from drug use and pregnancy from unprotected intercourse become *less* likely rather than more likely. Beatrix A. Hamburg, a child psychiatrist at Mount Sinai Hospital in New York City, says that adolescents "do lots of exploring at a time when their cognitive development has not yet reached the point where they can make judgments that will keep them out of trouble. They cannot really comprehend laws of probability."[216]

- *Underestimation of health risks:* Many people (not just young people) tend to underestimate their own health risks compared to those of others.[217,218] According to Robert Jeffery of the University of Minnesota, this optimism may have two bases.[219] One is the personal biases that support one's sense of psychological well-being.[220] The other is a tendency to overgeneralize from one's personal history that if nothing bad has happened yet it probably won't in the future.[221]

- *Immediate rewards favored over long-term rewards:* Health psychologist Nancy Adler says that, for adolescents, "The immediate experience is what matters to them, not worries about long-term consequences."[222] Perhaps one reason for this is that young people are more present-centered than future-centered, according to Stanford psychologist Philip Zimbardo.[223] For many adults too, of course, immediate rewards tend to outweigh longer term benefits, even in matters such as healthy eating, so adhering to healthy behavior is difficult.[224]

- *Need to impress peers*: Adolescents see their world in different terms than adults do. They fear not physical danger but social rejection from other adolescents. Adler found, for example, that when it comes to using condoms, adolescents are less concerned about pregnancy than in whether they think their peers use condoms and whether use of condoms might make them look "silly." In fact, this concern with others in their age groups can lead them to overestimate the number of people engaged in risky behavior (such as smoking) and underestimate the physical dangers, according to a study cited by Hamburg.

Ten sources of excitement. Economist Tibor Scitovsky, who thinks the search for excitement is an important form of human satisfaction, suggests a number of activities that people take up in trying to fulfill this need. An important precondition in all of them, he says, is challenge or threat and uncertainty—the possibility of failure and the less-than-certain expectation of being able to cope. Enjoyable excitement lies between the extremes of being unpleasant and unbearable on the one hand and boring and unsatisfying on the other.

1. Do-it-yourself activities and hobbies, including handicraft and artwork
2. Competitive games of skill, such as card games
3. Sports, especially competitive and dangerous sports
4. Gambling, an activity of nearly half of U.S. adults
5. Dangerous driving
6. Alcohol or drugs
7. Crime, as when children delight in defying adult authority and adults take pleasure in breaking the law
8. Violence experienced vicariously, as in viewing gut-wrenching movies
9. Violence experienced in actuality, as in participating in violent crime
10. Collective adventurous or hazardous action, ranging from business entrepreneurship to scientific expeditions to strikes to wars

We can be our own worst enemies when we could be our own best friends. For many people, other matters have a higher priority than their health: To avoid boredom. To feel passion. To find excitement. To achieve success. These secrets of the self exert a powerful attraction. Do they for you?

UNIT

13 Conquering Heart Disease and Cancer

In These Chapters:

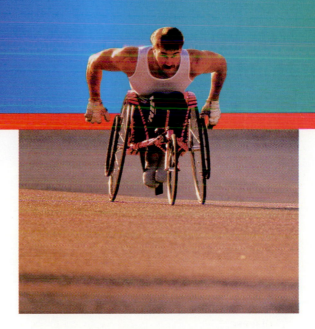

Can stress do things inside you without your knowing it?

It was a highly stressful job, involving continual conflict and negotiation with people inside and outside of a university bureaucracy, but to one of the authors it simply felt like the normal tensions of work. That is, until one day I volunteered to give blood at a "blood mobile" that appeared outside the office seeking donors for a community blood bank.

I lay back on a bunk within the van, my sleeve rolled up, feeling wonderfully virtuous about the selfless act I was about to perform of giving up a pint of blood. The technician put a cloth blood-pressure cuff around my arm, applied a stethoscope to the inside of my elbow, and pumped the rubber ball. So far, standard procedure, I thought.

A look of concern crossed her face as she eyed the dial. "I don't think you should be giving any blood today," she said, removing the cuff. "Your blood pressure is much too high."

I was shocked. Until then, I had felt I was perfectly normal. Sure, I didn't exercise as much as I should, and maybe my diet could be improved, and the job drove me wild, but *this*? I was too young to have high blood pressure!

Unfortunately, it is by such revelations that many people find out they are at high risk for being felled by a heart attack or similar condition. High blood pressure, or hypertension, has been called the Silent Killer precisely because you can't tell you have it. And, in point of fact, hypertension may or may not be related to having a tense (or even hyper-tense) job: the role of stress in the disease is not certain.

In the United States, the No. 1 cause of death for the population as a whole is heart disease. The No. 2 cause of death is cancer. Some things you cannot help: your predisposition toward getting heart disease or cancer may in part be hereditary. But family history is only part of it. People in other countries don't succumb to these diseases in the same way or at the same rate that Americans do. This means, then, that many of the risks have to do with *lifestyle*. And dedicating oneself a to healthy style of life is one of the fundamental arts of living.

30 The Way to a Healthy Heart

▶ Describe the cardiovascular system of blood, blood vessels, and heart and how they work. Explain how blood pressure is measured and its significance.

▶ Describe the five major groups of cardio-vascular disease.

▶ State what needs to be done in the event of a heart attack and how it may be treated.

▶ Discuss both predisposing and precipitating risk factors for heart disease.

▶ List the nine steps for preventing heart disease.

What would you say if you learned that a computer program suggests that adopting good heart-related health habits—stopping smoking, lowering cholesterol, and so on—would add only *a couple of years or so* to the average life span? You would probably say, "Why bother?"

Indeed, a study by Dr. Joel Tsevat and others, based on a computer program developed by two Boston medical researchers, found exactly this. Eliminating all deaths from heart disease, the computer said, would extend the average life expectancy of a 35-year-old man by 3.1 years and a woman by 3.3 years.[1] The average life span in the United States today is 75.

There are, however, two important points about this. First, although the average increases might be small, the gains for *individuals* could be dramatic—especially if healthier habits prevented deaths from heart attacks at age 40 or 50. Second, the study found that eliminating the No. 1 killer, heart disease, still left one open to death from a host of other ailments: cancer, pneumonia, strokes.

Thus, as we consider **cardiovascular disease**—any disease of the heart or blood vessels—and ways to avoid it, we need to keep in mind that it's just one life-threatening disorder on a list of several that we can take steps against.

The Cardiovascular System: Blood, Circulation, and Heart

The cardiovascular system consists of blood, blood vessels, and heart. Blood carries nourishment to the body's cells. The circulatory system consists of arteries, which take blood out to the body from the heart, and veins, which bring it back. The heart is a pump with four chambers; its contractions force blood into the arteries. Blood pressure, a measure of the force of the blood in the blood vessels, consists of systolic and diastolic pressures.

Have a heart, the expression goes. What if you didn't have a heart or the circulatory system that goes with it? You would then be sort of like a city with no food-delivery and trash-removal trucks. Your body would have no means of delivering nutrients and oxygen to the cells or of removing the waste products of metabolism from the cells.

The closed system of heart, blood vessels, and blood is called the **cardiovascular system.** Blood does not flow through your body like a meandering stream. It is pushed through by the force of your heart's contractions and carried throughout the body by means of the blood vessels that comprise your circulatory system.

Let us see how this works, starting with the blood.

The Blood What, exactly, is that red liquid that seeps from your finger when you accidentally cut yourself? Blood is the substance that carries nourishment to the cells in your tissues and protects you against disease. Specifically, it consists of cells of several types and a solution called **plasma,** in which the cells are suspended. That is, it includes:

- *Red blood cells—45%:* About 45% of the blood consists of **red blood cells,** whose purpose is to carry oxygen to the cells and carbon dioxide from the cells.

- *White blood cells—1%:* About 1% of the blood is **white blood cells,** whose purpose is to defend the body against a variety of organisms.

The Circulatory System The **circulatory system** consists of the heart and blood vessels. The system of blood vessels is called the **vascular system.** The heart pumps blood out through the arteries to the body and then back to the heart through the veins. (*See ● Figure 30.1.*)

The **arteries** are large-diameter blood vessels that carry oxygen-rich blood from the heart to smaller and smaller blood vessels, called **arterioles.** The arterioles in turn branch into **capillaries,** tiny, thin-walled blood vessels that connect the system of arteries with the system of veins. (*See ● Figure 30.2.*) The **veins** return

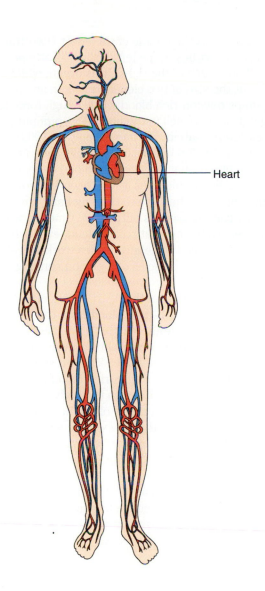

Heart

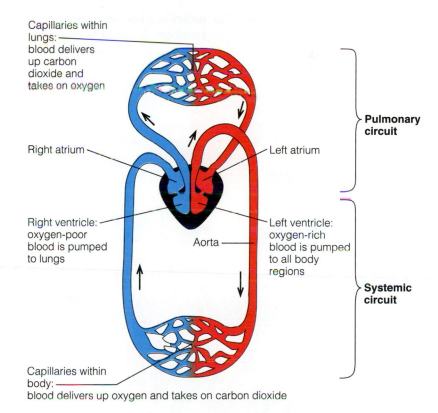

Capillaries within lungs: blood delivers up carbon dioxide and takes on oxygen

Right atrium

Left atrium

Pulmonary circuit

Right ventricle: oxygen-poor blood is pumped to lungs

Aorta

Left ventricle: oxygen-rich blood is pumped to all body regions

Systemic circuit

Capillaries within body: blood delivers up oxygen and takes on carbon dioxide

● **Figure 30.1 The circulatory system.** The human circulatory system, including the heart, arteries (*shown in red*), and veins (*shown in blue*).

● **Figure 30.2 Diagram of general pattern of circulation.** Oxygen-rich (oxygenated) blood (*shown in red*) is taken from the lungs and pumped by the left side of the heart out to the blood vessels, which carry it to all body tissues. Oxygen-poor (deoxygenated) blood (*shown in blue*) is picked up from the capillaries and pumped back into the right side of the heart and back to the capillaries of the lungs. The blood returning to the heart carries carbon dioxide, which the lungs also pick up and expel when you exhale.

- *Platelets—4%:* **Platelets** are cell fragments in the blood that release substances necessary for clot formation. Platelets clump together to help stop bleeding.
- *Plasma—50%:* About half the blood is made up of the watery substance called plasma, which contains 90% water and various salts, sugar, cholesterol, proteins, minerals, and other substances.

the blood from the body to the heart. The blood in the capillaries delivers oxygen and nutrients to the cells in the tissues. The capillaries also take up carbon dioxide and other waste products of metabolism from the cells, and these wastes are sent to the heart through the veins. Stretched end to end, all the vessels in the circulatory system would measure about 60,000 miles.[2]

The part of the circulatory system, both arteries and veins, that has to do with the lungs is called the **pulmonary circuit.** The part that has to do with the rest of the body is called the **systemic circuit.** (*Refer back to Figure 30.2.*)

The Heart The **heart** is a hollow, muscular pump with four chambers. Located between the two lungs in the middle of the chest (two-thirds of the heart lies to the left of the breastbone and one-third to the right), this organ, which is about the size of two clenched fists in an adult, pumps oxygen-rich blood with enough force to get it to every cell in the body. The pumping is relentless—about 70 times a minute, 100,000 times a day, 2.5 billion times in a 70-year life span, processing 75 gallons of blood every day of your life. Sometimes it has to work harder than others: when you're running hard, the heart can increase its output five times to what it does when you're at rest. Indeed, even when you're resting, the heart muscles work twice as hard as the leg muscles of a person running at top speed.[3]

The right side of the heart is concerned with taking oxygen-poor blood from the body by way of the two **venae cavae** (singular: **vena cava**), the primary veins, and returning it to the lungs. (*See ● Figure 30.3.*) The left side is concerned with taking oxygen-rich blood from the lungs and pumping it out to the body by way of the **aorta,** the main artery of the body. Blood does not flow directly between the left and right sides of the heart, which are divided by a thick wall. However, the two sides contract at the same time.

Like any other part of the body, the heart muscle itself also needs nourishment. The blood vessels that supply oxygen-rich blood to the heart muscle are the **coronary arteries.**

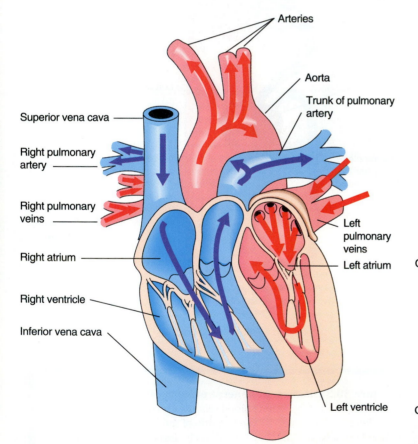

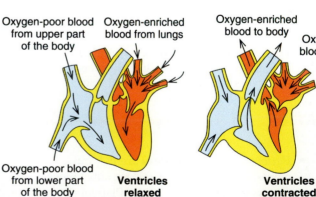

● **Figure 30.3 The heart.** (*Left*) Partial view of the interior. (*Right*) Blood flow through the heart during contraction and relaxation.

Each half of the heart (the right and left sides) has two holding chambers, an atrium and a ventricle. (*Refer back to Figure 30.3.*)

- *The atrium:* The upper chamber on each side of the heart is called an **atrium** (plural: **atria**). The right atrium receives oxygen-poor blood from the body. The left atrium receives oxygen-rich blood from the lungs. The blood from each atrium is then pumped through a valve into a corresponding lower chamber called a ventricle. The special **valves** between atria and ventricles prevent the blood from flowing in the wrong direction.

- *The ventricle:* The **ventricle** is a holding chamber and does not pump blood. Blood within each ventricle is pumped out of the heart through another valve to the arteries. Blood held within the right ventricle is pumped to the lung. Blood from the left ventricle is pumped to the body.

The contraction of the heart (your heartbeat) is actually a two-part process. First, muscles surrounding the top atria contract, forcing blood into the ventricles. Then, in quick succession, the heart muscle surrounding the ventricles contracts, forcing blood into the arteries.

When you feel your pulse, you are feeling the consequences of the contraction of the left ventricle. The resultant increased pressure of blood in the main arteries of the body causes these blood vessels to expand. You can feel the expansion with each heartbeat.

During the contraction phase, called **systole,** the heart forces blood into the arteries. During the relaxation phase, called **diastole,** the heart chambers fill with blood.

Blood Pressure Your **blood pressure** is the measure of the pressure or force of circulating blood against the walls of your blood vessels. Since the pressure changes when the heart contracts and relaxes, blood pressure is expressed as:

- *Systolic pressure:* **Systolic blood pressure,** the highest pressure, occurs when the heart contracts and blood is forced into the arteries.

- *Diastolic pressure:* **Diastolic blood pressure,** the lowest pressure, occurs when the heart is relaxed.

These pressures are expressed together as two figures—for example, 120/70, stated as "120 over 70." The 120 number is the systolic pressure, the 70 number the diastolic pressure. A blood pressure reading is taken with a device called a *sphygmomanometer* (pronounced "sfig-moe-man-*om*-e-ter"), or blood-pressure cuff, and a stethoscope. (*See • Figure 30.4.*)

An average blood-pressure reading for young adults is 120/80. Generally, any blood pressure under 140/90 is considered within the normal range. When blood pressure is low, people may feel faint or dizzy. It is not uncommon for children and young adults to have blood-pressure readings of 100/60 or less. Many feel fine, but they may notice dizziness if they move from a lying to a standing position too quickly.

Cardiovascular Diseases: The Things That Can Go Wrong

The five major groups of cardiovascular disease are (1) high blood pressure (hypertension); (2) coronary heart disease, which may lead to angina and heart attack; (3) stroke, impaired blood flow to the brain; (4) congenital heart disorders and rheumatic heart disease; and (5) other problems such as peripheral artery disease, congestive heart failure, and irregular heartbeat.

What mechanical or electrical machine has functioned for a century or more without failing? The answer is: none. Some human hearts, however, have gone that long.

Still, like machines, hearts do break down. Heart disease, or cardiovascular disease—all diseases of the heart and blood vessels—is the No. 1 cause of death in the United States. Coronary heart disease is the biggest killer of these; it alone kills more people in the United States than any other disease. **Stroke**—a blockage of the blood supply to the brain—is the No. 4 cause of death. (*See • Figure 30.5.*) Strokes commonly represent a form of cardiovascular disease. The threat of cardiovascular disease and death, then, is enormously high for Americans. Unhealthy lifestyle habits are a major contributor to the problem. To understand the need for assessing and possibly changing your

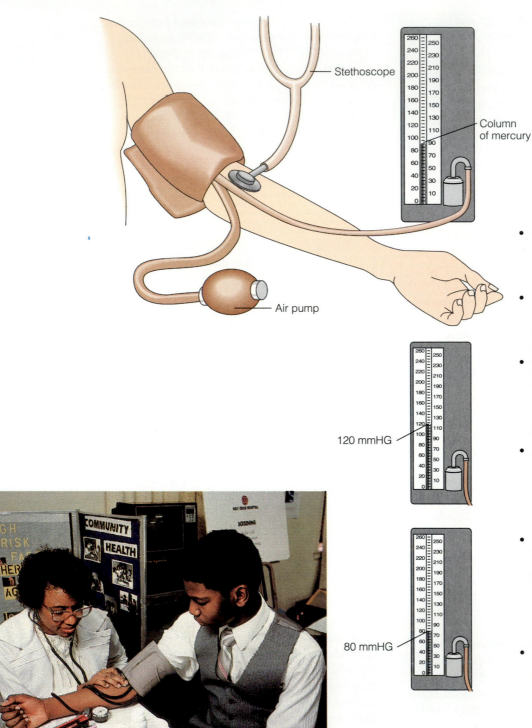

Stethoscope

Column
of mercury

120 mmHG

80 mmHG

Air pump

- A hollow cuff is wrapped around the upper arm and inflated with air to stop the flow of blood through the major artery in the arm.

- The person performing a blood-pressure test places one end of the stethoscope on the inside bend of the arm and the other ends in his or her ears.

- While looking at a blood-pressure gauge, which measures pressure in millimeters of mercury, the person doing the testing gradually releases air from the cuff and listens carefully.

- **Systolic pressure:** The number on the gauge (normally around 120 mmHG) that corresponds to the *first* sound of the heart beat is the *systolic blood pressure*, when the heart is in its contraction phase.

- **Diastolic pressure:** As the person continues releasing air from the cuff, the pulse suddenly becomes inaudible. The number on the gauge at this point (normally around 80 mmHG) is the *diastolic blood pressure*, when the heart is in its relaxation phase.

- An average reading for young adults is 120/80—120 systolic, 80 diastolic.

● **Figure 30.4 Taking blood pressure**

lifestyle for improved cardiovascular health, let us consider the common cardiovascular disorders.

In general, there are five major groups of cardiovascular diseases, according to the American Heart Association:

1. *High blood pressure:* High blood pressure (hypertension) results when there is marked resistance within the vascular system that forces the heart to pump harder.

2. *Coronary heart disease:* Coronary heart disease involves atherosclerosis, which severely narrows the vessels supplying blood to the muscle of the heart itself. This may lead to angina and heart attack.

3. *Stroke:* Stroke is the result of impaired blood flow to the brain.

4. *Diseases of the young—congenital heart disorders and rheumatic heart disease:* A congenital defect is one that is present at birth—in this case, an abnormality of the heart. Rheumatic heart disease is heart damage resulting from a streptococcal infection that begins as strep throat.

5. *Other problems:* Three other important problems are peripheral artery disease, congestive heart failure, and irregular heartbeat.

High Blood Pressure Your blood pressure normally varies depending on your body's demand for oxygen. It can also vary according to age: a baby's blood pressure may be 70/50. For a young adult, average blood pressure is 120/80.

High blood pressure (along with coronary heart disease) is one of the two most common forms of cardiovascular disease in the United States. How high is high? Today physicians agree that blood pressure readings that are *consistently above 140/90* constitute **hypertension.** This potentially life-threatening disease affects more than 60 million American adults and children.[4] The higher the blood pressure, the more serious the problem and the greater the need for treatment. (See ● *Table 30.1.*)

When having your blood pressure taken, it's recommended that a reading with abnormal results be repeated. A number of otherwise normal people, for example, are so nervous in a doctor's office that they have elevated blood pressure readings—a condition called *white-*

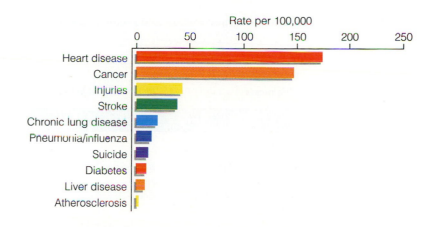

Rate per 100,000

Heart disease
Cancer
Injuries
Stroke
Chronic lung disease
Pneumonia/influenza
Suicide
Diabetes
Liver disease
Atherosclerosis

● **Figure 30.5 Leading causes of death.** Heart disease and stroke are among the major causes of death in the United States in 1987.

coat hypertension—that are not found at home or at work.[5] Thus, most health professionals recommend that the reading be repeated over a few weeks' time to establish your true level.

Some key aspects of hypertension are:

• *Primary and secondary hypertension:* Hypertension is of two types, primary and secondary.

• In **primary** (or **essential**) **hypertension,** the form seen in 90% of cases, the disease has no known cause, though it is probably related to both uncontrollable and controllable factors. Those factors that are uncontrollable include age (older people are more likely to have elevated blood pressures), family history, diabetes, and race (African Americans are twice as likely as whites to develop hypertension).[6] The probable controllable factors include diet (salt and unsaturated fats), weight (being overweight), alcohol and tobacco use, lack of exercise, and possibly stress. Primary hypertension is controllable but not curable.

Secondary hypertension is triggered by other primary diseases such as kidney disorders, disorders of the endocrine system such as hypothyroidism, and bloodvessel diseases such as arteriosclerosis, or hardening of the arteries.

● **Table 30.1 Categories of hypertension and recommended activity**

Range (mm Hg)	Diagnosis	Recommended activity
Diastolic:		
Under 85	Normal blood pressure	Recheck within 2 years.
85–89	High normal blood pressure	Recheck within 1 year.
90–104	Mild hypertension	Confirm within 2 months.
105–114	Moderate hypertension	Treatment should be undertaken.
Above 115	Severe hypertension	Treatment with medication should begin.
Systolic:		
Below 140	Normal blood pressure	Recheck within 2 years.
140–159	Borderline isolated systolic hypertension	Confirm within 2 months.
160–199	Isolated systolic hypertension	Confirm within 2 months and start treatment if blood pressure stays elevated.
Above 200	Isolated systolic hypertension	Begin treatment with medication.

Source: Adapted from: Moser, M. High blood pressure. Zaret, B. L., Moser, M., Cohen, L. S., & Subak-Sharpe, G. J. (Eds.) (1992), *Yale University School of Medicine heart book.* New York: Hearst Books, p. 152.

- *What having hypertension means:* Is hypertension by itself a serious health problem or is it simply a symptom of other, graver disorders? The answer is: both.

  You may not know you have hypertension—an estimated third of the 50 million Americans who have hypertension are unaware they have it.[7] As mentioned, hypertension is called the Silent Killer because it is not associated with symptoms such as headaches, dizziness, or other adverse effects. Nevertheless, it takes its toll on vital organs, speeds up the process of hardening of the arteries, forces the heart to work harder, may narrow the blood vessels to the brain, and may cause kidney damage.

- *Treatment:* Treatment for hypertension is of two types—lifestyle and drugs.

  Taking a pill is easy. Making lifestyle changes may be difficult. Most doctors will counsel their high-blood-pressure patients to lose weight, take up exercise, quit smoking, consume no more than two alcoholic drinks a day, switch to a low-fat and low-sodium diet, and practice stress reduction. Lifestyle changes can significantly reduce blood pressure for some people. In one study, for example, men with mild hypertension who took up moderate exercise for 10 weeks (20 minutes of aerobics and 30 minutes of weight training 3 times a week) lowered their blood pressure as much as they would have by taking antihypertensive medication.[8]

  Among the classes of drugs used to treat hypertension, two are particularly important. *Antihypertensive drugs* open up (dilate) some of the smaller blood vessels, thus reducing blood pressure. *Diuretic drugs* remove excess water from the bloodstream, lowering the volume of blood and thereby lowering the blood pressure. Many people who take medication for hypertension don't do so consistently. Reasons for noncompliance include misunderstandings about the disease, the lack of symptoms, and drug-related side effects. Drugs' adverse side effects include muscle weakness, impotence, depression, reduced sex drive, dizziness, and fainting.

It is important to take every available opportunity to have your blood pressure checked. If you receive a reading of 140/90 or higher, have it rechecked by a health care professional. Many of the controllable risk factors for hypertension are associated with other forms of heart disease.

Coronary Heart Disease: Atherosclerosis, Angina, and Heart Attack Known as **CHD, coronary heart disease** involves damage to the blood vessels to the heart. CHD is *the* leading cause of death of Americans today, killing 500,000 of us every year.[9] To explain how it happens, we first need to distinguish between *arteriosclerosis* and *atherosclerosis,* although you may hear the terms being used interchangeably.

Arteriosclerosis is considered an *impairment* but not a disease. Arteriosclerosis is "hardening of the arteries," a general condition often associated with aging in which the blood vessel walls thicken, harden, and become less elastic. In part this is because of buildups of fatty material from the diet. For some people, however, the rate of material building up is faster than others, and this is called atherosclerosis.

Atherosclerosis is a type of arteriosclerosis, but it is considered a *disease.* Atherosclerosis is characterized by deposits of **plaque** —deposits of fat, cholesterol, calcium, cell parts, and a blood-clotting material (fibrin)— on the inner lining of the arteries. Over time, the channels in the artery become narrowed, thus reducing the supply of blood to the tissues supplied by the affected arteries. A complete blockage may also occur. (*See* ● *Figure 30.6.*)

Atherosclerosis can occur in blood vessels throughout the body, but it is particularly dangerous when it happens in a coronary artery, which supplies blood—and hence oxygen and nutrients—to the heart muscle itself. When the opening of the coronary artery is narrowed by 50–70% of its normal diameter, one is considered to have *coronary heart disease.* At this point, a person is probably on the road to angina or a heart attack:

● *Angina:* **Angina,** or **angina pectoris,** is an intense pain in the chest behind the breastbone, owing to a diminished supply of oxygen to the heart. The pain may radiate to the arm and even the jaw. Angina can be triggered by emotional stress, exercise, a heavy meal, or exposure to cold.

Angina is not itself fatal. Indeed, 2.5 million Americans presently live with angina, and some have had it for years and never suffered a heart attack. However, angina is a warning, particularly if it becomes longer in duration, more severe, or more frequent.

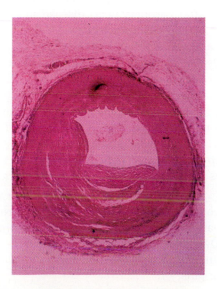
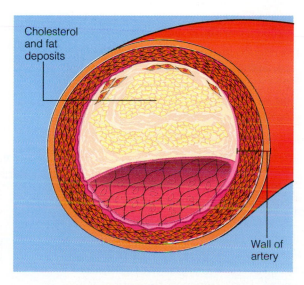

Cholesterol
and fat
deposits

Wall of
artery

● **Figure 30.6 The effects of atherosclerosis.** (*Left*) An artery partially blocked by the plaque of atherosclerosis. (*Right*) Diagram of atherosclerotic plaque.

Angina is treated with drugs. Nitroglycerin is frequently used because it is a **vasodilator**—it widens blood vessels. Other useful drugs lower blood pressure, slow the heart to reduce its need for oxygen, and reduce the chance of arterial spasms.

- *Heart attack:* A heart attack is called a **myocardial infarction (MI),** which literally means *death of heart muscle.* Although often caused by impaired blood supply to a part of the heart muscle, it may also have other causes, such as an electrical shock. The risk of fatality is significantly related to the extent and location of the damage.

When a heart attack is underway, it is important to act quickly. This means not ignoring its principal signs: severe chest pain or pressure lasting more than 2 minutes and usually 20 minutes or more—a pain that may radiate to the arms (especially the left arm), jaw, or neck—shortness of breath, sweating, nausea, dizziness, and fainting.

A myocardial infarction may come about in three ways:

(1) It may be by the slow accretion of atherosclerotic plaque within a coronary artery until the artery is so blocked (occluded) that oxygen and nutrients cease to reach the heart. This type is called a **coronary occlusion.**

(2) It may be due to a blood clot, called a **thrombus,** stuck to a blood vessel wall, that blocks the blood flow. This produces the kind of heart attack called a **coronary thrombosis**.

(3) It may result from a gathering of several circulating blood clots, each called an **embolus,** which collect in a narrowed coronary artery. This is called a **coronary embolism.**

Regardless of the cause, it is critical that a heart attack victim get medical aid *immediately. Sixty percent of deaths occur within an hour after first symptoms appear.*[10] Don't transport the patient yourself. Stay with the person and call for an ambulance. If the patient can be rushed to a hospital, he or she has a better chance of surviving now that treatment is possible with clot-dissolving drugs, which can get the blood flowing again.

Long-term treatment may involve the drugs used to treat angina, balloon angioplasty, coronary artery bypass graft, and other therapies that we shall describe.

The atherosclerosis that produces angina and heart attacks can occur in other blood vessels and produce stroke or affect the supply of blood to the legs (peripheral artery disease).

Stroke Like a myocardial infarction, a **stroke,** also known as a **cerebrovascular accident (CVA),** can be caused by a blockage in a blood vessel. In this instance, however, the blockage is in an artery carrying blood to the brain.

The resulting loss of oxygen to the brain can produce dramatic changes: The face, arm, and leg on one side of the body suddenly become weak or numb. There may be a loss of speech, difficult or slurred speech, or inability to understand speech. There may be a complete or partial loss or dimming of vision, or memory loss. People experiencing a stroke may feel unsteady, dizzy, or experience a sudden fall. Because brain cells can perish very quickly after a stroke, it is crucial when observing these warning signs to get the patient to a hospital quickly. Again, call an ambulance. Don't try to transport the person yourself.

Strokes are the third leading cause of death, after coronary heart disease and cancer. About 500,000 Americans have strokes each year, and about 150,000 of them die.[11] Strokes are also a major cause of disability. Often the impairment is permanent, or recovery can take a long time. Nor are strokes a misfortune of the old; they are a leading cause of death among women in their late 30s. (*See* • *Figure 30.7.*)

The term *stroke* actually represents a *group* of diseases. There are two broad categories of stroke, *ischemic* and *hemorrhagic:*

- *Ischemic:* **Ischemic strokes,** which account for about 70% of all strokes, are caused by lack of blood flow to the brain. Over a third of ischemic strokes have an unknown cause, but others have the following origins:

(1) A **cerebral thrombosis** is caused by a clot (thrombus) blocking blood flow in a brain artery. As with heart arteries, plaque builds up deposits on the inner lining of an artery, eventually obstructing the flow of blood.

(2) A **cerebral embolism** is caused by a wandering clot (embolus) that travels through the bloodstream and becomes wedged in an artery or vessel leading to the brain.

(3) A **lacunar stroke** results from blockage of the very small blood vessels (arterioles) reaching deep into the brain.

• *Hemorrhagic:* **Hemorrhagic strokes** are those in which blood seeps from a hole in a blood vessel wall. It accounts for 20–25% of all strokes. The hemorrhage may be of two types:

(1) A **cerebral hemorrhage** is a seepage of blood into the brain itself. The onset is signaled by severe headaches and a decrease in or loss of consciousness.

(2) A **subarachnoid hemorrhage** is a seepage of blood into the space around the brain. Symptoms include the sudden onset of an excruciating headache and perhaps a stiff neck, nausea and vomiting, change in consciousness, and seizures. The cause of this kind of hemorrhage is often an **aneurysm,** an outpouching or ballooning of a weakened area of the blood vessel, which may go unnoticed for years, then suddenly rupture.

Some kinds of stroke, particularly the ischemic kinds, have warnings in the form of "ministrokes" called **transient ischemic attacks (TIAs).** The symptoms are the same as those for a stroke—weakness or numbness on one side of the body, inability to speak, lack of coordination, and so on. The difference is that most TIAs last only a few minutes, so that people who have them tend to dismiss them as nothing. However, the event should be taken seriously: about a third of all TIA patients will go on to have a stroke.[12]

Anyone experiencing a stroke of any kind needs immediate medical help. Treatment depends on the underlying cause of the problem. Some patients undergo drug treatment, including use of anticoagulant (anticlotting) drugs and aspirin. Some require surgery to repair blood vessels.

Heart Disease in the Young Two of the most common heart problems found in the young are congenital heart disease and rheumatic heart disease:

• *Congenital heart disorders:* The word *congenital* means "present at birth." **Congenital heart disorders** are structural defects in the heart that develop while the fetus is in the womb. About 1% of newborn babies have some congenital heart malfunction, which means the condition is relatively rare. The cause of a congenital heart defect is often unknown, but can include rubella (German measles), chemical substances used by the mother, and inherited factors. Defects range from heart murmurs due to a failure of the heart valves to close properly to serious structural problems that require major surgery. In only half the cases is the problem severe enough to require surgery or medical treatment.[13]

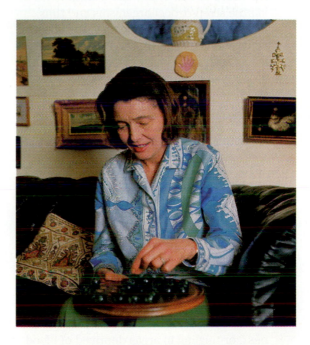

● **Figure 30.7 Stroke at 39.** Actress Patricia Neal had to learn how to walk and talk again after suffering a stroke at age 39. Part of her therapy involved manipulating dominoes and chinese puzzles. Within 3 years she resumed her career.

Maladies include holes in the wall dividing the lower chambers of the heart (the ventricular septum), damage to the heart valves, and transposition of the arteries to the body and to the lungs. Any of these can keep some blood from being pumped to the lungs where it is oxygenated (picks up oxygen for delivery to the rest of the body). Lack of oxygen in the blood leads to a bluish skin color called *cyanosis*; an infant with cyanosis is called a *blue baby*.

- *Rheumatic heart disease:* **Rheumatic heart disease** is one of the consequences of *rheumatic fever,* which develops in about 1% of acute streptococcal (strep) infections of the throat.[14] Rheumatic fever develops mainly in children ages 5–15. Symptoms are often nonspecific but may include skin rash, swollen joints, and fever. Rheumatic heart disease occurs in about half of these cases; it involves damage to the heart valves. Treatment is antibiotics to kill the streptococci organisms and thus prevent scarring of the heart valves. Prevention includes having any severe sore throat examined by a doctor and appropriately treated. The symptoms of strep throat include a sudden sore throat, fever, swollen glands, nausea, vomiting, and headache.

Three Other Cardiovascular Problems
Other problems are peripheral artery disease, congestive heart failure, and irregular heartbeat:

- *Peripheral artery disease:* **Peripheral artery disease**—also called *peripheral vascular disease*—is damage resulting from atherosclerosis or other problems such as diabetes that leads to restricted blood flow to the body's extremities, especially the legs and feet, but sometimes the hands. Symptoms include coldness, numbness, or tingling in areas deprived of blood flow, and cramps during exercise. This problem can lead to ulcerations, tissue death, and gangrene and may necessitate amputation of the affected limb.

  Treatment includes modifications in the diet, exercise, drug therapy, weight loss, and (because nicotine constricts the blood vessels) elimination of tobacco use. Surgery on the blood vessels is sometimes required.

- *Congestive heart failure:* **Congestive heart failure** occurs when the heart does not have the power to continue to pump blood normally. As blood returns to the heart and can't all be pumped out, the blood flow starts to back up. Fluid collects in the lungs, a condition called **pulmonary edema,** causing shortness of breath, which may worsen to struggling to breathe. Fluid accumulation also leads to swelling (edema) in other parts of the body, especially the ankles and legs.

  Congestive heart failure can result from any problem that impairs the ability of the heart to pump blood. Such underlying problems include lung disease, birth defects, rheumatic fever, heart attack, high blood pressure, or atherosclerosis. Treatment involves increasing the effectiveness or reducing the workload of the heart. Several kinds of drugs are commonly used, including vasodilators to relax smooth muscle and improve function of the ventricles, diuretics to remove excess body fluid, and digitalis to improve the effectiveness of the heart.

- *Irregular heartbeat:* Rheumatic fever, infections, drug use (including coffee, nicotine, and alcohol), coronary heart disease, and heart attacks can produce irregular heartbeats called **arrhythmias.** The electrical activity of the heart can be measured in an **electrocardiogram (ECG,** or **EKG** for the German spelling).

  The normal heart rate for adults at rest is 60–80 beats per minute. An abnormally slow rate, **bradycardia,** is below 60 beats per minute, though people who are physically fit have a bradycardia due to the efficiency with which their heart works. An abnormally high rate, **tachycardia,** is more than 100 beats per minute, though tachycardia is normal when exercising. In **ventricular fibrillation,** the ventricles are unable to pump blood because the cardiac muscle contracts haphazardly, and the ECG pattern is very uneven.

An arrhythmia is an irregular heartbeat. It may be corrected by use of drugs or, in some cases, by means of a **pacemaker,** which is surgically implanted in the chest. The pacemaker electrically stimulates the heart to beat at a normal rate.

Help for the Unhealthy Heart

Getting help for a heart attack means knowing how to recognize it and get emergency help, and understanding the tools for diagnosis, such as the electrocardiogram. Treatment may consist of bypass surgery, balloon angioplasty, or heart transplant, or a variety of lifestyle changes.

Every year, about half a million people die from heart attacks. What can you do to increase the survival chances for a friend or for yourself if suddenly you are presented with the classic symptoms of a heart attack?

The Signs of Heart Attack Heart attacks sometimes happen without warning, but they often have characteristic signs and symptoms: (1) steady, squeezing pressure or burning pain in the center of the chest lasting 2 minutes or more; (2) pain radiating from the center of the chest down the left or both arms or to the shoulders, neck, jaw, or back; (3) blue skin color; (4) sweating or clamminess; (5) dizziness or fainting; (6) shortness of breath; (7) nausea or vomiting; and (8) a sense of anxiety or feeling of dread.

Getting Emergency Help Individually, these signs may be symptoms of some disorder other than heart disease or heart attack. *However, people have died from heart attacks who might have been saved had treatment not been delayed because the signs were misinterpreted.* If you become aware of any of these symptoms, in yourself or someone else, you should *immediately call the 911 emergency number or Emergency Medical Service and ask for an ambulance.*

Don't try to drive the person to a hospital emergency room yourself, unless you are in an extremely remote location. The Emergency

Medical Service technicians will have life-support resources and equipment to use en route to the emergency room.

While you are waiting for help to arrive, be reassuring and make sure the person is comfortable. If vomiting occurs, have the person sit up rather than lie down to prevent stomach contents from getting into the lungs. Don't give the person any drugs, foods, or liquids.

If the individual loses consciousness, you may need to start cardiopulmonary resuscitation (CPR), if you have proper training. Once the person arrives at the emergency room or coronary care unit of the hospital, health professionals may use a *defibrillator* to administer an electrical shock that will stimulate the heart back to a normal rhythm. They may also administer anticoagulants, pain medication, oxygen, and other treatment as necessary in order to stabilize the person and prevent further progression of the problem.

Tools for Diagnosis If there is no medical emergency but doctors suspect a heart problem of some kind or want to routinely screen an individual for the possibility of heart diseases, they have a choice of diagnostic tools:

- *The electrocardiogram:* As mentioned, the purpose of the electrocardiogram (ECG or EKG) is to provide information about heart rhythms and other clues to a heart problem. In the procedure, electrodes, or leads, are attached to the patient's chest or ankles. The electrical activity of the heart is transmitted to an electrocardiograph, a machine that prints onto a continuous strip of paper.

- *Exercise stress testing:* The electrocardiogram just described is often called a "resting ECG," because it is administered while the patient is lying down. The **exercise stress test,** sometimes referred to as a treadmill test, is an electrocardiogram taken while the individual walks on a treadmill or pedals a stationary bicycle. The purpose of the test is to assess the action of the heart under conditions of increased oxygen demand and to elicit any symptoms, such as chest pain or ECG abnormalities, that might occur under these conditions.

- *The echocardiogram:* The **echocardiogram** is a one-, two-, or three-dimensional picture of the heart taken with sound waves. The procedure is used for diagnosing conditions that require information about the anatomy of the heart, such as valve disorders.

- *Nuclear cardiology:* In nuclear cardiology, a small amount of a nonharmful radioactive material is injected into the bloodstream. A radiation-detecting device is then used to follow its progress through the circulatory system. The results are then displayed by a computer as three-dimensional images of the heart.

- *Cardiac catheterization:* **Cardiac catheterization** is the process of inserting a thin tube into a blood vessel in the leg or arm, then passing it into or around the heart. Physicians may then take pressure readings or inject radiopaque dyes (visible on X rays) and see how they show up. (This type of X ray is called an *angiogram.*)

Treatment Most people with cardiovascular problems can be treated with drugs to lower blood pressure, control heart rhythms, relieve angina pain, or help the heart work better to overcome congestive failure. Other forms of treatment are coronary bypass surgery, balloon angioplasty, and heart transplants.

- *Bypass surgery:* **Bypass surgery** is designed to alleviate the problem of blocking or narrowing of one or all of the arteries in the heart itself. Because of their small diameter, the coronary arteries are particularly susceptible to blockage by plaque formation or a blood clot. In coronary bypass surgery, a section of a vein is taken from the arm or leg or a synthetic graft is used to bypass a blocked coronary artery. (See ● *Figure 30.8.*) When the procedure must be done for all coronary arteries, it is called a "triple bypass."

  Unfortunately, bypass surgery does not always solve the problem permanently. Because the underlying tendency for buildup is not resolved, some patients find that they may require a second bypass operation at some point in the future.

- *Balloon angioplasty:* Increasingly, bypass surgery is being replaced with **balloon angioplasty** (technically called percutaneous transluminal coronary angioplasty, or PTCA), which is less risky than bypass surgery. Using the process of cardiac catheterization, a deflated miniature balloon is inserted inside a coronary artery. When inflated, it compresses the plaque causing the blockage and widens the artery to increase the flow of blood.

  Balloon angioplasty is successful in 85% of cases. One problem, occurring in 4–7% of all cases, is a recurrence of the narrowing of the arteries within 6 months of the procedure.[15]

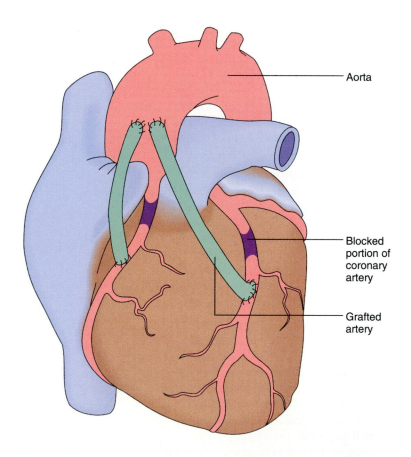

Aorta

Blocked portion of coronary artery

Grafted artery

● **Figure 30.8 Coronary bypass.** In this operation, two grafted arteries (*shown in green*) are used to bypass blocked portions of two coronary arteries.

- *Heart transplant:* Heart transplants consist of the surgical removal of a defective heart and its replacement by a heart taken from a donor. (Usually the donor is a person of similar size, under 35 years old, who has suffered brain death, as from an auto accident.) Tissue matching, by blood type, is done through regional organ banks, and the donor heart is flown to the hospital where the recipient is being prepared to receive it. Great care is taken to monitor possible rejection of the heart after the operation and to avoid infections.

   Approximately 85% of heart transplant patients are still alive after the first year and 65% after 5 years.[16] In recent years, there has also been excitement about the use of mechanical (artificial) hearts, such as the Jarvik heart. Although some physicians wonder whether an artificial heart will ever be more than a temporary means of keeping patients alive until donors are found, a 1991 study ordered by the Heart, Lung and Blood Institute predicts that self-contained mechanical pumps implanted in patients' bodies will be able to replace diseased human hearts within 20 years.[17]

Nonsurgical Treatment: Lifestyle Changes
In recent years, there has also been evidence that people with blocked coronary arteries can reverse the blockage without medication or surgery. In a study known as the Lifestyle Heart Trial, San Francisco physician Dean Ornish and his colleagues demonstrated that lifestyle changes alone—a strict vegetarian diet, mild daily exercise, and practice of stress-reduction techniques—could actually reverse the progression of atherosclerotic plaques in coronary arteries.[18,19]

The Risk Factors for Heart Disease

Risk factors that increase the chances of getting heart disease consist of predisposing factors, such as heredity, gender, age, and race or ethnic group. They also consist of precipitating factors, such as cigarette smoking, high blood pressure, blood cholesterol levels, exercise, diabetes, weight, personality, and stress.

The term *risk factors* may not set alarm bells ringing in your head, but this term signals caution. **Risk factors** are those traits and behaviors that increase one's chances of getting heart disease. (*See Self Discovery 30.1.*) Knowledge of these factors enables you to make better informed decisions about your lifestyle.

Some risk factors you cannot control, some you can:

- *Not controllable—predisposing risk factors:* Those that cannot be controlled are called *predisposing risk factors*. They include your heredity, gender, age, and race or ethnic group.

- *Controllable—precipitating risk factors:* Those that can be controlled are called *precipitating risk factors* and include cigarette smoking, high blood pressure, blood cholesterol levels, exercise, diabetes, weight, personality, and stress. The first three of these—smoking, hypertension, and cholesterol—are considered the Big Three controllable risk factors. All other risk factors mainly affect these three.

Predisposing Risk Factors: Age, Gender, Heredity, Race Nothing can be done to change predisposing risk factors, although if any of these indicate high risk for you, it might provide additional motivation for you to control the precipitating risk factors:

- *Age:* The risk of cardiovascular disorders increases as you get older. Half of those who have heart attacks are 65 or over, and 4 out of 5 people who die of heart attacks are over 65.

   Although nothing can be done to reduce age, paying attention to diet and fitness will delay the effects of aging.

- *Gender:* Men are more likely than women to develop cardiovascular disorders, particularly before age 40. Four times as many men as women develop atherosclerosis. Even so, coronary heart disease is the number one cause of death among American women, though mainly in later life.

SELF DISCOVERY 30.1

Is Your Heart at Risk?

For each of the five following categories—weight, systolic blood pressure, blood cholesterol level, cigarette smoking, and (for women only) estrogen use—indicate the response that best describes you and your lifestyle.

1. Weight. Study the following chart and find your weight category. Indicate the points in the right-hand column.

Weight category	Points
A	−2
B	−1
C	+1
D	+2

Your points: _____

**MEN
Weight category (lbs.)**

Your height	A	B	C	D
5′1″	up to 123	124–148	149–173	174 +
5′2″	up to 128	127–152	153–178	179 +
5′3″	up to 129	130–156	157–182	183 +
5′4″	up to 132	133–160	161–186	187 +
5′5″	up to 135	136–163	164–190	191 +
5′6″	up to 139	140–168	169–196	197 +
5′7″	up to 144	145–174	175–203	204 +
5′8″	up to 148	149–179	180–209	210 +
5′9″	up to 152	153–184	185–214	215 +
5′10″	up to 157	158–190	191–221	222 +
5′11″	up to 161	162–194	195–227	228 +
6′0″	up to 165	166–199	200–232	233 +
6′1″	up to 170	171–205	208–239	240 +
6′2″	up to 175	176–211	212–246	247 +
6′3″	up to 180	181–217	218–253	254 +
6′4″	up to 185	186–223	224–260	261 +
6′5″	up to 190	191–229	230–267	268 +
6′6″	up to 195	196–235	236–274	275 +

**WOMEN
Weight category (lbs.)**

Your height	A	B	C	D
4′8″	up to 101	102–122	123–143	144 +
4′9″	up to 103	104–125	126–146	147 +
4′10″	up to 106	107–128	129–150	151 +
4′11″	up to 109	110–132	133–154	155 +
5′0″	up to 112	113–136	137–158	159 +
5′1″	up to 115	116–139	140–162	163 +
5′2″	up to 119	120–144	145–168	169 +
5′3″	up to 122	123–148	149–172	173 +
5′4″	up to 127	128–154	155–179	180 +
5′5″	up to 131	132–158	159–185	186 +
5′6″	up to 135	136–163	164–190	191 +
5′7″	up to 139	140–168	169–196	197 +
5′8″	up to 143	144–173	174–202	203 +
5′9″	up to 147	148–178	179–207	208 +
5′10″	up to 151	152–182	183–213	214 +
5′11″	up to 155	156–187	188–218	219 +
6′0″	up to 159	160–191	192–224	225 +
6′1″	up to 163	164–196	197–229	230 +

2. Systolic blood pressure. Use the first number from your most recent blood pressure test. If you do not know your blood pressure, estimate it by circling the number corresponding to your weight category (A = −2, B = −1, etc.).

Blood pressure/ weight category	Points if male	Points if female
A 119 or less	−1	−2
B 120–139	0	−1
C 140–159	0	0
D 160 or higher	+1	+1

3. Blood cholesterol level. Use the number from your most recent blood cholesterol test. If you do not know your blood cholesterol, estimate it by circling the number that corresponds to your weight category.

Blood cholesterol/ weight category	Points if male	Points if female
A 199 or less	−2	−1
B 200–224	−1	0
C 225–249	0	0
D 250 or higher	+1	+1

(continued)

SELF DISCOVERY 30.1
(continued)

4. Cigarette smoking

Amount smoked	Points
Do not smoke	−1
Smoke less than a pack a day or smoke a pipe	0
Smoke a pack a day	+1
Smoke more than a pack a day	+2

5. (For women only) estrogen use. Answer these two questions:
  a. Have you ever taken birth-control pills or other hormone drugs containing estrogen for 5 or more years in a row?
  b. Are you age 35 or older and now taking birth-control pills or other hormone drugs containing estrogen?

Usage	Points
"No" to both questions	0
"Yes" to one or both questions	+1

Scoring

Total the points circled. Be careful to *add* the plus numbers and *subtract* the minus numbers. Then add 10 points to your total.

Interpretation

Total points	Amount of heart risk
0–4	Very low
5–9	Low to moderate
10–14	Moderate to high
15–19	High
20+	Extremely high

Source: American Heart Association, 1985.

It is speculated that male hormones (androgens) increase risk, whereas female hormones (estrogens) protect against atherosclerosis. This is supported by the fact that heart disease risk for women rises after menopause, when their bodies have stopped producing estrogen.

- *Heredity:* If you have close relatives who suffered heart attacks or strokes before age 50, it increases your chances of experiencing a similar problem. Some families have a history of very high levels of blood cholesterol, indicating an inherited tendency.

  The good news is that there is nothing inevitable about this, because prior generations did not have the benefit of the lifestyle changes many American have instituted nor the quality of medical care we have now. Still, if you have a family history of heart attacks or strokes, you should be especially careful to change controllable (precipitating) risk factors.

- *Race:* African Americans are twice as likely to have high blood pressure as whites.[20,21] (*See* • *Figure 30.9.*) This may be because of societal factors, such as stress, poverty, and high-fat diet. The chances of having a heart attack are similar among blacks and whites, but in African Americans heart attacks are more likely to be fatal.[22]

  Now let us turn to the controllable risk factors—the Big Three of cigarette smoking, high blood pressure, and blood cholesterol levels. We

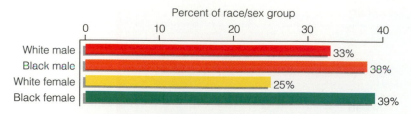

Percent of race/sex group

Hypertensives are defined as persons with a systolic level that is greater than or equal to 140 and/or a diastolic level that is greater than or equal to 90 or who report using antihypertensive medication.

● **Figure 30.9 High blood pressure and race.** Estimated percent of population with hypertension, by race and sex, U.S. adults ages 18–74.

will also consider other risk factors that affect the Big Three—namely, exercise, diabetes, weight, personality, and stress.

Cigarette Smoking: No. 1 Controllable Risk Factor By now people have gotten the message about the association between smoking and lung cancer. However, the bigger enemy strengthened by smoking is cardiovascular disease. Indeed, smoking is *the* No. 1 cause of heart disease in the United States. Moreover, of people who have heart attacks, smokers have less chance of surviving than nonsmokers do.[23]

Why is smoking so lethal? It seems that cigarette smoking accelerates atherosclerosis in three ways:[24]

1. *Carbon monoxide damage:* The carbon monoxide in smoke is poisonous, and over time it damages the lining of the blood vessels, making it easier for fatty deposits to adhere to the walls.

2. *Effect on cholesterol:* Smoking raises "bad" cholesterol and lowers "good" cholesterol, as we will describe, increasing the risk and severity of atherosclerosis.

3. *Increases blood clots:* Smoking increases the possibility of blood clots forming and blocking the arteries, thus raising the likelihood of heart attacks or stroke.

There is good news in this, however: the overall risk of having a heart attack starts to de-

cline within the *first day* after one stops smoking. Within 1 year of quitting, the risk of heart disease is cut in half.[25]

High Blood Pressure: No. 2 Controllable Risk Factor High blood pressure, or hypertension, is defined generally as a systolic level that is 140 millimeters of mercury (mm Hg) or higher and/or a diastolic level that is 90 mm Hg or higher. The result of high blood pressure is that the blood presses against the artery walls. This increases the work the heart has to do, weakening it over time.

Controlling hypertension is imperative, since it can result in heart disease, stroke, and kidney failure. Nearly one-third of people whose hypertension is not controlled die of heart disease. Another third die of stroke. Of the remaining, 10–15% die of kidney failure.[26] High blood pressure can be controlled with medication, exercise, and diet.

Blood Fats: No. 3 Controllable Risk Factor **Blood fats,** or **serum lipids,** include *cholesterol* and *triglycerides*. These are the culprits that are believed to play a role in the buildup of plaque in the lining of the blood vessels, producing atherosclerosis and heart disease.

Although it has been portrayed as being almost like poison, **cholesterol** is actually an organic substance that is vital to the functioning of the body. Cholesterol is found only in fats and oils produced by animals, never plants. The cholesterol found in the food you eat is referred to as **dietary cholesterol.** The cholesterol in your body is **blood cholesterol** or **serum cholesterol.**

Studies show that the level of cholesterol in the blood is a fairly reliable predictor of how likely an individual is to develop coronary heart disease and, to some extent, stroke.[27] Cholesterol levels are expressed in mg/dl, or milligrams of cholesterol per deciliter of blood. In general, experts consider cholesterol levels under 200 mg/dl to be normal, 200–239 to be borderline, and 240 and up to be dangerously high risk. About 1 out of 4 adults has a serum cholesterol level of 240 or more.

Cholesterol is carried within the circulatory system by *lipoproteins,* a word much in the news in the last few years. As the term suggests, a **lipoprotein** can be thought of as "lipid plus protein"; it is a compound of fat (lipid) and protein that serves to carry cholesterol and other fats (such as triglycerides) through the bloodstream. Several types of lipoprotein exist. These have come to be known as the "good" and "bad" forms of blood cholesterol.

- *"Bad" cholesterol—LDLs:* **Low-density lipoproteins,** abbreviated **LDLs,** transport blood cholesterol *to* the cells in the body. This form is considered the "bad" lipoprotein (or bad form of blood cholesterol) because some gets deposited in fatty streaks in blood vessels, forming buildups of plaque.

- *"Good" cholesterol—HDLs:* Abbreviated **HDLs, high-density lipoproteins** transport blood cholesterol *from* the cells in the body to the liver. This form is considered "good" lipoprotein (or good form of blood cholesterol) because it removes excess cholesterol from blood vessels.

Now to get down to basics: The consensus about the effects of diet on heart and blood-vessel disease seems to be as follows:[28]

- *High LDL and low HDL blood cholesterol levels mean increased risk of heart disease.* The higher the blood cholesterol levels of the low-density lipoproteins (LDLs) and the lower the levels of the high-density lipoproteins (HDLs), the greater the severity of atherosclerosis and the risk of coronary heart disease.

- *Eating saturated fats and dietary cholesterol increases blood cholesterol.* Avoid saturated fats—those found in meat and dairy products, palm and coconut oils, and cocoa butter. Saturated fats, and to some extent dietary cholesterol, promote the production of blood cholesterol in the body.

Weight Excess body fat appears to raise the risk of heart disease. The more the weight, the higher the risk. For instance, one study of 116,000 women found that the risk of heart disease was three times higher among the most obese group than among the leanest group.[29]

Diabetes Mellitus People who develop the disorder of the endocrine system called diabetes mellitus, especially that which begins later in life (Type 2 diabetes), have an increased risk of

coronary heart disease and stroke. Exercise and weight reduction can help to slow down the onset of diabetes.

Inactivity The evidence is convincing that regular exercise will reduce the likelihood of a heart attack and may improve the chances of survival if one does occur. Indeed, the authors of one study argued that inactivity should be classified as a primary rather than secondary risk factor for heart disease.[30] Exercise can certainly help control weight, perhaps improve the body's ability to use insulin, may raise the HDL (the "good" cholesterol), and lower blood pressure, among other positive effects.

"Type A" Personality and Stress People with **Type A personalities** are people who are hurried, deadline-ridden, and competitive, as well as hostile and antagonistic. **Type B personalities,** by contrast, are relaxed, unhurried, and carefree. In the early 1970s, San Francisco physicians Meyer Friedman and Ray Rosenman suggested that Type A behavior was linked to stress-related heart disease, whereas Type B personalities seemed less at risk.[31] However, it was also found that it was possible through counseling to reduce Type A behavior and reduce the number of heart attacks.[32]

Not all experts agree that Type A behavior is a true cardiovascular risk factor. Still, it has been shown that job stress can raise blood pressure and lead to other detrimental physical changes that often precede heart disease.[33] Physician Dean Ornish has shown that the use of yoga, visualization, and meditation—all stress-relieving techniques—along with changes in diet and exercise can actually reverse heart disease.[34-36]

Strategy for Living: Preventing Heart Disease

Nine steps for preventing heart disease are (1) quit smoking, (2) reduce dietary fat and cholesterol, (3) reduce sodium, (4) add fiber, (5) moderate alcohol use, (6) keep weight down, (7) exercise, (8) perhaps take aspirin, and (9) cope with stress.

A great part of the art of living is recognizing that your habits really do matter. Nowhere is this more apparent than in the link between your lifestyle and heart disease. In a way, having heart disease is a sign of *accelerated* aging: for many people, having heart disease means they let their bodies begin to run down sooner than nature intended because of certain choices they made about how they wanted to live.

Of course, when you're young you may not have any sense of urgency about the importance of quitting smoking, changing your diet, taking up exercise, and adopting other habits favorable to your heart's survival. What could induce you to make these changes? Perhaps it would be to ask some cardiologists not what advice they give their patients but what lifestyle changes they have made *themselves*. After all, who better than a heart doctor would know the daily changes required to prevent heart disease?

A 1990 survey of 400 cardiologists by the *Wall Street Journal* found that, based on their own example, the doctors rate the following as the best preventive steps for resisting heart disease: stopping smoking; altering diet to reduce cholesterol; limiting intake of salt; exercising; and taking aspirin.[37] Let us look at these and other steps.

Step 1: Quit Smoking Cardiologists are very strong on the subject of smoking. "I rarely see any patient with heart problems under the age of 65—unless they are smokers," said one.[38] Smokers have twice the risk of heart attack that nonsmokers have.

Step 2: Reduce Fat and Cholesterol in Your Diet You should get no more than 30% of your daily calories from fat in any form. No more than 10% should come from saturated fats.

To cut down fat, avoid fried foods. Broil, bake, or steam your food instead. If you use cooking oils, use those that contain polyunsaturated fats—corn, safflower, soybean, sunflower, or cottonseed oils. Eat less butter and cheese, less red meat, and more fish and poultry.

Step 3: Reduce Sodium (Salt) in Your Diet Sodium can affect high blood pressure. Thus, reduce your consumption of processed foods (such as potato chips, and canned vegetables and soups) and condiments (such as mustard, ketchup, and soy sauce), which are apt to be heavily salted. Don't add salt when cooking or eating food. Instead of salt, use herbs and spices as condiments.

Step 4: Add Fiber to Your Diet Fiber can reduce cholesterol levels, perhaps lower blood pressure, and make you feel "fuller" since it takes longer to digest. Fiber is found in whole grains, beans, legumes, fruits, and vegetables.

Step 5: Be Moderate in Your Alcohol Consumption Alcohol can raise the blood pressure. Drink only two alcoholic beverages or less a day.

Step 6: Keep Your Weight Down Being overweight can increase the chances of high blood pressure and other heart and blood-vessel diseases.

Step 7: Exercise Engaging in aerobic exercise—walking, jogging, bicycling, swimming, dancing—three times a week for about 30 minutes each time will lower blood pressure, maintain body weight, and reduce the risk of heart attack. (*See ● Figure 30.10.*)

Step 8: Consider Taking Aspirin Aspirin, the so-called wonder drug, may be a potent protector against fatal heart attacks and strokes. It seems that aspirin causes the blood to be less susceptible to clotting. In the United States, a daily dose of baby aspirin (81 milligrams) or alternate-day use of a regular, adult-sized aspirin tablet (325 milligrams) is recommended to head off more serious attacks among people who have already suffered a small stroke or who have evidence of reduced blood flow to the brain.

Many Americans without a history of blood-vessel disease (including cardiologists) also take half an adult aspirin or one baby aspirin daily to prevent heart attacks and strokes.[39,40] There is no advantage to taking more than one aspirin, which may lead to stomach distress, ulcers, and rectal bleeding. Nor should one take aspirin substitutes (such as Tylenol). Coated or buffered aspirin is less apt to cause internal distress. There is some concern about increased risk of stroke among aspirin users, and the evidence regarding stroke prevention remains inconclusive.

Step 9: Learn to Cope with Stress The stresses in our lives are ongoing and ever-changing. It is doubtful that we can ever get rid of all of them. However, we can learn to cope with the ones we have, using such relaxation techniques as progressive relaxation, meditation, visualization, and mental imagery.

800-HELP

American Heart Association. 800-527-6941

Heartlife. 800-241-6993 (in Arkansas, Hawaii, and Georgia call collect: 404-523-0826). Provides information about heart disease, pacemakers, medication, exercise, and nutrition

Suggestions for Further Reading

Ornish, Dean. (1990). *Dr. Dean Ornish's program for reversing heart disease: The only system scientifically proven to reverse heart disease without drugs or surgery*. New York: Ballantine. Presents evidence of the reversal of heart disease without drugs or surgery. The program explores the psychological, emotional, and spiritual as well as physical sides of recovery.

Schoenberg, Jane, & Stichman, Jo Ann. (1990). *Heart family handbook*. Philadelphia: Hanley & Belfus. Geared mainly to heart disease patients and their families.

Zaret, Barry L., Moser, Marvin, Cohen, Lawrence S., & Subak-Sharpe, Genell J. (Eds.) (1992). *Yale University School of Medicine heart book*. New York: Hearst Books. Comprehensive, practical lay reference guide from one of the country's finest medical schools.

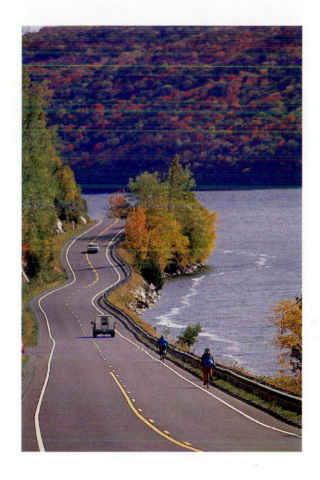

● **Figure 30.10 How much exercise?**

❝ *. . . To obtain a conditioning effect, a person must exercise three times a week for half an hour per session at a consistent intensity. One session is better than none, two is better than one, and three is still better than two. After three times a week, the gain in cardiovascular benefit, while still increasing, becomes progressively less. Additionally, when we start to exercise five, six, or seven times a week, orthopedic injuries become more of a problem. Therefore, there is a window of optimal frequency—three or four times each week, at which time the gain is near maximal while the injury risk is minor. More often becomes a threat to well-being—we wind ourselves too tightly.* ❞

—Walter M. Bortz II. (1991). *We live too short and die too long.* New York: Bantam Books, pp. 227–228.

31   Preventing and Conquering Cancer

▶ Explain what cancer is, how it is caused, how it spreads, and what its various types are.

▶ Describe the seven early warning signals and discuss several important cancers.

▶ Discuss how cancer is diagnosed and treated.

▶ Describe the predisposing risk factors and controllable risk factors for cancer.

▶ List the nine steps for preventing cancer.

Many diseases that were once thought to be practically synonymous with death—yellow fever, smallpox, scarlet fever—have been defeated or ameliorated by medical progress. However, cancer continues to hold some special horror in the public mind. Actor John Wayne, who died of lung cancer, called cancer "the Big C."

This is unfortunate, because cancer no longer has the inevitable outcome once associated with it. True, cancer is the No. 2 cause of death in the United States, accounting for 1 out of 5 deaths, and about 1 out of 3 Americans now living will eventually have cancer.[41] Even so, death rates have been steadily declining. Even better news, the potential is quite good for reducing cancer through prevention and early detection, as we shall show.

The first step in prevention is recognizing that cancer is not one disease but rather a constellation of more than 100 different diseases. What each has in common is the uncontrolled growth of abnormal cells.

Cancer: What It Is, What It Does

Cancer—abnormal cells spreading uncontrolled—is caused by initiators, promoters, and oncogenes. Cancer may spread in three ways—by direct extension, through the circulatory system, and through the lymphatic system. Tumors may be of four general types.

In only 9 months we grow from a single cell into a complete, functioning human being. In the 18 or so years following our birth, we develop into a more or less fully formed adult. Along the way, as we suffer life's cuts and bruises, our bodies produce new cells to repair the damage. These are the marvels of cellular growth.

Sometimes, however, cells don't follow this pattern. This is the beginning of the process called cancer.

What Is Cancer?   Cancer is a disease in which abnormal cells develop that can spread in an uncontrolled manner. Picture a cell that doesn't follow the rules. Something happens to make it **mutate**—change in a way that makes it lose its original ability to grow in orderly, regulated ways. The single abnormal cell divides into two abnormal cells, then four, and so on, eventually forming clusters of cells called **tumors.**

Tumors may be of two types:

• *Benign:* **Benign tumors** are abnormal in some way, but they usually are harmless, such as freckles, moles, or fatty lumps in the skin. They may be left alone or removed, but in any event they do not invade surrounding tissues.

• *Malignant:* **Malignant tumors** have two characteristics:

 (1) They grow and **infiltrate,** or invade, surrounding tissues.

 (2) In time, these malignant cells may also **metastasize,** spreading like seeds to other parts of the body, where they start other growths.

The only way to tell whether a tumor is benign or malignant is by examining the cells under a microscope. As you might expect, the sooner cancer is identified, the easier it is to treat.

The Causes of Cancer: Initiators, Promoters, and Oncogenes   Normal growth—the doubling and copying of cells—is governed by genes within the cells. However, some normal genes may be transformed, for whatever reason, into **oncogenes,** genes that promote the growth of cancer. These genes alter the regulation of cells so that the cells become abnormal.

What kind of changes transform these genes? According to one theory, "the multiple hit theory," all cancers arise from at least two changes or "hits" to the genes in the cell.[42] The hits may be *initiators,* which initiate the cancer process, or they may be *promoters,* which accelerate the growth of abnormal cells:

- *Initiators:* Initiators may include tobacco and tobacco smoke, excessive X rays, excessive exposure to sunlight, certain industrial agents or toxic substances, high-fat and low-fiber diet, obesity, certain hormones and drugs, and certain sexual practices (as in unprotected sexual contact against HIV/AIDS).

- *Promoters:* Promoters may include alcohol use, which is a factor in 4% of cancers (especially of the head, neck, and liver), and stress, which may weaken the immune system.

Heredity may also be a factor. As we shall explain, the risk of developing cancer comes down to three main factors: (1) your genetic makeup, (2) your environmental and occupational exposures to cancer-causing, or **carcinogenic,** agents, and (3) your personal lifestyle.

The Three Ways Cancer Spreads It is possible, but not usual, for tumors to grow in different parts of the body simultaneously. More commonly, a tumor begins in one place and then cancer cells travel from it to other areas. The spreading metatasis may take place in three ways:[43]

1. *Direct extension:* As the tumor grows in size, it invades tissues immediately next to it.

2. *Through the circulatory system:* Pieces of a tumor can grow through the walls of an artery or vein and enter the bloodstream, circulating through the body until they invade other organs.

3. *Through the lymphatic system:* Besides the blood vessel system (of arteries, veins, and capillaries), the body also has another circulatory vessel system, the **lymphatic system.** This consists of a separate system of tiny vessels (lymphatics), which carry a liquid called lymph, the purpose of which is to drain infectious, toxic, and other waste materials from the body. These materials are trapped in bean-shaped structures throughout the body called *lymph nodes,* where particles are destroyed. The lymph fluid is eventually returned to the bloodstream via the large vein that feeds into the heart called the *vena cava.*

Cancer cells can spread into the lymphatic system, perhaps eventually bypassing lymph nodes and getting directly into the body.

The Different Types of Tumors Physicians use an extensive classification system for types of malignant tumors, but for purposes of understanding we can say there are four general types of tumors, which correspond to four different kinds of tissues:

1. *Carcinomas:* **Carcinomas** are tumors that develop in an organ that secretes something. These are tumors found in the skin, glands, or membranes and include lung, breast, rectal, oral, testicular, and pancreatic cancers. About 85% of malignant tumors are carcinomas.

2. *Sarcomas:* **Sarcomas** are tumors of the connective tissues of the body—muscles, ligaments, bones, nerves, tendons, or blood vessels. Only 2% of malignant tumors are sarcomas.

3. *Leukemias:* **Leukemias** are tumors of the blood cells and blood-forming tissues, including the cells in the bone marrow.

4. *Lymphomas:* **Lymphomas** are tumors that develop in the lymph glands. Breast cancer, for instance, may initially spread from the breast to the lymph nodes in the armpit.

Although most tumors fall in these four areas, there are many concerns, from Hodgkin's disease to melanoma, whose names alone do not suggest the kinds of tissues from which they arise.

Cancers and Warning Signs

Cancer may be noticed by any of seven early warning signals. Several important

cancers are those of the lungs, breast, colon and rectum, prostate, blood and lymph systems, ovaries and uterus, oral cavity, skin, and testicles.

Some cancers have a higher risk of death than others. Every year the American Cancer Society reports the incidence and deaths associated with cancer in 12 different areas, covering about 40 organs and tissues. (*See* ● *Figure 31.1.*) Lung cancer and colon and rectum cancers are high on the list of deadly cancer for both men and women, breast cancer is the second most likely to kill for women, and prostate cancer the third most likely to kill for men.

General Warning Signs of Cancer The American Cancer Society has published a list, called *Seven Early Warning Signals* for cancer, whose first letters correspond to the word *C-A-U-T-I-O-N.* These are worth memorizing:

- *C:* Change in bowel or bladder habits
- *A:* A sore that does not heal
- *U:* Unusual bleeding or discharge
- *T:* Thickening or lump in breast or elsewhere
- *I:* Indigestion or difficulty in swallowing
- *O:* Obvious change in wart or mole
- *N:* Nagging cough or hoarseness

Unfortunately, many people don't pay much attention to these warning signs. However, *the earlier cancer is diagnosed, the better the chances for treatment and survival.*

Often cancer signs and symptoms are detected during a routine physical examination, such as a yearly checkup. This is better than their not being observed at all, but it is better yet to take any sign seriously and have it checked out.

Lung Cancer Lung cancer, the leading cause of cancer death in the United States, would be rare were it not for cigarette smoking. Most cases are associated with exposure to tobacco, both active smoking and passive smoking.

Identifying lung cancer early is difficult, because most signs don't appear until the disease has spread. As with any disease, however, the earlier the detection, the better the chances of reversing its course. If you're a smoker or have spent many years in smoking environments, be alert for persistent cough; change in volume, odor, or color of sputum; shortness of breath; and frequent upper respiratory infections.

Breast Cancer For women, breast cancer is nearly as serious as lung cancer: nearly 1 out of 9 American women will develop this disease. Some women are more at risk than others: women who consume alcohol moderately to

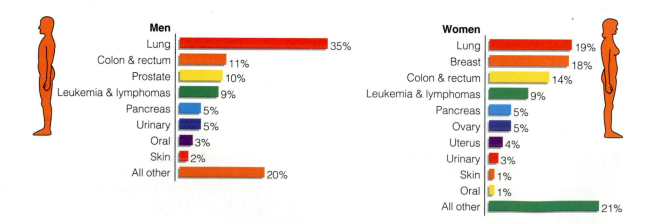

● **Figure 31.1 Risks of death, by cancer type.** The numbers express the percentage of fatalities among each type of cancer.

heavily; women with a family history of breast cancer, women who have had no children or who have had children late in life, women whose diets are high in saturated fats, women whose menstrual periods began when they were very young, and women whose menopause came later than usual.

In two-thirds of cases, the breast cancer produces no pain, but is experienced as a painless mass in the upper outside quadrant (quarter) of the breast. In another few cases, the mass is experienced as painful. Sometimes there is nipple discharge.

Colon and Rectum Cancer Lung cancer and breast cancer seem to grab all the headlines. However, cancer of the **colon,** part of the large intestine joining the rectum, and the **rectum,** the terminal part of the intestine, are nevertheless extremely common. Among cancers, colon and rectal cancer is the second cause of death of men, the third cause of death of women. A strong link is suspected between these cancers and a high-fat, low-fiber diet. Colon and rectal cancers may also tend to run in families.

Symptoms are bleeding from the rectum, blood in the stool, or a change in bowel habits.

Prostate Cancer The **prostate gland**, which secretes a fluid that is part of the male ejaculatory fluid, encircles the urethra just below the bladder. Cancer of the prostate is the third most common form of cancer in males, and probably 1 out of 11 men will develop this disease. There has been an increase in prostate cancer during the last 20 years, perhaps in part related to the North American high-fat diet.

Symptoms include difficulty urinating, blood in the urine, and low-back pain.

Leukemia and Lymphomas Leukemias are cancers of the blood system, lymphomas are cancers of the lymph system.

- *Leukemia:* There are several types of leukemia, but what all have in common is that they produce abnormal white blood cells that crowd out three substances of the blood: healthy white blood cells, making the body unable to fight infections; red blood cells, so the body cannot prevent anemia; and platelets, so the body cannot control bleeding.

Chronic leukemia often develops slowly and has few warning signs. Acute leukemia may offer several symptoms: fatigue, weight loss, susceptibility to infections, paleness, susceptibility to bruising, or nosebleeds.

- *Lymphoma:* Lymphomas provide several warning signs, including swollen lymph nodes, fever, weight loss, or night sweats.

Cancers of the Ovaries and Uterus Known as *gynecological cancers,* cancers of the ovaries and uterus together are responsible for about 9% of women's death by cancer every year.

- *Ovarian cancer:* The **ovaries** are the female reproductive organs. If the ovaries become cancerous, they may show no signs until later, although sometimes vaginal bleeding develops.

- *Uterine and cervical cancer:* The **uterus** is the pear-shaped muscle whose primary purpose is to contain the fetus until it is born. About 70% of uterine cancers affect the **endometrium,** the lining of the uterus. The other 30% of uterine cancers affect the **cervix,** the opening between the vagina and the uterus. Warning signs of either type include unusual vaginal discharge or bleeding between periods.

Oral Cancer Oral cancers occur anywhere between the lips and the throat—that is, anywhere in the oral cavity. Oral cancers may be associated with heavy smoking, excessive drinking, and use of chewing tobacco.

Symptoms include sores in the mouth that bleed easily or don't heal, a lump or thickening in the mouth or on the lips, whitish and hardened patches, persistent sore throat, and difficulty in chewing or swallowing.

Skin Cancer Most skin cancers, called basal-cell and squamous-cell carcinomas, are not considered very hazardous, because they are easily cured by medicine applied to the skin or by outpatient surgery. However, the skin cancer known as **melanoma** (which means "black tumor") is an exception. "Not only is melanoma the most malignant of all skin cancers," write one team of experts, "it is among the most malignant of *all* cancers."[44] Although it is not a common cancer, it is increasing yearly, with 27,600 cases reported in 1990.[45]

What distinguishes the two conditions?

- *Basal- and squamous-cell carcinomas:* These constitute about four-fifths of all skin cancers. The first symptom may be the appearance of a pale, waxlike, pearly nodule or a red, scaly patch.

- *Malignant melanomas:* These are most commonly found on the skin, but 10% arise in the eye. A melanoma often begins as a small, molelike growth that gradually increases in size, changes color, becomes ulcerated, and bleeds easily from the slightest injury. Typically, melanomas appear flat, asymmetrical with irregular borders, and with varied pigmentation (brown, black, red, white, or blue colors are common). They can appear on normal-looking skin or as a change in a mole.

Testicular Cancer Cancer of the **testicles** (sperm-producing organs) is not a common form of cancer, but it *is* a common form for men ages 20–34.[46] Fortunately, it is one of the most curable cancers if detected early.

Symptoms of testicular cancer include the presence of a small, painless lump on the side of the testicle, a change in shape of a testicle, or a dull ache or heaviness in the groin or scrotum.

Help for Cancer

Cancer may be diagnosed by physical examination, laboratory tests, imaging techniques, endoscopy, and biopsy. Treatment may be by surgery, radiation therapy, chemotherapy, or immunotherapy, along with complementary treatments.

Suppose, as a result of some worrisome signs, you suspect you have cancer. Or suppose you learn in the course of a regular physical examination that your physician "has some suspicions" and "wants to run some tests."

At first, you may be engulfed by the terrifying feeling that you are under a death sentence. You may plunge abruptly through an emotional constellation of shock, confusion, despair, anger, and depression.

It's important to know, however, that *cancer can be cured*—particularly if it is detected early. The challenge to a cancer patient is to decide to deal aggressively with the disease and to actively participate in fighting it.

Tools for Diagnosis A bit later in the chapter, we present strategies you can use to provide your own early-warning system against cancer. Here, however, let us look at the tools that physicians use to make a diagnosis.[47]

- *The physical examination:* A good physician will do an examination of the entire body, in particular touching and scrutinizing those parts that are most prone to develop cancers. These areas include:

  (1) The nose, throat, and larynx, to see if oral cancer is present.

  (2) The neck above the collarbone, under the arms, and in the groin—areas containing lymph nodes—to check for swellings that might indicate lymphomas.

  (3) The abdomen, to check for enlargement of abdominal organs, such as the liver and spleen.

  (4) The rectum and male genitals, using a rubber-gloved finger, to check for colon and rectal cancers and, in men, for an enlarged prostate gland. In men, the testicles are checked for signs of testicular cancer.

  (5) In women, the breasts and the pelvic areas; samples of cells are also collected from the cervix for a Pap smear to detect cancers of the cervix and uterus.

  (6) In men and women, the skin to check for signs of skin cancer and other signs of problems.

       The physician will also ask you about swallowing problems, hoarseness, bleeding, coughing of blood, and constipation, as well as about cancer among close relatives.

- *Laboratory tests:* The physician may ask you to go to a lab and have blood drawn for several tests. Some blood tests are nonspecific, but may show results that suggest the presence of a tumor. Other blood tests are fairly specific for particular kinds of cancer.

Besides blood tests, a physician may order tests of various body fluids, such as urine, or of the stools, to see if a hidden cancer is possible.

The Pap smear, mentioned above, is an example of a cytological test. Cytology is the study of cells. In the Pap smear, the cervix is scraped, and the cellular material removed, including cells shed from the ovaries and uterus, is put on slides, stained with dyes, and examined under a microscope. The cytologist can then make a diagnosis as to whether the cells are malignant.

• *Imaging techniques:* The original imaging technique was the X ray, and this is still used extensively. For example, perhaps the best tool for early detection of breast cancer is the diagnostic X ray exam called **mammography.** (*See ● Figure 31.2.*)

In recent years, the arsenal of imaging techniques has been expanded to include nuclear scans, computerized tomography (CT) scans, magnetic-resonance imaging (MRI) scans, and ultrasound scans.

• *Endoscopy:* Sometimes direct visualization is preferable to an imaging technique for diagnosis. Flexible fiber-optic "scopes" that can see around corners can be used to look inside body cavities, giving physicians a direct view of possible tumor areas.

• *Biopsies:* A **biopsy** is a procedure in which a specimen of tissue is removed from the body and then is examined under a microscope by a specialist (pathologist) to see if the cells fit the characteristic profile for cancer. Some biopsies can be performed with very thin needles and a local anesthetic. Other biopsies are performed during surgery that may be necessary to expose the potential tumor.

Treatment Once you have been diagnosed as having cancer, perhaps by your primary physician, internist, or (if you're a woman) a gynecologist, a treatment team will be assembled. This team will include not only internists—specialists in internal medicine—but also **oncologists,** internists with additional training in the treatment of cancer. They may be assisted by surgeons and radiation oncologists, who specialize in shrinking tumors with X rays or other high-energy particles.

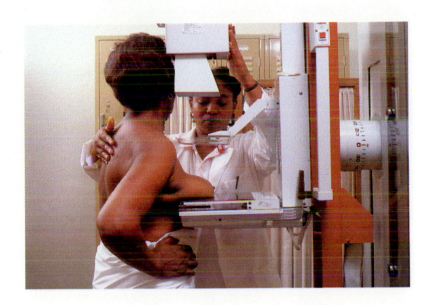

● **Figure 31.2 Mammography.** This diagnostic X ray technique is one of the best tools for early detection of breast cancer.

The kinds of treatment for cancer are *surgery, radiation therapy, chemotherapy,* and *immunotherapy*.

• *Surgery:* The oldest technique, surgery often works fine if (1) the tumor is in one location and the cancer has not spread, and (2) the tumor can be removed without damaging vital organs (such as the brain or the liver).

Surgery is particularly recommended for cancers of skin, gastrointestinal tract, breast, uterus, prostate, and testicles.

• *Radiation therapy:* **Radiation therapy** is the use of X rays, gamma rays, electrons, photons, or other high-energy particles to treat cancer. (*See ● Figure 31.3.*) Radiation therapy attempts to shrink a tumor by damaging the tumor cells so they cannot reproduce themselves. The process is painless. Experiencing radiation is like having a chest X ray, except the radiation is concentrated for several minutes instead of seconds.

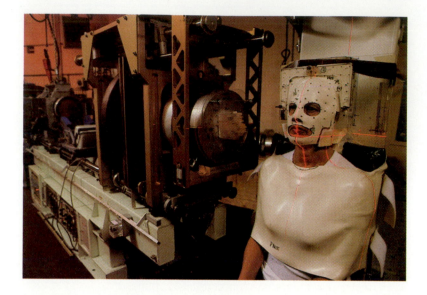

• **Figure 31.3 Radiation therapy.** Some parts of this cancer patient's body are shielded to prevent the radiation from damaging noncancerous areas.

It needs to be remembered that some healthy tissue may be destroyed along with the cancer cells. Possible side effects include nausea and vomiting, hair loss, and other localized reactions. Radiation therapy is particularly suited to cancers of the skin, larynx, uterus, cervix, and lymphoid tissue.

• *Chemotherapy:* **Chemotherapy** is actually a fairly broad term that means using drugs and medicines to fight *any* disease. However, people have come to associate the word with using drugs to fight cancer. Often these anticancer drugs destroy the ability of the cancer cells to reproduce.

Chemotherapy is generally used for cancers that are no longer at one place but have traveled through the blood and lymph systems to other parts of the body. The chemotherapy can also affect normal cells, as a result of which some patients temporarily experience fatigue, nausea, and hair loss. Although some people have moderate to severe side effects, most people tolerate them rather well. Moreover, side effects such as nausea can be alleviated with other drugs.

• *Immunotherapy:* **Immunotherapy** tries to use the body's own immune system to fight disease, especially by bolstering natural immune mechanisms (lymphocytes such as T-cells) to destroy the cancer cells. Immunotherapy consists mainly of using highly purified proteins (such as interferon and interleukin-2) to activate the immune system.

Several of these treatments may be applied simultaneously, as, for example, when radiation and chemotherapy are combined to produce a more powerful anticancer effect than is possible with one therapy alone.

Additional Treatment—and Questionable Therapies Cancer specialists will recommend not only the treatments we've just described but also what are called *complementary* or *adjunctive* treatments, because they are used along with standard therapies.[48] These include nutritional therapy, yoga, relaxation techniques, and the use of social-support systems. After all, fighting cancer can require a great deal of energy and overcoming a great many fears, and these additional therapies can only assist in that struggle.

However, sometimes these therapies are promoted as having the power to cure cancer on their own, without traditional medical treatments. Thus, certain diets are advertised as cancer cures, guided imagery or relaxation programs are said to promote the right healing attitude, and so on. Some treatments are even more far-fetched. In the 1970s, a substance prepared from apricot pits called Laetrile (and misleadingly referred to as vitamin B_{17}, even though it is not a vitamin) was offered as a cancer treatment, although it had been shown to have no effect. Today clinics throughout the United States and in Mexico offer "oxygenation," or "natural therapy," or "cellular detoxification and restoration," by such supposed methods as cleansing of the colon or vitamin therapy.[49]

One can certainly sympathize with the plight of cancer patients desperate for the certainty of a cure. However, unless a treatment method has been studied scientifically and properly (reviewed and approved by other knowledgeable researchers), it is not enough to have promises and testimonials. Indeed, such methods can actually be harmful, diverting money and energy, causing patients to neglect legitimate treatments, and raising false hopes.

Risk Factors for Cancer

Predisposing risk factors are age, gender, heredity, race, and viruses. Risk factors that can be controlled include tobacco, diet, sexual behavior, occupation, alcohol, environmental pollution, sunlight, and radiation.

As with heart disease, some risk factors for cancer are not controllable, but many are. (*See* ● *Figure 31.4.*) Uncontrollable, or *predisposing,* risk factors include age, gender, heredity, race, and viruses and infection. Controllable, or *precipitating,* risk factors include diet, smoking, sexual behavior, occupation, alcohol, environmental pollution, sunlight, radiation, and other matters. (*See Self Discovery 31.1.*)

Predisposing Risk Factors: Age, Gender, Heredity, Race, Viruses There is nothing that you can do about these uncontrollable risk factors, except to be especially alert to them:

- *Age:* Some forms of cancer seem to strike some age groups more than others: testicular cancer—ages 15–44; Hodgkin's disease—ages 20–40; endometrial cancer—ages 55–69. In general, however, the risk of cancer rises as one grows older.

- *Gender:* Some cancers are principally sex-specific, of course—testicular and prostate cancer in men, breast and gynecological cancers in women, although some men get breast cancer too. Oral cancer and Hodgkin's disease show up more in males than in females.

- *Heredity:* Some cancers seem to be found clustered in families: breast, ovarian, colon/rectum, prostate, stomach, and lung and leukemia. However, only about 2% of cancers are caused directly by heredity; many family histories of cancer may be the result of environmental rather than genetic factors.[50] Children with Down syndrome are more apt to develop leukemia than most

children.[51] Certain individuals may have genetic skin disorders (xeroderma pigmentosum and albinism) that predispose them to skin cancer.[52]

- *Race:* The role of race in cancer is seen quite specifically in skin cancers. Light-skinned people suffer a more adverse reaction to the sun's ultraviolet radiation.

  In general, cancer death rates are higher among blacks than among whites, and the average survival times are shorter.[53] However, this may be because of socioeconomic factors rather than race.

- *Viruses:* Viruses have been associated with certain cancers—of the blood, the liver, the cervix, the pharynx, and the lymph system. The AIDS virus, human immunodeficiency virus (HIV), can so weaken the immune system that an otherwise rare cancer called *Kaposi's sarcoma* occurs.

Although you cannot control your age, gender, heredity, race, or your exposure to certain viruses, there are many other risk factors you can do something about: tobacco, diet, sexual behavior, occupation, alcohol, environmental pollution, sunlight, and radiation.

Tobacco Despite the pronouncements of the cigarette-industry-sponsored Tobacco Institute, over 50,000 studies have shown the causal

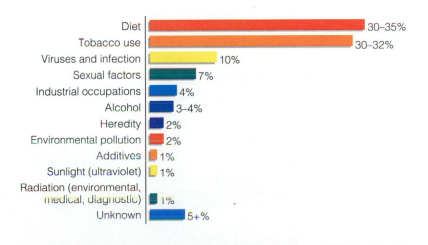

Diet	30–35%
Tobacco use	30–32%
Viruses and infection	10%
Sexual factors	7%
Industrial occupations	4%
Alcohol	3–4%
Heredity	2%
Environmental pollution	2%
Additives	1%
Sunlight (ultraviolet)	1%
Radiation (environmental, medical, diagnostic)	1%
Unknown	5+%

● **Figure 31.4 Cancer risk factors, with percentages**

SELF DISCOVERY 31.1

What Is Your Risk of Cancer?

For each of the following questions, circle the answer that best describes you and your lifestyle.

Males: Answer questions for the first three sections only—the lung, colon/rectal, and skin cancer sections.

Females: Answer all questions, but if you have had a complete hysterectomy then skip the questions for cervical and endometrial cancers.

Lung Cancer

1. Sex
   a. Male (2)   b. Female (1)
2. Age
   a. 39 or less (1)   b. 40–49 (2)
   c. 50–59 (5)   d. 60+ (7)
3. Smoking behavior
   a. smoker (8)   b. nonsmoker (1)
4. Type of smoking
   a. cigarettes or little   b. pipe and/or cigar,
      cigars (1)   but not cigarettes (3)
   c. ex-cigarette   d. nonsmoker (1)
      smoker (2)
5. Amount of cigarettes smoked per day
   a. 0 (1)   b. less than ½ pack (5)
   c. ½–1 pack (9)   d. 1–2 packs (5)
   e. 2+ packs (20)
6. Type of cigarette by amount of tar/nicotine
   a. high tar/nicotine (20 mg tar/1.3 mg nicotine) (10)
   b. medium tar/nicotine (16–19 mg tar/1.15 mg
      nicotine) (9)
   c. low tar/nicotine (15 mg or less tar/1.0 mg or less
      nicotine) (7)
   d. nonsmoker (1)
7. Duration of smoking
   a. Never smoked (1)   b. ex-smoker (3)
   c. up to 15 years (5) d. 15–25 years (10)
   e. 25+ years (20)
8. Type of industrial work
   a. mining (3)   b. asbestos (7)
   c. uranium and radio- d. none of these (0)
      active products (5)

Colon/Rectum Cancer

1. Age
   a. 39 or less (10)   b. 40–59 (20)
   c. 60 and over (50)
2. Has anyone in your immediate family ever had:
   a. colon cancer (20) b. one or more polyps
                            of the colon (10)
   c. neither (1)
3. Have you ever had:
   a. colon cancer (100) b. one or more polyps
                            of the colon (40)
   c. ulcerative colitis (20) d. cancer of the breast
                                  or uterus (10)
   e. none of the above (1)
4. Have you had bleeding from the rectum (other than
   obvious hemorrhoids or piles)?
   a. yes (75)   b. no (1)

Skin Cancer

1. Do you frequently work or play in the sun?
   a. yes (10)   b. no (1)
2. Do you work in mines, around coal tars, or around
   radioactivity?
   a. yes (10)   b. no (1)
3. Do you have fair and/or light skin?
   a. yes (10)   b. no (1)

Breast Cancer

1. Age
   a. 20–35 (10)   b. 35–49 (40)
   c. 50 and over (90)
2. Race
   a. black (20)   b. hispanic (10)
   c. oriental (5)   d. white (25)
3. Family history
   a. mother, sister, aunt, or grandmother with breast
      cancer (30)
   b. none (10)
4. Your history
   a. no breast disease (10)
   b. previous lumps or cysts (25)
   c. previous breast cancer (100)
5. Maternity
   a. first pregnancy before 25 (10)
   b. first pregnancy after 25 (15)
   c. no pregnancies (20)

Cervical Cancer

1. Age
   a. less than 25 (10) b. 25–39 (20)
   c. 40–54 (30)   d. 55 and over (30)
2. Race
   a. black (20)   b. hispanic (10)
   c. oriental (20)   d. white (10)
3. Number of pregnancies
   a. 0 (10)   b. 1–3 (20)
   c. 4 and over (30)
4. Viral infections
   a. herpes and other viral infections or ulcer forma-
      tions on the vagina (10)
   b. never had such infections (1)
5. Age at first intercourse
   a. before 15 (40)   b. 15–19 (30)
   c. 20–24 (20)   d. 25 and over (10)
   e. never (5)
6. Bleeding between menstrual periods after
   intercourse
   a. yes (40)   b. no (1)

(continued)

SELF DISCOVERY 31.1
(continued)

Endometrial Cancer

1. Age
   - a. 39 or under (5)
   - b. 40–49 (20)
   - c. 50 and over (60)
2. Race
   - a. black (10)
   - b. hispanic (10)
   - c. oriental (10)
   - d. white (20)
3. Births
   - a. none (15)
   - b. 1–4 (7)
   - c. 5 or more (5)
4. Weight
   - a. 50 or more pounds overweight (50)
   - b. 20–49 pounds overweight (15)
   - c. underweight for height (10)
   - d. normal (10)

5. Diabetes
   - a. yes (3)
   - b. no (1)
6. Estrogen hormone intake
   - a. yes, regularly (15)
   - b. yes, occasionally (12)
   - c. none (10)
7. Abnormal uterine bleeding
   - a. yes (40)
   - b. no (1)
8. High blood pressure
   - a. yes (3)
   - b. no (1)

Scoring

For each form of cancer, add up the numbers in parentheses following the answers you selected.

Interpretation

Numerical risks for skin cancer are difficult to state. A person with a dark complexion can work longer in the sun and be less likely to develop cancer than a light-complected person can. A person wearing a long-sleeved shirt and wide-brimmed hat may work in the sun and be less at risk than a person who wears a bathing suit for only a short time. The risk goes up greatly with age. Still, in general, the more questions to which you answered "yes," the greater your risks.

For other cancers, see the chart below.

Type of cancer	Very low risk	Low risk	Moderate risk	High risk	Very high risk
Lung/colon	6–24		25–49	50–74	75+
Rectum		13–29	30–69	70+	
Breast		45–100	100–199	200+	
Cervical		40–69	70–99	100+	
Endometrial		45–69	60–99	100+	

Source: American Cancer Society, 1981.

relationship between smoking and cancer. In the early 1900s, lung cancer was a rare disease, with probably no more than 500 cases a year. But after 1912, when milder tobaccos came on the market that could be inhaled without causing excessive coughing, smoking became much more commonplace—and so did lung cancer. In 1950, when the first report was published linking smoking and lung cancer, there were 18,000 lung cancer deaths, in 1990 an estimated 160,000 deaths.[54] No effective treatment for lung cancer is available. Nearly 90% of lung cancer patients die within 5 years of diagnosis.[55]

Cigarette smoking is the major determinant of lung cancer risk, although exposure to asbestos, ionizing radiation, and radon decay products increases the risk. Exposure to environmental (passive) tobacco smoke also increases the risk of lung cancer in people who have never smoked.

People who smoke pipes or cigars (and don't inhale) or who use smokeless tobacco (chewing tobacco and dipping snuff) do not show high rates of lung cancer. However, they do show high rates of oral cancer and of cancer of the esophagus.

Diet Researchers seem to have found a number of links between diet and cancer. The riskiest diets are those that are high in calories; that are high fat and low fiber; that contain pickled, salted, smoked, or grilled foods; that have additives such as nitrites and nitrates; and that are high in alcohol. (*See* ● *Figure 31.5.*)

- *High calories:* Obese people have a much higher risk of developing cancers of the uterus, breast, colon, stomach, gallbladder, and kidneys.

- *High fat/low fiber:* Diets that are high in fats—both saturated (hard, mostly animal) and unsaturated (liquid, mostly vegetable) —raise the risk of cancers of the colon, rectum, prostate, testicles, breast, uterus, and gallbladder. Diets that are low in fiber

seem to lead to the development of colon and rectum cancers.

- *Preserved and grilled foods:* Foods that are cured or smoked—such as smoked ham and sausage—may contribute to high rates of stomach cancer. Salted and pickled foods and nitrite- and nitrate-cured meats increase the risk of cancers of the stomach and esophagus. Foods grilled at high temperatures, as on barbecues, may have carcinogenic substances from the grease burning on the coals.

- *Low vitamins A and C:* People whose diets are low in vitamin A increase the risk of cancers of the larynx, esophagus, and lung. People with diets low in vitamin C increase the risk of cancers of the stomach and esophagus.

Sexual Factors The more sex partners you have, the more likely you are to be exposed to sexually transmitted diseases, including viruses that can cause cancers of the cervix, penis, and anus, as well as the head and neck. Women who have had their first sexual intercourse at an early age also have a higher risk of developing cervical cancer.

For women, childbearing reduces the risk of cancers of the breast, ovary, and uterus. Women who give birth before age 30 are less likely to have breast cancer in later life.

Occupation and Environment People who work around carcinogenic chemicals such as asbestos, coal products, cadmium, uranium, nickel, or nuclear wastes increase the risk of developing cancers. People living and working in areas with heavy air pollution may also be at greater risk.

Alcohol In about 4% of people (7% males, 3% females), alcohol can lead to cancers in the head, neck, larynx, liver, and pancreas.[56] Many people who drink also smoke, and the combination strongly raises the risk for developing oral cancers and cancer of the esophagus.

Sunlight Ultraviolet radiation is a high-energy, invisible part of the rays emitted by the sun. Even on cloudy days, these may affect your skin, and as the protective ozone layer becomes thinner, these rays are becoming more intense.

Key

Red = strongest links
Blue = weaker links
Green = weakest links

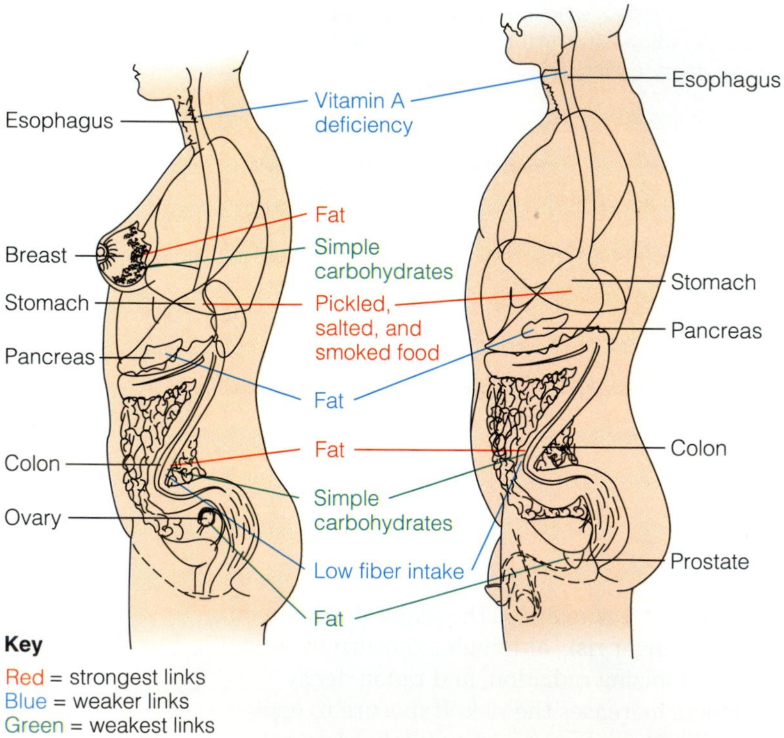

● **Figure 31.5 Diet and cancer.** Various studies with humans and laboratory experiments with rodents have suggested correlations between specific components of diets and specific cancers. Some diets have been shown to have stronger links than others.

The supposed beauty benefits of tanning, whether from the sun or from artificial tanning lights, are transitory at best and fatal at worst. After several years, tanning actually makes you look older, because of the leathery skin texture, wrinkles, and age spots. Worse, exposure to the sun may lead to basal-cell or squamous-cell cancers or even to the dangerous malignant melanoma, now the ninth most common cancer in the United States.

Strategy for Living: Preventing Cancer

Nine steps for preventing cancer are (1) quit tobacco use; (2) eat a low-fat, high-fiber diet; (3) moderate alcohol use; (4) control weight through exercise; (5) protect yourself from STDs; (6) reduce exposure to sunlight; (7) reduce exposure to environmental carcinogens; (8) do regular self-exams; and (9) get regular professional evaluations.

Cancer can totally disrupt your life. It can inflict great emotional and physical pain, be enormously time-consuming and expensive to treat, and can completely undo all your life's routines and plans—maybe even permanently. People knowing what most cancer patients go through should fully appreciate the chance to avoid having to undergo this kind of agony— in a word, for having the chance to exercise *prevention*.

Prevention against cancer has two parts: (1) taking steps to increase the chances that cancer never happens to you, and (2) taking steps to catch it in its earliest stages, when it is most curable.

Step 1: Avoid All Forms of Tobacco Use

Cure rates for cancer have increased steadily during the past half century—but not for lung cancer. Smoking is responsible for 85% of lung cancer cases, not to mention several other cancers. If you use smokeless tobacco, try to stop, to avoid oral cancer. If you find yourself continually breathing passive (sidestream) smoke, try to create a smoke-free environment for yourself, putting out signs that say THANK YOU FOR NOT SMOKING.

Step 2: Eat a Low-Fat, High-Fiber Diet

A cancer-fighting diet may mean changing a few old habits, but you'll be glad you did.

- *Reduce your fat intake:* Reduce the consumption of animal fats, especially red meats and dairy products. Trim excess fat from foods, cook with little or no fat, don't always butter your bread, and otherwise try to scale back your fat consumption.

- *Eat more fiber, cruciferous vegetables, and vitamins A and C:* You can get fiber from whole grains, cereals, vegetables, and fruits. Cruciferous vegetables, which help reduce the risk of several cancers (such as colon cancer) are those in the cabbage families (cabbage, brussels sprouts, turnips, and cauliflower). Vitamin A is found in dark-green and deep-yellow vegetables (such as cantaloupe, carrots, spinach, and sweet potatoes). Vitamin C is found in oranges, grapefruit, broccoli, and cauliflower, among other foods.

- *Avoid smoked or charcoal-broiled foods:* You can still grill or broil foods, but try to keep them away from smoke and flames, which produce carcinogens. Wrap food in foil or place it in a pan before grilling. Stay away from meats that have been smoked, salted, or pickled.

Step 3: Use Alcohol in Moderation

Heavy alcohol users have increased oral cancers and cancer of the esophagus. If you drink, be sparing—say, 1–2 glasses a day.

Step 4: Control Your Body Weight Through Exercise

Being overweight produces excess hormones that may promote cancer growth. Indeed, women who are obese are more apt to develop cancer of the breast, uterus, and ovary. The best way to control your weight is through aerobic exercise, such as walking, swimming, or bicycling, about 30 minutes three times a week.

Step 5: Protect Yourself from STDs

Use condoms, when appropriate, to protect yourself from sexually transmitted diseases. There are increased incidences of cancer of the cervix and of the penis among people with multiple sexual partners.

Step 6: Reduce Your Exposure to Sunlight
Every spring college students head for the beaches to "catch a few rays," returning to show off their "healthy" tans—yet more proof, as if any were needed, that for many people appearance is more important than safety. Perhaps, however, with the thinning ozone layer and the rise in skin wrinkling and melanoma cases, this standard will change.

Some tips:

- *Avoid sunlamps:* Tanning parlors and sunlamps do the same thing as the sun itself, despite some manufacturers' claims. They all increase your risk of skin cancer.

- *Know when UV rays are strongest:* Between 10 A.M. and 3 P.M. is the time of day when ultraviolet (UV) rays are strongest. This is a good time to stay out of the sun or wear wide-brimmed hats and long sleeves. Be aware that UV rays are also strongest at high altitudes, and that snow and water are powerful reflectors of the sun's rays.

- *Understand the uses of sunblock and use it:* Even overcast skies do not filter the sun's rays, and you should wear sunblock or sunscreen when you plan to be outside for more than a few minutes. You can be surprised at how much sun you get after only a half hour of walking or gardening.

  In using sunblock, follow these guidelines:

  (1) Use sunscreen lotion containing PABA (para-aminobenzoic acid).

  (2) Make sure it has a sun protection factor (SPF) of 15 or more, especially if you are blond, red-headed, freckled, or light-skinned. Sunblocks are labeled with SPF ratings ranging from a low of 8 to a high of 30. (See ● *Table 31.1.*)

  (3) Apply it an hour *before* going into the sun.

  (4) Sunblock wears off when you're swimming or sweating and thus needs to be reapplied from time to time.

Step 7: Reduce Your Exposure to Work and Environmental Carcinogens If you work in industrial surroundings, where you might be exposed to cancer-causing chemicals such as benzene and industrial asbestos, try to make an effort to use protective equipment, such as masks, gloves, and overalls. If possible, avoid contact with such carcinogens altogether.

Step 8: Do Regular Self-Exams for Early Detection The foregoing steps are intended to try to prevent cancer from developing, but these should be backed up with measures to ensure early detection should tumors develop. The first line of detection is self-examination, as follows:

- *Men—checking for testicular cancer:* Once a month, after a warm bath or shower (when the scrotum is relaxed), take 3 minutes to roll first one testicle, then the other, between thumbs and forefingers of both hands. Look or probe for lumps, tenderness, swelling, heaviness, or anything else unusual. (*See* ● *Figure 31.5.*)

  Testicular cancer is the most common malignancy among males ages 15–44. However, you cannot make the diagnosis yourself; that usually requires an X ray. Thus, any irregularity you find should be examined promptly by a physician.

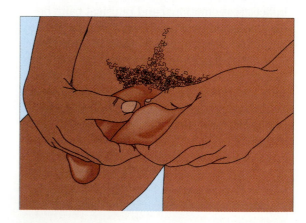

1. Roll each testicle between thumbs and forefingers of both hands.
2. Look or feel for pea-sized, painless lump. Also look for swelling, tenderness, or other irregularities.
3. If you find anything unusual, don't disregard it. Contact a physician immediately. Only a doctor can make an accurate diagnosis.

● **Figure 31.5 Testicular self-exam**

- *Women—checking for breast cancer:* A breast self-exam should be done once a month, at the same time if you are not menstruating (during pregnancy, or after menopause or a hysterectomy), or 2–3 days after your period, if you are menstruating. The self-exam should be done in three phases: (1) while in the shower or bath; (2) before a mirror; and (3) while lying down. (*See* ● *Figure 31.6.*)

    Many women's breasts normally feel lumpy. However, once you become familiar with these normal lumps, you will be in a position to notice any changes—lumps, hard knots, or thickenings. If you notice any, you should see a physician immediately.

- *Both males and females—monthly overall self-check:* Once a month, use a full-length mirror and a hand mirror to check yourself all over for suspicious lumps or patches on the skin, in the mouth, in and around the genitals, around the rectal area, and lymph nodes.

Step 9: Get Regular Professional Evaluations During physical examinations, the physician should use the following procedures and tests to check for cancer:

- *For lung cancer:* After age 40, an elective yearly chest X ray and a blood chemistry profile should be done to check for lung cancer, especially for smokers.

- *For colon cancer:* A simple test for colon cancer, which can be done in the physician's office, detects blood in the person's stool. Another standard yearly test, recommended after age 40, is a digital rectal exam, which is also a check for prostate cancer. After age 50, a sigmoidoscopy/colonoscopy (which uses a hollow, lighted tube) of the rectum and lower colon is recommended every 2–3 years.

- *For gynecological cancers:* Women should have a yearly pelvic examination, including a Pap test, to check for cervical, ovarian, and endometrial cancers.

- *For breast and testicular cancers:* A physician should in the course of a normal

● **Table 31.1 Sunscreen guide**

Type of skin (pigmentation)	History of sunburning or tanning	Sun protection factor (SPF)
Very fair skin; freckles; blond, red, or brown hair	Burns easily, never tans	15–30
Fair skin; blond, red, or brown hair	Burns easily, tans minimally	15–20
Light brown skin, brown hair and eyes	Burns moderately, tans gradually and evenly	8–15
Light brown skin, dark hair and eyes	Burns minimally, tans well	8–15
Brown skin, dark hair and eyes	Burns rarely, tans profusely	8–15
Brown-black skin, dark hair and eyes	Never burns, deeply pigmented	8–15

physical examination inspect a man's genitals for testicular and penile cancers and a woman's breast, chest, and armpits for breast cancers.

Women should be examined for breast cancer every 3 years between the ages of 20 and 40 and every year after age 40. A mammography, which can detect cancer lumps that are too small to feel, is recommended as follows for women whose family history does not show them to be members of high-risk breast-cancer groups: ages 35–39—one time; ages 40–49—once every 1 or 2 years; over age 50—once a year. Women in high-risk groups may need more frequent mammograms.

800-HELP

American Cancer Society. 800-ACS-2345.
National headquarters in Atlanta; supplies medical information on cancer

Cancer Information Service. 800-4-CANCER.
Hotline for the National Cancer Institute, Bethesda, MD

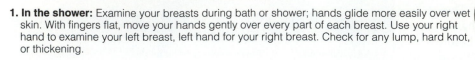
● **Figure 31.6 Breast self-exam**

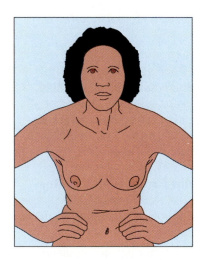

1. In the shower: Examine your breasts during bath or shower; hands glide more easily over wet skin. With fingers flat, move your hands gently over every part of each breast. Use your right hand to examine your left breast, left hand for your right breast. Check for any lump, hard knot, or thickening.

2. Before a mirror: While standing before a mirror, examine your breasts from three positions:
• Inspect your breasts with arms at your side.
• Next, raise your arms high overhead. Look for any changes in the contour of each breast: a swelling, dimpling of the skin, or change in the nipple.
• Then, rest your palms on your hips and press down firmly to flex your chest muscles.

  Left and right breast will not match exactly—few women's breasts do.

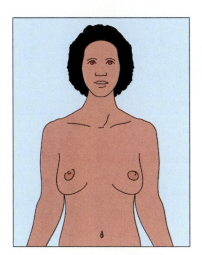
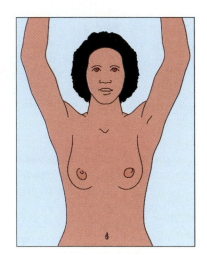
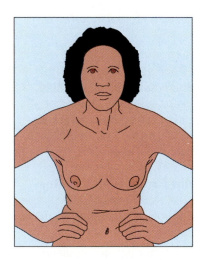

3. Lying down: To examine your right breast, put a pillow or folded towel under your right shoulder. Then do the following:
• Place your right hand behind your head—this distributes breast tissues more evenly on the chest.
• With your left hand, fingers flat, press gently in small circular movements around an imaginary clock face. Begin at the outermost top of your right breast for 12 o'clock, then move to 1 o'clock, and so on around the circle back to 12. A ridge of firm tissue in the lower curve of each breast is normal.

  Then move in an inch, toward the nipple, and keep circling to examine **every part of your breast**, including the nipple. This requires at least three more circles. Now slowly repeat this procedure on your left breast.
• Finally, squeeze the nipple of each breast gently between thumb and index finger. Any discharge, clear or bloody, should be reported to your doctor immediately.

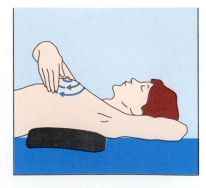
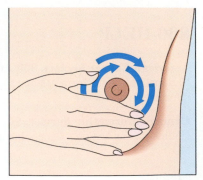
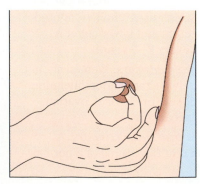

Belief and Healing: Can the Mind Help Cure Disease?

Answer the following yes or no:

___ **1.** Can humor cure illnesses?

___ **2.** Can the body cure itself?

___ **3.** Is there such a thing as miracle healing?

___ **4.** Are you emotionally responsible for your health?

All four questions have a one-word answer: maybe.

Only in the last decade or so has medicine in North America begun to pay attention to ideas that lie at the heart of traditional healing as practiced in other cultures—"ideas concerning the spiritual realm, mind-body interactions, the interplay among humanity, the environment, and the cosmos," as ethnobotanist Wade Davis describes them.[57] Let us consider what some of these aspects are.

Humor, Placebos, and Cancer Support Groups

Some time in the 1970s, magazine editor Norman Cousins returned home exhausted from a stressful overseas trip. He had great difficulty staying on his feet, and checked himself into a hospital. His physicians' diagnosis: a stress-induced, painful arthritis-type disease that was breaking down the connective tissue in his spine. Their prognosis: further deterioration of the spine, leading to paralysis and complete disability, with little chance of survival.

Thinking about his grim future, Cousins reasoned that if negative emotional experiences could cause physical harm, then positive emotions—must notably "hope, faith, laughter, confidence, and the will to live"—might improve health. With his doctor's approval, he checked into a hotel room, where for weeks he watched funny movies (Marx Brothers, Buster Keaton) and had someone read him funny stories.

In the early weeks, Cousins was in such pain that he was hardly able to sleep. Gradually, however, he found that 10 minutes of "genuine belly laughter" would relax him enough to give him 2 hours of pain-free sleep. Eventually, he gained complete recovery and went on to write about his experience in a medical journal, which led to more serious scientific study of the relationship between emotions and healing.[58–60]

The Placebo Effect Cousins himself, as well as other observers, thought that part of the reason for his recovery was the action of the **placebo effect**, the kind of healing that takes place when people get better who are given a **placebo**, a sugar pill or inert substance, and told it is a drug. Given a placebo, approximately 30–40% of people will experience relief of pain or even recover from various physical maladies.[61] But how important, really, is the emotional component?

Cancer Support Groups In the early 1980s, professor of psychiatry David Spiegel of Stanford University studied a group of 50 women with breast cancer being treated with conventional cancer therapies who had also taken part in weekly discussion groups in which they shared their feelings and learned simple techniques to reduce stress. His investigations showed the women were less depressed, felt less pain, and had a more positive outlook than women who did not receive such emotional support. However, Spiegel doubted the claims of "wish-away-cancer" proponents who said that a positive outlook could actually help the body combat the cancer.

He found out otherwise. In a landmark study published in 1989, he revealed that the patients who had only conventional treatment survived an average of 19 months after the study began, but the women in the support groups lived nearly twice as long—an average of 37 months.[62]

Can the Body Cure Itself?

When Robert M. was in his 20s, his physician told him that the cancer that had started in his testicles had spread to his lymph nodes, chest, and lungs, and that he had 3 months to live. Robert decided to take some life-affirming steps: he married his girlfriend, was ordained an Episcopal priest, and argued with his health care practitioners, insisting on explanations for everything. A month later, his physician was astounded to find that the X rays showed no trace of cancer in Robert's body. Thirty-three years later, Robert is still cancer-free.[63]

Spontaneous Remission Robert's experience is an an example of the phenomenon known as *spontaneous remission (SR)*—recoveries from cancer and other serious diseases that take place without medical treatment, or recoveries that take place after physicians have given up, or after only a very short course of treatment. SR is so rare—occurring in about 1% of all cancer cases—that medical practitioners tend to consider it a fluke, or to believe that patients never had the illness to begin with.[64]

However, a project called the Remission Project led by Brendan O'Regan of the Institute of Noetic Sciences in Sausalito, California, which has compiled a database on spontaneous remission of over 3000 papers from 860 medical journals in 20 different languages, suggests that SR is more prevalent than is generally believed.[65] It is possible, for instance, that SR is vastly underreported because patients who recover "naturally" from terminal disease are unlikely to return to the doctors who gave them little chance to live. Or the physicians are unlikely to write up such cases in medical journals. Or many patients may have conventional treatment (nearly all cancer patients do) that camouflages whatever mechanism is behind the SR effect.

Some reasons for SR may be biological, but others seem to be psychological. Psychiatrist Charles Weinstock, former director of New York's Psychosomatic Cancer Study Group, says that in some cases of SR in cancer patients, "there was a major, favorable change in the patient's life situation just preceding the cancer shrinkage."[66] For instance, a person may have witnessed the birth of a grandchild, seen the removal of career obstacles, had a reconciliation with a long-despised mother, or experienced religious conversion. "These people," says Weinstock, "suddenly found life more meaningful and satisfying. They no longer harbored a sense of hopelessness."

PNI: Studying Mind-Body Links To talk seriously about spontaneous remission, says oncologist Rose Papac, who in three decades of practice has witnessed 8–10 cases, is to walk "a thin line between doubt and quackery."[67,68] Nevertheless, the recent interest in the subject has given impetus to a relatively new field, known as *PNI*, short for **psychoneuroimmunology**—exploring the links between mind and body, and the immune system in particular.

Examples of people working in this field are psychologist Janice Kiecolt-Glaser and immunologist Ronald Glaser, who have found that emotional stress—as measured in medical students during final exam week—seems to dampen the body's immune strength. Moreover, they found, the lonelier the students were, the greater the decrease in immune function.[69,70]

A Crash Course in Miracles

In many societies besides our own, the healer is both physician and priest. The state of the body is considered inseparable from the state of the mind and spirit. "Sickness is [considered] disruption, imbalance, the manifestation of malevolent forces in the flesh," says ethnobotanist Davis. "Health is a state of balance, of harmony, and in most cultures it is something holy.[71] Thus, illness is treated by Native American shamans, Tibetan healers, African priests, and others for whom there is no rigid separation between the secular and the sacred.

Many readers may be dubious about the results of such "miracle" healers. However, there are plenty of people who believe in miraculous healing in Western society, and one location is particularly famous for miracles—Lourdes, France.

Miracle of Lourdes Lourdes first became famous when St. Bernadette witnessed an apparition of the Virgin Mary there in 1858. Since then millions of people have taken the waters of the shrine, many of them ill or infirm and hoping for a restorative miracle. Claims of healing are referred to the International Medical Commission to be declared official miracles. The commission has been organized since 1947 and has records since about the 1860s. The 25 European members, all Catholics, some pilgrimage medical officers, some not connected to the shrine, represent a range of medical specialties.

Claims of miracles are first scrutinized by the shrine's Medical Bureau, then rigorously investigated by one or two members of the commission, which then votes as a committee as a whole on whether the diagnosis was correct, according to a rigid set of criteria. After this, the commission considers whether the cure is not explainable by science.[72]

Since 1858, there have been approximately 6000 claims of miraculous healing, a rather small percentage considering the millions of people who have visited Lourdes. Of these 6000, only 64 have officially been declared miracles. Whether you think even these few rigorously evaluated cases of recovery at Lourdes actually came about through spiritual healing— or through a placebo effect or biological factors not in evidence—is up to you. The fact is that these 64 very ill people did recover.

Celebrating the Miraculous Retired Yale surgery professor Bernie Siegel struck a nerve with the public when his 1986 book *Love, Medicine, and Miracles* became a bestseller.[73] Says Siegel: "I've seen things I can't explain. Too often physicians reject what they can't explain. But it's your illness, not your doctor's."[74]

By "miracles," Siegel means that the medical literature is full of case reports of people surviving "incurable" diseases. However, both he and the aforementioned Brendan O'Regan of the Remission Project point out that until recently researchers have had a blind spot and not seemed to want to study this population of people with exceptional resistance to disease.[75]

Times have changed. For years, the medical establishment shunned so-called alternative medicine (including yoga, guided imagery, and the like). In 1992, however, the National Institutes of Health convened an Office for the Study of Unconventional Medical Practices to evaluate such treatments scientifically.[76]

The Uses of Hope: Are You Emotionally Responsible for Healing Yourself?

"Physicians walk a very fine line between promising more than we know and destroying a person's hope," says psychologist and cancer researcher Sandra Levy. "We know mental health helps. Currently, we cannot go beyond that."[77]

Many physicians think that there is a lot of confusion between cause and effect: just because one condition (positive outlook) is correlated with another (survival), it does not mean that the one *causes* the other. Still, can it hurt to hope against hope?

Certainly giving false hope is to be deplored, particularly when it causes patients to neglect conventional cancer treatment, or to pursue off-the-wall alternative therapies that verge on quackery, such as "psychic surgery" or apricot-pit extracts. It is also wrong to somehow give patients the idea that they are "emotionally responsible" for their disease, to play games of blame the victim.[78]

On the other hand, Siegel has a strong point in warning against "false despair," as when a doctor tells a patient he or she has only 3 months to live. "The physician's habitual prognosis of how much time a patient has left is a terrible mistake—it's a self-fulfilling prophecy," says Siegel. By not telling patients they will die in a short time and offering them options— visual imagery, for example—physicians at least give them the *opportunity* to get better.[79]

"In the absence of certainty, there is nothing wrong with hope," says Stephanie Simonton, original proponent of imagery for cancer patients. "Hope is simply a stance you take toward an unknown outcome, and none of us knows whether we're going to live another two weeks or another 20 years. I tell physicians the information they give patients affects that stance, so don't give them only half the story."[80]

14 Using Health Resources

In These Chapters:

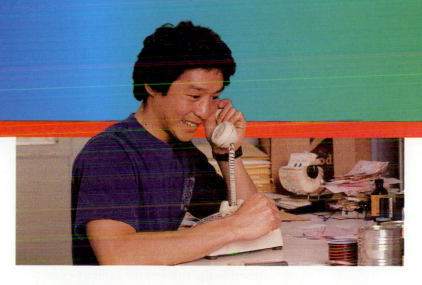

Where do you turn when you need help? Sometimes it's hard to know when you're in pain.

She had once been quite a good ice skater, but she had not done much of it for a few years. Then, in her mid-20s, she was invited to join some friends for outdoor skating on a frozen New Jersey pond. Unfortunately, instead of speed skates, she had only her old figure-skating skates, with grooves on the blade tips to permit quick stops.

As she soared across the ice, skating fast, she was mindful that, unlike indoor rinks, pond ice tends to build up ridges, which can catch a skate and send one sprawling. Suddenly she saw a series of ice ridges and tried to slow down, leaning far backward to try to keep her skates from catching. Unfortunately, she overcompensated and lost her balance—falling on her back with tremendous force, nearly knocking herself unconscious.

It was several minutes before she was able to pick herself off the ice, wondering if she had fractured her spine. Her friends helped her up. "Are you all right?"

"I don't know," she said, her body a screaming mass of pain.

"I know someone who can help," said a friend. "My chiropractor. He's close by."

Twenty minutes later she was lying in the chiropractor's office. Chiropractors must undergo several years of training and are licensed by the state, but they are not medical doctors and are permitted only to do spinal and joint manipulation.

The chiropractor took several minutes, probing the vertebrae and the lower back. Then he did something—she does not know what— that sent a tremendous jolt of pain through her back, almost worse than the fall on the ice.

"I think you'll be okay now," he said.

Did the chiropractor make any difference? This woman, a relative of one of the authors, still does not know. However, she reports she continued to ache for days afterward. Today she feels grateful that she was not permanently damaged. No X rays had been taken, which would have established whether there were broken bones. No physician had been consulted. The chiropractor had simply proceeded as he saw fit, making a diagnosis on the basis of look and feel, then applying treatment.

"I was lucky," she says now. "If I had to do it all over again, I would have asked my friends to take me to a hospital emergency room where I could get an X ray. I mean, what if there *had* been spinal fractures and he had done those manipulations on me?"

Some chiropractors are quite competent, at least within the confines of their specialty, but there are all kinds of people out there advertising themselves as healers. How can you tell who's competent, who's fraudulent? How do you know when you're not getting appropriate care even from conventional health practitioners, such as doctors and dentists? These are the important matters we consider in this chapter. First we examine the options available with conventional medicine, then those offered by alternative medicine.

32 Getting the Most Out of Conventional Health Care

▶ Explain the principal sources of health information and explain how patients can become their own experts.

▶ Discuss how health consumers can become active in and responsible for their own health care.

▶ Describe the roles of the primary-care physician and of specialist physicians.

▶ Summarize other health professionals who support them. Describe the various health care facilities available. Discuss how to choose a health care practitioner.

▶ Discuss how to prepare for and what to expect in a medical checkup and a dental checkup, a doctor's treatment recommendations, and surgery.

▶ Discuss what you need to be aware of for prescription and nonprescription drugs.

▶ Explain how the Canadian and American health care systems differ, what types of health insurance policies are available, and different health provider and governmental health programs.

You can't help but make decisions: *taking* action is a decision; so is *not* taking action.

When it comes to your health, then, you're making decisions all the time. Considering that health decisions can be life-and-death matters, is the thought you put into them proportional to their importance? Of course, many choices may not matter very much—which orange juice to buy, which toothpaste. But other health-related decisions truly are important—which doctor, which psychotherapist, which health insurance, which brand of prescription drug. Moreover, you have certain *medical rights* that you may not even be aware of but that you definitely should be. (*See Self Discovery 32.1.*)

Where Do You Get Your Health Information?

People get health information from friends and family, from folklore, from the mass media and advertising, from health practitioners and health groups, from public and private consumer protection agencies, and from health educators and information sources. It's important to learn how to tell if a health information source is credible or legitimate. As a patient, you may need to become your own expert—get a second opinion, get through technical language, find helpful organizations to help you, and learn how to use research tools.

Where do you get your information about health—and how can you evaluate your sources? Let's consider some possibilities:

• Friends, family, and folklore
• Mass media and advertising
• Health practitioners and health groups
• Public and private consumer protection agencies
• Health educators and data sources

Friends, Family, and Folklore If you're trying to find out who's a good dentist, gynecologist, or psychotherapist, it's natural to start by asking people you know and have trusted in other matters. In fact, this is probably the place where most of us start. There's nothing wrong with this—at least to begin your investigation. Certainly friends and family members can tell you if a health practitioner misdiagnosed them, caused them pain, or had an uncaring manner. On the other hand, being pleasant and earnest does not guarantee competence.

Family and friends may also pass along folklore, some old, some recent. Do you have a real itchy case of poison ivy? Go pick some jewelweed (wild touch-me-not), older relatives may advise, and rub the milky insides on your skin. Have a cold? Take megadoses of vitamin C, your friends may say, just as Nobel laureate Linus Pauling does. Folk wisdom is not limited to people you know well. Clerks in health-food stores, for example, will tout the benefits of this vitamin or that herb—although oftentimes they are just plain wrong or ignorant.

14.3

*Chapter 32
Getting the
Most Out of
Conventional
Health Care*

SELF DISCOVERY 32.1

What Are Your Medical Rights?

Answer true or false to each of the following statements:

	True	False

1. You can always leave a hospital you've signed into—even if you haven't paid the bill.

2. If you seek a second opinion about your illness from another physician and your first physician hears about it, he or she might drop you as a patient.

3. If a physician starts to give you some medication, as during an emergency, and you ask what it is, he or she doesn't have to tell you.

4. If you don't like the medical care you got or feel the charges are too high, you can withhold payment.

5. Even if you're injured, if you don't have medical insurance, a hospital emergency room can turn you away.

6. If nurses snap at you and physicians call you "Honey" or "Pal," there's not much you can do.

7. Not being insured, you're worried about the cost of certain treatment. That, however, is none of the doctor's concern.

8. Your worried family wants to ease your mind, so they ask the physician not to tell you the truth about your condition, though you would rather know. It is improper for the physician to go along with them.

9. Federal health facilities are required by law to give you copies of your medical records if you ask for them.

10. The hospital can restrict your spouse or partner to certain set visiting hours, although you might want that person to be with you day and night.

The answers

1. *True.* You can discharge yourself from a hospital at any time, even against medical advice and even if you haven't paid your bill.

2. *False.* The American Medical Association does not allow a physician to drop a patient.

3. *False.* It's your right to be fully informed about your treatment. Moreover, the physician can only recommend; you have the right to determine your treatment.

4. *True.* It's your right to withhold payment if you're dissatisfied with your treatment or feel the charges are excessive. The local medical society can help resolve any disputes, if necessary.

5. *False.* You have a legal right to treatment at an emergency room if your condition might cause serious illness, disability, or death, regardless of your ability to pay.

6. *False.* You have the right to be treated with respect and dignity. If you're not, make a complaint.

7. *False.* If you ask about costs, the doctor should be able to provide some sort of estimate.

8. *True.* Legally the physician must tell you what you want to know if you want to know it and if, in the doctor's opinion, the knowledge won't endanger your health (as if the news might make a patient commit suicide).

9. *True.* Federal facilities must give you your medical records if requested. However, only about half the states have statutes allowing this.

10. *False.* Unless the hospital determines your partner might be in the way (as during surgery), you have the right to have a spouse, relative, friend, or grown child with you 24 hours a day.

Mass Media and Advertising We are most comfortable with the familiar. Advertisers know this, which is why so much money is spent on promoting products—and why, it is said, we are bombarded with a staggering 400–3000 advertising messages *every day*.[1] When you think of a headache, no doubt you can name two or three *brand names* of aspirin or similar painkillers without a pause, so pervasive are the commercials and ads for such products. The fact that a product is familiar to us, however, does not make it superior to other products: generic aspirin packaged by a supermarket under its own name is probably every bit as good as, and certainly cheaper than, the brands we see advertised on television.

There is also a great deal of health information in the mass media that is presented as news, feature articles, books, or television or radio programs. One of the driving forces of journalism, however, is the constant pressure to convert dry, technical material into interesting, readable stories. Relatively few journalists have special training in medicine or science and so are unable to evaluate the reliability of information emanating from sources that may be biased. No wonder reporters unwittingly introduce inaccuracies, make important omissions, overemphasize the emotional side of scientific stories, or exaggerate or misinterpret risks.[2]

Health Practitioners and Health Groups If you look around your dentist's or doctor's office, it's possible you will see a variety of patient-education pamphlets. In addition, there are many professional associations, ranging from the American Heart Association to the American Dietetic Association, that publish informational pamphlets, audiotapes and videotapes, and other educational materials.

In general, the information in these materials is quite reliable. These professional associations can ill afford to be thought of as being "inaccurate" or "crackpot." The same may be said about information provided as insert material to pharmaceutical products, which are regulated by the Food and Drug Administration.

Public and Private Consumer Protection Agencies Several federal and state agencies, as well as private consumer advocacy groups

and voluntary health agencies, exist both to educate the public in health matters and to provide protection against the worst kinds of fraud or danger.

The principal consumer protection agencies are as follows:

- *Federal agencies:* There are numerous government agencies providing effective information to the public:

  The *Food and Drug Administration (FDA),* which has jurisdiction over advertising of prescription drugs and labeling of nonprescription drugs, has an ongoing public information program, including a magazine on health and safety issues, *FDA Consumer.*

  The *U.S. Department of Health and Human Services* issues a great many useful reports on health under the authority of the Surgeon General, the Public Health Service, the National Institutes of Health, Head Start Bureau, Centers for Disease Control and Prevention, and other agencies.

  Other federal offices, from the Federal Trade Commission, to the U.S. Postal Service, to the Environmental Protection Agency, also release educational information. In addition, federal departments such as the Department of Agriculture, the Department of Education, and the Department of the Interior publish health-related information.

- *State agencies:* State agencies charged with health, education, environmental protection, and consumer safety produce a great deal of health information. So, of course, do state-supported colleges and universities. State regulatory boards license physicians, nurses, and other health professionals and may investigate allegations of malpractice and other wrongdoings. State attorneys general are able to investigate and halt illegal advertising and services of unapproved drugs and health and safety matters.

- *Consumer advocacy groups:* Private organizations such as Consumers Union, the National Consumers League, and the Center for Science in the Public Interest also produce information designed to protect consumers.

14.5

Chapter 32
Getting the
Most Out of
Conventional
Health Care

Health Educators and Health Information Sources You're no doubt aware that health educators are employed in colleges and universities. You may not be aware that they are also employed in hospitals, corporations, and community agencies and generally serve as a good resource for health information.

A great deal of health information is also available in reference libraries and through computer software programs and computerized databases.

How Do You Tell Who's an Authority? Health knowledge essentially comes down to a question of authority or *credibility*.

When trying to determine whether a particular source is credible or legitimate, you need to ask:[3]

1. Does this source have the information or judgment you need, according to his or her past record?

2. If so, can you trust him or her to give you an honest, accurate assessment of your problem?

3. Are you in a position to understand the expert's reasoning so you don't merely have to accept his or her conclusion?

When experts disagree or when matters become complex, you may need to become your own expert by doing your own research. This is particularly true if the potential outcome of a particular decision—whether or not to have back surgery, for example—is problematic, serious, or associated with significant side effects.

Power to the Patient: Becoming Your Own Expert Suppose the doctor says that surgery designed to "fuse your spine" *may* help alleviate the back pain that has been giving you such agony for so long. However, the physician cautions, there are no guarantees, and indeed the surgery offers the risk of possible paralysis. The pain in your back is so great that it has profoundly diminished your enjoyment of life. On the other hand, you certainly don't want to *worsen* the situation by developing other problems. What do you do?

Your ally here is information, the more the better. When faced with major medical decisions, you need to gather as much information as you can from credible sources.

- *Get a second opinion:* When facing surgery, cancer treatments, treatment for heart disease, questions involving extended hospitalization, and other important issues, you need to obtain a second opinion from another specialist in the same field as the first. You may even want to get a third or fourth opinion.

- *Don't let the technical language stop you:* Don't be afraid of medical mumbo-jumbo; there is lots of medical information available in language written for lay people.

- *Learn how to find helpful organizations:* We won't go so far as to say that for every disease there's an organization, but there are many—probably 200 or more.[4] The American Cancer Society and the American Heart Association are among the best known. In addition, there are support groups and self-help groups, libraries and databases, as mentioned above.

- *Learn to use research tools:* The telephone book and library give you access to information you need. You can also use a computer with a modem that connects through the telephone to all kinds of networks of computerized libraries and databases.

Patient, Heal Thyself: Your Attitude Matters

Health consumers need to become active in and responsible for their own health care. As part of this, we need to learn preventive self-care and self-care treatment.

"Consumers will be the primary practitioners in the new health-care system," writes physician and medical editor Tom Ferguson. "Already, health-active, health-responsible individuals are improving and maintaining their own health and that of their families, actively seeking information on all the complex forces that make them ill or well."[5]

The Active and Responsible Health Consumer There are three classes of health consumers, according to John Fiorello of New

York's Health Strategy Group and cancer sur-geon Bernie Siegel—*passive patients, con-cerned consumers,* and *active and respon-sible consumers.*[6] During the past several years, there has been a rise in the last two cate-gories, and that trend is expected to continue. (See ● *Figure 32.1.*)

- *Passive patients:* Passive patients feel there is little they can do personally to im-prove their health or manage their illness. They rarely seek out information about their health condition or health in general. They may deteriorate even more quickly than their physicians predict.

- *Concerned consumers:* These patients see themselves as operating under the umbrella of the doctor's authority, although they sometimes ask questions and may occasion-ally obtain a second opinion. To health practitioners, they often act as "model pa-tients," rarely questioning their physician's decisions. "Indeed," says Ferguson, "they sometimes act as if they were more inter-ested in pleasing their doctor than in get-ting well."[7]

- *Health-active, health-responsible con-sumers:* Active and responsible health con-sumers are highly motivated to play an active role in their own health. They refuse

to relinquish key decisions having to do with their own care, they ask lots of ques-tions, they question their physicians' as-sessments and recommendations, and they seek additional health advice—including second, third, and more opinions and infor-mation from alternative therapies. They want to not only understand their treat-ment but also to be active participants in it.

Self-Care Comes First The foremost ex-pression of the new attitude of health-active, health-responsible consumers is the **self-care movement.** This is the trend toward more peo-ple taking responsibility for managing their health and preventing ill health. Involvement in self-care focuses in two primary areas:

- *Prevention:* Preventive self-care is based on a good foundation of knowledge and a healthful lifestyle that includes avoiding to-bacco and illegal drugs; keeping alcohol consumption moderate; taking measures to prevent sexually transmitted diseases and unintended pregnancy; getting regular ex-ercise; eating a diet low in fat and rich in fruits, grains, and vegetables; fastening seat belts, and driving soberly and defensively; brushing and flossing to prevent dental dis-ease; keeping the home environment safe; having periodic assessments for such mat-ters as cholesterol (blood test), cervical cancer (Pap smear), and breast cancer (mammogram and professional breast exam); and performing self-examinations, such as breast and testicular self-exams.[8]

- *Self-care treatment:* When you become aware of acute but nonserious conditions (colds, flu, sore throats), you usually first try to treat them on your own, by using the help of family and friends. If these steps aren't sufficient, *then* you would turn to a health professional for advice. If you're in-capacitated and unable to participate, your health care professional becomes the man-ager of your situation, often in collaboration with your family members.[9]

Obviously, self-care means self-education. You should learn everything from what the nor-mal range is for blood pressure, pulse rate, and respiration to how to buy nonprescription drugs. Most importantly, you must learn when

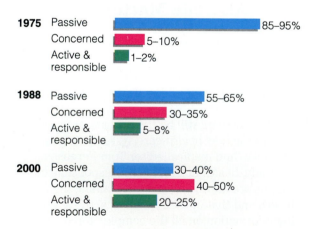

● **Figure 32.1 The rise of health-active consumers**

14.7

*Chapter 32
Getting the
Most Out of
Conventional
Health Care*

to seek the assistance of health care providers for a particular health problem.

Conventional Health Care: Practitioners and Facilities

The doctor who makes the first evaluation of you is the primary-care physician (usually a general practitioner, family practitioner, or internist), who in turn may refer you to specialist physicians. Other health care professionals include osteopaths, physician assistants, nurses (RNs or LPNs), and dentists, who are supported by audiologists, optometrists, podiatrists, pharmacists, and other medical specialists. A variety of conventional health care facilities are available, from hospitals to clinics to specialized "medicenters." It's important to learn how to choose a health care practitioner—someone you know is competent and whose manner and practices make you feel comfortable.

At some point even the most dedicated pursuer of informed self-care will need to seek professional advice. Who are the health professionals you might seek out? Let us consider those most likely to be found in the front line of your health defense: physicians, physician assistants, registered nurses, practical and vocational nurses, dentists, podiatrists, and optometrists.

Physicians The word *physician* is sometimes used in other medical specialties, but here we mean **medical doctors,** health professionals who have earned M.D. (Doctor of Medicine) degrees after 4 years of undergraduate education and graduation from a 4-year accredited medical-school program. Most new M.D.s then take a state medical-license examination, followed by a 1-year internship in a hospital. This may then be followed by 2–5 years of residency that lead to further examinations ("boards"), after which they may declare themselves "board-certified" in a medical specialty (such as pediatrics or cardiology).

Everyone should have a **primary-care physician,** the doctor who makes the primary evaluation, and does the primary treatment, for

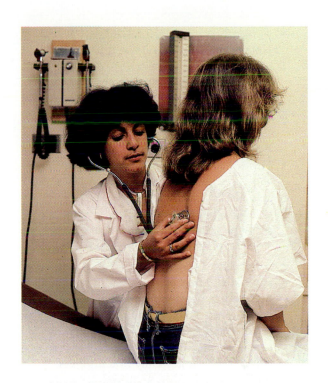

● **Figure 32.2 The primary-care physician**

"*Everyone should have a good, reliable doctor for the ordinary medical problems that come up from time to time. Using a specialist such as a gynecologist or a cardiologist for basic medical care is a mistake—and can be costly. Going to an emergency room is also a mistake, since emergency rooms will not have access to your medical records and are, in any case, oriented to handle emergencies, not ordinary medical problems. A primary-care physician ought to be competent to recognize and handle the full range of problems that individuals usually encounter, know your medical history, and keep your records on file.* "

—Editors of the University of California, Berkeley, *Wellness Letter.* (1991). *The wellness encyclopedia.* Boston: Houghton Mifflin, p. 429.

ordinary health problems. (*See* ● *Figure 32.2.*) Primary-care physicians are of three basic types—general practitioners, family practitioners, and internists:[10]

- *General practitioners:* **General practitioners (GPs)** treat the full range of medical problems, referring patients to specialists for consultation and problems (such as heart disease) requiring ongoing care. Earlier in this century, most doctors were GPs, but specialization has reduced their numbers drastically.

- *Family practitioners:* **Family practice** was recognized as a specialty by the American Medical Association in 1969. A practitioner qualifies by completing a 3-year residency that covers internal medicine, obstetrics, pediatrics, and orthopedics.

- *Internists:* **Internists** specialize in the diagnosis and nonsurgical treatment of adults with problems in their internal organs. They have more advanced training in the diagnosis and management of such matters as heart disease, diabetes, and cancer compared to GPs and family practitioners.

It needs to be pointed out that perhaps two-thirds of all women use their gynecologist as their primary-care physician; they may not be seeing any other doctor.[11]

Except for GPs, primary-care physicians are specialists, but they in turn will refer you to other M.D.s who specialize even further—such as in a particular organ (for example, cardiology, the heart), in children or the aged (pediatrics or geriatrics), or in emotional problems (psychiatry). (*See ● Figure 33.3.*)

Osteopaths **Osteopathy** is based on the principle that the body, once correctly adjusted, can make its own remedies against disease and other disorders. The adjustments consist of the same sorts of treatments available to conventional medicine—physical, medicinal, and surgical—while placing chief emphasis on physical manipulation of the body.

Osteopaths are physicians who have received the doctor of osteopathy (D.O.) after completing undergraduate education plus 4 years of training in one of the 15 schools of osteopathy in the United States. Today their practice is almost indistinguishable from that of conventional M.D.s except that they tend to focus more on problems of the musculoskeletal system.

Physician Assistants Because of the shortage of primary-care physicians, a new class of health-care practitioners has been created called **physician assistants (PAs).** They perform about 80% of what M.D.s can do—their medical duties range from basic primary care to high-technology surgical procedures—but always under the direction of a doctor.[12] Physician assistants complete a 2-year training program. They then usually pass a national certifying examination in order to be licensed.

Nurses Not all nurses are alike, and their responsibilities usually depend on their training. There are two levels of nursing training:

- *RNs:* **Registered nurses (RNs)** are the more highly trained, having earned either a 2-year associate degree (the *technical nurse*) or a 4-year bachelor's degree (the *professional nurse*). All nurses must pass a state examination in order to be licensed.

  Some RNs go on to take 2 more years of graduate study and become **nurse practitioners (NPs),** specializing in such areas as pediatrics, family health, public health, or school health.

- *LPNs/LVNs:* **Licensed practical nurses (LPNs),** also known as **licensed vocational nurses (LVNs),** usually have at least 2 years of high school and 12–18 months of training in a hospital-based program. They must also take a state board examination to be licensed.

RNs may specialize in various fields of medicine. They provide direct patient care, or supervise such care, in a variety of settings; educate patients, families, and others; and sometimes serve as researchers. With additional training, some have their own practice, particularly in the area of mental health counseling. LPNs work in hospitals, nursing homes, and home health settings under the supervision of RNs and physicians, where they give direct patient care such as bathing, oral hygiene, and changing of dressings.

Dentists **Dentists** are trained not only to diagnose and treat impairments of the teeth but also of the gums and oral cavity in general. A D.D.S. (Doctor of Dental Surgery) or D.M.D.

14.9

*Chapter 32
Getting the
Most Out of
Conventional
Health Care*

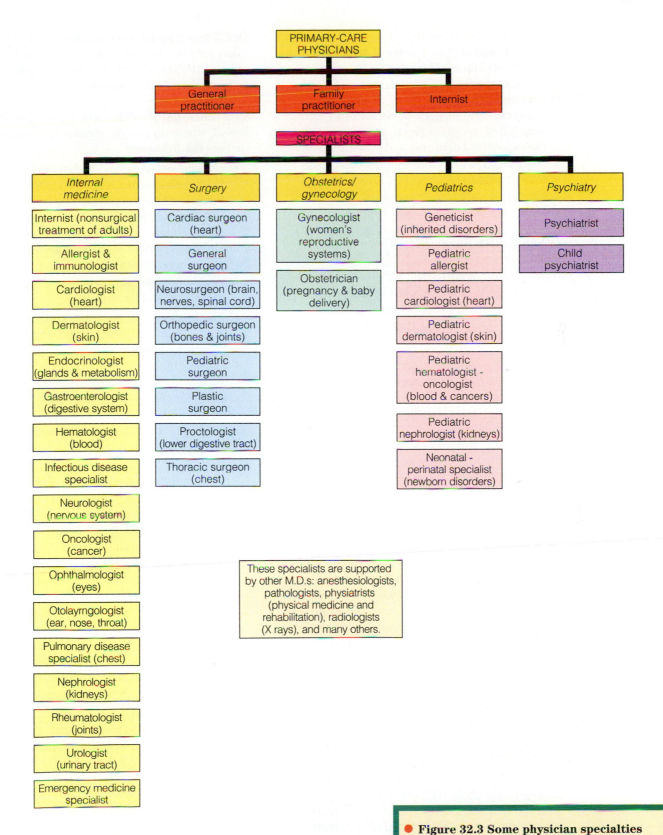

PRIMARY-CARE PHYSICIANS

General practitioner | Family practitioner | Internist

SPECIALISTS

Internal medicine
- Internist (nonsurgical treatment of adults)
- Allergist & immunologist
- Cardiologist (heart)
- Dermatologist (skin)
- Endocrinologist (glands & metabolism)
- Gastroenterologist (digestive system)
- Hematologist (blood)
- Infectious disease specialist
- Neurologist (nervous system)
- Oncologist (cancer)
- Ophthalmologist (eyes)
- Otolayrngologist (ear, nose, throat)
- Pulmonary disease specialist (chest)
- Nephrologist (kidneys)
- Rheumatologist (joints)
- Urologist (urinary tract)
- Emergency medicine specialist

Surgery
- Cardiac surgeon (heart)
- General surgeon
- Neurosurgeon (brain, nerves, spinal cord)
- Orthopedic surgeon (bones & joints)
- Pediatric surgeon
- Plastic surgeon
- Proctologist (lower digestive tract)
- Thoracic surgeon (chest)

Obstetrics/ gynecology
- Gynecologist (women's reproductive systems)
- Obstetrician (pregnancy & baby delivery)

Pediatrics
- Geneticist (inherited disorders)
- Pediatric allergist
- Pediatric cardiologist (heart)
- Pediatric dermatologist (skin)
- Pediatric hematologist - oncologist (blood & cancers)
- Pediatric nephrologist (kidneys)
- Neonatal - perinatal specialist (newborn disorders)

Psychiatry
- Psychiatrist
- Child psychiatrist

These specialists are supported by other M.D.s: anesthesiologists, pathologists, physiatrists (physical medicine and rehabilitation), radiologists (X rays), and many others.

● **Figure 32.3 Some physician specialties**

(Doctor of Medical Dentistry) degree requires a bachelor's degree plus 4 years of dental school. This is often followed by a year of internship, followed by passage of written and clinical examination for licensure. Some dentists go on to specialize in oral surgery, *periodontics* (gum disease), *orthodontics* (teeth straightening), or *prosthodontics* (dentures and other artificial appliances). Dentists may employ *dental hygienists* to clean teeth and educate patients about dental care and *dental assistants* to help them in various procedures.

Other Health Specialists There are more than 60 other types of health specialties, but those you are likely to deal with directly, without necessarily being referred by a primary-care physician, include the following:

- *Audiologists:* An **audiologist** screens for hearing problems and can fit a hearing-impaired person with a hearing aid.
- *Optometrists:* **Optometrists** assess the eyes for vision problems and diseases of the eye. They can prescribe corrective lenses. An optometrist is not a physician but holds an O.D. (Doctor of Optometry) degree.

  Evidence of complex vision problems or eye disease may require a referral to an *ophthalmologist,* an M.D. specializing in the eye. Prescriptions for lenses are filled by *opticians.*
- *Podiatrists:* A **podiatrist** specializes in disorders of the feet and legs. Podiatrists are the only health care practitioners besides M.D.s and dentists who may use drugs and surgery in their practice. The length of training for podiatrists is similar to that for M.D.s, but their degree is a D.P.M. (Doctor of Podiatric Medicine).
- *Pharmacists:* **Pharmacists** are trained and licensed to dispense medications in accordance with doctor's prescriptions and to give advice about medications.

There are a great many other *allied health care professionals* to whom you might be referred by a physician for specialized treatment. Examples are those with the word *therapist* in their job title—occupational, physical, recreational, respiratory, speech. Other specialists are nutritionists and dietitians, nurse-midwives (to assist in childbirth), radiologic technicians (for X rays), social workers, and psychologists. Many may be assisted by a variety of nurses' aides, orderlies, attendants, medical records personnel, and receptionists.

Conventional Health Care Facilities If you feel ill, where do you go? Health care facilities include the following:

- *College health service:* Many colleges and universities have a student health service. Some health centers may just be small medical dispensaries; others are fully accredited clinics. If you're reluctant to use such a service because you're worried about costs, you may be pleasantly surprised; the services are reasonably priced and, in some cases, covered by student fees.
- *Hospitals:* There are approximately 6000 hospitals in the United States that principally offer **inpatient care**—in-hospital care for the ill and injured. Many also have clinics offering **outpatient** or **walk-in care,** for those whose illnesses or injuries do not require overnight stays.

  There are three types of hospitals:

(1) *Public hospitals,* such as large city or county hospitals or military or Veterans Administration hospitals, are supported by tax dollars. At the local level, such hospitals serve all comers, which means that they assess and treat most of the poor. Some public hospitals are affiliated with academic medical centers and are called *teaching hospitals.* In recent years, the emergency rooms of public hospitals have been overwhelmed because they have to handle not just trauma (such as auto-accident and shooting victims) but also primary care for people who cannot afford other hospitals.

(2) *Private, for-profit hospitals,* which are in business to make money, generally accept only patients who have the ability to pay their expenses (or whose insurance companies do). Such hospitals, which offer fewer beds and more personalized care than do public hospitals, sometimes limit their services to specific disorders, such as drug and alcohol recovery.

14.11

*Chapter 32
Getting the
Most Out of
Conventional
Health Care*

(3) *Voluntary, nonprofit hospitals* are operated by charitable organizations or religious orders and are supported by patient fees and contributions. They usually offer more services than private hospitals do.

- *Clinics:* Clinics offer diagnosis and treatment for outpatient care. Although some are attached to hospitals or student health centers, others exist independently. *Community clinics,* for instance, have been established in rural and inner-city areas to serve residents who have difficulty getting to more centralized medical services.

- *Specialized walk-in "medicenters":* A recent trend has been the establishment of walk-in "medicenters" offering "shopping-mall medicine," consisting of specialized services once found only in a hospital. These so-called "doc-in-the-box" medicenters may be of several types:[13]

    (1) *"Urgicenters"* are freestanding emergency centers, which usually stay open evenings, see patients without an appointment, and handle minor emergencies.

    (2) *"Surgicenters"* offer same-day outpatient surgery for a range of procedures, including eye surgery, gynecologic and orthopedic operations, and ear, nose, and throat surgery. The main difference is that no overnight hospital stay is required.

    (3) *Women's centers* provide general medical care and obstetric and gynecological services, as well as screening for breast disease and osteoporosis. They also offer advice on such matters as childbirth, PMS, and eating disorders.

    (4) Other types of outside-the-hospital medicenters include birth centers, imaging centers—offering X rays, magnetic-resonance imaging (MRI), and computer-assisted tomography (CAT), pain and rehabilitation centers, and even local-care cancer-therapy centers.

- *Home care and house calls:* The physician house call, which disappeared for a number of years, seems to have returned. As many

as four-fifths of primary-care physicians see patients in their homes.[14] Nurses, health aides, and other health practitioners associated with home health agencies also provide home health care.

Choosing a Doctor How do you know your primary-care physician or a specialist is right for you? How do you know if he or she is competent—indeed, even safe? These are important questions, and they apply to other health practitioners as well—dentists and psychotherapists, for example. You should not rely on advertising or even a hospital's physician-referral service.

Here are some tips:

- *Ask people you trust:* Begin by asking family and friends and physicians *you* trust which physicians *they* trust.

- *Find out if the doctor is certified:* You can ask the doctor what kind of training and certification he or she has—medical school, board certification, and current hospital privileges. Or you can go to a large library and check out either the American Medical Association's *American Medical Directory* or the *Directory of Medical Specialists.* This will tell you whether the doctor is certified in his or her specialty—an indication of basic ability.

- *Find out if the doctor has a questionable record:* There are a handful of ways to find out if your doctor has been disciplined by state medical boards or has a malpractice record: You can call the state's medical licensing board and ask if he or she has been seriously disciplined. You can call the state's department of insurance to see if malpractice records are kept, if the doctor has been sued, and what the outcome of the suit was. You can look up your doctor's name in *9,479 Questionable Doctors,* a directory compiled and published by Public Citizen Health Research Group, which obtained information from public files.[15]

    In 1986, Congress created the National Practitioner Data Bank, a computer service listing physicians, nurses, and other health-care providers who have lost malpractice suits or had adverse actions taken against them by state boards, hospitals, or professional societies.[16]

- *Determine the doctor's practice and availability:* Questions to ask the doctor directly include: Are you in a solo or group practice? If alone, are there others who will cover when you are away and will they have access to my medical records? Find out how available the doctor is: Can you make time for me during an emergency or when I have questions and concerns about my health? What times can you be reached on the telephone? Do you make home visits, if needed?

- *Determine method of payment required:* Find out if you have to pay the fee directly, or if the doctor will bill the insurance company or accept Medicare or Medicaid payments.

A final factor is one of the most important: are you comfortable with your doctor's manner?

Caring—The All-Important Bedside Manner "Comfort always, cure rarely" was a motto of many physicians before the era of high-technology medicine, during times when cures were not possible.[17] Then, as science and specialization became more important, many doctors became more distant from their patients. A patient was sometimes referred to between doctors and nurses not by name but as "the gallbladder in room 203." Some surgeons became so far removed from the notion of extending comfort that they would bluntly tell patients immediately before an operation, "You have a 5% chance of dying or becoming a quadriplegic," reducing them to tears.[18]

During the last decade, there has been a rising tide of patient complaints about doctors' bedside manners. A 1990 survey by Miles Inc.'s pharmaceutical division, for instance, found that one in four U.S. patients had switched physicians at least once because the doctor made them feel uncomfortable, didn't relieve their anxiety, or failed to answer questions.[19] Another study found that general practitioners interrupted their patients an average of 18 seconds into their account of their problem and 80% didn't even hear all of the patient's chief complaints.[20]

As a result of patients' concerns that doctors are more adept at technology and jargon than compassion, many medical schools began to devote resources to training future doctors in

the art of TLC—tender loving care, of empathy and comforting.[21–23]

For you, looking for a new health practitioner, whether doctor or dentist, the lesson would seem plain—you want someone who will offer competence in managing your medical care and who will do the following:

- *Be accessible:* You want a health practitioner whose office you can get to easily and who is accessible by telephone.

- *Take time to listen:* You want someone who will listen to your complaint and not interrupt you 18 seconds into the interview. You should not be rushed through a visit. Even better, you hope your doctor will have a sensitive, empathetic manner.

- *Give you information in an understandable way:* According to one study, physicians spend less than 2 minutes of a 20-minute session imparting information. As a result, 60% of patients leave a doctor's office confused about instructions about medication or other aspects of their care.[24] Be sure your physician takes time to answer all your questions.

Physical Exams, Medical Tests, Dental Checkups, and Treatment

Before getting a medical checkup, you should make a few notes to help the physician. A physician makes a diagnosis based on three sources of information: the patient's medical history and description of symptoms, the physical examination, and the results of lab tests and medical procedures—blood tests, urinalysis, X ray, mammography, and electrocardiogram. Dental checkups should be done once or twice a year. Many patients don't follow a doctor's treatment recommendations because they don't understand or are intimidated. If surgery is recommended, you usually have time to make certain preparations.

You may expect certain things of your doctor or dentist, but he or she should also expect some things of you. The health-care partnership

14.13

*Chapter 32
Getting the
Most Out of
Conventional
Health Care*

doesn't work unless both participate. We can see how this works during the course of having a physical exam, getting medical tests, and following a treatment plan.

Preparing for a Medical Checkup In 1983, the American Medical Association recommended that healthy Americans over age 18 undergo a medical checkup every 5 years until age 40. After age 40, they recommend a physical every 1–3 years, depending on one's occupation, present health status, medical history, and other personal characteristics.[25] Other authorities suggest a complete physical every 1–3 years even for 18-year-olds; certain other tests, such as blood-pressure checks, blood-cholesterol measurement, and Pap tests, should be done every 1–3 years. (See ● *Table 32.1.*)

When preparing for a physical exam, or any

● **Table 32.1 Medical checkups: Your examination timetable.** The following are general recommendations for screening tests for healthy individuals. Because of your lifestyle, occupation, or family history, some additional tests or more frequent screening may be indicated. Discuss with your health care professional a schedule that meets your needs.

Age	Sex	Test	Frequency
18 and over	M/F	Complete physical	Every 1–3 years
	M/F	Blood pressure	Every 1–3 years
	M/F	Total cholesterol	Every 1–3 years
	M/F	Tetanus and diphtheria booster (Td)	Every 10 years
	F	Pelvic exam	Annually
	F	Pap smear[a]	Every 1–3 years
	F	Breast exam	Annually
35 and over	F	Baseline mammogram	Repeat in 5 years
	F	Kidney function: BUN and creatinine clearance	Every 5 years
40 and over	M/F	Visual acuity, glaucoma	Every 3 years
	M/F	Digital rectal[b]	Annually
	M/F	Hearing test	Every 3 years
	F	Mammogram	Annually
45 and over	M/F	Exercise electrocardiogram (Stress test)	Every 5 years
50 and over	M/F	Baseline sigmoidoscopy	Repeat every 3 years
	M/F	Fecal occult blood[c]	Annually
65 and over	M/F	Visual acuity, with glaucoma check	Annually
	M/F	Hearing	Annually
	M/F	Dipstick urinalysis	Annually
	M/F	Influenza vaccine	Annually
	M/F	Pneumococcal vaccine	One time only
	F	Thyroid function tests	Annually

[a]After a woman between the ages of 18 and 40 has had negative Pap smears for three consecutive years, the test may be performed less frequently at the discretion of her doctor. Starting at age 40, she should have a Pap smear annually.

[b]An examination of the lower bowel and, in men, the prostate, in which the physician inserts a gloved finger into the anal opening.

[c]A test for microscopic blood in the stool.

Source: Adapted from Editors of the University of California, Berkeley, *Wellness Letter*. (1991). *The wellness encyclopedia: The comprehensive family resource for safeguarding health and preventing illness.* Boston: Houghton Mifflin, p. 430.

appointment with a health care provider, the following are advocated:

- *Make notes of your concerns beforehand:* According to an analysis by the American Society of Internal Medicine, 70% of correct diagnoses *depend solely on what you tell your doctor.*[26] Thus, write down questions, worries, and symptoms and bring this "agenda" to your visit.

- *Be aware of your family's medical history:* If it is your first visit, it's important to be knowledgeable about your family's medical history as well as your own, such as a history of heart disease, cancer, or genetic abnormalities.

- *Bring along medications:* Bring along any medications (prescription or nonprescription) you are taking. Describe any treatments you are using.

- *Women note last menstrual period:* Women of reproductive age should note the first day of their last menstrual period. Such information will be needed to assess the possibility of pregnancy or reproductive-system problems.

It's important that you be as complete as possible, even if you think some details may be insignificant or embarrassing.

Having a Physical Exam A physician usually makes a diagnosis based on three sources of information:

1. The patient's medical history and description of symptoms and concerns

2. The physical examination

3. The results of various laboratory tests and procedures (such as X rays)

Whether you go in to see a physician just for a medical checkup or with a complaint about something troubling you, the physician will proceed to obtain information via these three avenues.

The traditional medical checkup is called a "history and a physical." In the first part, the health care provider will document your health **history,** which contains all health-related information, including past and present illnesses, allergies, and immunizations; prior hospitalizations and operations; and present medications. Sometimes you are asked to fill out a form describing your history in the reception room be-fore you see the provider, but he or she will clarify the information you provide during the interview. He or she may also ask about your **chief complaint,** the primary concern that caused you to seek medical care in the first place.

The provider will next do a physical examination. A complete examination includes the following:

- *Vital signs:* The provider will measure your **vital signs**—your temperature (which should be about 98.2), blood pressure (average is 120/70–138/88, depending on sex and age), pulse rate (average: 72 beats per minute), and breathing rate (about 12–20 breaths per minute). Irregularities may suggest the presence of heart or blood-vessel disease, thyroid disorders, kidney damage, or other problems.

- *Head and throat area:* The provider will examine eyes, ears, nose, and throat.

  After first inspecting the exterior of the eye for signs of redness (indicating possible infection) or paleness (indicating possible anemia), the provider will use a special lighted instrument (ophthalmoscope) to look at the interior of the eye for irregularities in the blood vessels that may indicate disease.

  The provider may do a minimal screening for vision problems, such as asking you to read a line or two from an eye chart, but otherwise will refer you to an ophthalmologist or optometrist for a more thorough eye examination. If you are over age 20 and have a family history of **glaucoma**—a disease characterized by increased pressure within the eyeball which can lead to gradual loss of vision—the health care provider will probably ask you to go to an ophthalmologist or optometrist to check for the presence of this disease.

  Using another lighted instrument (otoscope), the provider will look into your ears for signs of blockage or infection. He or she may also use a tuning fork or other device to get a rough idea of your hearing.

  Asking you to say "Ahhh," the health care provider will examine your throat, as well as your tongue, gums, and mouth in general, to check for any problems.

14.15

*Chapter 32
Getting the
Most Out of
Conventional
Health Care*

- *Neck and chest:* The health care provider will feel the front and sides of your neck to check for enlarged lymph glands (signaling infection) and abnormalities in the thyroid gland. With a stethoscope, he or she may listen to the arteries in the neck for signs of stroke, or blockage of blood flow.

  Also with the stethoscope, the provider will listen to your chest, checking first for abnormal heart sounds and rhythms, then for irregularities in lung sounds. Tapping on the chest with fingers will also signal whether there is fluid in the lungs, a sign of pneumonia. In addition, if you're a woman, the provider will check your breasts for lumps or other abnormalities.

- *Abdomen:* The health care provider will probe with his or her fingers the area around your stomach, feeling for the presence of masses or tenderness, which might indicate an enlarged spleen or liver, hernias (rupture of the intestine through abdominal wall), or other disorders.

- *Rectum, genital, and pelvic areas:* Wearing a glove, the provider will insert a finger into the rectum to check for abnormal growths and hemorrhoids. In males, this will reveal whether the prostate gland is enlarged, a sign of possible prostate cancer.

  The provider will check a male's genitals for sores or growths. By feeling the scrotum while asking you to cough, the physician may detect whether one type of hernia is present.

  Females will be given a pelvic examination, which will include a **Pap smear,** in which cells gently scraped from the cervix are sent to a laboratory and examined under a microscope for signs of cervical cancer.

- *Skin, hair, and extremities:* The doctor or other health care provider will examine your skin for signs of rashes, sores, lumps, discoloration, and other abnormalities. Hair and nails will be examined for clues to blood disorders.

  Ankles and feet will be scrutinized for signs of swelling that would suggest heart, liver, or kidney disorders. Pulses in feet and wrists will be checked for blood flow. Joints will be checked for redness, swelling, or de-

formity that suggests the existence of arthritis. Your kneecap may be tapped with a rubber hammer to check your reflexes, which can determine whether there are problems in the muscle or nervous system.

If the health provider's probing produces any pain or you feel some unusual sensations, you will be doing both of you a favor if you point it out. Don't be hesitant about saying, "Oh, by the way, I noticed . . ." if something in the examination triggers a memory of something you observed that was unusual. All this may provide significant information.

Medical Tests Taking a history and doing a physical examination are the first two sources of information a health professional relies on to get a picture of you; the third source is provided by medical testing. Depending on the provider's location, you may be able to have these done on the same day and in the same clinic, hospital, or offices as the location of the physical exam.

The principal medical tests are the following:

- *Blood tests:* Blood may be taken from a vein in your arm or from a finger prick. The sample is sent to a laboratory for analysis. (*See* ● *Figure 32.4.*)

  Blood tests are of three principal types:

(1) The **complete blood count (CBC),** which is the most commonly performed blood test, is useful in diagnosing certain illnesses, the major ones being anemia and leukemia.[27]

(2) The **blood-chemistry panel** is a test for kidney, bone, liver, pancreas, prostate, and some glandular functions. Such tests provide indications of diseases such as diabetes, gout, or kidney stones. The word *panel* means that a group of different tests is done using one sample of blood.

(3) The **cholesterol test**, according to many experts, is an indicator of risk of heart and blood-vessel disease. If your cholesterol level is optimum, below 200 milligrams per milliliter, and the level of "bad cholesterol" (low-density liproprotein, or LDL) is under 130, you are

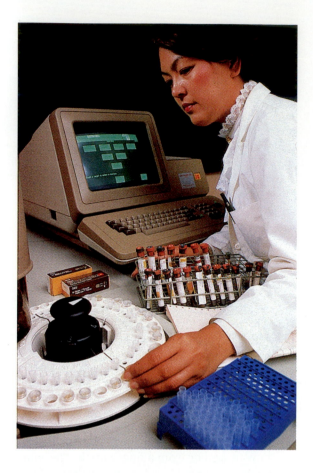

No lab test is foolproof. Healthy people sometimes have test results that are "false positive"—that is, in error.

If the results are abnormal, you should ask your health care provider whether the test should be repeated. Find out if any medications you are taking could affect the tests.

Medical test results also depend on the quality of the laboratory performing the test. Ask whether the lab is accredited or licensed. Accreditation is voluntary, but licensing is mandatory and is done by the state or the Department of Health and Human Services.

Lab work done in a physician's office on his or her own patients does not have to be licensed; generally such results aren't as accurate as those of licensed labs.

advised to repeat the test every 5 years. If it is borderline, you should repeat it every year.

- *Urinalysis:* When you have a blood test, many times you also may be requested to have a **urinalysis.** That is, a sample of your urine is examined by a laboratory for signs of bacteria, diabetes, or disorders of the urinary tract, kidneys, pancreas, or thyroid.

- *Chest X ray:* The chest X ray can detect an enlarged heart, pneumonia, or sinus infection. It can also detect lung cancer, and your physician will probably insist on this test if you are a smoker.

    The risk of genetic and immune system damage correlates with the total amount of radiation you receive over your lifetime.[28] X rays are no longer done routinely for healthy patients because their radiation adds to the cumulative lifetime total. Two exceptions, however, have been mammograms (breast X rays) and dental X rays.

    You should always ask if any X ray is really necessary or if a previous one can be used. Sometimes an alternative can be used (such as a CAT scan or magnetic-resonance imaging), although they cost more.

- *Mammography:* **Mammograms** are X rays (using a small amount of radiation) designed to detect breast abnormalities early. According to the American Cancer Society and most other organizations, women should get their first mammogram between ages 35 and 39, then every 1–2 years between 40 and 49, then annually thereafter. Recently, however, some studies have cast doubt on whether even good-quality mammograms benefit women under 50.[29]

- *Electrocardiogram:* A routine **electrocardiogram (ECG or EKG)** is sometimes called a "resting ECG." ECGs are assessment and diagnostic tools. While you are at rest, electrodes attached to your chest transmit electrical impulses from your heart to a stylus that records the impulses on paper. The electrocardiogram can detect an enlarged heart, abnormal heart rhythms, blood-vessel disease, and other problems. It can aid in the diagnosis of heart problems.

    A variation of the resting ECG is one conducted while you walk or run on a treadmill, called an **exercise stress test.**

14.17

*Chapter 32
Getting the
Most Out of
Conventional
Health Care*

The purpose of this test is to assess heart function under conditions of stress when the demand for oxygen to the heart muscle is increased.

Dental Checkups The American Dental Association recommends that adults have a dental exam at least once a year and have teeth professionally cleaned at least twice a year.

Besides a cleaning, a dental checkup should include a screening for four primary problems: oral cancer, jaw disorders, gum disease (using an instrument called a periodontal probe), and cavities and existing fillings. A full set of dental X rays should be taken every 5 years, and bitewing X rays (which show the tops of your teeth and under the gumline and are good for spotting bone loss caused by gum disease) should be taken yearly; individual X rays should be done as needed.[30]

Medical and Surgical Treatment After the history and physical exam, the health care provider will discuss any immediate findings with you. Some things may not be known, however, until your lab results come back, probably a few days later. At that point, the provider is likely to call you if there are any abnormalities and recommend a plan of action.

Two issues about treatment are particularly worth noting:

- *Noncompliance—the deadly epidemic:* Probably 125,000 lives are lost in the United States every year for a simple reason: people do not take their prescribed medication properly or at all.[31] Indeed, what the medical profession calls *noncompliance,* or ignoring the doctor's orders, has become a very expensive and unnecessary epidemic in the United States. *Half of all patients don't take their medication or take it incorrectly.*[32]

- *Preparing for surgery:* Since 80% of all surgeries performed are considered **elective surgery**—they are not emergencies, and the patient can generally choose when and where to have the operation—you actually have plenty of time to get ready for most operations and any hospital stay. There are a number of things you can do:[33,34]

(1) "Pre-donate" your own blood 2 weeks before the operation for use during your surgery.

(2) Make out a living will (described in Chapter 35), which describes what life-sustaining treatment you want in the unlikely event this comes up. Also appoint a relative or friend as a proxy or give them power of attorney to see that your wishes are carried out.

(3) Pack personal belongings that will make your stay more comfortable.

Prescription and Nonprescription Medications

Medications may be available by a doctor's or dentist's prescription or available "over-the-counter." Prescription drugs are often available under a brand name or less expensively under a generic name. In using medications, you need to be aware that prescription mistakes are made; that drugs may be misused, producing side effects, allergies, and adverse drug interactions; and that one can become inadvertently addicted. Nonprescription drugs may also be powerful, especially the pain relievers (aspirin, acetaminophen, and ibuprofen) and cold-and-allergy medications (antihistamines and decongestants). Pharmacists and physicians are the best sources of advice about the handling and hazards of medications.

Powders and potions have always been a powerful aspect of healing, and still are. Outside of medicine's mainstream, medicine men, *curanderos,* and folk healers may, for example, prepare a "foxglove tea" for patients with heart problems. The foxglove plant contains digitalis, a drug regularly prescribed by conventional doctors for heart patients.

Medications are of two types:

1. *Prescription:* **Prescription drugs** must be ordered by a licensed practitioner, most likely a medical doctor, osteopathic physician, or dentist. There are 2500 prescription drugs, ranging from tranquilizers to anti-hypertension pills.[35]

2. *Nonprescription:* **Nonprescription,** or **over-the-counter (OTC) drugs,** are medications that can be obtained legally without a prescription. There are 300,000 different nonprescription products (classified into 26 families), ranging from antacids to cold remedies to contraceptives.

In addition, there are medical and health *devices*, ranging from canes to heart pacemakers. Drugs are regulated by the Food and Drug Administration (FDA); other medical devices and health products are regulated by the Federal Trade Commission (FTC).

Prescription Drugs Of the 2500 or so drugs available by prescription, only 200 are among the majority of those prescribed and renewed.[36]

There are a number of considerations to be aware of regarding prescription drugs:

- *Be aware of generic versus brand-name drugs:* A pharmaceutical company that develops a drug can patent and sell it exclusively for 17 years (and perhaps extend the patent protection for 5 more years). During this time, the drug is sold under its **brand name,** the specific patented name assigned to a drug by its manufacturer. *Inderal,* for example, is the brand name of a leading blood-pressure drug, *Valium* of a leading tranquilizer.

   After the patent expires, other drug companies can apply to the FDA to market their own versions under the drug's **generic name,** the common or nonproprietary name for the drug. The generic name for *Inderal,* for example, is propranolol.

   The significance to you, as a consumer, is this: *the same chemical can have an incredible price spread.* For instance, it was found in 1989 that 100 tablets of *Inderal* (the brand name) can cost as much as $43.25. By contrast, 100 tablets of propranolol (the generic name) cost as little as $1.99—a price 21 times cheaper![37]

   Some states or insurance companies require pharmacists to substitute a less expensive generic drug for the brand-name drug (unless the physician has checked the "dispense as written" box on the prescription). All other states merely permit the pharmacist to make the substitution, if the physician approves.

- *Be aware of prescription mistakes:* Physicians write 827 million new prescriptions and 729 million refills every year—and not all of them are correct.[38,39]

   The most common serious mistake made by physicians is prescribing a drug to which the patient is allergic. Other errors include prescribing antibiotics for the wrong patient, ordering overdoses or underdoses of drugs, and mixing up the names of drugs.

   Clearly, then, it's important to inform your doctor about any allergies, dietary restrictions (including reactions to alcohol), other drugs you're taking, and pre-existing health conditions (such as if you are pregnant, breast-feeding, or diabetic).

- *Be aware of the dangers of drug misuse:* If you had a bacterial infection, would you borrow a friend's **antibiotic,** a drug designed to destroy bacteria? If you were feeling depressed, would you accept Valium from a roommate or family member? Many people may see nothing wrong with doing this, but the reason that certain drugs are *prescribed* in the first place—particular drugs are ordered in particular dosages for a particular person—is that they can produce serious consequences, as follows:

   (1) **Side effects** are secondary, and usually adverse, reactions produced by a drug, such as nausea, dizziness, or more serious responses. FDA approval does not guarantee that drugs are free of risk.[40] Indeed, it has been found that over half the new drugs approved by the FDA in a 10-year period had such adverse side affects as heart, kidney, or liver failure; blindness; and birth defects.[41]

   (2) An **allergy** is a hypersensitivity to a particular substance. Some drugs—such as penicillin, barbiturates, or anticonvulsants—can produce allergic reactions. The worst of these is **anaphylaxis,** an extreme allergic reaction resulting in shock, drop in blood pressure, nausea and vomiting, unconsciousness, and possibly life-threatening collapse and death. This constitutes a medical emergency that requires im-

14.19

*Chapter 32
Getting the
Most Out of
Conventional
Health Care*

mediate intervention by a health care professional.

(3) *Drug interactions* may occur when two drugs (prescription and/or nonprescription) mix in ways that one might not have immediately foreseen. One powerful—and often tragic—example of this is the mixture of tranquilizers and alcohol, which can produce unconsciousness, and even death. Another example is the interaction between tranquilizers and cold medications, which may cause extreme drowsiness.

- *Be aware of inadvertent addiction:* While the nation continues to focus on illegal drug use, thousands of Americans have become hooked on psychoactive (mood-altering) drugs that are perfectly legal—and prescribed by their doctors. This seems to be particularly true for older people. One 1989 federal report estimated that 2 million older adults were addicted or at risk of addiction to sleeping pills or tranquilizers.[42] (*See ● Figure 32.5.*)

Nonprescription Drugs Prescription drugs are powerful, but so are many nonprescription drugs. Indeed, the FDA has permitted many marketers to repackage active ingredients formerly available only by prescription and to sell them as over-the-counter (OTC) drugs. This has been the case, for example, with the painkiller Advil, the antihistamine Benadryl, and the athlete's-foot remedy Tinactin.[43] Although perfectly legal, this might suggest something about OTC drugs: they are not to be taken lightly.

Although nonprescription medications have a reputation for being harmless, they are not. Every year hundreds of thousands of Americans are hospitalized because of adverse reactions to OTC drugs, and many die. Indeed, some over-the-counter pain and allergy pills, especially in combinations, can be more dangerous than the aches and pains they are designed to treat.

The dangers of the principal OTC medications are as follows:

- *Pain relievers:* There may be more than 100 brands of pain relievers, but essentially they are of three types: *aspirin, acetaminophen,* and *ibuprofen.* For occasional relief of minor aches, pains, and headaches,

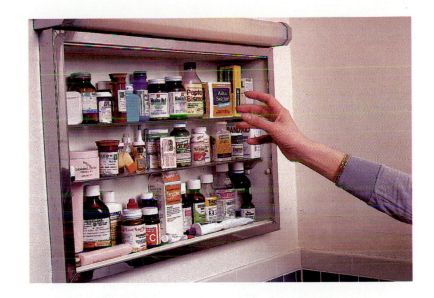

● **Figure 32.5 Inadvertent addiction.** People of all ages may be at risk for becoming "inadvertently addicted"—addicted by accident—to legally prescribed psychoactive drugs, such as sleeping pills and tranquilizers, but the problem may be especially pervasive among older adults.

"*A number of factors place the older person at special risk: Aging and retirement can set the stage . . . leaving a person anxious or depressed due to illness, loss of a spouse, or diminished self-esteem. Health problems can compound the situation because many older people see several specialists and may be taking multiple medications. They may also end up taking several brand-name versions of the same drug without realizing it, thus increasing the risk of addiction. And . . . because bodily functions slow with age, the same amount of any drug—including alcohol—can have a greater effect and last longer. Yet physicians often prescribe the same dosage they would for a younger patient.*"

—Sue Chastain. (1992, February–March). The accidental addict: Are you hooked on your prescriptions? *Modern Maturity,* p. 39.

a medication containing any one of these drugs should do the trick (although some drugs work better for some purposes than others, as we discuss).[44] However, all three have potential side effects:

(1) *Aspirin* (Anacin, Bayer, Bufferin) is effective against minor pains and low fevers. It also has an anti-inflammatory effect that makes it effective against arthritis. Unfortunately, many heavy users of aspirin, such as the 20 million Americans who take daily doses for arthritis, suffer stomach irritation. Twenty percent develop severe gastric ulcers, and an estimated 100,000 die from hemorrhages each year.[45] Aspirin can also cause kidney and liver damage among elderly users. It should not be given to children or adolescents with the flu since it can trigger Reye's syndrome, a rare disorder that can result in severe brain damage. Incidentally, when taken by someone who's been drinking, in order to avoid a hangover, aspirin actually *increases* blood-alcohol concentrations.[46]

(2) *Acetaminophen* (Tylenol, Datril, Panadol) causes fewer complications than aspirin. Instead of suppressing prostaglandins, it simply blocks pain receptors in the brain. Useful for relieving minor to moderate headache and muscle pains and reducing fever, acetaminophen does not reduce inflammation and so may not be useful in arthritis. Overuse and use by alcoholics may lead to irreversible liver damage.[47–50]

(3) *Ibuprofen* (Advil, Motril, Nuprin) works the same way aspirin does, suppressing the output of prostaglandins. It not only relieves mild to moderate pain, including headache and muscle pain, but is especially useful against menstrual pain, dental pain, soft-tissue strains and sprains, and (in high doses under a doctor's supervision) as an anti-inflammatory agent against arthritis. The possible side effects, however, are the same as for aspirin. Children should not be given ibuprofen at all, unless a physician approves.

- *Cold-and-allergy medications:* Driving with a blood-alcohol concentration equivalent to 0.1 gram per deciliter is not only a crime, it makes you 20 times more likely to cause a fatal traffic accident. However, in most states it's perfectly legal to drive with an equivalent dose of a cold-and-allergy-fighting antihistamine (50 milligrams of diphenhydramine, or Benadryl), which a study by pharmacologist Fran M. Gengo found made drivers' reaction times more than *twice* as slow as normal.[51]

Two types of cold-and-allergy medications, *antihistamines* and *decongestants*, have some potent side effects:

(1) **Antihistamines** (the one called *diphenhydramine* is found in Actifed, Allerest, Benadryl, and Dimetapp) are useful medications for hay fever and similar allergies, but not for the common cold. Antihistamines block the chemical messenger histamine; when it's released by cells in the nasal tissues it makes the nose itch and run. However, histamine also has another purpose—as an alerting agent within the central nervous system. When you take an antihistamine, therefore, you fight not only nose itch but also fight alertness. Besides drowsiness, important side effects of antihistamines include dizziness, poor coordination, and impaired judgment—exactly what you don't need when you're driving.

Antihistamines containing diphenhydramine, found in many cold and allergy medications, also have a dehydrating (drying) effect and should be used with caution by people with asthma, glaucoma, hypertension, or cardiovascular disease. The drying effects are intensified when antihistamine is combined with antidepressants called MAO (monoamine oxidase) inhibitors. Alcohol combined with antihistamines can create severe drowsiness and impaired coordination.

(2) **Decongestants** are intended to fight mucus production by constricting the blood vessels in the nose. Spray decongestants, if used sparingly, are considered the most effective. Oral decongestants can constrict blood vessels throughout the body, making such drugs unsafe for people with high blood

14.21

*Chapter 32
Getting the
Most Out of
Conventional
Health Care*

pressure, thyroid disease, or diabetes. Besides blood-pressure elevation, side effects include anxiety, restlessness, and hallucinations.

Pharmacist Assistance Pharmacists are not just glorified clerks who hand out drugs on doctors' orders. They can provide a valuable service when you've forgotten (or been reluctant) to ask your physician about medications, whether prescription or nonprescription. Indeed, one survey by the National Consumers League found that 88% of Americans think of pharmacists as their primary or secondary source of information about drugs.[52] Unfortunately, many consumers don't take advantage of this free service.

When you are buying a drug, whether prescription or nonprescription, ask your pharmacist the following:

- *Purpose:* What *is* this drug? What does it do? Why should I take it? What if I don't take it? How long will it take to get favorable results?

- *Hazards:* What are the possible adverse reactions? What are its side effects? How will it react with other medications? Can I drink alcohol while taking it? Will it go with the particular diet I'm on? Are there foods I should avoid?

- *Handling:* What time of day should I take it? Can I take it on an empty stomach? How should it be stored? How long should I take it? How do I get refills? Can I substitute a generic for a brand name?

If your pharmacist asks you questions about your health, you should be as honest as with a physician. Be sure to describe any other drugs (including over-the-counter drugs) you're taking, any allergies you have, and any special diet you're on. "It's not just a matter of putting pills in a bottle," says one pharmacist about his role. "I see myself as a health consultant."[53]

Paying for Health Care

Canada and the United States have different experiences in health care. All Canadians have health coverage and choice of health services. Millions of Americans do not have health insurance, although the American health care system offers the finest new technology. U.S. health insurance covers either fee-for-service medicine or prepaid medicine. Three types of insurance policies are basic protection, major medical, and comprehensive major medical. Individual and group insurance policies are available. Some health organizations offer "managed care," which limits fees; two types are health-maintenance organizations and preferred provider organizations. Government programs offer Medicaid and Medicare.

By this point, you know a few things about how to judge quality health care and how to promote your own health interests. But can you *afford* quality health care? Are you covered in the event you should fall seriously ill? In this section, we explore one of the most serious matters you may have to confront: paying for health care.

The Canadian and American Experiences Because most readers of this book are probably either American or Canadian, it is instructive to briefly characterize the health care systems of both countries.

- *The Canadian experience:* All Canadians are currently entitled to a full range of medical and hospital services. In reality, there are 12 programs, administered by the 10 provinces and two territories, each of them subsidized by contributions from Canada's federal treasury.[54] The program is available to a highly mobile population everywhere in the country, and does not limit residents of one province from moving permanently to another province. Citizens pay a fee, of around $400–$500 (U.S.) a year; usually employers make the contribution for their employees, and the government pays for those on welfare.

  Canadians have freedom of choice in selecting physicians; patients are not assigned doctors from approved lists. If a patient is dissatisfied with a doctor, he or she simply chooses another. The same is true of choice of hospitals. Primary and emergency care, universally insured, are readily available.

The government's insurance covers all health costs except dental care, eyeglasses, ambulance service, private hospital rooms, and prescription drugs. If individuals want to take out extra insurance—to cover private rooms in hospitals, for example—they may do so.

Are there delays and waiting lists, as some critics of the system have complained? Some, particularly for nonemergency heart surgery and hip replacement. However, the waiting is hardly serious, say defenders of the system, citing government statistics: 96% of Canadians over the age of 15 get their care within 7 days of requesting it.[55] (The wait for coronary-bypass surgery for British Columbians was found to be 14 weeks.[56]) The majority of Canadians themselves are satisfied with their health system, and so are Canadian doctors.[57,58]

As for costs, the Canadian system seems to provide good value. In 1990, the Canadians spent an average of $1730 per capita on health care (compared to $2566 per capita spent in the United States), but life expectancy is longer, infant mortality less, and death from heart disease less.[59] (*See* ● *Table 32.2.*) A 1990 study found little difference in death rates for a variety of procedures in the two countries, despite wide differences in costs.[60]

● *The American experience:* The American experience in health care has not been as positive, at least overall. Whereas the Canadian system provides basic health coverage for every resident, the number of U.S. citizens with no health insurance—37 million—exceeds the entire population of Canada.[61] As a result, it is said, 50% of personal bankruptcies in the United States has been attributed to medical costs.[62]

● **Table 32.2 Health statistics: Canada and the United States**

	Canada	United States
Life expectancy	77.1	75.3
Infant mortality	7.2 per 1000 live births (8th in the world)	10 per 1000 live births (17th in the world)
Death from heart disease	348 per 10,000	434 per 10,000
Per capita health care expenditure, 1990 (in U.S. dollars)	$1730	$2566
Health expenditure as percentage of 1991 GDP (Gross Domestic Product)	10%	12.4%
Doctors per 1000 people	2.2	2.3
Open-heart-surgery units per million people, 1990*	1.23	3.26
Radiation therapy units per million people, 1990*	0.54	3.97
Average days in-patient care, 1989	13	9.2
Cost of standard quadruple coronary artery bypass, 1991	$12,236 (Montreal)	$25,439
Average net income for a doctor, 1990 (U.S. dollars)	$105,000	$164,000
Average annual malpractice premium	$7500	$57,000
Total taxes paid as percent of national income, 1989	46.9%	36.9%

*This is a comparison of available technology, not of its use. For instance, each radiation therapy unit in the United States might not be used as often as those in Canada because the United States has so many more.

Sources: American Medical Association, American Hospital Association, Canadian Medical Association, Department of National Health and Welfare–Canada, Organization for Economic Cooperation and Development, U.S. General Accounting Office.

14.23
*Chapter 32
Getting the
Most Out of
Conventional
Health Care*

Still, for those who can afford it, the American system offers the finest technology and scientific medicine in the world.

Costs, however, have been astronomical. It is ironic that, in spending per capita, Canada's is the *second* most expensive medical system in the world (at $1730 per person), because the United States' is the *first* (at $2566)—yet half the American health care (by cost) is consumed by only 5% of the population.[63] The share of the national output of wealth, the gross domestic product (GDP), expended by the United States on health is 12.4%—and rising—compared to Canada's 10%.[64] Yet the United states has a lower life-expectancy and higher infant-mortality rate not only compared to Canada but also compared to Japan, Britain, France, Italy, and Germany.

There are a great many possible reasons why the American health system costs so much but fails to deliver for so many of its citizens. Some argue that lawyer-inspired litigation has led to skyrocketing settlements for malpractice lawsuits by patients against doctors.[65] This in turn has led to rising premiums doctors must pay for malpractice insurance and has led physicians to practice "defensive medicine" by ordering all kinds of extra tests and procedures. Some say the imposition of extra paperwork and second-guessing of doctors' judgments by insurance companies has driven costs up.[66] Some argue that the United States is technology-happy—that because one hospital orders an MRI unit (a $4 million expenditure), competing hospitals in the same city decide they each have to have one, too.[67] Some say American doctors are overpaid, and that their salaries constitute a gigantic expense.[68] Some say that medicine in the United States is run as a for-profit business rather than as a social service, as in other countries.[69] And some say the burden of social problems on health care—homicides, serious assaults, and drug offenses—and the highest rate of AIDS infection in the developed world imposes demands on American medicine that far exceed those of any other industrialized countries.[70]

Perhaps as you read this, the American health care system will be on its way to reform. We anticipate, however, that many of the existing arrangements will remain in place. Let us,

therefore, consider the various types of health insurance, types of health organizations, and government-financed insurance plans.

Health Insurance If you get sick, *really* sick, and have no health insurance, the United States is not the place to be. You're likely to end up owing thousands of dollars to doctors and hospitals. Students who finish or drop out of school—or who cut back their course loads to part-time—may find themselves no longer covered by their parents' or partner's health plan and exposed to considerable financial risks. Health insurance is too important to be ignored.

There are two basic approaches to paying for health care:

- *Fee-for-service:* **Fee-for-service medicine** means that the physician or hospital performs treatment and presents you and/or the insurance company with a bill. This used to be the most common arrangement in the United States.

- *Prepaid:* **Prepaid medicine** means that you (or your employer) pay for specified kinds of medical services ahead of time. This arrangement, being favored more and more, is characteristic of *managed-care organizations: health-maintenance organizations* (HMOs) and *preferred-provider organizations* (PPOs), as we will describe.

Three Types of Insurance Policies Assuming for the moment that you are interested in fee-for-service medicine, there are three kinds of coverage—*basic protection, major medical (catastrophic),* and *comprehensive major medical:*

- *Basic protection:* A **basic-protection** health-insurance policy covers hospital, surgical, and medical care. It usually does not cover visits to physicians' offices and may exclude other costs, such as prescription drugs. An **exclusion** refers to conditions or circumstances for which the policy does not pay benefits. An example of an exclusion is a **pre-existing condition,** a health problem you had before becoming insured.

  A basic-protection policy is a good one to have if you're healthy and rarely need medical attention. In addition, you can get regular medical insurance, which covers physicians' fees for nonsurgical care.

One form of basic-protection policy reimburses you for 80% of covered charges once you have met the deductible. The **deductible** is the amount you must pay before the insurance company starts paying. For instance, you might have to pay $2500 for medical bills in one year, but after that the policy pays for 80% of the charges covered by the policy.

The arrangement whereby you and the insurance company share the costs—as when you pay 20% and it pays 80% beyond the deductible—is known as **co-insurance.**

- *Major medical or catastrophic:* A **major-medical** or **catastrophic** policy is for those who can't afford basic coverage, and everyone should *at least* have one of these, since it will protect you from financial catastrophe should you experience a medical catastrophe. These policies are designed to protect against medical expenses arising from serious injury or prolonged illness.

  The deductible for such policies is apt to be high—you may have to pay the first $10,000 or more before the insurance company pays. However, hospitals are likely to arrange credit terms for you to pay off the $10,000 if they know the rest is covered by insurance.

- *Comprehensive major medical insurance:* A **comprehensive major medical insurance** policy combines both the basic-care and the major-medical features into one policy.

Individual Versus Group Policies Health insurance may be purchased as an *individual policy* or as a *group plan.*

- *Individual policies:* Individual policies, which are arranged directly between you and an insurance company, are usually (but not necessarily) more expensive than group plans and provide less coverage. With individual plans, the insurers may inquire about your health and turn you down if they consider you a bad risk. On the other hand, with an individual policy, the insurer can't drop the coverage unless it does so for every other individual in the state with the same policy.[71]

- *Group policies:* Group plans are available through the organization you work for. They are usually cheaper and offer more coverage than individual policies, but the main drawback is that they expire when you leave the job. However, under 1986 legislation, you have the right to continue coverage under your old employer's plan for up to 18 months, although you have to pay the premiums yourself.

  Group policies are also available to members of professional associations (for example, the American Bar Association), social and religious organizations (for example, B'nai B'rith), unions, and even small-business owners.

Managed Care: HMOs and PPOs The term **managed care** has come into the language as shorthand for the idea of limiting fees charged by health care providers and controlling the use of medical services. The concept means essentially that health care costs less, but there is less flexibility than under the old fee-for-service medicine. Two types of managed care are HMOs and PPOs.

- *Health-maintenance organizations:* A **health-maintenance organization (HMO)** is an organization in which, in return for a fixed monthly fee by patients or their employers, salaried physicians and other health professionals deliver medical services, usually under one roof. Because the HMO receives the same amount of money whether members are sick or well, an important goal is to keep people healthy by providing preventive services. In addition, HMOs try to deliver care less expensively by controlling use of hospitals and surgery and limiting referrals to specialists.[72] If you join an HMO, you get to choose your primary-care physician from a list of participating doctors, and you need a referral by this physician in order to see a specialist. If you go outside the HMO, you have to pay all the costs yourself.

- *Preferred-provider organizations:* A **preferred-provider organization (PPO)** is a network of doctors and hospitals that has

14.25

*Chapter 32
Getting the
Most Out of
Conventional
Health Care*

agreed to treat members of a sponsoring organization—union, employer, insurance company—at a discount (perhaps 15–20% less) from their usual charges. If you join a PPO, you can go to any physician in the network you want. If you go outside the network, the sponsor (for example, your employer) will not reimburse you for as much.

Besides these two basic models, there are a number of variations. For example, *independent-practice associations* (*IPAs*) are groups of doctors who follow the HMO model but offer services out of their own offices rather than out of a central facility. Another version is the *opt-out HMO,* which allows you to go outside the HMO for medical services, and your employer's plan will pay some of the cost, usually 60% or 70%.

Government Programs: Medicaid and Medicare There are two principal government programs (outside those available to civilian and military government employees) that are available to those who qualify—Medicaid and Medicare.

- *Medicaid:* **Medicaid** is a program run by each state but subsidized by the federal government that covers a range of health services for people who are receiving public assistance and are unable to pay for themselves.

- *Medicare:* **Medicare** is a federal program designed for those 65 and over or people who are chronically disabled. Part A of the program is a hospital-insurance program and is financed by the contributions you made during your working life through Social Security taxes. Part B, for which the subscriber must pay a monthly fee, is supplementary insurance that covers several kinds of physicians' fees and other services not covered by Medicare A.

Strategy for Living A strong message of this book is that there is only one ultimate watchdog for your health: you. It's fair to say that all the other advice in this book about how to take care of yourself could be wasted if your find yourself without health insurance and suddenly in need of high-priced health care.

For most citizens of Canada (and Germany and Japan), this is no problem: even if you lose your job, health insurance covers you. In the United States, however, an enormous segment of the population, perhaps 26%, is uninsured at some point in a year. Some of them are people between jobs or students temporarily without coverage, but their exposure is serious nonetheless. All it takes is being a passenger in someone else's car that is hit by an uninsured motorist to completely change your life. Until the day, then, that there is universal health care for all Americans, you should be as watchful about your insurance coverage as you should about any other aspect of your health.

800-HELP

Ask-A-Nurse. 800-535-1111. A national information and referral service, dispensing advice that can save on unnecessary patient visits to hospitals

Health Reference Center. 800-227-8431. A commercial database of 4000 consumer and medical publications. Call to find the center nearest to you and ask about fees.

Information Center for Individuals with Disabilities. 800-462-5015

National Health Information Center. 800-336-4797. Refers callers to appropriate organizations for information about every disease and disability, including rare ones. Also offers toll-free 800 numbers for other hotlines.

National Organization for Rare Disorders. 800-999-NORD. Supplies the public with reports on any of 950 diseases, including current research and new clinical trials.

Second Surgical Opinion Hotline. 800-638-6833 (in Maryland, 800-492-6603). Provides information on how to get a second opinion on surgery.

Suggestion for Further Reading

Editors of the University of California, Berkeley, *Wellness Letter.* (1991). *The wellness encyclopedia: The comprehensive family resource for safeguarding health and preventing illness*. Boston: Houghton Mifflin. A well-written guide for health consumers and patients.

33   Alternative Therapies and Quackery

▶ Explain some of the more accepted therapies to conventional medicine: chiropractic, acupuncture and acupressure, biofeedback, hypnosis, and mental imagery.

▶ Describe the three categories of alternative therapies, some of which may be somewhat questionable: bodywork or hands-on; chemical, herbal, and dietary; and "mind over matter."

▶ Discuss the hazards of quackery and health fads.

For 124 years, physicians accepted 98.6 degrees Fahrenheit as the normal body temperature for healthy adults. They were wrong.

In 1992, researchers found that the *actual* average body temperature for healthy adults was . . . 98.2.[73]

If conventional medicine can be mistaken about something as fundamental as ordinary human temperature, might it not be missing the boat in other areas as well? Many patients think so. Indeed, because of dissatisfaction with traditional medicine, there has been a rising interest in what is called *alternative medicine* or *alternative health care*. In fact, a 1991 *Time*/CNN poll of a sample of 500 Americans found that 30% had tried some form of unconventional therapy. It also found that 62% who had never sought alternative therapy said they would do so if conventional treatment failed, and 84% of those who had already visited an alternative therapist said they would go back.[74]

Some Accepted Alternatives to Conventional Medicine

Alternative therapies to conventional medicine range from the helpful to the dangerous. Some more accepted alternative therapies are chiropractic, acupuncture and acupressure, biofeedback, hypnosis, and mental imagery.

Conventional medicine, it has been pointed out, is best at crisis intervention.[75] When you are stricken with a virus, are found to have a tumor, or are pulled from a car wreck, the drugs, surgery, and high technology of conventional medicine are exactly what you want. However, physicians with traditional training do not seem to be as well equipped to handle the illnesses related to lifestyle and aging—stresses, back pain, obesity, osteoporosis. These kinds of maladies, which creep up on you over a lifetime rather than all at once, are less susceptible to being fixed by 15 minutes in a doctor's office and a couple of prescriptions. Yet our expectations are that we should be able to do *something* about them. Hence the rise in popularity of alternative therapies. (*See* ● *Figure 33.1.*)

What do we mean by alternative therapies? In general, what alternative therapies share, according to one writer, "is an emphasis on wellness over disease, prevention over treatment, and a belief that they can heal the mind and spirit as well as the body."[76]

Here we consider a few alternative therapies: chiropractic, acupuncture, biofeedback, hypnosis, and mental imagery.

Chiropractic A therapy that attempts to treat disease by manipulating the body joints, **chiropractic,** is the third largest primary health care profession in the Western world.[77] It is based on the ideas of an Iowa "healer" named D. D. Palmer, who theorized in 1895 that small spinal misalignments—what he called "subluxations"—cause virtually all human diseases by interfering with the flow of nerve energy from the brain to the rest of the body. Although today most chiropractors believe that disease can also result from viruses, bacteria, and lifestyle factors, they still focus principally on the vertebrae as the key to good health. The subluxation theory remains unproved.

Chiropractors may use X rays in making diagnoses, but they may not use drugs or surgery in treatment. Chiropractic treatment principally consists of spinal manipulation. According to one 1991 study led by physician Paul Shekelle for the Rand Research Institute, chiropractic technique is considered unorthodox for treatment of anything other than acute low-back pain that has been present for 3 weeks or less, assuming X rays do not reveal any fractures, tumors, or abnormalities.[78]

Acupuncture and Acupressure Traditional in China, where it has been practiced for more than 4500 years, **acupuncture** is a therapy in which fine-gauge needles are inserted at specific points in the body. (See ● *Figure 33.2.*) **Acupressure** is a similar technique, except that gentle finger pressure is used instead of needles. In a variant, it has been discovered that pregnant women can eliminate or reduce symptoms of morning sickness by wearing wristbands (marketed under the name Sea Band) with a button that presses on the inside of the wrist.[79] Common to both acupuncture and acupressure is the belief that the various "acupuncture points" of the body, through which healthful energy (*chi,* or the life force) is supposed to flow, are connected to specific organs and body functions.

The main role of acupuncture in the United States is the management of pain. Stimulating the points in the body triggers the release of **endorphins,** mood-elevating, painkilling chemicals produced by the brain. Acupuncture has also been used in drug and alcohol treatment with some success. However, whether the technique can successfully treat acne, insomnia, arthritis, ulcers, or shingles, as some claim, has yet to be demonstrated.[80]

Biofeedback Biofeedback is the process of using an electronic device to teach you how to monitor and modify your physiological and mental state. With some training, subjects can learn to use brainwave biofeedback to produce relaxation and heart-rate biofeedback to slow the heart rate through breathing control and other techniques.

Biofeedback is used to treat dozens of ailments, from hypertension to chronic pain, asthma to epilepsy, drug addiction to Raynaud's disease (a condition in which fingers become white and painful when exposed to cold). There are 1800 certified biofeedback therapists in the United States, and several insurance companies now cover the procedure.[81]

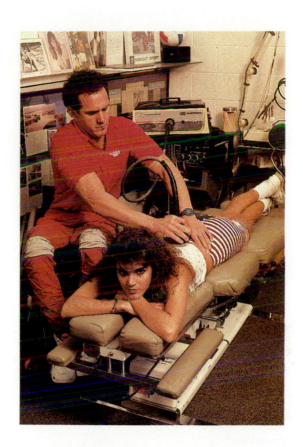

● **Figure 33.1 Why the popularity of alternative therapies?**

❝ *. . . Our health expectations have risen to heights that are perhaps impossible to satisfy. The steady lengthening of life expectancy, the banishment of numerous lethal infectious diseases, the development of cures for several cancers, the breakthroughs in surgery—all great triumphs of medicine and public health—have encouraged us to think there must be a fix for whatever ails us. . . .*

And, yes, modern doctoring has failed to keep many of its promises. A visit to any hospital is an unsettling reminder that scientific medicine remains virtually helpless in the face of a great deal of human suffering. Even ordinary problems are sometimes beyond the reach of the ordinary M.D. And if stress really causes or aggravates all the disorders currently blamed on it, the typical annual visit to a harried physician is hardly the cure—especially when the doctor first keeps you waiting for an appointment, then forgets your name, yet expects you to write a sizable check on your way out. ❞

—Sharon Begley. (1992, April). Alternative medicine: A cure for what ails us? *American Health,* p. 40.

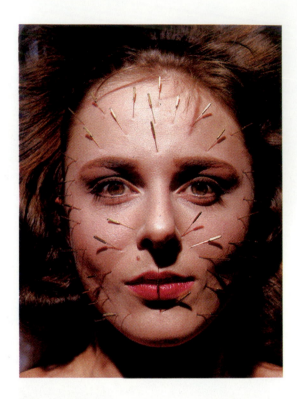

❝*In the U.S. the technique [of acupuncture] was virtually un-known outside Chinese neighborhoods until New York Times journalist James Reston needed an emergency appendectomy while on assignment in China in 1971. Reston reported that an acupuncturist's needles effectively blocked his pain following the operation. Now 21 states license acupuncturists, and many insurance companies will cover the treatments. In 24 states, however, only physicians may perform the technique. Acupunc-ture seems to be most effective in relieving arthritis and chronic pain. . . . In addition, studies show, it is useful in eas-ing the misery of smokers, alcoholics, and other addicts trying to kick their habit.*❞

—Janice M. Horowitz & Elaine Lafferty. (1991, November 4). Why new age medicine is catching on. *Time*, pp. 68–76.

Hypnosis Hypnosis, or more specifically *hyp-notherapy,* is now practiced by 15,000 health professionals, according to the American Soci-ety of Clinical Hypnosis, and it has been recom-mended for further study by the American Medical Association.[82] The technique has been

found to succeed in reducing pain, as in den-tistry; diminishing fears and phobias; helping to overcome smoking, overeating, and nail biting; and easing the breathing of asthmatics and the tremors of Parkinson's disease. It's best to look for someone with professional credentials in psychology, medicine, or dentistry who uses hypnotherapy as part of a larger practice.

Mental Imagery In **mental imagery,** also known as **guided imagery** or **creative visual-ization,** you essentially visualize or daydream your condition and any change you wish to make. Sometimes a therapist or a tape record-ing is used to help "guide" the imagery.

Mental imagery can help people reduce their muscle tensions and focus on their prob-lems without heightening their anxiety. The technique has also been put to use for patients battling serious illness in hopes of improving the immune response.

Unconventional Therapy and Medical Re-spectability Various kinds of meditation and de-stressing techniques in particular have be-gun to find their way into conventional medi-cine. The uses of massage, yoga, and muscle relaxation, for instance, have attracted the at-tention of heart specialists after studies by Dean Ornish showed that lifestyle changes that included stress reduction could actually reverse heart and blood-vessel disease. Indeed, the Na-tional Institutes of Health has even established an Office for the Study of Unconventional Med-ical Practices to scientifically evaluate healing arts once regarded as too bizarre to be useful.[83]

Some Other Alternatives to Conventional Medicine

Alternative therapies, some of which are highly questionable, have three general approaches: bodywork or hands-on; chemi-cal, herbal, and dietary; and "mind over matter." Bodywork includes the Alexander technique, Shiatsu, Feldenkrais, Rolfing, and Reflexology. Chemical and dietary in-cludes homeopathy, naturopathy, herbal medicine, Ayurvedic medicine, Zen macro-biotics, iridology, and aromatherapy. Mind-over-matter approaches include crystal healing, color therapy, and faith healing.

It is one thing to see a licensed acupuncturist or biofeedback therapist on the recommendation of your doctor. It is quite another to try to assess the bewildering number of claims of unconventional schools of healing ranging from homeopathy and herbalism to crystal healing and psychic surgery. Let us try to make some sense out of these offerings. (*See* ● *Table 33.1.*)

In general, alternative medicine may be classified according to three approaches:

- Bodywork or hands-on
- Chemical, herbal, and dietary
- Mind over matter

Bodywork or Hands-On Approaches This category includes chiropractic, acupuncture and acupressure, and all forms of manipulation or massage. Behind most bodywork treatments is the idea that manipulating your body can also bring harmony to your mind. A sample of some bodywork or hands-on approaches:

- *Alexander technique:* The **Alexander technique** is a gentle technique in which you stand in place and practitioners touch you lightly along the back and neck, gently correcting your posture. By improving posture and carriage, the theory goes, the technique relieves muscle tension and pain. In addition, practitioners claim that several sessions can ease stress, depression, headaches, asthma, and digestive problems, although the Alexander technique does not directly cure disease.

- *Shiatsu:* **Shiatsu** is a Japanese therapeutic massage. Oriental medicine maintains that when energy is blocked from flowing through the body, illness results. Whereas the acupuncturist uses needles to manipulate certain "acupuncture points" in the body, the shiatsu therapist uses thumbs, knuckles, and the like to "get energy moving again."

- *Feldenkrais:* Developed by a Russian-born Israeli, Moshe Feldenkrais, who saw the brain as a computer and the body as a terminal, the **Feldenkrais** technique attempts to use manipulations of the limbs and joints to reprogram the mind.

- *Rolfing:* Developed by Ida Rolf, a biochemist, **Rolfing** consists of a deep and sometimes painful massage to realign the

● **Table 33.1 The range of alternative therapies.** Those that are more mainstream and that have more credibility appear toward the left. Those that are more questionable appear toward the right.

Have credibility		Dubious
Chiropractic	Alexander technique	Feldenkrais
Acupuncture & acupressure	Shiatsu	Rolfing
Biofeedback	Homeopathy	Reflexology
Hypnosis	Naturopathy	Zen macrobiotics
Mental imagery	Herbal medicine	Iridology
	Ayurvedic medicine	Aromatherapy
		Crystal healing
		Color therapy
		Faith healing

body. Rolfers hold that the body gets out of shape with the downward pull of gravity and with emotional and physical trauma. By restructuring the body through vigorous massage, they say, they give it better flexibility and alignment, which will restructure the emotions.

- *Reflexology:* Originating in China 5000 years ago but known in the United States only since a half century ago, **reflexology** is the idea that manipulating areas of the feet (and hands) can affect the rest of the body. For instance, if you have a cold, a reflexologist would concentrate on the parts of the foot that correspond to the eyes, nose, ears, chest, and diaphragm.

  Medical authorities say there is no basis to the theory or the claims of reflexology.

There is a whole host of other forms of bodywork, ranging from Swedish massage to Hellerwork to therapeutic touch. Almost all these activities lack the science to back up their claims, although their supporters point to plenty of testimonials and anecdotal evidence. While there may be nothing wrong with having a conventional massage to remove the kinks and muscular tensions of the body (although an inept massage therapist can do a lot of damage), you should stay away from practitioners who claim their activities will do more.

Chemical, Herbal, and Dietary Approaches
Chemicals, potions, herbs, and foods of all sorts have long been the basis of various alternative therapies, as follows:

- *Homeopathy:* **Homeopathy,** based on theories developed in the late 1700s by German physician Samuel Hahnemann, operates on the principal of "like cures like." That is, a homeopathic physician treats a disease with tiny doses of natural substances (highly diluted with water) that in larger amounts would cause the same symptoms as the ailment.

    Skeptics insist that whatever effectiveness homeopathy has is the result of the patient's beliefs in the therapy—in other words, the famed placebo effect.[84] However, one reason for the popularity of homeopathy is that, unlike conventional medicine, homeopathic physicians focus on the individual, spending considerably more time on finding a unique cure for each person.[85]

- *Naturopathy:* Practitioners of **naturopathy** believe that diseases represent the body's efforts to purify itself and that treatment consists of helping the body by ridding it of toxins. Naturopathic physicians tend to favor a mixed bag of "natural" remedies: medicinal herbs, vitamin megadoses, homeopathy, hypnotherapy, acupuncture, guided imagery, and psychological counseling.

- *Herbal medicine:* **Herbal medicine,** or **herbology,** is the use of herbs and botanical products to treat disease. Around 2500 plants and herbs have been used over the centuries for medicinal purposes. For example, quinine, from the bark of a South American tree, is still used for malaria. The Reishi mushroom is supposed to counter the adverse effects of chemotherapy.

    Plant remedies are available without prescription, are relatively inexpensive, and, because they are all-natural, are usually considered safe. "Unfortunately," points out one writer, "a few *aren't* safe, and since the Food and Drug Administration (FDA) regulates herbs as food and not as drugs, consumers have had no way of knowing which herbs have therapeutic value and which don't."[86]

- *Ayurvedic medicine:* **Ayurvedic medicine** is a 4000-year-old Indian system that classifies people according to body type and uses mostly herbs and massage as therapies. For instance, a 20-minute drip of a warm mixture of herbs and oils is supposed to aid those suffering from insomnia, hypertension, and digestive problems.

- *Zen macrobiotics:* The **Zen macrobiotic diet** consists of a sequence of 10 diets, based on Buddhist principles of balancing yin (passive energy) and yang (active energy). Each diet becomes more restricted, the last one consisting only of cereals. Nutritionists have found it to be severely deficient in nutrients, and it has produced certain malnutrition diseases (such as kwashiorkor) that are usually nonexistent in North America.

- *Iridology:* Devised over 100 years ago by a Hungarian physician, **iridology** is a diagnostic method that is based on the theory that each area of the body is represented by a corresponding area of the iris, the colored area surrounding the pupil of the eye. Abnormalities in a body area appear as an abnormality in a corresponding area in the iris. Treatment of abnormalities is usually with a mixture of vitamins, minerals, herbs, and other botanic products.

    Iridology has so far failed to prove itself as an effective diagnostic technique.

- *Aromatherapy:* In **aromatherapy,** practitioners use essential oils from plants and flowers as odors to influence people's moods. They may also massage these substances into the skin. While it may be true that breathing orange essence can induce relaxation, there is no scientific proof that using thyme and lavender will heal wounds.

What is interesting about the preceding therapies is that many have *some* basis in fact. Herbs used in Eastern medicine, for instance, contain some of the active ingredients used in the conventional drugs of Western medicine.

Mind-Over-Matter Approaches Biofeedback, hypnotherapy, and guided imagery are all types of "mind over matter" therapies that have been found useful by conventional medicine. Others are a variety of stress-busting techniques, ranging from transcendental meditation to **yoga,** a 6000-year-old Indian philosophy that combines meditation, posture, exercise, and diet. Beyond these, however, are a whole range of alternative therapies, from crystal healing to psychic surgery, that many conventional health professionals find to be useless or even dangerous. Some examples:

- *Crystal healing:* **Crystal healing** purports to release tension by deriving healing energy from quartz and other colorful minerals. There seems to be no scientific basis for the approach.

- *Color therapy:* **Color therapy** consists of shining colored light on the body to alter its "aura."

- *Faith healing:* Faith healing actually covers a variety of practices, ranging from prayer to "laying on of hands" to so-called **therapeutic touch,** in which practitioners move their hands over a person's "energy fields" to unblock energy flow, thus supposedly hastening the patient's healing powers. Most investigations of faith healing have failed to show that it really works, and in a great many cases the practitioners have proved to be frauds.[87,88]

Strategy for Living: Dealing With Quackery and Fads

Quackery is the practice of fake solutions to health problems and may be quite dangerous. A health fad is a fashionable practice followed for a short time, which may or may not be dangerous. One needs to guard against frauds and fads.

The very human desire to be well and free of pain has a long history that is matched only by the ready answers provided by charlatans, faith healers, and quacks. We in the late 20th century may think we're above buying electric "galvanic" gadgets to "restore lost manhood" or "eye batteries" to do away with eyeglasses. (*See* ● *Figure 33.3.*) However, the presence of health-food stores in suburban shopping centers, holistic "wellness weekends" at rural retreats, and popular big-city Whole Life Expos are proof that many people continue to be

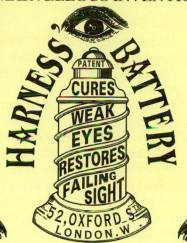

● **Figure 33.3 Duck that quack!** The ads for fraudulent products from times past (such as this one from the late 1880s) seem amusing to us now. But how do we recognize the quacks and frauds of our time?

“ *Be wary if immediate, effortless, or guaranteed results are promised.*

- *Look for telltale words and phrases such as "breakthrough," "miracle," "secret remedy," "exclusive," and "clinical studies prove that. . . ."*

- *Beware of promotions for a single product claimed to be effective for a wide variety of ailments.*

- *Don't forget that, unlike scientists and health professionals, quacks do not subject their products to the scrutiny of scientific research. The quack simply thrusts a product onto the market in order to get your money.*

- *If it sounds too good to be true—it probably is. ”*

—Food and Drug Administration and Council of Better Business Bureaus (1988). *Quackery targets teens.* HHS Pub. No. (FDA) 88-1147. Rockville, MD: Department of Health and Human Services.

obsessed with methods of fitness and longevity that fall outside the mainstream of conventional medicine.[89] It's important, then, that we know what's useful and what isn't. Let us consider the twin subjects of *quackery* and *health fads*.

Quackery: The "P. T. Barnum Effect"
Quackery is the practice of fake solutions or cures to health problems. In other words, quackery is fraud. The facts of medical science are often dry, uninteresting, and inconclusive. The promises of quacks, however, are usually dramatic, eye-catching, and billed as quick, easy, and safe. The problem is that these promises cost money, may be dangerous—and seldom deliver the change or cure being sought.

Some forms of quackery seem almost harmless, such as astrology, numerology, psychic readings, tarot cards, and handwriting analysis. However, the spreading acceptance of such ancient/New Age ideas makes scientists shiver. Writer Christopher Joyce calls this kind of acceptance the *P.T. Barnum effect*—named for the circus showman whose immortal words were, "There's a sucker born every minute." The Barnum effect, says Joyce, applies when two things happen: (1) people believe that vague, flattering statements apply personally to them, and (2) cash changes hands.[90]

More usually, though, quackery is *not* outlandish, says psychiatrist Stephen Barrett, a board member of the National Council Against Health Fraud. "Quacks rarely resemble the shady characters selling snake oil in Westerns," he says. "Quackery's modern promoters use scientific terms and quote (or misquote) scientific references. Some even have reputable scientific training."[91]

Quackery includes tanning pills, breast developers, steroids and growth hormones, and hair removal/hair growth practices.[92] It includes fake pharmaceuticals, pills that look like the real thing.[93] It includes weight-loss programs, an area of particular concern to the Federal Trade Commission; you should steer away from any diet that claims to be "easy," "effortless," "guaranteed," "miraculous," "magical," "exotic," "secret," "exclusive," or "ancient."[94] It includes certain self-esteem-boosting and performance-enhancing techniques, such as so-called self-help "subliminal learning" tapes, which claim to help you relax, lose weight, stop smoking, study

better, and improve your sex life. None of these claims has been substantiated.[95,96]

Health Fads A health *fad*—a practice followed for a time with excessive zeal—may or may not be as dangerous as quackery. However, often the very fact that something is a fad suggests that people are gravitating in great numbers to a new idea that may simply be an old idea with a different spin on it.

Some recent fads have been basically good, although their flaws weren't immediately apparent. For example, the running and jogging craze, which developed into the aerobic-dance fad, may have produced a lot of fit cardiovascular systems but also a lot of high-impact-induced shin splints and cracked bones in the feet.

Perhaps the best way to guard against being victimized by frauds and fads is to be knowledgeable about health and health care resources and assertive in exercising your consumer's right to know. In addition, you might follow a few strategies suggested by psychiatrist and health-fraud expert Stephen Barrett:[97]

- *Take a close look at the practitioner:* Not all diplomas and certificates are valid, nor are all scientific-sounding groups respectable.

- *Turn on your "hype detector":* Be wary of advertising hype, testimonials, medical endorsements (reputable physicians rarely endorse commercial products), talk-show guests, and health-food industry propaganda.

- *Know your own needs:* Don't let desperation cloud your judgment. Be wary of pseudomedical jargon, paranoid accusations against the medical establishment, and methods characterized as "alternative" (including the ones discussed in this chapter).

800-HELP

American Chiropractic Association. 800-368-3083

Consumer Product Safety Commission. 800-636-8326. This federal agency provides information on unsafe products.

Intellectual Health: Critical Thinking and the Art of Living

What, finally, will make the difference as to whether you prevail in life? Your drive? discipline? good nature? faith? It might be all of these, and then something else: your intellect.

State whether you agree or disagree with the following by answering yes or no.

___ **1.** Since it's clear that traditional Western medicine is not always able to cure various kinds of cancer, you might as well see what the alternative therapies have to offer.

___ **2.** Because condoms sometimes break, there's no point in using them to protect against HIV.

___ **3.** I wouldn't want a doctor who was rumored to like child pornography to be my surgeon; he or she couldn't be very good at performing surgery.

___ **4.** If we allowed marijuana to become legal, sooner or later there would be a lot more people ending up on hard drugs.

The answers to all of these should be no, for all of these statements are examples of incorrect reasoning, as follows: (1) jumping to conclusions; (2) irrelevant reason; (3) irrelevant attack on a person; (4) slippery slope. We explain these concepts below.

Intellectual health has to do with thinking or cognition and covers such activities as speaking, writing, analyzing, and judgment. It is one of the five dimensions of the definition of health (the others being physical, emotional, social, and spiritual). Developing the faculties of your intellectual health is crucial in helping to evaluate the claims of prospective healers, whether traditional or alternative.

A good way to expand your range intellectually is to learn to think critically. *Critical thinking* means actively seeking to understand, analyze, and evaluate information in order to solve specific problems. Critical thinking, in other words, is simply clear thinking. "Clear thinkers aren't born that way. They work at it," says one writer. "Before making important

choices, they try to clear emotion, bias, trivia and preconceived notions out of the way so they can concentrate on the information essential to making the right decision."[98]

The Hazards of Uncritical Thinking

Uncritical thinking is all around us. People run their lives on the basis of horoscopes, numerology, and similar nonsense. They pick lottery tickets based on their spouse's birth date. They believe in "crystal healing" and "color therapy." They think so-called outside experts—actually, cranks or quacks—will do what medicine cannot: cure cancer with apricot-pit extract, alleviate arthritis with copper bracelets, end blindness with prayer.

These are not just bits of harmless goofiness, like wearing your "lucky" shirt to your final exam. "We live in a society that is enlarging the boundaries of knowledge at an unprecedented rate," points out James Randi, a debunker of claims made by supporters of the paranormal, "and we cannot keep up with more than a small portion of what is made available to us. To mix our data input with childish notions of magic and fantasy is to cripple our perception of the world around us. We must reach for the truth, not for the ghosts of dead absurdities."[99]

By the time we are grown up, our minds have become "set" in various patterns of thinking that affect the way we respond to new situations and new ideas. These mindsets are the result of our personal experiences and the various social environments in which we grew up. Such mindsets determine what ideas we think are important and, conversely, what ideas we ignore. "Because we can't pay attention to all the events that occur around us," points out one book on clear thinking, "our minds filter out some observations and facts and let others through to our conscious awareness."[100] Herein lies the danger: ". . . we see and hear what we subconsciously want to, and pay little attention to facts or observations that have already been rejected as unimportant."

The Reasoning Tool: Deductive and Inductive Arguments

The tool for breaking through the closed habits of thought called mindsets is reasoning. *Reasoning*—giving reasons in favor of this assertion or that—is essential to critical thinking and solving life's problems. Reasoning is put in the form of *arguments,* which consist of one or more *premises,* or reasons, logically supporting a result or outcome called a *conclusion.*

An example of an argument is as follows:

Premise 1: All students must pass certain courses in order to graduate.

Premise 2: I am a student who wants to graduate.

Conclusion: Therefore, I must pass certain courses.

Note the tip-off word "Therefore," which signals that a conclusion is coming. In real life, such as arguments on radio and TV shows, in books and magazines and newspapers, and the like, the premises and conclusions are not so neatly labeled. Still, there are clues: the words *because, since,* and *for* usually signal premises. The words *therefore, hence,* and *so* signal conclusions. Not all groups of sentences form arguments. Often they form anecdotes or other types of exposition or explanation.[101]

The two main kinds of correct or valid arguments are inductive and deductive:

- *Deductive argument:* A deductive argument is defined as follows: *If its premises are true, then its conclusions are true also.* In other words, if the premises are true, the conclusions cannot be false.

- *Inductive argument:* An inductive argument is defined as follows: *If the premises are true, the conclusions are PROBABLY true, but the truth is not guaranteed.* An inductive argument is sometimes known by

logicians as a "probability argument."

An example of a *deductive argument* is as follows:[102]

Premise 1: All students experience stress in their lives.

Premise 2: Reuben is a student.

Conclusion: Therefore, Reuben experiences stress in his life.

This argument is deductive—the conclusion is *definitely* true if the premises are *definitely* true.

An example of an *inductive argument* is as follows:[103]

Premise 1: Stress can cause illness.

Premise 2: Reuben experiences stress in his life.

Premise 3: Reuben is ill.

Conclusion: Therefore, stress may be the cause of Reuben's illness.

Note the word *may* in the conclusion. This argument is inductive—the conclusion is not stated with absolute certainty; rather, it only suggests that stress *may* be the cause. The link between premises and conclusion is not definite because there may be other reasons for Reuben's illness.

Some Types of Incorrect Reasoning

Patterns of incorrect reasoning are known as *fallacies.* Learning to identify fallacious arguments will help you avoid patterns of faulty thinking in your own writing and thinking and identify it in others'.

Jumping to Conclusions Also known as *hasty generalization,* the fallacy called *jumping to conclusions* means that a conclusion has been reached when not all the facts are available.

Example: You might believe that, because traditional Western medicine is not always able to cure various kinds of cancer, you might as well see what the alternative therapies (such as promoters of apricot-pit extracts) have to offer. However, what you don't know is that alternative therapies have an even *worse* record at curing cancer than high-tech medicine does.

Irrelevant Reason or False Cause The faulty reasoning known as *non sequitur* (Latin for "it does not follow") might be better called *false cause* or *irrelevant reason*. Specifically, it means that the conclusion does not follow logically from the supposed reasons stated earlier. There is no *causal* relationship.

Example: Because you know that condoms sometimes break, you think there's no point in using them to protect against HIV. This is irrelevant, because condoms do not *always* break and, in your case, may *never* break while you are using them.

Irrelevant Attack on a Person or an Opponent Known as an *ad hominem* argument (Latin for "to the person"), the *irrelevant attack on an opponent* attacks a person's reputation or beliefs rather than his or her argument.

Example: You may decide you wouldn't want a surgeon who was rumored to be interested in child pornography because you think he or she couldn't be very good at surgery. However, the interest in pornography may have no bearing on his or her present ability to do surgery.

Slippery Slope The *slippery slope* is a failure to see that the first step in a possible series of steps does not lead inevitably to the rest.

Example: Believing that, if we allowed marijuana to become legal, sooner or later there would be a lot more people ending up on hard drugs is a slippery-slope argument. Although it *may* be true that marijuana is a "gateway drug" that could lead some users to progress to stronger and more dangerous narcotics, it is not inevitable.

Appeal to Authority The *appeal to authority* argument (known in Latin as *argumentum ad verecundiam*) uses an authority in one area to pretend to validate claims in another area in which the person is not an expert.

Example: You see the appeal-to-authority argument used all the time in advertising.

But what, for example, does an Olympic skating star know about nutrition?

Circular Reasoning The *circular reasoning* argument rephrases the statement to be proven true and then uses the new, similar statement as supposed proof that the original statement is in fact true.

Example: You declare that you can drive safely at high speeds with only inches separating you from the car ahead because you have driven this way for years without an accident.

Straw Man Argument The *straw man argument* is when you misrepresent your opponent's position to make it easier to attack, or when you attack a weaker position while ignoring a stronger one. In other words, you sidetrack the argument from the main discussion.

Example: Saying "You don't care about being spontaneous" is a way of misrepresenting a person who is concerned about using condoms as protection.

Appeal to Pity The *appeal to pity* argument appeals to mercy rather than making an argument on the merits of the case itself.

Examples: The joke of the boy who kills his parents and then throws himself on the mercy of the court because he is an orphan is one example. So is the appeal to the dean not to expel you for cheating because your parents are poor and made sacrifices to put you through college.

Questionable Statistics Statistics can be misused in many ways as supporting evidence. The statistics may be unknowable, drawn from an unrepresentative sample, or otherwise suspect.

Examples: Stating that in the past 10,000 years people have been far less happy or healthy than they are today is an example of unknowable or undefined use of statistics. Stating how much money is lost to taxes because of illegal drug transactions is speculation because such transactions are hidden or underground.

UNIT

15 Aging Well and Coping with Death

In These Chapters:

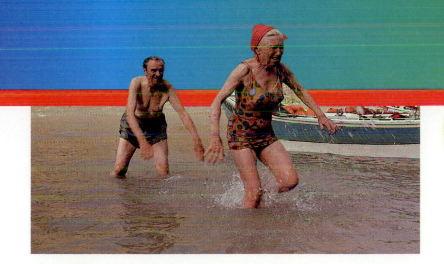

Life isn't a mountain that has a summit.

Nor is it a game that has a final score.

So says John W. Gardner, founder of the public-interest group Common Cause. Rather, he says, "Life is an endless unfolding, and if we wish it to be, an endless process of self-discovery, an endless and unpredictable dialogue between our own potentialities and the life situations in which we find ourselves."[1]

Life, then, is a continual series of tests —but there are no answers in the back of the book. We discover its meaning through ourselves.

What will you be like as you grow older? Will you become increasingly grouchy as you advance in years? Or will you mellow with age? Although the study of personality during older age is new, research seems to show that much of our personality remains consistent as we age. In your older years, you are likely to be much as you've been so far, particularly in terms of intellect and satisfaction. You will be what you are, you are what you were.[2-7]

Still, change is always possible. Thus, if there are personality traits you and those around you are not happy about, you can probably modify them. You can also take the steps now to live both longer and well. A healthy lifestyle begun at age 30 can extend the average person's life expectancy of 70-plus years by another 15 years. Not just any old 15 years, as one writer points out, but "15 *healthy* years. The same smart behaviors that help you live long can also help you live well."[8]

Historian Page Smith thinks that the two most "interesting and significant ages" are youth and old age, the intervening years quite often being surrendered to reproduction and capital accumulation. Youth, he says, is a marvelous time, in part because life lies ahead and the possibilities are dazzling. With old age, "You know the price of all good life. You have run the course, or at least the most demanding part of it. Moreover, you are not inclined to take the world for granted."[9]

The world is not taken for granted because older people know what is next. Still, for most people, whether young or old, death is not something they worry about, fear, or even think about very much.[10] However, aging and drawing closer to death present an opportunity. As Smith says, our reflections on our youth "becomes a crucial element in an expanded consciousness of the infinite, incommensurable power and beauty and strange variety of life, so that we literally live in wonder all our latter days."[11]

34   Successful Aging

▶ Explain the difference between life span
and life expectancy, distinguish between
the "time-bomb" and "spacecraft" models
of aging, and describe three possible ways
age and vitality may be extended.

▶ Discuss the various physical changes that
are typical of growing older and explain
what disorders are often associated with
aging but are not inevitable.

▶ Identify the psychosocial changes associated with aging.

▶ Discuss what can be done to avoid disability in later life.

How old do you feel? Not how old are you
in actual years, but how old are you
psychologically?

When the question was put by a marketing-
research firm to 1000 adults of all ages, most
people said that, regardless of their actual age,
they felt and acted as if they were in their
mid 30s.[12]

If "you're only as old as you feel," as the expression goes, the next question should be:
How closely can you *function* to your psychological age?

How Long Will You Live?

**Life span is the maximum years a person
can live; life expectancy is the average age
people are expected to live to be. The
"time bomb" model of aging holds that the
human organism is programmed to die
upon reaching a certain specific age. The
"spaceship" model holds that humans can
do things to increase their life expectancy.
Three possible ways to extend age may be
to fight cell damage with antioxidants,
eat less, or administer human growth
hormone.**

At 100 years and 5 months old, Claire Willi
still takes a dance class every day. At 101, Harry
Schneider is so sharp he can recall the weekly

salaries of his youth.[13] Jeanne Calment of
France, the world's oldest citizen at 117, according to the *Guinness Book of Records,* attributes her longevity to a healthy lifestyle and
happy-go-lucky character.[14]

According to Guinness, only one person
in 2 billion lives to be more than 115. Still, both
the number and percentage of **centenarians**
—people 100 and over—is increasing throughout the world. The United States Census counted 35,808 people 100 years old and older
in 1990—double the number 10 years
previously.[15]

Most Americans would like to live to be
100.[16] Is that possible, if we're really serious
about it? How long *can* a human live?

The oldest living things are trees: individual
redwood trees can live over 3000 years, and
bristlecone pines, on the eastern slope of the
Sierra Nevada Mountains, even longer. People,
of course, don't even come close. Although from
time to time we hear of such long-lived people
as 130-year-old Chinese (who attribute their
longevity to a diet rich in lizards), there is always an absence of documentation.[17]

Life span and life expectancy are two different things:

- *Life span:* **Life span** refers to the maximum number of years that a human being
  can live. The apparent *maximum* life span
  is 120 years, based on the evidence. The
  average biological limit to life is considered
  to be 85 years.[18]

- *Life expectancy:* **Life expectancy** refers
  to the *average* age that people born at a
  certain time are expected to live to be. For
  example, the average life expectancy for
  newborns in America has risen to 75 years
  today from 47 in 1900.[19]

  Life expectancy increases with age:
  the older you already are, the better your
  chances of living longer. Thus, a 35-year-old
  woman is expected to live to age 80, but a
  65-year-old woman to age 84.

Today **gerontologists,** specialists in the
study of aging, are concerned not only with decline, which is what most of us associate with
aging, but also with *vitality* and *resilience.*
What is it, they ask, that enables some people to
play tennis in their 80s, run marathons in their
90s, and take dance classes in their 100s?

There are several theories about aging, some of them rather technical, all of them fascinating. Here, however, let us consider some of those with practical applications to possibly extending your own life.

The Time-Bomb Versus Spaceship Models of Aging In general, there are two basic models of aging:

- *Time bomb:* The *time-bomb model* assumes, as age researcher James R. Carey puts it, "when you attain a certain age, you self-destruct."[20,21] This point of view has been represented by gerontologist James Fries, who says there is essentially a "death gene" that takes effect about age 85, give or take 7 years—with some exceptions who hang on past 100. In this view, the body is programmed to run down and end at a certain time.[22–26] Some propose that a centralized clock controlling aging is located in the pineal gland in the brain.[27]

- *Spaceship:* The other model, says Carey, is the *spaceship model:* a spaceship engineered to reach a particular goal may be capable of going a little further. Carey and James W. Curtsinger and colleagues have grown fruit flies and found that, past a certain age, their life expectancy actually increases.[28,29] In other words, it was not true that the older flies got, the more likely they were to die. With a few individuals, once the flies achieved a certain age, their life expectancies increased, and they died at unusually advanced ages.

  Demographer James Vaupel, who studied extremely elderly people in Scandinavia, argues that a rise in life expectancy can also be found in humans.[30] "I think it's possible to increase life expectancy from 75 to maybe 100 within the lifetimes of people alive today," Vaupel said.[31] Life expectancy would rise, in Vaupel's opinion, with prevention or cure of major diseases such as cancer and AIDS.

Assuming that the time-bomb model of inevitable dying around age 85 is not true, what measures might you take to try to resist aging? Let us consider three possibilities: *countering exposure to free radicals, eating low-calorie diets,* and *human growth hormone injections.*

Fighting Cell Damage with Antioxidants Some researchers assume that age limits are not genetically predetermined but are affected by gradual damage to the body's cells by *free radicals,* renegade oxygen atoms that rob electrons from molecules and cause destructive chemical reactions. These free radicals are produced by the body's exposure to radiation, heat, air pollution, and sunlight. The cellular damage is said to result in heart attacks, emphysema, Alzheimer's, and other diseases.

To slow development of these diseases, it is proposed, people should get not only the usual recommended daily allowances of vitamins and minerals but also special vitamins called **antioxidants.** Antioxidants consist of *vitamin C* (found in oranges, broccoli, and tomatoes), *vitamin E* (leafy green vegetables, vegetable oils, wheat germ), and *beta carotene* (carrots, leafy green vegetables, sweet potatoes).

Is there anything to this theory of free radicals and antioxidants? Research by Charles Hennekens of 87,000 nurses, 333 doctors, and 1300 elderly persons found that those with higher levels of vitamin E or beta carotene had the lowest risk of heart disease.[32]

Eating Less and Living Longer If you like to eat, you won't like this: studies have shown that animals and insects whose normal calorie intake has been reduced 30–50% lengthen their life spans 40–60%.[33–35] One of the foremost proponents of this idea in humans is gerontologist Roy Walford, who personally eats a calorie-restricted diet that he believes could take him to age 120 or beyond.[36–38] The goal is a weight 10–25% below what is considered normal.

Other experts on aging, however, wonder whether the results of animal experiments can be applied to humans.[39] For example, geneticist George Roth speculates that short-lived species such as insects and rodents could have biological mechanisms that enable them to withstand famine years and still live long enough to reproduce. Long-lived species, such as humans, which can reproduce over a number of years, might not need this life-prolonging safeguard.[40–42]

Human Growth Hormone: The Fountain of Youth? The hormone called **human growth hormone (HGH),** which is produced by the pituitary gland at the base of the brain, helps stimulate normal bone growth in children and maintain healthy tissue in adults. However, after age 30 or so, there is a decline in the hormone, leading to thinning of the skin, decrease in lean body mass, and other signs of aging.

In 1990, researchers reported that a synthetically produced HGH transformed the body components of several men ages 61–81, all of them HGH-deficient, by as much as *20 years*.[43] For example, lean body mass increased by 9% and fat tissue decreased by 14%. The drug did not, however, improve failing eyesight or hearing or improve degenerating brain cells. Nor did it affect the life span.

Needless to say, the report about human growth hormone reducing signs of aging generated as much public excitement as would the discovery of the Fountain of Youth, with physicians receiving thousands of phone calls from older patients. However, HGH is not for everyone. Experts point out that administering the substance to someone who is not deficient could risk development of diabetes, hypertension, excess fluid in body joints, growth of cancerous tumors, and enlargement of face and hands.[44,45] Moreover, HGH is not a life-*extension* drug even in those people for whom it is suitable.

Life Span or Health Span? Is increased longevity actually desirable? Certainly not at the price of ill health.

Gerontologist Edward Schneider, for one, finds the debate about longevity and various aging theories "interesting and important" but not as critical as the steps that can be taken to increase the *healthy* years of life. For instance, he says, it's more important that teenage women be persuaded to take in more calcium and exercise more to build up their bone mass, so they'll have less risk of getting the bone-crumbling disease osteoporosis in their later years.[46]

To see what the future might be for your "health span," let us consider some of the physical and psychosocial changes associated with aging.

Physical Changes of Aging

Aging changes physical appearance and the senses (sight, hearing, taste, touch) and slows the metabolism. Reduction in the vital capacity of the lungs and loss of muscle strength and joint flexibility may be offset by diet and exercise. Diseases such as osteoporosis and arthritis are not inevitable with aging. Intellectual powers do not diminish with age, except for one form of memory, and Alzheimer's is a disease, not a normal part of aging. Slower reaction times are normal. Sexuality might slow but need not stop. Some difficulties experienced in menopause, the end of menstruation, can be eased with hormone therapy.

How does it feel to be old? If you're a young person, you can try doing as students in a college class on aging and human development did: put on earplugs to reduce hearing, use or discard glasses to impair eyesight, and wrap your joints in elastic bandages to simulate stiffness.[47] Or you can do as medical residents do in a program training them in better communication skills with the elderly: besides wearing wax earplugs and fastening splints to your joints, put raw peas in your shoes to simulate corns and calluses, don rubber gloves to dim the sense of touch, even smear Vaseline on contact lenses to blur your vision.[48]

Both the students and the residents found a few hours of these activities an eye-opening exercise, changing many of their assumptions about aging. Do you think you might have some mistaken preconceptions here?

People differ in how they age, and a lot of it is controllable, especially through diet and exercise. However, after age 30, even the healthiest person is, in that well-known phrase, going to "start slowing down." Let us consider what happens physically.

Appearance: Skin, Hair, and Shape The stages of life are reflected in our faces, as well as in other parts of our bodies. (*See* ● *Figure 34.1*.) "Looking old" is, of course, not looked on favorably in our ageist society, and many people

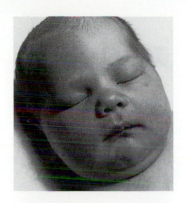
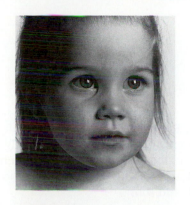
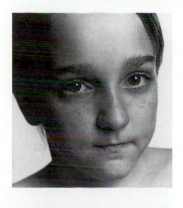
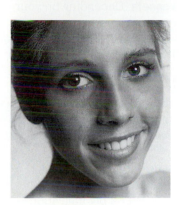
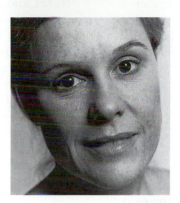
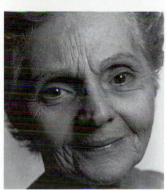

● **Figure 34.1 The appearance of age.** The stages of life are reflected in our faces.

dread these changes. There are perhaps three general areas of appearance that are affected by age:

- *Skin:* Thirty years of living—laughing, worrying, squinting—will begin to tell in the form of smile and frown lines. Ten years later, the wrinkles will be more evident and there will be more of them as the skin becomes drier and less elastic. By age 50, the skin may sag in the cheeks and beneath the chin as gravity begins to take over. By the 60s and 70s, bags will appear under the eyes and nose and earlobes will start to lengthen.

  Skin also roughens as you age, but a lot of the wrinkles and spots are up to you—cigarette smoking and exposure to the sun are the two biggest enemies.[49] Still, the dark patches of skin known as "age spots" are visible in about 25% by age 60 and the percentage increases as people get older.

- *Hair:* Hair begins to go gray in your 30s. Hair is also thickest in your 20s, but some people (about 12% of men) also become bald while in their 20s, depending on how unlucky they've been in their genetic programming (37% of men are bald by age 35, 45% by age 45).[50]

  About 50 million men and 30 million women suffer from **pattern baldness,** gradual thinning from the roots.[51] For men cosmetic options are available, and a hair-stimulating drug works in some; in women, hormone therapy may help.[52]

- *Shape:* As people grow older, many find they need roomier clothes. After age 25—depending on your diet and exercise practices—even if you don't gain weight the shape of your body may change as fat begins to replace lean muscle. By age 40, you may weigh 20 pounds more than you did 20 years before. Depending on their heredity, diet, and exercise, men begin to deposit fat in and around their upper chest and abdomen, women around the hips and thighs.

Sensory Changes: Taste, Touch, Sight, and Hearing One of the advantages of growing older is that you may be able to stand the hot peppers and sauces better. Of the four categories of taste—salty, bitter, sweet, and sour—all begin to decline as a result of the loss of taste buds. Thus, a 60-year-old may need three times the flavorings to experience a particular taste as someone half that age. The sense of touch, and consequently the ability to feel temperature and pain, is also lessened.

The two major senses that diminish are eyesight and hearing:

- *Eyesight:* Although it doesn't happen to everyone, one of the more irritating signs that you're getting older is the need for eyeglasses. By their late 40s, most people become **farsighted,** unable to see things clearly close up, because the ocular lens does not expand and contract readily. This is when most people find they need reading glasses. On the other hand, some **nearsighted** people, who earlier had difficulty seeing things at a distance, find their distance vision improves, as the phenomenon of farsightedness somewhat counteracts their nearsightedness.

  By age 60, only a third as much light reaches the retina as at age 20, resulting in a decreased ability to distinguish detail and see in the dark. Also, as people get into their 60s, they may develop **cataracts,** a clouding of the lens of the eye. Some older people, especially those with a family history of the disease, may also develop **glaucoma,** the buildup of fluid in the eye, which can damage the optic nerve and cause blindness.

- *Hearing:* By the mid-30s, people's ability to hear high-pitched sounds declines, and sounds must be louder to be heard as well by someone 35 as by someone 25, on average. Nowadays, the decline in hearing is being found at younger ages because of prolonged or repeated exposure to electronic amplification and urban noise.

Metabolism One of the reasons the body so easily gains weight as you age is that your metabolism—the rate at which your body uses energy—slows down. The slowing process begins gradually after adolescence and accelerates dramatically in later life. Every 10 years, the rate at which food is converted into energy slows by about 3%.[53]

Heart and Blood Vessels Depending on your level of fitness, your resting heartbeat can remain about the same all your life, although the amount of blood pumped with each beat lessens. With age, circulation also tends to slow, owing to the buildup of fat and cholesterol within the blood vessels, and the blood pressure rises. Two of the major disorders of old age are heart disease and stroke.

Lungs and Respiration By age 75, a man's **vital capacity**—the amount of air that can be expelled from the lungs after a big inhalation—is half that at 17. A woman's vital capacity is a third of that of her 20s. This is a consequence of reduced elasticity in the tissues surrounding the chest and the capillaries within the lungs. By 85, even though lung size has doubled, capacity is only half that of a 30-year-old. Still, the ability to *use* oxygen depends on your physical fitness: athletic runners in their 60s are able to use their oxygen better than nonathletic people in their 20s.

Muscles, Bones, and Joints: Coping with Osteoporosis and Arthritis People who continue to exercise and stay physically active experience less loss of muscle strength and mass than those who don't. Still, by age 60, a man may have lost up to 20% of his muscle strength and women more than that. In addition, in losing 3–5% of our muscle mass each year, we become more susceptible to strains and cramps—which is why warm-ups and cool-downs become more important before and after exercise.

In addition, as back muscles weaken and discs between the small bones making up the spine, the **vertebrae,** deteriorate, we lose height. Most people are an inch shorter in old age than they were in young adulthood.

In your 20s, after your bones have stopped growing, they begin to lose calcium and other minerals, so that they become more brittle and heal less quickly. Joints also weaken and become susceptible to cartilage damage, especially if you continue high-impact activities such as teeth-rattling forms of aerobic exercise. Two particularly significant disorders of aging are osteoporosis and arthritis:

- *Osteoporosis:* **Osteoporosis** is a condition common in older people in which the bones become soft and porous, increasing the risk of fracture. Half of all women over 50 will have an osteoporosis-related fracture at some time, and by age 75 one-third of all men are affected by the disease.[54] Women who have otherwise normal menstrual periods may lose bone rapidly if they do not ovulate during every monthly cycle, according to one study.[55] This means that women who regularly miss ovulation may have to take progesterone supplements to preserve their bones. Another possibility why American women are unusually prone to osteoporosis is that when they lose weight they also lose bone.[56]

  Older women can strengthen bones by taking the recommended daily allowance (800 milligrams) of calcium accompanied by vitamin D.[57,58] In addition, a combination therapy of estrogen and progesterone can also reduce the risk of some spine and hip fractures, according to a study by Swedish researchers.[59,60] New drugs seem to increase bone mass and prevent bone loss in the spine.[61,62] Contrary to popular belief, moderate exercise alone will not prevent bone loss in older women; exercise should be combined with estrogen and calcium.[63]

  The best advice for young women seems to be to take calcium supplements and get enough exercise in the form of aerobic activity and weight training. Make sure the exercise is of a *weight bearing* type; swimming, for example, won't build bone mass.

- *Osteoarthritis:* **Osteoarthritis,** a disintegration of the cartilage between bones, which produces pain, stiffness, and lack of mobility, affects about 16 million Americans, most of them 60 and older.[64] Research links it to a genetic defect.[65] However, it may also be affected by sports injuries or similar accidents to the joints. Obesity also puts extra weight on the joints and may produce arthritis of the knees.[66]

The Brain: Intellectual Power, Memory, and Alzheimer's By age 30, less blood is traveling to the brain than at younger ages. The brain also shrinks as it ages, losing about 10% of its weight.[67] Although the shrinkage may result in some loss of mental vigor, according to neuropathologist Robert D. Terry, "normal elderly people are largely intact intellectually."[68] Still, it has been long accepted that the aging brain declines, bringing a loss of intellectual powers. Is this true?

- *Normal memory decline—for one kind of memory:* Police and juries may place a lot of trust in people's ability to recall events. Are they right?

  Actually, memory can be quite complex on a psychological level, regardless of age, because remembering is an act of *reconstruction,* not *reproduction.*[69] For instance, 13% of people ages 18–44 have trouble sometimes or frequently remembering names, and this rises to 35% for ages 45–54.[70] If you're over 30, you're losing your memory; psychologist and memory expert Thomas H. Crook says that losing 6–8% memory for each decade is normal.[71–73] The kind of memory affected by this loss is *episodic memory*—memory about specific events, such as what happened at yesterday's meeting.

  The loss of episodic memory—in which older people have more trouble than they used to remembering what happened a few minutes, hours, or days ago—is called **age-associated memory impairment (AAMI).** AAMI varies tremendously from person to person. It also can be reversed. Whereas young people may repeat a string of numbers or words until they learn them, many older people—anxious that they are losing their memory—give up after only a few tries. However, retention can be helped by practice and by analyzing surroundings, people's names, and so on, so that key details can be remembered later.[74]

- *Kinds of memory that do not decline with age:* Episodic memory is only one kind of memory; there are other kinds, and older people (in good health) do not lose these. *Semantic memory*—factual knowledge—does not decline with age. Nor does *implicit memory,* remembering skills one mastered to the point they seem automatic, such as how to swim.[75] Indeed, psychologist David Mitchell, an expert on memory, says, "semantic memory is the seat of wisdom. When you make decisions and judgments, you draw on this store of knowledge." Moreover, he says, "Semantic memory does not decline with age."[76] This is good news indeed.

- *Memory impaired by illness:* Older people lose their memories for many reasons, many of them reversible. Examples range from clinical depression to head injury to poor circulation.*

These may be serious problems, but with the help of a health care professional something may be done about them. Unfortunately, a form of brain disease called *dementia* corresponds to memory problems that are more likely irreversible.

- *Dementias:* The two most common forms of dementia are *vascular dementia* and *Alzheimer's disease.*[77] It is possible for both forms to be present in the same person.

In **vascular dementia,** changes in the blood vessels of the brain cause death of brain tissue due to a stroke. Besides memory impairment, the signs of a stroke include vision problems, speech problems, and weakness on one side of the body.

In **Alzheimer's disease,** nerve cell changes in parts of the brain result in the death of a large number of brain cells. The disease afflicts 4 million Americans and accounts for 50% of dementia cases in people over age 65.[78]

Unlike vascular dementia, symptoms for Alzheimer's disease begin slowly and become worse. It is invariably fatal and is one of the leading causes of death in the United States.[79] Over a period of 5–15 years, the disease progressively destroys patients' memories and robs them of their ability to reason and recognize reality. It gradually takes away their speech and makes them incontinent.[80] People around them worry they may wander away and get lost. (*See* ● *Figure 34.2.*)

A great difficulty is that Alzheimer's family members may fear they will inherit the flawed gene that is theorized to cause most, if not all, cases of the disease.[81,82] As a result, some people may refuse to recognize that a family member has the disease.[83]

Families are also the other victims of Alzheimer's. As the disease progresses, care-givers have to do everything, including cleaning, dressing, and feeding. They must make sure the patient doesn't wander off or cause self-harm. Money is often a problem, keeping many families from turning to nursing home care. Moreover, a spouse may be witnessing someone's personality deteriorate at the same time his or her own health is failing.[84–87] The dilemma for the caregiver is needing more support from friends and family but having less time to seek it. One solution has been the formation of support groups, such as those of the Alzheimer's Association.

The media are full of headlines, first promising, then disappointing, about the frustrating search for a drug treatment or a cure for Alzheimer's. Until one of those is found, treatment is mainly with psychotherapy in the early stages, antidepressant or antipsychotic drugs, and "reminiscence therapy," which encourages patients to recall important events in their lives.[88]

What is important to realize is that Alzheimer's is far from being a normal part of aging. It is a disease, one that has symptoms that resemble those of other disorders. Thus, just forgetting where you put your glasses doesn't mean you have it, perhaps unless you can't remember what your glasses are for.

As far as other problems of aging and the brain, the brain does not degenerate with age. Experts say it's often a matter of "use it or lose it," just as with so many of our physiological processes. For instance, anatomy professor

---

*Ten of the most common causes of reversible memory loss that are not the result of surgery: clinical depression, fluid imbalance (as when people don't get enough water on hot days), drug overdose (not just from alcohol but tranquilizers, painkillers, heart and diabetes medications, and others), malnutrition, low blood sugar, anemia and lung disease, head injury, small stroke, poor blood circulation, and severe hypothyroidism.

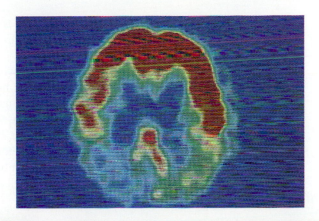

Marian Diamond found that rats in stimulating environments (sharing cages with other rats and with ever-changing toys) developed more branches and connections in the nerve cells in their brains compared with those of understimulated rats.[89,90] Likewise, "mental gymnastics" or other challenges may keep the human brain creative and productive.[91]

The Nervous System: Reaction Time Although the mind may stay active in its thought processes as we grow older, some **neurons,** or nerve cells, of the brain will begin to be lost, affecting reaction times. What do these changes—along with deteriorating eyesight and hearing—mean for such daily activities as continuing to drive?

Some women who used to count on their husbands or on public transportation to get around have found that learning to drive gives them more flexibility.[92] Older drivers have proportionately fewer car crashes (per 100,000 population) than younger ones. Yet it is also true that, per mile driven, two sets of age groups have the highest rankings for fatalities, accidents, and costs to insurance companies: those ages 16–24, and those 65 and older.[93–95]

Age and Sexuality Aging might slow down sexual functioning, but it need not stop it, if a person is in good health. Men need more direct and longer stimulation to obtain an erection and women may need more foreplay to lubricate adequately.[96] The sex drive itself does not decrease with menopause. Indeed, many older women find that with no children at home and the threat of pregnancy removed, lovemaking after menopause is more relaxed and spontaneous than it was before.[97]

"Myths about seniors and sexuality abound," says one writer. "They can't have sex. They don't want to have sex. They shouldn't have sex."[98] These are indeed myths, for romance and sex aren't just for the young. It turns out, according to a study by sociologist Andrew M. Greeley of 5738 people, that 37% of married people over 60 make love once a week or more and 16% make love several times a week. More important, perhaps, sexually active married men are happier at 60 than 20-year-old single males sleeping around. Men and women engaging in frequent sex after 60 report the happiest

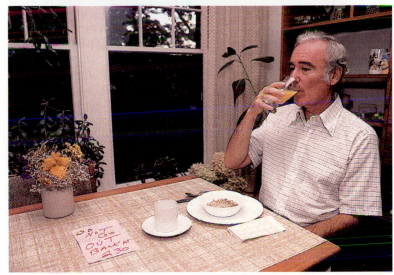

● **Figure 34.2 Alzheimer's disease.** *Top:* Brain scan of a person with Alzheimer's. The scan by positive emission tomography (PET scan) shows areas, in blue, in which brain activity has been reduced. *Bottom:* An Alzheimer's patient. A caretaker is clearly afraid he will wander off. At a later point, a note such as this will be insufficient.

"*Once it sets in, Alzheimer's offers no reprieve. Whether it afflicts a forgotten movie goddess or the neighbor who quietly faded behind the upstairs curtains years ago, the disease proceeds relentlessly, stripping victims of their humanity before it takes their lives. As it destroys brain cells, first memory goes, then cognition, then physical functioning. Finally, only a shell of the person is left, evoking every child's nightmare of a parent's decline to incompetence.*"

—David Gelman, Mary Hager, & Vicki Quade. (1989, December 18). The brain killer. *Newsweek,* p. 54.

marriages, and they are also more likely to report they are living exciting lives, says Greeley.[99] (*See ● Figure 34.3.*)

Sexuality "is something that grows with experience," says Robert N. Butler, former head of the National Institute on Aging. "The romance of many older people can be very tender, very sensitive. It may have a lot of physicality. It may have intercourse. It may not."[100] Sexuality, in other words, involves the total human being, emotionally and intellectually as well as physically.[101]

Sexual Changes in Men As men age, they may experience a gradual decline in sexual performance. The urgency of the sex drive may decrease, so that sex is still important but may be reduced in frequency. Erections may take longer to achieve: more physical stimulation may be needed and more elaborate fantasies necessary to produce arousal. The erection may not be as firm as it was in earlier years. There is longer time between orgasms, and more frequent loss of erection during intercourse. The volume of semen decreases. Yet the majority of

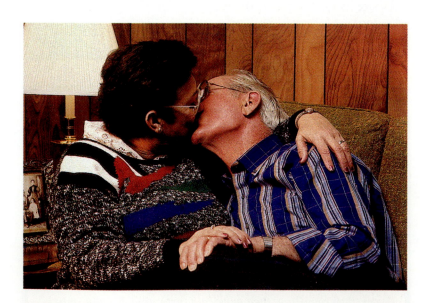

● **Figure 34.3 Sex after 60.** Men and women engaging in frequent sex after 60 report the happiest marriages. More than a third of married couples over 60 make love once a week or more.

men are still interested in sex even into their 70s and beyond and are capable of fathering children in later life (as evidenced by the offspring fathered by Charlie Chaplin and Bing Crosby in later life).[102]

Sexual Changes in Women The physiological equivalent of male erection in women is vaginal lubrication. As women get older, the vagina lubricates more slowly, and there is less lubrication.

Menopause Usually between ages 45 and 55, but sometimes earlier, women experience **menopause**—or "the change of life." During this period, their cycles of ovulation and menstruation come to an end. Actually, the process begins with women in their mid-30s, when the ovaries begin to make less of the female hormones estrogen and progesterone, raising the risk for heart disease and osteoporosis. About 3–5 years before the last menstrual period, there is the beginning of the **climacteric,** when periods change, becoming less regular and often either lighter or heavier.

During menopause, some women (about 1 in 10) experience **hot flashes,** sudden, intense sensations of heat in the upper part or all of the body. Most hot flashes last 2–5 minutes, but some last as long as 30 minutes or more. They may be as mild as a light blush or as severe as red blotches, heavy sweating, and cold shivering. They may occur rarely or as often as every hour. Some women get moody and depressed, but the vast majority do not.[103–105]

Hormone replacement therapy—that is, taking estrogen and progesterone—can ease some of the problems associated with menopause, including women's risk of cardiovascular disease as a result of decreased estrogen. Some women take estrogen alone; this is **estrogen replacement therapy.** Use of estrogen poses a dilemma for women.[106–109] Besides easing hot flashes and preventing osteoporosis, estrogen has been found to prevent heart disease in post-menopausal women.[110] On the other hand, the use of estrogen also seems to have some risks, including increasing the possibility of cancer and gallbladder disease. One 10-year study of over 121,000 female nurses found that those taking estrogen had an increased risk of breast cancer.[111] Some researchers also found women taking estrogen may become dependent on the hormone in much the same way as people become dependent on drugs, because it improves their mood and sense of well-being.[112]

Hormone replacement therapy is clearly not for every woman. Some alternatives include vitamin E and clonidine, a drug used to treat high blood pressure, either of which may reduce hot flashes.[113] Aerobic and weight-bearing exercise, like walking and cycling, also can strengthen bones and lower the risk of heart problems.

With the interest in menopause in recent years has come an interest in the possibility of a *male menopause*. Is there such a thing? Actually, the jury is still out on this question. Some studies have suggested that levels of testosterone drop gradually with age, perhaps by 30–40% between the ages of 48 and 78.[114] Nobody knows, however, if boosting blood levels of testosterone would put extra lustiness into older men.[115]

Does Greater Longevity Mean Being Sicker Longer? Some disabilities make it difficult for older people to have sex. Then again, points out one sex therapist, some older people are afraid to attempt love making due to their health problems.[116] Patients recovering from heart disease, for example, are afraid they will collapse during sex. People suffering from the pain of arthritis are reluctant to attempt "the more athletic forms of sexual expression."

More than 10 million Americans, most over age 65, have to deal with **urinary incontinence**—urinary seepage owing to lack of bladder control.[117] As a result of this embarrassment, many older people stop having sex for fear they will urinate during the act. However, almost all of those troubled by urinary incontinence can be helped or cured with bladder control training, scheduled urination, pelvic muscle exercises, drugs to fight infection or to treat underlying physical problems, and surgery.[118]

These and other health problems of the elderly simply did not get much public attention when most people lived only into their 40s, as they did in 1900. However, because of the good news—namely, that Americans are living longer—we also have some bad news: people are sicker longer. Still, as psychology writer

Daniel Goleman points out, "lengthened life means that, on average, people will have more years of being well before becoming ill."[119]

As we will show, many kinds of illness associated with growing older can be forestalled. Before we describe these, however, let us look at some of psychological and social changes associated with growing older.

Psychosocial Changes of Aging

The "midlife crisis" is only one of many psychosocial turning points associated with growing older. Ideas that older workers aren't adaptable or that retired people are either wealthy or poor are myths. Some older people's attitudes affect their mental health, leading to depression, medication and alcohol abuse, and suicide, though these are by no means inevitable. Growing older brings new relationships with one's parents and new challenges for dealing with change and loss.

When is the happiest time of life? Probably youth, one might judge by the efforts of those who don't have it and are trying to get it back. In addition, of course, advertising and the mass media reinforce this with a seeming obsession with youth culture. Interestingly, however, when older people are asked what are the best years of a person's life, they don't say the teenage years but rather the *retirement* years. (*See ● Figure 34.4.*) Independent observers have also found old people feel psychologically better than young people, with fewer worries and higher self-esteem.[120]

Still, just as people in their younger years have some distinctive psychosocial problems—determining a career, deciding on a permanent companion, and so on—so do people in their middle and older years.

Middle Adulthood and Old Age "I remember now that the toughest birthday I ever faced was my fortieth," stated writer and director Norman Corwin, at age 82. "It was a big symbol because it said goodbye, goodbye, goodbye to youth. But I think that when one has passed through that age it's like breaking the sound barrier."[121]

Age of respondent

"I think the best years are..."

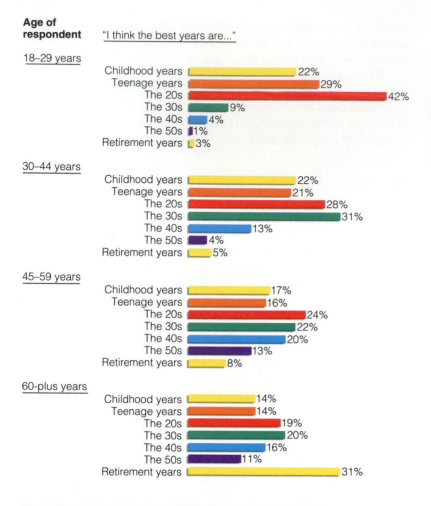

18–29 years

Childhood years	22%
Teenage years	29%
The 20s	42%
The 30s	9%
The 40s	4%
The 50s	1%
Retirement years	3%

30–44 years

Childhood years	22%
Teenage years	21%
The 20s	28%
The 30s	31%
The 40s	13%
The 50s	4%
Retirement years	5%

45–59 years

Childhood years	17%
Teenage years	16%
The 20s	24%
The 30s	22%
The 40s	20%
The 50s	13%
Retirement years	8%

60-plus years

Childhood years	14%
Teenage years	14%
The 20s	19%
The 30s	20%
The 40s	16%
The 50s	11%
Retirement years	31%

● **Figure 34.4 The best years of our lives.** "People feel differently about what years are the best time of a person's life. Which of these do you think are the best time of life?" People of different ages who were asked this question in a Roper Organization poll gave quite different answers. Interestingly, among older people, the best time was not the younger years but the retirement years.

Much has been made of the "midlife crisis," when people have done all the "right things"—marriage, family, hard work, career advancement—but on hitting the Big 40 find themselves asking, "Is this all there is?" As Daniel Levinson writes, "Adults hope that life begins at 40—but the great anxiety is that it ends there."[122] Levinson reported that 80% of all adults experience a midlife transition, a reas-

sessment of their personal goals. At this important turning point, the midlife crisis theory is, many people supposedly become very depressed, despairing, and anxious and begin to worry that they've wasted their lives and have been heading in the wrong direction.

There are indeed turning points in life, but sociologist John Clausen finds that many were childhood events and most came *before* the middle years.[123] Asked by Clausen whether there was any time in their lives when they felt so disappointed with work or lacked satisfaction to such an extent that they thought they would "throw things over," more than 85% of the people who had passed through middle age identified one or more turning points. The most traumatic were divorce or death of a spouse, getting married, having children, and choice of first career job. "Turning points during college" were also cited as significant.

The main concerns of most middle-aged adults are earning a living, trying to make a valuable contribution, raising children, and, for many, caring for their own elderly parents. A number of doctors surveyed in 1990 thought that many Americans in their 40s and 50s were under such severe financial strains, as a result of taking care of both their adult children and their aged parents, that they were damaging their own health.[124]

However, many middle-aged adults view their lives positively. A 1989 survey of Americans themselves, not of their doctors, asked several age groups whether they found life "exciting, pretty routine, or dull." Of those ages 36–41, 53% found life exciting, compared to 46% of young adults (ages 18–23) and 33% of those over 65.[125] People in another survey said that the middle years are years of positive growth, with as many as 89% associating this period with compassion, caring, and purposeful contribution.[126]

Midlife changes happen to almost everyone, but what a person makes of them depends on what he or she wants out of it. "For some, a little change is enough; the pull of security is stronger," says one writer. "For others, change stimulates quantum leaps in growth—and that's where the adventure lies."[127]

When does middle age end and old age begin? In one national study, a majority of 1200 people surveyed said midlife was the period between 46 and 66.[128] But 30% of those over 76 said they considered themselves middle-aged! Whatever the definition of old age, many of the changes that people experience as they grow older are probably determined by society rather than by biology, with people being expected to be productive during their 40s and 50s and to retire in their 60s.[129]

Some older people speak of inner feelings of youthfulness despite physical infirmities and weaknesses that remind them of their actual age. "I feel so young inside," says one, "and yet my old body requires that I acquiesce in a role that life demands of us all."[130]

Aging, Work, and Money We have seen that episodic memory may begin to falter as one gets older, and reaction times may be slower. However, judgment, accuracy, and general knowledge actually improve with age—qualities of experience that are celebrated in many cultures. Moreover, creative abilities may improve with age. Indeed, most artists, musicians, and writers really begin to hit their strides at midlife and continue on into their later years. Examples are author Marion Hart, who not only continued writing but learned to fly at age 54 and made seven nonstop solo flights across the Atlantic, the last time in 1975 at age 83; dancer and choreographer Martha Graham, who performed on stage until she was 75 and choreographed her 180th work at age 95; and painter Grandma Moses, who took up painting in her 70s and had her first one-woman show when she was 80.

Despite these productive qualities, there are two stereotypes about older people that have to do with their work performance and financial abilities:

- *Myth—older workers aren't as adaptable:* A 1989 survey of 400 firms conducted for the American Association of Retired Persons found that personnel managers appreciate the work habits and "work ethic" characteristics of older employees, including commitment to quality, company loyalty, coolness in crisis, and practical knowledge.[131] Although these managers questioned the ability of those over 50 to adapt to new technology, a 1991 study concluded that older workers could be retrained in new technologies. Indeed, older

workers learned to use computers as quickly as younger people. They also stay on the job longer and take fewer sick days, and were often better salespeople than younger workers.[132,133] Even so, some employers still continue to discriminate against older workers, and many older persons said they avoid searching for a job because they think nobody will hire them.

The federal Age Discrimination in Employment Act is intended to combat this kind of **ageism**—discrimination against older people—but it is not always easy to prove that discriminatory practices have been going on.[134,135]

- *Myths—retired people are poor/are wealthy:* Retired women workers receive less in the way of Social Security and pension benefits than men do—76 cents for every dollar paid to retired male workers, according to a report by the Older Women's League. The principal reason is that women who take time off to have a child or take care of an ill spouse are unfairly penalized.[136]

Does this mean that retired men are not financially needy—or that they are also? We keep getting two views—that millions of older adults could be thrown into poverty by cuts in Social Security, or that older Americans are getting an outsize share of government funds, forcing the nation to shortchange others, particularly the young.[137,138] The facts are that the poorest 20% of elderly households have an average net worth of about $3400. The top 20%—for whom the ads for cruise ships are intended—are worth almost 90 times as much.[139] In other words, there is no single answer about the financial abilities of the aging.

From a health standpoint, it certainly makes a difference which income and education group one is in. Researchers have found that of four groups, the health of those with low education and income deteriorated most rapidly in later life and the health of those with high education and income declined comparatively slowly.[140–143]

As you might expect, the biggest difference between Americans over 65 and other adults is that they don't work: retirement frees up 25 hours a week for men and 18 hours for women, on the average.[144]

Mental Health If you live to be older, you are more apt to have health problems. Epidemiologist Robert M. Kaplan estimates that, over a lifetime, men lose a total of 12 well years of life to illness, and women lose 16.[145] (The differences in years may reflect the fact that men are more susceptible to fatal diseases, such as heart attacks, early in life, while women are susceptible to chronic but not life-threatening diseases, such as arthritis.) What is important for mental health, however, is that people's *attitude* toward their disabilities makes a great deal of difference. Some people do very well managing severe problems, while others feel overwhelmed by relatively minor ones, according to epidemiologist Deborah Wingard.[146,147]

Among some of the important mental-health indicators are depression, medication and alcohol abuse, and suicide:

- *Depression:* **Depression**—persistent feelings of sorrow and apathy—is considered a major health problem among older Americans. Doctors may not notice because older patients are apt to complain about physical symptoms rather than their mental states.[148] Yet, according to physician Arnold Friedhoff, who headed a National Institutes of Health panel on the subject, 15% of elderly adults show signs of depression and nearly two-thirds go untreated.[149] The good news, however, is that 80% of depressed older people can be treated successfully, using combinations of counseling and anti-depressant drugs.

  The stacking of difficulties encountered in later life—the transition of retirement, health deterioration, the death of friends, financial problems, living alone—can be the most brutal in life, says Marvin Rosenberg, a therapist specializing in gerontology.[150] The stress may be manifested in the kind of behavior thought to be merely typical of old age, such as irritability or withdrawal.

- *Medication and alcohol abuse:* Misuse of prescription and over-the-counter drugs has been called a major problem among the elderly, according to a 1990 report of the National Academy of Sciences.[151] Indeed, one in five people over 60 has had an adverse reaction to a prescription drug, causing serious problems for 43% of them, according to another survey.[152] Often the problem is that doctors prescribe doses too high for the slower metabolisms of older people or there are cross reactions among multiple drugs. Also, some older people use long-lasting sleeping pills or tranquilizers, which can lead to drowsiness, amnesia, and dementia-like side effects that can land them in a nursing home or lead to falls and hip fractures.[153–155]

  Alcohol abuse is a serious problem with people in their 60s and beyond, as it is with other age groups. The rate of alcoholism among the elderly is estimated at 2–5%, and even higher in hospitals and health facilities. Because the elderly population is the fastest growing in the United States, there will probably be more elderly alcoholics in the next few decades.[156,157] Some symptoms of alcohol abuse, such as insomnia, depression, anxiety, and loss of memory, may be misunderstood as simply conditions seen among nonalcoholic older patients. Elderly alcoholics also have a high incidence of adverse drug reactions and health problems not caused by alcohol.

- *Suicide:* There is a public perception that older Americans who kill themselves do so because they are sick, broke, or alone, but this has been challenged by a study that shows that mental illness, especially depression, is the main cause of suicide.[158,159] Whatever the reason, rates of suicide among Americans aged 65 and over rose 21% in the years 1980–1986.[160] Two other studies are even more alarming: one by the National Institutes of Mental Health says the suicide rate among people 65 and older is 36% higher than among young adults; the other, by the American Association for Retired Persons, says white males over 65 have a suicide rate four times the national average.[161]

Some psychiatrists suggest that an older person might tend to think of suicide after experiencing a series of personal losses—such as physical health, job, spouse, or partner.

Life's Changes and Losses: Your Relationship to Your Parents Growing up means constantly experiencing a series of losses—of childhood friends, of pets, of familiar places, even of some of our dreams. In growing older, even as we *gain* strength and competence and experience, our losses grow heavier: couples divorce or dissolve their relationships, siblings move away, children leave home, jobs don't deliver what they promise, parents die. For the elderly, life's disappointments can be even more severe. There is the loss of job or career, the loss of physical ability and mobility, the loss of friends and spouses, and perhaps the loss of familiar places.

Among the changes and losses that young-adult and middle-aged children need to be aware of is their relationship to their parents. Emerging from adolescence into adulthood involves learning to interact with parents from your own vantage point, says psychoanalyst John Oldham. Then, as you become middle-aged, you perceive your parents as being less "magically omnipotent." Finally, as parents grow old and die, children may idealize them once more. As people grow older themselves, they are more apt to see that their parents did their best and to forgive them their limitations and mistakes.[162]

In some families, there are adult children who never quite detach from their parents, either financially or emotionally. This may occur at the end of adolescence, when children are resisting the transition to adulthood, or during middle age, when grown children are facing a crisis at home or at work.[163] It is best, however, if each generation can maintain a relationship of independence yet interdependence with the other.

Among the most difficult changes faced by people during their lives is the role shift in which children end up taking care of their parents. Some of the problems associated with this are as follows:

- *Care-giver stress:* Single elderly people prefer to live alone rather than share homes with family members.[164] Nevertheless, many end up living with their offspring. This can put a tremendous strain on the care-givers, most of whom are women, especially as the person being taken care of gets older.[165] The stresses can become se-

vere for those in midlife who must care for both children and dependent parents simultaneously.[166] Even the *elderly,* however, are more often having to care for their own elderly parents.[167]

- *Elder abuse:* Strains between adult children and their parents can become so great that they can lead to **elder abuse,** which may consist of physical or psychological abuse or neglect, by children or other caretakers.[168–170] Sometimes this takes the extreme form of "granny dumping," in which elderly and often confused Americans are simply abandoned on the doorsteps of public buildings, often by their children, who have come to regard their aging parents as a nuisance or because they have inadequate resources.

- *Nursing homes, care managers, and other options:* Children of aging parents may feel they have to take their parents into their homes or else put them in nursing homes. However, there are a variety of options in between. These include senior daycare, eldercare in apartment-like living situations (some including lifetime health-care plans), and private-care managers.[171–176]

Strategy for Living: Build Yourself to Last

Most people would like to live a long time, if in good health. To avoid disabilities in later life, one should learn to manage stress, stay physically active, eat right, maintain normal weight, avoid tobacco, go easy on alcohol, and stay involved socially.

How long will you live? Probably genetics or heredity has a lot to do with it—although to the surprise of scientists doing long-term study of centenarians in Georgia, they can't prove it with the data they have so far.[177] Indeed, the characteristics of parents and other family members of these 100-year-old seniors covered a wide range. If you sense your life might be short because others in your family did not live long, this finding should brighten your outlook. For instance, Mary Elliott lost her mother when she was 14 and outlived a brother and sister, two husbands, and two daughters, one of whom died at 77 when Elliott herself was 102.

Many people would like to live a long time but are afraid of being crippled by disabilities. In a 1991 survey conducted for the Alliance for Aging Research, two-thirds of Americans said they wanted to live to be 100 years old. However, 75% stated they were worried about losing control of their lives in their older years. Nearly 80% said they feared ending up in a nursing home.[178]

This kind of concern about disabilities in the later years is something you can begin to alleviate now—by building yourself to last. The following paragraphs offer a crash course in longevity and vitality.

Manage Stress Think how much of people's lives is organized around the matter of trying to avoid or reduce stress. For instance, people drink, smoke, and use drugs because they say life is too stressful, although in point of fact these diversions only aggravate the stresses.

As long as you live, there will never come a time in which you are completely without stress. To be alive, to experience change, is to experience stress. The only real question is, will you handle it, or will it handle you?

How can stress be effectively handled? The answer is: with practice. Building what is called *mental toughness,* or resilience, comes with practice. This includes learning to use the stress-management techniques we have described in Unit 2.

Stay Physically Active Among the truest words ever uttered are these: "Use it or lose it." Being physically active seems to be the closest thing there is to an anti-aging pill. Even people who take up exercise in later life show benefits in increased strength and stamina.

It's best, however, if you stay active throughout your entire life. Physically the payoffs are increased energy, stamina, flexibility, strength, and endurance. Mentally the rewards may be even better—a positive outlook and greater alertness. Older people who are physically active score higher on intelligence tests than the less active do. The benefits of exercise also extend to avoiding those very things Americans say they fear most in old age—disabilities.

Exercise reduces osteoporosis and heart and blood-vessel diseases, including stroke.

Eat Right Eating is indeed one of life's pleasures. But food need not be greasy and sugary to be pleasurable. We all have a few foods that "we really don't care for" (the stereotypical picture is of a child rejecting spinach). The trick is to make those foods we don't care for those that are high in fat. Some people have a handful of personal eating rules just to keep things simple: they won't eat red meat more than once a week, or they stay away from any food that comes from a four-footed animal (which includes cheese and other dairy products). Or in restaurants they always ask for sauces and salad dressings to be served "on the side." Such dietary proscriptions still leave a lot of room for eating in a way that need not be boring or complicated. Salads, breads, chicken, fish, and raw fruits and vegetables will help you stay away from fat and give you the fiber, vitamins, and minerals that will help you ward off heart disease, diabetes, obesity, cancer, and other afflictions of older people.

Maintain Normal Weight As you age, your metabolism slows down. If you eat and exercise the same as you did in youth, you will automatically gain weight. While there's probably nothing wrong with gaining ½ pound a year after age 20, you should avoid putting on much more than that. Obesity not only doesn't help your appearance and self-esteem, it leads to premature aging and places you at risk for many health problems.

Avoid Tobacco If you smoke, you're essentially trading a minute of life for every minute you smoke. That may not sound like a lot to give up, but it works out to 12 years less to a pack-a-day smoker, on average. Moreover, despite the image of virility and vitality projected in cigarette ads, smokers usually begin to go into physical decline years before their deaths, showing everything from prematurely wrinkled skin to loss of sex drive to hacking coughs to more colds to the serious consequences of cancer and respiratory diseases.

Go Easy on the Alcohol You may be aware that heavy alcohol use impairs the liver and kidneys and is a factor in the majority of traffic deaths. What you may not know is that heavy drinking in effect pickles the brain. If you drink 8 drinks a day for more than 20 years, according to University of Florida researchers, you may experience a 40% reduction in chemicals vital to learning and memory.[179] This will most certainly produce the kind of diminished intellectual capacity that many people fear in conjunction with aging.

Stay Involved Socially Compared to the 1950s, adult Americans in the 1970s are less likely to be married, more likely to be living alone, less likely to belong to voluntary organizations, and less likely to visit informally with others. These trends, say three sociologists, will only be accelerated in the 21st century, with fewer older people having spouses or children —the very people most elders turn to for relatedness and support.[180] Yet people with few or poor-quality relationships are the very ones who are less healthy, both psychologically and physically, and more likely to die sooner. It's important, therefore, that you not isolate yourself from social relationships.

Your First and Last Day of Life Today could be the last day of your life—a fact of which many older people are well aware. This knowledge also compounds the meaning in the somewhat corny but altogether true expression, "Today is the first day of the rest of your life."

"We love youth," says clinical psychologist Mark Gerzon and author of *Coming Into Our Own: Understanding Adult Metamorphosis.* "In America we're all in love with staying young. That works until a certain point in life. But if you only love what's young, eventually you'll start to hate yourself."[181] The second half of your life does not mean there is no change or growth. On the contrary, it can be a time of reinvention, self-renewal, and altruism—giving something back to the community. As many have discovered, Act II of their lives may be the best part. (See ● *Figure 34.5.*)

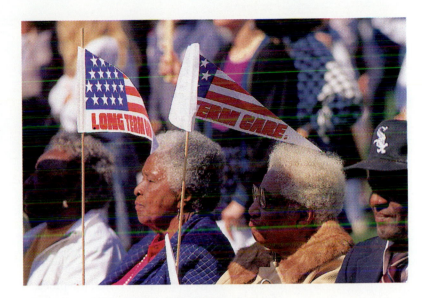

● **Figure 34.5 Act II: Is the best yet to come?** The second half of life can be a time of reinvention, self-renewal, and altruism.

800-HELP

Alzheimer's Disease and Related Disorders Association. 800-621-0379 (in Illinois, 800 572-6037). Provides phone numbers of local support groups for families of patients with Alzheimer's disease or vascular dementia

Arthritis Foundation Information Line. 800-283-7800. Provides information about osteoarthritis

National Council on the Aging. 800-424-9046. National information and consulting center for the aged

Simon Foundation for Continence. 800-23-SIMON. Provides help for problems of urinary incontinence

Suggestion for Further Reading

Solomon, David H., Salend, Elyse, Rahman, Anna Nolen, Liston, Marie Bolduc, & Reuben, David B. (1992). *A consumer's guide to aging.* Baltimore: Johns Hopkins University Press. Tips on physical and mental health, medical care, personal finances, relationships and other subjects for people over 50.

35 The End of Life

▶ Describe how people seem to handle feelings about death and the value of personal death awareness.

▶ Discuss the different definitions of death, the definition of a coma and of a persistent vegetative state, and the questions of right to die and euthanasia.

▶ Explain the different kinds of advance directives and their benefits.

▶ Discuss several death-related situations, including near-death experiences, stages of adjustment to death, pain relief, hospices, feelings during impending death, and after-death practicalities, such as death certificates and funeral arrangements.

▶ List the four stages of mourning, describe different ways people react to grief, and discuss how you can help a person in bereavement.

"I f you have a lot of unfinished business," said terminal cancer patient Howard Eckel, "maybe that's where the pain comes from dying."[182]

What is *your* unfinished business? What is it that you would devote your remaining life energy to? Your *life energy* is your portion of time here on earth, the hours of life available to you.[183] Those hours could end at any time, as though you turned the next page and found the rest of the book blank. How you use your finite, irretrievable life time represents the purpose of your presence here on earth.

Thus, death is at the core of discovering the art of living. Despite its unpleasant associations and details, death needs to be thought about because it forces you to come to terms with what you want to do with your own life and how you want to deal with those close to you, whose lives someday also will end.

In this chapter, we deal with the following important areas:

• Facing your feelings about death

• Defining death and considering decisions about ending life

• Making plans for your hospitalization and your death

• The process of dying

• Dealing with others' deaths

• Preparing for your own end

Your Feelings About Death

Feelings about death are often characterized by denial of the fact of death. Personal death awareness, however, represents an opportunity to put one's life in meaningful perspective.

"It's an honor to be with someone when he or she dies."

Is this a sentiment you could express? It was uttered by the friend of a failing cancer patient, a single person who wished not to die alone and had asked her friend to be with her. In other words, the patient honored her friend by singling her out and asking her to be there during one of the most intimate of all acts.[184]

Death and Denial We live in a society that conditions us to deny death. Most Americans no longer die at home. Seventy percent, in fact, die in hospitals, nursing homes, and extended-care facilities.[185] Often in such places death is considered the enemy, and people cling to their degenerating bodies in hopes of some miraculous medical turnaround. Children and the rest of us are exposed to enacted death thousands of times a day on television; however, we are rarely at the bedside when a grandparent or relative dies. Moreover, with the rise in cremations and the decline in open-casket funerals, it is possible to go through one's whole life without seeing a dead person. If, at some point, death rudely inserts itself into our lives, it may register itself simply by a person's *absence*—literally, here today, gone tomorrow, as when someone is killed in a car crash.

When we do have to think seriously about death, whether others' or our own, it evokes "a murky swirl of emotions: terror, sadness, anxiety," as one writer describes it. "The more we try to counteract the natural deterioration of the body and the more attached we become to our accomplishments and our possessions, the more we dread our own demise."[186] And the more we are apt to deny that it can happen to us. While a reasonable amount of denial is useful and helps us get through day-to-day difficulties, excessive denial of death—as in driving fast without seat belts or smoking cigarettes— can actually hasten our own end. To examine your own feelings about death, you may wish to take the accompanying Self Discovery. (*See Self Discovery 35.1.*)

Personal Death Awareness: An Opportunity One writer makes the interesting observation that the recent interest in *danger sports* —mountain climbing, hang gliding, skydiving, and the like—"may all be ways we have of tricking ourselves into the present." Focusing on death is a way of becoming fully alive, for wherever attention and awareness is, that is where our experience of life arises. He goes on:

> *Many say they "feel so alive" when doing these sports because they demand attention. Perhaps that is why so many who are dying also say they have never felt so alive. When we take death within us we stop reinforcing our denial, our judging, our anger, or continuing our bargaining. We don't push our depression away.*[187]

Personal death awareness—accepting the fact that you are going to die—thus becomes an opportunity to confront your life, to put it into meaningful perspective. Some matters you might want to try to deal with:

- *How would I like my epitaph to read?* Many gravestones or monuments have no **epitaphs,** or inscriptions, just birth and death dates. Some epitaphs may seem a bit general ("faithful husband, loving father"), but they nevertheless express the best memories the survivors have of the person. How would you like to be remembered on your monument? Your proposed death inscription could actually become your words to *live* by.

- *What would I want an obituary or eulogy to say about me?* Writing your own **obituary notice**—a short biographical account of the sort published under "Death Notices" in the newspaper—can be quite useful. It becomes a statement of your life purpose and how you would like to be remembered.

A similar exercise is to write your own imaginary **eulogy,** the kind of speech of praise given about the deceased at a memorial service.

- *Make a list to avoid aimlessness:* All life journeys end at the same place. The difficulty is to figure out what events, depending on the choices available to you, you want your journey to include. If aimlessness suits you, that's fine, but realize that aimlessness is a choice like any other. Perhaps making a list of all the things you'd like to do and places you'd like to see will help you focus. Or listing the two or three important things you'd like to do if you only had a year to live. Don't forget to include people in your plans—how you would like to treat and be treated by people important to you. And in focusing on the future, don't neglect the present: enjoying sunsets, birds, music, a meal with a friend—simple pleasures.

Some day the tomorrows will stop rolling in. Within the limits of your mortality, you must determine the art of living for yourself.

What Are the Definitions of Death, and Who Decides Who Dies?

Death is defined in different ways: cessation of heart and lungs, cellular death, brain death, and cortical death. In between life and death are the coma and the persistent vegetative state. This state raises the question of who should decide when a person should die and whether suicide should be allowed. Euthanasia, or "mercy killing," may be either passive or active.

Technology has changed all our ways of dealing with death. Technology, for instance, may force us to think about death even before birth. Laura Campo and Justin Pearson knew from prenatal tests that their infant would not be born with a fully formed brain—what medical ethicists call a "brain absent" baby—yet with a brain stem that still permitted heartbeat and breathing.[188] How should parents, physicians, and lawyers deal with such an event? The

How Do You Feel About Death?

This questionnaire is not designed to test your knowledge. Instead, it should encourage you to think about your present attitudes toward death and how these attitudes may have developed.

Answer the questions to the best of your knowledge by circling the appropriate letter.

1. Who died in your first personal involvement with death?
   a. Grandparent, great-grandparent
   b. Parent
   c. Brother or sister
   d. Other family member
   e. Friend or acquaintance
   f. Stranger, or public figure
   g. Animal

2. To the best of your memory, at what age were you first aware of death?
   a. Under 3
   b. 3–5
   c. 6–10
   d. 11 or older

3. When you were a child, how was death talked about in your family?
   a. Openly
   b. With some sense of discomfort
   c. Only when necessary, with an attempt to exclude children
   d. As though it were a taboo subject
   e. Never recall any discussion

4. Which of the following best describes your childhood conceptions of death?
   a. Heaven-and-hell concept
   b. After-life
   c. Death as sleep
   d. No physical or mental activity
   e. Mysterious and unknowable
   f. Something other than the above
   g. No conception, or can't remember

5. To what extent do you believe in life after death?
   a. Strongly believe in it
   b. Tend to believe it
   c. Uncertain
   d. Tend to doubt it
   e. Convinced it does not exist

6. Regardless of your belief about life after death, what is your wish about it?
   a. I strongly wish there were a life after death.
   b. I am indifferent.
   c. I definitely prefer that there not be a life after death.

7. Has there been a time in your life when you wanted to die?
   a. Yes, mainly because of great physical pain
   b. Yes, mainly because of great emotional upset
   c. Yes, mainly to escape an intolerable social or interpersonal situation
   d. Yes, mainly because of great embarrassment
   e. Yes, for a reason other than above
   f. No

8. What does death mean to you?
   a. The end, the final process of life
   b. The beginning of a life after death; a transition, a new beginning
   c. A joining of the spirit with a universal cosmic consciousness

   d. An endless sleep; rest and peace
   e. Termination of this life but with survival of the spirit
   f. Don't know
   g. Other (specify)

9. What aspect of your own death is the most distasteful to you?
   a. I could have no experiences.
   b. I am afraid of what might happen to my body after death.
   c. I am uncertain as to what might happen if there is life after death.
   d. I could no longer provide for my dependents.
   e. It would cause grief to my relatives and friends.
   f. All my plans and projects would come to an end.
   g. The dying process may be painful.
   h. Other (specify)

10. How is your present physical health?
    a. Excellent
    b. Very good
    c. Moderately good
    d. Moderately poor
    e. Extremely bad

11. How is your present mental health?
    a. Excellent
    b. Very good
    c. Moderately good
    d. Moderately poor
    e. Extremely bad

12. Based on your present feelings, what is the probability of your taking your own life in the near future?
    a. Extremely high (I feel very much like killing myself)
    b. Moderately high
    c. Between high and low
    d. Moderately low
    e. Extremely low (very improbable)

13. In your opinion, at what age are people most afraid of death?
    a. Up to 12 years
    b. 13–19 years
    c. 20–29 years
    d. 30–39 years
    e. 40–49 years
    f. 50–59 years
    g. 60–69 years
    h. 70 years and over

14. When you think of your own death (or mortality), how do you feel?
    a. Fearful
    b. Discouraged
    c. Depressed
    d. Purposeless
    e. Resolved, in relation to life
    f. Pleasure in being alive
    g. Other (specify)

questions mount as more sophisticated medical devices permit critically ill persons, even those in a coma, to be kept alive for years, so that "the definition of death edges closer to life," as one writer points out.[189]

Definitions of Death Religions consider death to be a spiritual event, the moment when the soul leaves the body. However, death is also a medical and legal event—and the definition keeps changing. Consider:

- *Heart and lungs cease:* Not so long ago, a physician had to let a person's heart stop, completely on its own, before death could be declared.[190] At the same time, or shortly before, the lungs would also have ceased to function. The lack of heartbeat and breathing, determined by feeling for a pulse or listening through a stethoscope, is one of the classic clinical signs of death.

- *Cellular death:* In earlier eras, some cultures considered putrefaction the only acceptable proof of death.[191] This, of course, takes time, for cells can live on for a little while. Indeed, they often do, if an organ is transplanted to another human's body. Still, the presence of **rigor mortis,** when the body shows rigidity, indicates that the body has experienced **cellular death**—the cells in tissues and organs are no longer functioning.

- *Brain death:* The brain can continue to function for a short time (perhaps 10 minutes or less) after the heartbeat ceases. However, a person who has suffered irreversible loss of all brain functions may be considered legally dead—declared **brain-dead**—even if the heart is still beating.

  Brain death is indicated by the absence (flat line) of brain-wave activity on a device called an electroencephalograph. An **electroencephalograph (EEG)** is an instrument that records the electrical activity of the brain, as recorded from electrodes attached to the scalp. To declare a person brain-dead, a physician must find brain-wave activity absent on the first measurement and then again 24 hours later.

- *Cortical death:* **Cortical death,** also called *cerebral* or *cognitive death,* is a new criterion of death that is being discussed but has not been legally accepted. Cortical death means that the person is brain-dead, but the **brain stem,** or **medulla**—the part of the brain that controls breathing and heartbeat—is still functioning. If adopted as a definition, cortical death would mean that a person is dead because, even though breathing, heartbeat, blood pressure, temperature, and other signs were normal, the person would not show any detectable brain waves. That is, there would be no evidence of functioning of the **cerebral cortex,** that part of the brain responsible for higher brain functions such as thought, memory, love, and voluntary muscle movement.[192]

Campo and Pearson, parents of the "brain absent" baby mentioned above, knew in advance that their infant would meet the definition of cortical death, but they chose to continue the pregnancy because they wanted to donate their daughter's organs for transplants. Lower courts overruled them because the functioning brain stem meant the baby was not legally brain dead.[193]

Persistent Vegetative State: Loss of Consciousness and Personhood About 2 million people die in the United States every year, more than half when some life-sustaining treatment is ended.[194] Nancy Cruzan was 25 years old when her car overturned on a country road, and it was 15 or 20 minutes before paramedics could restart her heart; in the meantime her brain was severely damaged from lack of oxygen. For almost 8 years, Cruzan was kept alive by a feeding tube implanted in her abdomen. Though she could breathe, her mind was obliterated. After several years of legal efforts by her parents, the U.S. Supreme Court ruled that the feeding tube could be disconnected, and Cruzan died at the

age of 33.[195–200] As we discuss, the court's ruling gives tremendous urgency to the matter of having a "living will" or other advanced directive about what you want to have done should you become incapacitated. Cruzan, doctors said, was in a persistent vegetative state, which is not the same as a coma:

- *Coma:* A **coma** is a state of profound unconsciousness. People sometimes awaken from a coma.

- *PVS:* Patients in a **persistent vegetative state (PVS)** are completely paralyzed and show no signs of awareness or reflexes. Yet they have sleep/wake cycles, are often able to breathe on their own after being on artificial respiration, and have all the normal vital signs. They do not, however, show evidence of consciousness.[201] There are 15,000–25,000 PVS people, according to a report in the *Journal of the American Medical Association.*[202]

Doctors would say that Nancy Cruzan and other PVS victims are not actually alive but are already dead under the definition of cortical death. "Once consciousness is irreversibly lost, the person is lost," says one psychiatrist, Stuart Youngner, who is a leading advocate of the definition of cortical death. "What remains is a mindless organism."[203] The loss of personhood, he says, "leaves only a body that has outlived its owner."

Reporter Mark Dowie, who investigated the matter of PVS and cortical death, asked everyone he interviewed a troubling question: How do we know that PVS victims are not experiencing some form of consciousness, even bliss, that cannot be described by existing technology? The unanimous answer is, we don't.

In that case, asks Dowie, do we have the right to declare them dead, simply to remove the emotional and economic burden of keeping them alive?[204] Once again, such questions mean that, in order to guard our close relatives from years of emotional turmoil and economic catastrophe, as happened with Nancy Cruzan's family, it is imperative that we communicate clear instructions *while we are alive* on what we want done should we find ourselves in a PVS or similar state.

The Right to Die: Who Should Decide?
Mary Henderson's body was under attack by a

bacterial infection, gram-negative sepsis, that kills as many as 100,000 Americans each year. Her family gathered by her hospital bed at 3 P.M. as she began fading toward death. Then around midnight an experimental drug arrived, released under the Food and Drug Administration's "compassionate use" exemptions, and was administered. Four hours later every objective sign of her condition improved, and eventually Henderson went home.[205]

Seemingly miraculous cures do happen. Patients in comas do sometimes come out of them. Resuscitation does bring back patients whose hearts have stopped.

On the other hand, many doctors think that resuscitation is wasteful, painful, and brutal to patients who are chronically sick, very elderly, or near the end of life.[206] An 86-year-old severely brain-damaged woman in Minnesota, whom doctors argued had no hope of recovery and should be removed from life-support systems, remained in a vegetative state from May 1990 to July 1991 (when she died of natural causes) because her husband won a court order to keep her on a respirator, saying she would have wanted to live, for religious reasons.[207,208] A 6-year-old severely brain-damaged girl, incurably ill and in great pain, was kept alive for 10 months through repeated operations and resuscitation, against doctors' recommendations, because the girl's mother refused to grant permission for a do-not-resuscitate order.[209]

From one viewpoint, marvelous medical technology prolongs living. From another, it prolongs dying. But who should decide who has the right to live or die—the patient's family, the physicians, the courts? While many doctors believe that consulting with the family is important, they also believe that giving the family ultimate authority in do-not-resuscitate and similar life-support measures is a mistake. (*See ● Figure 35.1.*)

Medical ethicist Bruce Hilton states that a key word in the discussion about whether to remove life-support equipment is *futile*. "If the treatment isn't working, and clearly isn't going to," he says, "doctors have no legal, moral, or professional obligation to keep it up."[210] If the medical treatment is futile, the physician is under no obligation to continue it even if the patient wants to go on, although extending futile treatment may sometimes be justified for a short time.

How do doctors *know* that a patient will or won't survive? They don't always, of course. However, into this very question of life and death brought about by medicine's success with technology has come a new piece of technology: the APACHE III computer program. Doctors in hospital intensive-care units (ICUs) use the computerized system to predict their patients' likelihood of survival. To use APACHE, the physician answers 27 questions posed by the

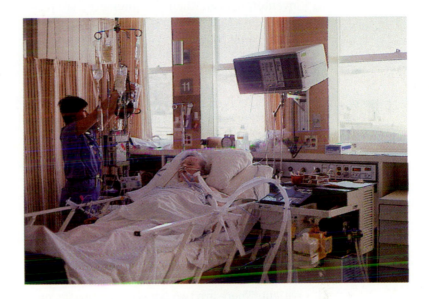

● **Figure 35.1 A patient on life support: Who decides the right to die?** Respirators, feeding tubes, intravenous fluids, and other technology can prolong living or prolong dying. Who should decide if and when such life-sustaining equipment should be removed—the family, the physicians, or the courts?

"*Typically, nobody knows what the patient would want because everyone was so good at denying their mortality. Family members are divided because they still don't want to face it. And you have heart-rending waiting-room scenes with hopeful loved ones rising and falling on the ebb and flow of the doomed patient's good days and bad days. What's a success or failure at the end of life? Everyone is distraught and afraid. And we're living in a horror movie that doesn't end after two weeks, let alone two hours.*"

—Poughkeepsie, New York, physician Donald E. Berman. Quoted in: Malcolm, A. H. (1991, November 29). Decisions about life and death. *New York Times*, p. A16.

software, describing the patient's medical history, treatment, lab results, vital signs, and severity of illness on arrival at the ICU. APACHE provides two daily numbers, expressed as percentages, estimating the patient's chances of dying in the ICU or later in the hospital. The program also predicts the patient's length of stay and tells how much intervention is normally used in this kind of case. Finally, the computer addresses the issue of futility: it asks if treatment is making a difference.[211–213]

No one claims that APACHE is perfect. Its inventor, William Knaus, an intensive-care physician, says that it never gives either zero or 100% estimates of mortality. The system, he says, "never describes hopelessness or complete safety."[214]

According to the Patient Self-Determination Act, hospitals must advise patients admitted for any reason that they have a right to sign "advance directives" for health care decisions, such as whether they wish to be kept on life-support. We describe this in detail in the section "Choosing Death." Of course, a patient who is brought to an emergency room unconscious is in no position to sign an advance directive.

Euthanasia: The Question of Mercy Sometimes called "mercy killing," **euthanasia** is any method of causing the death of a desperately ill patient. There are two types of euthanasia, passive and active:

- *Passive euthanasia—allowing someone to die:* **Passive euthanasia** is withholding life-sustaining aid or lifesaving techniques. Physicians or nurses who disconnect respirators or tube feeders, who don't use drugs that might continue life, or who don't practice lifesaving techniques such as cardiopulmonary resuscitation (CPR) are practicing passive euthanasia.

- *Active euthanasia—intentionally inflicting death:* **Active euthanasia,** sometimes called "assisted suicide," involves a physician or other person (such as a relative) administering depressant drugs, potassium chloride, carbon monoxide, or other lethal methods of ending life. This is murder when it is not done by the patient's own hand.

   In recent years, physician Jack Kevorkian became famous for helping set up the equipment and chemicals ("suicide machines") by which severely ill patients, such as victims of Alzheimer's disease or multiple sclerosis, could press a button and take their own lives.[215–221] Most such incidents took place in Michigan, which for a time had no law specifically barring assistance in a suicide.

The American Hospital Association estimates that 70% of the 6000 deaths that occur in the United States every day are already somehow timed or negotiated, with medical technology withdrawn or not applied at all—what could be called forms of passive euthanasia.[222] Yet some physicians have admitted, nearly always anonymously, that they actually helped patients commit suicide.[223,224] One who spoke for the record was Timothy Quill, who said that he had prescribed enough barbiturates to kill a 45-year-old leukemia patient and had told her the size of a lethal dose.[225] A New York grand jury declined to indict the doctor for the crime of aiding in a suicide, which carries a prison sentence of up to 15 years.[226] In the Netherlands, where euthanasia was illegal but widely tolerated until it was legalized in 1993, a study showed that about 1.8% of all deaths were deliberately caused by doctors acting on their patients' orders, typically cancer patients in their early 60s.[227,228]

The public has repeatedly expressed support for euthanasia. A January 1991 Gallup poll found that 59% of American adults sampled say a terminally ill patient has the right to end his or her life "under any circumstances." Two-thirds thought a doctor has the "moral right" to end a patient's life if the patient and his or her family agree.[229] Other polls also show that the majority of Americans support doctor-assisted suicide and euthanasia.[230–232]

As might be expected, physicians in many circumstances are torn between their Hippocratic oath to prolong life in all instances and their concern with alleviating pain and suffering if hope is nonexistent.[233–237]

Suicide Perhaps severe or terminal illness has always been a reason for suicide, but in recent years it has even taken the form of a self-help movement, making sales of Derek Humphry's controversial guide to suicide, *Final Exit,* a bestseller.[238] No one knows what proportion of suicides are motivated by illness, but, to take one example, the American Hospital Association says that every year 12,000 of the 80,000 patients on artificial kidney machines voluntarily quit, bringing about a self-inflicted end within 2 weeks.[239]

Leaders of the country's largest Christian groups, the Roman Catholic Church and the Southern Baptist Convention, are opposed to all forms of euthanasia or suicide. However, religious advocates, mostly from liberal and mainline Protestant churches, express affirmation for individual choice in such matters.[240] The courts, at least in one Florida case, state that dying people have a right to refuse food and need not have a court's approval to stop forced feeding.[241]

For some ill patients, the *timing* of their suicide can be a tricky business. Questions arise: What if you're not as sick as the doctors think you are? How sure can you be, at a given moment, that you want to die?[242] Janet Adkins, a victim of Alzheimer's disease, was assisted by physician Jack Kevorkian to comfortable and compassionate death. A different tale is told by the widower of another Alzheimer's victim. He wrote that his wife began to show symptoms of the disease when she was 66 years old, and within 2 years "her condition had reached what I would call the crucial stage." He continues:

> That is when a victim understands what is almost certainly ahead and can still make well-informed judgments. Such a person can look back on a good life, can abhor the thought of becoming a non-person to family and friends and can strongly and wisely wish for a quick and painless death. This relatively brief period provides an opportunity that, if not taken, will often make one's spouse and children regretful and angry that there was no socially approved way to help that person die with dignity.[243]

In less than a year, the man reported, his wife could no longer make an informed judgment at all. "She declined, spending much of the last 5 years of her 14-year bout with Alzheimer's in a nursing home as a near vegetable." Her death, at 80, was a very delayed blessing.

Choosing Death: The Importance of Making Plans

To avoid becoming a not-quite-living burden to yourself or your family, it's advisable to write an advance directive giving instructions about resuscitation and use of life-support equipment. This can take the form of a living will, a health-care proxy, or a durable power of attorney. Organ-donor cards and wills should also be considered.

It should be apparent by now that modern medicine can extend our lives but it could also make the end of our lives a living—or not-quite-living—hell, both for ourselves and for our families.

Death is not the exclusive experience of old people, of course. Automobile accidents and AIDS have cut short the lives of many in the prime of life. Thus, it's important that everyone, even young people, should give clear instructions—*in writing and in as much detail as possible*—to their family, friends, and doctors about what types of treatment they do and do not want. These instructions, known as **advance directives** or **medical directives**, allow you not only to specify how much or how little treatment you want but also to designate a family member or friend to make decisions on your behalf if you become too ill to speak for yourself.

Under the Patient Self-Determination Act, virtually all hospitals, nursing homes, and health-maintenance organizations must inform all patients over age 18 of their right to fill out an advance directive. (You are not required to have one, only to be advised of your *right* to have one.)

Advance directives may include living wills, health-care proxies, and durable power of attorney for health care. These documents vary from state to state, and it's important to comply with state law. (See ● *Figure 35.2.*) In some cases, patients who have said they did *not* want "heroic treatment" have nevertheless been kept on life-support systems.[244] This is because the living wills in many states become effective only when you are in a "terminal" condition, which might exclude people with PVS; other states

A Living Will

This living will applies to New York State. Forms for other states are available from Choice in Dying, 200 Varick St., 10th floor, New York, NY 10014.

I, _____ , being of sound mind, make this statement as a directive to be followed if I become permanently unable to participate in decisions regarding my medical care. These instructions reflect my firm and settled commitment to decline medical treatment under the circumstances indicated below.

I direct my attending physician to withhold or withdraw treatment that serves only to prolong the process of my dying, if I should be in an incurable or irreversible mental or physical condition with no reasonable expectation of recovery.

These instructions apply if I am (a) in a terminal condition; (b) permanently unconscious, or (c) if I am conscious but have irreversible brain damage and will never regain the ability to make decisions and express my wishes.

I direct that treatment be limited to measures to keep me comfortable and to relieve pain, including any pain that might occur by withholding or withdrawing treatment.

While I understand that I am not legally required to be specific about future treatments, if I am in the condition(s) described above I feel especially strongly about the following forms of treatment:

I do not want cardiac resuscitation.
I do not want mechanical respiration.
I do not want tube feeding.
I do not want antibiotics.
I do not want maximum pain relief.
Other directions (insert personal instructions):

These directions express my legal right to refuse treatment, under the law of New York State. I intend my instructions to be carried out, unless I have rescinded them in a new writing or by clearly indicating that I have changed my mind.

Signed: _____ Date: _____
Witness: _____
    Address: _____
Witness: _____
    Address: _____

● **Figure 35.2 Advance directive.** Example of a living will. This is for New York State.

allow the withdrawal of tube feeding only under very limited conditions, regardless of a patient's preference.

In this section we discuss:

- Living wills
- Health-care proxies
- Durable power of attorney for health care
- Organ-donor cards
- Wills

Living Will A **living will** specifies what treatments you would or would not want if you were to become irreversibly incapacitated and dependent on life-sustaining equipment. (*Refer back to Figure 35.2.*) Some people may want to specify that they actually want *any* type of treatment available, and it's important that this be spelled out: the issue here is about choice, not about "pulling the plug."[245]

Some living-will forms allow you to state that you do not want "heroic" treatment measures taken, but it's better to be specific. You can state whether you do or don't want cardiac resuscitation, mechanical respiration, tube feeding, kidney dialysis, or antibiotics. You can ask for painkilling drugs, or to be allowed to die at home.[246] Specifically, the measures you can decide about are the following:

- *Cardiac resuscitation:* Cardiac resuscitation includes measures to stimulate a stopped heart or to regulate aberrant heart rhythms—including the use of chest compressions, electrical shocks, intravenous insertion of a pacemaker, and medications like epinephrine.

  Some doctors think that cardiac resuscitation is misapplied and overused, because only 5–15% of patients on whom resuscitation is attempted will survive to leave the hospital.[247] Nevertheless, under existing law physicians are obliged to make the effort even when they think it's useless, as on people with widespread cancer—unless the patient has formally signed a "Do Not Resuscitate" (DNR) form or indicated this instruction in a living will.

  In some localities, paramedics will respect the wishes of people—usually those in the last stages of life—wearing leg or arm bands that say "Do Not Resuscitate."

- *Mechanical respiration:* Mechanical respiration or artificial ventilation is used if a patient stops breathing or is not able to get enough oxygen to the organs. Generally, a respirator is used that forces oxygen into the lungs through a tube inserted through the nose or mouth.

- *Tube feeding:* For patients incapable of feeding themselves, nutrition is given intravenously or through a feeding tube into the stomach.

What Would You Want Done to Keep You Alive?

Consider what your choice would be for each category of treatment in these four scenarios. Reading from left to right across each line, write yes or no for whether you would want the treatment listed to be applied in the situation described above (scenarios I, II, III, and IV).

	I Coma or persistent vegetative state, with no chance of regaining awareness	II Coma with small chance of recovery and greater chance of surviving with brain damage	III Irreversible brain damage or disease	IV Irreversible brain damage or disease, and terminal illness
Cardiopulmonary resuscitation				
Mechanical breathing				
Artificial nutrition and hydration				
Major surgery				
Kidney dialysis				
Chemotherapy				
Minor surgery				
Invasive diagnostic tests				
Blood or blood products				
Antibiotics				
Pain medications				

Source: Linda Emanuel, M.D., Massachusetts General Hospital, Boston, and Ezekiel Emanuel, M.D., Beth Israel Hospital, Boston. Presented in: Schultz, E. E. (1990, June 29). Ruling draws the worried to 'living wills.' *Wall Street Journal*, p. C1.

- *Antibiotics and painkillers:* Antibiotics and certain other medicines previously prescribed may be continued or withheld, according to your wishes. You can also state whether or not you want maximum pain relief.

To help you decide what kind of measures you would want done under what circumstances, you may wish to take the accompanying Self Discovery. (*See Self Discovery 35.2.*)

Because living wills vary from state to state, you should get one from a local hospital, financial planner, stationery store, or at no charge from Choice in Dying, 200 Varick St., 10th floor, New York, NY 10014. The document should be signed in the presence of two witnesses, neither a potential heir or the attending doctor, nurse, or health care facility employee. Some states insist the living will be notarized. Give copies to your immediate family, doctor, and anyone else involved. To keep the documents legally binding, they should be signed (and if necessary notarized) again every couple of years.[248] You can also send your living will to Choice in Dying to be recorded in their computerized Living Will Registry, in return for which you will get a wallet-size plastic mini-will with the registry number printed on it.

In some counties, people are permitted to wear "Do Not Resuscitate" arm or leg bands.

UNIFORM DONOR CARD

of_____

Print or type name of donor

In the hope that I may help others, I hereby make this anatomical gift, if medically acceptable, to take effect upon death. The words and marks below indicate my wishes:

I give: (a)_____any needed organs or parts
     (b)_____only the following organs or parts

_____

Specify the organ(s), tissue(s), or part(s)

for the purposes of transplantation, therapy, medical research or education;

     (c)_____my body for anatomical study if needed.

Limitations or special wishes, if any:_____

● **Figure 35.3 Organ-donor card**

"*Dear Abby: Last May, our 22-year-old son, Michael, was involved in a motorcycle accident. He was pronounced brain dead three days later. Because of an article he had read in your column, he carried an organ donor card in his wallet.*

The lord took our precious son 10 days later, but we were comforted knowing that Michael gave two blind people the gift of sight, and a young father who had been on a kidney machine for three years is now living a normal life. . . ."

Michael's Father

—Letter to columnist "Dear Abby" (Abigail Van Buren). (1990, April 23). Gifts of life from son's death. *San Francisco Chronicle*, p. F10.

Health-Care Proxy A **health-care proxy** form appoints a health-care agent—a friend or family member—to act for you in health care matters if you become incapacitated. It is often included within a living will. You should also indicate someone else as a backup, in case your first choice cannot be available. Laws regarding health-care proxies also vary from state to state and may give only limited powers, such as the ability to act for a person with terminal illness but not a person in a coma or with Alzheimer's disease.

Durable Power of Attorney The document for **durable power of attorney for health care decisions** is a more inclusive document than the health-care proxy and permits your representative to act for you in most health care matters, including those you might not have considered. This document allows you to control your own affairs through your own agent—again, a friend or family member—instead of relying on a court to appoint a conservator. This form, which should be completed along with a living will, is also available from Choice in Dying.

Organ-Donor Forms There is currently a great need for organs, so great, in fact, that in California half the patients who are waiting for transplants die because they don't get an organ. Many of these are children.[249]

Because of medical technology, many parts of the body can be transplanted: heart, lungs, kidneys, liver, pancreas, corneas, ligaments, tendons, bone, skin, heart valves, veins, and the tiny bones of the middle ear.[250] Although you can do everything possible to avoid your demise as a result of an auto or motorcycle accident, murder, or other tragedy, it might comfort your survivors to know that, simply by carrying an organ-donor card in your wallet, you have enabled a person with a bad heart to survive or a child to see. An organ-donor card is available at state motor-vehicle departments (or from The Living Bank, POB 6725, Houston, TX 77265). It should be filled out, signed in the presence of two witnesses, and attached to the back of your driver's license or identification card. (See ● *Figure 35.3.*)

Will Some people become quite involved with "taking care of their affairs" in the event of their death, getting into estate planning, living trusts, and the like. Things need not be this complicated. However, you *should* have a will, particularly if there are family changes through marriage, divorce, the birth of a child, or death of a prospective heir. If you die without a will—what is called "intestate"—then the state's laws take over, and the decisions that are made about disposal of your property or other wishes might not be as you would have liked.

If you own property, are married, or have children, you should probably hire a lawyer to do the will. By telephoning different lawyers, you can find out what the rates are—often they are not expensive. Or, you can do a **holographic will,** which is written entirely in ink in your own hand, specifying who you wish to have your property and who should raise your children. You can also specify what funeral arrangements you want, if any. Designate a family member or friend as the executor, who will carry out your wishes.

Surviving Others' Mortality: Dying and Death

Because you may be present when someone you know dies, you should be knowledgeable about a number of death-related situations: near-death experiences, Kübler-Ross's five stages of adjustment to death, telling dying people the truth, giving relief from pain, dying in a hospice or at home, and dealing with feelings during impending death. You may also be associated with certain practicalities after death: death certificate, autopsy, organ donation, and funeral arrangements.

It is possible that you yourself will be blessed with a sudden, virtually painless end. But before that day, you may well be caught up in the dying of family members or friends—involved in events that you can't control and that are tremendously saddening but that call upon you to give comfort as well. There are important lessons here.

In this section, we will describe the following:

- Near-death experiences
- The emotional stages of dying
- The final days—including pain relief, hospice care, and autopsies
- Grieving, including for children
- Death rituals, including funerals and wakes

Near-Death Experience What is it like, really like, to die? Since most people die only once, we can't be sure. There is, however, a highly exclusive group of people who have had a **near-death experience (NDE),** mainly people whose hearts had stopped but who were brought back, usually through the intervention of medical technology.

A study by Kenneth Ring of over 100 NDEers found that all shared some core experiences: an out-of-body experience, during which one seems to float above one's body and to view surrounding activities and hear conversations; a feeling of well-being and peace; a movement into darkness or a tunnel; discovering a bright light and deciding to enter that light; making a decision to either move toward death or to return to life to complete unfinished business; a feeling of sadness upon leaving this blissful dimension.[251] People also report meeting dead relatives, historical religious figures, or beings of light and undergoing a reevaluation of the events in their lives.[252]

According to Ring, "while the process of dying may be scary as we contemplate the end of everything, what we enter into at the moment of death is so magnificent, so beautiful, so full of love, that it's a very powerful source of hope and comfort."[253] Some believe that the near-death experience is a glimpse of the afterlife or of past lives.[254] Some neurologists consider NDEs hallucinations of a dying brain.[255] Researchers Justine Owens, Ian Stevenson, and Emily Cook reported that the experiences of 30 people who merely thought they were going to die were remarkably similar to the experiences of 28 people who were in fact desperately ill, which suggests both physiological and psychological causes.[256]

We cannot be sure that a near-death experience is truly like death itself. Still, it may be reassuring to hear that a nationwide Gallup poll conducted in 1982 found that fully a third of the 8 million Americans who reported having had a near-death experience "recall being in an ecstatic or visionary state."[257] Death, then, may not only be nontraumatic but actually an experience of transcendent joy.

The Emotional Stages of Dying The final act may bring "intense feelings of joy, love, and peace," as Raymond Moody put it in his book *Life After Life*.[258] But getting there, particularly if it is a slow process, as for someone with a terminal illness, can be agonizing. Based on observations of dying patients, psychiatrist Elisabeth Kübler-Ross described five stages of feelings or behavior that she says constitute adjustment to death.[259] (*See* ● *Figure 35.4.*)

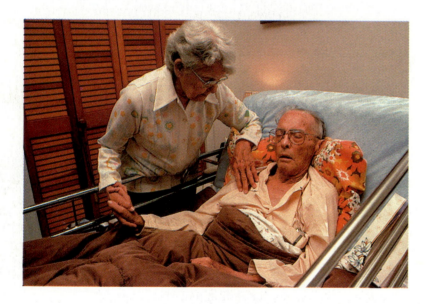

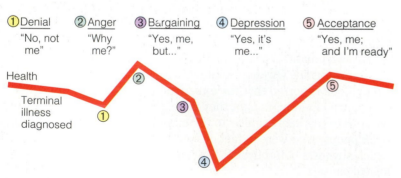

● **Figure 35.4 Kübler-Ross's five stages of adjustment to death**

1. *Stage 1—Denial* ("*No, not me; it cannot be true*"): Told that he or she is going to die, a terminally ill patient will first show *denial*—disbelief. Patients will refuse to acknowledge their condition, and may visit several physicians and perhaps alternative healers (such as faith healers). Denial may actually be helpful because it allows patients to gather their resources for the grim days to come.

2. *Stage 2—Anger* ("*Why me?*"): Patients now begin to feel resentment, that they've been cheated. In *anger* they vent their fears, frustration, and rage about their impending death against relatives, doctors, and nurses.

    If you are trying to give comfort to a dying person, this is where you can offer solace and patience.

3. *Stage 3—Bargaining* ("*Get me through this, God* [*or Doctor*], *and I'll give half my money to the church* [*or hospital*]"): In this stage, the patient may try to *bargain*—perhaps with God, a religious leader, or even the doctor—in which in return for the extension of life he or she will promise good behavior. Some people undergo religious conversions at this time.

4. *Stage 4—Depression* ("*All I can do is wait for the bitter end*"): The stage of *depression* is one of grieving for one's anticipated death—and for the loss of friends and loved ones and of unfinished work. Sighing, crying, and prolonged periods of silence are to be expected.

    If you are trying to offer comfort to someone dying you can be helpful by simply listening, not trying to cheer him or her up. If the patient shows signs of wanting to be alone, you should respect this wish.

5. *Stage 5—Acceptance* ("*This is the final rest before the long journey*"): In *acceptance*, the final stage, the person is psychologically ready to die, seeing the moment as inevitable. He or she does not wish to be moved by news of the outside world, even news of a new treatment that might prolong life. Kübler-Ross says this stage "is almost void of feelings. It is as if the pain has gone, the struggle is over, and there comes a time for 'the final rest before the long journey' as one patient phrased it."[260]

If the person asks to see only a few friends or visitors, as he or she begins separating from the present, you can honor those wishes. If you are the principal companion, you may be the one the dying person wishes to have for support.

Just as life is not simple, neither is death. Not all people proceed through these stages in just this way. Some people skip some stages, some stages may occur at the same time, some may not occur in the order given here. And throughout the process, denial may return from time to time. The way people face death is very much the way they face life: the same skills, or lack of them, that they bring to bear on life's other problems will apply here.

Family and close friends may well go through many of the same kinds of emotions as the dying person: denial, anger, bargaining, depression, and finally acceptance. If someone close to you is in the process of dying, you should be alert to these feelings within yourself as well.

Leveling: Telling the Patient the News At one time, in the 1950s, doctors were encouraged to withhold bad news from terminal patients and to tell a relative instead. The reasoning was that, if told directly, the patient might be so shocked, agitated, or depressed that he or she might have a heart attack, stop eating, or commit suicide. Now doctors realize that withholding information impairs their communication with their patients, prevents patients from making choices, puts nurses and family on the spot, and opens themselves to malpractice suits. Worse, says ethicist Bruce Hilton, this silence leaves patients to perform their great leave-taking, perhaps the most important moment of their lives, all alone.[261]

Many patients are less worried about dying than they are about being abandoned or suffering intractable pain, says one physician. When reassured on these two counts, they deal well with approaching death.[262] The National Institute on Aging also found that patients are less afraid of death than they are of pain and chronic disability.[263]

Dying and Pain Perhaps the greatest fear associated with dying is the prospect of having to endure nearly endless, unrelieved pain. A great deal of the time, however, pain is not present. A study of older men and women found that 61% were free of pain on the day they died and over half died in their sleep without pain.[264] Moreover, the majority were in good health the year preceding their deaths.

Terminal patients often do experience a fair amount of physical pain, but nowadays physicians are more conscious of this. Instead of giving painkilling drugs only when the patient asks for it, as was once common practice, doctors now usually prescribe drugs that are delivered in ongoing, timed doses.

Hospices and Homes A **hospice** is a facility or program designed to provide medical and emotional care for terminally ill people. It may be part of a hospital, but more often it is a separate facility entirely or an at-home program because most hospitals are designed to give short-term treatment rather than long-term maintenance. In recent years, there have also been specialized hospices for AIDS patients.[265,266] The staff consists of physicians and nurses, social workers, mental-health and spiritual counselors, and others as needed. Volunteers are widely used, and visiting hours flexible. The hospice tries to make the patient's last days as comfortable and pain-free as possible.

Many people find dying at home a welcome alternative to clinical settings, where they would end their lives in a building full of strangers. However, most families don't have the experience our forebears had of "sitting with the dying"—of having the physical and emotional strain of cleaning, changing, and comforting someone they love. Care-givers need to learn how to use formal support, such as hospice services, home health aides, and social workers, and how to find support systems to meet their own needs so they can effectively administer to the patient.[267]

Dealing with Feelings During Impending Death Care-givers are whipsawed by emotions, many of which correspond to those that people in bereavement must handle. If, for instance, it is your parent that is dying, it can lead you and other family members to reassess your relationships with the dying parent and with each other. "It is a chance to resolve loose ends before it is too late," says one writer. "Knowing that they will soon die often makes parents more willing to discuss topics that had previously been avoided and to reconnect with estranged children."[268] Even close-knit families have many things they wish to settle. Public-health professor Robert Veninga says many people wish they had been able to thank their parents before they died.[269]

Parents who are seriously ill themselves may also have to deal with telling their young children about their disease. The temptation may be to avoid discussing serious illness or impending surgery—to protect children and not worry them. However, children prefer to know rather than be threatened by the unknown.[270]

After Death: The Practicalities After a person dies, there are a number of matters that close family members will have to deal with—all, unfortunately, at a time of considerable emotional turmoil.

- *Death certificate:* A physician or medical examiner will need to fill out and sign a death certificate, which indicates the cause of death and the disposition of the body. The death certificate must be filled out and filed with local authorities. This certificate is needed for survivors to collect on the deceased's life insurance.

- *Autopsy:* If there is uncertainty about the cause of death, an autopsy will be performed to gather evidence, in case there is a criminal or legal proceeding. An **autopsy** is a medical examination of the body after death, which may include the removal of some organs for study.

- *Arrange for donations of organs, if necessary:* If there is no autopsy and the deceased has filled out the Uniform Donor Card or its equivalent, arrange as quickly as possible with a medical school or organ bank to have the organs recovered for surgical transplantation to someone else.

- *Notify all who need to know:* If you are in charge of handling the death arrangements, you or someone you designate will need to telephone family members, close friends, employer, and all others who should be notified personally. You should write an obituary, including time and place of any

memorial service, and send it to the newspapers.

- *Make arrangements for disposition of the body:* Unless the deceased has made arrangements to donate his or her body to a medical school for the purpose of advancing medical science, most people opt to be disposed of in two principal ways:

  (1) *Burial,* the method of disposition of perhaps 80% of bodies, requires the purchase of a cemetery plot, or the body may be *entombed* in above-ground cemetery structures called mausoleums.[271] Most graves are lined with concrete, brick, metal, or other materials, which helps protect ground water.

  (2) *Cremation* is now used in about 17% of deaths, up from 11% in the early 1980s.[272] **Cremation** consists of burning a body at very high temperature (up to 2200°F) until what's left are large bone fragments, which are usually pulverized into sand-like grains (called the *cremains*) for storage in an urn. Ashes may be scattered (state laws permitting), buried, or entombed in vault-like areas called niches. At $200–$500, cremation is considerably cheaper than burial, which averages $5179 when embalming, funeral services, and burial plot and marker are included.[273] (With services and burial plot and marker, cremation averages $2380.)

Funeral Services and Memorial Societies
In 41 states, a family—or another group with the family's consent—has the right to handle all the death arrangements of their deceased without a funeral director. Still, as one woman who herself handled the burial arrangements for her husband pointed out, "Not everyone is inclined—or even able—to build a casket, transport a body, or even, at a time of grief, assemble the information needed for a death certificate or an obituary."[274] Funeral directors (morticians) provide these services.

Besides helping to take care of the paperwork of death certificates and obituaries, funeral directors offer the following services:

- *Embalming:* Once promoted as a defense against the spread of disease (long since discredited), **embalming** is the process of injecting fluids containing formaldehyde into the circulatory system to replace blood. Embalming came about because, at a time when refrigeration was not available, it preserved bodies for later viewing by family members and friends. This is still its principal purpose.

  The average cost of embalming, which is optional (except under certain circumstances), is $226. Other preparations for viewing, such as hairdressing and cosmetology, average $91.

- *Rituals—visiting hours, funeral service, and burial ceremony:* The funeral home will make available a private room for visiting hours or calling hours, in which family and friends may view the body (if the casket is open) or pay their respects to the deceased.

  A funeral service or religious service may take place a few days after death either in a church or in a chapel within the funeral home. After this, the body is then usually transported by hearse, followed by a processional of mourners, to the cemetery, where there is a graveside service.

It is easy for many families to spend great sums of money on embalming, caskets, and burial—where the biggest profits are for the mortician—at a time when they are ill-prepared emotionally to do competitive shopping. As a result, many thoughtful people have joined together to form nonprofit **memorial societies,** which help members make simple, priceworthy burial or cremation arrangements in advance.

Many people also specify in advance that they prefer to have a *memorial service* rather than (or even in addition to) a funeral. This enables the community of mourners to concentrate on the person's life rather than death.

Individualizing Ritual Some death rituals are quite formal, others are less so. In New Orleans, many families in the black community hire a jazz band to lead mourners from the church service to the cemetery. (*See* ● *Figure 35.5.*) Elsewhere families may charter a boat and invite friends of the departed to join them in scattering ashes at sea. In urban ghettos, on the site where lives have ended violently, temporary memorials of flowers and candles spring up. In graveyards, personalized monuments—etched with guitars, flowers, teddy bears, or photographs of the departed—have become widespread and are now referred to as "cemetery art."[275] Or friends will plant a tree or donate money to save a redwood in memory of the deceased. Through such practices, the dead live on in the minds of the survivors.

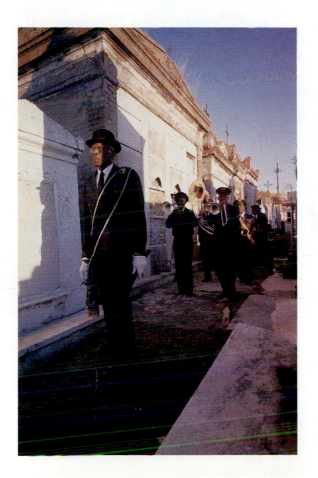

● **Figure 35.5 A New Orleans funeral.** A jazz band leads mourners from church to cemetery.

Grief: Understanding Our Losses

Grief and loss may bring about four stages of mourning—shock, longing, depression and despair, and recovery. Different people respond to grief in different ways, as in anticipatory grief or grieving for the loss of a child, or "bereavement overload" when several loved ones die close together in time. You can help the bereaved to recover by listening and empathizing and by being aware that bereavement takes lots of time.

For some survivors, black crepe and funerals may provide the solace they need to help them through their bereavement. For others, grief really only *begins* with the person's death—particularly if the survivor lost a child or a long-time companion. (*See ● Figure 35.6.*) Young adults are usually spared this agony, but in recent years many have been in a state of shock as the AIDS epidemic has decimated neighborhoods, professions, families, and circles of friends.[276]

Grief and Loss Even if we have never lost someone close to us, we have all been exposed

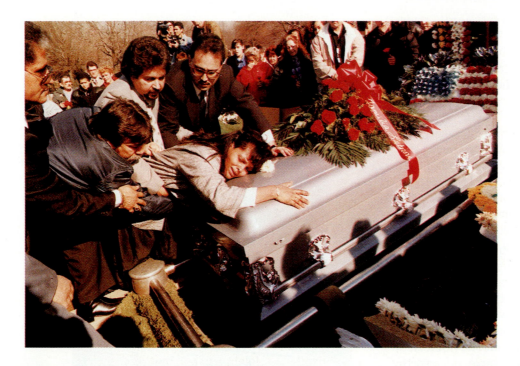

● **Figure 35.6 The agony of grief.** The conventional trappings of mourning, such as funerals, may help some people with bereavement, but for others grief may last for months or years.

66*What is there to say about grief? Grief is a tidal wave that overtakes you, smashes down upon you with unimaginable force. . . .*

Grief means not being able to read more than two sentences at a time. It is walking into rooms with intentions that suddenly vanish. . . .

*Grief makes what others think of you moot. It shears away the masks of normal life and forces brutal honesty before propriety can stop you.*99

—Stephanie Ericsson. (1991, September/October). The agony of grief. *Utne Reader*, pp. 75–78.

to grief because we have all been exposed to *loss*. Some of the losses, says Lillian Chance, a psychiatric nurse specializing in grief counseling, are obvious: "a separation, the end of a romantic relationship, a job loss, a physical infirmity, aging, moving, a child leaving home." Other losses in life are more intimate: "the loss of a cherished dream, of a beloved pet, of innocence, or trust in a friend. . . ."[277]

Any change or turning point in your life—even positive ones, such as marrying or committing to someone, gaining a career opportunity, or, as Chance says, experiencing the "loss of a self-destructive substance abuse"—can bring on the process and feelings of grief.

The Stages of Mourning To be sensitive to a grieving person's needs or your own feelings of loss, it helps to understand that four distinct stages of mourning have been observed, although they do not follow an orderly schedule:[278,279]

- *Stage 1—shock:* Some people during the shock phase seem dazed and distant, others calm and rational. A degree of numbness, disbelief, and detachment nearly always occurs at first. One may feel swept up by a sense of unreality, asking "What happened?" or "Did it really happen?" Becoming involved in the immediate problems associated with the death—taking care of funeral arrangements, out-of-town guests, and the various documents—can postpone the feeling of letdown.

- *Stage 2—longing:* In this stage, the bereaved person has an intense longing to be with the departed person. His or her mind is filled with yearnings, memories, and dreams about the deceased. Some forms of denial or guilt may be present: it's normal to wish the loss had never happened.

- *Stage 3—depression and despair:* The third stage, depression and despair, is expressed in despondency, sudden anger, and disordered thinking. A bereaved person may act irrationally, suddenly changing neighborhoods or buying unaffordable things. Anger may be directed against the departed for "disappointing or deserting" the bereaved.

- *Stage 4—recovery:* The second and third stages can average 18–24 months, although everyone's grief period is different. In the last stage of mourning, recovery, the survivor finally puts the death into perspective and is able to move on. This means realizing there is no returning to normal but creating a new form of normality. It means also recognizing what was not lost, the good that is left in one's life.

Different Responses to Loss Despite these stages, not all people respond to grief in the same way, although generally all start with a period of shock and numbness. Some of the variations are as follows:[280]

- *Anticipatory grief:* When someone is dying of a terminal illness, it allows for **anticipatory grief,** when both the dying person and family and friends can cry and share their affection. This may actually strengthen the attachments during the period before death, thus intensifying the feeling of loss afterward. However, the feelings of the bereaved may be less conflicting.

- *Grief for loss of children:* Experiencing the loss of a child is one of the very hardest things anyone can go through.

  If the loss is of a baby in the first year of life, as in **sudden infant death syndrome (SIDS),** or "crib death," when an apparently healthy infant is unexpectedly found dead in its bed, the parents may be wracked with guilt as well as sadness.

  If the child who died was old enough to have a distinct personality, and if his or her death was violent and sudden (as such deaths often are), the loss is particularly powerful. There may be strong feelings not only of sorrow but also of guilt and anger, which may cause parents (and siblings) to inflict pain on each other, just at a time when they most need each other's support. A self-help group for parents of dead children, The Compassionate Friends, finds that many married couples are driven apart by their different reactions.

  Even when a child is fully grown, the loss never really heals for many parents and siblings. One father who lost his 17-year-old daughter in a freak auto accident says that even 2 years later he cannot handle her death. When he has lunch with friends and the conversation turns to children and how they're doing at college, he has to get up and leave the table. "Not that they're doing anything wrong—it's perfectly natural for them to talk about their kids," he says. "But Meg would have been a student at Ohio U. this year, and I am unable to sit there and listen."[281] The feelings of devastation are even more intense if the child or young person committed suicide.[282]

- *Grief for loss of parents:* "It happens without you even consciously thinking about it," 44-year-old Ernestina Higuera said. "Maybe you'll be driving to work . . . , and suddenly you start crying in the car."[283] She is talking about experiencing the death of her parents, both in their 80s, 3 years before.

  According to one researcher, Andrew Scharlach, at least 25% of adults still cry or become upset when they think of their deceased parent—even 1–5 years after the parent's death. More than 20% continue to be preoccupied with thoughts of the parent.[284] Especially profound responses among adult children include (1) an overwhelming sense of feeling orphaned, and (2) the sense that one no longer fits the role of a child. As Scharlach says, "As long as a parent is alive, there is somebody between us and what we fear." The death of a parent, particularly the second parent, can also profoundly change the relationships of adult siblings toward each other as they reevaluate the meaning of family and their roles within it.[285]

- *Differences in grieving between men and women:* Men and women tend to express their grieving differently, although the pain is as strong for both. In general, women tend to use their social-support systems and men do not, mainly because women have more friends than men do and tend to use them as supports.[286] Because men tend to keep their grief to themselves, they are more likely to feel lonely and depressed than women in similar circumstances.

  When one partner in a marriage dies, often the other does soon after. Indeed, mortality rates for widowed people in every age group are higher than for married peo-

ple.[287] Men are at greater risk, particularly if the wife dies suddenly rather than after a long illness—perhaps, speculates sociologist Ken R. Smith, women usually fill the care-giver's role and men are not prepared for the loss of their nurturers.[288] In some instances, however, widowed men have gotten together to meet weekly and help each other get started again.[289] On the other hand, as widows many women become more independent, finding satisfaction in careers and friends and living as individuals rather than as one-half of a pair.[290]

- *The grief of children:* How do you explain the inexplicable to a child under 12 (or even under 18) whose parent recently died? One out of 20 American children suffers the loss of a parent, and others suffer bereavements of other sorts, from the loss of a pet to friends moving away.[291]

  According to behavioral scientist Phyllis R. Silverman, most children come through the first 1–2 years after a parent's death quite well, but 20% may be at risk for behavioral and emotional problems in the first year. Preschoolers may have two ideas at once: that they won't see the person again but also that they can undo it with wishful thinking. Slightly older children may not show much sadness at the time, then fall apart a few years later when they realize, for example, that their father won't be present for their high-school graduation.

  Protecting children by not talking about the dead person is a mistake because it makes the child think you don't miss the person very much. Moreover, although children can't always talk about how they feel, they need to talk about who the person was; they need opportunities to remember, says Silverman. In addition, the loss of a parent is almost a double loss for a child because the surviving parent is temporarily unavailable to the child in at least some ways. Children who experience the death of a sibling or parent may feel responsible or angry and worry about the surviving parent.[292]

- *Bereavement overload:* **Bereavement overload** is a state of feeling overwhelmed emotionally when one experiences the death of several loved ones over a short period of time and is unable to reach acceptance of the first death before having to mourn the second.[293] Until recently, this was most apt to happen to the elderly, but the AIDS epidemic has caused the same thing to happen in environments such as offices in which younger people are together.[294,295]

It's important to understand that everyone who loses someone close is at risk for psychological and physical illness: a child whose parent dies or a husband whose wife dies is particularly vulnerable.[296]

Helping the Bereaved to Recover What can you do to help a bereaved person? Here are some suggestions:

- *Listen and empathize:* The first two tasks of grief are to accept the reality of the loss and experience the pain.[297] Thus, you can be aware that powerful emotions are at work and that, if the feelings are bottled up and never dealt with, the person could be in a continual state of depression and anxiety. Thus, you should be prepared to listen and empathize. Indeed, you should try to detect if the bereaved person is hiding his or her feelings.

- *Be aware bereavement takes lots of time:* Months and even years may pass before the bereaved person can finally be said to have passed into the stage of recovery. Throughout he or she may demand sympathy and social support—and you should be prepared to offer it. Do not discourage saving photographs, talking about shared experiences, or visiting the gravesite. Indeed, **anniversary reactions**—expressions of grief and sorrow on birthdays or the anniversary of the death, which may initiate a new burst of mourning—are to be expected.

Eventually, the bereaved person should be able to confront the loss and, just as important, recognize what was *not* lost. At that point, the bereaved may have developed a deeper appreciation of human relationships.[298]

Strategy for Living: The Will to Live and a "Good Death"

The will to live may postpone death.

One study shows that some people seem to actually tell death to wait, that the *will to live* matters. For instance, it is folk wisdom to say that people often stave off death for important occasions. However, two studies found sharp drops in death rates among Chinese women before the Harvest Moon Festival and Jewish men before Passover.[299] The delayed deaths were most noticeable in stroke, heart disease, and cancer cases. Perhaps the most famous example of a person delaying death was that of Thomas Jefferson, author of the Declaration of Independence. He died July 4, 1826, exactly 50 years after the document's signing and only after he had asked his physician, "It is the Fourth?" and received the assurance, "It soon will be."

Most people want to die a "good death," a swift, pain-free, dignified death surrounded by people they love. In the meantime, there are things to do, people to be close to, a world to see—the parts that constitute our "will to live." Think about what is in your life that would make you want to postpone your mortality for a "good death."

800-HELP

HOSPICELINK. 800-331-1620. Provides information on hospices and referrals to local hospices. Also offers supportive listening

The Living Bank Organ Donor Registry and Referral Service. 800-528-2971. Sends information to anyone interested in becoming an organ donor

National Funeral Director Association Funeral Service Consumer Arbitration Program. 800-662-7666. Acts as liaison or arbitrator between consumers and funeral services

The Sudden Infant Death Syndrome Alliance. 800-221-7437. Provides information on "crib death"

United Network for Organ Sharing. 800-24-DONOR. Provides information on becoming an organ donor

Developing Resilience: Just Do It

Check which of the following you would agree with:

__ **1.** My life does not belong to me, I belong to it.

__ **2.** Life is difficult.

__ **3.** Things happen to others; I was not singled out by the universe.

__ **4.** Feelings can't be controlled, behavior can be.

All of these are expressions of certain outlooks on life—subjective interpretations. Although there are no "right answers," how you feel about these expressions may have an important bearing on your resiliency—that is, on your ability to bounce back from life's travails. *Resiliency* is defined as your ability to cope with disruptive, stressful, or challenging life events in a way that provides you with additional protective and coping skills.[302]

1. "My Life Does Not Belong to Me, I Belong to It"

This awareness, stated by Spanish philosopher José Ortega y Gasset, is brutally thrust on some people. For instance, Richard Carmichael had a routine but comfortable life working at a computer job for an insurance firm, jogging in the evenings, and sometimes shooting pool with friends. Then he inexplicably started dropping things and falling down and learned he had multiple sclerosis, a chronic, debilitating, incurable disease of the nervous system. Becoming one in five Americans suffering from a chronic illness, Carmichael soon realized that he could never go back to his old life. Indeed, he was uncertain that he even had the strength to continue.[303]

Coming to terms with chronic illness, points out psychiatry professor JoAnn LeMaistre, is like dealing with grief. (Indeed, as with grief, patients react to chronic illness in stages: crisis, isolation, anger, reconstruction, intermittent depression, and renewal.) However, she says, there is one important difference: "When you lose someone or something dear to you, a chapter has finally closed and you must face that finality. Chronically ill people, however, must deal with a grave assault on their identity as well as future threats to whatever sense of their selves remains. In fact, for many people, becoming chronically ill feels a lot like having died."[304]

Even without chronic illness, everyone has imperatives in his or her life or must sometimes face disasters or traumatic life changes, so that life indeed seems to own us rather than we own it. What are or have been such imperatives or crises for you? How did you or do you deal with them?

2. "Life Is Difficult"

These three words, with which psychiatrist M. Scott Peck begins *The Road Less Traveled*, have become familiar to many people in the more than 500 weeks the book has been on the best-seller lists.[305] The message of the mass media and many other voices of our society, however, is that the purpose of life is to be *happy*—fulfilled, comfortable. "If we're not," says Peck, "we feel there must be something wrong with us."[306]

This, he says, is a dreadful lie. The purpose of life, Peck thinks, is not to achieve happiness. Rather, he suggests, "We are here to learn." Indeed, one of the things we need to learn is that life, in fact, *is* difficult. And, surprisingly, once we understand and accept this, Peck says, "then life is no longer difficult."

A task of all human beings is to learn to endure. However, the challenge is to go beyond that and not just to endure but to *prevail*—to go forward despite the stresses of pain, uncertainty, and limitations and to overcome the obstacles. Among the terms psychologists use to describe people who seem to be more stress-resistant than others is *psychological hardiness*.[307,308] Hardiness is a combination of three personality traits—*commitment*, *challenge*, and *control*. Commitment means that you understand and pursue your goals and values. Challenge means you take charge and even seek out and solve problem situations. Control means you have a reasonably strong belief that your destiny is affected by your own actions rather than by fate and luck. With these three characteristics—which can be learned—life's difficulties become not threats but hurdles to be triumphed over.

3. "These Things Happen to Others; I Was Not Singled Out by the Universe"

Learning this lesson, says psychology professor Salvatore Maddi, is the first step in what he calls "hardiness training."[309] It's important to put into perspective, he says, the traumas of your life, such as an abusive childhood, poverty, parental discord or divorce, the death of a parent or sibling, or severe physical or mental illness in your family. Another writer suggests that building resilience begins with understanding that "falling apart" following significantly stressful events is a necessary prelude to personal renewal.[310]

Resilient people have been found to share six qualities, according to psychology professor Raymond Flannery, who has studied 1200 men and women who have triumphed over great stress.[311,312] Besides the commitment and challenge attributes mentioned above, such people maintain a sense of humor and make sensible lifestyle choices (in diet, exercise, and relax-

ation). Two other qualities are (1) they are guided by the principles of the great religions of the world, such as the golden rule, even if they don't go to church, and (2) they gain emotional support from being with others.

Human development professor Emmy Werner, who has studied resilience, suggests that people wanting to build their stress resistance seek out support by joining a club or church or seeking out friends and mentors.[313,314] She also advises those who have experienced setbacks early in life to take advantage of "second chance" opportunities for education, employment, and skills training.

4. "Feelings Can't Be Controlled, Behavior Can Be"

This statement reflects parts of a Japanese philosophy known as Morita, or Constructive Living (CL), a "lifeway" or practical strategy for dealing with life's difficulties. Constructive Living is based on three action-oriented principles: (1) Accept your feelings. (2) Know your purpose. (3) Do what needs to be done.[315,316]

The CL philosophy assumes that feelings can't be determined or controlled, but behavior can be, according to David Reynolds. "Mentally healthy people get done what needs to get done, regardless of how they're feeling," says Reynolds, who is one of CL's leading American proponents. "If we did only what we felt like doing, we'd never get anything done."

People familiar with Nike's slogan can easily relate to the CL doctrine: *Just Do It.* Or, as another writer puts it, "Life is short, after all, and we have things to do."[317]

In These Chapters:

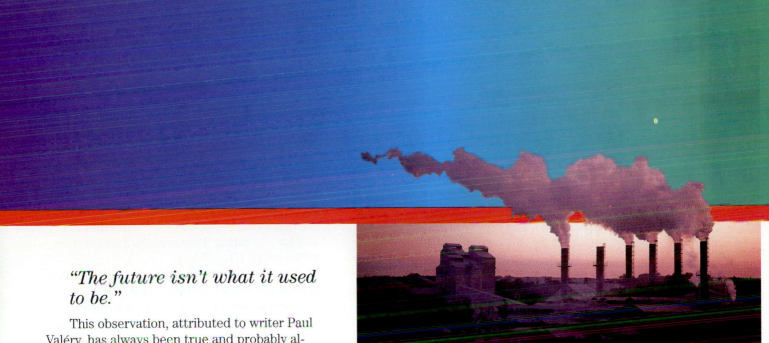

"The future isn't what it used to be."

This observation, attributed to writer Paul Valéry, has always been true and probably always will be. We sense this because, from time to time, we see something that reminds us of the past and at the same time reminds us of how we then *thought* the future was going to be.

It is as though with a time traveler's vision one can look through a shopping center and see the fruit trees that used to be there, or look at a superhighway and see the country road now buried underneath. We think: "I once thought that orchard and that rural road would be there forever!" In our mental landscape, we often prefer that the future not be radically different from the present.

Once in a while we also see reminders of ways we thought we would handle future threats, as when coming across a faded nuclear fallout shelter sign. Considering the awesome power of nuclear weapons, those shelters probably would not have done much good. Fortunately, *that* future didn't turn out as we anticipated either.

These ruminations give rise to an important thought: do we control the environment around us, or does it control us? Our environment presents us with two challenges—personal and global:

- *Handling personal environmental challenges to your health:* Unless you are pretty much removed from human society, you will always be exposed to environmental threats to your health: noise, radiation, chemicals, impurities in the air and water. How do you defend yourself against such personal irritants as high-decibel electronic noise, indoor chemicals that make your eyes water, or strange-tasting water? Fortunately, there *are* things you can do to control these threats, and the first chapter of this unit shows you how.

- *Handling global environmental challenges to your health:* The kinds of worldwide environmental problems that fill the headlines—billions of people overrunning the planet, widespread poverty and famine, careless handling of toxic and nuclear wastes, acid rain, global warming, ozone holes over Antartica, war—may eventually affect you personally, if they don't now. These threats may look very much like a case of the environment controlling you. What is one person, for instance, going to do about the growing population problem, which has such an impact on so many other environmental problems? Fortunately, there are things you—in concerted action with others—can do to minimize these threats, too.

The future will never turn out as planned because people in combination with the effects of technology make tomorrow always unpredictable. That does not mean that we should give up and live only for today. The best reason why not was stated by scientist Charles F. Kettering:

We should all be concerned about the future because we will have to spend the rest of our lives there.

36   Personal Environmental Challenges

▶ Explain the effects of noise and how the decibel scale works.

▶ Describe the controversy about possible hazards from electromagnetic fields.

▶ Discuss ionizing radiation and radioactivity.

▶ Explain the factors behind sick building syndrome and environmental illness.

▶ Explain the effects of air pollution on health.

▶ Discuss the problems of solid waste disposal, especially of toxic and nuclear wastes.

When we hear the words "environment" and "pollution," we may be accustomed to thinking of supertanker oil spills, old tires and trash in vacant lots, the sunset as an orange ball sinking through a brown haze. Certainly, you may think, these things might have some long-range effects on your health. However, it may be hard to get excited about them, because they seem to have no *immediate* connection to your life.

Actually, though, environmental health begins as an *extremely* personal matter. Consider, for instance, the impact of noise.

Noise Pollution

The intensity of sound is measured in decibels, whereby each 10-point increase on the decibel scale is 10 times as loud. Exposure to excessive noise produces hearing loss and stress. Premature hearing loss is being found more among younger Americans, often because of amplified music.

Mike Negron, 20, who lives near Fordham University in the Bronx, New York, didn't get it. So what if his car had a stereo system consisting of four 300-watt SuperPro speakers, a 280-watt Sherwood amplifier, and a pair of powerful tweeters. "I don't play it loud," he said. Nevertheless, Bronx police seized Negron's car for noise violation when they measured sound coming from it exceeding the legal threshold of 80 decibels measured at 50 feet.[1] A **decibel** is a unit for measuring the intensity of sound. (*See* ● *Figure 36.1.*)

How much is 80 decibels? Actually, it's only as loud as a ringing alarm clock 2 feet away, or a vacuum cleaner, or a car alarm, or a minibike, yet it's the beginning of the danger zone for loss of hearing. (The U.S. Navy is trying to reduce noise aboard hospital ships to below 65 decibels because doctors complain they cannot hear their patients' hearts using stethoscopes.)[2] Truly loud music, such as that heard in the front row at a rock concert, might be 120 decibels (the same as a jackhammer at 3 feet); a blaring stereo might be 130 decibels (equal to a jet engine at 100 feet). Nevertheless, if Negron's "boombox car" registered 80 decibels at 50 feet away, imagine what it was like inside the car: amplified car stereos can hit 140 decibels at full volume—like standing near a jet taking off.

What's important to note is that, on the decibel scale, 20 is not twice as loud as 10 but rather *10 times as loud.* That is, each 10-decibel increase represents a tenfold increase in the intensity of sound. Thus, *50 decibels is 1000 times louder than 20 decibels.*

The Effects of Noise   A study of remote African tribes on the Sudanese-Ethiopian border found that men in their 70s could hear sounds as faint as a whisper across a distance the length of a football field.[3] By contrast, one in three Americans over 65 has a hearing loss great enough to make communication difficult. Now hearing loss is being found among people much younger: in one study, 6 of 10 first-year students at the University of Tennessee at Knoxville were found to have hearing loss of the kind formerly found mainly among elderly people.[4] In a survey in Fountain Valley, California, researchers testing hearing found failure rates of 13% among high-school seniors, a significant increase from 10 years earlier.[5] Once damaged, the destruction of the sensory cells in the ear can never be restored. To see if you might have a problem with your hearing, try the Self Discovery. (*See Self Discovery 36.1.*)

Exposure to excessive noise has two principal effects:

- *Hearing loss:* The U.S. Public Health Service says almost half of the 81 million Americans with hearing loss owe their impairment to noise exposure.[6]

  A person who has a 50-decibel loss cannot hear sounds that have a loudness of 50 decibels or less. A 16- or 25-decibel loss is considered a slight loss, causing problems only if listening conditions are poor, as at a noisy party. A loss of 26–40 decibels is a mild hearing loss; background noise and distant speech are hard to hear. A loss of 41–55 decibels is a moderate hearing loss; conversation can be heard at a distance of 3–5 feet, but understanding speech is a strain, and full-time use of a hearing aid is necessary. A loss of 56 decibels or more becomes much more difficult to deal with.

  What is it like to have a hearing loss? Among the problems faced by the hearing-impaired are the following:[7]

  (1) *Frustration*, because they miss a lot of what's said and have to ask people to repeat themselves

  (2) *Fear of embarrassment*, because they make inappropriate responses during conversation

  (3) *Tension*, because they must be constantly alert for fear of missing something important

  (4) *Exhaustion*, because listening is not a passive activity; it requires that they actively attempt to fill in what they miss and predict what will be said

- *Stress:* Prolonged noise above 100 decibels (subway, video arcade) is uncomfortable for most people. However, you may have noticed that a noise need not be loud to keep you from falling asleep. Because you can't control the traffic noise, the bass on your neighbor's stereo, the building air-conditioning, or whatever, it becomes upsetting.

  Noise increases tension. As the "fight-or-flight" mechanisms are triggered, adrenaline rises, increasing heart rate and blood pressure. Various studies have linked prolonged exposure to noise of 85 decibels (heard on a crowded school bus) up to 115 decibels (Sony Walkman) with an "assort-

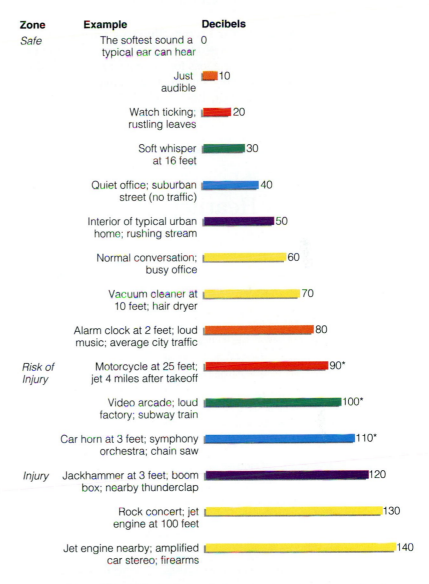

Zone	Example	Decibels
Safe	The softest sound a typical ear can hear	0
	Just audible	10
	Watch ticking; rustling leaves	20
	Soft whisper at 16 feet	30
	Quiet office; suburban street (no traffic)	40
	Interior of typical urban home; rushing stream	50
	Normal conversation; busy office	60
	Vacuum cleaner at 10 feet; hair dryer	70
	Alarm clock at 2 feet; loud music; average city traffic	80
Risk of Injury	Motorcycle at 25 feet; jet 4 miles after takeoff	90*
	Video arcade; loud factory; subway train	100*
	Car horn at 3 feet; symphony orchestra; chain saw	110*
Injury	Jackhammer at 3 feet; boom box; nearby thunderclap	120
	Rock concert; jet engine at 100 feet	130
	Jet engine nearby; amplified car stereo; firearms	140

*Note: The maximum exposure allowed on the job by federal law, in hours per day, is as follows: 90 decibels—8 hours; 100 decibels—2 hours; 110 decibels—1/2 hour.

● **Figure 36.1 How loud is loud?** An increase of 10 decibels represents a tenfold increase in acoustic energy or intensity of sound, but the human ear perceives these 10 decibels as a doubling of loudness. Thus, the 100 decibels of a subway train sounds a great deal more than twice as loud as the 50 decibels of a rushing stream.

ment of physical, mental, and social problems ranging from hypertension to helplessness, from learning disabilities to birth defects," says one report.[8]

Strategy for Living: Shutting Out Noise

Workers exposed to factory noise may not experience hearing loss for as long as 10 years.[9] Musicians playing amplified music may run the risk a lot sooner. In 1984, punk-rock musician Kathy

Peck woke up after a concert with a ringing in her ears that wouldn't go away. Today Peck, who has lost 40% of her hearing and wears a hearing aid, is active in an organization called HEAR (Hearing Education and Awareness for Rockers), which urges rock musicians and concertgoers to wear earplugs.[10] Even home stereos, headset radios and tape players, and car stereo systems can be dangerous when played at the levels that many people prefer.

Here are some tips for preventing premature hearing impairment:

- *Turn it down!* "People with more than moderate hearing loss can probably no longer appreciate the nuances of the very music that brought about their disability," points out one writer.[11] Walkabout stereos, such as Sony Walkmans, are commonly operated by some people at levels of around 107 decibels. This is about twice as loud as 100 decibels, which federal law prohibits workers from enduring longer than 1 hour a day.

  People wearing headphones often turn up the volume to block out the sounds of noisy surroundings. However, if it's loud enough to be heard by a person next to you, according to experts' rule of thumb, it can cause damage if used more than 2 hours a day, or even less for some individuals.[12]

- *Watch out for loud environments—and deal with them:* You know you're in a too-loud place when you have trouble hearing someone a few feet away, when you have to raise your voice to be heard—or when afterward your ears are ringing or you have a temporary hearing loss.

  If you find yourself in a loud place (bowling alley, disco), get out after a couple hours, if only to take a short walk. If you engage in a noisy activity in which, for safety reasons, you can't protect your ears, such as motorcycling or snowmobiling, take breaks to give your ears a rest.[13]

- *Use earplugs—even at concerts:* Record producer Jeff Baxter was a guitarist in the 1970s with the rock groups Steely Dan and the Doobie Brothers. He was noted for blocking out the booming sound of onstage amplifiers with an earmuff-style headset—

SELF DISCOVERY 36.1

How's Your Hearing?

Answer each of the following statements "true" or "false."

	True	False
1. Sounds are loud enough, but not clear.	____	____
2. Soft sounds, such as my watch ticking, birds singing, and voices from another room, are very difficult to hear or simply cannot be heard anymore.	____	____
3. People often seem to be mumbling or talking too fast.	____	____
4. Understanding what is being said is very difficult when there is any background noise.	____	____
5. Group conversations are difficult to follow.	____	____
6. Loud sounds may seem more annoying than before.	____	____
7. My hearing is good when I'm fresh and rested, but seems to deteriorate quickly.	____	____
8. My family tells me that the television or stereo is uncomfortably loud for them.	____	____

If you answered true to one or more of these questions, it's possible you may have a hearing loss, even one that you're not conscious of. To take it to the next step, call 800-322-EARS (in Pennsylvania, 800-345-EARS) to be referred to a number in your area that offers a simple hearing test by phone. The 800 number operates Monday through Friday 9 A.M. to 5 P.M., Eastern Standard Time. The local numbers operate 24 hours a day.

When you call the local number, a recording will play four tones for each ear and a message. You should hear all the tones. If not, you may need to have your hearing checked by a professional. This service is provided by Occupational Hearing Service, which can also make referrals to audiologists and ear, nose, and throat doctors. You can also call the American Speech-Language-Hearing Association at 800-638-8255.

Source: Deborah Huning, certified audiologist. Cited in: Anonymous. (1992, June). Danger signs of hearing problems. *Men's Health*, p. 10.

the reason, he says, that he still has his hearing today and so is able to produce records.[14]

Baxter says that people can enjoy the experience of being surrounded by sound at a very loud concert but still protect their hearing by wearing foam earplugs, which let sound pass through but cut down on the volume.

- *Minimize the sound of the environment:* If you live in a noisy place, you can dampen sound by using fabric, rugs, curtains, and acoustic tile. Noisy appliances, such as blenders or computer printers, can be put on rubber pads or covered with sound-proofing material. If street noise or loud neighbors bother you, you can try turning on the fan in your air conditioner or buying "white noise" machines, which give off a sound similar to that which you hear on a TV channel that's not receiving. Static-like white noise acts as a masking device, drowning out unwanted sounds.

It's important to note that susceptibility to noise varies. Some people can tolerate sound that would damage the hearing of someone else. The sound level of a radio that you find acceptable may drive other people on the beach or in the neighborhood to distraction.

Electromagnetic Fields

Electromagnetic fields are fields of electrical and magnetic energy, which travel in waves across the electromagnetic spectrum, with low-frequency waves at one end and high-frequency waves at the other end. Prolonged exposure to high-frequency waves, such as X rays, may be dangerous to health. There is speculation that exposure to low-frequency waves, such as those put out by power lines, computers, and cellular phones, may also be hazardous.

In the 1980s, large numbers of people suddenly became aware that one of the foundations of our high-tech society—electromagnetic waves—might adversely affect our health. The subject took on more urgency with the prospect that the world stood on the brink of what some called "the wireless revolution," with computers and telephones becoming untethered from connecting cords and operating on waves of electromagnetic radiation transmitted through the air.

The Effects of Electromagnetic Fields

Electromagnetic fields are fields of electrical energy and magnetic energy, which travel in waves. These waves cover an *electromagnetic spectrum,* with low-frequency waves at one end and high-frequency waves at the other. If we were to represent this spectrum in terms of appliances and machines, it would start with video-display terminals and hair dryers at the low-frequency end and range up through electric heaters, walkie-talkies, cellular phones, radar, microwave ovens, infrared "nightscope" binoculars, ultraviolet-light tanning machines, X ray machines, and gamma-ray machines for food irradiation at the high-frequency end. (*See ● Figure 36.2.*)

The higher the wave frequency, the greater the energy. Thus, we know that X rays, which are very high frequency, have so much energy that they can ionize atoms (release electrons from atoms). They can also cause cancer, which is why physicians and dentists recommend limiting your exposure to X rays. This has been known for years. What is a relatively recent concern, however, is whether *low*-frequency waves may be harmful. Does exposure to high-voltage power lines, video-display terminals, microwave ovens, and cellular phones lead ultimately to ill health? The answer is: so far no one is sure.

In the United States, a 1991 study by John M. Peters and Stephanie J. London suggested that childhood leukemia is approximately doubled in homes with higher concentrations of nearby electric power lines. It also appeared to be somewhat higher in homes reporting frequent use of appliances such as electric hair dryers and black-and-white television sets.[15] Two 1992 long-term epidemiological studies in Sweden showed clear associations between exposure to extra-low frequency fields and brain cancer and leukemia.[16] A 1992 study in Finland found a correlation between extra-low frequency fields and miscarriages in women who use video-display terminals at work.[17]

The foregoing studies investigated the effects of extra-low frequency (ELF) fields and health. Even less is known about radio frequency (RF) fields and microwave fields, which are higher on the electromagnetic spectrum. (*Refer back to Figure 36.2.*) In January 1993, a man alleged in a lawsuit that use of a cellular phone caused his wife's fatal brain cancer, although this has not been substantiated in other cases.[18] Two 1990 studies by biophysicist Stephen Cleary showed that normal human blood cells and one type of cancer cell grew abnormally after 2-hour exposures to the frequency at which microwave ovens operate or a lower frequency.[19]

The risk to your health from electromagnetic radiation seems far less than that from not giving up smoking or failing to engage in a regular program of aerobic exercise. Still, it may be that, in the term used by the Environmental Protection Agency, we should all exercise *prudent avoidance*—do the easy things but not change our whole lives or spend a fortune to minimize exposure to electromagnetic fields.[20,21]

Strategy for Living: Reducing Electromagnetic Radiation Most people move in and out of extremely low frequency (ELF) fields throughout the day, and probably brief exposures will not put anyone at risk. However, in the interests of "prudent avoidance," it might be wise to avoid prolonged exposure within a field. Thus, you might want to analyze where you and any children for whom you are responsible spend most of your time in one place. The following are some tips for reducing ELF:[22–24]

- *Reduce children's exposure.* For example, keep them 5 feet away from color TVs.
- *Distance yourself from appliances.* For example, move clocks and fans 3 feet away from your bed.
- *Avoid ELF-producing devices at work.* Stay an arm's length from video display terminals.

If you're particularly concerned about ELF fields, have your home measured with a gauss-meter (available for about $100). Some utilities will do this for you.

Hazardous Radiation

High-intensity radiation, called *ionizing radiation*, can form ions, or electrical charges, that can damage living tissue. Overexposure to radioactive particles can produce radiation sickness. Sources of radiation, which is measured in rads and rems, are medical and dental X rays and radioactive elements, radon, nuclear reactors, and nuclear weapons plants.

The word *radiation* is a scary word to many people, evoking memories of the nuclear age's worst consequences (the World War II atom-bombing of Hiroshima) and terrible acci-

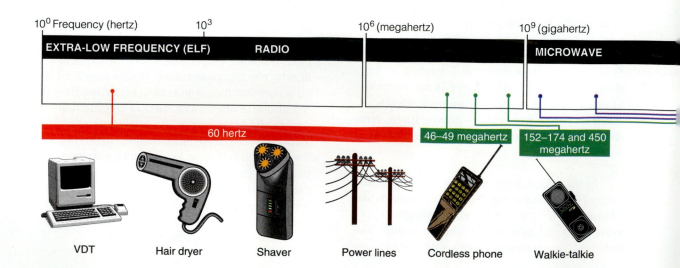

VDT	Hair dryer	Shaver	Power lines	Cordless phone	Walkie-talkie

dents (the 1979 near-meltdown of the nuclear power plant at Pennsylvania's Three Mile Island). In point of fact, however, we are surrounded by radiation all the time—from the sun, mineral deposits, industrial wastes, and other things. Most of this exposure produces negligible health risks. What we are concerned about in this section, however, is the kind that *does* produce health risks.

Radiation is simply energy sent or emitted in the form of waves or particles. Thus, it includes the low-intensity electromagnetic radiation we just described of radio waves, microwaves, infrared light, and ordinary light; this is called **nonionizing electromagnetic radiation.** However, radiation also includes high-intensity **ionizing radiation,** fast-moving particles or high-energy radiation (such as gamma rays) capable of dislodging electrons from atoms they hit. The significance of ionizing radiation is that it can form charged **ions**—atoms with positive (+) or negative (−) electrical charges—that can react with and damage living tissue.

Radiation: How Much Is Too Much? In small doses, ionizing radiation such as X rays can benefit your health. High doses, however, whether from radiation for cancer therapy or from a nuclear accident, are harmful, perhaps even fatal. Of particular concern are radioactivity, which emanates from substances such as uranium, and radiation sickness, which can be fatal:

- *Radioactivity:* **Radioactivity** refers to the emission of harmful rays or particles from the nucleus of an atom. Radioactive materials emit three kinds of particles or rays:

  (1) *Alpha particles* cannot pass through skin and are not considered hazardous unless the substance is eaten or breathed.

  (2) *Beta particles* penetrate the body slightly; if the radioactive substance is eaten, it can affect bones and the thyroid gland.

  (3) *Gamma rays,* which can pass through the human body, are the most hazardous.

- *Radiation sickness:* The result of overexposure to radioactive materials is **radiation sickness,** characterized by low white-

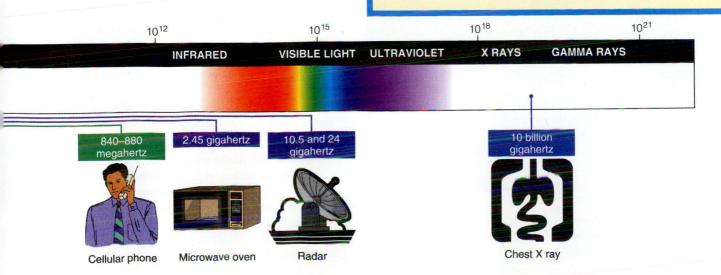

● **Figure 36.2 The electromagnetic spectrum.** Electromagnetic waves are produced by rhythmic variations, or cycles, in electrical and magnetic fields. *Hertz* is a unit for measuring the frequency, or cycle, of the waves. In the United States, the electricity sent out from power plants is 60 hertz. The higher the wave frequency, the greater the energy.

10^{12} 10^{15} 10^{18} 10^{21}

INFRARED   VISIBLE LIGHT   ULTRAVIOLET   X RAYS   GAMMA RAYS

840–880 megahertz

2.45 gigahertz

10.5 and 24 gigahertz

10 billion gigahertz

Cellular phone   Microwave oven   Radar   Chest X ray

How Much Annual Radiation Are You Exposed to?

Follow the directions to fill in the column at right to find out your estimated annual dose of radiation, in millirems (mrems):

	Millirems
Natural Radiation	
1. Cosmic rays from space:	
At sea level (U.S. average)	40
Add 1 mrem for every 100 feet you live above sea level	___
2. Radiation in rocks and soil (U.S. average)	55
3. Radiation from air, water, and food (U.S. average)	25
Radiation from Human Activities	
4. Medical and dental X rays and treatments (U.S. average)	80
5. Add 40 if you live in a stone or brick building	___
6. Add 40 if you work in a stone or brick building	___
7. Add 40 if you smoke one pack of cigarettes per day	___
8. Nuclear weapons fallout (U.S. average)	4
9. Add 2 for each 1500 miles of air travel per year	___
10. Add 4 for each 2 hours of exposure to television per day	___
11. Add 4 for each 2 hours of exposure to computer screen per day	___
12. Occupational exposure (U.S. average)	0.8
13. Add 76 if live next to nuclear power plant with boiling water reactor	___
14. Add 4 if live next to nuclear power plant with pressurized water reactor	___
15. Add 0.6 if live within 5 miles of nuclear power plant	___
16. Exposure to normal operation of nuclear power plants, fuel processing, and research facilities (U.S. average)	0.1
17. Miscellaneous radiation exposure—industrial wastes, some watch dials, smoke detectors (U.S. average)	2
Your total points:	___

Interpretation

The average annual exposure for people in the United States is 230 mrems—130 from natural radiation and 100 from human activities. Your exposure could be higher, depending on occupation, location of residence, health behavior, medical tests, and the like.

The International Commission on Radiation Protection recommends a person receive no more than 100 mrems from human-made sources in a year. Do you see ways you might reduce your risk?

Source: Adapted from G. Tyler Miller, Jr. (1990). *Living in the environment: An introduction to environmental science* (6th ed.). Belmont, CA: Wadsworth, p. 296.

It's difficult to know how much radiation you are being exposed to, because, as we mentioned, so much of it is natural radiation, as well as radiation from human activities. Radiation exposure is measured in rads and rems.

- *Rads:* A **rad** is a measure of the amount of radiation absorbed by an organism. A rad is used to measure dosages of radiation in treating cancer. A normal chest X ray is about $1/10$ of a rad. Between 50 and 150 rads will produce radiation sickness; 650 rads will kill one outright.

- *Rems:* A **rem** is a measure of the relative danger of exposure to ionizing radiation. Smaller doses are millirems (mrems), which are thousandths of a rem. The average annual exposure per person in the United States to ionizing radiation is 230 millirems, of which 130 comes from natural radiation and the rest from human activities. You should not receive more than 100 millirems from human-made sources in a year. (*See Self Discovery 36.2.*)

Sources of Radiation Let us now consider some important human-made sources of radiation. We must hasten to mention, however, that radioactive hazards are not considered to include **irradiated food,** food that has been exposed to low doses of ionizing radiation, such as gamma rays. Irradiation is designed to rid foods of harmful microorganisms, much as canning does, and make them stay fresh longer. At least 20 nations already irradiate produce and spices, and the World Health Organization encourages the practice, which can help eradicate salmonella and trichinosis and prevent spoiling.[25] The Food and Drug Administration approved the use of irradiation for pork in 1985 and fruits and vegetables in 1986, and other foods are being tested.

Some more legitimate sources of worry about radiation are the following:

- *Medical and dental X rays—do the minimum:* You might wonder why the dental assistant makes such a production about putting a lead apron on you and then vanishing from the room while the X ray machine clicks. You might especially wonder why, if the dose you get from a full set of dental X rays is equivalent to the amount of

blood-cell counts, nausea, weight loss, immune deficiencies, hair loss, bleeding from mouth and gums, and ultimately death.

natural "background" radiation you might pick up just being outside over 11 days' time.[26] However, your dentist is just being cautious: although the risk is small, it's always a good idea to minimize the dose.

Guarding against too much exposure is even more important for chest and other medical X rays. Every time someone suggests an X ray might be a good idea—and it may only be because physicians are trying to protect themselves in the event of a malpractice suit—you should ask, "Why is this necessary?" The reason for being concerned is that X ray exposure is *cumulative* and no exposure is by itself absolutely safe.

- *Radioactive elements used for medical treatment:* A number of radioactive elements are useful for medical diagnosis and treatment. For example, radioactive iodine (iodine 131) is used in tests of thyroid disorders. Cobalt 60, iodine 125, cesium 137, and radium 226 are used to treat cancer.[27] If, of course, you are being treated for a disease as serious as cancer, the effects of the radioactive elements might seem to be of secondary concern. Nevertheless, they are potentially harmful to health.

- *Radon—radioactive gas beneath the house:* **Radon** is an odorless, colorless radioactive gas given off by underground uranium deposits. At one time, there was a good deal of worry that radon seeping up into homes along water and sewage pipes or through foundation cracks could be inhaled and that its radioactive particles could damage lung tissue and lead to cancer.[28-30] More recently, some scientists have argued that the risks have been overblown and that the EPA's original estimates for lung cancer caused by radon have been too high.[31,32]

  Radon self-tests ($10–$50) are available through hardware stores and supermarkets, although some are better than others. There are also companies that test for radon, although few are licensed by the states. The gas can be reduced by sealing cracks in basement floors and ventilating crawl spaces, although repairs may be expensive.

- *Nuclear reactors—should you move if you live near one?* In 1991, nine countries generated a third or more of their electricity from nuclear reactors.[33] In the United States, the 110 reactors now in operation generate about 20% of the nation's electricity.[34]

  Are such plants safe? In 1979, as a result of operator mistakes, design flaws, and mechanical failures, the nuclear power plant at Three Mile Island, Pennsylvania, was destroyed when it overheated to 2500° Fahrenheit; cleanup at the site continued for 14 years.[35] However, no increase in cancer rates near the plant associated with the accident has been found.[36] In 1986, the Chernobyl nuclear plant in Ukraine (in what was then the Soviet Union) erupted in a volcano of deadly radioactivity, causing the evacuation of 116,000 people from the 18-mile zone around the plant and requiring 600,000 people to work on the cleanup. In the aftermath, there have been reports of a soaring increase in thyroid cancer rates.[37-39]

  Less serious accidents have since been reported at other American nuclear power plants. The nonprofit advocacy group Public Citizen said that in 1990 the commercial nuclear reactors in the United States had 1921 safety-related incidents that had to be reported to the Nuclear Regulatory Commission (NRC). However, the NRC said the numbers were lower than in previous years, showing steady safety improvements.[40,41] In 1990, the National Cancer Institute found no increased risk of death from cancer for people living near nuclear power plants or other nuclear installations.[42]

  One major problem is that over the next 25 years, more than half of the nation's nuclear plants will turn 40, and their operating licenses will expire when they do.[43,44] At that point, many of the plants will need to be torn down and their radioactivity-permeated remains somehow disposed of safely—a societal problem of awesome proportions.

- *Nuclear weapons plants:* Knowledge about radioactivity and radiation safety standards has changed through the Nuclear

Age. As a 17-year-old sailor in 1946, Henry Tingle watched a nuclear bomb test a dozen miles away on the Pacific atoll of Bikini without so much as sunglasses for protection, then was sent the next day to "decontaminate" ships at ground zero. Today he has suffered two bouts of cancer and is trying to get government compensation.[45] Tingle is just one of perhaps 300,000 U.S. military personnel who took part in atmospheric testing or occupied the atomic-bombed cities of Hiroshima and Nagasaki.

In addition, increased incidents of cancer have been found among the 600,000 employees who since 1942 have worked in federal nuclear research centers and weapons plants, such as Tennessee's Oak Ridge National Laboratory.[46,47] Some Nevada, Utah, and Arizona "down-winders" of open-air nuclear testing and Colorado uranium miners of the 1950s have also established relationships between cancer and their exposure to radioactive materials.[48-50] Even in the 1990s, serious safety problems were being turned up at nuclear weapons plants in Colorado and Oklahoma, and the Occupational Safety and Health Administration in 1991 found more than 600 safety violations and basic defects at these and other government weapons facilities.[51-53]

Strategy for Living: Reducing Exposure to Radioactivity In 1990, the Nuclear Regulatory Commission revised radiation exposure rules. Effective January 1993, the rules state that the maximum exposure to the general population from atomic facilities should be no more than 100 millirems a year (a fifth of what was allowed in the previous 30 years). Atomic workers are to be exposed to no more than 5 rems a year (as opposed to as much as 20 rems previously).[54]

Some radiation matters you have some control over, such as the amount of X rays and other radioactive medical treatments to which you are exposed. You can have the basement of your house checked for radon levels. If living close to a nuclear power plant bothers you, conceivably you could move. Dealing with other radioactive hazards—nuclear-waste dumps, stockpiled nuclear weapons, decaying nuclear power plants in Eastern Europe—is not so sim-

ple and requires political efforts. We describe these in the next chapter.

Indoor Pollution and Environmental Illness

Indoor air pollution may cause headaches, dizziness, and other symptoms of so-called sick building syndrome. Pollution in buildings may derive from carbon monoxide, formaldehyde, asbestos, and lead. Household chemicals may also turn houses into unhealthy toxic-waste sites. Some people experience an extreme sensitivity to chemicals called *environmental illness*.

If you live over a dry cleaner, you will not be happy to know that many of the apartments—even as high as the 12th floor—over these establishments in New York City show unacceptable levels of a primary dry-cleaning chemical (perchloroethylene) that has been connected to cancer in animals.[55] If you work in an office and have been getting headaches and nausea there, it may or may not brighten your day to know it could be caused not by your job but by the chemicals in the new carpet.[56] This is the new world of *sick buildings, toxic houses,* and *environmental illness,* terms that were hardly known a few years ago.

Sick Buildings and Chemicals The malaise called **sick building syndrome (SBS),** which is recognized by the World Health Organization, is illness that comes from indoor air pollution. Symptoms may consist of some or all of the following: stinging eyes, hoarseness, headaches, nausea, runny nose, dizziness, and lethargy.[57,58] As in other work-related illness, however, people's feelings about their jobs and working conditions could play a role. Perhaps the tip-off as to whether the fault is in the building is whether the symptoms get worse as the workday wears on but improve in the evenings and on weekends.

SBS health problems may occur in older buildings with deficient ventilation and ancient air-conditioning systems or in new, tightly sealed, energy-efficient buildings. Sometimes the condition may be traced to a single contaminant, such as a fungus or tobacco smoke.[59] However, chemical engineer Richard Shaughnessy, who directs an indoor-air research program, says that everything contributes: "Copiers, ventilation systems, the air brought in from outdoors, the number of people in a work space."[60]

Houses, too, may cause SBS, if they have been weatherized to save energy, thereby seal-ing in air pollutants. The culprit pollutants may be natural, like radon gas, or they may be in such building materials as particleboard, the chemicals in wood adhesives and carpet fibers, paint and wood finishes, and insulation. (*See ● Figure 36.3.*)

Among some of the principal polluters of buildings are the following:

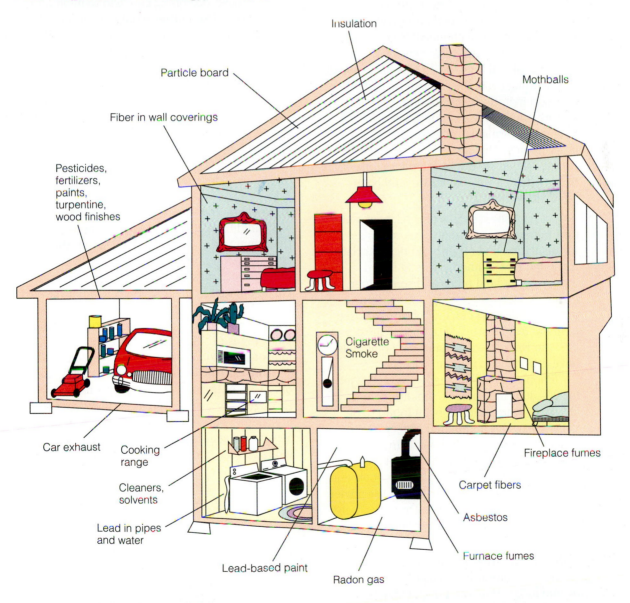

● **Figure 36.3 The sick building.** Scientists have given the name "sick building syndrome" to illness that comes from indoor air pollution. Here are some of the sources.

- *Carbon monoxide:* **Carbon monoxide** is a colorless, odorless gas that can be produced by furnaces, water heaters, space heaters, and gas stoves as a result of incomplete combustion. At high doses, the gas can be fatal, but at low doses it can produce headache, nausea, dizziness, and fatigue, although most people are quickly restored by breathing pure oxygen.

- *Formaldehyde:* Once used widely as an adhesive in particleboard and plywood, **formaldehyde** is a chemical that, in high concentrations, can cause cancer in laboratory animals. In humans, low levels can lead to breathing problems, dizziness, and eye and skin irritations. Although most manufacturers of wooden building materials no longer use formaldehyde, it is present in older homes. The best advice is to avoid pressed-wood products, keep humidity and temperature levels moderate, and have adequate ventilation.

- *Asbestos:* **Asbestos** is a fibrous, heat-resistant mineral that for many years was used for insulation and other building materials. Although now banned, it is still found around household pipes and some older furnaces. However, except for janitors, maintenance workers, and others exposed to fibers from disturbed asbestos, most people who work in well-maintained buildings have little to worry about.[61,62]

    People exposed to asbestos on the job for 20–30 years, such as pipefitters and shipyard workers, have been found to develop chest and abdominal cancers, lung diseases, and other illnesses.[63] In recent years, researchers thought that old asbestos should be removed from schools and public buildings. Today, however, the advice seems to be: Leave it alone. Or, if it is damaged or crumbling, have certified experts remove it.[64,65]

- *Lead:* A soft, gray-blue metal, **lead** used to be in most paint and all gasoline. Although by and large eliminated from those products, it is still found in the paint of old houses; indeed, perhaps three-quarters of all occupied housing units built before 1980 contain lead paint.[66] Young children live in 3.8 million homes that have peeling deteriorated lead-based paint or lead in dust.[67]

Lead is also found in old water pipes and in new homes where lead leaches from solder used to link copper and brass plumbing fixtures.[68–70] Finally, lead is found in materials that have nothing to do with buildings: car batteries, soldered cans of imported products, food (lead occurs naturally in soil), some imported table wines, and ceramic tableware and old china.[71–75]

Lead poisoning can lead to mental retardation and other mental disorders. It can also damage the liver and lead to paralysis of the extremities, sometimes followed by convulsion and collapse. Its effects cannot be reversed. The impairment to intellectual development from prenatal and early childhood exposure to lead occurs in children of all socioeconomic backgrounds.[76] In 1992, the federal government required that virtually all young children on Medicaid be screened for lead poisoning.[77]

Houses as Toxic-Waste Sites Besides being sick buildings themselves, houses may also be their own toxic-waste dumps. Indeed, the average American household generates 15 pounds of hazardous waste a year.[78] These are ordinary consumer goods ranging from shoe polish to oven cleaner, house paint to turpentine, weed killer to motor oil. Car owners who do their own oil changes produce as much as 400 million gallons of waste oil every year—equal to 36 of the Alaskan *Exxon Valdez* oil-tanker spills—but only 12% of that is disposed of properly, as through a service station or recycler. The rest of it is simply poured into the ground, streams, or sewers—1 gallon of oil can make a million gallons of water undrinkable.[79]

According to the Environmental Protection Agency, products designated as hazardous must use "signal words" on labels: DANGER, POISON, WARNING, CAUTION. Typically they fall into five categories: (1) paints and solvents; (2) vehicle fluids; (3) pesticides; (4) household cleaners and polishes; (5) miscellaneous—including batteries, pharmaceuticals, and some cosmetics.

Household toxic waste leads to two problems. First, if left around the house, it may be a respiratory hazard, a fire hazard, and a poison or skin and eye danger to children. Second, if thrown in the garbage or poured in the ground or down a storm drain, it could end up in the groundwater or nearby lakes.

Environmental Illness If you smell fumes from some paints, automobile exhaust, or ammonia, do you get blurred vision and headaches? Does your speech begin to slur? Does a magazine "scent strip"—the perfume advertising insert—make you ill? The National Academy of Sciences has suggested that about 15% of the population has a heightened sensitivity to chemicals.[80]

With some people, chemical sensitivity is so extreme that they are suspected of having the syndrome known as **environmental illness (EI),** or **multiple-chemical sensitivities,** violent reactions to the numerous chemicals and toxins that are a part of everyday life. (From 1945 to 1988, production of synthetic organic chemicals went from under 1 billion pounds to 273 billion pounds.)[81]

Although many health professionals do not accept the existence of EI as such, there is no disagreement that there are many patients who have multiple-chemical sensitivities.[82] Symptoms may range from fatigue, hives, and forgetfulness to severe headaches, joint pain, and a paralyzing disorientation that makes people incapable of speaking. One study suggested that symptoms of EI were the results of a mental disorder; however, clinical ecologists, physicians specializing in the disorder, say the study was sloppily executed.[83] They also say that the psychological explanation ignores the similarity of symptoms and exposure problems being reported.[84]

What causes EI? According to clinical ecologists, patients' vulnerability "may be caused by initial overdose or acute exposure to chemicals, by biochemical differences in the individual, by overall stress load, by viral or bacteriologic accompaniment, or by complex biological processes in the body which we don't yet fully understand."[85] It's also likely that pollutants often interact with each other so that two pollutants together make you far sicker than they would independently. For example, animal studies show that the toxicity of one chemical can add to the toxicity of another (the additive effect, as when the urine of rats exposed to lead and arsenic shows twice the level of toxicity as that of rats exposed to only one of the chemicals.)[86]

EI is a difficult matter to treat. One Seattle-area man spent $700,000 (including consultants' fees) on remodeling the interior of his new condominium to make it free of irritants: a furnace/air-conditioning system with triple filters, special glues, nontoxic grout, custom paints, special upholstery and cabinetry, and a double layer of vapor barriers to seal the apartment.[87]

Strategy for Living: Dealing with Indoor Chemicals If we spend 90% of the time *indoors,* as has been reported, what can we do to make our indoor environment safer?[88] Here are a few tips:

- *Deal with your sick building:* If you suspect you are the victim of sick building syndrome, the first thing to do is obvious: get as much ventilation and fresh air as possible. See whether the air is actually moving around existing ventilation systems. See if office machines are near functioning vents. Open vents that have been sealed to conserve energy. Ask the building maintenance supervisor if filters and drain pans have been cleaned or replaced, if pesticides or renovation work are near the air supply. Use a desk ionizer.

  Suspect tobacco smoke, toxins in old building materials, and fungus if there is water in the ductwork. Suspect fumes from carpeting and upholstery. Suspect old paint, which may be lead-based. Suspect heavy chemicals used by the janitorial service.

  Get a plant: as NASA scientists found out, certain houseplants absorb formaldehyde and other health-threatening pollutants. (Efficient plants include the peace lily, gerbera daisy, English ivy, chrysanthemum, bamboo palm, mother-in-law's tongue, Janet Craig dracaena, moss cane, and marginata dracaena.)[89,90]

- *Dispose of household toxins—properly:* What are you supposed to do with hazardous waste? If you can't reuse them yourself or give such things as paints, pesticides, and cleaners to a garden club, local theater troupe, school, or homeless project, you should at least dispose of them properly. If your house connects with a wastewater plant (not a septic tank), you can dump *some* materials down a laundry sink or bathroom toilet—if you do it slowly and don't mix materials—but call the local water authority to be sure.[91]

The following should be taken to a household-hazardous-waste event (some communities have an annual toxic roundup or collection drive): paints, strippers, stains/finishes, wood preservatives, metal primers, pesticides, furniture polish, batteries, motor oil, prescription drugs.[92]

A word about lead: there is no way to tell by looking whether a piece of ceramic-ware is safe, but you can be sparing in your use of old or handcrafted china or china with a corroded glaze or dusty chalky glaze.

Water Pollution: Fear at the Faucet?

Unsafe drinking water can produce intestinal distress such as gastroenteritis. Water pollutants may include infectious microorganisms, pesticides, lead, and chemicals such as PCBs and heavy metals. Chlorine and fluoride have been found to be beneficial.

Water symbolizes purity. Indeed, in a classic example of marketing imitating life, we have seen a series of popular "clear" products: first bottled waters, then clear soft drinks, most recently clear beer.[93]

But is the water we drink, in fact, pure? Madeline Moore, of Quinlan, Texas, lost seven teeth after her dentist found her gums riddled with disease—the result, she said, of the town's water coming from a quarry that was formerly used as a dump. The Safe Drinking Water Act was passed in 1974, but in 1990 the General Accounting Office of Congress found that neither the states nor the Environmental Protection Agency were adequately enforcing it and reporting water violations.[94] In 1992, a study by the National Water Education Council said the nation might have to spend $500 billion over the next 20 years to ensure clean water as crumbling water-supply and sewer systems are repaired or improved to meet federal requirements.[95]

The Effects of Unsafe Drinking Water A good indicator of the infection potential of a particular tap water is whether or not people who drink it get **gastroenteritis,** inflammation of the lining membranes of the stomach and intestines. The symptoms of gastroenteritis include vomiting, diarrhea, nausea, and cramps —what people have come to accept as the "one-day flu" and as "normal." However, this condition may represent the activity of a class of viruses called enteroviruses, some of which (poliovirus, hepatitis A, Coxsackie virus) are linked to long-term, serious illness. In one experiment in Canada, it was found that Montreal residents had a 30–35% greater chance of getting gastroenteritis from drinking regular tap water than those drinking highly filtered tap water.[96]

Types of Pollutants Besides viruses, bacteria, protozoa, and parasitic worms, which enter the water supply through human sewage and human wastes, other water pollutants consist of oxygen-demanding organic wastes, inorganic plant nutrients, sediment and silt, and excessive inputs of heated water used to cool electric power plants.[97] Perhaps more serious, from the personal control standpoint, are radioactive substances and organic and inorganic chemicals. A few chemicals of particular concern are as follows:

- *Pesticides:* A **pesticide** is any poisonous substance used to kill pests or vermin. The advantages of pesticides are that they increase food supplies and lower food costs and even save lives (as when used against malaria-bearing mosquitos). The disadvantages are that eventually they fail and lead to even larger populations of pest species. In addition, every year at least 1 million people are poisoned by pesticides and 3000–20,000 of them die. Moreover, pesticides leach into groundwater, and traces show in the food most Americans eat.[98] (*See ● Figure 36.4.*) In 1987, the National Academy of Sciences reported that 30–90% of pesticides may cause cancer in humans.[99]

- *Lead:* As a result of the presence of lead pipes in houses built before 1930 and the solder on copper pipes installed in the 1980s, lead levels have been found in unhealthily high levels in the water in many cities. Among the 660 large public water

systems sampled by the Environmental
Protection Agency, those serving 130 cities,
including New York, Detroit, and Washington, D.C., were found to contain excessive
levels of lead.[100]

- *Chlorine:* **Chlorine** is used as a disinfectant in water purification. About three-fourths of the water supply in the United States is chlorinated, although the degree of chlorination varies, depending on the source of the water and the contaminants in it. One study found that chlorinated drinking water has been linked to small increases in the rates of rectal and bladder cancer.[101] However, the small risk is greatly outweighed by chlorination's diminishing the risks of microbial contamination of drinking water.

- *Fluoride:* In Honolulu, Los Angeles, and San Antonio, Texas, the population doesn't drink fluoridated water, but in 41 of the other 50 largest cities they do.[102] **Fluoride** is an element added to the water supply, and today 17–40% of all cavity reduction is directly linked to fluoridated water. Despite the fact that it has been nearly half a century since fluoridation was first approved for citywide use in the United States, some people have worried that it might cause cancer. However, in 1991, federal officials found no evidence for this and concluded that the tooth-decay-fighting benefits outweighed any possible risk.[103]

- *PCBs:* **PCBs,** abbreviation for *polychlorinated biphenyls,* are hydrocarbon compounds once used in electrical transformers to dissipate heat, although the Environmental Protection Agency ordered the removal of such transformers by 1990. Many industrial wastes containing PCBs have been dumped into landfills, and there is some worry that the chemicals may have found their way into groundwater. The long-term effects of low levels of PCBs on people is unknown, but in laboratory animals they have produced liver and kidney damage, birth defects, and tumors.[104]

- *Heavy metals:* **Heavy metals** (called "heavy" because they are of relatively high atomic weight) include not only lead but also mercury, cadmium, and arsenic.

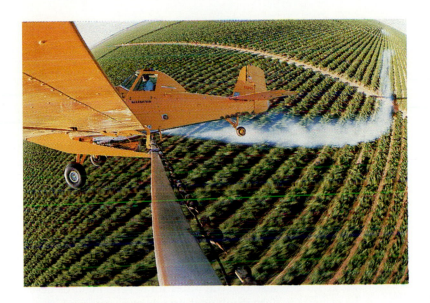

● **Figure 36.4 Chemicals and groundwater.** The agricultural use of chemicals, as from pesticides sprayed from airplanes, is a major contributor to pollution of the environment, including the water supply.

❝*Ground water is being increasingly contaminated by thousands of different chemicals, ranging from agricultural pesticides and household cleaners to industrial wastes. . . . Once polluted, ground water is virtually impossible to clean, so the contamination of this huge and vital water supply may be irreversible. We are conducting a massive but unwilling experiment on human exposure to low levels of water-borne toxic chemicals, and the result may be disastrous health consequences in the form of widespread poisonings, cancers, and birth defects.*❞

—Ian Robertson. (1987). *Sociology* (3rd. ed.). New York: Worth, p. 616.

Mercury is a heavy metallic element found in many house paints and industrial wastes. The element is released into rivers, where it changes form (from inorganic mercury to methyl mercury), is ingested by fish, and then consumed by human beings. When absorbed in sufficient doses it seriously alters the central nervous system and can cause death.

Strategy for Living: Getting a Safe Drink of Water If your tap water smells funny or is orange or red in color, you might want to switch to bottled water. Be aware, however, that bottled water may be purer than tap water, but some city-manufactured bottled waters may contain more bacteria than plain tap water. You should also know the distinction between *distilled* water, which is not chlorinated (and is frequently contaminated with bacteria), and *sterile* water, which is chlorinated.[105]

Some other tips:[106]

- *Let the water run first:* In the morning, run the water for at least half a minute before taking a drink. This will remove some of the lead and other contaminants. You can also boil the water for several minutes before drinking it. In addition, you can buy a home water-treatment unit.

- *Find out how good your water is:* Call the water department and ask for a free copy of its latest water-quality report. If you're really concerned, you can have your water tested by an independent laboratory.

Note: If you're out hiking or camping, don't drink directly from a stream, which may be contaminated with *Giardia lamblia* protozoans, which can produce severe diarrhea. Boil the water for 10 minutes first. These days, no North American stream water can be assumed to be fit to drink, even in remote wilderness areas.[107]

Air Pollution: 15,000 Quarts a Day

Smog and other forms of air pollution can cause respiratory distress, lung abnormalities, cancers, and heart risks.

When UCLA shot-putter Greg Winkler, 21, laced up his shoes on a September day in 1988 and headed for the track, it was the first time he had gone running since arriving in Los Angeles from northern California. As he broke into a trot, he immediately got a strange sensation: his chest was as tight as a drum; his lungs felt like they would burst.

"Heart attack," he thought.

"Smog," his doctor told him later.

Winkler, who had had no previous health problems, had exercise-induced asthma, prompted by the famous L.A. air pollution.[108]

Air pollution can actually be of several forms, ranging from dust in the desert to smoke from fires to coal soot to smog from automobiles and industry. (Air pollution also encompasses acid rain, as we describe in Chapter 37.) However, the pollution probably most identified with our own time is **smog**—a grayish or brownish fog or haze caused by the presence of smoke or other pollutants in the air.

The Effects of Smog "Most environmental risks are through inhalation," says air-pollution researcher Robert Phalen. "Each day, you drink 2 quarts of liquid, you eat 2 quarts of food, but you inhale 15,000 quarts of air."[109]

Should you be worried about what you're inhaling? In recent years, air pollution has been found everywhere—down in the Grand Canyon, damaging trees in Yosemite National Park, obscuring the view from the Blue Ridge Mountains in Virginia.[110–112] Air pollution casts a concealing cloak of haze over most states east of the Mississippi, routinely reducing visibility more than 80% in city and countryside alike.[113] Wood stoves have been declared a health menace.[114,115] Luxury cars such as Lamborghinis and Rolls-Royces have been criticized for producing five times as much carbon dioxide as conventional subcompacts.[116] Texas puts out more carbon dioxide than Britain or Italy, and California more than France and Mexico together.[117] Where will it all end?

Actually, there *have* been improvements, as we shall describe. However, if you're currently dissatisfied with the air you breathe, it's important to understand that it's not just a minor irritant. A number of studies have established relationships between polluted air and ill health:

- *Ozone and respiration:* **Ozone,** one of the most hazardous air pollutants, is formed when hydrocarbons from automobile exhaust and nitrogen oxides from industrial processes combine under sunlight. Even in healthy individuals, ozone can cause sensations of chest tightness, shortness of breath, decreased lung capacity, coughing, and nose and throat irritation. It aggravates emphysema and other respiratory illnesses.[118]

- *Smog and cancer:* Loma Linda University researchers who studied 6000 Californians found that smog increases cancer risks, particularly among women. Women living in the Los Angeles Basin were found to have a 37% greater chance of getting all cancers because of particle pollution.[119]

- *Smog and lung abnormalities:* Pathologist Russell Sherwin found that 30 of 107 young Los Angeles residents who died from accidents or violence had severe lung abnormalities caused by air pollution.[120]

- *Carbon monoxide and heart risks:* Exposure to carbon monoxide—the pollutant emitted in auto exhaust and by industrial smokestacks—can provoke dangerous heartbeat irregularities in people suffering from coronary artery disease, according to one study.[121]

Strategy for Living: Can You Survive Smog? The good news is that there *are* some improvements. For instance, as a result of tough motor-vehicle emission controls, air pollution has dropped by 50% in much of southern California since 1982, and dangerous peak levels have dropped by more than 25%, according to a 1992 report by the California Air Resources Board.[122] The goal is blue skies over Los Angeles by the year 2007. Here and in other smoggy cities, individual actions will count, as we will describe.

If you live in a smoggy area and are concerned about guarding your health, what do you do? For people who have asthma, bronchitis, emphysema, or other respiratory problems, it is a particularly serious matter. Children, too, suffer more because their lungs are smaller and they take in more air than adults do. In general, the best advice is as follows:

- *Minimize efforts on smoggy days:* On days when there are air-pollution alerts, you should avoid exercise and stay indoors as much as possible. When exercising on regular days, stay away from heavy traffic areas.

- *Don't smoke:* Cigarette smoke and smog have a more deleterious effect on your lungs together than either do by themselves.

In the long run, there are aspects of air pollution that may not be affecting you right now but that have the most serious consequences for our planet: acid rain, global warming, the greenhouse effect, destruction of the ozone layer. These are matters that won't be solved by staying indoors; as we describe in the next chapter, they require political action.

Land Pollution

Solid waste in landfills tends not to be biodegradable or to turn to compost. Despite misconceptions, most solid waste is paper. Dumps are now being more closely regulated, especially toxic-waste dumps. The disposal of nuclear waste is a particularly difficult problem, because this dangerous material can endure for thousands of years.

"One of the critical problems of our time is *stuff*," writes columnist Molly Ivins. "Nobody seems to understand how they come to have so much stuff."[123] Many college students may have fewer accumulations than other people do. However, a look around you may turn up, as one person found, "old magazines, out-of-fashion or threadbare clothing, half-dead running shoes, extra kitchenware, broken furniture, old notebooks," and so on.[124] What do you do with this?

Who Is Harmed by Land Pollution? Unused possessions and junk—much of which can be given away or recycled—are not difficult to deal with, given a little time. What's harder are the nastier aspects of garbage. For instance, a supervisor of gardeners in city parks says she is always grateful for the efforts of her staff whenever she sees someone running across the grass barefoot: "I thank goodness someone has been there to pick up the broken glass and the needles."[125] Besides tending to shrubs and flowers, urban gardeners must pick up potentially infectious hypodermic needles, which could expose them or park users to hepatitis B or the AIDS virus, and human waste, which could carry a range of infectious diseases. These hazards are the result of present public policy toward drug addicts and the homeless, many of whom use public parks.

All the sources of pollution we have mentioned so far—noise, electromagnetic, radiation, indoor, water, and air—can directly affect your health. However, pollution of the land may seem less likely to threaten your well-being. This may only be because many people are fortunate enough to lead lives that avoid exposure to the health hazards of garbage. There are important exceptions, however: minorities and low-income people say that their neighborhoods are apt to become industrial dumping grounds and benefit least from cleanup programs because they are poor and powerless.[126,127] In June 1992 their assertions received official recognition when the Environmental Protection Agency found evidence that minorities suffer disproportionate exposure to dangerous air pollutants as well as emissions from hazardous waste dumps.[128]

In the long run, however, the health of *all* of us may be at risk from land pollution, because the substances that are disposed of on or beneath the land can ultimately get into the water we drink and the air we breathe, which means they can also get into the food we eat. Let us see what the problems are.

Garbage and Landfills For more than two decades, archaeologist William L. Rathje has sorted through numerous garbage cans and landfills—what scholars call the *solid-waste stream.* **Solid waste** is any unwanted or discarded material that is not a liquid or a gas. In that time, he has uncovered 40-year-old hot dogs, a head of lettuce perfectly preserved after 25 years, and an order of guacamole that was almost as unchanged as the day it was thrown out with a nearby newspaper dated 1967.[129] One important discovery Rathje has made is that a great deal of garbage dumped in landfills tends *not* to be **biodegradable**—that is, to be broken down by bacteria into basic elements and compounds. Nor does a lot of it turn to **compost,** in which organic matter becomes a humus-like product that can be used as a soil conditioner. Biodegradation occurs, but it takes place over centuries rather than decades. The problem with landfills, say Rathje and his coauthor, is that they "are not vast composters; rather, they are vast mummifiers."[130]

In recent years, a number of other interesting facts have come to light regarding Americans and their garbage:

- *Garbage doesn't lie, people do:* Rathje's field of **garbology**—the study of trash, refuse, rubbish, and litter—has produced some interesting insights. By comparing surveys of food consumption with the contents of the same respondents' trash containers, it has been discovered that people consistently understate the amount of junk food they eat, underreport their alcohol consumption by 40–60%, overstate the quantities of fruit and diet soda they consume, and embellish their accounts as to the amount of recycling they do. Heads of households, conscious of their roles as "good providers," exaggerate the amount of food their families consume.[131]

- *Misconceptions about what fills the landfills:* Most people, says Rathje, believe that landfill contents are 20–30% fast-food packaging, 30–40% polystyrene foam (which makes up coffee cups and packing "peanuts"), and 25–45% disposable diapers—filling up perhaps 75% of landfills.[132] One result of this belief was that in 1990 McDonald's switched from foam to paper for its hamburger boxes.[133,134]

  In fact, fast-food packaging has been found to make up a tiny one-quarter of 1%. Polystyrene products accounted for a mere 0.9%.[135] The 16 billion disposable diapers thrown away every year made up only 0.8%. Moreover, it was found that the energy used to manufacture and launder cloth diapers—including the gasoline burned by diaper-service delivery trucks—exceeded that of disposables.[136–138]

  The largest component of landfills is, as is appropriate to the information age, paper. (*See ● Figure 36.5.*) From 35% of refuse volume in 1970, paper has become 50%.[139] The most common kind of paper is newspaper, which occupies 10–15% of landfill volume. Yard waste, consisting of grass clippings and leaves, and construction debris make up two other major categories.

- *Complex choices about waste disposal:* In older times, people simply threw garbage in the streets (Troy), or outside the city gates (Paris), or in the river (London). One hundred years ago, pigs were turned loose in New York City to eat garbage in the streets.

A few years later, New Yorkers began having their garbage carted away to a dump.

Today having a town dump has become a lot more complicated. Many people don't like landfills because they look unsightly, consume valuable municipal space, pollute groundwater and surface water, and emit gases (such as methane) that threaten the atmosphere. Environmentalists also say landfills discourage recycling and waste reduction.[140]

Federal regulations now require town dumps to close unless they met new regulations by 1993. These rules, designed to prevent dumps from polluting air and groundwater, require that new landfills be built with plastic and clay liners and other expensive environmental equipment. As a result, the 6500 old community dumps will be closed in the next few years, and solid waste will be concentrated in 1000 or so modern—and much larger—landfills.[141]

One mountain of garbage called "Mount Trashmore" in south Florida is half a mile long and 150 feet high. New York City's Fresh Kills Landfill, the largest municipal garbage dump on the planet, is expected to evolve into a 505-foot mountain of trash by 2005.[142] As urban centers in the East have run out of landfills, they have shipped their garbage to less-congested states, which now are also running out of room and are trying to obstruct the transport of millions of tons of other people's garbage.[143]

Landfills are only one option of disposal, but they are the largest. Burning is attractive because it can reduce the volume of waste by 90% and the heat can be used to make steam to generate electricity; however, burning raises problems of safety and environmental nuisance.[144] Despite incineration, composting, and recycling, the amount of garbage going into landfills amounts to 130 million tons a year. By the end of the century, however, the Environmental Protection Agency projects less use of landfills and more use of recycling and converting of solid waste to energy.[145] (See
● Figure 36.6.)

Toxic Waste People don't like having dumps nearby. They especially hate being near **toxic-**

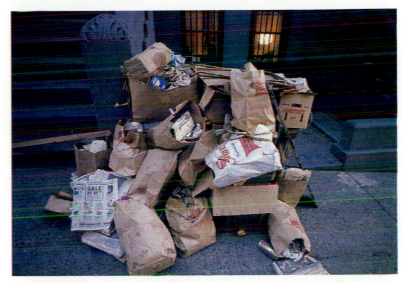

Paper: Includes packaging, newspaper, telephone books, glossy magazines, & mail-order catalogs — 50%

Organic: Includes wood, yard waste, & food scraps — 13%

Plastic: Includes milk jugs, soda bottles, food packaging, garbage bags, & polystyrene foam — 10%

Metal: Includes iron as well as aluminum & steel cans for food & beverages — 6%

Glass: Includes beverage bottles, food containers, & cosmetics jars — 1%

Miscellaneous: Includes construction and demolition debris, tires, textiles, rubber, & disposable diapers — 20%

● **Figure 36.5 What's in the garbage?** When trash ends up in a landfill, it's not polystyrene and disposable diapers that take up most of the volume. Half of it is paper.

waste dumps—containing everything from chemicals to motor oils to, in special cases, radioactive materials. Any time officials contemplate opening a new dump, particularly one for toxic waste, they are confronted with the phenomenon of NIMBYism. **NIMBY** stands for Not

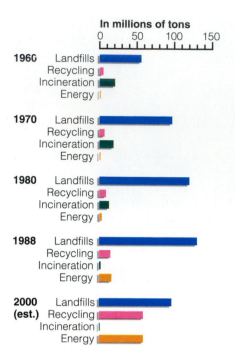

In millions of tons

| | 0 | 50 | 100 | 150 |

1960 Landfills / Recycling / Incineration / Energy

1970 Landfills / Recycling / Incineration / Energy

1980 Landfills / Recycling / Incineration / Energy

1988 Landfills / Recycling / Incineration / Energy

2000 (est.) Landfills / Recycling / Incineration / Energy

● **Figure 36.6 Getting rid of trash.** Use of landfills has grown, incineration has decreased. Recycling and conversion of solid waste to energy are expected to be popular modes of disposal in the future.

In My Back Yard. The term NIMBY, says one writer, "is usually applied broadly to people who don't want to bear social burdens or risks of any kind. Yet technological fears are a separate category deserving special attention."[146] In other words, although NIMBYism can be selfish and irresponsible, it also can promote social responsibility, as we shall explain.

There are two problem areas with nonnuclear toxic waste:

- *Cleaning of old toxic-waste dumps:* In 1980, Congress passed what came to be known as the Superfund program, to be used by the Environmental Protection Agency to clean up abandoned or inactive hazardous-waste dump sites. In the past decade, the EPA has spent $11 billion on emergency measures at 400 abandoned

sites and full-scale cleanups at 60 others; however, the cleanup has only begun.[147] The Congressional Office of Technology has estimated that the final list might include 10,000 sites and take 50 years to clean up.[148]

People living near old toxic-waste sites, such as leaking underground storage tanks, inactive uranium dumps, and abandoned mine lands, naturally worry that the chemicals will find their way into air and water. However, analysts believe the risks are overestimated. The EPA estimates that roughly 1000 cancer cases a year can be linked to public exposure to hazardous waste—not a negligible problem but far behind other cancer risks such as exposure to chemicals in the workplace or to radon gas leaking underneath houses.[149]

- *Relocating hazardous wastes to new dumps:* It will take a while, but probably some day contaminated dumps and buildings, of the kind found on land owned by chemical factories, will either be cleaned up or at least isolated from doing harm. But what should be done with the toxic waste being generated now? Trucks and trains carry toxic waste from one state to another and even one country to another.

Industrialized nations in North America and Europe, finding disposal of such waste more restricted and more costly at home, are exporting it. Not so long ago a favored location was Africa, where a ton of toxic waste could be disposed of for as little as $2.50 compared to $2000 in the United States. More recently, more and more has gone to Latin America. Despite millions of tons of dangerous cargo moving around the world, no global monitoring system exists to police hazardous-waste exports.[150,151]

Nuclear Waste Radioactive waste is in a class by itself. A 1992 Environmental Protection Agency study concluded that 45,361 sites across the United States, including factories and hospitals, are *potentially*—the qualifier is important—contaminated by radioactivity.[152] Many of the locations are not likely to be dangerous, but some include highly radioactive liquids and solids from nuclear reactors and nuclear-weapons plants.

Until 1993, only three repositories (in Nevada, South Carolina, and Washington) existed for permanent disposal of low-level radioactive waste from medical facilities and research laboratories. However, because the three states objected to being dumping grounds for the nation's low-level waste, federal law decreed that states now have to make other arrangements, either within their own boundaries or by entering into regional compacts with other states. Every year enough low-level waste is produced in the United States to fill a dozen Olympic-size swimming pools.[153]

The government classifies radioactive-waste materials into five groups, of which low-level is the least problematic. Above that are uranium mill-tailings, spent fuel, transuranic (elements heavier than uranium), and high-level. Most troublesome are these higher-level nuclear wastes, probably the most difficult garbage problem we face. Some of it comes from the nation's 110 nuclear reactors, most of which store radioactive wastes in indoor water pools originally designed to hold small quantities for only a few years.[154–156] This means that when the plants themselves reach the end of their 40-year operating licenses, they cannot really shut down; the control rooms, miles of plumbing, and deep pools of water holding the spent fuel must be monitored 24 hours a day. Tearing down and disposing of decommissioned plants themselves, whose walls and equipment are permeated with radioactivity, is another problem for which there seems to be no present solution. Eventually, however, all these reactors will probably have to come down.[157]

The same difficulty exists at the government's 17 nuclear weapons-production reservations. Nuclear wastes are stored in pools of water or above ground in sealed casks. There has been deep concern, however, because the government's own experts have said that catastrophic explosions are possible at million-gallon waste tanks at the Hanford bomb plant in Washington State, to name just one.[158] In addition, the end of the Cold War has meant that both the United States and Russia are having to think about how to retire nearly 40,000 nuclear warheads and hundreds of tons of bomb materials like plutonium 239 and uranium 235.[159,160]

What we have not mentioned so far is *how long* these radioactive materials remain dangerous. The amount of time over which the radioactive potency of any substance diminishes to half its original value is called the **half-life.** Radioactive phosphorus-32, used in hospitals, has a half-life of 14 days. Tritium has a half-life of 12.26 years. Carbon 14 has a half life of 5780 years. Even after achieving its half-life, a material can still be dangerous. Weapons-grade uranium will continue to emit radiation for *billions* of years.[161]

Are there no solutions for choosing sites for solid-waste dumps, particularly for radioactive materials? Advocates of nuclear technology say that high-level wastes can be safely disposed of permanently deep in the Earth in rock or salt formations that have not moved or had moisture in them for millions of years.[162]

This may be so, but the U.S. Energy Department has concluded that it cannot withdraw radioactive material from civilian power plants and store it in a permanent underground repository by 1998, as the law requires it to.[163,164] An enormous reactor-waste burial site had been built in Yucca Mountain, Nevada, 100 miles from Las Vegas, because it was argued there had not been a major earthquake in the area in perhaps 10,000 years. However, following a 1992 earthquake that caused $1 million worth of damage to a building just 6 miles from the site, Nevada residents were successful in getting officials to postpone taking fuel until 2010.[165] Opponents also have delayed movement of nuclear waste into sites in Idaho and New Mexico.[166–168]

In the meantime, a growing number of people support "intermediate storage" for 50–100 years or however long it takes to find the best disposal method. Decommissioned nuclear plants, for instance, could be simply mothballed rather than dismantled and transported to a burial site. The British government has announced it will mothball reactors for at least 130 years.[169]

Other possibilities include nuclear burial at sea, reprocessing and recycling of nuclear waste, using a process (transmutation) to accelerate the radioactive decay (half-life) and reduce the radioactive danger, even using jimsonweed to digest plutonium and a bacterium called GS-15 to transform uranium waste water into a solid form that can be easily filtered out.[170–173]

Strategy for Living: Dealing with Land Pollution At least one writer believes that NIMBY-ism against solid-waste dumps, toxic-waste dumps, and nuclear weapons plants comes about because opponents' skepticism is understandable: given the experience of the past 40 years, people no longer believe that science and government offer progress or protection from unwanted hazards.[174] When NIMBYists have the facts, they may well be a political power that can force risky industries and government to take better precautions.

From the standpoint of safeguarding your personal health from garbage and toxic waste, here are some tips:

- *Cleaning up public litter:* When picking up public or roadside litter, as around your house, wear heavy clothing and durable gloves that fit tightly at the wrist. A mask may be desirable if odors are a problem. Wash your hands frequently and clean them with alcohol-saturated towelettes. The same sorts of advice apply if you are disposing of household chemicals.

- *Dealing with a nearby waste facility:* If your neighbor is an industry or even an individual (such as someone who works on cars) that you suspect may be polluting the ground or the water supply in a way that may be endangering you, you may find you have a choice: You can move. Or you can take some form of political action.

At this point, you may see why we started this unit on environmental health with a chapter about those forms of environmental pollution that are also health matters you can personally and individually do something about. With land-pollution problems, it is possible to see that the environmental problems that affect you are not always amenable to individual solutions. You need to join forces with others.

800-HELP

American Speech-Language-Hearing Association. 800-638-8255 (in Maryland, 301-800-8682). Offers advice on hearing protection, hearing aids, and audiologists

Dial A Hearing Screening Test. 800-222-EARS (in Pennsylvania, 800-345-EARS). Refers you to a number in your area that offers a simple screening test by phone

Environmental Protection Agency Resource Conservation and Recovery Act Hotline. 800-424-9346 (in Washington, DC, 202-382-3000). Referrals to local government agencies for disposal of hazardous waste

National Institute of Occupational Safety and Health (NIOSH). 800-35NIOSH. Will provide information on where to go for a health hazard evaluation of your office or workplace

National Pesticides Telecommunications Network. 800-858-7378. Makes disposal recommendations for pesticides, herbicides, and paint

Radon Information Hot Line. 800-767-7236. Advice on measuring and dealing with this radioactive gas when it occurs beneath houses

Safe Drinking Water Hot Line. 800-426-4791. Call for testing information about drinking water

Suggestions for Further Reading

Dadd, Debra Lynn. (1986). *The nontoxic home.* Los Angeles: Jeremy P. Tarcher.

Wolfson, Richard (1991). *Nuclear choices: A citizen's guide to nuclear technology.* Cambridge, MA: MIT Press. Stresses connections between nuclear technologies, so you can make your own choice about nuclear policy.

37 Global Environmental Challenges

▶ Describe the principal concerns behind four overriding world environmental problems: population growth, poverty, pollution, and war.

▶ Discuss the personal health benefits of voluntarism.

N*o man is an island, entire of itself; every man is a piece of the continent, a part of the main. . . .*
He might have said "man or woman" when he wrote this in 1624, but poet John Donne made the point nevertheless: we and our individual problems are not inseparable from those of others.

Toxic wastes, dwindling rain forests, holes in the ozone, and global warming may seem to be environmental problems that are far from your personal concerns. They may also seem to be insurmountable. Yet in recent years people acting together have made a tremendous difference. They have halted nuclear power development, reduced air and water pollution, and saved millions of acres of wilderness. Although some of our problems seem so overwhelming as to warrant cynicism, the examples of environmental achievement should inspire us to realize that individuals—in the company of others—*do* make a difference.

The Four Horsemen of Our Time: Population, Poverty, Pollution, and War

There are perhaps four overriding world environmental problems affecting our health. The first is excessive population growth, which needs to be reduced so the fertility rate equals the replacement rate. The second is poverty, along with hunger and disease, which must be remedied with sustainable development. The third is pollution brought about by acid rain, rainforest deforestation, the greenhouse effect and global warming, and the disappearing ozone layer, which require international action. The fourth is war, which requires regulation on proliferation of nuclear weapons.

In the Bible, Revelation 6.1–8, the allegorical figures known as the Four Horsemen of the Apocalypse are war, famine, pestilence, and death. Although these scourges remain with us today, let us suggest the Four Horsemen for our time: *population, poverty, pollution,* and *war.*

Population Human sexual intercourse occurs more than *100 million times a day* around the world, resulting in 1 million conceptions, according to the World Health Organization.[175] Those 100 million sexual acts a day end up at the end of the year as nearly 100 million more people on the planet. This means the world *annually* gains slightly more people than live in all of Mexico.[176] Or of Great Britain, Ireland,

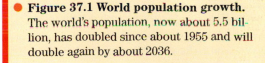

Figure 37.1 World population growth. The world's population, now about 5.5 billion, has doubled since about 1955 and will double again by about 2036.

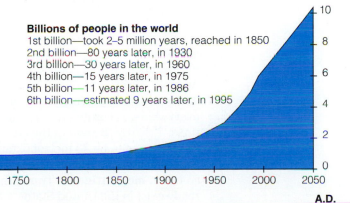

Billions of people in the world
1st billion—took 2–5 million years, reached in 1850
2nd billion—80 years later, in 1930
3rd billion—30 years later, in 1960
4th billion—15 years later, in 1975
5th billion—11 years later, in 1986
6th billion—estimated 9 years later, in 1995

1350 1400 1450 1500 1550 1600 1650 1700 1750 1800 1850 1900 1950 2000 2050

A.D.

Iceland, Belgium, Denmark, Norway, Sweden, and Finland *combined*.[177] Where is this all leading us?

- *World population growth:* The yearly population-growth number is not standing still—it is getting larger. Because of this kind of arithmetic, since famed biologist Paul Ehrlich wrote his book *The Population Bomb* in 1968 (in which he warned of the dangers of overpopulation), the world has gone from 3.5 billion people to about 5.5 billion today. By 2025—certainly within the lifetime of many people reading these pages—it will be 8.5 billion, says a report by the United Nations Population Fund.[178] By 2036, Ehrlich and population groups predict, it will be more than *twice* what it is today—11 billion.[179,180] (*See* ● *Figure 37.1.*) Two-fifths of the world's population is in China and India, and they account for one in three of the new people added each year.[181]

- *U.S. population growth:* What about the United States, which has a slower growth rate than other countries? Between 1950 and 1992, we grew from 150 million to 255 million. The U.S. Census Bureau now estimates that there will be 275 million by the end of this century and *383 million* by 2050.[182] This is a stunning 50% increase in only six decades. (This increase assumes fertility rates averaging 2.1 births per woman as well as legal and illegal immigration of between 880,000 and 1.4 million a year for the next six decades.) Next time you can't find a parking place or any space at a beach or campground, think what this awesome 50% increase will mean for the quality of life in North America.

- *The rise of megacities and edge cities:* Where will these people go? Probably where most of them go now: to the cities. For instance, in 1950, only 42% of Latin Americans were city dwellers; today almost 73% are, creating shantytowns and slums everywhere, according to the United Nations.[183,184] By the end of the century, there are expected to be 23 metropolitan areas of the world with 10 million people or more—so-called **megacities.**[185] Two of these already exist in the United States—the New York area, with 18 million people, and the

Los Angeles area, with 14.5 million. Regardless of what country they're in, megacities have much in common. (*See* ● *Figure 37.2.*)

In the United States, decades of movement from small towns and farms have resulted in 50% of the nation's population living in urban and suburban areas, up from 30% in 1950, according to the Census Bureau.[186] There are now 39 metropolitan areas with 1 million people or more. Indeed, demographers now speak of these metropolises as "metropolitan systems" that spread well beyond the central cities, including, in the United States, what one writer calls "edge cities" (nearly 125 of them, each bigger than Memphis), with their own city centers.[187]

- *What Americans think:* Most Americans find such rapid population growth, both at home and in the world, extremely troubling. A 1992 poll commissioned by the World Population Crisis Committee, a population-stabilization organization, found Americans expressed the following concerns regarding overpopulation:[188]

(1) Concern for environmental degradation and poverty. More than 85% of all Americans believe that rapid population growth is ruining the world's environment and will continue to contribute to environmental degradation and poverty if nothing is done.

(2) Worries about immigration and jobs. More than three-quarters felt rising world population would cause more illegal immigrants to come to the United States. The same number said they thought American jobs would move to countries where people would work for less.

(3) Belief in family-planning assistance. The survey found that most Americans want the government actively involved in international family planning. Sixty-seven percent believed the United States should resume financing for International Planned Parenthood (cut off in 1984). Fifty-five percent said the United States should pay directly for overseas abortion services.

No challenge is more urgent, says Werner Fornos, president of the nonprofit Population Institute, than stabilizing world population. The knowledge and technology exist to reach the objective. Only the will is missing.[189]

The highest priority is *population stabilization*. As Fornos and many others point out, population and family-assistance must be accelerated from all sources. The goal is to stabilize populations so that the **fertility rate**—the average number of children a woman will bear—equals the **replacement rate,** in which the number of persons born in a generation equals, rather than exceeds, the number dying. The goal should be a fertility rate of 2.4, according to Fornos, the level required for stabilizing population at present death rates. The world can achieve that goal by the year 2000, according to the World Bank, if the proportion of couples in developing countries using contraception rises from the current 40% to 72%.[190]

Poverty, Hunger, and Disease If the world were a village of only 1000 people, North Americans would make up only 60 of them.* Moreover, of those 1000 people, 60 would control half the total income. In addition, 500 would be hungry, 600 would live in shantytowns, and 700 would be illiterate.[191]

These kinds of figures make it plain how shockingly unequal the distribution of the world's wealth, food, housing, and education is. The poorest fifth of the world's population disposes of only 4% of the world's wealth, while the richest fifth disposes of 58%.[192] Incredibly, it seems, the world is actually producing enough food to feed all of the human race, according to the United Nations Food and Agricultural Organization.[193] The difficulty is one of distribution, so that starvation and malnutrition affect as many as half a billion people today.[194] The problems of poverty and hunger, which in turn expose people to disease, are aggravated by the fact that people of underdeveloped nations tend to have more children.

*The rest: 80 South Americans, 86 Africans, 210 Europeans, and 564 Asians. The 1000 villagers would also include 300 Christians (183 Catholics, 84 Protestants, 33 Orthodox), 175 Moslems, 128 Hindus, 55 Buddhists, 47 Animists, and 210 without any religion or atheist.

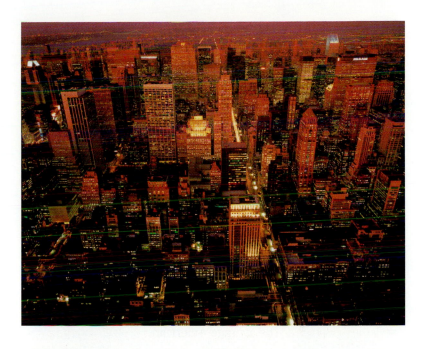

● **Figure 37.2 Megacities.** By the year 2000, there are expected to be 23 cities in the world with 10 million people or more. Janice Perlman, founder of The Mega-Cities Project at New York University, points out that developed (first-world) and underdeveloped (third-world) cities have much in common.

❝*Moving people around, moving garbage around, housing low-income people and matching people with jobs are universal problems. Every third-world city has a first-world city in it; every first-world city has a third-world city in it.*❞

—Janice E. Perlman. Quoted in: Roberts, S. (1990, June 25). 'Mega-cities' join to fight problems. *New York Times*, p. A13.

Some observers have pointed out a certain arrogance that exists among the West's more affluent nations. If poor people are to stop having so many children, for example, they must be aware that the children they do have will survive. This means making available health, education, and employment opportunities that we North Americans take for granted. However, if people in developing countries were able to live as we do, the result would be ecological disaster.

Sustainable development—striking a balance between ecological and economic concerns—is supposed to be the answer, but many people in North America and Europe regard sustainable development as something poorer nations need to practice but they themselves don't.[195]

In point of fact, says Paul Ehrlich, one American does 20–100 times more damage to the planet than one person in a developing country, and one rich American causes 1000 times more destruction.[196] People who drive gas-guzzling luxury cars, air-condition their homes, and eat food produced through high-intensity agriculture do far more damage than subsistence farmers, he says. Yet this criticism doesn't mean Americans need adopt a peasant lifestyle. In Sweden, for instance, the average person consumes about 60% as much energy as the average American.

Pollution: Acid Rain, Global Warming, and the Ozone Layer If Ehrlich is right, are we in North America (and others in the richest parts of the world) responsible for most of Earth's pollution problems? In 1992, the Worldwatch Institute in Washington, D.C., issued a study that echoed Ehrlich's views. The study states that the consumption by the richest fifth of the world is responsible for releasing virtually all ozone-depleting chemicals and two-thirds of greenhouse gases and pollutants that cause acid rain, as well as a large share of pesticides and radioactive waste.[197] Worse, the study said, the actions of the "consumer class" inspire poor countries to want to adopt the consumer lifestyle, as evidenced by the global spread of shopping malls.

The people of the developing world also contribute to global pollution, although much of it represents the desperation of poverty. For example, the United Nations says that half the world's population depends on wood to heat homes and to cook, pulling down trees and even shrubs. Many other impoverished people clear land for marginal farming. As a result, natural forests have all but disappeared in Haiti, Greece, and El Salvador.[198–200] The resulting deforestation contributes to increased levels of carbon dioxide, one of the principal greenhouse gases responsible for global warming, as we discuss in the list that follows.

What are the major pollution problems that need to be confronted to make Earth livable? The following are key:

- *Industrial pollution in Eastern Europe:* We have described the problems of disposing of toxic chemicals and nuclear waste in North America. The former USSR, including Russia and its former satellites such as East Germany and Poland, are mired in pollution and archaic industries and pose an environmental menace to the rest of the world.[201–205] Poisoned air, water, and land; dying forests; aging nuclear reactors; radioactive waste dumps—the poisoning of one-sixth of the Earth's land mass must somehow be dealt with. One statistic shows the seriousness of the problem: although the United States contributed 17.6% of greenhouse omissions in 1989, the former USSR contributed 13.6%.[206]

- *Acid rain and destruction of forests:* **Acid rain** is rain (or snow, fog, or clouds) containing sulfuric acid and nitric acid. The acid rain comes about because water droplets in the air mix with the burning of sulfur-content fuels (such as coal) and nitric oxide from auto emissions, as well as other industrial processes. The clouds or precipitation may be carried several miles, doing severe damage well outside the country of origin.

  Acid rain is a serious problem in the northeastern United States and southeastern Canada, caused largely by emissions from coal- and oil-burning plants in industrial parts of the United States; in northern and central Europe; and elsewhere. Besides damaging car finishes, buildings, statues, lakes, rivers, fish, and crops, acid rain has been destructive to forests. The same burning of fossil fuels and resulting forest damage combined with deforestation—heavy overall losses of forest acreage—may be having a consequence far beyond what people anticipated a generation ago: a global warming.

- *Destruction of tropical forests:* There are 10 billion acres of forests left in the world, including 5 million acres of tropical rain forest, of which more than half is in Latin America.[207] Today tropical forests are half the size they were a century ago, and the destruction has proceeded especially rapidly in recent years: forests more than 324,000 square miles—equal to two Californias in land area—were destroyed in Latin America alone in the years 1981–1990.[208] (Canada's once-vast rain forest has also been logged off at a rate that experts say means the forest will be gone within a generation.)[209] Most of the destruction (often through burning) of Latin American tropical rain forest has come about because of the "three C's," says anthropology and biology professor William Durham—coca (for cocaine), cattle, and colonization.[210] However, impoverished people hunting fuel, loggers, gold miners, and American oil companies are also responsible.[211]

Destruction of the rain forest has three possible consequences that should concern us:

(1) Fewer forests mean fewer plants to absorb carbon dioxide, the most important of the gases accumulating in the atmosphere that seem to be causing the greenhouse effect.[212]

(2) There are perhaps 10 million species on Earth today, from one-celled microbes to redwood trees to whales. Normally extinction is slow, 1–10 species a year. With the loss of tropical forests, perhaps 50,000 species disappear every year. As one writer put it, "One of the great mass extinctions in history appears to be underway."[213]

(3) Tropical forests serve as potentially invaluable sources of raw materials for drugs and vaccines. Recently, taxol, one of the most important new cancer drugs in 15 years, was discovered in the bark of the endangered Pacific yew tree in old-growth forests of the Pacific Northwest.[214,215] For thousands of years plants have been the primary source of medicine, and in the United States one in four prescriptions still comes from plants. Of 121 prescription drugs used widely around the world, nearly three-quarters came from following up folklore claims.[216] Currently

Western companies are trying to tap the knowledge of people in rain-forest cultures to develop leads for new medicines.[217] In addition, recent studies have shown that systematic harvesting of products—fruits, pigments, oils—from the Amazon rain forest can be more profitable than cutting down the trees for lumber and running cattle on the land.[218]

- *The greenhouse effect and global warming:* The burning of rain forests and fossil fuels and the rapid deforestation of the planet may be bringing about the greatest climatic change in human history: global warming from the greenhouse effect.

The buildup of carbon dioxide and other gases from these events—called "greenhouse gas"—can make the atmosphere act like a window pane in a gardener's greenhouse. "Greenhouse gas" is made up of four other gases:

(1) *Carbon dioxide* (56%), mostly from fossil fuels

(2) *CFCs* or chlorofluorocarbons (23%), the gas that (now being phased out under a 1987 international agreement in Montreal) was used in refrigeration, air conditioning, and spray cans

(3) *Methane* (14%), released largely by cattle and rice farming and by leaks from natural-gas pipelines

(4) *Nitrous oxides* (7%), produced by cattle and in engines

The **greenhouse effect** occurs when the "greenhouse gas" makes the atmosphere act like glass in a greenhouse, increasing the warming effects of sunlight: it lets in the sun's light and retains more heat than normal, causing the world's climate to warm up. (See ● *Figure 37.3.*)

So why worry about a little global warming? The problem is that if the average temperatures in the world were to increase by only 7°F (4°C), as they might 100 years from now, sea levels could rise by 2 feet because of melting glaciers and Antarctic ice sheets, flooding coastal areas—a threat to coastal cities and agricultural lowlands everywhere.[219]

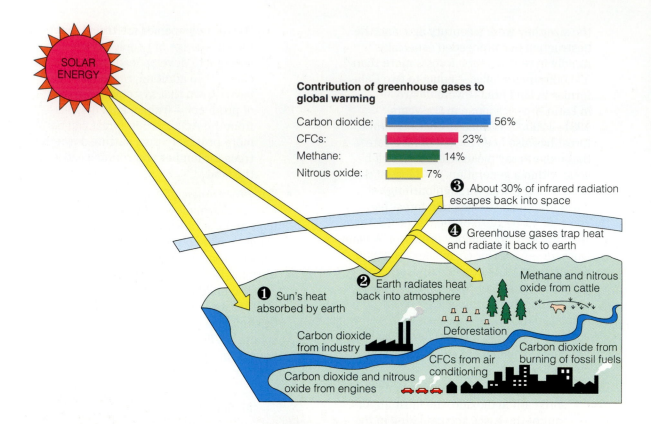

Contribution of greenhouse gases to global warming

Carbon dioxide:	56%
CFCs:	23%
Methane:	14%
Nitrous oxide:	7%

❸ About 30% of infrared radiation escapes back into space

❹ Greenhouse gases trap heat and radiate it back to earth

❶ Sun's heat absorbed by earth

❷ Earth radiates heat back into atmosphere

Methane and nitrous oxide from cattle

Deforestation

Carbon dioxide from industry

CFCs from air conditioning

Carbon dioxide from burning of fossil fuels

Carbon dioxide and nitrous oxide from engines

● **Figure 37.3 The greenhouse effect.** Like a window pane in a gardener's greenhouse, the collection of gases (carbon dioxide, CFCs, methane, nitrous oxide) collectively called "greenhouse gas" lets in light but retains heat, causing the earth's climate to warm up.

● *The thinning ozone layer:* **Ozone** is a form of oxygen that reacts readily with other substances and, on close exposure, can be harmful to living things. High up in the atmosphere, however, the **ozone layer** serves the important task of giving us a shield against excessive ultraviolet radiation from the sun, which has been found to cause skin cancer, cataracts, and suppression of the immune system in human beings. It also harms wildlife and crops.

Since 1967, however, there has been a 10% reduction in ozone over the middle latitudes of Europe and North America. Worse, there has been a loss of ozone at the poles, particularly over Antarctica, where a loss of 50% has been reported—a so-called ozone hole.[220] Satellite measurements in late 1992 showed the ozone hole over Antarctica to be the largest on record— almost three times larger in area than the United States.[221] People living in the southernmost part of South America, not far from the ozone hole, have reported cattle and sheep blinded by temporary cataracts and of ranch hands whose eyes and skin have been damaged.[222,223]

In late 1992, environmental officials from 93 countries agreed to eliminate the use of ozone-depleting chemicals *4–9 years earlier* than a previous target date in order to try to save Earth's protective layer.[224] Earlier, in 1987, signatories to the Montreal Protocol had agreed to reduce CFCs (used in refrigeration, air conditioners, and aerosol spray cans) and carbon tetrachloride (used in dry cleaning and fumigation) by half by 1998.[225] In the November 1992 meeting, they agreed to phase out *all* of these chemicals by January 1, 1996. They also moved up the elimination of halons (used in firefighting foam) and methyl chloroform (used in dry cleaning) from 2000 to 1994. In addition, they agreed to an accelerated phaseout schedule of HCFCs (hydrochlorofluorocarbons), used as a substitute for CFCs but also found to be dangerous.

Will the kinds of measures being taken against acid rain, global warming, and the vanishing ozone work? Or will the climate continue to be thrown out of kilter? In 1957, the late Roger Revelle of the University of California wrote of the changing atmosphere that humankind "is inadvertently conducting a great geochemical experiment."[226] The experiment is continuing.

War After considering the foregoing, we might agree with the secretary general of the United Nations, when he opened the Earth Summit meeting in Rio de Janeiro in June 1992, that the concept of world security is becoming less and less a military matter and that nations need to embark on "new collective security" by redirecting military spending toward environmental protection.[227]

We have been fortunate, despite some close calls, to have endured more than 40 years without nuclear war between the United States and its allies on the one hand and the Soviet bloc on the other. Yet there has been appalling loss of life from other kinds of wars. For example, Lentz Peace Research laboratory researchers in St. Louis, who have been keeping a computerized database on war deaths, found that there were more wars in 1987—26—than in any year in recorded history and they were responsible for 2.2 million deaths—84% of which were civilian casualties.[228]

Wars are of two principal kinds—nuclear and nonnuclear:

- *Nuclear war:* There has been only one hostile use of nuclear weapons since the birth of the atomic age. This was by the United States against Japan, when two atom bombs were dropped on Hiroshima and Nagasaki in August 1945. (*See* ● *Figure 37.4.*)

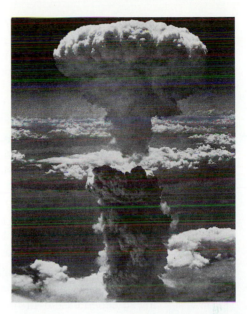

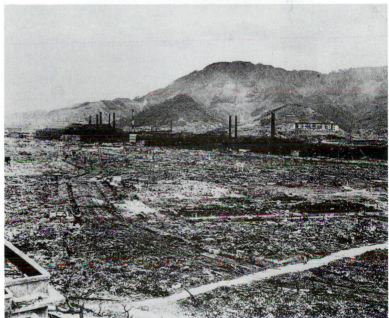

● **Figure 37.4 Nuclear weapons.** (*Top*) A mushroom cloud from an atomic-bomb test. (*Bottom*) Nagasaki after the A-bomb attack.

The bomb that destroyed Hiroshima was equivalent to 13 kilotons, or the explosive power of 13,000 tons of TNT. The first hydrogen bomb, tested by the United States in 1952, was calculated to be 700 times as great as the Hiroshima bomb. A single nuclear submarine can carry firepower equivalent to eight times *all* the firepower of World War II.

Since the end of the Cold War, concern has focused on the following issues:

(1) Who will get control of the remaining nuclear warheads in the former Soviet Union's far-flung arsenal, despite the arms cuts agreed to by the United States and Russia? Three independent states neighboring Russia (Ukraine, Belarus, and Kazakhstan) hold nuclear weapons in their territories.[229,230]

(2) What can be done to curtail the proliferation of nuclear weapons—including so-called basement-built atom bombs—to other countries or terrorist groups?[231,232]

It seems clear that vigilance will be required throughout our lifetimes.

• *Nonnuclear war:* So-called "conventional wars" are ongoing. In 1986, Ruth Leger Sivard published a table listing all wars in the 20th century with deaths of 100,000 or more.[233] The table, which covered conflicts throughout the world, listed 43 wars or conflicts, with a total loss of 83,642,000 lives.

What's important about this table is that it listed only *major* conflicts between 1900 and 1986. If the death toll in minor wars—those with deaths *under* 100,000— had been included, the total number of fatalities would probably have been over 100 million. And the 20th century still had another 14 years to run.

There may well be, say, 15 wars going on right now throughout the world. Most of the casualties will probably be civilian and from less developed nations. Civilians in advanced nations are generally not affected (except tourists or journalists in the war zones). However, if the past is any guide, it is the governments and companies of the rich countries—led by the United States—that sell the armaments to the poor countries, which use the arms against their countries' own populations, their minorities, and their neighbors.[234–236]

The Art of Living: Make Your Life Larger Than Yourself

To avoid catastrophic events in the future, immediate cooperative action is required. This can be done by adopting personal styles of living that are environmentally sound, such as avoiding overconsumption. People who do volunteer work not only benefit others but may also dramatically increase their life expectancy and vitality, as well as put purpose into their lives.

Is it too late to save the Earth? If a special computer model (called *World3*) can predict the future, the answer may be: yes, it is too late.[237] This model, which plotted future scenarios for the planet, based on population growth trends, use of energy and resources, food production, pollution, and so on, found that—without any major intentional changes— the future presents an extremely unhappy picture: famine, deforestation, species extinction, polluted water, global warming, depletion of the ozone layer, and social and political instability.

However, the authors of this computer model believe change is possible and collapse can be averted—provided action is *immediate*. The changes will require, however, that we and the rest of the world learn to live with limits on our consumption. Population growth, poverty, and pollution cannot be ended by indefinite material growth.

What can you do? Part of the art of living, it might be said, is to *make your life mean something more than just living for yourself.*

Personal Action Many people have begun a quiet revolution in their own lives.[238] They take a stand on the population issue by having few or no children themselves, by adopting children, and by supporting the decisions of friends and relatives who have two, one, or no children. They don't overconsume, following the adage "Use it up, wear it out. Make it do, or do without." They are avid recyclers. They use their votes and their influence to support reproductive planning, abortion, and land-use planning that preserves agricultural land and open space. They also come to terms with their feelings about money.

In *Your Money or Your Life,* Joe Dominguez and Vicki Robin point out that money is something we choose to trade our "life energy" for. They write:

> Our life energy is our allotment of time here on earth, the hours of precious life available to us. When we go to our jobs we are trading our life energy for money. . . .
>
> This definition of money gives us significant information. Our life energy is more real in our actual experience than money. You could even say money equals our life energy. So, while money has no intrinsic value, our life energy does—at least to us. It's tangible, and it's finite. Life energy is all we have. It is precious because it is limited and irretrievable and because our choices about how we use it express the meaning and purpose of our time here on earth.[239]

It thus becomes important, they point out, to decide whether you receive satisfaction and value in proportion to the life energy expended and whether the expenditure of life energy is in alignment with your values and purpose.

Many people have learned to live on less and enjoy it more.[240] Many are choosing to clean out the clutter in their homes, buy fewer gadgets, consume fewer disposable goods, avoid expensive cars and house payments, ride bicycles to work, use solar power, share child care with neighbors, or grow their own vegetables.

The rewards can be less consumer debt, less stressful work life, less worry about living costs, and less concern about *buying things* as a means of satisfying the soul.

Voluntarism and Its Rewards for Health

Many people are so cynical about the state of our society that, as one writer put it, they "feel too jaded to lift a finger, other than to change channels with the remote control."[241] It may be that the focus on the self has led people into "cocooning," withdrawing into comfortable private worlds. Yet sociologist Todd Gitlin points out, "The more people withdraw energy from their public lives, the more unsatisfying it becomes to participate."[242]

Actually, helping others can benefit the helper as much as the person being helped. In 1988, when Allan Luks was director of New York City's Institute for the Advancement of Help, he surveyed 3300 volunteers and found that 95% experienced significant reductions in stress after helping acts.[243] James House and his colleagues at the University of Michigan's Survey Research Center studied 2700 people for more than a decade to see how their social relationships affected their health. They found that *doing regular volunteer work, more than any other activity, dramatically increased life expectancy and probably vitality.*[244]

"To make ourselves healthier and to make the world a better place," says Luks, "we need to stop trying to protect ourselves and start opening up more. It's not easy, though. People need a push sometimes."[245]

Sometimes people become helpers because of a personal tragedy. Wayne Bates became the "Ralph Nader of the Railways," championing railroad safety, after his brother was seriously injured in a train accident.[246] Richard Eustice, 30, who experienced the first symptoms of rheumatoid arthritis at age 19, volunteers during his vacation at a summer camp for children with arthritis.[247]

Anger, points out David Walls in *The Activist's Almanac,* can also make a difference. Many activists begin with a sense of anger—at social injustice, at discrimination, or at the needless destruction of nature.[248] Anger may make one finally take the steps to join an organization and to effect social change. These steps, says Walls, can range from "checkbook activism," for those with a little money but not much time; to letter writing, telephoning, fundraising, and other activities, for those who have some time and want to meet others; to computer networking with other activists; to devoting full time to activism as a career.

Helping others helps your own health. Yet health, it has been pointed out, is not a goal in itself; it is a means to serving a purpose in life.

Thus, we come full circle.

800-HELP

National Volunteer Hotline. 800-HELP-664

Understanding the Effects of Sexism, Racism, and Poverty on Health

Answer the following true (T) or false (F):

___ **1.** From a health standpoint, women are the "weaker sex."

___ **2.** White Americans live longer than Americans of other races.

___ **3.** Money makes a difference: people with money are in better health than people without money.

___ **4.** Health is health, and it makes no difference what your level of education is.

The answers are (1) false, (2) true, (3) true, (4) false.

Gender and Health

For centuries, women were declared "the weaker sex." Although women may not equal men in muscular strength, by almost any other health yardstick they can hardly be declared "weaker."

The Biological Advantages for Women The average American man dies 7 years sooner than the average American woman. Indeed, throughout the course of life, men have a higher death rate: in the United States, more infants are born male than female (106 boys for every 100 girls), but by the mid-20s there are even numbers of each sex, and after the age of 65 there are only 85 males for every 100 females.[249] Men also suffer over 30 hereditary disorders (such as hemophilia) that women don't, seem to be less resistant to disease, and on the whole seem to be less hardy than women. In general, when given the same care as males, females tend to have biological advantages that ensure better survival rates than males.[250]

Men also may doom themselves for social reasons. Although males have traditionally had greater access to wealth and power, the price of this advantage, one sociologist suggests, is "the tremendous stress associated with a life of competition, repressed feelings, and fear of failure,"

all of which may have life-shortening consequences.[251] Compared to women, American men have three times the suicide rate, three times the rate for severe mental disorders, and six times the alcoholism rate. They are also more apt to have hypertension, ulcers, and asthma, which may be linked to stress.

Sexism and Health: The Socioeconomic Disadvantages for Women Whatever biological advantages females may have seem to be diminished by socioeconomic disadvantages. Throughout the world, *sexism*—the belief that one sex is superior to the other, justifying unequal treatment—prevails against women. In North America, men are favored in higher education, job specialization, and promotion. Elsewhere on the planet the favoritism of men over women is revealed in nearly all statistics. For instance, women perform two-thirds of the world's work, but receive only 10% of the income and own a scant 1% of the land.[252] The number of rural women living in poverty in developing countries has increased 50% in the past two decades, and they far outnumber men in a similar position, according to a United Nations agency.[253]

Some of the worst indicators are in the areas of health. In most of Asia and North Africa, points out one writer, "the failure to give women medical care similar to what men get and to provide them with comparable food and social services results in fewer women surviving than would be the case if they had equal care."[254] In these parts of the world, women suffer higher rates of disease and neglect in health care and medical attention relative to men. The result, says this writer, "is a lower proportion of women than would be the case if they had equal care."

These differences may be less pronounced in North America than elsewhere in the world, although they certainly apply to women in poverty.[255] Still, there have been many signs of the neglect of women's health in the United

States. For instance, in 1990, the General Accounting Office, the investigative arm of Congress, declared that the National Institutes of Health—which funds about 40% of the nation's health research—was failing to follow its own policy of actively including women in medical research studies.[256] (*See accompanying* ● *table*.) A notable example of this exclusion was a study of 22,071 doctors that began in 1981 to determine whether aspirin could prevent heart attacks; no women were included. Another 1990 study found that, of 2297 coronary artery bypass patients, 4.6% of the women died during or immediately after the operation, compared with 2.6% of the men, because physicians waited too long to order the procedure.[257]

Since then, remedial efforts have been undertaken. In 1991, the National Institutes of Health began strongly promoting the inclusion of more women in medical studies and launched "the most definitive, far-reaching study of women's health ever undertaken."[258] Nevertheless, the correction of this "oversight" is so recent as to suggest that the problem of giving equal importance to women's health as to men's has only begun.

Race and Health

If women, who make up half the population in the United States, seem to get less than their full measure of health care, what might be the situation with racial minorities? In polls sponsored by the American Jewish Committee in 1964 and 1989, in which adults nationwide were asked to rate the "social standing" of various ethnic groups, it has been found that tolerance of ethnicity seems to be rising and anti-Semitism dropping. Groups whose standings were perceived to have improved most significantly were the Japanese, Chinese, and African Americans.[259]

This increase in tolerance is good news. Still, death rates and other health indicators are widely at variance for different racial groups. Black Americans, for instance, have a shorter life expectancy than whites and are less likely than whites to survive certain diseases.[260] (*See accompanying* ● *table*.) Indeed, life expectancy for African Americans has dropped

● **Examples of studies biased against females**

Subject of study	Number of men in study	Number of women in study
Benefits of taking an aspirin a day to lower risk of heart attack	22,071	0
Possible benefits of fish diet while recovering from heart attack (British study)	2,033	0
Hard-charging "Type A" behavior and heart disease	3,154	0
Smoking and increase in risks of developing cataracts	838	0
Connection between high cholesterol, lack of exercise, and smoking and risk of heart disease	12,866	0

● **Differences in death rates for blacks and whites.** Age-adjusted rates per 100,000 in 1988

Cause of death	Blacks	Whites
Tuberculosis	2.1	0.3
Asthma	3.5	1.1
Liver disease	14.5	8.4
Diabetes	21.2	9.0
Stroke	51.5	27.5
Cancer	171.3	130.0
Heart disease	226.6	161.5

for several years in a row, to 69.2 years in 1988, while the figure for whites has been rising, to 75.6 in that year.[261] The differences are largely due to heart disease and the sharp increase in homicides and deaths related to acquired immune deficiency syndrome among blacks. In addition, Native Americans, Native Alaskans,

Puerto Ricans, and other Hispanics have been found to be in generally poorer health than whites, Asian Americans, and Cuban Americans.

Why do African Americans, for instance, have shorter lives? Race by itself is probably not the reason, although there is a danger that statistics can mislead people to think it is. Theories of black genetic inferiority, although discredited, still linger in many people's minds, as epidemiologist Richard Cooper points out.[262] Such thinking is an example of *racism,* the belief that racial differences produce an inherent superiority or inferiority of a particular race.

Some statisticians point out that educational attainment—which is correlated with high income, job stability, and health care—makes a difference: black college-educated people and white college-educated people show zero or very few health differences.[263] Demographer Richard Rogers also says that racial differences in mortality disappear when data about blacks is controlled for age, sex, marital status, family size, income, and education.[264] That is, in general, those who lead shorter lives are poor rather than rich, single rather than married, from large families rather than small ones, and are less educated rather than with college experience. Blacks tend to be on the wrong end of all of these—poor, single, from large families, and with less education.

The ill health of blacks definitely reflects economic differences; one third of blacks are below the poverty line (defined as an annual income of less than $13,924 for a family of four in 1991).[265] Blacks are three times more likely than whites to die of diabetes, a disease that is the byproduct of obesity, which can be controlled with good medical care. Blacks are also more likely than whites to have injuries and accidents—3.2 times more likely to die in a residential fire, for example, which is more apt to happen in poorly constructed low-income housing. Finally, blacks are more likely candidates for death from heart disease, stroke, and cancer, all linked to lifestyle habits such as smoking and high-fat diets—factors that reflect the fact that low-income people take longer to adapt to new health practices, suggests Rogers. Other factors are lack of medical attention and access to preventive care.[266,267]

Low income is only a partial explanation, however. Another is simply racial discrimination. Some psychologists have suggested, for instance, that the high levels of hypertension among African Americans reflects the stresses of living in a society where race is still a barrier.[268] Moreover, it is possible that some health care professionals just do not treat blacks' medical problems as seriously as those of whites. For instance, one study found that older black patients on Medicare get heart bypass operations only about a fourth as often as similar whites.[269] (That this may be due to racism is disputed, however; blacks may show different patterns of heart disease—such as hypertensive cardiomyopathy, resulting from hypertension—that cannot be fixed with bypass surgery.)[270] Other studies have found that blacks hospitalized for pneumonia receive less intensive treatment than whites do and that blacks undergoing dialysis for kidney disease are far less likely than whites to receive a kidney transplant.[271]

In New York City's central Harlem, reported an article in the *New England Journal of Medicine,* a black man has less chance of living to age 65 than a man living in Bangladesh. Said the authors, "A major political and financial commitment will be needed to eradicate the root causes of this high mortality: vicious poverty and inadequate access to the basic health care that is the right of all Americans."[272] The treatment of blacks represents perhaps the greatest inequities, but the same goals for better health care apply to many other minorities as well.

Money and Health

"What's the No. 1 cause of poor health?" asks medical ethicist Bruce Hilton. "Germs, you say? Viruses? Stress? Overeating?" If you said *None of the above,* you're right. "The No. 1 cause of illness," he says, "is poverty."[273]

One of the most vivid examples of this was illustrated by a 3-year study released in 1992 by Boston City Hospital, which showed that the number of emergency room visits by underweight children ages 2 months to 6 years increased by 30% after the coldest months of the year. This rise in medical emergencies, say physicians, seems to be the result of a "heat-or-eat" dilemma: poor families go without adequate nutrition in winter months in order to pay their heating bills. "Parents well know that children freeze before they starve," said one pediatrician, "and in winter some families have to divert their already inadequate food budget to buy fuel to keep the children warm."[274] Clearly, people with higher incomes don't have to make such decisions about health tradeoffs.

Nearly one in eight Americans lives in a family with an income below the Federal poverty level, and nearly a quarter of children younger than age 6 are in such families.[275] Lack of money affects health care in all kinds of ways. The government report *Healthy People 2000* says that "Health disparities between poor people and those with higher incomes are almost universal for all dimensions of health."[276] This is most graphically demonstrated in figures showing the relationship between annual income and limitation in major activity because of health problems. The poor experience higher rates of ill health in nearly every category: infant mortality, developmental limitations, chronic disease (heart disease, cancer, HIV infection, tuberculosis), and injury and traumatic death (murder, suicide).

In the 1980s, the United States underwent a major economic change, with the rich getting richer and the poor getting poorer. The top 20% of the population received nearly 43% of the income, but the bottom 40% received only about 16%.[277,278] In 1991, there were more poor people (35.7 million) than at any time since 1964.[279]

Of course, other countries have poor people, too, but many countries distribute their resources in a way that translates into higher living standards for their citizens. For instance, the average citizen of Brazil earns slightly more ($4718 versus $4542) per year than the average citizen of Costa Rica, but the Costa Rican lives longer, is better educated, and has cleaner water and better sanitation than the Brazilian. As a result, Costa Rica has a score of .852 out of a possible 1.000, according to the 1993 *United Nations Human Development Report*, whereas Brazil has only .730. By this same index, the United States has .976, putting its "human development score" in sixth place in the world, behind Japan (.983), Canada (.982), Norway (.978), Switzerland (.978), and Sweden (.976). However, the U.N. report observes there is a broad gap between the living standards of white Americans and those of other races.[280] In sum: it is not the total wealth of a country that is important so much as how that wealth is translated into health care and education for everyone.

Education and Health

A good income correlates with good health. But there is something even better: a good education.

According to a study of 125,000 people by the National Center of Health Statistics, those with little education are far more likely to have bad health.[281] For instance, compared to high school graduates, people who didn't finish high school were more than twice as apt to have heart problems, hypertension, ulcers, or visual or hearing problems; 2½ times more likely to have diabetes or arthritis; and 5 times more likely to have emphysema.

College graduates came out best. Only 1 in 13 college graduates were found to be limited in daily activity because of some chronic condition, compared with 1 in 4 people with less than a high school education. About 18% who didn't finish high school are hospitalized each year, nearly 2½ times as many as college graduates.

Interestingly, the study found that the correlation between education and health even transcends income levels. That is, among people in the same income group, people with less education were much less healthy than those with better educations and had to make greater use of medical services.

It has already been known that, as a rule, graduating from college pays off financially. The average monthly pay for a high school graduate, according to a 1993 Census Bureau report, was $1077, compared with $2116 for a person with a bachelor's degree. A master's degree was worth $2822 a month, a doctorate $3855, and a professional degree (such as medicine or law) $4961.[282] Additional health, then, would seem to be an added bonus for those with education.

Notes

Explanation of abbreviations:

AH: American Health
AIM: Annals of Internal Medicine
AJPH: American Journal of Public Health
JAMA: Journal of the American Medical Association
LAT: Los Angeles Times
MMWR: Morbidity & Mortality Weekly Report
NEJM: New England Journal of Medicine
NYT: New York Times
PT: Psychology Today
SFC: San Francisco Chronicle
SFE: San Francisco Examiner
WSJ: Wall Street Journal

UNIT 1: LEARNING HOW TO LIVE

1. Hilton, B. (1990, August 12). Taking a broader look at disease. *SFE*, D-16.
2. McCoy, R. (1991, January). Yesterday's children. *Arizona Highways*, 14–21
3. Hocking-Vigie, P. (1992, May 17). 117-year-old woman's secret? Attitude. *LAT*, A6.
4. Reuters. (1990, November 2). Is life expectancy now stretched to its limit? *NYT*, A16.
5. United Press International. (1990, April 6). Japanese live the longest. *SFC*, B3–B4.
6. Vachon, R. A. (1991, May 15). Living and breathing, yes, but not healthier (letter). *NYT*, A14.
7. Fries, J. F., & Crapo, L. M. (1981). *Vitality and aging*. New York: Freeman.
8. Breslow, L. (1990). A health promotion primer for the 1990s. *Health Affairs*, 9, 6–21.
9. Eberst, R. M. (1984). Defining health: A multidimensional model. *Journal of School Health*, 54, 99–104.
10. Eberst, 1984, 100.
11. Garfield, C. (1986). *Peak performers: The new heroes of American business*. New York: Morrow.
12. Garfield, 1986, 288–89.
13. Vickery, D. M. (1978). *Life plan for your health*. Reading, MA: Addison-Wesley.
14. Hilton, B. (1990, July 8). Stitch in time is still a penny earned. *SFE*, D-15.
15. Koop, C. E. (1990, July 11). Prevention still best and cheapest cure. *SFC*, Briefing section, 9; reprinted from *LAT*.
16. Associated Press. (1990, June). Experts say new generation is in trouble already. *SFC*, A1.
17. U.S. Department of Health and Human Services, Public Health Service (1990). *Healthy people 2000: National health promotion and disease prevention objectives*. DHHS Pub. No. (PHS)91–50213. Washington, DC: U.S. Government Printing Office, 16–20.
18. Brody, J. E. (1991, January 31). In pursuit of the best possible odds of preventing or minimizing the perils of major disease. *NYT*, B6.
19. Shirreffs, J. H. (1990). Expanded responseability: A prescription for health promotion. *Health Education*, 21, 29–35.
20. Shirreffs, 1990, 34.
21. Shirreffs, 1990, 34.
22. Cole, R. Quoted in: Stein, R. (1990, June 29). Changes and chances. *SFC*, B3.
23. Hymer, S. Cited in: Larkin, M., & Duane, M. (1986, April 10). Why it's healthy to take risks. *SFC*, 27; reprinted from *NYT*.
24. Schulman, D. Cited in: Larkin & Duane, 1986, 27.
25. Ziegler, D. J. Cited in: Larkin & Duane, 1986, 27.
26. Longman, D. G., & Atkinson, R. H. (1992). *College learning and study skills* (2nd ed.). St. Paul, MN: West, 4.
27. Douglass, M., & Douglass, D. (1980). *Manage your time, manage your work, manage yourself*. New York: American Management Association.
28. Beneke, W. M., & Harris, M. B. (1972). Teaching self-control of study behavior. *Behavior Research & Therapy*, 10, 35–41.
29. Zechmeister, E. B., & Nyberg, S. E. (1982). *Human memory: An introduction to research and theory*. Pacific Grove, CA: Brooks/Cole.
30. Bromage, B. K., & Mayer, R. E. (1986). Quantitative and qualitative effects of repetition on learning from technical text. *Journal of Educational Psychology*, 78, 271–78.
31. Longman & Atkinson, 1992, 148–53.
32. Lindgren, H. C. (1969). *The psychology of college success: A dynamic approach*. New York: Wiley.
33. Palkovitz, R. J., & Lore, R. K. (1980). Note taking and note review: Why students fail questions based on lecture material. *Teaching of Psychology*, 7, 159–61.
34. Palkovitz & Lore, 1980, 159–61.
35. Robinson, F. P. (1970). *Effective study* (4th ed.). New York: Harper & Row.
36. Langan, J., & Nadell, J. (1980). *Doing well in college: A concise guide to reading, writing, and study skills*. New York: McGraw-Hill, 93–110.
37. Langan & Nadell, 1980, 104.

UNIT 2: HANDLING STRESS

1. Selye, H. (1974). *Stress without distress*. New York: Lippincott, 27.
2. Lazarus, R. S., & Folkman, S. (1982). Coping and adaptation. In W. D. Gentry (Ed.), *Handbook of behavioral medicine*. New York: Guilford.
3. Lazarus, R. S. (1981, July). Little hassles can be hazardous to health. *PT*, 61.
4. Folkman, S., Lazarus, R. S., Pimley, S. et al. (1987). Age differences in stress and coping processes. *Psychology & Aging*, 2, 171–84.
5. Charney, D. Cited in: Goleman, D. (1990, August 22). Flashback terror: It's biological. *SFC*, "Briefing" section, 7; reprinted from *NYT*.
6. Bartlett, K., Associated Press. (1990, March 25). After a fall, pain is both her constant companion and her jailer. *LAT*, A2.
7. Selye, 1974, 28–29.
8. Selye, 1974.
9. Holmes, T. H., & Rahe, R. H. (1967). The social readjustment rating scale. *Journal of Psychosomatic Research*, 11, 213–18.
10. Sarason, I. G., Johnson, J. H., & Siegel, J. M. (1978). Assessing the impact of life changes: Development of the Life Experiences Survey. *Journal of Consulting & Clinical Psychology*, 46, 932–46.
11. Friedman, M., & Rosenman, R. H. (1974). *Type A behavior and your heart*. Greenwich, CT: Knopf.
12. Friedman, M., Thoreson, C. E., Gill, J. J. et al. (1986). Alteration of Type A behavior and its effect on cardiac recurrences in post myocardial infarction patients: Summary results of the recurrent coronary prevention project. *American Heart Journal*, 112, 653–65.
13. Dembroski, T. M., & Costa, P. T. (1988). Assessment of coronary-prone behavior: A current overview. *Annals of Behavioral Medicine*, 10, 60–63.
14. Dembroski, T. M., MacDougall, J. M., Costa, P. T. Jr. et al. (1989). Components of hostility as predictors of sudden death and myocardial infarction in the Multiple Risk Factor Intervention Trial. *Psychosomatic Medicine*, 51, 514–22.
15. Dembroski, T. M., & Costa, P. T. Jr. (1987). Coronary prone behavior: Components of the Type A pattern and hostility. *Journal of Personality*, 55, 211–35.

16. Kobasa, S. (1979). Stressful life events, personality and health: An inquiry into hardiness. *Journal of Psychology & Social Psychology*, 37, 1–11.
17. Kobasa, S. C., Maddi, S. R., & Kahn, S. (1981). Hardiness and health: A prospective study. *Journal of Personality & Social Psychology*, 22, 368–78.
18. Vaux, A. (1988). *Social support: Theory, research, and intervention*. New York: Praeger.
19. Colby, B. N. (1987). Well-being: A theoretical program. *American Anthropologist*, 89, 879–95.
20. Wittmeyer, I. W. Cited in: Doheny, K. Health & Fitness News Service. (1990, October 3). Illness 'all in your head'? Maybe not. *SFC*, B3.
21. Hinkle, L. E. Jr. (1987). Stress and disease: The concept after 50 years. *Social Science & Medicine*, 25, 561–66.
22. Sandler, R. S. (1990). Epidemiology of irritable bowel syndrome in the United States. *Gastroenterology*, 99, 409–15.
23. Everhart, J. Cited in: Patlak, M. (1990, September 23). Scientists learning how stress produces 'gut feelings.' *SFE*, D-14, D-16.
24. Williams, C. Cited in: Patlak, 1990, D-14.
25. Krueger, E., & Krueger, G. R. (1991). How does the subjective experience of stress relate to the breakdown of the human immune system. *In Vivo*, 5, 207–15.
26. Shavit, Y., Terman, G. W., Martin, F. C., Lewis, J. W., Liebeskind, J. C., & Gale, R. P. (1985). Stress, opioid peptides, the immune system, and cancer. *Journal of Immunology*, 135, 834S–37S.
27. Kiecolt-Glaser, J., & Glaser, R. Major life changes, chronic stress, and immunity. (1988). *Advances in Biochemical Psychopharmacology*, 44, 217–24.
28. Kiecolt-Glazer, J. et al. (1987) Stress, health, and immunity: Tracking the mind/body connection. Presentation at American Psychological Association meeting, New York, August 1987.
29. Kannel, W. B. (1990). CHD risk factors: A Framingham study update. *Hospital Practice*, 25, 119.
30. Eliot, R., & Breo, D. (1984). *Is it worth dying for?* New York: Bantam.
31. Dunkel-Schetter, C. Cited in: Roan, S. (1990, August 17). Stress affects premature births. *SFC*, B6; reprinted from *LAT*.
32. Levin, J. S., & DeFrank, R. S. (1988). Maternal stress and pregnancy outcomes: A review of the psychosocial literature. *Journal of Psychosomatic Obstetrics & Gynaecology*, 9, 3–16.
33. Rothberg, A. D., Shuenyane, E., Lits, B., & Strebel, P. M. (1991). Effect of stress on birth weight in two Johannesburg populations. *South African Medical Journal*, 79, 35–38.
34. Maslach, C. (1982). Understanding burnout: Definitional issues in analyzing a complex phenomenon. In W. S. Paine (Ed.), *Job stress and burnout: Research, theory and intervention perspectives*. Beverly Hills, CA: Sage.
35. MacBride, A. (1983). Burnout: Possible? Probable? Preventable? *Canada's Mental Health*, 31, 2–3, 8.
36. Girdano, D. A., & Everly, G. S. Jr. (1986). *Controlling stress and tension*. Englewood Cliffs, NJ: Prentice-Hall.
37. McCulloch, A., & O'Brien, L. (1986). The organizational determinants of worker burnout. *Children & Youth Services Review*, 8, 175–90.
38. Srnec, P. (1991). Children, violence, and intentional injuries. *Critical Care Nursing Clinics of North America*, 3, 471–78.
39. Bell, C. C., Taylor, C. K., Jenkins, E. J. et al.

(1988). Need for victimization screening in a Black psychiatric population. *Journal of the National Medical Association, 80*, 41–48.

40. Jenkins, E. J., Bell, C. C., Taylor, J. et al. (1989). Circumstances of sexual and physical victimization of Black psychiatric outpatients. *Journal of the National Medical Association, 81*, 246–52.

41. Bell, C., & Jenkins, E. Cited in: Anonymous. (1990, October 3). 1 in 4 kids had seen slayings. *SFC*, B4; reprinted from *Washington Post*.

42. Fields, R. Cited in: Drexler, M. (1990, July 1). Children of violence. *SFC, This World*, 23; reprinted from *Boston Globe Magazine*.

43. Jaffe, P., Wolfe, D., Wilson, S. et al. (1986). Similarities in behavioral and social maladjustment among child victims and witnesses to family violence. *American Journal of Orthopsychiatry, 56*, 142–46.

44. Burris, C. A., & Jaffe, P. (1984). Wife battering: A well-kept secret. *Canadian Journal of Criminology, 26*, 171–77.

45. Jaffe, P., Wolfe, D. A., Wilson, S. et al. (1986). Emotional and physical health problems of battered women. *Canadian Journal of Psychiatry, 31*, 625–29.

46. Jaffe, P. Cited in: Fine, S. (1990, May 5). Feelings of battered women similar to POWs', experts say. *The Globe & Mail* (Toronto), A7.

47. Kilpatrick, D. Cited in: Goleman, D. (1990, May 3). Second assault on crime victims: Long-term mental troubles. *NYT*, B7.

48. Kleinman, S. Cited in: Goleman, 1990, B7.

49. National Institute of Justice. Cited in: Goleman, 1990, B7.

50. Spiller, R. J. (1990, May/June). Shell shock. *American Heritage*, 75–87.

51. Blake, D. D., Keane, T. M., Wine, P. R. et al. (1990). Prevalence of PTSD symptoms in combat veterans seeking medical treatment. *Journal of Traumatic Stress, 3*, 15–27.

52. Burge, S. K. (1988). Post-traumatic stress disorder in victims of rape. Special Issue: Progress in traumatic stress research. *Journal of Traumatic Stress, 1*, 193–210.

53. Gersons, B. P. (1989). Patterns of PTSD among police officers following shooting incidents: A two-dimensional model and treatment implications. *Journal of Traumatic Stress, 2*, 247–57.

54. Goodwin, J. (1988). Post-traumatic symptoms in abused children. *Journal of Traumatic Stress, 1*, 475–88.

55. Kleinman, 1990. Cited in Goleman, 1990, B7.

56. Rinear, E. E. (1988). Psychosocial aspects of parental response patterns to the death of a child by homicide. *Journal of Traumatic Stress, 1*, 305–22.

57. Trice, A. D. (1988). Posttraumatic stress syndrome-like symptoms among AIDS caregivers. *Psychological Reports, 63*, 656–58.

58. American Psychiatric Association. (1987). *Diagnostic and statistical manual of mental disorders* (3rd ed.—Revised). Washington, DC: American Psychiatric Association, 250–51.

59. Tannen, D. (1990). *You just don't understand: Women and men in conversation*. New York: Morrow, 15.

60. Gilligan, C. (1982). *In a different voice*. Cambridge, MA: Harvard University Press, 173.

61. Tannen, 1990, 24–25.

62. Syme, S. L. (1982, July/August). People need people. *AH*.

63. Seeman, T. E., & Syme, S. L. (1987). Social networks and coronary artery disease: A comparison of the structure and function of social relations as predictors of disease. *Psychosomatic Medicine, 49*, 341–54.

64. Gallup Organization, Associated Press. (1990, January 12). Working at the wrong job. *SFC*, C1. [October 1989 survey for National Occupational Information Coordinating Committee.]

65. Leigh, J. P., & Waldon, H. M. (1991).

Unemployment and highway fatalities. *Journal of Health Politics, Policy & Law, 16*, 135–56.

66. Franks, P. J., Adamson, C., Bulpitt, P. F. et al. (1991). Stroke death and unemployment in London. *Journal of Epidemiology & Community Health–London, 45*, 16–18.

67. Sherman, C. (1982, July/August). The ills of unemployment. *AH*.

68. Hawton, K., Fagg, J., & Simkin, S. (1988). Female unemployment and attempted suicide. *British Journal of Psychiatry, 152*, 632–37.

69. Charlton, J. R., Bauer, R., Thakhore, A. et al. (1987). Unemployment and mortality: A small area analysis. *Journal of Epidemiology & Community Health, 41*, 107–13.

70. Dooley, D., Catalano, R., Rook, K. et al. (1989). Economic stress and suicide: Multilevel analyses: I. Aggregate time-series analyses of economic stress and suicide. *Suicide & Life-Threatening Behavior, 19*, 321–36.

71. Hochschild, A., & Machung, A. (1989). *The second shift: Working parents and the revolution at home*. New York: Viking Penguin.

72. Anonymous. (1987, October). The perils of burnout. *Newsweek on Campus*.

73. Timmrick, T. C., & Braza, G. (1980). Stress and aging. *Geriatrics, 25*, 113.

74. Turner, R. J., & McLean, P. D. (1989). Physical disability and psychological distress. *Rehabilitation Psychology, 34*, 225–42.

75. Reich, J. W., Zautra, A. J., & Guarnaccia, C. A. (1989). Effects of disability and bereavement on the mental health and recovery of older adults. *Psychology & Aging, 4*, 57–65.

76. Anonymous. (1990, September 1). Despite rights law, the disabled say there's a long way to go. *SFC*, A16; reprinted from *LAT*.

77. Young, E. (1990, August 3). Survey likens homeless to combat vets. *SFC*, B7. [Report of Staff, *By No MEANS*.]

78. Jung, J., & Khalsa, H. K. (1989). The relationship of daily hassles, social support, and coping to depression in Black and White students. *Journal of General Psychology, 116*, 407–17.

79. Ulbrich, P. M., Warheit, G. J., & Zimmerman, R. S. (1989). Race, socioeconomic status, and psychological distress: An examination of differential vulnerability. *Journal of Health & Social Behavior, 30*, 131–46.

80. Feagin, J., Associated Press. (1990, September 22). Even upper-income blacks suffer race bias, study shows. *SFC*, A8.

81. Aldwin, C., & Greenberger, E. (1987). Cultural differences in the predictors of depression. *American Journal of Community Psychology, 15*, 789–813.

82. Ebbin, A. J., & Blankenship, E. S. (1988). Stress-related diagnosis and barriers to health care among foreign students: Results of a survey. *Journal of American College Health, 36*, 311–12.

83. Levine, R. (1989, December). The pace of life. *PT*, 42–46.

84. Gallup, G. Jr., & Newport, F. (1990, October 8). Americans love—and hate—their TVs. *SFC*, B9.

85. Goleman, D. (1990, October 18). TV: More evidence of a 'plug-in drug.' *SFC*, B3–B4; reprinted from *NYT*.

86. Anonymous. (1987, August). "Dear Diary." *AH*.

87. Mee, C. L. Jr. (Ed.). (1987). *Managing stress from morning to night*. Alexandria, VA: Time-Life.

88. Zajonc, R. B. (1985). Emotion and facial efference: A theory reclaimed. *Science, 228*, 15–21.

89. Adelmann, P. K., & Zajonc, R. B. (1989). Facial efference and the experience of emotion. *Annual Review of Psychology, 40*, 249–80.

90. Zajonc, R. Cited in: Goleman, D. (1989, June

29). Put on a happy face—it really works. *SFC*, C10; reprinted from *NYT*.

91. Goleman, 1989, C10.

92. Donahue, P. A. (1989). Helping adolescents with shyness: Applying the Japanese Morita therapy in shyness counselling. *International Journal for the Advancement of Counselling, 12*, 323–32.

93. Zastrow, C. (1988). What really causes psychotherapy change? *Journal of Independent Social Work, 2*, 5–16.

94. Braiker, H. B. (1989, December). The power of self-talk. *PT*, 24.

95. Cousins, N. (1979). *Anatomy of an illness*. New York: Norton.

96. Dillon, K. M., Minchoff, B., & Baker, K. H. (1985–86). Positive emotional states and enhancement of the immune system. *International Journal of Psychiatry in Medicine, 15*, 13–18.

97. Long, P. (1987, October). Laugh and be well? *PT*, 28–29.

98. Siegel, B. (1986). *Love, medicine, and miracles*. New York: Harper & Row.

99. Reifman, A., & Dunkel-Schetter, C. (1990). Stress, structural social support, and well-being in university students. *Journal of American College Health, 38*, 271–77.

100. Leerhsen, C. et al. (1990, February 5). Unite and conquer. *Newsweek*, 50–55.

101. Spiegel, D., Bloom, J. R., Kramer, H. C. et al. (1989). Effect of psychosocial treatment on survival of patients with metastatic breast cancer. *Lancet, 2*, 888–91.

102. Ragland, J. Cited in: Busey, M. (1990, October). Industrial-strength stress dissolvers. *Men's Health*, 78–80.

103. Snyder, M. (1988). Relaxation. In J. J. Fitzpatrick, R. L. Taunton, & J. Q. Benoliel (Eds.), *Annual review of nursing research, 8*, 111–28. New York: Springer.

104. Benson, H. (1975). *The relaxation response*. New York: Avon.

105. Benson, H., & Proctor, W. (1984). *Beyond the relaxation response*. New York: Times.

106. Alexander, C. N., Langer, E. J., Newman, R. I. et al. (1989). Transcendental meditation, mindfulness, and longevity: An experimental study with the elderly. *Journal of Personality & Social Psychology, 57*, 950–64.

107. Goleman, D. (1989, January 15). Mind over blood pressure. *SFC, This World*, 14; reprinted from *NYT*.

108. Alexander et al., 1989.

109. Miller, L. (1989, November). What biofeedback does (and doesn't) do. *PT*, 23.

110. Sandroff, R. (1989, August). Is your job driving you crazy? *PT*, 45.

111. Meichenbaum, D. H. (1988). Stress inoculation training. *Counseling Psychologist, 16*, 69–90.

112. Gallup Poll (1990, November 5). People feel time is running out. *SFC*, B3.

113. Bureau of Labor Statistics. Cited in: Kilborn, P. T. (1990, June 3). Tales from the digital treadmill. *NYT*, sec. 4, 1, 3.

114. Louis Harris survey. Cited in: Kilborn, 1990, 1.

115. Davidson, J. (1989, August). Global vacations: U.S. comes out short. *PT*, 20.

116. Rosow, J. Cited in: Kilborn, 1990, 1.

117. Hall, C. T. (1991, January 21). U.S. workers losing spending power. *SFC*, C1.

118. Peterson, K. S. (1989, November 24–26). Kids think being a grown-up will be fun. *USA Today*, 1A.

119. Gallup Poll, 1990.

120. Ruffin, J. Cited in: Kilborn, 1990, 3.

121. Margolick, D. (1990, August 17). More lawyers are less happy at their work, a survey finds. *NYT*, B8.

122. Berglas, S. (1989, April). The success syndrome. *AH*, 57.

123. Steinberg, L., & Greenberger, E. (1990, July 13). How work is taking a toll on America's teenagers. *SFC*, A29; reprinted from *Washington Post*.

124. Smith, L., & Sipchen, B. (1990, August 13). Workers crave time with kids. *SFC*, B3, B5; reprinted from *LAT*.

125. Pesin, J. Quoted in: Trost, C., & Hymowitz, C. (1990, June 18). Careers start giving in to family needs. *WSJ*, B1–B2.

126. Trost & Hymowitz, 1990, B1–B2.

127. Lacher, I. (1990, October 21). Bound for glory. *LAT*, E1, E13–E15.

128. Weiss, R. Quoted in: Lacher, 1990, E1.

129. Weiss, R. Quoted in: Lacher, 1990, E13.

130. Leider, D. (1988, July/August). Purposeful work. *Utne Reader*, 52; excerpted from *On Purpose: A Journal About New Lifestyles and Workstyles*, Winter 1986.

131. Gallup Organization. Cited in: Associated Press. (1990, January 12). Working at the wrong job. *SFC*, C1.

132. Bolles, R. (1992). *What color is your parachute?* Berkeley, CA: Ten Speed Press.

133. Bolles, R. Cited in: Minton, T. (1991, January 25). Job-hunting requires eyes and ears of friends. *SFC*, D5.

134. Needleman, J. (1991). *Money and the meaning of life*. New York: Doubleday.

135. Needleman, J. Quoted in: Carman, J. (1990, June 26). Talking about money on PBS. *SFC*, E1.

UNIT 3: PSYCHOLOGICAL HEALTH

1. National Institute of Mental Health, Epidemiological Catchment Area Study. Cited in: Marbella, J. (1989, October 17). Mental ills widespread, study says. *SFC*, D3; reprinted from *Baltimore Sun*.

2. Erikson, E. H. (1963). *Childhood and society* (2nd ed.). New York: Norton.

3. Piaget, J. (1923/1957). *The language and thought of the child* (M. Gabain & R. Gabain, Trans.). New York: Humanities. (Original work published 1923).

4. Kohlberg, L. (1969). Stage and sequence: The cognitive-developmental approach to socialization. In D. A. Goslin (Ed.), *Handbook of socialization theory and research*. Chicago: Rand McNally.

5. Kohlberg, L., & Hersh, R. H. (1977). Moral development: A review of the theory. *Theory into Practice, 16*, 53–59.

6. Allport, G. W., & Odbert, H. S. (1936). Traitnames: A psycho-lexical study. *Psychological Monographs, 47*(1).

7. McCrae, R. R., & Costa, P. T. Jr. (1986). Clinical assessment can benefit from recent advances in personality psychology. *American Psychologist, 41*, 1001–1003.

8. Watson, J. B. (1928/1972). *Psychological care of infant and child*. Salem, NH: Ayer. (Originally published 1928.)

9. Bandura, A. (1986). *Social foundations of thought and action: A social-cognitive theory*. Englewood Cliffs, NJ: Prentice-Hall.

10. Leonard, G. (1983, December). Abraham Maslow and the new self. *Esquire*, 331–32.

11. Rogers, C. R. (1980). *A way of being*. Boston: Houghton Mifflin.

12. Shapiro, D. (1983). Cited in: R. Walsh & D. H. Shapiro (Eds.), *Beyond health and normality*. New York: Van Nostrand Reinhold, 273.

13. Maslow, A. H. (1968). *Toward a psychology of being* (2nd ed.). Princeton, NJ: Van Nostrand Reinhold.

14. Maslow, A. H. (1970). *Motivation and personality* (2nd ed.). New York: Harper & Row.

15. Garfield, C. (1986). *Peak performers: The new heroes of American business*. New York: Morrow.

16. Harre, R., & Lamb, R. (Eds.). (1983). *The encyclopedia dictionary of psychology*. Cambridge, MA: MIT Press.

17. Schneiderman, L. Cited in: Sylvester, D. A. (1990, April 10). Schools join self-esteem movement. *SFC*, A1, A4.

18. Wallerstein, J. S., & Kelly, J. B. (1990). *Surviving the breakup: How children and parents cope with divorce*. New York: Basic.

19. Curry, S., Marlatt, A., & Gordon, J. R. (1987). Abstinence violation effect: Validation of an attributional construct with smoking cessation. *Journal of Consulting & Clinical Psychology, 55*, 145–49.

20. Rotter, J. B. (1966). Generalized expectancies for internal versus external control of reinforcement. *Psychological Monographs, 80*(Whole No. 603).

21. Findley, M. J., & Cooper, H. M. (1983). Locus of control and academic achievement: A literature review. *Journal of Personality & Social Psychology, 44*, 419–27.

22. Lefcourt, H. M. (1982). *Locus of control: Current trends in theory and research*. Hillsdale, NJ: Erlbaum.

23. McGinnis, A. Quoted in: Maushard, M. (1990, October 22). How to get happy: What makes optimists tick. *SFC*, B5; reprinted from *Baltimore Evening Sun*.

24. McGinnis, A. L. (1990). *The power of optimism*. San Francisco: Harper & Row.

25. Tellegen, A. Quoted in: Swanbrow, D. (1989, July/August). The paradox of happiness. *PT*, 37–39.

26. Ornstein, R., & Sobel, D. (1989). *Healthy pleasures*. Reading, MA: Addison-Wesley.

27. Ornstein, R. E., & Sobel, D. S. (1989, May). Healthy pleasures. *AH*, 53–62.

28. Szent-Györgyi, A. Quoted in: von Oech, R. (1983). *A whack on the side of the head*. Menlo Park, CA: Creative Think, 7.

29. von Oech, 1983, 21.

30. Hyatt, C., & Gottlieb, L. (1987). *When smart people fail*. New York: Simon & Schuster, 20.

31. Garfield, C. Quoted in: Rozak, M. (1989, August). The mid-life fitness peak. *PT*, 32–33.

32. Harre & Lamb, 1983, 359.

33. Curtis, R. C., & Miller, K. (1986). Believing another likes or dislikes you: Behaviors making the beliefs come true. *Journal of Personality & Social Psychology, 51*, 284–90.

34. Keaton, D. Quoted in: Garis, L. (1991, January). Diane Keaton. *Mirabella*, 38–43.

35. Peplau, L. A., & Perlman, D. (1982). *Loneliness: A sourcebook of current theory, research and therapy*. New York: Wiley.

36. Page, R. M. (1990). Loneliness and adolescent health behavior. *Health Education, 21*, 14–18.

37. Beck, A. T., & Young, J. E. (1978, September). College blues. *PT*, 80–92.

38. Spitzberg, B. H., & Hurt, H. T. (1987). The relationship of interpersonal competence and skills to reported loneliness across time. *Journal of Social Behavior & Personality, 2*, 157–72.

39. Zimbardo, P. (1977). *Shyness: What it is; what to do about it*. Reading, MA: Addison-Wesley, 12.

40. Zimbardo, 1977, 14.

41. Kagan, J. Cited in: Bass, A. (1990, October 14). Shy? So are more adults than you'd think. *SFE*, E-15; reprinted from *Boston Globe*.

42. Solomon, J. (1990, May 4). Executives who dread public speaking learn to keep their cool in the spotlight. *WSJ*, B1.

43. National Foundation for Depressive Illness. Cited in: Gertz, K. R. (1990, November). Mood probe. *Self*, 165–68, 204–206.

44. Ray, M., & Myers, R. (1986). *Creativity in business*. Garden City, NY: Doubleday.

45. Averill, J. R. (1983). Studies on anger and aggression: Implications for theories of emotion. *American Psychologist, 38*, 1145–60.

46. Tavris, C. (1982). *Anger: The misunderstood emotion*. New York: Touchstone, 189.

47. Ebbesen, E. B., Duncan, B., & Konecni, V. J. (1975). Effects of content of verbal aggression on future aggression: A field experiment. *Journal of Experimental Social Psychology, 11*, 192–204.

48. Tavris, 1982, 223.

49. Styron, W. (1990). *Darkness visible: A memoir of madness*. New York: Random House, 15.

50. American Psychiatric Association. (1987). *Diagnostic and statistical manual of mental disorders* (3rd ed.—Revised). Washington, DC: American Psychiatric Association.

51. Popp, R. (1991, January 7). S.F. cop mugged 256 times retires. *SFC*, B1.

52. Kalat, J. W. (1990). *Introduction to psychology* (2nd ed.). Belmont, CA: Wadsworth.

53. Robins, L. N., Helzer, J. E., Weissman, M. M. et al. (1984). Lifetime prevalence of specific psychiatric disorders in three sites. *Archives of General Psychiatry, 41*, 949–58.

54. Holden, C. (1991). Depression: The news isn't depressing. *Science, 254*, 1450–52.

55. Lobel, B., & Hirschfeld, R. M. A. (1985). *Depression: What we know*. DHHS Pub. No. (ADM)85-1318) Washington, DC: National Institute of Mental Health.

56. Styron, 1990, 56.

57. Jacobsen, F. M., Sack, D. A., Wehr, T. A. et al. (1987). Neuroendocrine 5-hydroxytryptophan in seasonal affective disorder. *Archives of General Psychiatry, 44*, 1086–91.

58. Wurtman, R. J., & Wurtman, J. J. (1989). Carbohydrates and depression. *Scientific American, 260*, 68–75.

59. Keller, M. (Ed.). (1988). Unipolar depression. In *Psychiatry Update: Annual Review of Psychiatry*. Washington, DC: American Psychiatric Association.

60. Robins et al., 1984.

61. Holden, 1991.

62. Beardslee, W. R., Bemporad, J., Keller, M. B. et al. (1983). Children of parents with major affective disorder: A review. *American Journal of Psychiatry, 140*, 825–32.

63. Freedman, A. M. (1989). Overview: Depression in health and illness. *Journal of Clinical Psychiatry, 50*, 3–5.

64. Shuchman, M. (1990, November 15). Depression hidden in deadly disease. *NYT*, B8.

65. Freedman, 1989.

66. Freedman, 1989.

67. Price, K. P., Tryon, W. W., & Raps, C. S. (1978). Learned helplessness and depression in a clinical population: A test of two behavioral hypotheses. *Journal of Abnormal Psychology, 87*, 113–21.

68. Benassi, V. A., Sweeney, P. D., & Dufour, C. L. (1988). Is there a relation between locus of control orientation and depression? *Journal of Abnormal Psychology, 97*, 357–67.

69. Wells, K. B., Hays, R. D., Burnham, M. A. et al. (1989). Detection of depressive disorder for patients receiving prepaid or fee-for-service care. *JAMA, 262*, 3298–302.

70. Keller, 1988.

71. Wenzlaff, R. M., Wegner, D. M., & Roper, D. W. (1988). Depression and mental control: The resurgence of unwanted negative thoughts. *Journal of Personality & Social Psychology, 55*, 882–92.

72. Wenzlaff, R. M. Quoted in: Adler, V. (1989, January/February). Accentuate the positive. *AH*, 50.

73. Klerman, G. Cited in: Anonymous. (1987, May 4). Depression [cover story]. *Newsweek*, 48–54.

74. Low, B. P., & Andrews, S. F. (1990). Adolescent suicide. *Medical Clinics of North America, 74*, 1251–64.

75. Low & Andrews, 1990.

76. Blumenthal, S. J., & Kupfer, D. J. (1986). Generalizable treatment strategies for suicidal behavior. *Annals of the New York Academy of Sciences, 487*, 327–40.

77. Peterson, L. G., Peterson, M., O'Shanick, G. J. et al. (1985). Self-inflicted gunshot wounds: Lethality of method versus intent. *American Journal of Psychiatry, 142*, 228–31.

78. Kalat, 1990, 515.

79. Wolpe, J., & Rowan, V. C. (1988). Panic disorder: A product of classical conditioning. *Behaviour Research & Therapy, 26*, 441–50.

80. Ledwidge, B. (1980). Run for your mind: Aerobic exercise as a means of alleviating anxiety and depression. *Canadian Journal of Behavioral Science, 12*, 126–40.

81. Myers, J. K., Weissman, M. M., Tischler, G. L. et al. (1984). Six-month prevalence of psychiatric disorders in three communities. *Archives of General Psychiatry, 41*, 959–67.

82. Öst, L.-G., & Hugdahl, K. (1981). Acquisition of phobias and anxiety response patterns in clinical patients. *Behaviour Research & Therapy, 19*, 439–47.

83. Seligman, M. E. P. (1971). Phobias and preparedness. *Behavior Therapy, 2*, 307–20.

84. Wolpe, J. (1961). The systematic desensitization treatment of neuroses. *Journal of Nervous & Mental Disease, 132*, 189–203.

85. Avery, P. (1989, February). Good news for dental phobics: Special clinics help uptight patients. *AH*, 46–48.

86. Hughes, H. Quoted in: Fowler, R. D. (1986, May). Howard Hughes: A psychological autopsy. *PT*, 22–33.

87. Perse, T. (1988). Obsessive-compulsive disorder: A treatment overview. *Journal of Clinical Psychiatry, 49*(2), 48–55.

88. Vann, J. R. (1990). Obsessive-compulsive disorder: Suffering in silence. *Journal of American College Health, 39*, 47–48.

89. Greist, J. H. et al. (1989). *Obsessive-compulsive disorder: A guide.* Madison, WI: Anxiety Disorders and Lithium Information Centers, Department of Psychiatry, University of Wisconsin.

90. Robins et al., 1984.

91. Nicol, S. E., & Gottesman, I. I. (1983). Clues to the genetics and neurobiology of schizophrenia. *American Scientist, 71*, 398–404.

92. Quinnett, P. G. (1989, April). The key to successful therapy. *PT*, 46–47.

93. Smith, D. (1982). Trends in counseling and psychotherapy. *American Psychologist, 37*, 802–809.

94. Freud, S. (1900/1950). *The interpretation of dreams.* (A. A. Brill, Trans.) New York: Modern Library. (Original work published 1900.)

95. Myers, D. G. (1989). *Psychology* (2nd ed.). New York: Worth, 478.

96. Rogers, C. R. (1961). *On becoming a person: A therapist's view of psychotherapy.* Boston: Houghton Mifflin.

97. Rogers, C. R., 1980.

98. Meador, B. D., & Rogers, C. R. (1984). Person-centered therapy. In R. J. Corsini (Ed.), *Current psychotherapies* (3rd ed.). Itasca, IL: Peacock, 167.

99. Perls, F. (1969). *Ego, hunger and aggression: The beginning of Gestalt therapy.* New York: Random House.

100. Ellis, A. (1962). *Reason and emotion in psychotherapy.* Secaucus, NJ: Citadel Press.

101. Ellis, A. (1987). The impossibility of achieving consistently good mental health. *American Psychologist, 42*, 364–75.

102. Ellis, A. (1984). Rational-emotive therapy. In Corsini, 219.

103. Beck, A. T., Rush, A. J., Shaw, B. F. et al. (1979). *Cognitive therapy of depression.* New York: Guilford Press.

104. Myer, D. G. (1989). *Psychology* (2nd ed.). New York: Worth, 490. [Describes Rabin, A. S., Kaslow, N. J., & Rehm, L. P. (1986). Aggregate outcome and follow-up results following self-control therapy for depression. Paper presented at the American Psychological Association convention.]

105. Berne, E. (1964). *Games people play.* New York: Grove.

106. Eysenck, J. J. (1952). The effects of psychotherapy: An evaluation. *Journal of Consulting Psychology, 16*, 319–24.

107. Bergin, A. E., & Lambert, M. J. (1978). The evaluation of therapeutic outcomes. In S. L. Garfield & A. E. Bergin (Eds.), *Handbook of psychotherapy and behavior change: An empirical analysis* (2nd ed.). New York: Wiley.

108. Smith, M. L., Glass, G. V., & Miller, R. L. (1980). *The benefits of psychotherapy.* Baltimore: Johns Hopkins Press, 183.

109. Elkin, I. (1986). Outcome findings and therapist performance. Paper presented at the American Psychological Association convention.

110. Singer, J. L. (1981). Clinical intervention: New developments in methods and evaluation. In L. T. Benjamin, Jr. (Ed.), *The G. Stanley Hall Lecture Series,* (Vol. 1). Washington, DC: American Psychological Association.

111. Frank, J. D. (1982). Therapeutic components shared by all psychotherapies. In J. H. Harvey & M. M. Parks (Eds.), *The Master Lecture Series: Vol. 1: Psychotherapy research and behavior change.* Washington, DC: American Psychological Association.

112. Goldfried, M. R., & Padawer, W. (1982). Current status and future directions in psychotherapy. In M. R. Goldfried (Ed.), *Converging themes in psychotherapy: Trends in psychodynamic, humanistic, and behavioral practice.* New York: Springer.

113. Strupp, H. H. (1986). Psychotherapy: Research, practice, and public policy (How to avoid dead ends). *American Psychologist, 41*, 120–30.

114. Bachrach, A. J., Erwin, W. J., & Mohr, J. P. (1965). The control of eating behavior in an anorectic by operant conditioning techniques. In L. P. Ullmann & L. Krasner (Eds.), *Case studies in behavior modification.* New York: Holt, Rinehart & Winston, 153–63.

115. Watson, D. L., & Tharp, R. G. (1989). *Self-directed behavior: Self-modification for personal adjustment.* Pacific Grove, CA: Brooks/Cole.

116. Bowers, K. S. (1984). Hypnosis. In N. Endler & J. M. Hunt (Eds.), *Personality and behavioral disorders* (2nd ed.). New York: Wiley.

117. Kihlstrom, J. F. (1979). Hypnosis and psychopathology: Retrospect and prospect. *Journal of Abnormal Psychology, 88*, 459–73.

118. Udolf, R. (1981). *Handbook of hypnosis for professionals.* New York: Van Nostrand Reinhold.

119. Yalom, I. D. (1985). *The theory and practice of group psychotherapy* (3rd ed.). New York: Basic.

120. Rossi, P. H., Wright, J. D., Fisher, G. A. et al. (1987). The urban homeless: Estimating composition and size. *Science, 239*, 21.

121. Kolata, G. (1985). A guarded endorsement for shock therapy. *Science, 228*, 1510–11.

122. Scovern, A. W., & Kilmann, P. R. (1980). Status of electroconvulsive therapy: Review of the outcome literature. *Psychological Bulletin, 87*, 260–303.

123. Michener, J. Quoted in: Brim, G. (1988, September). Losing and winning. *PT, 22*, 48–52.

124. Tillich, P. (1958). *Love, power, and justice.* New York: Oxford University Press.

125. Needleman, J. Quoted in: Lattin, D. (1990, April 24). Strong Bay Area interest in 'New Age' mysticism. *SFC*, A1.

126. Gallup Poll. Cited in: Roof, W. C. (1990, July 20). The Episcopalian goes the way of the dodo. *WSJ*, A14.

127. Roof, 1990.

128. Cult Awareness Network. Quoted in: Irving, C. (1990, March 4). Cults prey on university students. *SFE*, B-1.

129. Nader, L. Quoted in: Irving, 1990, B-8.

130. Puig, L. C. (1990, February 11). Kidnaped in the name of love. *SFC, This World*, 13.

131. Needleman, J. Quoted in: Carman, J. (1990, June 26). Talking about money on PBS. *SFC*, E1.

132. Fowler, J. W. (1981). *Stages of faith: The psychology of human development and the quest for meaning.* New York: Harper & Row.

133. Fowler, J. W. (1986). Faith and the structuring of meaning. In C. Dykstra & S. Parks (Eds.), *Faith development and Fowler.* Birmingham, AL: Religious Education Press.

UNIT 4: CAFFEINE, TOBACCO AND ALCOHOL

1. Levenson, H. S., & Bick, E. C. (1977). Psychopharmacology of caffeine. In M. E. Jarvik (Ed.), *Psychopharmacology in the practice of medicine.* New York: Appleton-Century-Crofts, 451–63.

2. Dews, P. Quoted in: Bashin, B. J. (1988, February 28). The jolt in java. *SFC, This World*, 12–13.

3. Lecos, C. W. (1988). Caffeine jitters: Some safety questions remain. *FDA Consumer.* HHS Pub. No. (FDA)88-2221. Rockville, MD: U.S. Government Printing Office.

4. Bashin, 1988, 12.

5. Weidner, G., & Itvan, J. (1985). Dietary sources of caffeine (letter). *NEJM, 313*, 1421.

6. Gilbert, R. M. (1984). Caffeine consumption. *Progress in Clinical Biological Research, 158*, 185–213.

7. Ray, O., & Ksir, C. (1990). *Drugs, society, and human behavior* (5th ed.). St. Louis: Times Mirror/Mosby.

8. Leonard, T. K., Watson, R. R., & Mohs, M. E. (1987). The effects of caffeine on various body systems: A review. *Journal of the American Dietetic Association, 87*, 1048–53.

9. Ashton, C. H. (1987). Caffeine and health. *British Medical Journal, 295*, 1293–94.

10. Leonard, Watson, & Mohs, 1987.

11. Carroll, C. R. (1989). *Drugs in modern society.* Dubuque, IA: Wm. C. Brown.

12. Neims, A. Cited in: Bashin, 1988, 12.

13. Ray & Ksir, 1990.

14. Gilliland, K., & Andress, D. (1981). Ad lib caffeine consumption, symptoms of caffeinism, and academic performance. *American Journal of Psychiatry, 138*, 512–14.

15. Clements, G. L., & Dailey, J. W. (1988). Psychotropic effects of caffeine. *American Family Physician, 37*, 162–72.

16. Kenny, M., & Darragh, A. (1985). Central effects of caffeine in man. In S. D. Iversen (Ed.), *Psychopharmacology: Recent advances and future prospects.* Oxford: Oxford University Press, 278–88.

17. Gilliland & Andress, 1981.

18. Bruce, M. S., & Lader, M. (1989). Caffeine abstention in the management of anxiety disorders. *Psychological Medicine, 19*, 211–14.

19. Mathew, R. J., & Wilson, W. H. (1990). Behavioral and cerebrovascular effects of caffeine in patients with anxiety disorders. *Acta Psychiatrica Scandinavica, 81*, 17–22.

20. Ray & Ksir, 1990.

21. Carroll, 1989.

22. van Dusseldorp, M., & Katan, M. B. (1990). Headache caused by caffeine withdrawal among moderate coffee drinkers switched from ordinary to decaffeinated coffee: A 12 week double blind trial. *British Medical Journal, 300*, 1558–59.

23. Ray & Ksir, 1990.

24. van Dusseldorp & Katan, 1990.

25. Carroll, 1989.

26. Klag, M. Cited in: Friend, T. (1991, March 15–17). Coffee tied to increase in heart risk. *USA Today*, 1A. [Study reported at 1991 American Heart Association meeting, Florida.]

27. LaCroix, A. Z., Mead, L. A., Liang, K. et al. (1986). Coffee consumption and the incidence of coronary heart disease.

28. Rosenberg, L., Palmer, J. R., Kelly, J. P. et al. (1988). Coffee drinking and nonfatal myocardial infarction in men under 55 years of age. *American Journal of Epidemiology, 128,* 570–78.

29. Tverdal, A., Stensvold, I. Solvoll. K. et al. (1990). Coffee consumption and death from coronary heart disease in middle-aged Norwegian men and women. *British Medical Journal, 300,* 566–69.

30. Grobee, D. E., Rimm, E. B., Giovannucci, E. (1990). Coffee, caffeine, and cardiovascular disease in men. *NEJM, 323,* 1026–32.

31. Willet, W. Study reported in: Kolata, T. (1990, October 11). Study disputes coffee's tie to heart disease risk. *NYT,* B7.

32. Shirlow, M. J., Berry, G., & Stokes, G. (1988). Caffeine consumption and blood pressure: An epidemiological study. *International Journal of Epidemiology, 17,* 90–97.

33. Sharp, D. S., & Benowitz, N. L. (1990). Pharmacoepidemiology of the effect of caffeine on blood pressure. *Clinical Pharmacological Therapeutics, 47,* 57–60.

34. Ashton, 1987.

35. Myers, M. G. (1991). Caffeine and cardiac arrhythmias. *AIM, 114,* 147–50.

36. Myers, M. G., & Harris, L. (1990). High dose caffeine and ventricular arrhythmias. *Canadian Journal of Cardiology, 6*(3), 95–98.

37. National Institutes of Health. (1989). Caffeine may be associated with reduced fertility. *JAMA, 261,* 1864.

38. Joesoef, M. F., Beral, V., Rolfs, R. T. et al. (1990). Are caffeinated beverages risk factors for delayed conception? *Lancet, 335,* 136–37.

39. Aaronson, L. S., & Macnee, C. L. (1989). Tobacco, alcohol, and caffeine use during pregnancy. *Journal of Obstetric, Gynecologic, & Neonatal Nursing, 18,* 279–87.

40. Caan, B. J., & Goldhaber, M. K. (1989). Caffeinated beverages and low birthweight: A case-control study. *AJPH, 79,* 1299–300.

41. Fenster, L., Eskenazi, R., Windham, G. C. et al. (1991). Caffeine consumption during pregnancy and fetal growth. *AJPH, 81*(4), 458–61.

42. Brooke, O. G., Anderson, H. R., Bland, J. M. et al. (1989). Effects on birth weight of smoking, alcohol, caffeine, socioeconomic factors, and psychosocial stress. *British Medical Journal, 298,* 795–801.

43. Rossignol, A. M., & Bonnlander, H. (1990). Caffeine-containing beverages, total fluid consumption, and premenstrual syndrome. *AJPH, 80,* 1106–10.

44. Lubin, F., & Ron, E. (1990). Consumption of methylxanthine-containing beverages and the risk of breast cancer. *Cancer Letters, 53*(2–3), 81–90.

45. Phelps, H. M., & Phelps, C. E. (1988). Caffeine ingestion and breast cancer: A negative correlation. *Cancer, 61*(5), 1051–54.

46. Ray & Ksir, 1990.

47. Joesoef et al., 1990.

48. LaVecchia, C., Gentile, A., Negri, E. et al. (1989). Coffee consumption and myocardial infarction in women. *American Journal of Epidemiology, 130,* 481–85.

49. Grobbee et al., 1990.

50. Edmondson, B., & Fost, D. (1991, July). The frontier is still here. *American Demographics,* 50–52.

51. Edmondson & Fost, 1991.

52. American Medical Association, Council on Scientific Affairs. Reported in: Reuters (1990, June 29). Warning on the rise in tobacco use. *SFC,* A4.

53. Johnston, L. D., O'Malley, P. M., & Bachman, J. G. (1990). *Illicit drug use, smoking, and drinking by America's high school students, college students, and young adults: 1975–1989.* Rockville, MD: National Institute on Drug Abuse.

54. DiFranza, J. R., & Tye, J. B. (1990). Who profits from tobacco sales to children *JAMA, 263,* 2784–87.

55. DiFranza & Tye, 1990.

56. Kilbourne, J. (1988). Cigarette ads target women, young people. *Alcoholism & Addiction, 9,* 22–23.

57. U.S. Bureau of the Census, U.S. Department of Commerce. (1990). *Statistical abstract of the United States 1990.* Washington, DC: U.S. Department of Commerce, 123.

58. Fielding, J. E. (1987). Smoking and women: Tragedy of the majority. *NEJM, 317,* 1343–45.

59. Chronicle Wire Services. (1990, October 2). Cigaret ads for women assailed. *SFC,* A28.

60. Johnston, O'Malley, & Bachman, 1990.

61. Pierce, J. P., Fiore, M. C., Novotny, T. E. et al. (1989). Trends in cigarette smoking in the United States: Educational differences are increasing. *JAMA, 261,* 56–60.

62. U.S. Department of Health and Human Services. (1990). *Smoking and health: A national status report.* Rockville, MD: U.S. Department of Health and Human Services.

63. Istvan, J., & Matarazzo, J. D. (1984). Tobacco, alcohol, and caffeine use: A review of their interrelationships. *Psychological Bulletin, 95,* 301–26.

64. Bradstock, M. K., Marks, J. S., Forman, M. R. et al. (1987). Drinking-driving and health lifestyle in the United States: Behavioral risk factors surveys. *Journal of Studies on Alcohol, 48,* 147–52.

65. Peele, S., Brodsky, A., & Arnold, M. (1991). *The truth about addiction and recovery: The life process program for outgrowing destructive habits.* New York: Simon & Schuster, 101.

66. Sachs, D. Quoted in: Goodkind, M. (1989, Spring). The cigarette habit. *Stanford Medicine,* 12–14.

67. Kilbourne, 1988.

68. Carroll, 1989.

69. Nesbitt, P. D. (1972). Chronic smoking and emotionality. *Journal of Applied Social Psychology, 2,* 187–96.

70. U.S. Surgeon General. (1988). *Nicotine addiction: The health consequences of smoking.* Rockville, MD: U.S. Department of Health and Human Services, Office on Smoking and Health.

71. Peele, Brodsky, & Arnold, 1991.

72. Marsh, A. (1984). Smoking: habit or choice? *Population Trends, 37,* 19–20. Quoted in: Peele, Brodsky, & Arnold, 1991, 102.

73. Kilbourne, 1988, 22–23.

74. Kilbourne, 1988, 23.

75. U.S. Surgeon General, 1988.

76. Kozlowski, L. T., Wilkinson, D. A., Skinner, W. et al. (1989). Comparing tobacco cigarette dependence with other drug dependencies: Greater or equal 'difficulty quitting' and 'urges to use,' but less 'pleasure' from cigarettes. *JAMA, 261,* 898–901.

77. Blum, K. (1984). *Handbook of abusable drugs.* New York: Gardner Press.

78. Hughes, J. R., Grist, S. W., & Pechacek, T. F. (1987). Prevalence of tobacco dependence and withdrawal. *American Journal of Psychiatry, 144,* 205–208. Cited in: Maisto, S. A., Galizio, M., & Connors, G. J. (1991). *Drug use and misuse.* Fort Worth, TX: Holt, Rinehart and Winston, 147.

79. Gallagher, J. E. (1990, March 5). Under fire from all sides. *Time,* 41. [Describes report of U.S. Senator Edward Kennedy during Senate hearings in which a new regulatory group was proposed to curb tobacco.]

80. Weil, A., & Rosen, W. (1983). *Chocolate to morphine: Understanding mind-active drugs.* Boston: Houghton Mifflin, 50.

81. Russell, M. A. (1990). The nicotine addiction trap: A 40-year sentence for four cigarettes. *British Journal of Addiction, 85,* 293–300.

82. World Health Organization. Cited in: Anonymous. (1990). World no-tobacco day. *MMWR, 39*(13), 218.

83. Centers for Disease Control. (1991). Smoking-attributable mortality and years of potential life

lost—United States, 1988. *MMWR, 40*(4), 62.

84. Novotny, T. Quoted in: Snider, M. (1991, February 1–3). More smokers dying, though fewer smoke. *USA Today,* 1A.

85. Centers for Disease Control. Reported in: Associated Press. (1991, February 1). Death toll from smoking is worsening. *NYT,* A9.

86. Gilliam, H. (1991, June 2). Taking the risk: A sensible guide to environmental dangers. *SFC, This World,* 11.

87. Dinman, B. D. (1980). The reality and acceptance of risk. *JAMA, 244,* 1226–28.

88. Gilliam, 1991.

89. Ockene, J. K., Kuller, L. H., Svendsen, K. H. et al. (1990). The relationship of smoking cessations to coronary heart disease and lung cancer in the Multiple Risk Factor Intervention Trial (MRFIT). *AJPH, 80,* 954–58.

90. 1990 U.S. Surgeon General's report on smoking. Reported in: Perlman, D. (1990, September 26). Big benefits for smokers who can kick the habit. *SFC,* A2.

91. Office on Smoking and Health. (1989). *Reducing the health consequences of smoking: 25 years of progress. A report of the Surgeon General.* DHHS Pub. No. (CDC)89-8411. Washington, DC: U.S. Department of Health and Human Services.

92. U.S. Bureau of the Census, U.S. Department of Commerce. (1990).

93. Benfield, J. R. Cited in: Anonymous. (1991, May–June). Lung cancer and women. *The Futurist,* 6.

94. McLemore, T. L., Adelberg, S., Lieu, M. C. et al. (1990). Expression of cypial gene in patient with lung cancer: Evidence for cigarette smoke–induced altered gene regulation in primary pulmonary carcinomas. *Journal of the National Cancer Institute, 82,* 1333–39.

95. Willett, W. C., Green, A., Stampfer, M. J. et al. (1987). Relative and absolute excess risks of coronary heart disease among women who smoke cigarettes. *NEJM, 317,* 1303–09.

96. La Vecchia, C., Franceschi, S., Decarli, A. et al. (1987). Risk factors for myocardial infarction in young women. *American Journal of Epidemiology, 125,* 832–43.

97. Abbott, R. D., Yin, Y., Reed, D. M. et al. (1986). Risk of stroke in male cigarette smokers. *NEJM, 315,* 717–20.

98. 1990 Surgeon General's report. Cited in: Perlman, 1990.

99. Tosteson, A. N. A., Weinstein, M. C., Williams, L. W. et al (1990). Long-term impact of smoking cessation on the incidence of coronary heart disease. *AJPH, 80,* 1481–86.

100. Office of Smoking and Health, 1989.

101. Associated Press. (1991, May 16). Smokers with tans get even more wrinkles. *SFC,* B3.

102. Kadunce, D. P., Burr, R., Gress, R. et al. (1991). Cigarette smoking: Risk factor for premature facial wrinkling. *AIM, 114,* 840–44.

103. Glina, S., Reichelt, C., Leao, P., & Reis, J. (1988). Impact of cigarette smoking on papaverine-induced erection. *Journal of Urology, 140,* 523–24.

104. Berg, A. T., Shapiro, E. D., & Capobianco, L. A. (1991). Group day care and the risk of serious infection disease. *American Journal of Epidemiology, 133,* 154–63.

105. Midgette, A. S., & Baron, J. A. (1990). Cigarette smoking and the risk of natural menopause. *Epidemiology, 1,* 474–80.

106. Stevenson, J. C., Lees, B., Devenport, M. et al. (1989). Determinants of bone density in normal women: Risk factors for future osteoporosis? *British Medical Journal, 298,* 924–28.

107. Hellberg, D., Nilsson, S., Haley, N. J. et al. (1988). Smoking and cervical intraepithelial neoplasia: Nicotine and cotinine in serum and cervical mucus in smokers and nonsmokers. *American Journal of Obstetrics & Gynecology, 158,* 910–13.

108. Layde, P. N., & Broste, S. K. (1989). Carcinoma of the cervix and smoking. *Biomedicine & Pharmacotherapy, 43*, 161–65.

109. Licciardone, J. C., Brownson, R. C., Chang, J. C. et al. (1990). Uterine cervical cancer risk in cigarette smokers: A meta-analytic study. *American Journal of Preventive Medicine, 6*, 274–81.

110. Goldbaum, G. M., Kendrick, J. S., Hogelin, G. C. et al. (1987). The relative impact of smoking and oral contraceptive use on women in the United States. *JAMA, 258*, 1339–42.

111. Mason, J. O., Tolsma, D. D., Peterson, H. B. et al. (1988). Health promotion for women: Reduction of smoking in primary care settings. *Clinical Obstetrics & Gynecology, 31*, 989–1002.

112. Coste, J., Job-Spira, N., & Fernandez, H. (1991). Increased risk of ectopic pregnancy with maternal cigarette smoking. *AJPH, 81*, 199–201.

113. Ray & Ksir, 1990.

114. Mason et al., 1988.

115. Ray & Ksir, 1990.

116. Beaulac-Baillargeon, L., & Desrosiers, C. (1987). Caffeine-cigarette interaction on fetal growth. *American Journal of Obstetrics & Gynecology, 157*, 1236–40.

117. Olsen, J., Pereira, A., & Olsen, S. F. (1991). Does maternal tobacco smoking modify the effect of alcohol on fetal growth? *AJPH, 81*, 69–73.

118. Miller, L. G. (1990). Cigarettes and drug therapy: Pharmacokinetic and pharmacodynamic considerations. *Clinical Pharmacy, 9*(2), 125–35.

119. Handlin, D. Reported in: Goldfarb, B. (1990, October 22). Smokers need more time in recovery room. *USA Today*, 1D. [Describes report at October 1990 meeting of American Society of Anesthesiologists.]

120. Sears, C. (1990, January/February). Oral cancer: Room for improvement. *AH*, 26.

121. Logan, R. F., & Kay, C. R. (1989). Oral contraception, smoking, and inflammatory bowel disease: Findings in the Royal College of General Practitioners Oral Contraception Study. *International Journal of Epidemiology, 18*(1), 105–107.

122. Royce, R. A., & Winkelstein, W. Jr. (1990). HIV infection, cigarette smoking and CD4+ T-lymphocyte counts: Preliminary results from the San Francisco Men's Health Study. *AIDS, 4*, 327–33.

123. Botkin, J. R. (1988). The fire-safe cigarette. *JAMA, 260*, 226–29.

124. Patetta, M. J., & Cole, T. B. (1990). A population-based descriptive study of housefire deaths in North Carolina. *AJPH, 80*, 1116–17.

125. U.S. Surgeon General, 1988, 16.

126. Christen, A. G., McDonald, J. L., Olson, B. L. et al. (1989). Smokeless tobacco addiction: A threat to the oral and systemic health of the child and adolescent. *Pediatrician, 16*(3–4), 170–77.

127. Novotny, T. E., Pierce, J. P., Fiore, M. C. et al. (1989). Smokeless tobacco use in the United States: The adult use of tobacco surveys. *Nci Monographs, 8*, 25–28.

128. Glover, E. D., Laflin, M., & Edwards, S. W. (1989). Age of initiation and switching patterns between smokeless tobacco and cigarettes among college students in the United States. *AJPH, 79*(2), 207–20.

129. Glover, E. D., Laflin, M., Flannery, D. et al. (1989). Smokeless tobacco use among American college students. *Journal of American College Health, 38*, 81–85.

130. Winn, D. M. (1988). Smokeless tobacco and cancer: The epidemiologic evidence. *Ca: A Cancer Journal for Clinicians, 38*, 236–43.

131. Benowitz, N. L., Porchet, H., Sheiner, L. et al. (1988). Nicotine absorption and cardiovascular effects with smokeless tobacco use: Comparison with cigarettes and nicotine gum. *Clinical Pharmacology & Therapeutics, 44*(1), 23–28.

132. Brownson, R. C., diLorenzo, T. M., Van Tuinen, M. et al. (1990). Patterns of cigarette and smokeless tobacco use among children and adolescents. *Preventive Medicine, 19*(2), 170–80.

133. Grady, D., Ernster, V. L., Stillman, L. et al. (1991). Short term changes a surprise with smokeless tobacco. *Journal of the American Dental Association, 122*(1), 62–64.

134. Creath, C. J., Sheldon, W. O., Wright, J. T. et al. (1988). The prevalence of smokeless tobacco use among adolescent male athletes. *Journal of the American Dental Association, 116*(1), 43–48.

135. Christen et al., 1989.

136. Ray & Ksir, 1990.

137. Hoffman, D., Djordjevic, M. V., & Brunnemann, K. D. (1991). New brands of oral snuff. *Food & Chemical Toxicology, 29*, 65–68.

138. National Institutes of Health. (1988). NIH consensus statement: Health implications of smokeless tobacco use. *Biomedicine & Pharmacotherapy, 42*(2), 93–98.

139. Christen et al., 1989.

140. Winn, 1988.

141. Christen et al., 1989.

142. Grady et al., 1991.

143. Clark, G. C. (1990). Comparison of the inhalation toxicity of kretek (clove cigarette) smoke with that of American cigarette smoke. *Archives of Toxicology, 64*(7), 515–21.

144. Council on Scientific Affairs. (1988). Evaluation of the health hazard of clove cigarettes. *JAMA, 260*, 3641–44.

145. Ray & Ksir, 1990.

146. Guidotti, T. L., Laing, L., & Prakash, U. B. (1989). Clove cigarettes: The basis for concern regarding health effects. *Western Journal of Medicine, 151*(2), 220–28.

147. Bruno, K. (1990, January/February). The perils of passive smoke. *AH*, 15–17.

148. Ray & Ksir, 1990.

149. U.S. Public Health Service. (1986). *The health consequences of involuntary smoking: A report of the Surgeon General*. DHHS Pub. No. (CDC)87-8398. Washington, DC: U.S. Government Printing Office.

150. U.S. Environmental Protection Agency. Reported in: Associated Press. (1991, May 30). Secondhand smoke blamed for 53,000 deaths each year. *NYT*, A14.

151. Associated Press. (1990, December 6). Criticized panel backs the condemnation of second-hand smoke. *NYT*, A14.

152. Wells, A. J. (1991). Breast cancer, cigarette smoking, and passive smoking (letter). *American Journal of Epidemiology, 133*, 208–10.

153. Cowley, G. (1990, June 11). Secondhand smoke: Some grim news. *Newsweek*, 59.

154. Greenberg, R. A., Bauman, K. E., Strecher, V. J. et al. (1991). Passive smoking during the first year of life. *AJPH, 81*, 850–52.

155. U.S. Public Health Service, 1986.

156. Associated Press, 1990.

157. U.S. Public Health Service, 1986.

158. Ray & Ksir, 1990.

159. Novello, A. Quoted in: Perlman, 1990, A2.

160. Peele, Brodsky, & Arnold, 1991, 99.

161. LaCroix, A. Quoted in: Associated Press. (1991, June 6). Study says old smokers live longer by quitting. *SFC*, A5.

162. LaCroix, A. Z., Lang, J., Scherr, P. et al. (1991). Smoking and mortality among older men and women in three communities. *NEJM, 324*, 1619–25.

163. Carmody, T. P. (1990). Preventing relapse in the treatment of nicotine addiction: Current issues and future directions. *Journal of Psychoactive Drugs, 22*(2), 211–38.

164. Goodkind, M. (1989, Spring). The cigarette habit. *Stanford Medicine*, 13.

165. Okene, J. K. (1989). Promoting cessation. *Journal of the American Medical Women's Association, 44*(2), 60–63.

166. Fortman, S. Cited in: Goodkind, 1989, 14.

167. Fiore, M. C., Novotny, T. E., Pierce, J. P. et al. (1990). Methods used to quit smoking in the United States: Do cessation programs help? *JAMA, 263*, 2760–65.

168. Fiore et al., 1990.

169. Cohen, S., Lichtenstein, E., Procaska, J. O. et al. (1989). Debunking myths about self-quitting: Evidence from 10 prospective studies of persons who attempt to quit smoking by themselves. *American Psychologist, 44*, 1355–65.

170. Glynn, T. J. (1990). Methods of smoking cessation—finally, some answers (editorial). *JAMA, 263*, 2795–96.

171. Ray & Ksir, 1990.

172. Gourley, S. G., & McNeil, J. J. (1990). Antismoking products. *Medical Journal of Australia, 153*(11–12), 699–707.

173. Hughes, J. R., Gust, S. W., Keenan, R. M., Fenwick, J. W., & Healey, M. L. (1989). Nicotine vs placebo gum in general medical practice. *JAMA, 2*, 1300–1305.

174. U.S. Department of Health and Human Services (1988). *The health consequences of smoking: Nicotine addiction. A report of the Surgeon General*. Rockville, MD: Centers for Disease Control.

175. Higgins, L. C. (1990). Arm patch may help kick the butt. *Medical World News, 31*, 29.

176. Spiegel, D. Cited in: Goodkind, 1989.

177. Williamson, D. F., Madans, J., Anda, R. F. et al. T. (1991). Smoking cessation and severity of weight gain in a national cohort. *NEJM, 324*, 739–45.

178. Skoog, K. Quoted in: Associated Press. (1991, January 30). Weight gain by ex-smokers points to success. *SFC*, B3.

179. Kozlowski, L. T., Wilkinson, D. A., Skinner, W. et al. Pope, M. (1989). Comparing tobacco cigarette dependence with other drug dependencies: Greater or equal 'difficulty quitting' and 'urges to use,' but less 'pleasure' from cigarettes. *JAMA, 261*, 898–901.

180. Roine, R., Gentry, R. T., Hernandez-Munoz, R. et al. (1990). Aspirin increases blood alcohol concentrations in humans after ingestion of ethanol. *JAMA, 264*, 2406–08.

181. Maisto, S. A., Galizio, M., & Connors, G. J. (1991). *Drug use and misuse*. Fort Worth, TX: Holt, Rinehart and Winston, 207–208.

182. Kinney, J., & Leaton, G. (1987). *Loosening the grip: A handbook of alcohol information* (3rd ed.). St. Louis: Times Mirror/Mosby, 21.

183. National Institute on Drug Abuse. (1990, December). Summary of findings from the 1990 National Household Survey on Drug Abuse. *NIDA Capsules*. Issued by the Press Office of the National Institute on Drug Abuse, Rockville, MD.

184. Addiction Research Foundation, Toronto, in pamphlet, "Know the Score." Cited in: Maisto, Galizio, & Connors, 1991, 208.

185. Kinney & Leaton, 1987, 41–42.

186. Herd, D. (1989). The epidemiology of drinking patterns and alcohol-related problems among U.S. blacks. In *Alcohol use among U.S. ethnic minorities*. Rockville, MD: National Institute on Alcohol Abuse and Alcoholism, 3–50.

187. Caetano, R. (1989). Drinking patterns and alcohol problems in a national sample of U.S. Hispanics. In *Alcohol use among U.S. ethnic minorities*. Rockville, MD: National Institute on Alcohol Abuse and Alcoholism, 147–62.

188. Vaillant, G. E. (1983). *The natural history of alcoholism: Causes, patterns, and paths to recovery*. Cambridge, MA: Harvard University Press, 61.

189. Vaillant, 1983.

190. Peele, Brodsky, & Arnold, 1991, 55.

191. Kinney & Leaton, 1987, 71.

192. Bedell, T. (1991, February). Saintly suds. *Men's Health*, 58–61.

193. Miller, A., & Springen, K. (1990, March 5). This safe suds is for you. *Newsweek*, 42.

194. Stampfer, M. J., Colditz, G. A., Willett, W. C. et al. (1988). A prospective study of moderate alcohol consumption and the risk of coronary disease and stroke in women. *NEJM, 319*, 267–73.

195. Rimm, E. B., Giovannucci, E. L., Willett, W. C. et al. (1991). The prospective study of alcohol consumption and risk of coronary disease in men. *Lancet, 338*, 464–68.

196. Barnett, R. (1989, November). A good drink. *AH*, 66–69.

197. Maisto, Galizio, & Connors, 1991, 213–14.

198. Centers for Disease Control. (1990). Alcohol-related mortality and years of potential life lost—United States, 1987. *MMWR, 39*(11), 173–77.

199. Vegega, M. E., & Klein, T. M. (1991). Alcohol-related traffic fatalities among youth and young adults—United States, 1982–1989. *JAMA, 265*, 1930.

200. Centers for Disease Control, 1990.

201. Vegega & Klein, 1991.

202. Caudill, B. Reported in: King, P. (1989, December). Heavy drinkers often take the wheel. *PT*, 12.

203. Kinney & Leaton, 1987, 25.

204. Centers for Disease Control, 1990.

205. Kinney & Leaton, 1987, 25.

206. Pollock, D. A., Boyle, C. A., DeStefano, F. et al. (1987). Underreporting of alcohol-related mortality on death certificates of young U.S. Army veterans. *JAMA, 258*, 345–48.

207. Centers for Disease Control, 1990.

208. Mello, N. K. (1987). Alcohol abuse and alcoholism: 1978–1987. In H. Y. Meltzer (Ed.), *Psychopharmacology: The third generation of progress*. New York: Raven Press, 1515–20.

209. Wilsnack, S. C., Klassen, A. D., & Wilsnack, R. W. (1984). Drinking and reproductive dysfunction among women in a 1981 national survey. *Alcoholism: Clinical and Experimental Research, 8*, 451–58.

210. Plant, M. A. (1990). Alcohol, sex and AIDS. *Alcohol & Alcoholism, 25*, 293–301.

211. Parsons, O. A. (1986). Alcoholics' neuropsychological impairment: Current findings and conclusions. *Annals of Behavioral Medicine, 8*, 13–19.

212. U.S. Department of Health and Human Services (1987). *Alcohol and health*. Rockville, MD: U.S. Department of Health and Human Services.

213. Maisto, Galizio, & Connors, 1991, 211.

214. Maisto, Galizio, & Connors, 1991, 209, table.

215. Willett, W. C., Stampfer, M. J., Colditz, G. A. et al. E. (1987). Moderate alcohol consumption and the risk of breast cancer. *NEJM, 316*, 1174–80.

216. Graham, S. (1987). Alcohol and breast cancer. *NEJM, 316*, 1211–12.

217. Carroll, 1989, 127.

218. Carroll, 1989, 128.

219. Streissguth, A. P., & LaDue, R. A. (1987). Fetal alcohol: Teratogenic causes of developmental disabilities. *Monographs of the American Association on Mental Deficiency, 8*, 1–32.

220. Streissguth, A. P., Aase, J. M., Clarren, S. K. et al. (1991). Fetal alcohol syndrome in adolescents and adults. *JAMA, 265*, 1961–67.

221. Serdula, M., Williamson, D. F., Kendrick, J. S. et al. (1991). Trends in alcohol consumption by pregnant women, 1985 through 1988. *JAMA, 265*, 876–79.

222. Weddle, C. D., & Wishon, P. M. (1987). Children of alcoholics: What should we know today? *Children Today, 15*(1), 8–12.

223. Schoenborn, C. A. (1991). Exposure to alcoholism in the family: United States, 1988. *Advance Data from Vital and Health Statistics of the National Center for Health Statistics*. Washington, DC: U.S. Department of Health and Human Services.

224. Kinney & Leaton, 1987, 178.

225. Anonymous child. Quoted in: Woodside, M. (1986). Children of alcoholics: Breaking the cycle. *Journal of School Health, 56*, 448.

226. Woodside, 1986.

227. Mull, S. S. (1990). Help for the children of alcoholics. *Health Education, 21*, 42–45.

228. Starling, B. P., & Martin, A. C. (1990). Adult survivors of parental alcoholism: Implications for primary care. *Nurse Practitioner, 15*(7), 16–24.

229. Smith, A. Quoted in: Kohr, J. (1988). Grandchildren of alcoholics. *Alcoholism & Addiction, 9*, 44.

230. Harwood, H. J., Napolitana, D. M., Kristiansen, P. L., & Collins, J. J. (1984). *Economic costs to society of alcohol and drug abuse and mental illness: 1980*. Research Triangle Park, NC: Research Triangle Institute.

231. Stark, L. (1987, Spring). A century of alcohol and homelessness: Demographics and stereotypes. *Alcohol Health & Research World*, 8–13.

232. Weiner, E. (1990, August 21). Northwest pilots are found guilty of drunken flying. *NYT*, A1, A12.

233. Modell, J. G., & Mountz, J. M. (1990). Drinking and flying—the problem of alcohol use by pilots. *NEJM, 323*, 455–61.

234. Vaillant, 1983.

235. Pinkney, D. S. (1990, May 11). Specialists give new definition of alcoholism. *American Medical News*, 28.

236. Maisto, Galizio, & Connors, 1991, 217.

237. Gallup, G. Jr., & Gallup, A. (1988, April 25). Gallup poll: Most feel alcoholism is a disease. *SFC*, A8.

238. Blum, K., Nobele, E. P., Sheridan, P. J. et al. (1990). Allelic association of human dopamine D_2 receptor gene in alcoholism. *JAMA, 263*, 2055–60.

239. Gordis, E., Tabakoff, B., Goldman, D. et al. (1990). Finding the gene(s) for alcoholism (editorial). *JAMA, 263*, 2094–95.

240. Waldholz, M. (1991, July 15). New studies lend support to 'alcoholism gene' finding. *WSJ*, B1, B4.

241. Schuckit, M. A. (1987). Biology of risk of alcoholism. In H. Y. Meltzer (Ed.), *Psychopharmacology: The third generation of progress*. New York: Raven Press, 1527–33.

242. Donovan, J. M. (1986). An etiologic model of alcoholism. *The American Journal of Psychiatry, 143*, 1–11.

243. Johnson, V. E. (1980). *I'll quit tomorrow: A practical guide to alcoholism treatment*. New York: Harper & Row. Described in: Kinney & Leaton (1987), 153–58.

244. Johnson, V. E. (1986). *Intervention: How to help someone who doesn't want help*. Minneapolis: Johnson Institute.

245. Institute of Medicine (1989). *Prevention and treatment of alcohol problems: Research opportunities*. Washington, DC: National Academy Press.

246. Institute of Medicine (1990). *Broadening the base of treatment for alcohol problems*. Washington, DC: National Academy Press. 252. 247. Stipp, D. (1991, July 8). Heroin medication may help alcoholics avoid relapses. *WSJ*, B1–B2.

248. Anonymous. (1991, August 4). A drug for drying out lowers alcohol levels. *NYT*, sec. 1, pt. 2, 51.

249. Anonymous. (1987). Aversion therapy: Council on Scientific Affairs. *JAMA, 258*, 2562–66.

250. Wegscheider-Cruse, S. (1989). *Another chance: Hope and health for the alcoholic family*. Palo Alto, CA: Science & Behavior.

251. Robertson, N. (1988). *Getting better: Inside Alcoholics Anonymous*. New York: Morrow, 88.

252. Gallup, G. Jr., & Gallup, A. (1988, April 25). Gallup poll: Most feel alcoholism is a disease. *SFC*, A8.

253. Peele, Brodsky, & Arnold, 1991, 9.

254. Holden, C. (1987). Alcohol abuse: Do programs really work? *Science, 236*, 20–22.

255. Chiauzzi, E. (1989, December). Breaking the patterns that lead to relapse. *PT*, 18–19.

256. Anonymous NIAAA official, quoted in: Holden, 1987.

257. Klerman, G. L. (1989). Treatment of alcoholism (editorial). *NEJM, 320*, 394–95.

258. Gallagher, W. (1988, June). If you can't teetotal... *AH*, 48–49.

259. Helzer, J. Cited in: Gallagher, 1988.

260. Name withheld. (1991, January 12). Recovering from alcoholism is tough work (letter). *NYT*, 16.

261. Peele, Brodsky, & Arnold, 1991, 364.

262. Lily, C. [a pseudonym]. (1989, August 6). A long time coming: A skeptic encounters the Twelve Steps. *SFC, This World*, 12.

263. Chiauzzi, 1989, 18.

264. Marlatt, G. A. (1985). Relapse prevention: Theoretical rationale and overview of the model. In G. A. Marlatt & J. R. Gordon (Eds.), *Relapse prevention: Maintenance strategies in the treatment of addictive behaviors*. New York: Guilford, 39.

265. Chiauzzi, 1989, 18–19.

266. Peele, Brodsky, & Arnold, 1991, 271.

267. Marlatt, G. A. (1985). Cognitive assessment and intervention procedures for relapse prevention. In Marlatt & Gordon (Eds.), *Relapse prevention*, table 4-2. Described in: Peele, Brodsky, & Arnold, 1991, 271–72.

UNIT 5: DRUG AND OTHER DEPENDENCIES

1. Zinberg, N. E. Cited in: Hurley, D. (1989, July/August). Cycles of craving. *PT*, 56.

2. Hurley, 1989, 56.

3. Weil, A., & Rosen, W. (1983). *Chocolate to morphine: Understanding mind-active drugs*. Boston: Houghton Mifflin, 1.

4. Csikszentmihalyi, M. (1990). *Flow: The psychology of optimal experience*. New York: HarperCollins, 66.

5. Flynn, J. C. (1991). *Cocaine: An in-depth look at the facts, science, history and future of the world's most addictive drug*. New York: Carol, 50.

6. Csikszentmihalyi, 1990, 4.

7. Flynn, 1991, 14.

8. Schuster, C. Cited in: Medical Tribune News Service (1991, January 25). High school seniors report less drug use. *SFC*, A12.

9. Gallup Organization. (1990, December 13). Young people in poll call drugs top problem. *SFC*, A14.

10. Elam, S. M., Rose, L. C., & Gallup, A. M. (1991). The 23rd annual Gallup Poll of the public's attitudes toward the public schools. *Phi Delta Kappan, 73*(1), 55

11. Moskowitz, J. M., & Jones, R. (1988). Alcohol and drug problems in the schools: Results of a national survey of school administrators. *Journal of Studies on Alcohol, 49*, 299–305.

12. Bachman, J. G., Wallace, J. M. Jr., O'Malley, P. M. et al. (1991). Racial/Ethnic differences in smoking, drinking, and illicit drug use among American high school seniors. *AJPH, 81*, 372–77.

13. Pope, H. G., Ionescu-Pioggia, M., Aizley, H. G. et al. (1990). Drug use and life style among college undergraduates in 1989: A comparison with 1969 and 1978. *American Journal of Psychiatry, 147*, 998–1001.

14. Associated Press. (1990, July 11). Drug use declining in U.S. work force, testing lab reports. *NYT*, A14.

15. Shedler, J., & Block, J. (1990, May). Adolescent drug use and psychological health. *American Psychologist*, 612–24.

16. Perlman, D. (1990, May 14). Furor over report on teenage drug use. *SFC*, A10.

17. Shedler, J., & Block, J. Quoted in: Perlman, 1990.

18. World Health Organization (1981). Nomenclature and classification of drug- and alcohol-related problems: A WHO memorandum. *Bulletin of the World Health Organization, 59,* 227.

19. Carroll, C. R. (1989). *Drugs in modern society.* Dubuque, IA: Wm. C. Brown.

20. Girdano, D. A., & Dusek, D. E. (1988). *Drug education: Content and methods* (4th ed.). New York: Random House.

21. Weil & Rosen, 1983.

22. Maisto, S. A., Galizio, M., & Connors, G. J. (1991). *Drug use and misuse.* Fort Worth, TX: Holt, Rinehart and Winston.

23. McCarty, D. (1985). Environmental factors in substance abuse: The microsetting. In M. Galizio & S. A. Maisto (Eds.), *Determinants of substance abuse: Biological, psychological, and environmental factors.* New York: Plenum Press, 247–82.

24. Combs, B. J., Hales, D. R., & Williams, B. K. (1980). *An invitation to health: Your personal responsibility.* Menlo Park, CA: Benjamin/Cummings, 79.

25. Flynn, 1991, 14.

26. Flynn, 1991, 74.

27. Balster, R. L. (1988). Pharmacological effects of cocaine relevant to its abuse. In D. Clouet, K. Asghar, & R. Brown (Eds.), *Mechanisms of cocaine abuse and toxicity.* NIDA Research Monograph 88, 1-13. Washington, DC: U. S. Government Printing Office.

28. Chychula, N. M., & Okore, C. (1990). The cocaine epidemic: A comprehensive review of use, abuse and dependence. *Nurse Practitioner, 15*(7), 31–39.

29. Streissouth, A. P., Grant, T. M., Barr, H. M. et al. (1991). Cocaine and the use of alcohol and other drugs during pregnancy. *American Journal of Obstetrics & Gynecology, 164*(5 Pt 1), 1239–43.

30. Tallarida, R. J. (1984). *The top 200—1984: The most widely prescribed drugs in America.* Philadelphia: Saunders.

31. Gillin, J. C. (1991). The long and short of sleeping pills (editorial). *NEJM, 324,* 1735–36.

32. National Institute on Drug Abuse (1986). *Highlights of the 1985 National Household Survey on Drug Abuse.* Rockville, MD: National Institute on Drug Abuse.

33. Okrie, T. R. (1989). Three positive shifts away from marijuana use, 1979–1988. *Journal of School Health, 59*(1), 34–36.

34. Kozel, N. J., & Adams, E. H. (1986). Epidemiology of drug abuse: An overview. *Science, 234,* 970–74.

35. Johnson, B. A. (1990). Psychopharmacological effects of cannabis. *British Journal of Hospital Medicine, 43,* 114–16.

36. Jones, R. T. (1980). Human effects: An overview. In R. C. Peterson (Ed.), *Marijuana research findings: 1980.* Rockville, MD: National Institute on Drug Abuse, 54–80.

37. Maisto, Galizio, & Connors, 1991.

38. Johnson, 1990.

39. McGlothin, W. H., & West, L. J. (1968). The marihuana problem: An overview. *American Journal of Psychiatry, 125,* 370–78.

40. Abraham, H. D. (1983). Visual phenomenology of the LSD flashback. *Archives of General Psychiatry, 40,* 884–89.

41. Maisto, Galizio, & Connors, 1991.

42. Carroll, 1989.

43. Young, T., Lawson, G. W., & Gacono, C. B. (1987). Clinical aspects of phencyclidine (PCP). *The International Journal of Addictions, 22,* 1–15.

44. Maisto, Galizio, & Connors, 1991, 341.

45. Smith, D. E., & Gay, G. R. (Eds.). (1972). *It's so good don't even try it once: Heroin in perspective.* Englewood Cliffs, NJ: Prentice-Hall.

46. Jaffe, J. H., & Martin, W. R. (1985). Opioid analgesics and antagonists. In A. G. Gilman, L. S. Goodman, & A. Gilman (Eds.), *Goodman and Gilman's The pharmacological basis of therapeautics* (7th ed.) New York: Macmillan, 491–531.

47. Treaster, J. B. (1991, April 28). A more potent heroin makes a comeback in a new, needleless form. *NYT,* Sec. 4, 4.

48. Treaster, J. B. (1991, February 4). Search for better heroin high is fatal allure of synthetics. *NYT,* C11.

49. Rangel, C. B. (1990, August 14). The killer drug we ignore. *NYT,* A19.

50. Beck, J., & Morgan, P. A. (1986). Designer drug confusion: A focus on MDMA. *Journal of Drug Education, 16,* 287–99.

51. Kleber, H. D. Quoted in: Smith, L. (1991, May 6). Getting junkies to clean up. *Fortune,* 108.

52. Schaef, A. W. (1987). *When society becomes an addict.* San Francisco: Harper & Row, 4.

53. Schaef, 1987, 57.

54. Schaef, 1987, 18.

55. Sullivan, B. (1990, August 12). Becoming the 'thoroughly diseased society.' *SFE,* D-1; reprinted from *Chicago Tribune.*

56. Hickey, J. E., Haertzen, C. A., & Henningfield, J. E. (1986). Simulation of gambling responses on the Addiction Research Center Inventory. *Addictive Behaviors, 11*(3), 345–49.

57. Blaszczynski, A. P., Buhrich, N., & McConaghy, N. (1985). Pathological gamblers, heroin addicts and controls compared on the E.P.Q. "Addiction scale." *British Journal of Addiction, 80*(3), 315–19.

58. Shaffer, H. J., & Gambino, B. (1989). The epistemology of "addictive disease": Gambling as predicament. *Journal of Gambling Behavior, 5*(3), 211–29.

59. Walker, M. B. (1989). Some problems with the concept of "gambling addiction": Should theories of addiction be generalized to include excessive gambling? *Journal of Gambling Behavior, 5*(3), 179–200.

60. Weil & Rosen, 1983, 168.

61. Farmer, J. J. (1989, October 15). Legal gambling: America's biggest growth industry. *SFE,* A-2.

62. Welles, C. (1989, April 24). America's gambling fever. *Business Week,* 112–20.

63. Custer, R. L. Cited in: Welles, 1989.

64. Powers, L. (1989, July 16). Nevada has over twice as many compulsive gamblers. *Reno Gazette-Journal,* 1E.

65. Welles, 1989.

66. Walters, L. S. (1990, June 18). Teen gambling is the latest addiction of choice. *SFC,* B5; reprinted from *Christian Science Monitor.*

67. Associated Press. (1989, June 23). 1 in 20 college students are compulsive gamblers—survey. *Reno Gazette-Journal,* 6D.

68. American Psychiatric Association. (1987). *Diagnostic and statistical manual of mental disorders* (3rd ed.—Revised). Washington, DC: American Psychiatric Association.

69. Volberg, R. A., & Steadman, H. J. (1988). Refining prevalence estimates of pathological gambling. *American Journal of Psychiatry, 145,* 502–05.

70. O'Connor, J. J. (1990, June 29). The urge to gamble, and how to fight addiction. *NYT,* B10.

71. Roy, A., Adinoff, B., Roehrich, L. et al. (1988). Pathological gambling: A psychobiological study. *Archives of General Psychiatry, 45*(4), 369–73.

72. Roy, A., De Jong, J., & Linnoila, M. (1989). Extraversion in pathological gamblers: Correlates with indexes of noadrenergic function. *Archives of General Psychiatry, 46*(8), 679–81.

73. Lorenz, V. Quoted in: Goleman, D. (1989, October 15). Gambling—the odds are it's biological. *SFC, Sunday Punch, SFC,* 5; reprinted from *NYT.*

74. Peck, C. P. (1986). A public mental health issue: Risk-taking behavior and compulsive gambling. *American Psychologist, 41,* 461–65.

75. Will, G. F. (1989, May 8). In the grip of gambling. *Newsweek,* 78.

76. Siskin, B., Staller, J., & Rorvik, D. (1989). *What are the chances? Risks, odds, and likelihood in everyday life.* New York: Plume.

77. Wagenaar, W. Cited in: Goleman, 1989.

78. de la Pena, N., & Miller, A. (1990, April 1). Going for broke. *Newsweek,* 40–41.

79. O'Guinn, T., & Faber, R. Cited in: Goleman, D. (1991, July 17). Reining in a compulsion to spend. *NYT,* B1, B8.

80. Goleman, 1991, B8.

81. Mundis, J. (1986, January 5). A way back from deep debt. *New York Times Magazine,* 23.

82. Machlowitz, M. (1980). *Workaholics.* Reading, MA: Addison-Wesley.

83. Topolnicki, D. (1989, July/August). Workaholics: Are you one? *PT,* 25.

84. Topolnicki, 1989, 25.

85. Pietropinto, A. (1986, May). The workaholic spouse. *Medical Aspects of Human Sexuality,* 89–96.

86. Topolnicki, 1989, 25.

87. Kaminer, W. (1990, February 11). Chances are you're codependent too. *New York Times Book Review,* 1, 26–27.

88. Cermak, T. Cited in: Kinney, J., & Leaton, G. (1991). *Loosening the grip: A handbook of alcohol information* (4th ed.). St. Louis: Times Mirror/Mosby, 177–78.

89. Vinciguerra, V. , Moore, T., Brennan, E. (1988). Inhalation marijuana as an antiemetic for cancer chemotherapy. *New York State Journal of Medicine, 88,* 525–27.

90. Chang, A. 1979 study described in: Hecht, B. (1991, July 15 & 22). Out of joint. *New Republic,* p. 10.

91. Doblin, R., & Kleiman, M. A. R. (1991) Marijuana as an antiemetic medicine: a survey of oncologists' experiences and attitudes. *Journal of Clinical Oncology, 9,* 1314–18.

92. Flynn, 1991, 19–20.

93. Weisberger, B. A. (1990, May/June). Reflections on the dry season. *American Heritage,* 28.

94. Weisberger, 1990, 30.

95. Stark, P. (1990, August 12). Not all drug lords are outlaws. *NYT,* sec. 4, 21.

96. Morris, D. (1990, November/December). Dutch tolerance. *Utne Reader,* 118–19; reprinted from *Building Economic Alternatives.*

97. Benoit, E. (1989, October 3). Drugs: The case for legalization. *Financial World,* 34.

98. Mauer, R. (1990, October 25). Alaskans to vote on marijuana use. *NYT,* A10.

99. Ayres, B. D. Jr. (1991, March 23). 11 held and 3 fraternities seized in drug raids at U. of Virginia. *NYT,* 1, 7.

100. Hinds, M. deC. (1991, March 29). Stunned and divided, U. of Virginia reflects on drug raid at fraternities. *NYT,* A8.

101. Associated Press. (July 15, 1991). Mandatory heavy terms in drug cases assailed. *SFC,* A4.

102. Krauss, C. (1991, July 14). U.S. reports gains in drug war, but the battles keep on shifting. *NYT,* sec. 1, 6.

103. Centers for Disease Control. Reported in: Hilts, P. J. (1991, August 7). AIDS panel backs efforts to exchange drug users' needles. *NYT,* A1, A14.

104. Glasser, I. (1990, December 18). Now for a drug policy that doesn't do harm (letter). *NYT,* A22.

105. Gugliotta, G., & Isikoff, M. (1990, October 28). Drug use is down, but violent crime is up. *SFC, This World,* 19; reprinted from *Washington Post.*

106. Treaster, J. B. (1991, February 1). Bush proposes more anti-drug spending. *NYT,* A10.

107. Glasser, 1990, A22.

108. Associated Press. (1990, December 18). Drug-related felony convictions increase by 69% in state courts. *NYT*, A18.

109. Cohen, S. Associated Press. (1990, November 18). Narcotics cases clogging up courts, delaying civil matters and overcrowding jails. *LAT*, A8.

110. Meddis, S. V. (1991, April 25). Drug busts boost jail populations. *USA Today*, 12A.

111. Anonymous. (1991, April 1). U.S. aggressively seizing drug case assets. *SFC*, A3; reprinted from *Washington Post*.

112. Treaster, J. B. (1990, May 6). Is the fight on drugs eroding civil rights? *NYT*, 5.

113. Thompson, T. (1990, May 8). Drug war stepping on 4th Amendment stop-and-search rights. *SFC*, A16; reprinted from *Washington Post*.

114. Harris, R. (1990, April 24). War on drugs may be a war on blacks. *SFC*, A12; reprinted from *LAT*,

115. Anonymous. (1991, July 15). Postal service steps up efforts against drugs. *NYT*, A12.

116. Anonymous. (1991, August 22). Pentagon's role in war on drugs called wasteful, ineffective. *SFC*, B8; reprinted from *Washington Post*.

117. Kraar, L. (1990, March 12). How to win the war on drugs. *Fortune*, 70.

118. Freed, K. (1991, May 1). Drug scene in Panama worse than ever before. *SFC*, Briefing section, 1, 4; reprinted from *LAT*.

119. Lippin, T. (1991, January). Drug wars versus development. *Technology Review*, 17–19.

120. Hilts, P. J. (1990, September 20). Experts tell U.S. to expand drug-treatment programs. *NYT*, A1.

121. Glasser, 1990, A22.

122. Gould, S. J. (1990, April). The war on drugs. *Harper's Magazine*, 24; reprinted from *Dissent*.

123. Magura, S. (1990, October 22). The British experience (letter). *NYT*, A14.

124. Kilpatrick, J. J. (1989, December 18). Legalize drugs? It's a bad idea. *SFC*, A18.

125. Eisenberg, I. (1991, May 26). A way out of the drug war. *SFC*, *This World*, 16.

126. Kalett, E. (1990, October 22). Legalizing drugs would only increase abuse (letter). *NYT*, A14.

127. Smith, L. (1991, May 6). Getting junkies to clean up. *Fortune*, 106.

128. Murray, C. (1990, May 21). How to win the war on drugs. *New Republic*, 25.

UNIT 6: NUTRITION AND WEIGHT MANAGEMENT

1. American Dietetic Association survey, October 9, 1991. Reported in: Associated Press. (1991, October 10). People know they could improve diet. *SFC*, D4.

2. Anonymous. (1993, April). 14 dietary habits you can stop feeling guilty about. *Tufts University Diet & Nutrition Letter*, 3–6.

3. Featherstone, J. D. B. (1987). The mechanism of dental decay. *Nutrition Today*, 22, 10–16.

4. Williams, G. III (1991, October). Reading in a dim light will ruin your eyes, and other popular misconceptions. *AH*, 56–61.

5. Miller, S. A., & Frattali, D. (1989). Saccharin. *Diabetes Care*, 12(Suppl. 1), 75–80.

6. Dews, P. B. (1987). Summary report of an international aspartame workshop. *Food Chemistry Toxicology*, 25, 549–52.

7. Klurfeld, D. M. (1987). The role of dietary fiber in gastrointestinal disease. *Journal of the American Dietetic Association*, 87, 1172–77.

8. U.S. Public Health Service (1990). *Healthy people 2000: National health promotion and disease prevention objectives*. DHHS Pub. No. (PHS)91-50212. Washington, DC: U.S. Government Printing Office, 112. 1

9. U.S. Public Health Service (1988). *The Surgeon General's report on nutrition and health*. DHHS Pub. No. (PHS) 88-50210. Washington, DC: U.S Government Printing Office.

10. Cohen, L. A. (1987). Diet and cancer. *Scientific American*, 257, 42–48.

11. Cohen, 1987.

12. U.S. Public Health Service, 1988.

13. Glomset, J. (1985). Fish, fatty acids, and human health. *NEJM*, 312, 1253–54.

14. Phillipson, B. E., Rothrock, D. W., Connor, W. E. et al. (1985). Reduction of plasma lipids, lipoproteins, and apoproteins by dietary fish oils in patients with hypertriglyceridemia. *NEJM*, 312, 1210–16.

15. Kromhout, D., Bosschieter, E. B., & Coulander, C. D. (1985). The inverse relation between fish consumption and 20-year mortality from coronary heart disease. *NEJM*, 312, 1205–09.

16. U.S. Public Health Service, 1988.

17. Saltman, P., Gurin, J., Mothner, I. et al. (1987). *The California nutrition book*. Boston: Little, Brown, 216–17.

18. Pauling, L. C. (1970). *Vitamin C and the common cold*. San Francisco: Freeman.

19. Chalmers, T. C. (1975). Effects of ascorbic acid on the common cold. *American Journal of Medicine*, 58, 532–36.

20. Cameron, E., & Pauling, L. (1976). Supplemental ascrobate in the supportive treatment of cancer: Prolongation of survival times in terminal human cancer. *Proceedings of the National Academy of Science USA*, 73, 3685–89.

21. Creagan, E. T., Moertel, C. G., O'Fallon, J. R. et al. (1979). Failure of high-dose vitamin C (ascorbic acid) therapy to benefit patients with advanced cancer. *NEJM*, 301, 687–90.

22. Bruce, W. R., Eyssen, G. M., Ciampi, A. et al. (1981). Strategies for dietary intervention studies in colon cancer. *Cancer*, 47, 1121–25.

23. Root, E. J., & Longenecker, J. B. (1983). Brain cell alterations suggesting premature aging induced by dietary deficiency of vitamin B_6 and/or copper. *American Journal of Clinical Nutrition*, 37, 540–42.

24. Jones, D. Y., & Kumanyika, S. K. (1983). Premenstrual syndrome: A review of possible dietary influences. *Journal of the Canadian Dietetic Association*, 44, 194–203.

25. Anonymous. (1982). Possible vitamin B_6 deficiency uncovered in persons with the "Chinese restaurant syndrome." *Nutrition Reviews*, 40, 15–16.

26. Anonymous. (1985, November). More B_6 toxicity reported. *Nutrition Forum*, 84.

27. Brody, J. (1987). *Jane Brody's nutrition book: A lifetime guide to good eating for better health and weight control by the personal health columnist of The New York Times* (rev. ed.). New York: Bantam, 156.

28. Probber, J. (1987, November 30). The secrets of taste and smell. *SFC*, B4; reprinted from *NYT*.

29. Beauchamp, G. K. (1987). The human preference for excess salt. *American Scientist*, 75, 27–33.

30. Soemantri, A. G., Pollitt, E., & Kim, I. (1985). Iron deficiency anemia and educational achievement. *American Journal of Clinical Nutrition*, 42, 1221–28.

31. U.S. Public Health Service, 1988.

32. U.S. Public Health Service, 1988.

33. U.S. Public Health Service, 1988.

34. U.S. Public Health Service, 1988, 15.

35. Holmes, J. H. (1964). Thirst and fluid intake problems in clinical medicine. In M. J. Wayner (Ed.), *Thirst*. New York: Macmillan.

36. Bailey, L. et al. (1988). Food consumption. *National Food Review*, 11, 1–11.

37. Houts, S. S. (1988). Lactose intolerance. *Food Technology*, 3, 110–13.

38. Kreutler, P. A., & Czjka-Narins, D. M. (1987). *Nutrition in perspective* (2nd ed.). Englewood Cliffs, NJ: Prentice Hall.

39. Costill, D., & Miller, J. (1980). Nutrition for endurance sports: carbohydrate and fluid balance. *International Journal of Sports Medicine*, 1, 2–14.

40. Costill & Miller, 1980.

41. Select Committee on Health Aspects of Irradiated Beef. (1979). *Evaluation of the health aspects of certain compounds found in irradiated beef*. Bethesda, MD: Life Sciences Research Office, Federation of American Societies for Experimental Biology.

42. Whitney, E. N., & Hamilton, E. M. N. (1987). *Understanding nutrition*. St. Paul: West, 47–49.

43. Madigan, E. (1991, May 15). Agriculture food chart's ups and downs (letter). *NYT*, A14.

44. U.S. Senate Select Committee on Nutrition and Human Needs. (1977). *Dietary goals for the United States* (2nd ed.). Washington, D.C.: U.S. Government Printing Office.

45. U.S. Department of Agriculture and the Department of Health and Human Services. (1985). *Nutrition and your health: Dietary guidelines for Americans* (2nd ed.). Home and Garden Bulletin No. 232. Washington, D.C.: U.S. Government Printing Office.

46. U.S. Department of Health and Human Services. (1980). *Promoting health/preventing disease: Objectives for the nation*. Washington, D.C.: U.S. Government Printing Office.

47. U.S. Public Health Service, 1988.

48. National Research Council. (1989). *Diet and health: Implications for reducing chronic disease risk*. Washington, DC: National Academy Press.

49. Hegarty, V. (1988). *Decisions in nutrition*. St. Louis: Times Mirror/Mosby.

50. National Research Council, 1989.

51. U.S. Department of Agriculture and the Department of Health and Human Services, 1985.

52. National Research Council, 1989.

53. U.S. Department of Agriculture and the Department of Health and Human Services, 1985.

54. U.S. Department of Agriculture and the Department of Health and Human Services, 1985.

55. U.S. Public Health Service, 1988.

56. National Research Council, 1989.

57. National Research Council, 1989.

58. National Research Council, 1989.

59. National Research Council, 1989.

60. U.S. Department of Agriculture and the Department of Health and Human Services, 1985.

61. National Research Council, 1989.

62. Truswell, A. S. (1987). Evolution of dietary recommendations, goals and guidelines. *American Journal of Clinical Nutrition*, 75, 1060–72.

63. Princeton Survey Research Associates. 1990 survey. Cited in: Kobren, G. (1990, August 21). Most in survey would change their bodies if possible. *SFC*, B4; reprinted from *Baltimore Sun*.

64. Langlois, J. H., Roggman, L. A., Casey, R. J. et al. (1987). Infant preferences for attractive faces: Rudiments of a stereotype? *Developmental Psychology*, 23, 363–69.

65. Hatfield, E., & Sprecher, S. (1986). *Mirror, mirror... The importance of looks in everyday life*. Albany, NY: State University of New York Press.

66. Dion, K. K. (1986). Stereotyping based on physical attractiveness: Issues and conceptual perspectives. In C. P. Herman, M. P. Zanna, & E. T. Higgins (Eds.), *Physical appearance, stigma, and social behavior: The Ontario symposium on personality and social psychology* (Vol. 3). Hillsdale, NJ: Erlbaum.

67. Brigham, J. C. (1980). Limiting conditions of the "physical attractiveness stereotype": Attributions about divorce. *Journal of Research & Personality*, 14, 365–75.

68. Clifford, M. M., & Walster, E. H. (1973). The effect of physical attractiveness on teacher expectation. *Sociology of Education, 46,* 248–58.

69. Adams, G. R., & Huston, T. L. (1975). Social perception of middle-aged persons varying in physical attractiveness. *Developmental Psychology, 11,* 657–58.

70. Clifford & Walster, 1973.

71. Cash, T., & Janda, L. H. (1984, December). The eye of the beholder. *PT,* 46–52.

72. Quinn, R. P. (1978). Physical deviance and occupational mistreatment: The short, the fat, and the ugly. Master's thesis, University of Michigan Survey Research Center, University of Michigan, Ann Arbor.

73. Margolin, L., & White, L. (1987). The continuing role of physical attractiveness in marriage. *Journal of Marriage & the Family, 49,* 21–27.

74. Katchadourian, H. (1987). *Fifty: Midlife in perspective.* New York: Freeman.

75. Murstein, B. L. (1986). *Paths to marriage.* Newbury Park, CA: Sage.

76. Bronstein-Burrows, P. (1981). *Introductory psychology: A course in the psychology of both sexes.* Paper presented at the meeting of the American Psychological Association.

77. Wolf, N. (1991). *The beauty myth: How images of beauty are used against women.* New York: Morrow, 184.

78. Britton, A. G. (1988). Thin is out, fit is in. *AH, 7,* 66–71.

79. Britton, 1988, 66.

80. Princeton Survey Research Associates, 1990 survey. Cited in: Kobren (1990), B4.

81. Britton, 1988, 71.

82. Hutchinson, M. (1985). *Transforming body image: Learning to love the body you have.* Freedom, CA: Crossing Press.

83. Rodin, J. (1992, January/February). Body mania. *PT,* 56–60.

84. Yager, J. Cited in: Cook, L. C. (1989, August). The ideal body: Gay vs. straight. *PT,* 67.

85. Gallup Organization, December 1990 survey. Cited in: Sietsema, T. (1991, January 2). Fat's back. *SFC,* Food section, 1, 5.

86. Anonymous. (1991). Great bodies come in many shapes. *University of California, Berkeley, Wellness Letter, 7,* 2.

87. Wolf, 1991, 17.

88. Abernathy, P. Cited in: Sietsema, 1991, 5.

89. Stallones, R. A. (1980). The rise and fall of ischemic heart disease. *Scientific American, 243,* 53–59.

90. Bray, G. A. (1980). Definition, measurement, and classification of the syndromes of obesity. In G. A. Bray (Ed.), *Obesity: Comparative methods of weight control.* Westport, CT: Techomic.

91. Bray, G. A. (1979). *Obesity in America.* Washington, DC: U.S. Department of Health, Education, and Welfare.

92. Consensus Development Conference Statement. (1985). *Health implications of obesity.* Bethesda, MD: National Institutes of Health.

93. U.S. Public Health Service, 1990, 403.

94. Knittle, J. L., & Hirsch, J. (1968). Effect of early nutrition on the development of rat epididymal fat pads: Cellularity and metabolism. *Journal of Clinical Investigation, 47,* 209.

95. Grinker, J. A. (1982). Physiological and behavioral basis for human obesity. In D. W. Pfaff (Ed.), *The physiological mechanisms of motivation.* New York: Springer-Verlag.

96. Nisbett, R. E. (1972). Hunger, obesity, and the ventromedial hypothalamus. *Psychological Review, 79,* 433–55.

97. Bennett, W., & Gurin, J. (1982). *The dieter's dilemma: Eating less and weighing more.* New York: Basic, 6.

98. U.S. Public Health Service, 1990.

99. Anonymous (1991). The easy road to fitness. *University of California, Berkeley, Wellness Letter, 7,* 6.

100. Alt, C. Quoted in: MacVean, M., Associated Press. (1991, October 7). In search of realism: Model nearly died striving for ideal. *Albuquerque Journal,* B1.

101. Herzog, D. B., & Copeland, P. M. (1985). Eating disorders. *NEJM, 313,* 295–303.

102. U.S. Public Health Service, 1988, 510.

103. Storrow, H. A. (1984). Eating disorders. In R. J. Corsini (Ed.), *Encyclopedia of psychology* (Vol. 1). New York: Wiley, 407.

104. *British Journal of Psychiatry* study. Cited in: Arbetter, S. R. (1989). Emotional food fights. *Current Health 2, 15,* 4–10.

105. Yates, A., Leehey, K., & Shisslak, C. M. (1983). Running—an analogue of anorexia? *NEJM, 308,* 251–55.

106. Comerci, G. D. (1990). Medical complications of anorexia nervosa and bulimia nervosa. *Medical Clinics of North America, 74,* 1293–1310.

107. Hsu, L. K. G. (1980). Outcome of anorexia nervosa: A review of the literature. *Archives of General Psychiatry, 37,* 1041–46.

108. Hsu, L. K. G. (1988). The outcome of anorexia nervosa: A reappraisal. *Psychology & Medicine, 18,* 807–12.

109. Lustic, M. J. (1985). Bulimia in adolescents: A review. *Pediatrics, 76,* 685–90.

110. Halmi, K. A., Flak, J. R., & Schwartz, E. (1981). Binge-eating and vomiting: A survey of a college population. *Psychology & Medicine, 11,* 697–706.

111. Schotte, D. E., & Stunkard, A. J. (1987). Bulimia vs. bulimic behaviors on a college campus. *JAMA, 258,* 1213–15.

112. Kolodny, N. J. (1987). *When food's a foe: How to confront and conquer eating disorders.* Boston: Little, Brown.

113. Moore, D.-J. (1989, November/December). I invented bulimia. *Medical Self Care,* 32.

114. Quoted in: Moore, 1989, 32.

115. Yoder, B. (1990). *The recovery resource book.* New York: Fireside, 156.

116. Herman, C. P., & Polivy, J. (1984). A boundary model for the regulation of eating. In A. J. Stunkard & E. Stellar (Eds.), *Eating and its disorders.* New York: Raven, 141–56..

117. Fernstrom, J. D., & Wurtman, R. J. (1972). Brain serotonin content: Physiological regulation by plasma neutral amino acids. *Science, 178,* 414–16.

118. Wurtman, J. J., & Wurtman, R. J. (1983). Studies on the appetite for carbohydrates in rats and humans. *Journal of Psychiatric Research, 13,* 213–21.

119. Arbetter, 1989, 8.

120. Johnson, C. (1982). Bulimia: An analysis of moods and behavior. *Psychosomatic Medicine, 44* 34–51.

121. Harris, R. T. (1983). Bulimarexia and related serious eating disorders with medical complications. *AIM, 99,* 800–07.

122. Cooper, P. J., & Fairburn, C. G. (1986). The depressive symptoms of bulimia nervosa. *British Journal of Psychiatry, 148,* 268–74.

123. Siegel, M., Brisman, J., & Weinshel, M. (1988). *Surviving an eating disorder.* New York: Harper & Row.

124. Waldinger, R. J. (1986). *Fundamentals of psychiatry.* Washington, DC: American Psychiatric Press.

125. Saltman et al., 1987, 148.

126. Saddler, J. (1991, October 17). FTC targets thin claims of liquid diets. *WSJ,* B1.

127. Saltman et al. 1987.

128. Brody, J. E. (1991, June 27). Study links yo-yo dieting to an increased death rate. *NYT,* A9.

129. Gallup poll. Cited in: Brownell, K. (1988, March). The yo-yo trap. *AH,* 78–84.

130. Lissner, L., Odell, P. M., D'Agostino, R. B. et al. (1991). Variability of body weight and health outcomes in the Framingham population. *NEJM, 324,* 1839–44.

131. Brownell, 1988.

132. Brownell, K. D. Cited in: Brody, J. D. (1991, July 3). Personal health: Regardless of the weight-loss program you follow, successful dieting is really in the mind. *NYT,* B6.

133. Brownell, K. D. (1989, June). When and how to diet. *PT,* 40–46.

134. Meade, J. (1991, February). Drop a fast 10 pounds. *Men's Health,* 55–56, 92.

135. Kayman, S., Bruvold, W., & Stern, J. S. (1990). Maintenance and relapse after weight loss in women: Behavioral aspects. *American Journal of Clinical Nutrition, 52,* 800–07.

136. Anonymous. (1991). The four keys to losing weight and keeping it off. *Johns Hopkins Medical Letter, Health After 50, 3,* 7.

137. Rodin, J. (1990). Comparative effects of fructose, aspartame, glucose, and prewater loads on calorie and macronutrient intake. *American Journal of Clinical Nutrition, 51,* 428–35.

138. Rolls, B. J. (1991). Effects of intense sweeteners on hunger, food intake, and body weight: A review. *American Journal of Clinical Nutrition, 53,* 872–78.

139. Saltman et al. 1987, 156–58.

140. Gallup Organization. (1990, July 9). Top worries about daily diet: Sample survey of 772 adults. *Nation's Restaurant News,* 14.

141. Gallup Organization. (1991, November 4). People still eat steak but worry about it. *SFC,* D4.

142. Associated Press. (1990, October 17). Americans still eat too much fat. *SFC,* B3. [Report on U.S. Department of Agriculture draft report on nation's eating habits, presented at American Dietetic Association meeting, Denver, October 15, 1990.]

143. Arieff, I., Reuters. (1991, April 15). Americans leery of dietary advice. *SFC,* B3. [Report of 1990 telephone survey by National Cholesterol Education Program, run by National Institutes of Health.]

144. Associated Press. (1991, June 5). American men resisting change to low-fat diet. *SFC,* B6. [Report of March 1991 telephone survey of 506 men by R. H. Bruskin Associates for American Dietetic Association.]

145. Gallup Organization. (1991, November). Should ice cream cartons carry warning labels? And other questions from our Gallup poll. *In Health,* 45–47.

146. Associated Press. (1991, May 3). 2 out of 3 Americans are overweight, survey finds. *SFC,* A4. [Report of Louis Harris survey for *Prevention* magazine.]

147. Associated Press. (1991, April 27). People fib about food. *SFC,* C1. [Report of study by Walter Mertz, presented at annual meeting of the Federation of American Societies for Experimental Biology, Atlanta.]

148. Associated Press. (1991, October 10). People know they could improve diet. *SFC,* D4. [Report of American Dietetic Association, October 9, 1991 survey.]

149. Gibson, R., & Deveny, K. (1991, November 13). Americans' ignorance about nutrition hinders efforts to improve nation's diet. *WSJ,* B1, B4. [Report of American Dietetic Association survey.]

150. Abbott, C. J., United Press International (1990, December 4). Americans think they eat right. *SFC,* B3. [Report of U.S. Diet and Health Knowledge Survey.]

151. Gallup Organization, 1991, November, 45–47.

152. Garrison, J. (1991, July 21). Athletes' eating habits—a growing concern. *SFE,* A-1, A-13.

153. Heyl, K. Quoted in: Barks, J., & Muller, E. J. (1990). October). Food of the guards. *Men's Health, 5,* 26–30, 86.

154. Williams, L. (1991, August 28). Eating leaner to be meaner. *NYT,* B6.

155. Clark, N. (1990). *Sports nutrition guide-*

book. Champaign, IL: Leisure Press.

156. Applegate, L. (1991). *Power foods: High-performance nutrition for high-performance people.* Emmaus, PA: Rodale.

157. Siano, J. (1991, May 18). An auto racer's accessories: Diet and exercise. *NYT*, 29.

158. Lloyd, B. (1991, November 2). What you eat tells how you'll finish. *NYT*, 34.

159. Applegate, L. (1991, February). Fast-track snacks. *Men's Health*, 40–41.

160. Applegate, L. (1991, August). Unwrap some energy. *Men's Health*, 20–21.

161. Brody, R. (1990, February). How much protein is enough? *Men's Health*, 86.

UNIT 7: PHYSICAL FITNESS

1. Bechtel, S. (1990, October). The Mayflower boys. *Men's Health*, 94–95.

2. Mason, M. J. (1991). *Making our lives our own.* New York: HarperCollins.

3. Melpomene Institute for Women's Health Research staff and researchers. (1990). *The bodywise woman: Reliable information about physical activity and health.* New York: Prentice Hall Press.

4. Nagler, W. Quoted in: Sims, S. M. (1990, April). Dr. Nagler says 'keep moving.' *Self*, 165–68, 211.

5. Taylor, H. (1991, October). Has the fitness movement peaked? *American Demographics*, 10–11.

6. Centers for Disease Control (1990). Coronary heart disease attributable to sedentary lifestyle—selected states, 1988. *JAMA*, *264*, 1390, 1392.

7. Dietz, W. H. Jr., & Gormaker, S. L. (1985). Do we fatten our children at the television set? Obesity and television viewing in children and adolescents. *Pediatrics*, *75*, 807–12.

8. Singer, D. G. (1983, July). A time to reexamine the role of television in our lives. *American Psychologist*, 815–16.

9. Fahey, V. (1992, December/January). TV by the numbers. *In Health*, 35.

10. Cooke, P. (1992, December/January). TV or not TV. *In Health*, 33–43.

11. Fahey, 1992, 35.

12. Tucker, L. A., & Friedman, G. M. (1989). Television viewing and obesity in adult males. *AJPH*, *79*, 516–18.

13. Tucker, L. A., & Bagwell, M. (1991). Television viewing and obesity in adult females. *AJPH*, *81*, 908–11.

14. Anonymous. (1990). Inactivity, diet, and the fattening of America. *Journal of the American Dietetic Association*, *90*, 1247–52.

15. Tucker & Bagwell, 1991.

16. Anonymous. (1991, November). Better health with a twist of the wrist. *Prevention*, 116.

17. Ornstein, R., & Sobel, D. (1989). *Healthy pleasures.* Reading, MA: Addison-Wesley, 103.

18. Specter, M. (1989, January 15). Schools miss the mark on fitness. *SFC, This World*, 11; reprinted from *Washington Post*.

19. Brown, R. S. Quoted in: Cardozo, C. (1990, September). The new feel-great prescription: Even a few minutes of exercise can enhance creativity, self-esteem, and chase away the blues. *Self*, 122, 124–25.

20. Perry, P. (1987, March). Are we having fun yet? *AH*, 59–63.

21. Hopson, J. L. (1988, July/August). A pleasurable chemistry. *PT*, 29–33.

22. Flippin, R. (1989, October). Beyond endorphins: The latest research on runner's high. *AH*, 78–83.

23. Greist, J. H., Eischens, R. R. et al. (1978). Running out of depression. *The Physician & Sportsmedicine*, *6*(12), 49–56.

24. Monahan, T. (1986). Exercise and depression: Swapping sweat for serenity? *The Physician & Sportsmedicine*, *14*(9), 192–97.

25. Morgan, W. P., & O'Connor, P. J. (1987). Exercise and mental health. In R. K. Dishman (Ed.), *Exercise adherence*. Champaign, IL: Human Kinetics.

26. Farmer, M. E., Locke, B. Z., Moscicki, E. K. et al. (1988). Physical activity and depressive symptoms: The NHANES I epidemiologic follow-up study. *American Journal of Epidemiology*, *128*, 1340–51.

27. Tucker, L. A., Cole, G. E., & Friedman, G. M. (1986). Physical fitness: A buffer against stress. *Perceptual & Motor Skills*, *63*, 955–61.

28. Sime, W. E. (1984). Psychological benefits of exercise. *Advances*, *1*, 15–29.

29. Roth, D. L., & Holmes, D. S. (1987). Influence of aerobic exercise training and relaxation training on physical and psychological health following stressful life events. *Psychosomatic Medicine*, *49*, 355–65.

30. Rippe, J. M. Quoted in: Cardozo, 1990, 124.

31. Thayer, R. E. (1988, October). Energy walks. *PT*, 12–13.

32. Thayer, R. E. (1987). Energy, tiredness, and tension effects of a sugar snack versus moderate exercise. *Journal of Personality & Social Psychology*, *52*(1), 119–25.

33. Mott, P. (1990, October 7). Mental gymnastics. *LAT*, E1, E18–E19.

34. Gondola, J. C. Cited in: Cardozo, 1990, 124.

35. McCleary, K. (1991, December/January). The no-gimmick weight-loss plan. *In Health*, 83.

36. Ornstein & Sobel, 1989, 106.

37. Paffenbarger, R. S., Hyde, R. T., Wing, W. L. et al. (1986). Physical activity, all-cause mortality, and longevity among college alumni. *NEJM*, *314*, 605–13.

38. Leon, A. S., Connett, J., Jacobs, D. R. et al. (1987). Leisure-time physical activity levels and risk of coronary heart disease and death. *JAMA*, *258*, 2388–95.

39. Ornish, D., Brown, S. E., Scherwitz, L. W. et al. (1990). Can lifestyle changes reverse coronary heart disease? The Lifestyle Heart Trial. *Lancet*, *336*, 129–33.

40. Pritikin, N. (1984, March). Given the right diet, a champion can be made at any age. *Runner's World*, 120.

41. Martin, J. E., Dubbert, P. M., & Cushman, W. C. (1990). Controlled trial of aerobic exercise in hypertension. *Circulation*, *81*, 1560–67.

42. Kelemen, M. H., Effron, M. B., Valenti, S. A. et al. (1990). Exercise training combined with antihypertensive drug therapy. *JAMA*, *263*, 2766–71.

43. Somers, V., Conway, J., Johnston, J. et al. (1991). Effects of endurance training on baroreflex sensitivity and blood pressure in borderline hypertension. *Lancet*, *337*, 1363–68.

44. Medical Tribune News Service. (1991, September 25). Exercise lowers children's blood pressure. *SFC*, D5. [Report of study by Schoolchild Study Group, Odense, Denmark.]

45. Gilders, R. M., Voner, C., & Dudley, G. A. (1989). Endurance training and blood pressure in normotensive and hypertensive adults. *Medicine & Science in Sports & Exercise*, *21*, 629–36.

46. Blumenthal, J. A., Siegel, W. C., & Appelbaum, M. (1991). Failure of exercise to reduce blood pressure in patients with mild hypertension: Results of a randomized controlled trial. *JAMA*, *266*, 2098–2104.

47. Blumenthal, J. A. Quoted in: Brody, J. E. (1991, October 16). Reputed effect of exercise challenged. *NYT*, A10.

48. Frisch, R. E., Wyshak, G., Albright N. L. et al. (1985). Lower prevalence of breast cancer and cancers of the reproductive system among former college athletes compared to non-athletes. *British Journal of Cancer*, *52*, 885–91.

49. Lee, I.-M., Paffenbarger, J. Jr., & Hsieh, C. (1991). Physical activity and risk of developing colorectal cancer among college alumni. *Journal of the National Cancer Institute*, *83*, 1324–29.

50. Lee, I.-M. Quoted in: Associated Press. (1991, September 18). Exercise may cut cancer risk. *SFC*,

A3.

51. Horton, E. Quoted in: Chang, K. (1991, July 18). Exercise can prevent adult diabetes, study says. *SFC*, A4.

52. Helmrich, S. P., Ragland, D. R., Leung, R. W. et al. (1991). Physical activity and reduced occurrence of non-insulin-dependent diabetes mellitus. *NEMJ*, *325*, 147–52.

53. Kirkpatrick, M. K., Edwards, R. N., & Finch, N. (1991). Assessment and prevention of osteoporosis through use of a client self-reporting tool. *Nurse Practitioner*, *16*(7), 16–26.

54. Whitten, P., & Whiteside, E. J. (1989, April). Can exercise make you sexier? *PT*, 42–44.

55. Bortz, W. Quoted in: Chinnici, M. (1991, April). How to protect your body from time. *Self*, 128–29.

56. Nieman, D. Cited in: Drexler, M. (1991, July 14). Tuning up immunity. *SFC, This World*, 14–15; reprinted from *Boston Globe Magazine*.

57. Dishman, R. K. (1982). Compliance/adherence in health-related exercise. *Health Psychology*, *1*, 237–67.

58. Dishman, R. K., & Ickes, W. (1981). Self-motivation and adherence to therapeutic exercise. *Journal of Behavioral Medicine*, *4*, 421–38.

59. Biddle, S., & Smith, R. A. (1991, September). Motivating adults for physical activity: Towards a healthier present. *Journal of Physical Education, Recreation & Dance*, 39–48.

60. American College of Sports Medicine (1990). *Achieving and maintaining physical fitness.* Indianapolis, IN: American College of Sports Medicine.

61. Raskin, D. (1991, January 28). Updated guidelines to improve fitness. *NYT*, B7.

62. American College of Sports Medicine (1990). The recommended quantity and quality of exercise for developing and maintaining cardiorespiratory and muscular fitness in healthy adults. *Medicine & Science in Sports & Exercise*, *22*, 265–74.

63. Borg, G. (1973). Perceived exertion: A note on history and methods. *Medicine and Science in Sports*, *5*, 90–93.

64. Borg, G. (1982). Psychophysical bases of perceived exertion. *Medicine & Science in Sports & Exercise*, *14*, 380.

65. Higdon, H. (1991, December). Cross over to cross training. *AH*, *10*(10), 46–51.

66. Flippin, R. (1991, July/August). Mix-and-match aerobics. *AH*, 88.

67. Kaufmann, E. (1989, December). The new rhythms of fitness. *AH*, 45–49.

68. Johnson, E., *Albuquerque Journal*. Quoted in: Clancy, M., Reuters. (1991, July 21). Pueblo Indians sprinting toward sun, face new day. *SFE*, B-8.

69. Cuerdon, D. (1991, August). A good ride. *Men's Health*, 47–50.

70. Sharp, R. (1991, January/February). Know your sport: Swimming. *AH*, 30–33.

71. Rimer, S. (1990, April 29). Swimming for fitness and solitude. *New York Times Magazine*, 59–60, 84.

72. Bauer, S. (1990, April 29). 'Blading'—with a hoot and a holler. *New York Times Magazine*, pt. 2, 20–21, 34.

73. Brody, J. E. (1991, May 2). Roller blading: A new sport that can be fun as well as an aerobic activity to enhance fitness. *NYT*, B8.

74. Fisher, L. (1991, September). Step right. *AH*, 66–70.

75. Gordon, J., & Quade, V. (1991, April 29). Jam up for jelly bellies. *Newsweek*, 57.

76. Rogers, E. (1989, April). Emotional rescue. *AH*, 44.

77. McKee, S. (1991, April). The balance of power. *AH*, 62–67.

78. Frontera, W., Meredith, C., O'Reilly, K. et al. (1988). Strength conditioning in older men: Skeletal muscle hypertrophy and improved func-

tion. *Journal of Applied Physiology, 64,* 1038–44.

79. DeWitt, J., & Roberts, T. (1991, September). Pumping up an adult fitness program. *Journal of Physical Education, Recreation, & Dance,* 67–71.

80. McKee, 1991, 62–67.

81. Bensimhon, D. (1991, October). Exercise for dumbbells: How to use hand weights for a total-body workout. *Men's Health,* 28–29.

82. Thaxton, N. A. (1988). *Pathways to fitness: Foundations, motivation, applications.* New York: Harper & Row, 244.

83. Garrick, J. Quoted in: Raskin, D. (1990, October 15). Hitting the open trail for a varied workout. *NYT,* B8.

84. Morrow, J., & Harvey, P. (1990, November). Exermania! *AH,* 31–32.

85. Cobb, K. (1989, October). When is too much of a good thing bad? *AH,* 79–84.

86. Morrow, J., & Harvey, P. (1990, November). How do you compare to the marathoners? *AH,* 31.

87. Cobb, 1989, 81.

88. Morgan & O'Connor, 1987.

89. Dishman, R. K. (Ed.), *Exercise adherence.* Champaign, IL: Human Kinetics.

90. Smith, L. Quoted in: Welch, D. (1991, April). How many sports shoes do you really need? *Self,* 163, 184.

91. Wischnia, B. (1991, April). A shoe for all seasons. *Men's Health,* 68–70.

92. McNerney, J. E. (1991, November 2). Smart runners make smart shoe choices. *NYT,* 34.

93. Thaxton, 1988, 342–43.

94. Thaxton, 1988, 343–44.

95. Halim, A. (1980). Fluid and electrolyte balance and physical training in hot climates. *Journal of Sports Medicine, 20,* 350.

96. Costill, D., & Miller, J. (1980). Nutrition for endurance sports: carbohydrate and fluid balance. *International Journal of Sports Medicine, 1,* 2–14.

97. Thaxton, 1988.

98. American National Red Cross. (1973). *Standard first aid and personal safety.* New York: Doubleday, 160–65.

99. Horvath, S. M. (1981). Impact of air quality on exercise performance. In D. I. Miller (Ed.), *Exercise & Sports Sciences Reviews, 9,* 267.

100. Thaxton, 1988, 330.

101. Balke, B. (1960). Work capacity at altitude. In W. R. Johnson (Ed.), *Science and medicine of exercise and sports.* New York: Harper & Row, 339.

102. Klein, F. C. (1991, January 6). Confessions of a steroid-abusing lineman. *WSJ,* A12.

103. Hough, D. O., & Kovan, J. R. (1990, November). Is your patient a steroid abuser? *Medical Aspects of Human Sexuality,* 26–34.

104. Janofsky, M. (1990, November 6). 2 U.S. track stars face 2-year ban for drug use. *NYT,* A1, B12.

105. Franklin, D. (1990, July 1). Stuck on steroids. *SFC, This World,* 14; reprinted from *In Health.*

106. Cowart, V. S. (1990). Blunting 'steroid epidemic' requires alternatives, innovative education. *JAMA, 264,* 1641.

107. Buckley, W. E., Yesalis, C. E. III, Friedl, K. E. et al. (1988). Estimated prevalence of anabolic steroid use among high school seniors. *JAMA, 260,* 3441–45.

108. Fultz, O. (1991, May). 'Roid rage. *AH,* 60–65.

109. Miller, R. W. (1987, November 17–21). Athletes and steroids: Playing a deadly game. *FDA Consumer,* 17–21.

110. Hough & Kovan, 1990, 26–34.

111. Hough, D. O. (1990). Anabolic steroids and ergogenic aids. *American Family Physician, 41,* 1157.

112. Anonymous. (1991). Anabolic steroids: The

bulk of the questions remain resolved. *Modern Medicine, 59,* 10–13.

113. Council on Scientific Affairs. (1988). Drug abuse in athletes: Anabolic steroids and human growth hormone. *JAMA, 259,* 1703–05.

114. Lombardo, J. A., Longcope, C., & Voy, R. O. (1985, August 15). Recognizing anabolic steroid abuse. *Patient Care, 19,* 28.

115. Klein, F. C. (1991, August 28). The scales tell the steroid story. *WSJ,* A8.

116. Smith, T. W. (1991, July 3). N.F.L.'s steroid policy is too lax, doctor warns. *NYT,* B7–B8.

117. Thaxton, 1988, 345–46.

118. Lamberg, L. (1990, November). The boy who ate his bed...and other mysteries of sleep. *AH,* 56–60.

119. Dement, W. (1992, March). The sleepwatchers. *Stanford,* 56.

120. Aldrich, M. S. (1990). Narcolepsy. *NEJM, 323,* 389–94.

121. Dement, W. C., Carskadon, M., & Ley, R. (1973). The prevalence of narcolepsy. *Sleep Research, 2,* 147.

122. Roth, B. (1980). *Narcolepsy and hypersomnia.* Basel: Springer-Verlag, 94–95.

123. Angier, N. (1990, May 15). Sleepiness epidemic blankets nation. *SFC,* A1; reprinted from *NYT.*

124. Chollar, S. (1989, April). Dreamchasers. *PT,* 60–61.

125. Gackenbach, J., & Bosveld, J. (1989, October). Take control of your dreams. *PT,* 27–32.

126. Home, J. A. Quoted in: Israeloff, R. (1990, November 15). Feeling a bit drowsy? Join the club. *SFC,* B3–B4; reprinted from *Working Woman.*

127. Krueger, J. M., & Dinarello, C. A. Reported in: Moffat, A. S. (1988, July/August). "Get a good night's rest." *AH,* 54.

128. Nordheimer, J. (1991, September 8). It's Sunday afternoon, and in counterpoint to Friday highs, blues settle in. *NYT,* 15.

129. Kolata, G. (1990, May 3). Light resets body rhythms for the night worker. *NYT,* A10.

130. Czeisler, C. A., Johnson, M. P., Duffy, J. F. et al. (1990). Exposure to bright light and darkness to treat physiologic maladaptation to night work. *NEJM, 322,* 1253–59.

131. Locitzer, K. (1989, July/August). Are you out of sync with each other? *PT,* 66.

132. Dinges, D. F., & Broughton, R. J. (Eds.) (1989). *Sleep and alertness: Chronobiological, behavioral, and medical aspects of napping.* New York: Raven Press.

133. Schroepfer, L. (1991, February). An army of fatigued. *Men's Health,* 26–27.

134. Carlinsky, D. (1990, March 14). Not everyone needs eight-hour slumber. *SFC,* B3–B4.

135. Kates, W. (1990, March 30). America is not getting enough sleep. *SFC,* B3.

136. Maas, J. Cited in: Kates, 1990, B3.

137. Allen, R. P. et al. Cited in: Rovner, S. (1990, September 25). Teen sleepyheads aren't really lazy: School hours deprive them of sleep. *SFC,* B3, B6; reprinted from *Washington Post.*

138. Angier, 1990, A1.

139. Lafavore, M. (1991, August). Good nights: 5 ways to sleep better. *Men's Health,* 56.

140. Williams, T. F. (1990, July 1). Scientists looking at sleep disorders have made some eye-opening discoveries. *LAT,* A9.

141. Lamberg, 1990, 59.

142. Jacobs, G. D. (1992, January). The zzzzzz plan. *Prevention,* 44–47, 114–20.

143. Lipman, D. S. (1990, November). Snore no more! *Prevention,* 39–46.

144. Novaco, R. Cited in: Huey, J. (1992, January 13). New frontiers of commuting. *Fortune,* 56–58.

145. Schor, J. B. (1991, November/December). Workers of the world, unwind. *Technology Review,* 25–32.

146. Hugick, L., & Leonard, J. (1991, September 2). The Gallup poll: Job satisfaction drops. *SFC,* D3, D5.

147. Schor, J. B. Quoted in: Gower, T. (1991, October 17–23). *Metropolis* (Santa Clara Valley, Calif.), 14–18; reprinted from *Boston Phoenix.*

148. Cooper, C. Quoted in: Worthy, F. S. (1987, April 27). You're probably working too hard. *Fortune,* 133–40.

149. Schor, 1991.

150. Sanger, D. E. (1990, March 20). Death by overwork—study of Japan offices. *SFC,* A15–A16; reprinted from *NYT.*

151. Fuchs, V. R., & Reklis, D. M. (1992). America's children: Economic perspectives and policy options. *Science, 255,* 41–45.

152. University of Maryland study. Cited in: Labich, K. (1991, May 20). Can your career hurt your kids? *Fortune,* 38–68.

153. Gallup poll. Cited in: Schwartz, J. (1991, July). Workers want 40 hours in 4 days. *American Demographics,* 11.

154. Laurence, L. (1990, December). Active rest. *Self,* 115–16.

155. McCarthy, P. (1992, January/February). Soothing the savage exerciser. *AH,* 98.

156. Loehr, J. (1991). *Mental toughness training for sports.* New York: New American Library/Dutton.

157. Canter, M. (1991, April). The tough don't choke. *Men's Health,* 44–45.

158. Csikszentmihalyi, M. (1991). *Flow: The psychology of optimal experience.* New York: HarperCollins.

159. Dement, 1992.

160. Johnson, L. C. (1982). Sleep deprivation and performance. In W. B. Webb (Ed.), *Biological rhythms, sleep and performance.* New York: Wiley.

161. Gillberg, M. (1984). The effects of two alternative timings of a one-hour nap on early morning performance. *Biological Psychology, 19*(1), 45–54.

162. Davis, C. (1991, November). Clockwise exercise. *In Health,* 90–92.

163. Dolnick, E. (1992, February/March). Snap out of it. *Health,* 86–90.

164. Thayer, R. E. (1989). *The biopsychology of mood.* New York: Oxford University Press.

165. Harris survey. Cited in: Bloom, M. (1991, June). Beat the clock. *AH,* 44, 51.

166. Bloom, 1991.

167. Kate, N. T. (1991, June). What makes triathletes run? *American Demographics,* 15.

UNIT 8: INTIMACY AND SEXUALITY

1. Gallagher, W. (1988, March). Worried women, lonely men. *AH,* 48.

2. Burns, D. D. (1985). *Intimate connections.* New York: Signet, 29.

3. Storr, A. (1989). *Solitude: A return to the self.* New York: Free Press.

4. Brody, J. E. (1992, February 5). Maintaining friendships for the sake of good health. *NYT,* B8.

5. Robertson, M. (1991, July 22). What are friends for? *SFC,* E3–E4.

6. Fielbert, M. Cited in: Robertson, M. (1991, July 22). Friendship gender gap. *SFC,* E4.

7. Rubin, L. B. (1984). *Intimate strangers: Men and women together.* New York: Harper Perennial Library.

8. Anonymous. (1989, January-February). Just friends. *PT,* 10.

9. Schroepfer, L. (1990, December). Boy friends. *AH,* 84.

10. Claes, M. E. (1992). Friendship and personal adjustment during adolescence. *Journal of Adolescence, 15*(1), 39–55.

11. Ishii-Kuntz, M. (1990). Social interaction and psychological well-being: Comparison across stages of adulthood. *International Journal of Aging & Human Development, 30*(1), 15–36.

12. Stein, J. (Ed.) (1973). *The Random House dictionary of the English language*. New York: Random House.

13. Schaefer, M. T., & Olson, D. H. (1981). Assessing intimacy: The pair inventory. *Journal of Marital & Family Therapy, 7,* 47–60.

14. Jorgensen, S. R., & Gaudy, J. C. (1980). Self-disclosure and satisfaction in marriage: The relationship examined. *Family Relations, 29,* 281–87.

15. Asbell, B., & Wynn, K. (1991). *What they know about you*. New York: Random House.

16. Montagu, A. (1971). *Touching: The human significance of the skin*. New York: Columbia University Press.

17. Rice, F. P. (1989). *Human sexuality*. Dubuque, IA: Wm. C. Brown.

18. Shea, J. A., & Adams, G. R. (1984). Correlates of male and female romantic attachments: A path analysis study. *Journal of Youth & Adolescence, 13,* 27–44.

19. Rubin, L. (1973). *Liking and loving*. New York: Holt, Rinehart & Winston.

20. Hatfield, E., & Sprecher, S. (1986). *Mirror, mirror..The importance of looks in everyday life*. Albany: State University of New York Press.

21. Dutton, D., & Aron, A. (1974). Some evidence for heightened sexual attraction under conditions of high anxiety. *Journal of Personality & Social Psychology, 30,* 510–17.

22. Hatfield, E., & Walster, G. W. (1978). *A new look at love*. Reading, MA: Addison-Wesley.

23. Beck, A. (1989). *Love is never enough*. New York: HarperPerennial.

24. Viorst, J. (1979). Just because I'm married, does it mean I'm going steady? In B. J. Wishart & L. C. Reichman (Eds.), *Modern sociological issues*. New York: Macmillan, 283–89.

25. Norwood, R. (1985). *Women who love too much*. Los Angeles: J. P. Tarcher.

26. Peele, S., & Brodsky, A. (1976). *Love and addiction*. New York: New American Library.

27. Saxton, L. (1977). *The individual, marriage, and the family* (3rd ed). Belmont, CA: Wadsworth.

28. Sternberg, R. (1988). *The triangle of love*. New York: Basic.

29. Timmreck, T. C. (1990). Overcoming the loss of a love: Preventing love addiction and promoting positive emotional health. *Psychological Reports, 66,* 515–28.

30. Rhoades, R. A. (1990). Break it off: Identifying a destructive love relationship. *Today's OR Nurse, 12*(9), 13–16.

31. Phillips, D. (1980). *How to fall out of love*. New York: Fawcett.

32. Wholley, D. (1988). *Becoming your own parent*. New York: Doubleday.

33. Saluter, A. F. (1990). Singleness in America. Studies in marriage and the family. *Current Population Reports*, Series P-23, No. 162. Washington, DC: U.S. Department of Commerce, Bureau of the Census.

34. United Press International (1990, August 13). Many single women aren't desperate to wed. *SFC*, B5. [Report of F. Kaslow, The thirty-something women: Companionship, children, and career choices. Presented at August 1990 American Psychological Association meeting, Boston, MA.]

35. Farrell, C. (1992, June 29). Where have all the families gone? *Business Week*, 90–91.

36. Curran, J. P. (1982, October). Dating anxiety. *Medical Aspects of Human Sexuality*, 160–75.

37. Curran, 1982, 165.

38. Whyte, M. Quoted in: United Press International. (1990, May 4). Dating a lot won't net good marriage. *SFC*, B7.

39. Staff, *American Demographics*. (1990, May 4). Traditional households are fading worldwide. *WSJ*, B1.

40. Rindfuss, R. Cited in: Larson, J. (1991, November). Cohabitation is a premarital step.

41. Bumpass, L. L., & Sweet, J. A. (1989). National estimates of cohabitation. *Demography, 26,* 615–25.

42. Thornton, A. (1988). Cohabitation and marriage in the 1980s. *Demography, 25,* 497–508.

43. Rindfuss, 1991, 20.

44. Associated Press. (1992, September 3). Why live-ins get divorced. *SFC*, B3. [Report of study by W. Axinn & A. Thornton in August 1992 *Demography*]

45. Bennett, N. Cited in: Hall, H. (1988, July/August). Marriage: Practice makes perfect? *PT*, 15.

46. Hall, 1988.

47. Hamilton, D. (1992, November 19). Lovers who choose not to marry. *Point Reyes* (California) *Light*, 6.

48. Baker, J. N., & Lewis, S. D. (1990, March 12). Lesbians: Portrait of a community. *Newsweek*, 24.

49. Blumstein, P., & Schwartz, P. (1983). *American couples*. New York: Morrow.

50. Stroock, A. (1990, May 14). Gay divorces complicated by lack of laws. *SFC*, A4.

51. Sullivan, A. (1989, August 28). Here comes the groom. *New Republic*, 20–22.

52. Dean, C. R. (1991, September 28). Legalize gay marriage. *NYT*, 15.

53. Ames, K., Sulavik, C., Joseph, N. et al. (1992, March 23). Domesticated bliss. *Newsweek*, 62–63.

54. Patterson, C. Cited in: Tuller, D. (1992, November 23). Lesbian families—study shows healthy kids. *SFC*, A13.

55. Gross, J. (1991, February 11). New challenge of youth: Growing up in gay home. *NYT*, A1, A12.

56. National Center for Health Statistics. (1989, April 28). Births, marriages, divorces, and deaths for 1988. *Monthly Vital Statistics Report*, U.S. Department of Health and Human Services, vol. 37, no. 12, suppl. DHHS Pub. No. (PHS)89-1120.

57. Umberson, D. (1989, May). Marital benefits for men vs. women. *Medical Aspects of Human Sexuality*, 56.

58. Hu, Y. R., & Goldman, N. (1990). Mortality differentials by marital status: An international comparison. *Demography, 27*(2), 233–50.

59. Wilson, B. F. (1991, October). The marry-go-round. *American Demographics*, 52–54.

60. U.S. Census Bureau. Cited in: Teegardin, C. (1992, July 20). Americans steer clear of altar, census says. *SFC*, D5.

61. National Center on Health Statistics. Cited in: McLeod, R. G. (1992, October 1). Births, marriages decline—just like in Depression. *SFC*, A1.

62. Umberson, 1989.

63. Bozzi, V. (1988, March). Brains and beauty merge. *AH*, 116.

64. Olson, D. H. Quoted in: Kochakian, M. J. (1992, October 27). Study finds many marriages unhappy. *SFC*, D3; reprinted from *Hartford Courant*.

66. Olson, quoted in Kochakian, 1992.

66. Gottman, J. et al. Cited in: Brody, J. E. (1992, August 13). Science finds a way to predict who will divorce. *SFC*, D3; reprinted from *NYT*.

67. Cleek, M., & Pearson, A. (1985). Perceived causes of divorce: An analysis of interrelationships. *Journal of Marriage & the Family, 47,* 179–83.

68. U.S. Census Bureau. Cited in: Anonymous. (1991, October 4–6). Liz leads at the altar. *USA Today*, 1A.

69. U.S. Census Bureau. Cited in: Staff, *American Demographics*. (1990, August 3). Romance in America, and how it pans out. *WSJ*, B1.

70. Arbetter, S. R. (1989). The way it is: The remarried family. *Current Health 2, 17,* 17–19.

71. National Center for Health Statistics. Reported in: Associated Press. (1990, April 4). Marriage can be habit-forming. *SFC*, A7.

72. Crooks, R., & Baur, K. (1990). *Our sexuality* (4th ed.). Redwood City, CA: Benjamin/Cummings, 522.

73. Weiten, W., Lloyd, M. A., & Lashley, R. L. (1991). *Psychology applied to modern life:*

American Demographics, 20–21.

Adjustment in the 90s (3rd ed.). Pacific Grove: CA: Brooks/Cole.

74. Eisler, R. M., Skidmore, J. R., & Ward, C. H. (1988). Masculine gender-role stress: Predictor of anger, anxiety, and health-risk behaviors. *Journal of Personality Assessment, 52*(1), 133–41.

75. Gillespie, B. L., & Eisler, R. M. (1992). Development of the feminine gender role stress scale: A cognitive-behavioral measure of stress, appraisal, and coping for women. *Behavior Modification, 16*(3), 426–38.

76. Arrighi, H. M., Guess, H. A., Metter, E. J. et al. (1990). Symptoms and signs of prostatism as risk factors for prostatectomy. *Prostate, 16,* 253–61.

77. Fowler, F., Wennberg, J., Timothy, R. et al. (1988). Symptom status and quality of life following prostatectomy. *JAMA, 259,* 3018–22.

78. Barry, M. J. (1990). Epidemiology and natural history of benign prostatic hyperplasia. *Urologic Clinics of North America, 17,* 495–507.

79. Avant, R. F. (1988). Dysmenorrhea. *Primary Care; Clinics in Office Practice, 15,* 549–59.

80. Izzo, A., & Labriola, D. (1991). Dysmenorrhea and sports activities in adolescents. *Clinical & Experimental Obstetrics & Gynecology, 18,* 109–16.

81. Osofsky, H. J. (1990). Efficacious treatments of PMS: A need for further research. *JAMA, 264,* 387.

82. Sedney, M. (1987) Development of androgyny: Parental influences. *Psychology of Women Quarterly, 11,* 311–26.

83. Crooks & Baur, 1990.

84. Crooks & Baur, 1990.

85. Centers for Disease Control. Cited in: Associated Press. (1992, November 23). Risky sex declining among teens. *SFC*, C4.

86. Crooks & Baur, 1990.

87. Crooks & Baur, 1990.

88. Crooks & Baur, 1990.

89. Pauly, I., & Edgerton, M. (1986). The gender identity movement: A growing surgical-psychiatric liaison. *Archives of Sexual Behavior, 15,* 315–30.

90. Green, R. (1974). *Sexual identity conflict in children and adults*. New York: Basic.

91. Pauly, I. (1974). Female transsexualism: Part II. *Archives of Sexual Behavior, 3,* 509–26.

92. Tollison, C. D., & Adams, H. E. (1979). *Sexual disorders: Treatment, theory, and research*. New York: Gardner Press.

93. Lundstrom, B., Pauly, I., & Walinder, J. (1984). Outcome of sex reassignment surgery. *Acta Psychiatrica Scandinavica, 70,* 289–94.

94. Kinsey, A., Pomeroy, W., & Martin, C. (1948). *Sexual behavior in the human male*. Philadelphia: Saunders.

95. Bloch, H., Donley, M., & Lafferty, E. (1992, August 17). Bisexuality: What is it? *Time*, 49–51.

96. Barinaga, M. (1991). Is homosexuality biological? *Science, 253,* 956–57.

97. Bailey, J. M., & Pillard, R. C. Cited in: Bishop, J. E. (1991, December 17). Study of brothers of gay men suggest genetic tendency for homosexuality. *WSJ*, B4.

98. LeVay, S. (1991). A difference in hypothalamic structure between heterosexual and homosexual men. *Science, 253,* 1034–37.

99. Allen, L. S., & Gorski, R. A. (1992). Sexual orientation and the size of the anterior commissure in the human brain. *Proceedings of the National Academy of Sciences of the United States of America, 89,* 7199–7202.

100. Gallup Organization. (1992, June 12). Poll finds most disapprove of gay lifestyle. *SFC*, A27.

101. Masters, W., & Johnson, V. (1966). *Human sexual response*. Boston: Little, Brown.

102. Kaplan, H. (1979). *Disorders of sexual desire*. New York: Brunner/Mazel.

103. Masters & Johnson, 1966.
104. Masters & Johnson, 1966.
105. World Health Organization. *Reproductive health: A key to a brighter future*. Cited in: Associated Press. (1992, June 25). U. N. agency on sex: Pitfalls and promise. *NYT*, A4.
106. Klein, M. (1992, June). The answer guy. *Men's Health*, 84–85.
107. Friday, N. (1991). *Women on top: How real life has changed women's sexual fantasies*. New York: Simon & Schuster, 191.
108. Zilbergeld, B. (1992). *The new male sexuality*. New York: Bantam.
109. Sue, D. (1979). Erotic fantasies of college students during coitus. *Journal of Sex Research, 15*, 299–305.
110. Crooks & Baur, 1990.
111. Kinsey, Pomeroy, & Martin, 1948.
112. Kinsey, A., Pomeroy, W., Martin, C. et al. (1953). *Sexual behavior in the human female*. Philadelphia: Saunders.
113. Follingstad, D., & Kimbrell, D. (1986). Sexual fantasies revisted: An expansion and further clarification of variables affecting sex fantasy production. *Archives of Sexual Behavior, 15*, 475–86.
114. Hunt, M. (1974). *Sexual behavior in the 1970s*. Chicago: Playboy Press.
115. Crooks & Baur, 1990.
116. Huey, C., Kline-Graber, G., & Graber, B. (1981). Time factors and orgasmic response. *Archives of Sexual Behavior, 21*, 111–18.
117. Crooks & Baur, 1990.
118. Crooks & Baur, 1990, 296.
119. Hass, A. (1979). *Teenage sexuality*. New York: Macmillan.
120. Kinsey, Pomeroy, Martin, & Gebhard, 1953.
121. Byer, C. O., & Shainberg, L. W. (1991). *Dimensions of human sexuality* (3rd ed.). Dubuque, IA: Wm. C. Brown.
122. Hunt, 1974.
123. Harold, E., & Way, L. (1983). Oral-genital sexual behavior in a sample of university females. *Journal of Sex Research, 19*, 327–29.
124. Consumers Union. (1989, March). Can you rely on condoms? *Consumer Reports*, 135–41.
125. Hunt, 1974.
126. Kinsey, Pomeroy, & Martin, 1948.
127. Westoff, C. (1974). Coital frequency and contraception. *Family Planning Perspectives, 6*, 136–41.
128. Trussell, J., & Westoff, C. F. (1980). Contraceptive practice and trends in coital frequency. *Family Planning Perspectives, 12*, 246–49.
129. Greenblatt, C. S. (1983). The salience of sexuality in the early years of marriage. *Journal of Marriage & the Family, 45*, 289–99.
130. National Opinion Research Center, University of Chicago. (1990, February). Report on sexual behavior. Presented to February 1990 American Association for the Advancement of Science Meeting, New Orleans. Cited in: Petit, C. (1990, February 19). Sex survey says Americans are faithful—once a week. *SFC*, A1.
131. National Opinion Research Center, 1990.
132. Marin, P. (1983, July). A revolution's broken promises. *PT*, 50–57.
133. Byer & Shainberg, 1991.
134. Kaminer, W. (1992, November 29). Exposing the new authoritarians: Censorship under the guise of protecting women. *SFE*, D-1, D-4, D-5; exerpted from *The Atlantic* (1992, November).
135. Martin, G. (1991, August 11). The body trade. *SFC, This World*, 7–10.
136. Goldberg, L. (1991, November 10). Walking away from the wild side. *SFE*, C-5.
137. Masland, T., Nordland, R., Liu, M. et al. (1992, May 4). Slavery. *Newsweek*, 30–39.
138. Schmetzer, U. (1991, December 8). Sex slave business flourishes in Asia. *SFE*, A-1, A-12; reprinted from *Chicago Tribune*.

139. Hoigard, C., & Finstad, L. (1992). K. Hanson, N. Sipe, & B. Wilson (trans.), *Backstreets: Prostitution, money, and love*. University Park, PA: Pennylvania State University Press.
140. Anonymous. (1992, April 23). Sex for sale (editorial). *The Times* (London), 13.
141. Knopf, J., & Seiler, M. (1990). *Inhibited sexual desire*. New York: Morrow.
142. Josselson, R. (1992). *The space between us*. San Francisco: Jossey-Bass.
143. Bechtel, S. (1991, August). Burning down the house. *Men's Health*, 78–80.
144. Carnes, P. (1983). *Out of the shadows: Understanding sexual addiction*. Minneapolis: CompCare.`
145. Levin, R., & Levin, A. (1975, September). Sexual pleasure: The surprising preferences of 100,000 women. *Redbook*, 51–68.
146. Sternberg, R. J., & Soriano, L. J. (1984). Styles of conflict resolution. *Journal of Personality & Social Psychology, 47*, 115–26.
147. Weiten, Lloyd, & Lashley, 1991.
148. Weiten, Lloyd, & Lashley, 1991, 179.
149. Burns, D. D. (1989). *The feeling good handbook*. New York: Plume.
150. Burns, 1989, 371.
151. Beck, 1989.
152. Burns, 1989, 379.
153. Crooks & Baur, 1990, 268.

UNIT 9: SAFER SEX, BIRTH CONTROL, AND ABORTION

1. Anonymous. Quoted in: Adler, J., Wright, L., McCormick, J. et al. (1991, December 9). Safer sex. *Newsweek*, 52–56.
2. Workman, B. (1991, May 2). Sex at Stanford not always safe, poll finds. *SFC*, A20.
3. D.B. (1989, April). Conception misconceptions. *PT*, 10–11.
4. Fisher, J. D. Cited in: Adler et al., 1991.
5. Montefiore, S. S. (1992, October). Love, lies and fear in the plague years... *PT*, 30–35.
6. Merson, M. H., World Health Organization. Cited in: Altman, L. K. (1992, July 21). Women worldwide nearing higher rate for AIDS than men. *NYT*, B8.
7. Merson, M. H. Quoted in: Chase, M. (1992, February 13). HIV is spreading to heterosexuals at growing rate. *WSJ*, B3.
8. Ekstrand, M. L., & Coates, T. J. (1990). Maintenance of safer sexual behaviors and predictors of risky sex: The San Francisco Men's Health Study. *AJPH, 80*, 973–77.
9. Kolata, G. (1991, May 15). Drop in casual sex tied to AIDS peril. *NYT*, A12.
10. Kagay, M. R. (1991, June 18). Fear of AIDS has altered behavior, poll shows. *NYT*, B1, B8.
11. Workman, 1991.
12. Klitsch, M. (1990). Teenagers' condom use affected by peer factors, not by health concerns. *Family Planning Perspectives, 22*, 9.
13. Catania, J. A., Coates, T. J., Stall, R. et al. Prevalence of AIDS-related risk factors and condom use in the United States. *Science, 258*, 1101–06.
14. Alan Guttmacher Institute. Cited in: Barringer, F. (1993, April 1). 1 in 5 in U.S. have sexually caused viral disease. *NYT*, A1, B9.
15. Alan Guttmacher Institute. Cited in: Barringer, 1993.
16. Adler et al., 1991.
17. Montefiore, 1992.
18. Cochran, S. D., & Mays, V. M. Sex, lies, and HIV (letter). *NEJM, 322*, 774–75.
19. Cochran, S. Quoted in: Roberts, M. (1988, December). Dating, dishonesty and AIDS. *PT*, 60.
20. Katzenstein, L. (1991, January/February). When he has AIDS—and she doesn't know. *AH*, 58–62.
21. Carlsen, W. (1990, June 22). Herpes award allowed to stand. *SFC*, A4.

22. United Press International. (1991, January 13). HIV-infected man faces assault charges for sex. *SFE*, B-4.
23. Rosenfeld, S. (1992, February 2). Sex moves from the bedroom to the courtroom. *SFE*, A-1, A-10.
24. Hoffman, J. (1992, August 11). A question of law: How much must lovers tell? *NYT*, A10.
25. Katzenstein, 1991.
26. Hall, T. (1992, May 20). No sex is good sex. *SFC*, D3–D4; reprinted from *NYT*.
27. Harlap, S., Kost, K., & Forrest, D. (1991). *Preventing pregnancy, protecting health: A new look at birth control choices in the United States*. New York: Alan Guttmacher Institute.
28. Family Health International of North Carolina survey. Cited in: Royland, F. D. (1992, March 10). Condoms break up to 20 percent of the time. *SFC*, D3; reprinted from *Baltimore Sun*.
29. Centers for Disease Control. (1988). Leads from the MMWR. Condoms for prevention of sexually transmitted diseases. *JAMA, 259*, 1925–27.
30. Kost, K., Forrest, J. D., & Harlap, S. (1991). Comparing the health risks and benefits of contraceptive choices. *Family Planning Perspectives, 23*, 54–61.
31. Forrest, J. D. (1987). Has she or hasn't she? U.S. women's experience with contraception. *Family Planning Perspectives, 19*, 133.
32. Kost, Forrest, & Harlap, 1991.
33. Starr, C., & Taggart, R. (1989). *Biology: The unity and diversity of life* (5th ed.). Belmont, CA: Wadsworth.
34. Hatcher, R., Guest, F., Stewart, F. et al. (1990). *Contraceptive technology: 1990–1992* (15th ed.). New York: Irvington.
35. Byer, C. O, & Shainberg, L. W. (1991). *Dimensions of human sexuality*. Dubuque, IA: Wm. C. Brown.
36. Consumers Union. (1989, March). Can you rely on condoms? *Consumer Reports*, 135–41.
37. Hatcher et al., 1990.
38. Hatcher et al. 1990.
39. Hatcher et al., 1990.
40. Kost, Forrest, & Harlap, 1991.
41. Hatcher et al., 1990.
42. Hatcher et al., 1990.
43. Siegler, A., Hulka, J., & Peretz, A. (1985). Reversibility of female sterilization. *Fertility Sterilization, 43*, 499–510.
44. Jarow, J., Budin, R. E., Dym, M. et al.(1985). Quantitative pathologic changes in the human testis after vasectomy. *NEJM, 20*, 1252–56.
45. Hilts, P. J. (1990, December 16). Birth-control backlash. *New York Times Magazine, 41*, 55, 70–74.
46. Kaeser, L. (1990). Contraceptive development: Why the snail's pace? *Family Planning Perspectives, 22*, 131–33.
47. Leary, W. E. (1992, February 1). U.S. Panel backs approval of first condom for women. *NYT*, 7.
48. Turner, R. (1990). Vaginal ring is comparable in safety and efficacy to other low-dose, progestogen-only methods. *Family Planning Perspectives, 22*, 236–37.
49. Silvestre, L., Dubois, C., Renault, M. et al. (1990). Voluntary interruption of pregnancy with mifepristone (RU 486) and a prostaglandin analogue. *NEJM, 322*, 645–48.
50. Glasier, A., Thong, K. J., Dewar, M. et al. (1992). Mifepristone (RU 486) compared with high-dose estrogen and progestogen for emergency postcoital contraception. *NEJM, 327*, 1041–44.
51. Hilts, P. J. (1992, November 15). Sale of abortion pill soon is discounted. *NYT*, sec. 1, 14.
52. Tanouye, E. (1992, July 20). Abortion-rights forces plan to pursue return of pills despite justices' ruling. *WSJ*, B4.
53. World Health Organization. Cited in: Prendergast, A. (1990, October). Beyond the pill. *AH*, 37–44.

54. Gregg, S. R. (1981, February 16). Tailoring contraceptives to patients. *Medical World News*, 47–61.

55. Turner, R. (1991). Weekly testosterone injections suppress sperm production, may provide effective contraception. *Family Planning Perspectives*, *23*, 86–87.

56. National Center for Health Statistics. (1989, September 26). Advanced report of final mortality statistics, 1987. *Monthly Vital Statistics Report*, vol. 38, no. 5, sppl. DHHS Pub. No. (PHS)89-1120. Washington, DC: U.S. Department of Health and Human Services.

57. Kolata, G. (1992, January 5). In late abortions, decisions are painful and options few. *NYT*, sec. 1, 1, 12.

58. Lasker, J., & Borg, S. (1990). *When pregnancy fails: Families coping with miscarriage, ectopic pregnancy, stillbirth, and infant death* (2nd ed.). New York: Bantam.

59. Adler, N. E., David, H. P., Major, B. N. et al. (1990). Psychological responses after abortion. *Science*, *248*, 41–44.

60. Lunneborg, P. (1992). *Abortion: A positive decision*. South Hadley, MA: Bergin & Garvey.

61. Dagg, P. K. (1991). The psychological sequelae of therapeutic abortion—denied and completed. *American Journal of Psychiatry*, *148*(5), 578–85.

62. Rosenblatt, R. (1992). *Life itself: Abortion in the American mind*. New York: Random House.

63. Vail-Smith, K., Durham, T. W., & Howard, H. A. (1992). A scale to measure embarrassment associated with condom use. *Journal of Health Education*, *23*, 209–14.

64. Alberti, R. E., & Emmons, M. L. (1970). *Your perfect right: A guide to assertive behavior*. San Luis Obispo, CA: Impact.

65. Alberti, R. E., & Emmons, M. L. (1975). *Stand up, speak out, talk back!* New York: Pocket.

66. Jakubowski-Spector, P. (1973). Facilitating the growth of women through assertive training. *Counseling Psychologist*, *4*, 75–86.

67. Weiten, W., Lloyd, M. A., & Lashley, R. L. (1991). *Psychology applied to modern life: Adjustment in the 90s* (3rd ed.). Pacific Grove, CA: Brooks/Cole.

68. Horner, M. J. (1972). Toward an understanding of achievement related conflicts in women. *Journal of Social Issues*, *28*, 157–76.

69. Freundl, P. C. (1981, August). Influence of sex and status variables on perceptions of assertiveness. Paper presented at meeting of the American Psychological Association, Los Angeles.

70. Smye, M. D., & Wine, J. D. (1980). A comparison of female and male adolescents' social behaviors and cognitions: A challenge to the assertiveness literature. *Sex Roles*, *6*, 213–30.

71. Castleman, M. (1989, September/October). What should you do? How to request safe sex. *Medical Selfcare*, 11–12.

72. Weiten, Lloyd, & Lashley, 1991.

73. Bower, S. A., & Bower, G. H. (1976). *Asserting yourself: A practical guide for positive change*. Reading, MA: Addison-Wesley, 222–23.

74. Zimbardo, P. G. (1977). *Shyness: What it is, what to do about it*. Reading, MA: Addison-Wesley, 185.

UNIT 10: FAMILY MATTERS

1. Galinsky, E. (1981). *Between generations: The six stages of parenthood*. New York: Berkley.

2. Alpert, J. L., & Richardson, M. S. (1980). Parenting. In L. W. Poon (Ed.), *Aging in the 1980s*. Washington, DC: American Psychological Association.

3. Guttmann, D. (1987). *Reclaimed powers*. New York: Basic.

4. Vaillant, G. E. (1977). *Adaptation to life*. Boston: Little, Brown.

5. Schwartz, J. (1992, February). Healthy families make smarter children. *American Demographics*, 13–14.

6. National Commission to Prevent Infant Mortality. Cited in: Associated Press. (1992, March 29). Panel says nation is lagging in children's health. *NYT*, sec. 1, 16.

7. Keith, L. G., Papiernik, E., & Luke, B. (1991). The costs of multiple pregnancy. *International Journal of Gynaecology & Obstetrics*, *36*, 109–14.

8. Luke, B., Witter, F. R., Abbey, H. et al. (1991). Gestational age-specific birthweights of twins versus singletons. *Acta Geneticae Medicae Et Gemollologiae*, *40*, 69–76.

9. Hack, M., & Fanaroff, A. A. (1989). Outcomes of extremely-low-birth-weight infants between 1982 and 1988. *NEJM*, *321*, 1642–47.

10. Fuchs, V. R., & Reklis, D. M. (1992). America's children: Economic perspectives and policy options. *Science*, *255*, 41–45.

11. Centers for Disease Control. (1990). Fatal injuries to children—United States, 1986. *JAMA*, *264*, 952–53.

12. Short, K. (1992, May). Health insurance coverage: 1987–1990. *Current Population Reports*, Series P-70, No. 29. Washington, DC: U.S. Department of Commerce, Bureau of the Census.

13. U.S. Public Health Service. (1990). *Healthy people 2000: National health promotion and disease prevention objectives*. DHHS Pub. No. (PHS)91-50212. Washington, DC: U.S. Government Printing Office.

14. Fuchs & Reklis, 1992.

15. Lewis, P. (1990, October 1). World leaders endorse U.N. plan to improve the lives of children. *NYT*, A1, A11.

16. Anonymous. (1990, October 1). Excerpts from the United Nations declaration on children. *NYT*, A10.

17. Anonymous. (1990, September 29). U.N. summit: The plight of the world's children. *NYT*, 6.

18. McGrew, M. C., & Shore, W. B. (1991). The problem of teenage pregnancy. *Journal of Family Practice*, *32*, 17–25.

19. Passell, P. (1991, September). When children have children. *NYT*, C2.

20. McGrew & Shore, 1991.

21. Furstenberg, F., Brooks-Gunn, J., & Morgan, S. (1987). Adolescent mothers and their children in later life. *Family Planning Perspectives*, *19*, 142–51.

22. Furstenberg, F. F. Jr., Levine, J. A., & Brooks-Gunn, J. (1990). The children of teenage mothers: Patterns of early childbearing in two generations. *Family Planning Perspectives*, *22*, 54–61.

23. McNeil, J., U.S. Census Bureau. Cited in: McLeod, R. M. (1992, February 20). New federal study says middle class is shrinking. *SFC*, A2.

24. Population Reference Bureau. (1992, August). *New realities of the American family*. Cited in: Anonymous. (1992, August 31). Family matters. *Newsweek*, 6.

25. National Center for Health Statistics (1992). Family structure and children's health: United States, 1988. *Vital & Health Statistics*, Series 10, No. 178. Hyattsville, MD: National Center for Health Statistics.

26. Bachu, A. (1991, October). Fertility of American women: June 1990. *Current Population Reports*, Series P-20, No. 454. Washington, DC: U.S. Department of Commerce, Bureau of the Census.

27. Bumpass, L. L. Cited in: Pear, B. (1991, December 4). Bigger number of new mothers are unmarried. *NYT*, All.

28. Berger, K. S. (1988). *The developing person through the life span* (2nd ed.). New York: Worth.

29. Weitzman, L. J. (1985). *The divorce revolution: The unexpected social and economic consequences for women and children in America*. New York: Free Press.

30. Shellenbarger, S. (1992, January 20). Child-support rules shake parents, firms. *WSJ*, B1.

31. Furstenberg, F. F. Jr., & Nord, C. W. (1985). Parenting apart: Patterns of childbearing after marital disruption. *Journal of Marriage & the Family*, *47*, 893–912.

32. Furstenberg, F. F. Jr., Nord, C. W., Peterson, J. L. et al. (1983). The life course of children of divorce: Marital disruption and parental contact. *American Sociology Review*, *48*, 656.

33. Anonymous. (1988). Recent U.S. fertility patterns continue: Birthrates climb among older women, childlessness rises. *Family Planning Perspectives*, *20*, 44–45.

34. Berkowitz, G. S., Skovron, M. L., Lapinski, R. H. et al. (1990). Delayed childbearing and the outcome of pregnancy. *NEJM*, *322*, 659–64.

35. Hardie, A., Cox News Service. (1991, September 2). Aging boomers having babies. *SFC*, D1, D5.

36. Shellenbarger, S. (1992, May 27). Family issues hit home with single fathers. *WSJ*, B1.

37. Harris, S. (1991, October 27). More gays, lesbians are raising families. *Oakland Tribune*, C-4.

38. Newberger, C. M., Melnicoe, L. H., & Newberger, E. H. (1986). The American family in crisis: Implications for children. In J. D. Lockhart (Ed.), *Current Problems in Pediatrics*. Chicago: Year Book Medical, 1986, 674–721.

39. Newberger, Melnicoe, & Newberger, 1986.

40. Springer, I. (1991, June). Only a mother. *AH*, 83.

41. Bauerlein, M. (1991, September/October). Why doesn't the U.S. have a family policy? *Utne Reader*, 17–19.

42. Trost, C. (1990, March 15). Workers should get 1-year parental leaves, panel says. *WSJ*, B1, B6.

43. Hughes, K. A. (1991, February 6). Pregnant professionals face subtle bias at work as attitudes toward them shift. *WSJ*, B1, B6.

44. Hughes, K. A. (1991, February 6). Mothers-to-be sue, charging discrimination. *WSJ*, B1, B6.

45. Bernstein, A. (1992, August 10). The mommy backlash. *Business Week*, 42–43.

46. Wadman, M. K. (1992, July 16). Mothers who take extended time off find their careers pay a heavy price. *WSJ*, B1, B8.

47. Brott, A. A. (1992, September 20). Paternity leave given a wide berth. *SFE*, A-6.

48. Shellenbarger, 1992.

49. O'Connell, M., & Bachu, A. (1990, July). Who's minding the kids? *Current Population Reports*, Series P-70, No. 20. Washington, DC: U.S. Department of Commerce, Bureau of the Census.

50. Dawson, D. A., & Cain, V. S. (1990, October 1). Child care arrangements: Health of our nation's children, United States, 1988. *Advance Data from Vital and Health Statistics of the National Center for Health Statistics*, No. 187. Washington, DC: U.S. Department of Health and Human Services.

51. Shellenbarger, S. S. (1992, January 7). Parents' heavy burden of child-care costs. *WSJ*, B1.

52. Kraizer, S., Witte, S., Fryer, G. E. Jr., et al. (1990). Children in self-care: A new perspective. *Child Welfare*, *49*(6), 571–81.

53. Labich, K. (1991, May 20). Can your career hurt your kids? *Fortune*, 38–56.

54. Miller, A. B. (1990). *The daycare dilemma: Critical concerns for American families*. New York: Plenum.

55. Desai, S., Chase-Lansdale, P. L., & Michael, R. T. (1989). Mother or market? Effects of maternal employment on the intellectual ability of 4-year-old children. *Demography*, *26*, 545–61.

56. Schellhardt, T. P. (1990, September 19). It still isn't dad at home with sick kids. *WSJ*, B1.

57. Recer, P. (1992, November 22). Executive moms more content than careerists. *SFE*, A-10.

[Report of E. Roskies presented at November 21, 1992, conference on workplace stress cosponsored by National Institute for Occupational Safety and Health and the American Psychological Association, Washington, D.C.]

58. Bernstein, A. (1991, August 5). Do more babies mean fewer working women? *Business Week*, 49–50.

59. Gallup, G. H. Jr., & Newport, F. (1990, June 4). Parenthood—a (nearly) universal desire. *SFC*, B3–B4.

60. Exter, T. (1991, August). The costs of growing up. *American Demographics*, 59.

61. Gallup & Newport, 1990.

62. Ambry, M. K. (1992, April). Childless chances. *American Demographics*, 55.

63. Belsky, J. Cited in: Dunatov, A.-M. (1992, June). Childless by choice. *AH*, 87.

64. Ireland, M. Quoted in: Dunatov, 1992.

65. Dunatov, 1992.

66. Ireland, M. Quoted in: Dunatov, 1992.

67. Guttmacher, A. F. (1983). *Pregnancy, birth, and family planning* (rev. ed.). New York: New American Library.

68. McCary, S. P., & McCary, J. L. (1984). *Human sexuality* (3rd ed.). Belmont, CA: Wadsworth.

69. Crooks, R., & Baur, K. (1990). *Our sexuality* (4th ed.). Redwood City, CA: Benjamin/Cummings.

70. Marchbanks, P. A., Peterson, H. B., Rubin, G. L. et al. (1989). Research on infertility: Definition makes a difference. The Cancer and Steroid Hormone Study Group. *American Journal of Epidemiology*, 130, 259–67.

71. Rice, F. P. (1989). *Human sexuality*. Dubuque, IA: Wm. C. Brown.

72. Rice, 1989.

73. Rice, 1989.

74. Bates, G. W., & Boone, W. R. (1991). The female reproductive cycle: New variations on an old theme. *Current Opinion in Obstetrics & Gynecology*, 3, 838–43.

75. Elmer-Dewitt, P. (1991, September 30). Making babies. *Time*, 56–63.

76. Carey, B. (1991, July/August). Sperm, Inc. *In Health*, 51–56.

77. Gaines, J. (1990, October 7). A scandal of artificial insemination. *New York Times Magazine, The Good Health Magazine*, 23, 28–29.

78. Luke, B., Witter, F. R., Abbey, H. et al. (1991). Gestational age-specific birthweights of twins versus singletons. *Acta Geneticae Medicae Et Gemellologiae*, 40, 69–76.

79. Luke, B., & Keith, L. G. (1992). The contribution of singletons, twins and triplets to low birth weight, infant mortality and handicap in the United States. *Journal of Reproductive Medicine*, 37, 661–62.

80. Ames, K., Denworth, L., Wright, L. et al. (1991, September 30). And donor makes three. *Newsweek*, 60–61.

81. Sauer, M. V., Paulson, R. J., & Lobo, R. A. (1990). A preliminary report on oocyte donation extending reproductive potential to women over 40. *NEJM*, 323, 1157–60.

82. Sauer, M. V., Paulson, R. J., & Lobo, R. A. (1992). Clinical trial of oocyte donation in women of advanced reproductive age. *JAMA*, 268, 1275–79.

83. Quigley, M. M. (1992). The new frontier of the reproductive age (editorial). *JAMA*, 268, 1320–21.

84. Bachrach, C. A., Stolley, K. S., & London, K. A. (1992). Relinquishment of premarital births: Evidence from national survey data. *Family Planning Perspectives*, 24, 27–32.

85. Gubernick, L. (1991, October 14). How much is that baby in the window? *Forbes*, 90–98.

86. McManus, I. C. (1991). The inheritance of left-handedness. *Ciba Foundation Symposium*, 162, 251–67.

87. Coren, S. (1992). *The left-hander syndrome: The causes and consequences of left-handedness*. New York: Free Press.

88. Associated Press. (1993, February 16). Threats to left-handed invisible in new study. *NYT*, B6.

89. Hepper, P. G., Shahidullah, S., & White, R. (1991). Handedness in the human fetus. *Neuropsychologia*, 29, 1107–11.

90. Coren, 1992.

91. National Foundation for the March of Dimes. (1977). Birth defects: Tragedy and hope.

92. Anonymous. (1990, July). The telltale gene. *Consumer Reports*, 483–88.

93. Rivers, R., & Williamson, N. (1990). Sickle cell anemia: Complex disease, nursing challenge. *RN*, 53, 24–27.

94. Barrett, J. M., Abramoff, P., Kumaran, A. K. et al. (1986). *Biology*. Englewood Cliffs, NJ: Prentice-Hall.

95. Schmeck, H. M. Jr. (1990, April 29). Battling the legacy of illness. *New York Times Magazine, The Good Health Magazine*, 36-37, 46-50.

96. National Center for Health Statistics. Cited in: Anonymous. (1990, December). Older mothers: chromosome defects. *AH*, 11.

97. Handyside, A. H., Kontogianni, E. H., Hardy, K. et al. (1990). Pregnancies from biopsied human preimplantation embryos sexed by Y-specific DNA amplication. *Nature*, 344, 768–70.

98. Gargan, E. A. (1991, December 13). Ultrasonic tests skew ratio of births in India. *NYT*, A12.

99. Schmeck, 1990.

100. Bishop, J. E. (1990, February 1). New cystic-fibrosis test for carriers raises moral issue. *WSJ*, B1.

101. Bishop, J. E., & Waldholz, M. (1990, September). Misfortune telling. *AH*, 64–71.

102. Angier, N. (1989, March). The gene dream. *AH*, 103–08.

103. Schmeck, 1990.

104. Carey, J., Hamilton, J. O'C., Jereski, L. et al. (1990, May 28). The genetic age. *Business Week*, 68–83.

105. Hubbard, R. C., McElvaney, N. G., Birrer, P. et al. (1992). A preliminary study of acrosolized recombinant human deoxyribonuclease I in the treatment of cystic fibrosis. *NEJM*, 326, 812–15.

106. Drumm, M. L., Pope, H. A., Cliff, W. H. et al. (1990). Correction of the cystic fibrosis defect in vitro by retrovirus-mediated gene transfer. *Cell*, 62, 1227–33.

107. Ahlborg, G. Jr., & Bodin, L. (1991). Tobacco smoke exposure and pregnancy outcome among working women: A prospective study at prenatal care centers in Orebro County, Sweden. *American Journal of Epidemiology*, 133, 338–47.

108. Williams, M. A., Lieberman, E., Mittendorf, R. et al. (1991). Risk factors for abruptio placentae. *American Journal of Epidemiology*, 134, 965–72.

109. Savitz, D. A., Whelan, E. A., & Kleckner, R. C. (1989). Self-reported exposure to pesticides and radiation related to pregnancy outcome—results from National Natality and Fetal Mortality Surveys. *Public Health Reports*, 104, 473–77.

110. Kulhanjian, J. A., Soroush, V., Au, D. S. et al. (1992). Identification of women at unsuspected risk of primary infection with herpes simplex virus type 2 during pregnancy. *NEJM*, 326, 916–20.

111. Althaus, F. (1990). Folic acid supplementation during early pregnancy appears to lessen risk of neural tube defects. *Family Planning Perspectives*, 22, 140–41.

112. Tamura, R., Goldenberg, R. L., Freeberg, L. E. et al. (1992). Maternal serum folate and zinc concentrations and their relationships to pregnancy outcome. *American Journal of Clinical Nutrition*, 56, 365–70.

113. Carlsen, E., Giwercman, A., Keiding, N. et al. (1992). Evidence for decreasing quality of semen during past 50 years. *British Medical Journal*, 305, 609–13.

114. Fraga, C. G., Motchnik, P. A., Shigenaga, M. K. et al. (1991). Ascorbic acid protects against endogenous oxidative DNA damage in human sperm. *Proceedings of the National Academy of Sciences of the United States of America*, 88, 11003–6.

115. Emanuele, M. A., Tentler, J., Emanuele, N. V. et al. (1991). In vivo effects of acute EtOH on rat alpha and beta luteinizing hormone gene expression. *Alcohol*, 8, 345–48.

116. Brody, J. E. (1991, December 25). Possible links are being explored between babies' health and fathers' habits and working conditions. *NYT*, 15.

117. Zhang, J., Cai, W. W., & Lee, D. J. (1992). Occupational hazards and pregnancy outcomes. *American Journal of Industrial Medicine*, 21, 397–408.

118. Blakeslee, S. (1991, April). Father figures: The male link to birth defects. *AH*, 55–57.

119. Waldrop, J. (1991, September). The birthday boost. *American Demographics*, 4.

120. Rogers, J. L. Cited in Waldrop, 1991.

121. Roenneberg, T., & Aschoff, J. (1990). Annual rhythm of human reproduction: Environmental correlations. *Journal of Biological Rhythms*, 5, 217–39.

122. Mediamark Research. Cited in Waldrop, 1991.

123. Leifer, M. (1980). *Psychological effects of motherhood: A study of first pregnancy*. New York: Praeger.

124. McCary, J. L., & McCary, S. P. (1982). *McCary's human sexuality* (4th ed.). Belmont, CA: Wadsworth.

125. Carpenter, M. (1979). Physicians ponder popularity of pregnancy self-test kits. *Medical News*, 14, 18.

126. Rice, 1989.

127. Guttmacher, 1983.

128. Guttmacher, 1983.

129. Westbrook, M. T. (1978). The effects of the order of a birth on women's experience of childbearing. *Journal of Marriage & the Family*, 40, 165–72.

130. Meyerowitz, J. H. (1970). Satisfaction during pregnancy. *Journal of Marriage & the Family*, 32, 38–42.

131. Leifer, 1980.

132. Antle, K. (1978). Active involvement of expectant fathers in pregnancy: Some further considerations. *Journal of Obstetric, Gynecologic, & Neonatal Nursing*, 7, 7–12.

133. Lipkin, M. J., & Lamb, G. S. (1982). The couvade syndrome: An epidemiologic study. *AIM*, 96, 509–11.

134. Conner, G. K., & Denson, V. (1990). Expectant fathers' response to pregnancy: Review of literature and implications for research in high-risk pregnancy. *Journal of Perinatal & Neonatal Nursing*, 4, 33–42.

135. Longobucco, D. C., & Freston, M. S. (1989). Relation of somatic symptoms to degree of paternal-role preparation of first-time expectant fathers. *Journal of Obstetric, Gynecologic, & Neonatal Nursing*, 18, 482–88.

136. Jackson, B. (1984). *Fatherhood*. London: George Allen and Unwin.

137. Gelles, R. J. (1975). Violence and pregnancy: A note on the extent of the problem and needed services. *Family Coordinator*, 24, 81–86.

138. Kitzinger, S. (1983). *The complete book of pregnancy and childbirth*. New York: Knopf.

139. May, K. A. (1982). Factors contributing to first-time father's readiness for fatherhood: An exploratory study. *Family Relations*, 31, 353–61.

140. Kotre, J., & Hall, E. (1990). *Seasons of life:*

Our dramatic journey from birth to death. Boston: Little, Brown, 4.

141. National Center for Health Statistics. (1990). *Health, United States, 1989, and prevention profile.* DHHS Pub. No. (PHS)90-1232. Hyattsville, MD: U.S. Department of Health and Human Services.

142. U.S. Public Health Service. (1990). *Healthy people 2000: National health promotion and disease prevention objectives.* DHHS Pub. No. (PHS)91-50212. Washington, DC: U.S. Government Printing Office.

143. Scott, J. (1990, December 31). Low birth weight's high cost. *LAT*, A1, A20.

144. Franks, A. L., Kendrick, J. S., Olson, D. R. et al. (1992). Hospitalization for pregnancy complications, United States, 1986 and 1987. *American Journal of Obstetrics & Gynecology, 166*, 1339–44.

145. Guttmacher, 1983.

146. Repke, J. T., Villar, J., Anderson, C. et al. (1989). Biochemical changes associated with blood pressure reduction induced by calcium supplementation during pregnancy. *American Journal of Obstetrics & Gynecology, 160*, 684–90.

147. King, J. C. (1991). New National Academy of Sciences guidelines for nutrition during pregnancy. *Diabetes, 40*(suppl. 2), 151.

148. Scholl, T. O., Hediger, M. L., Khoo, C. S. et al. (1991). Maternal weight gain, diet and infant birth weight: Correlations during adolescent pregnancy. *Journal of Clinical Epidemiology, 44*, 423–28.

149. Hall, D. Quoted in: Longstreet, D. (1992, June). Expecting the best. *AH*, 89.

150. American Health Magazine. (1991, July 29). Pregnancy stress may affect birth weights. *SFC*, D3. [Report of study by Marci Lobel et al. at UCLA Medical Center.]

151. Klebanoff, M. A., Shiono, P. H., & Rhoads, G. G. (1990). Outcomes of pregnancy in a national sample of resident physicians. *NEJM, 323*, 1040–45.

152. Milunsky, A., Ulcickas, M., Rothman, K. J. (1992). Maternal heat exposure and neural tube defects. *JAMA, 268*, 882–85.

153. Imperiale, T. F., & Petrulis, A. S. (1991). A meta-analysis of low-dose aspirin for the prevention of pregnancy-induced hypertensive disease. *JAMA, 266*, 260–64.

154. Caan, B. J., & Goldhaber, M. K. (1989). Caffeinated beverages and low birthweight: A case-control study. *AJPH, 79*(9), 1299–1300.

155. Fenster, L., Eskenazi, R., Windham, G. C. et al. (1991). Caffein consumption during pregnancy and fetal growth. *AJPH, 81*(4), 458–61.

156. Anonymous. (1989). One in five pregnant women are smokers, new U.S. study shows. *Family Planning Perspectives, 21*, 141.

157. Mason, J. O., Tolsma, D. D., Peterson, H. B. et al. (1988). Health promotion for women: Reduction of smoking in primary care settings. *Clinical Obstetrics & Gynecology, 31*, 989–1002.

158. Moore, K. (1989). *Before we are born* (3rd ed.). Philadelphia: Saunders.

159. McLaren, N., & Nieburg, P. (1988, August). Fetal tobacco syndrome and other problems caused by smoking during pregnancy. *Medical Aspects of Human Sexuality*, 69–75.

160. Niebyl, J. (1988, September). Smoking presents many risks to mother and fetus. *Medical Aspects of Human Sexuality*, 10–24.

161. Coleman, S., Piotrow, P. T., & Rinehart, W. (1979, March). Tobacco: Hazard to health and human reproduction. *Population Reports*, Series L (1).

162. Mason, J. O., Tolsma, D. D., Peterson, H. B. et al. (1988). Health promotion for women: Reduction of smoking in primary care settings. *Clinical Obstetrics & Gynecology, 31*, 989–1002.

163. Ray, O., & Ksir, C. (1990). *Drugs, society, and human behavior* (5th ed.). St. Louis: Times Mirror/Mosby.

164. Weitzman, M., Gortmaker, S., Walker, D. K. et al. (1990). Maternal smoking and childhood asthma. *Pediatrics, 85*, 505–11.

165. Carroll, C. R. (1989). *Drugs in modern society.* Dubuque, IA: Wm. C. Brown.

166. Carroll, 1989.

167. Streissguth, A. P., & LaDue, R. A. (1987). Fetal alcohol: Teratogenic causes of developmental disabilities. *Monographs of the American Association on Mental Deficiency, 8*, 1–32.

168. Streissguth, A. P., Aase, J. M., Clarren, S. K. et al. (1991). Fetal alcohol syndrome in adolescents and adults. *JAMA, 265*, 1961–67.

169. Streissguth, A. P., Barr, H. M., & Martin, D. C. (1983). Maternal alcohol use and neonatal habituation assessed with the Brazelton scale. *Child Development, 54*, 1109–18.

170. Mukherjee, A. B., & Hodgen, G. D. (1982). Maternal ethanol exposure induces transient impairment of umbilical circulation and fetal hypoxia in monkeys. *Science, 218*, 700–702.

171. Weiner, N. (1992, March 22). Unfair warning? *SFC, This World*, 7, 11.

172. Ostrea, E. M. Jr., & Chavez, C. J. (1979). Perinatal problems (excluding neonatal withdrawal) in maternal drug addiction: A study of 830 cases. *Journal of Pediatrics, 94*, 292–95.

173. Scher, J., & Dix, C. (1983). *Will my baby be normal? Everything you need to know about pregnancy.* New York: Dial Press.

174. Fried, P. A., Watkinson, B., Grant, A. et al. (1980). Changing patterns of soft drug use prior to and during pregnancy: A prospective study. *Drug & Alcohol Dependency, 6*, 323.

175. Hingson, R., Alpert, J., Day, N. et al. (1982). Effects of maternal drinking and marijuana use on fetal growth and development. *Pediatrics, 70*, 539–46.

176. Coles, C. D., Platzman, K. A., Smith, I. et al. (1992). Effects of cocaine and alcohol use in pregnancy on neonatal growth and neurobehavioral status. *Neurotoxicology & Teratology, 14*, 22–33.

177. Janke, J. R. (1990). Prenatal cocaine use: Effects on perinatal outcome. *Journal of Nurse-Midwifery, 35*, 74–77.

178. Mayes, L. C., Granger, R. H., Bornstein, M. H., & Zuckerman, B. (1992). The problem of prenatal cocaine exposure. *JAMA, 267*, 406–408.

179. Gupta, C., Yaffe, S. J., & Shaprio, B. H. (1982). Prenatal exposure to phenobarbital permanently decreases testosterone and causes reproductive dysfunction. *Science, 216*, 640–42.

180. O'Brien, T. E., & McManus, C. E. (1978). Drugs and the fetus: A consumer's guide by generic and brand name. *Birth & the Family Journal, 5*, 58–86.

181. Brent, R. L. (1986). The complexities of solving the problem of human malformations. In J. L. Sever & R. L. Brent (Eds.), *Teratogen update: Environmentally induced birth defect risks.* New York: Liss.

182. Stewart, A., & Kneale, G. W. (1970). Radiation dose effects in relation to obstetric X-rays and childhood cancers. *Lancet, 1*, 1495.

183. Jacobson, J. L., Jacobson, S. W., Fein, G. G. et al. (1984). Prenatal exposure to an environmental toxin: A test of multiple effects. *Developmental Psychology, 20* 523–32.

184. Raloff, J. (1986). Even low levels in mom affect baby. *Science News, 130*, 164.

185. U.S. Public Health Service. (1990). *Healthy people 2000: National health promotion and disease prevention objectives.* DHHS Pub. No. (PHS)91-50212. Washington, DC: U.S. Government Printing Office.

186. Public Health Service, 1990.

187. Wallenbrock, M. A., Sekar, K. C., & Toubas, P. L. (1992). Prediction of the acute response to surfactant therapy by pulmonary function testing. *Pediatric Pulmonology, 13*, 11–15.

188. Pritchard, J., MacDonald, D., & Gant, N. (1985). *Williams Obstetrics* (17th ed.). New York: Appleton-Century-Crofts.

189. Beck, M. (1988, August 15). Miscarriages. *Newsweek*, 46–52.

190. Guttmacher, 1983.

191. Neugebauer, R., Kline, J., O'Connor, P. et al. (1992). Determinants of depressive symptoms in the early weeks after miscarriage. *AJPH, 82*, 1332–39.

192. Moore, K. (1989). *Before we are born* (3rd ed.). Philadelphia: Saunders.

193. Centers for Disease Control. (1988, October 21). Ectopic pregnancy—United States, 1984 and 1985. *MMWR*, 666–69.

194. Coste, J., Job-Spira, N., & Fernandez, H. (1991). Increased risk of ectopic pregnancy with maternal cigarette smoking. *AJPH, 81*, 199–201.

195. Pritchard, MacDonald, & Gant, 1985.

196. Larsen, J. W. (1986). Congenital toxoplasmosis. In J. L. Sever & R. L. Brent (Eds.), *Teratogen update: Environmentally induced birth defect risks.* New York: Liss.

197. Byer, C. O., & Shainberg, L. W. (1991). *Dimensions of human sexuality* (3rd ed.). Dubuque, IA: Wm. C. Brown.

198. Grossman, J. H. (1986). Congenital syphilis. In J. L. Sever & R. L. Brent (Eds.), *Teratogen update: Environmentally induced birth defect risks.* New York: Liss.

199. Berger, K. S. 1988). *The developing person through the life span* (2nd ed.). New York: Worth.

200. Greenwood, S. (1989, March/April). Prenatal testing update. *Medical Selfcare*, 19–20.

201. Haddow, J. E., Palomaki, G. E., Knight, G. J. et al. Prenatal screening for Down's syndrome with use of maternal serum markers. *NEJM, 327*, 588–93.

202. Anonymous. (1992, August 19). A simpler screening for Down risks. *NYT*, B6. [Report of study led by N. J. Wald.]

203. Kolata, G. (1992, July 15). As fears about a fetal test grow, many doctors are advising against it. *NYT*, B7.

204. Remez, L. (1989). Chorionic villus sampling is useful alternative to amniocentesis, despite slightly higher risk. *Family Planning Perspective, 21*, 188–89.

205. Jackson, L. G., Zachary, J. M., Fowler, S. E. (1992). A randomized comparison of transcervical and transabdomianl chorionic-villus sampling. The U.S. National Institute of Child Health and Human Development Chorionic-Villus Sampling and Amniocentesis Study Group. *NEJM, 327*, 594–98.

206. Kotre & Hall, 1990, 18.

207. Bean, C. (1974). *Methods of childbirth.* New York: Dolphin.

208. Brazelton, T. B. (1991, March 26). What newborns really look like. *SFC*, B5.

209. Kennell, J., Klaus, M., McGrath, S. et al. (1991). Continuous emotional support during labor in a US hospital: A randomized controlled trial. *JAMA, 265*, 2197–2201.

210. Health Insurance Association of America. Cited in: Weinhouse, B., & Burgower, B. (1990, August 30). Answers to questions about birth styles. *SFC*, B3, B5.

211. Crooks & Bauer, 1990.

212. Rosenblatt, R. A., Bovbjerg, R. R., Whelan, A. et al. (1991). Tort reform and the obstetric access crisis: The case of the WAMI states. *Western Journal of Medicine, 154*, 693–99.

213. Declercq, E. R. (1992). The transformation of American midwifery: 1975 to 1988. *AJPH, 82*, 680–84.

214. Kay, B. J., Butter, I. H., Chang, D. et al. (1988). Women's health and social change: The case of lay midwives. *International Journal of Health Services, 18*, 223–36.

215. Kennell et al., 1991.

216. Kennell, J. Quoted in: Winslow, R. (1991, May 1). Third World birthing practice is safer, less costly than U.S. way, study finds. *WSJ*, B9.

217. Otis, C.H. (1990, November/December). Midwives still hassled by medical establishment. *Utne Reader*, 32, 34.

218. Fahey, V. (1992, June). Shopping for a midwife. *Health*, 58.

219. Armstrong, P., & Feldman, S. (1989, January/February). Midwives: Tapping every woman's strength. *AH*, 75–80.

220. U.S. Bureau of the Census. (1991). *Statistical Abstract of the United States* (111th ed.). Washington, DC: U.S. Government Printing Office.

221. Lieberman, E., & Ryan, K. H. (1989). Birthday choices. *NEJM*, 321, 1824–25.

222. Belkin, L. (1992, March 25). Births beyond hospitals fill an urban need. *NYT*, A1, A17.

223. Duran, A. M. (1992). The safety of home birth: The farm study. *AJPH*, 82, 450–53.

224. Albers, L. L., & Katz, V. L. (1991). Birth setting for low-risk pregnancies: An analysis of the current literature. *Journal of Nurse-Midwifery*, 36, 215–20.

225. Tyson, H. (1991). Outcomes of 1001 midwife-attended home births in Toronto, 1983–1988. *Birth*, 18, 14–19.

226. Thorp, J. M. Jr., & Bowes, W. A. Jr. (1989). Episiotomy: Can its routine use be defended? *American Journal of Obstetrics & Gynecology*, 160, 1027–30.

227. Bromberg, M. H. (1986). Presumptive maternal benefits of routine episiotomy: A literature review. *Journal of Nurse-Midwifery*, 31, 121–27.

228. Larsson, P. B., Platz-Christensen, J. J., Bergman, B. et al. (1991). Advantage or disadvantage of episiotomy compared with spontaneous perineal laceration. *Gynecologic & Obstetric Investigation*, 31, 213–16.

229. Wilson, R. J., Bacham, C. T., & Carrington, E. R. (1975). *Obstetrics and Gynecology*. St. Louis: Mosby.

230. Whipple, B., Josimovich, J. B., & Komisaruk, B. R. (1990). Sensory thresholds during the antepartum, intrapartum, and postpartum periods. *International Journal of Nursing Studies*, 27, 213–21.

231. Leventhal, E. A., Leventhal, H., Shacham, S. et al. (1989). Active coping reduces reports of pain from childbirth. *Journal of Consulting & Clinical Psychology*, 57, 365–71.

232. Felton, G., & Segelman, F. (1978). Lamaze childbirth training and changes in belief about personal control. *Birth and Family Journal*, 5, 141–50.

233. Lamaze, F. (1970). *Painless childbirth*. Chicago: Regency.

234. Leboyer, F. (1975). *Birth without violence*. New York: Alfred Knopf.

235. Mosedale, L. (1991, April). Fathers in the delivery room. *Self*, 104, 106–108.

236. Block, C. R., Norr, K. L., Meyering, S. et al. (1981). Husband gatekeeping in childbirth. *Family Relations*, 30, 197–204.

237. Szeverenyi, P., Hetey Ane, H., Munnich, A. et al. (1989). Anxiety and the presence of the father at childbirth. *Orvosi Hetilap*, 130, 783–88.

238. Miller, B. C., & Bowen, S. L. (1982). Father-to-newborn attachment behavior in relation to prenatal classes and presence at delivery. *Family Relations*, 31, 71–78.

239. Nortzon, F. C., Placek, P. J., & Taffel, S. M. (1987). Comparisons of national cesarean-section rates. *NEJM*, 316, 386–89.

240. Winslow, R. (1990, January 2). C-sections tied to economic factors in study. *WSJ*, B4.

241. Anonymous. (1992, May 13). Caesareans decline, but rate is called too high. *NYT*, C12.

242. Anonymous. (1991, February). Too many cesareans. *Consumer Reports*, 120–26.

243. Stafford, R. S. (1991). The impact of non-clinical factors on repeat cesarean section. *JAMA*, 265, 59–63.

244. Joseph, G. F. Jr., Stedman, C. M., & Robichaux, A. G. (1991). Vaginal birth after cesarean section: The impact of patient resistance to a trial of labor. *American Journal of Obstetrics & Gynecology*, 164, 1441–44.

245. Stichler, J. P., & Alfonso, D. D. (1980). Cesarean birth. *American Journal of Nursing*, 80, 466–68.

246. Anonymous. (1991, February). The effects on mother and child. *Consumer Reports*, 122.

247. Klaus, M., & Kennel, J. (1982). *Parent-infant bonding* (2nd ed.). St. Louis: Mosby.

248. Salk, L. (1974). *Preparing for parenthood*. New York: Bantam.

249. Harlow, H. F., & Suomi, S. J. (1970). Nature of love—simplified. *American Psychologist*, 25, 161–68.

250. Brody, J. E. (1991, December 11). Caring for a baby's delicate skin, even with products made for newborns, can be tricky. *NYT*, B9. 251. Bartlett, K., Associated Press. (1990, March 11). Changes seen in diaper industry. *Las Vegas Review-Journal*, 1F.

252. Meier, B. (1990, December 22). To save infants, labels warn of bed hazards. *NYT*, 16.

253. Brody, J. E. (1990, October 25). New vaccines protect infants and toddlers from HIB infection. *NYT*, B7.

254. Anonymous. (1992). Sudden infant death syndrome—United States, 1980–1988. *MMWR*, 41, 515–17.

255. Wigfield, R. E., Fleming, P. J., Berry, P. J. et al. (1992). Can the fall in Avon's sudden infant death rate be explained by changes in sleeping position? *British Medical Journal*, 304, 282–83.

256. American Academy of Pediatrics, Committee on Fetus and Newborn (1975). Report of the Ad Hoc Task Force on Circumcision. *Pediatrics*, 56, 610–11.

257. National Center for Health Statistics. Cited in: Rosenberg, D. (1992, July). Circumcision circumspection. *Technology Review*, 17.

258. Wiswell, T. E., Smith, F. R., & Bass, J. W. (1985). Decreased incidence of urinary tract infections in circumcised male infants. *Pediatrics*, 75, 901–903.

259. Wiswell, T. E., & Roscelli, J. D. (1986). Corroborative evidence for the decreased incidence of urinary tract infections in circumcised male infants. *Pediatrics*, 78, 96–99.

260. Roberts, J. A. (1990). Is routine circumcision indicated in the newborn? An affirmative view. *Journal of Family Practice*, 31, 185–88.

261. Schoen, E. J. (1990). The status of circumcision of newborns. *NEJM*, 322, 1308–12.

262. Thompson, R. S. (1990). Is routine circumcision indicated in the newborn? An opposing view. *Journal of Family Practice*, 31, 189–96.

263. Tedder, J. L. (1987). Newborn circumcision. *Journal of Obstetric, Gynecologic, & Neonatal Nursing*, 16(1), 42–47.

264. Robson, W. L., & Leung, A. K. (1992). The circumcision question. *Postgraduate Medicine*, 91, 237–42.

265. Anonymous. (1989). American Academy of Pediatrics. Report of the Task Force on Circumcision. *Pediatrics*, 84, 388–91.

266. Ryan, A. S., Rush, D., Krieger, F. W. et al. (1991). Recent declines in breast-feeding in the United States, 1984 through 1989. *Pediatrics*, 88, 719.

267. Macfarlane, A. (1977). *The psychology of childbirth*. Cambridge, MA: Harvard University Press.

268. Medical Tribune News Service. (1991, September 9). Breast-milk benefits extend to adulthood. *SFC*, D3.

269. Sears, C. (1991, December). Baby bottle blues. *AH*, 17.

270. Lucas, A., Morley, R., Cole, T. J. et al. (1992). Breast milk and subsequent intelligence quotient in children born preterm. *Lancet*, 339, 261–64.

271. Karjalainen, J., Martin, J. M., Knip, M. et al. (1992). A bovine albumin peptide as a possible trigger of insulin-dependent diabetes mellitus. *NEJM*, 327, 302–307.

272. Freed, G. L., Fraley, J. K., & Schanler, R. J. (1992). Attitudes of expectant fathers regarding breast feeding. *Pediatrics*, 90, 224–27.

273. Dix, D. N. (1991). Why women decide not to breastfeed. *Birth*, 18, 222–25.

274. Hopkins, J., Marcues, M., & Campbell, S. B. (1984). Postpartum depression: A critical review. *Psychological Bulletin*, 95, 498–515.

275. Beck, C. T., Reynolds, M. A., & Rutowski, P. (1992). Maternity blues and postpartum depression. *Journal of Obstetric, Gynecologic, & Neonatal Nursing*, 21, 287–93.

276. Coll, C. G. Quoted in: Kutner, L. (1991, November 7). First comes the baby, then anger and frustration when not all goes according to expectations. *NYT*, B4.

277. Goodman, S. (1992, August 20). Inside a newborn's world: Babies' social instincts are remarkably sophisticated. *SFC*, D3–D4.

278. Bernstein, L. (1990, June 27). Babies' senses sharper. *SFC*, B3, B5.

279. Goleman, D. (1992, August 22?). Study finds babies at 5 months grasp simple mathematics. *NYT*, A1, A9.

280. Blakeslee, S. (1992, February 4). Babies learn sounds of language by 6 months. *NYT*, B6.

281. Goodman, S. (1991, December–1992, January). Presumed innocents. *Modern Maturity*, 25–28.

282. Webster-Stratton, C. Cited in: Brody, J. E. (1991, December 3). Better conduct? Train parents, then children. *NYT*, B5, B8.

283. Gelles, R. J. (1978). Violence toward children in the United States. *American Journal of Orthopsychiatry*, 48, 580–92.

284. McCormick, K. F. (1992). Attitudes of primary care physicians toward corporal punishment. *JAMA*, 267, 3161–65.

285. Forward, S. (1989). *Toxic parents: Overcoming their hurtful legacy and reclaiming your life*. New York: Bantam.

286. Warejcka, M. (1992, June 7). Defining a crime: A fine line between discipline, abuse. *Reno Gazette-Journal*, 4A.

287. Cantwell, H. B. (1980). Child neglect. In C. H. Kempe & R. E. Helfer (Eds.), *The battered child* (3rd ed.). Chicago: University of Chicago Press.

288. Wolock, I., & Horowitz, B. (1984). Child maltreatment as a social problem: The neglect of neglect. *American Journal of Orthopsychiatry*, 54, 530–43.

289. U.S. Department of Health and Human Services (1989, March). *Child abuse and neglect: A shared community concern*. DHHS Pub. No. (OHDS)89-30531. Washington, DC: Clearinghouse on Child Abuse and Neglect Information.

290. Greven, P. (1991). *Spare the child: The religious roots of punishment and the psychological impact of physical abuse*. New York: Knopf.

291. Warejcka, M. (1992, June 7). Fallon faces a soaring child abuse rate. *Reno Gazette-Journal*, 4A.

292. Nevada Division of Child and Family Services. Cited in: Anonymous. (1992, June 7). Family stress factors: Top 6 factors involved with Nevada's child abuse. *Reno Gazette-Journal*, 4A.

293. Bijur, P. E., Kurzon, M., Overpeck, M. D. et al. (1992). Parental alcohol use, problem drinking, and children's injuries. *JAMA*, 267, 3166–71.

294. Lowry, J. (1991, September 15). Report calls child abuse a 'national emergency.' *SFE*, A-

4. [Report on second annual report of U.S. Advisory Board on Child Abuse and Neglect, released September 15, 1991.]

295. National Center on Child Abuse and Neglect (1988). *Study Findings: Study of National Incidence and Prevalence of Child Abuse and Neglect: 1988.* Washington, DC: U.S. Department of Health and Human Services, Office of Human Development Services, Administration for Children, Youth and Families, Children's Bureau, National Center on Child Abuse and Neglect.

296. U.S. Department of Health and Human Services, 1989.

297. Pelton, L. H. (1978). Child abuse and neglect: The myth of classlessness. *American Journal of Orthopsychiatry, 48,* 608–17.

298. Whipple, E. E., & Webster-Stratton, C. (1991). The role of parental stress in physically abusive families. *Child Abuse & Neglect, 15,* 279–91.

299. LaMar, D. F. (1992). *Transcending turmoil: Survivors of dysfunctional families.* New York: Plenum Press, 3.

300. Northcraft, K. Quoted in: Rogers, T., Associated Press. (1991, January 2). Why some people transcend their traumatic childhoods. *SFC,* B1, B4.

301. Bachmann, G. A., Moeller, T. P., & Benett, J. (1988). Childhood sexual abuse and the consequences in adult women. *Obstetrics & Gynecology, 71,* 631–42.

302. Anonymous. (1990, July 21). Childhood abuse cause of later ills. *SFC,* C1; reprinted from *NYT.* [Moeller, T., & Bachmann, G. Presentation at 1990 meeting of American College of Obstetricians and Gynecologists.]

303. Martin, B. (1975). Parent-child relations. In F. D. Horowitz (Ed.). *Review of child development research* (Vol. IV). Chicago: University of Chicago Press.

304. Heide, K. M. (1992, September/October). Why kids kill parents. *PT,* 62–66, 76–77.

305. Lemily, N. Quoted in: Malcolm, A. H. (1991, November 12). A woman's quiet fight against child abuse. *NYT,* B12.

306. Boyer, D., & Fine, D. (1992). Sexual abuse as a factor in adolescent pregnancy and child maltreatment. *Family Planning Perspectives, 24,* 4–11.

307. Marshall, L. L., & Rose, P. (1990). Premarital violence: The impact of family of origin violence, stress, and reciprocity. *Violence & Victims, 5*(1), 51–64.

308. Department of Criminal Justice, Indiana University. (1990). Childhood victimization and violent offending. *Violence & Victims, 5*(1), 19–35.

309. Dodge, K. A., Bates, J. E., & Pettit, G. S. (1990). Mechanisms in the cycle of violence. *Science, 250,* 1678–83.

310. Koestner, R., Franz, C., & Weinberger, J. (1990). The family origins of empathic concern: A 26-year longitudinal study. *Journal of Personality & Social Psychology, 58*(4), 709–17.

311. Spock, B. (1992). *Dr. Spock's baby and child care* (6th ed.). New York: Pocket.

312. Spock, B. Quoted in: Goleman, D. (1991, April 18). Parents' warmth is found to be key to adult happiness. *NYT,* B1, B6.

UNIT 11: INFECTIOUS AND SEXUALLY TRANSMITTED DISEASES

1. Sontag, S. (1978). *Illness as metaphor.* New York: Farrar, Straus & Giroux, 3.

2. Frank, A. W. (1991). *At the will of the body.* Boston: Houghton Mifflin.

3. Kilbourne, E. D. (1990). New viral diseases: A real and potential problem without boundaries. *JAMA, 264,* 68–70.

4. Freundlich, N. (1991, January 21). The microbes are back—with a vengeance. *Business Week,* 80–82.

5. Wright, K. (1990). Bad news bacteria. *Science, 249,* 22–24.

6. Nash, J. M. (1992, August 31). Attack of the superbugs. *Time,* 62–63.

7. Skolnick, A. (1991, January 2). New insights into how bacteria develop antibiotic resistance. *JAMA, 265,* 14–16.

8. Rasche, R. E. (1991). Mapping malaria. *Today, 16,* 26–28.

9. Rosenthal, E. (1991, February 12). Outwitted by malaria, desperate doctors seek new remedies. *NYT,* B5, B8.

10. Suro, R. (1992, March 22). The cholera watch. *New York Times Magazine,* 32–35.

11. Epstein, P. R. (1992). Cholera and the environment. *Lancet, 339,* 1167–68.

12. Mitchell, C. J., Niebylski, M. L., Smith, G. C. et al. (1992). Isolation of eastern equine encephalitis virus from *Aedes albopictus* in Florida. *Science, 257,* 526–27.

13. Jaret, P. (1986, June). The wars within. *National Geographic,* 702–34.

14. American College of Allergy and Immunology. Cited in: Brody, J. E. (1991, April 11). Old advice as well as new hope for millions who are allergic to the pollens of springtime. *NYT,* B8.

15. Brody, J. E. (1992, June 24). Learn to recognize, avoid and treat the ubiquitous enemy known as poison ivy. *NYT,* B7.

16. Gorman, C. (1992, June 22). Asthma: Deadly...but treatable. *Time,* 61–62.

17. Sampson, H. A., Mendelson, L., & Rosen, J. P. (1992). Fatal and near-fatal anaphylactic reactions to food in children and adolescents. *NEJM, 327,* 380–84.

18. Firestein, G. S. (1992). Mechanisms of tissue destruction and cellular activation in rheumatoid arthritis. *Current Opinion in Rheumatology, 4,* 348–54.

19. Perlman, D. (1990, May 24). MS clue found—Cells that attack brain. *SFC,* A2. [Report in 5/23/92 *Nature* of Stanford and Australian researchers.]

20. Anonymous. (1991, January). Myasthenia gravis: The 'weakening' disorder. *Mayo Clinic Health Letter,* 6.

21. Associated Press. (1990, June 29). English scientists lose a cold war. *SFC,* B1.

22. Marlin, S. D., Staunton, D. E., Springer, T. A. et al. (1990). A soluble form of intercellular adhesion molecule-1 inhibits rhinovirus infection. *Nature, 344,* 70–72.

23. Brody, J. E. (1992, January 1). Setting the record straight on how to live with the minor discomforts of winter. *NYT,* 13.

24. Anonymous. (1989, January). Cold remedies: Which ones work best? *Consumer Reports,* 8–11.

25. Cohen, S., Tyrrell, D. A., & Smith, A. P. (1991). Psychological stress and susceptibility to the common cold. *NEJM, 325,* 606–12.

26. Macknin, M. L., Mathew, S., Medendorp, S. V. (1990). Effect of inhaling heated vapor on symptoms of the common cold. *JAMA, 264,* 989–91.

27. Graham, N. M., Burrell, C. J., Doublas, R. M., Debelle, P., & Davies, L. (1990). Adverse effects of aspirin, acetaminophen, and ibuprofen on immune function, viral shedding, and clinical status in rhinovirus-infected volunteers. *Journal of Infectious Diseases, 162,* 1277–82.

28. Pauling, L. C. (1970). *Vitamin C and the common cold.* San Francisco: Freeman.

29. Chalmers, T. C. (1975). Effects of ascorbic acid on the common cold. *American Journal of Medicine, 58,* 532–36.

30. Advisory Committee on Immunization Practices. (1987). Prevention and control of influenza. *MMWR, 36,* 373–87.

31. Gunn, W. Quoted in: Associated Press. (1990, November 10). Doctors, warning of flu danger, say ignoring risk could be fatal. *NYT,* 9.

32. Le, C., & Chang, R. S. (1988). In T. W. Hudson, M. A. Reinhart, S. D. Rose et al. (Eds.), *Clinical preventive medicine: Health promotion and disease prevention.* Boston: Little, Brown, 615–17.

33. Le & Chang, 1988.

34. Gunn. Quoted in: Associated Press, 1990.

35. Ruben, F. L. (1987). Prevention and control of influenza: Role of vaccine. *American Journal of Medicine, 82,* 31–34.

36. Beck, M., & Wilson, L. (1990, February 5). Feeling bad, getting worse. *Newsweek,* 57.

37. Altman, L. K. (1991, December 3). Gaps shown in flu fight. *NYT,* A1, B6.

38. Levine, D. (1992, November). Prevent the flu. *AH,* 11–12.

39. Anonymous. (1991). Infectious mononucleosis. *Postgraduate Medicine, 89,* 54.

40. Shafran, S. D. (1991). The chronic fatigue syndrome. *American Journal of Medicine, 90,* 730–39.

41. Katzenstein, L. (1992, May). Sick & tired. *AH,* 51–56.

42. Kaufman, W. (1992, May). Virus hunter. *AH,* 33–35.

43. Schlueberberg, A., Straus, S. E., Peterson, P. et al. (1992). NIH conference. Chronic fatigue syndrome research: Definition and medical outcome assessment. *AIM, 117,* 325–31.

44. Garelik, G. (1992, May). Desperately seeking solutions. *AH,* 54–55.

45. Felts, W. M., & Knight, S. M. (1992). The nature and prevention of viral hepatitis: What health educators should know. *Journal of Health Education, 23,* 267–74.

46. Navarro, M. (1992, March 6). Health officials see increase in hepatitis among gay men. *NYT,* A9.

47. Centers for Disease Control. (1990). Recommendations for IG prophylaxis for hepatitis A. *MMWR, 39,* 3–5.

48. Anonymous. (1992). Hepatitis A: A vaccine at last. *Lancet, 339,* 1198–99.

49. Kingsley, L. A., Rinaldo, C. R., Lyter, D. W. et al. (1990). Sexual transmission efficiency of hepatitis B virus and human immunodeficiency virus among homosexual men. *JAMA, 264,* 230.

50. Brody, J. E. (1991, September 11). U.S. seeks vaccination of babies to avert the growing danger of hepatitis B. *NYT,* B8.

51. Carey, W. D. (1990). Interferon for chronic hepatitis. *Cleveland Clinic Journal of Medicine, 57,* 218–19.

52. Perrillo, R. P., Schiff, E. R., Davis, G. L. et al. (1990). A randomized, controlled trial of interferon alpha-2b alone and after prednisone withdrawal for the treatment of chronic hepatitis B. *NEJM, 323,* 295–301.

53. Felts & Knight, 1992.

54. Brody, 1991 (September 11).

55. Schucat, A., & Broome, C. V. (1991). Toxic shock syndrome and tampons. *Epidemiologic Reviews, 13,* 99–112.

56. Beck, M., Crandall, R., & Hager, M. (1990, July 23). A mean strain of strep. *Newsweek,* 57.

57. Brody, J. E. (1990, November 15). Resurgence of rheumatic fever puts focus on treatment of strep throat. *NYT,* B8.

58. Bisno, A. (1991, September 12). Group A streptococcal infections and acute rheumatic fever. *NEJM, 325,* 783–93.

59. Gable, C., Holzer, S. S., Engelhart, L. et al. (1990) Pneumococcal vaccine: Efficacy and associated cost savings. *JAMA, 264,* 2910–15.

60. Shapiro, E. D., Berg, A. T., Austrian, R. et al. (1991). The protective efficacy of polyvalent pneumococcal polysaccharide vaccine. *NEJM, 325,* 1453–60.

61. Anonymous. (1990). Pneumonia. *Postgraduate Medicine, 88,* 48.

62. Cowley, G., Leonard, E. A., & Hager, M. (1992, March 16). Tuberculosis: A deadly return. *Newsweek,* 53–57.

63. Specter, M. (1992, October 11). Neglected for years, TB is back with strains that are dead-

lier. *NYT*, sec. 1, 1, 20.

64. Rosenthal, E. (1992, October 12). Doctors and patients are pushed to their limits by grim new TB. *NYT*, A1, A18.

65. Rosenthal, E. (1992, October 13). TB, easily transmitted, adds a peril to medicine. *NYT*, A1, B9.

66. Specter, M. (1992, October 14). TB carriers see clash of liberty and health. *NYT*, A1, A22.

67. Altman, L. K. (1992, October 15). Quest for TB treatment leads to an old answer. *NYT*, A1, B5.

68. Flynn, N. Tuberculosis. In Hudson et al. (Eds.), 1988, 620–27.

69. Benenson, A. S. (Ed.). (1990). *Control of communicable disease in man*. Washington, DC: American Public Health Association.

70. Benjamin, R. Quoted in: Craffey, B. (1992, June 14). A killer returns. *SFE, Image*, 6–13.

71. Altman, L. K. (1992, January 25). For most, risk of contracting tuberculosis is seen as small. *NYT*, 1, 9.

72. Reichman, L. B. Cited in: Altman, 1992, 9.

73. Russell, S. (1992, July 22). Study says shelters host high risk of TB. *SFC*, A11. [Zolopa, A. Preliminary results of two-year TB and AIDS screen project, reported at 8th International Conference on AIDS, Amsterdam, July 22, 1992.]

74. Centers for Disease Control. (1991). Deaths among homeless persons—San Francisco, 1985–1990. *MMWR*, *40*, 877–80.

75. Ciesielski, S. D., Seed, J. R., Esposito, D. H., & Hunter, N. (1991). The epidemiology of tuberculosis among North Carolina migrant farm workers. *JAMA*, *265*, 1715–19.

76. Centers for Disease Control. (1992). Transmission of multidrug-resistant tuberculosis among immunocompromised persons in a correctional system—New York, 1991. *MMWR*, *41*, 507–509.

77. Rosenthal, E. (1991, November 16). Doctors see a growing tuberculosis threat in prisons and shelters. *NYT*, 10.

78. Altman, L. K. (1991, December 7). Americans aren't being protected against tuberculosis, panel says. *NYT*, 6.

79. Specter, 1992 (October 11).

80. Medical Tribune News Services. (1991, December 26). HIV-positive people develop TB faster. *SFC*, A8. [Report by W. W. Stead.]

81. Associated Press. (1992, October 18). Doctors telling of wider risks in spread of TB. *NYT*, 16.

82. Altman, 1992 (January 25).

83. Cowley, Leonard, & Hager, 1992.

84. Specter, 1992 (October 11).

85. Specter, 1992 (October 11).

86. Rosenthal, E. (1992, August 1). Drug-resistant TB is seen spreading within hospitals. *NYT*, 1, 9.

87. Rosenthal, E. (1992, August 13). Scientists identify what is making TB resistant to drugs. *NYT*, A1, A9.

88. Pershing, D. H., Telford, S. R. 3d, Rys, P. N. et al. (1990). Detection of *Borrelia burgdorferi* DNA in museum specimens of *Ixodes dammini* ticks. *Science*, *249*, 1420–23.

89. Cunha, B. A. (1990). Lyme disease: Strategies for this summer. *Emergency Medicine*, *22*, 75–97.

90. Harbit, M. D., & Willis, D. (1990). Lyme disease: Implications for health educators. *Health Education*, *21*, 41–43.

91. Centers for Disease Control. (1991). Lyme disease surveillance—United States, 1989–1990. *MMWR*, *40*, 417–21.

92. Fultz, O. (1991, June). The tick that ate summer. *AH*, 52–57.

93. Travis, J. (1992). Biting back at Lyme disease. *Science*, *256*, 1623.

94. Magid, D., Schwartz, B., Craft, J., & Schwartz, J. S. (1992). Prevention of Lyme disease after tick bites: A cost-effective analysis. *NEJM*, *327*,

534–41.

95. Edelman, R. (1991). Perspective on the development of vaccines against Lyme disease. *Vaccine*, *9*, 531–32.

96. Reuters. (1990, December 15). Last small pox viruses to be destroyed. *SFC*, A19.

97. Lee, F. R. (1991, October 16). Poor record seen in immunizations. *NYT*, B12.

98. Freeman, P., & Robbins, A. (1991, July 10). An epidemic of inactivity. *NYT*, A15.

99. Rosenthal, E. (1991, April 24). Measles resurges, and with far deadlier effects. *NYT*, A1, A18.

100. Maniace, L. (1991, June). The perils of pertussis. *AH*, 8.

101. Gershon, A. A. (1990). Immunization practices in children. *Hospital Practice*, *25*, 91–107.

102. Camfield, P. (1992). Brain damage from pertussis immunization: A Canadian neurologist's perspective. *American Journal of Diseases of Children*, *146*, 327–31.

103. Farizo, K. M., Cochi, S. L., & Patriarca, P. A. (1990). Poliomyelitis in the United States: A historical perspective and current vaccination policy. *Journal of American College Health*, *39*, 137–43.

104. Anonymous. (1991, May 27). New worries about old diseases. *Newsweek*, 68.

105. Smith, D. W. (1989). Polio and postpolio sequelae: The lived experience. *Orthopaedic Nursing*, *8*(5), 24–28.

106. Agre, J. C., Rodriquez, A. A., & Sperling, K. B. (1989). Symptoms and clinical impressions of patients seen in a postpolio clinic. *Archives of Physical Medicine & Rehabilitation*, *70*, 367–70.

107. Smith, H. (1990). Mumps. *The Practitioner*, *234*, 903–904.

108. Hudson, W. T. (1988). Rubella and pregnancy. In Hudson et al. (Eds.), 124–29.

109. Black, S. B., & Shinefield, H. R. (1992). Immunization with ogligosaccharide conjugate Haemophilus influenzae type b (HbOC) vaccine on a large health maintenance organization population: Extended follow-up and impact on Haemophilus influenzae disease epidemiology. The Kaiser Permanente Pediatric Vaccine Study Group. *Pediatric Infectious Disease Journal*, *11*(8), 610–13.

110. Kennedy, D. H. (1990). Measles. *The Practitioner*, *234*, 895–900.

111. Centers for Disease Control. (1990). Public health burden of vaccine-preventable diseases among adults: Standards for adult immunization practice. *MMWR*, *39*, 725–29.

112. Hilton, E., Singer, C., Kozarsky, P. et al. (1991). Status of immunity to tetanus, measles, mumps, rubella, and polio among U.S. travelers. *AIM*, *115*, 32–33.

113. Centers for Disease Control, 1990, *MMWR*, *39*, 725–29.

114. Anonymous. (1990). Immunization: Important for adults, too! *Patient Care*, *26*, 124–25.

115. Kennedy, 1990.

116. Smith, 1990.

117. Ellis, M. (1990). Rubella. *The Practitioner*, *234*, 906–10.

118. Centers for Disease Control. (1991). Human rabies—Texas, Arkansas, and Georgia, 1991. *MMWR*, *40*, 765–69.

119. Strum, C. (1991, November 15). Rabies infection spreads north via raccoons. *NYT*, A12.

120. Marx, J. (1986). AIDS virus has a new name—perhaps. *Science*, *232*, 699–700.

121. Centers for Disease Control. (1992). The second 100,000 cases of acquired immunodeficiency syndrome—United States, June 1981–December 1991. *MMWR*, *41*, 28–29.

122. Brundage, J. F. (1991). Epidemiology of HIV infection and AIDS in the United States. *Dermatologic Clinics*, *9*, 443–52.

123. Peaceman, A. M., & Gonik, B. (1991).

Sexually transmitted viral disease in women. *Postgraduate Medicine*, *89*, 133–40.

124. Mann, J. M. (1992). AIDS—the second decade: A global perspective. *Journal of Infectious Diseases*, *165*, 245–50.

125. Centers for Disease Control. (1991). The HIV/AIDS epidemic: The first 10 years. *MMWR*, *40*, 357.

126. Mann, J. (1990, June 30). The global lessons of AIDS. *New Scientist*, 30.

127. Anonymous. (1991, November 17). The long road from HIV to AIDS. *NYT*, sec. 4, 1.

128. Associated Press. (1992, September 3). Women seek to expand list of illnesses in defining AIDS. *NYT*, A6.

129. Blattner, W. A. (1991). HIV epidemiology: past, present, and future. *Faseb Journal*, *5*, 2340–48.

130. Byer, C. O., & Shainberg, L. W. (1991). *Dimensions of human sexuality* (3rd ed.). Dubuque, IA: Wm. C. Brown.

131. Giesecke, J., Scalia-Tomba, G., Hakansson, C. et al. (1990). Incubation time of AIDS: Progression of disease in a cohort of HIV-infected homo- and bisexual men with known dates of infection. *Scandinavian Journal of Infectious Diseases*, *22*, 407–11.

132. Anonymous. (1992). Still a mystery but 'not likely' a virus. *JAMA*, *268*, 1236–37.

133. Snell, J. J., Supran, E. M., Esparza, J. et al. (1990). World Health Organization quality assessment programme on HIV testing. *Aids*, *4*, 803–806.

134. Moore, R. D., Hidalgo, J., Sugland, B. W. et al. (1991). Zidovudine and the natural history of the acquired immunodeficiency syndrome. *NEJM*, *324*, 1412–16.

135. Kolata, G. (1991, November 4). Patients turning to illegal pharmacies. *NYT*, A1, A10.

136. Garrison, J. (1992, February 2). Experts glum as new drugs for AIDS flop. *SFE*, A-1, A-10.

137. Girard, M. (1990). Prospects for an AIDS vaccine. *Cancer Detection & Prevention*, *14*, 411–13.

138. Kurth, R., Binninger, D., Ennen, J. et al. (1991). The quest for an AIDS vaccine: The state of the art and current challenges. *Aids Research & Human Retrovirus*, *7*, 425–33.

139. Antoni, M. H., Schneiderman, N., Fletcher, M. A. et al. (1990). Psychoneuroimmunology and HIV-1. *Journal of Consulting & Clinical Psychology*, *58*, 38–39.

140. LaPerriere, A. R., Antoni, M. H., Schneiderman, N. et al. (1990). Exercise intervention attenuates emotional distress and natural killer cell decrements following notification of positive serologic status for HIV-1. *Biofeedback & Self Regulation*, *15*, 229–42.

141. Leerhsen, C., Foote, D., Gordon, J. et al. (1991, November 18). Magic's message. *Newsweek*, 58–62.

142. Lambert, B. (1992, August 9). Alison L. Gertz, whose infection alerted many to AIDS, dies at 26. *NYT*, sec. 1, 19.

143. Padian, N. S., Shiboski, S. C., & Jewell, N. P. (1991). Female-to-male transmission of human immunodeficiency virus. *JAMA*, *266*, 1664–67.

144. Staver, S. (1990, June 1). Women found contracting HIV via unprotected sex. *American Medical News*, 4–5.

145. Kerr, D. L. (1991). Women with AIDS and HIV infection. *Journal of School Health*, *61*, 139–40.

146. Eckholm, E., & Tierney, J. (1990, September 16). AIDS in Africa: A killer rages on. *NYT*, sec. 1, 1, 10.

147. Eckholm, E. (1990, September 16). What makes the 2 sexes so vulnerable to epidemic. *NYT*, 1, 11.

148. Centers for Disease Control, 1992, *MMWR*, *41*, 28–29.

149. Centers for Disease Control, 1991, *MMWR*, *40*, 357.

150. Kimmel, M., & Levine, M. (1991, May 10). AIDS is a disease of men involved in risky behavior. *SFC*, A25.

151. Addiction Research Foundations. Reported in: Reuters. (1991, July 10). Needle swap credited for Canada's drop in AIDS. *SFC*, A9.

152. Coates, R. A., Rankin, J. G., Lamothe, F. et al. (1992). Needle sharing behaviour among injection users (IDUs) in treatment in Montreal and Toronto, 1988–1989. *Canadian Journal of Public Health, 83*, 38–41.

153. Kaplan, E. H., & Heimer, R. (1992). HIV prevalence among intravenous drug users: Model-based estimates from New Haven's legal needle exchange. *Journal of Acquired Immune Deficiency Syndromes, 5*, 163–69.

154. Anonymous. Quoted in: Thompson, D. (1992, May 25). Getting the point in New Haven. *Time*, 55–56.

155. American Foundation for AIDS Research. Cited in: Navarro, M. (1992, May 14). Needle swaps to be revived to curb AIDS. *NYT*, A1, B10.

156. Kolata, G. (1991, December 25). Hemophiliacs, hard hit by H.I.V., are angrily looking for answers. *NYT*, 1, 7.

157. Sandler, S. G., & Popovsky, M. A. (1990, July). New technologies for a safer blood supply. *Technology Review*, 23–31.

158. Nelson, K. E., Donahue, J. G., Munoz, A. et al. (1992). Transmission of retroviruses from seronegative donors by transfusion during cardiac surgery. *AIM, 117*, 554–59.

159. Symonds, R. J., Holmberg, S. D., Hurwitz, R. L. et al. (1992). Transmission of human immunodeficiency virus type 1 from a seronegative organ and tissue donor. *NEJM, 326*, 726–32.

160. Kerr, 1991.

161. Blanche, S., Rouzious, C., Moscato, M. L. et al. (1989). A prospective study of infants born to women seropositive for human immunodeficiency virus type 1. HIV Infection in Newborns French Collaborative Study Group. *NEJM, 320*, 1643–48.

162. Van de Perre, P., Simonon, A., Msellati, P. et al. (1991). Postnatal transmission of human immunodeficiency virus type 1 from mother to infant: A prospective cohort study in Kigali, Rwanda. *NEJM, 325*, 593–98.

163. Holmberg, S. D., & Curran, J. W. (1990). The epidemiology of HIV infection in industrialized countries. In K. K. Holmes, P. Maroh, P. F. Sparling et al. (Eds.), *Sexually transmitted diseases* (2nd ed.). New York: McGraw-Hill, 1990, 343–53.

164. Koop, C. E. Quoted in: Hilts, P. J. (1991, September 20). Experts oppose AIDS tests for doctors. *NYT*, A11.

165. Saddler, J. (1991, December 3). OSHA sets broader rules to protect health-care workers from infections. *WSJ*, B6.

166. Lambert, W. (1991, November 19). Discrimination afflicts people with HIV. *WSJ*, B1, B8.

167. Reuters. (1992, August 18). AIDS survey finds many feel abused. *SFC*, A2.

168. Krieger, L. M. (1992, August 16). AIDS often spells poverty. *SFE*, A-1, A-7.

169. Kimmel, M., & Levine, M. (1991, May 10). AIDS is a disease of men involved in risky behavior. *SFC*, A25.

170. Winkelstein, W. Jr., Samuel, M., Padian, N. S. et al. (1987). Selected sexual practices of San Francisco heterosexual men and risk of infection by the human immunodeficiency virus. *JAMA, 257*, 1470.

171. Joseph, J. G., Montgomery, S. B., Emmons, C.-A. et al. (1987). Perceived risk of AIDS: Assessing the behavioral and psychosocial consequences in a cohort of gay men. *Journal of Applied Social Psychology, 17*, 231–50.

172. Fineberg, H. V. (1988). Education to prevent AIDS: Prospects and obstacles. *Science, 239*, 592–96.

173. Bauman, L. J., & Siegel, K. (1987). Misperception among gay men of the risk for AIDS associated with their sexual behavior. *Journal of Applied Social Psychology, 17*, 329–50.

174. Centers for Disease Control. (1991, January). *HIV/AIDS Surveillance Report*, 1–22.

175. Kerr, 1991.

176. Brody, J. E. (1992, August 12). 30 million Americans have genital herpes, a lifelong illness that thrives on secrecy. *NYT*, B6.

177. Davies, K. (1990). Genital herpes: An overview. *Journal of Obstetric, Gynecologic & Neonatal Nursing, 19*, 401–406.

178. Corey, L., & Holmes, K. K. (1983). Genital herpes simplex virus infections: Current concepts in diagnosis, therapy, and prevention. *AIM, 98*, 973–83.

179. Brock, B. V., Selke, S., Benedetti, J. et al. (1990). Frequency of asymptomatic shedding of herpes simplex virus in women with genital herpes. *JAMA, 263*, 418–20.

180. Mertz, G. J., Benedetti, J., Ashley, R. et al. (1992). Risk factors for the sexual transmission of genital herpes. *AIM, 116*, 197–202.

181. Koutsy, L. A., Stevens, C. E., Holmes, K. K. et al. (1992). Underdiagnosis of genital herpes by current clinical and viral-isolation procedures. *NEJM, 326*, 1533–39.

182. Lynch, P. J. (1988). Psychiatric, legal, and moral issues of herpes simplex infections. *Journal of the American Academy of Dermatology, 18*, 173–75.

183. Brown, Z. A., Benedetti, J., Ashley, R. et al. (1991). Neonatal herpes simplex virus infection in relation to asymptomatic maternal infection at the time of labor. *NEJM, 324*, 1247–52.

184. Subak-Sharpe, G. J. (Ed.). (1984). Genital herpes. In *The physician's manual for patients*. New York: Times, 370–72.

185. Apuzzio, J. J., & Leo, M. V. (1991). Herpes in the pregnant woman. *Medical Aspects of Human Sexuality, 25*, 54–58.

186. Mertz et al., 1992.

187. Longo, D. J., & Clum, G. A. (1989). Psychosocial factors affecting genital herpes recurrences: Linear versus mediating models. *Journal of Psychosomatic Research, 33*, 161–66.

188. Futterman, A. D., Kemeny, M. E., Shapiro, D. et al. (1992). Immunological variability associated with experimentally-induced positive and negative affective states. *Psychological Medicine, 22*, 231–38.

189. Rand, K. H., Hoon, E. F., Massey, J. K. et al. (1990). Daily stress and recurrence of genital herpes simplex. *Archives of Internal Medicine, 150*, 1889–93.

190. Longo, D. J., Clum, G. A., & Yaeger, N. J. (1988). Psychosocial treatment for recurrent genital herpes. *Journal of Consulting & Clinical Psychology, 56*, 61–66.

191. Goldsmith, M. F. (1989). 'Silent epidemic' of 'social disease' makes STD experts raise their voices. *JAMA, 261*, 3509–10.

192. Bauer, H. M., Ting, Y., Greer, C. E. et al. (1991). Genital human papillomavirus infection in female university students as determined by a PCR-based method. *JAMA, 265*, 472–77.

193. Gordon, A. N. (1990, February). New STD menace: HPV infection. *Medical Aspects of Human Sexuality*, 20–24.

194. Daling, J. R., Weiss, N. S., Hislop, T. G. et al. (1987). Sexual practices, sexually transmitted diseases, and the incidence of anal cancer. *NEJM, 317*, 973–77.

195. Nuovo, G., & Pedemonte, B. (1990). Human papillomavirus types and recurrent cervical warts. *JAMA, 263*, 1223–26.

196. Bergman, A. (1991, December). HPV infection in men: Severing the link to cervical cancer. *Medical Aspects of Human Sexuality*, 20–30.

197. Carlson, J. W., Hill, P. S., & Robertson, A. W. (1990, August). Evaluation and treatment of human papillomavirus infection in men. *Medical Aspects of Human Sexuality*, 58–62.

198. Waldholz, M. (1992, September 24). Cost may limit use of Pfizer drug against chlamydia. *WSJ*, B4.

199. Martin, D. H. (1990). Chlamydial infections. *Medical Clinics of North America, 74*, 1367–87.

200. White, D. M., & Felts, W. M. (1989a). Knowledge of chlamydial infection among university students. *Health Education, 20*, 23–26.

201. White, D. M., & Felts, W. M. (1989b, Spring). Chlamydial infection: The quiet epidemic. *Our Sexuality Update, 1*, 4–5.

202. Jones, R. B., Rabinovitch, R. A., Katz, B. P. et al. (1985). Chlamydia trachomatis in the pharynx and rectum of homosexual patients at risk for genital infection. *AIM, 102*, 757–62.

203. Washington, A., Arno, P., & Brooks, M. (1986). The economic cost of pelvic inflammatory disease. *JAMA, 255*, 1735–38.

204. Chow, J. M., Yonekura, L., Richwald, G. A. et al. (1990). The association between *Chlamydia trachomatis* and ectopic pregnancy: A matched-pair, case-control study. *JAMA, 263*, 3164–67.

205. McCormack, W., Rosner, B., McComb, D. et al. (1985). Infection with *Chlamydia trachomatis* in female college students. *American Journal of Epidemiology, 121*, 107–15.

206. Wolner-Hanssen, P., Eschenbach, D. A., Paavonen, J. et al. (1990). Decreased risk of symptomatic chlamydial pelvic inflammatory disease associated wtih oral contraceptive use. *JAMA, 263*, 54–59.

207. Holmes, K. K. (1981). The *Chlamydia* epidemic. *JAMA, 245*, 1718–23.

208. Martin, D., Kotitsky, L., Eschenbach, D. et al. (1982). Prematurity and perinatal mortality in pregnancies complicated by maternal *Chlamydia trachomatic* infections. *JAMA, 247*, 1585–1615.

209. White & Felts, 1989b.

210. Holmes, K., & Stamm, W. (1981, October). Chlamydial genital infections: A growing problem. *Hospital Practice*, 105–17.

211. Rice, F. P. (1989). *Human sexuality*. Dubuque, IA: Wm. C. Brown.

212. Waldholz, 1992.

213. Schwebke, J. R. (1991, March). Gonorrhea in the '90s. *Medical Aspects of Human Sexuality*, 42–46.

214. Platt, R., Rice, P., & McCormack, W. (1983). Risk of acquiring gonorrhea and prevalence of abnormal adnexal findings among women recently exposed to gonorrhea. *JAMA, 250*, 3205–09.

215. Zenilman, J. M. (1990). Update on gonorrhea. *Hospital Medicine, 26*, 21–37.

216. Gilbaugh, J. H. Jr., & Guchs, P. C. (1979). The gonococcus and the toilet seat. *NEJM, 301*, 91–93.

217. Rein, M. F. (1982, February). Asymptomatic gonorrhea in men. *Medical Aspects of Human Sexuality*, 103–107.

218. Starcher, E., Kramer, M., Carlota-Orduna, B. et al. (1983). Establishing efficient interview periods for gonorrhea patients. *AJPH, 73*, 1381–84.

219. Zenilman, 1990.

220. Anonymous. (1990, August). Resistant gonorrhea on the rise. *Medical Aspects of Human Sexuality*, 37.

221. Schwarcz, S. K., Zenilman, J. M., Schnell, D. et al. (1990). National surveillance of antimicrobial resistance in *Neisseria gonorrhoeae*. *JAMA, 264*, 1413–17.

222. Altman, L. K. (1990, November 13). Syphilis fools a new generation. *NYT*, B7.

223. Anonymous. (1991). Primary and secondary syphilis—United States, 1981–1990. *MMWR, 40*, 314–23.

224. Goldsmith, M. F. (1988). Sex tied to drugs equals STD spread. *JAMA, 260*, 2008.

225. Byer & Shainberg, 1991.

226. Rice, 1989.

227. Handsfield, H. H. (1990). Old enemies: Combating syphilis and gonorrhea in the 1990s (editorial). *JAMA, 264,* 1451–52.

228. Rosen, T. (1990, January). The reemergence of syphilis. *Medical Aspects of Human Sexuality,* 20–22.

229. Stamm, W. E., Handsfield, H. H., Rompalo, A. M. et al. (1988). The association between genital ulcer disease and acquisition of HIV infection in homosexual men. *JAMA, 260,* 1429.

230. Hillier, S., & Holmes, K. K. (1990). Bacterial vaginosis. In Holmes et al., 457–59.

231. Chapel, T. A. (1982, August). Dissemination of trichomoniasis. *Medical Aspects of Human Sexuality,* 145–49.

232. Tortora, G., Funke, B. R., & Case, C. L. (1989). *Microbiology* (3rd ed.). Menlo Park, CA: Benjamin/Cummings.

233. Plant, M. A. (1990). Alcohol, sex and AIDS. *Alcohol & Alcoholism, 25,* 293–301.

234. Munzell, M. (1992, August 23). Dancing with death. *SFE, Image,* 23–27.

235. Tanner, W. M., & Pollack, R. H. (1988). The effects of condom use and erotic instructions on attitudes toward condoms. *Journal of Sex Research, 25,* 537–41.

236. Di Costanzo, D. (1992, August). The abc's of cleansing. *Self,* 134–35, 165.

237. Lister, P. (1992, March). Save your skin. *Self,* 123, 168.

238. Britton, A. G. (1992, November). Potions and lotions. *Self,* 131–32, 193.

239. Perrine, S. (1993, January/February). Class action. *Men's Health,* 50–55.

240. Perrine, 1993, 52.

241. Smith, S., & Smith, C. (1988). *The college student's health guide.* Los Altos, CA: Westchester.

242. Perrine, 1993.

243. Sharp, D. (1992, December/January). Watch your mouth—If you want to keep your teeth. *In Health,* 68–71.

244. Ramirez, A. (1990, May 13). Growth is glacial, but the market is big, and so is the gross. *NYT,* sec. 5, 11.

245. Sharp, 1992.

UNIT 12: NONINFECTIOUS ILLNESS AND PERSONAL SAFETY

1. Labbe, E. Quoted in: Bahr, R. (1991, August). Stack the deck. *Men's Health,* 82–84.

2. Vitulli, W. F. Quoted in: Bahr, 1991.

3. Bahr, 1991.

4. U.S. Public Health Service. (1990). *Healthy people 2000: National health promotion and disease prevention objectives.* DHHS Pub. No. (PHS)91-50212. Washington, DC: U.S. Government Printing Office.

5. Haffner, S. M., Stern, M. P., Hazuda, H. P. et al. (1990). Cardiovascular risk factors in confirmed prediabetic individuals: Does the clock for coronary heart disease start ticking before the onset of clinical diabetes? *JAMA, 263,* 2893–98.

6. Centers for Disease Control. (1990). Perinatal mortality and congenital malformations in infants born to women with insulin-dependent diabetes mellitus—United States, Canada, and Europe, 1940–1988. *MMWR, 39,* 363–65.

7. Mulder, E. J., & Visser, G. H. (1991). Growth and motor development in fetuses of women with type-1 diabetes. I. Early growth patterns. *Early Human Development, 25*(2), 91–106.

8. Ramos-Arroyo, M. A., Rodriguez-Pinilla, E., & Cordero, J. F. (1992). Maternal diabetes: The risk for specific birth defects. *European Journal of Epidemiology, 8,* 503–508.

9. Porth, C. (1986). *Pathophysiology* (2nd ed.). Philadelphia: Lippincott.

10. Stein, J. (Ed.). (1989). *Internal medicine: Diagnosis and therapy, 1988–1989.* Boston: Little, Brown.

11. Coleman, R., Lombard, M., Sicard, R. et al.

(1989) *Fundamental immunology.* Dubuque, IA: Wm. C. Brown.

12. Bankhead, C. D. (1990). Diabetes risk groups elucidated. *Medical World News, 31,* 19–20.

13. Public Health Service, 1990.

14. Carey, B. (1991, January/February). Dodging diabetes. *In Health,* 18.

15. Pryse-Phillips, W., Findlay, H., Tugwell, P. et al. (1992). A Canadian population survey on the clinical, epidemiologic and societal impact of migraine and tension-type headache. *Canadian Journal of Neurological Sciences, 19,* 333–39.

16. Perlman, D. (1990, May 24). MS clue found—Cells that attack brain. *SFC,* A2.

17. Anderson, D. W., Ellenberg, J. H., Leventhal, C. M. et al. (1992). Revised estimate of the prevalence of multiple sclerosis in the United States. *Annals of Neurology, 32,* 333–36.

18. Wolf, P. (1991). The phenotype: Seizures and epilepsy syndromes. *Epilepsy Research—Supplement, 4,* 19–29.

19. Farnham, A. (1992, December 14). Backache. *Fortune,* 132–41.

20. Public Health Service, 1990.

21. Garg, A., & Moore, J. S. (1992). Epidemiology of low-back pain in industry. *State of the Art Reviews: Occupational Medicine, 7,* 593–608.

22. Public Health Service, 1990.

23. Stipp, D. (1989, September 26). Low-back pain gives up some secrets. *WSJ,* B1.

24. Anonymous. (1990). Proper lifting. *Mayo Clinic Health Letter, 8*(11), 4.

25. Gutfield, G. (1991, October). Building a defensive back. *Men's Health,* 70–75.

26. Gutfield, 1991.

27. Abyad, A., & Boyer, J. T. (1992). Arthritis and aging. *Current Opinion in Rheumatology, 4,* 153–59.

28. Anonymous. (1990). Crohn's disease. *Mayo Clinic Health Letter, 8*(11), 4–5.

29. Gumaste, V. V., & Zimmerman, M. J. (1990). Diagnosis: Ulcerative colitis. *Hospital Medicine, 26,* 31–48.

30. Bronson, G. (1990, November/December). Mitigated gall. *Assets,* 92–93.

31. Anonymous. (1990). Gallbladder removal. *Mayo Clinic Health Letter, 8*(11), 1–2.

32. Bankhead, C. D. (1990). One-day cholecystectomy popular. *Medical World News, 31*(13), 48–49.

33. The Southern Surgeons Club. (1991). A prospective analysis of 1518 laparoscopic cholecystectomies. *NEJM, 324,* 1073–78

34. Anonymous. (1990, December 17). It's the dialysis machine that sets his place apart. *NYT,* B4.

35. Pak, C. Y. (1991). Etiology and treatment of urolithiasis. *American Journal of Kidney Diseases, 18,* 624–37.

36. Brody, J. E. (1992, July 8). Treating kidney stones becomes faster and safer. *NYT,* B8.

37. Gorman, C. (1992, June 22). Asthma: Deadly...but treatable. *Time,* 61–62.

38. Buist, A. S., & Vollmer, W. (1990, October 3). Reflections on the rise in asthma morbidity and mortality. *JAMA, 264,* 1719–20.

39. Weiss, K., & Wagener, D. (1990, October 3). Changing patterns of asthma mortality: Identifying target populations at high risk. *JAMA, 264,* 1683–87.

40. Ogushi, F., Hubbard, R. C., Vogelmeier, C. et al. (1991). Risk factors for emphysema: Cigarette smoking is associated with a reduction in the association rate of lung alpha 1-antitrypsin for neutrophil elastase. *Journal of Clinical Investigation, 87,* 1060–65.

41. Harris poll for Teledyne Water Pik. Cited in: Anonymous. (1991, November). Preach yes, practice no. *AH,* 22.

42. Berczuk, C. (1992, July 5). Are you afraid to go to the dentist? *Parade,* 12–13.

43. Wyngaarden, J. P. (1989). *Cecil-textbook of medicine* (29th ed.). Philadelphia: Saunders.

44. United Press International. (1990, June 9). Americans keeping their teeth longer, dental study finds. *SFC,* A8.

45. Brody, J. E. (1990, October 18). With cavities on decline, flossing is key weapon in battle for dental health. *NYT,* B8.

46. Addy, M., Dummer, P. M., Hunter, M. L. et al. (1990). The effect of toothbrushing frequency, toothbrushing hand, sex and social class on the incidence of plaque, gingivitis and pocketing in adolescents: A longitudinal cohort study. *Community Dental Health, 7,* 237–47.

47. Sicilia, A., Noguerol, B., Hernandez, R. et al. (1990). Relationship of dental treatment and oral hygiene to caries prevalence and need for periodontal treatment [Spanish]. *Avances En Odontoestomatologia, 6,* 343–49.

48. Papas, A. Quoted in: Bensimhon, D. (Ed.). (1991, October). Ask Men's Health. *Men's Health,* 16.

49. Hughes, R. (1993, January/February). Breaking the gum disease cycle. *AH,* 17.

50. Bedell, T. (1991, December). Floss, anyone? *Men's Health,* 20–21.

51. Gilliam, H. (1991, June 2). Taking the risk. *SFC, This World,* 7–11.

52. Siskin, B., Staller, J., & Rorvik, D. (1990, October). Chances are. *Men's Health,* 90.

53. Gilliam, 1991, 11.

54. Centers for Disease Control. Cited in: Kinsley, M. (1991, August 12). Red peril. *New Republic,* 4, 42.

55. Davis, B. (1992, August 6). Risk analysis measures need for regulation, but it's no science. *WSJ,* A1, A7.

56. Dinman, B. D. (1980). The reality and acceptance of risk. *JAMA, 244,* 1226–28.

57. Dinman, 1980.

58. Gilliam, 1991.

59. Gilliam, 1991.

60. Farley, C. J. (1991, March 28). Guarding against day-to-day, often deadly, risks. *USA Today,* 6D.

61. National Safety Council. (1988). *Accident facts.* Chicago: National Safety Council.

62. Kunz, J., & Finke, A. (Eds.). (1987). *The American Medical Association family medical guide* (rev. ed.). New York: Random House.

63. National Safety Council, 1988.

64. Coren, S. (1992). *The left-hander syndrome: The causes and consequences of left-handedness.* New York: Free Press.

65. National Safety Council, 1988.

66. National Safety Council, 1988.

67. Blyskal, J. (1993, January/February). Crash course: How to steer clear of your next auto accident. *AH,* 74–79.

68. Zane, M. (1992, January 28). More drivers running the signals. *SFC,* A1.

69. Brody, J. E. (1990, July 5). Why drivers fall asleep, and how to avoid becoming a statistic. *NYT,* B8.

70. Deutsch, G. (1990, October). Cruise control. *Men's Health,* 47, 82.

71. Associated Press. (1992, July 23). Drivers keep themselves busy. *SFC,* D3.

72. Ramirez, A. (1992, May 14). The life you save may be on the phone. *NYT,* D5.

73. Centers for Disease Control. Cited in: Associated Press. (1992, February 13). U.S. survey shows seat belt use is on the rise. *SFC,* D7.

74. Cory, D. (1989, November 12). Seat belt study assesses savings in medical costs and injuries. *NYT.*

75. Traffic Safety Now. (1987). *Buckle up.* Detroit: Traffic Safety Now, Inc.

76. Cushman, J. H. Jr. (1991, April 27). Officials say little is done to cut crashes in fog. *NYT,* 8.

77. Public Policy Research Institute, University of California, Irvine. (1987). *Orange County annual survey: 1987 final report.* Irvine, CA: University of California.

78. Berger, T. Cited in: Greenwald, J. (1992,

April). Driving yourself sane. *Health*, 86–89.

79. Meier, B. (1991, November 2). Auto safety vs. fuel economy: Questions of size and design. *NYT*, 12.

80. Hamilton, J. (1991, November/December). Safe by design. *Sierra*, 36–39.

81. Cushman, J. H. Jr. (1992, January 14). Auto roll-overs are new target of a U.S. push. *NYT*, A16.

82. Anonymous. (1991, September.) A tip for the taxi. *University of California, Berkeley, Wellness Letter*, 6.

83. Anonymous. (1992, December). Nonfatal vision. *Men's Health*, 27.

84. Sosin, D. M., Sacks, J. J., & Holmgreen, P. (1990). Head injury-associated deaths from motorcycle crashes: Relationship to helmet-use laws. *JAMA*, *264*, 2395–99.

85. Miller, T. C. (1992, July 28). Motorcycle fatalities decline. *SFC*, A15–A16.

86. Braddock, M., Schwartz, R., Lapidus, G. et al. (1992). A population-based study of motorcycle injury and costs. *Annals of Emergency Medicine*, *21*, 273–78.

87. Muelleman, R. L., Mlinek, E. J., & Collicott, P. E. (1992). Motorcycle crash injuries and costs: Effect of a reenacted comprehensive helmet use law. *Annals of Emergency Medicine*, *21*, 266–72.

88. Williams, M. (1991). The protective performance of bicyclists' helmets in accidents. *Accident Analysis & Prevention*, *23*, 119–31.

89. Thompson, R., Rivara, F., & Thompson, D. (1989, May 25). A case-control study of the effectiveness of bicycle safety helmets. *NEJM*, *320*, 1361–67.

90. Centers for Disease Control. (1988). Public health surveillance of 1990 injury control objectives for the nation. *MMWR Surveillance Summary*, *37*, 1–68.

91. Rand Corporation. Cited in: Otten, A. L. (1991, May 17). Accidents take big toll on health, earnings. *WSJ*, B1.

92. Baker, S. P., & Harvey, A. H. (1985). Fall injuries in the elderly. *Clinical Geriatric Medicine*, *1*, 501–12.

93. Cummings, S. R., Kelsey, J. L., Nevitt, M. C. et al. (1985). Epidemiology of osteoporosis and osteoporotic fractures. *Epidemiologic Reviews*, *7*, 178–208.

94. Centers for Disease Control, 1988.

95. McNeil, D. G. Jr. (1991, December 22). Why so many more Americans die in fires. *NYT*, sec. 4, 3.

96. Brodzka, W., Thornhill, H. L., & Howard, S. (1985). Burns: Causes and risk factors. *Archives of Physical Medicine & Rehabilitation*, *66*, 746–52.

97. U.S. Preventive Services Task Force. (1990). Counseling to prevent household and environmental injuries. *American Family Physician*, *42*, 135–42.

98. National Fire Protection Association. Cited in: McNeil, 1991.

99. McNeil, 1991.

100. McNeil, 1991.

101. Brody, J. E. (1991, October 30). Have smoke detectors? Do they work? Thinking about the unthinkable: a home fire. *NYT*, B9.

102. National Safety Council. (1985). *Accident facts*. Chicago: National Safety Council.

103. Associated Press. (1992, October 28). The first step in CPR is now to call for help. *NYT*, B6.

104. Robinson, A. G. (1991, April). Painful mistakes. *Men's Health*, 32.

105. Centers for Disease Control, 1988.

106. Spyker, D. A. (1985). Submersion injury: Epidemiology, prevention, and management. *Pediatric Clinics of North America*, *32*, 113–25.

107. Wintemute, G. J., Kraus, J. F., Teret, S. P. et al. (1988). The epidemiology of drowning in adulthood: Implications for prevention.

American Journal of Preventive Medicine, *4*, 343–48.

108. Wintemute et al., 1988.

109. Powers, R. D. (1990). Taking care of bite wounds. *Emergency Medicine*, *22*, 131–39.

110. Serrin, W. (1991, January 28). The wages of work. *Nation*, 80.

111. Serrin, 1991.

112. Lacayo, R. (1991, September 16). Death on the shop floor. *Time*, 28–29.

113. Associated Press. (1991, November 20). Big jump in on-the-job injuries, illnesses. *SFC*, A6.

114. Nobel, C. (1992, February/March). Keeping OSHA's feet to the fire. *Technology Review*, 42–51.

115. Nobel, 1992.

116. Monthly Labor Review. (June 1991). Cited in: Anonymous. (1991, October). Careful with that knife. *American Demographics*, 18.

117. National Safety Council. Cited in: Milbank, D. (1991, March 29). Companies turn to peer pressure to cut injuries as psychologists join the battle. *WSJ*, B1, B3.

118. Siegel, M. Cited in: Fernandez, E. (1992, October 23). Study says smoky air endangers waitresses. *SFE*, A-1, A-22.

119. Greenwood, S. (1989, November/December). Workplace hazards. *Medical SelfCare*, 19–20.

120. Hopkins, A. (1990). The social recognition of repetition strain injuries: An Australian/American comparison. *Social Science & Medicine*, *30*, 365–72.

121. Mandel, S. (1990). Overuse syndrome in musicians: When playing an instrument hurts. *Postgraduate Medicine*, *88*, 111–14.

122. Thompson, J. S., & Phelps, T. H. (1990). Repetitive strain injuries: How to deal with 'the epidemic of the 1990s.' *Postgraduate Medicine*, *88*, 143–49.

123. Hembree, D., & Sandoval, R. (1991, August). RSI has become the nation's leading work-related illness. How are editors and reporters coping with it? *Columbia Journalism Review*, 41–46.

124. Kilborn, P. T. (1990, June 24). Automation: Pain replaces the old drudgery. *NYT*, sec. 1, 1, 11.

125. Horowitz, J. M. (1992, October 12). Crippled by computers. *Time*, 70–72.

126. Roel, R. E. (1991, July/August). Wrist watch. *AH*, 72–75.

127. Associated Press. (1990, November 16). Job illness rose by 43,000 for 1989. *NYT*, A13.

128. Fingerhut, L. A., & Kleinman, J. C. (1990). International and interstate comparisons of homicide among young males. *JAMA*, *263*, 3292–95.

129. U.S. Department of Justice. (1986). *Criminal victimization in United States, 1984: A national crime survey report*. Pub. No. (NCJ)100435. Washington, DC: U.S. Department of Justice.

130. Mercy, J. A., & O'Carroll, P. W. (1988). New directions in violence prediction: The public health arena. *Violence & Victims*, *3*, 285–301.

131. Reuters. (1992, March 27). Canada worries about climbing murder rate. *SFC*, A10.

132. Fingerhut & Kleinman, 1990.

133. Fingerhut & Kleinman, 1990.

134. Spivak, H., Hausman, A. J., & Prothrow-Stith, D. (1989). Practitioners' forum: Public health and the primary prevention of adolescent violence: The violence prevention project. *Violence & Victims*, *4*, 203–12.

135. Page, R. M., Kitchin-Becker, S., Solovan, D. et al. (1991). Interpersonal violence: A priority issue for health education. *Journal of Health Education*, *23*, 286–91.

136. Page et al., 1991, 287.

137. Messner, S. F. (1988). Research on cultural and socioeconomic factors in criminal violence. *Psychiatric Clinics of North America*, *11*, 511–25.

138. Ropp, L., Visintainer, P., Uman, J. et al. (1992). Death in the city: An American childhood tragedy. *JAMA*, *267*, 2905–10.

139. Page et al., 1991.

140. U.S. Department of Health and Human Services. (1987). *Alcohol and health*. DHHS Pub. No. (ADM)87-1519. Washington, DC: Department of Health and Human Services.

141. Page et al., 1991.

142. Bell, C. A. (1991). Female homicides in United States workplaces, 1980–1985. *AJPH*, *81*, 729–32.

143. Eckholm, E. (1992, March 8). Ailing gun industry confronts outrage over glut of violence. *NYT*, sec. 1, 1.

144. Hilts, P. J. (1992, June 10). Gunshot wounds become second-leading cause of death for teen-agers. *NYT*, A14.

145. National Safety Council, 1985.

146. Blumenthal, D. (1991, March 30). How to keep guns safely. *NYT*, 4.

147. Associated Press. (1990, July 9). Justice Dept. says pistols used in 44 percent of murders. *SFC*, A4.

148. Kilborn, P. T. (1992, March 9). The gun culture: Fun as well as life and death. *NYT*, A1.

149. Eckholm, E. (1992, April 3). Thorny issue in gun control: Curbing responsible owners. *NYT*, A1, A15.

150. Reuters. (1991, November 8). Canada's Parliament votes for gun control legislation. *NYT*, A6.

151. Marcus, J. (1992, September 13). Crime reports reveal dangers on campuses. *SFE*, A-4.

152. Trost, C. (1992, September 30). Carjacking spreads to nation's suburbs, raising fear there are no safe havens. *WSJ*, B1, B10.

153. McDowell, E. (1992, October 28). Threat of crime rises on the main highways. *NYT*, A7.

154. San Jose State University Police Department. (1989). *Safety and security at San Jose State*. San Jose, CA: San Jose State University, Police Department, Investigations/Crime Prevention Unit.

155. Terry, D. (1992, April 3). Failed by law, women seek bodyguards' help. *NYT*, A10.

156. Brody, J. E. (1992, March 18). Each year, six million American women become victims of abuse without ever leaving home. *NYT*, B6.

157. Todd, J. S. (1992, December). A terrible national secret. *Living Well*, 108.

158. Herman, J. L. (1992). *Trauma and recovery*. New York: Basic.

159. Sonnenberg, S. M. (1988). Victims of violence and post-traumatic stress disorder. *Psychiatric Clinics of North America*, *11*, 581–90.

160. Brody, 1992 (March 18).

161. Kutner, L. (1991, November 14). A large number of teen-age girls have become caught up in abusive relationships. *NYT*, B4.

162. Saunders, D. B. Cited in: Anonymous. (1992, September/October). Men of mean. *PT*, 18.

163. Brody, 1992 (March 18).

164. Miedzian, M. (1991). *Boys will be boys: Breaking the link between masculinity and violence*. New York: Doubleday.

165. Gray, A., Jackson, D. N., & McKinlay, J. B. (1991). The relation between dominance, anger, and hormones in normally aging men: Results from the Massachusetts Male Aging Study. *Psychosomatic Medicine*, *53*, 375–85.

166. Brody, 1992 (March 18).

167. Irving, C. (1991, August 18). Why battered women stay with abusers. *SFE*, A-5. [Graham, D., & Rawlings, E. Paper presented to American Psychological Assocation convention, San Francisco, August 17, 1991.]

168. Brody, 1992.

169. U.S. Department of Justice. Cited in: French, M. (1992). *The war against women*. New York: Summit.

170. Sward, S. (1991, May 18). Struggling with a universal scourge. *SFC*, A1, A6.

171. Lewin, T. (1992, June 7). When women bat-

ter men. *SFC, Sunday Punch*, 6; reprinted from *NYT*.

172. Coleman, D. H., & Straus, M. A. (1986). Marital power, conflict, and violence in a nationally representative sample of American couples. *Violence & Victims*, 1, 141–57.

173. National Center for Prevention of Child Abuse. Cited in: Toufexis, A. (1992, November 23). When kids kill abusive parents. *Time*, 60–61.

174. U.S. Department of Health and Human Services. (1989). *Child abuse and neglect: A shared community concern.* DHHS Pub. No. (HDS)89-30531. Washington, DC: Clearinghouse on Child Abuse and Neglect Information.

175. U.S. Department of Health and Human Services, 1989.

176. U.S. Department of Health and Human Services, 1989.

177. Hinds, M. deC. (1992, November 6). Child sex-abuse: Hard to prove, to much dismay. *NYT*, B12.

178. Thomas, J. N., Rogers, C. M., Lloyd, D. et al. (1985). *Child sexual abuse: Implications for public health practice.* Rockville, MD: Division of Maternal and Child Health, U.S. Department of Health and Human Services.

179. Turner, R. (1991). One in seven 6th–12th graders had an unwanted sexual encounter, including one in five females. *Family Planning Perspectives*, 23, 286–87.

180. Maltz, W. (1990, December). Adult survivors of incest: How to help them overcome the trauma. *Medical Aspects of Human Sexuality*, 42–47.

181. Maltz, 1990.

182. Gorman, C. (1991, October 7). Incest comes out of the dark. *Time*, 46–47.

183. Darnton, N., Springen, K., Wright, L. et al. (1991, October 7). The pain of the last taboo. *Newsweek*, 70–72.

184. Tavris, C. (1993, January 3). Beware the incest-survivor machine. *New York Times Book Review*, 16.

185. U.S. Supreme Court, *Meritor Savings Bank v. Vinson.* Cited in: Goldstein, L. (1991, November). Hands off at work. *Self*, 110–13.

186. U.S. Merit Systems Protection Board. Cited in: Deutschman, A. (1991, November 4). Dealing with sexual harassment. *Fortune*, 145–48.

187. Anonymous. (1991, October 12). Proving harassment is tough in court, lawyers say. *SFC*, C10; reprinted from *NYT*.

188. Karl, T. Cited in: O'Toole, K. (1991, November–December). How to handle harassment. *Stanford Observer*, 8.

189. U.S. Merit Systems Protection Board, 1991.

190. Anonymous. (1989, April). Offering resistance: How most people respond to rape. *PT*, 13.

191. Stanford Rape Education Project. Cited in: Anonymous. (1991, January–February). Men, women interpret sexual cues differently. *Stanford Observer*, 15.

192. National Victim Center. Cited in: Anonymous. (1992, May 4). Unsettling report on an epidemic of rape. *Time*, 15.

193. Celis, W. 3d. (1991, January 2). Growing talk of date rape separates sex from assault. *NYT*, A1, B7.

194. Celis, 1991, B7.

195. Stanford Rape Education Project, 1991.

196. Coffe, J. (1993, January–February). To escape rape. *AH*, 18.

197. Schroepfer, L. (1992, November). When the victim is a woman. *AH*, 20.

198. Gross, J. (1991, May 28). Even the victim can be slow to recognize rape. *NYT*, A6.

199. Darden, D. (1990, May). How bored are you? *Self*, 237.

200. McGiboney, G. W., & Carter, C. (1988). Boredom proneness and adolescents' personalities. *Psychological Reports*, 63, 741–42.

201. Anonymous. Quoted in: Kiechel, W. III.

(1984, March 5). Chairmen of the bored. *Fortune*, 175–76.

202. Csikszentmihalyi, M. (1975). *Beyond boredom and anxiety.* San Francisco: Jossey-Bass.

203. Csikszentmihalyi, M. (1990). *Flow: The psychology of optimal experience.* New York: HarperCollins.

204. Goleman, D. (1986, March 4). Concentration is likened to euphoric states of mind. *NYT*, 21–22.

205. Alderson, J. W. (1990, May). Boredom. *Self*, 236–37, 262, 272.

206. Scitovsky, T. (1980, October). Why do we seek more and more excitement? *Stanford Observer*, 13.

207. Zuckerman, M. Cited in: Weiss, R. (1987, November 12). Finding out why we take chances. *SFE*, E1, E4; reprinted from *Science News*.

208. Greydanus, D. E. (1987). Risk-taking behaviors in adolescence. *JAMA*, 258, 2110.

209. Blum, R. (1987). Contemporary threats to adolescent health in the United States. *JAMA*, 257, 3390–95.

210. Goleman, D. (1987, December 2). Why teenagers are reckless. *SFC*, B8; reprinted from *NYT*.

211. Robinson, T. N., Killen, J. D., Taylor, C. B. et al. (1987). Perspectives on adolescent substance use: A defined population study. *JAMA*, 258, 2072–76.

212. MacDonald, N. E., Wells, G. A., Fisher, W. A. et al. (1990). High-risk STD/HIV behavior among college students. *JAMA*, 263, 3155–59.

213. Katz, J. (1990). *Seductions of crime: Moral and sensual attractions in doing evil.* New York: Basic.

214. Zuckerman, M. Cited in: Goleman, 1987, December 2.

215. Irwin, C. Cited in: Goleman, 1987, December 2.

216. Hamburg, B. A. Cited in: Goleman, 1987, December 2.

217. Weinstein, N. D. (1984). Why it won't happen to me: Perceptions of risk factors and susceptibility. *Health Psychology*, 3, 431–57.

218. Weinstein, N. D. (1987). Unrealistic optimism about illness susceptibility: Conclusions from a community-wide sample. *Journal of Behavioral Medicine*, 10, 481–500.

219. Jeffery, R. W. (1989). Risk behaviors and health: Contrasting individual and population perspectives. *American Psychologist*, 44, 1194–1202.

220. Taylor, S. E., & Brown, J. D. (1988). Illusion and well-being: A social psychological perspective on mental health. *Psychological Bulletin*, 103, 193–210.

221. Weinstein, 1987.

222. Adler, N. Quoted in: Goleman, 1987, December 2.

223. Zimbardo, P. Cited in: Goleman, D. (1986, December 30). Perception of time emerges as key psychological factor. *NYT*, 15–16.

224. McReynolds, W. T., Green, L., & Fisher, E. B. Jr. (1983). Self-control as choice management with reference to the behavioral treatment of obesity. *Health Psychology*, 2, 261–76.

UNIT 13: CONQUERING HEART DISEASE AND CANCER

1. Tsevat, J., Weinstein, M. C., Williams, L. W. et al. (1991). Expected gains in life expectancy from various coronary heart disease risk factor modifications. *Circulation*, 83, 1194–1201.

2. Zaret, B. L., Moser, M., Cohen, L. S. et al. (Eds.) (1992). *Yale University School of Medicine heart book.* New York: Hearst.

3. Zaret et al., 1992.

4. American Heart Association. (1991). *1991 Heart and stroke facts.* Dallas: American Heart Association.

5. McGrady, A., & Higgins, J. Jr. (1990, February). Effect of repeated measurements of blood pressure on blood pressure in essential hypertension: Role of anxiety. *Journal of Behavioral Medicine*, 93, 93–101.

6. American Heart Association, 1991.

7. Cohen, L. S. (1992). What can go wrong. In Zaret et al. (Eds.), 11–20.

8. Kelemen, M. H., Effront, M. B., Valenti, S. A. et al. (1990). Exercise training combined with antihypertensive drug therapy: Effects on lipids, blood pressure, and left ventricular mass. *JAMA*, 263, 2766–71.

9. Cohen, 1992.

10. Cohen, 1992.

11. Brass, L. M. (1992). Stroke. In Zaret et al. (Eds.), 215–33.

12. Brass, 1992.

13. Kleinman, C. S. (1992). Heart disease in the young. In Zaret et al. (Eds.), 247–62.

14. Kleinman, 1992.

15. Kuntz, R. E., Piana, R., Pomerantz, R. M. et al. (1992). Changing incidence and management of abrupt closure following coronary intervention in the new device era. *Catheterization & Cardiovascular Diagnosis*, 27, 183–90.

16. Baldwin, J. C., Elefteriades, J. A., & Kopf, G. S. (1992). Heart surgery. In Zaret et al. (Eds.), 313–29.

17. Associated Press. (1991, July 24). Total mechanical heart expected in 20 years. *SFC*, A3.

18. Ornish, D. M., Brown, S. E., Scherwitz, L. W. et al. (1990). Can lifestyle changes reverse coronary heart disease? The Lifestyle Heart Trial. *Lancet*, 336, 129–33.

19. Ornish, D. (1990). *Dr. Dean Ornish's program for reversing heart disease: The only system scientifically proven to reverse heart disease without drugs or surgery.* New York: Ballantine.

20. Kittner, S. J., White, L. R., Losonczy, K. G. et al. (1990). Black-white differences in stroke incidence in a national sample. *JAMA*, 264, 1267–70.

21. Murray, R. F. (1991). Skin color and blood pressure. *JAMA*, 265, 639–40.

22. Ostfeld, A. (1992). Racial and ethnic differences in heart disease. In Zaret et al. (Eds.), 273–80.

23. Black, H. R. (1992). Cardiovascular risk factors. In Zaret et al. (Eds.), 23–26.

24. Zahler, R., & Piselli, C. (1992). Smoking, alcohol, and drugs. In Zaret et al. (Eds.), 71–84.

25. Zahler & Piselli, 1992.

26. Luckmann, J., & Sorenson, K. (1987). *Medical-surgical nursing: A psychophysiologic approach* (3rd ed.). Philadelphia: Saunders.

27. U.S. Public Health Service. (1989). *Report of the expert panel on dection, evaluation, and treatment of high blood cholesterol in adults.* DHHS Pub. No. (NIH)89-2925. Washington, DC: U.S. Department of Health and Human Services.

28. U.S. Public Health Service (1988). *The Surgeon General's report on nutrition and health.* DHHS Pub. No. (PHS)88-50210. Washington, DC: U.S Department of Health and Human Services.

29. Manson, J. E., Tosteson, H., Ridker, P. M. et al. (1990). A prospective study of obesity and risk of coronary heart disease in women. *NEJM*, 326, 1406–16.

30. Ekelund, L G., Haskell, W. L., Johnson, J. L. et al. (1988). Physical fitness as a predictor of cardiovascular mortality in asymptomatic North American men. The Lipid Research Clinics Mortality Follow-up Study. *NEJM*, 319, 1379–84.

31. Friedman, M., & Rosenman, R. H. (1974). *Type A behavior and your heart.* Greenwich, CT: Knopf.

32. Friedman, M., Thoreson, C. E., Gill, J. J. et al. (1986). Alteration of Type A behavior and its effect on cardiac recurrences in post myocardial infarction patients: Summary results of the

recurrent coronary prevention project. *American Heart Journal, 112*, 653–65.

33. Schnall, P. L., Pieper, C., Schwartz, J. E. et al. (1990). The relationship between 'job strain,' workplace diastolic blood pressure, and left ventricular mass index. *JAMA, 263*, 1929–35.

34. Ornish, D. M., Scherwitz, L. W., Doody, R. S. et al. (1983). Effects of stress management training and dietary changes in treating ischemic heart disease. *JAMA, 249*, 54–59.

35. Ornish, D. M. (1983). *Stress, diet, & your heart*. New York: New American Library (Signet).

36. Ornish et al., 1990.

37. Koten, J., & McWethy, V. L. (1990, May 11). Do as we do. *WSJ*, R26.

38. Koten & McWethy, 1990.

39. Willard, J. E., Lange, R. A., & Hillis, L. D. (1992). The use of aspirin in ischemic heart disease. *NEJM, 327*, 175–200.

40. Brody, J. E. (1991, October 31). Lower dose of aspirin is safe and effective, new study finds. *NYT*, A17.

41. Public Health Service. (1990). *Healthy people 2000: National health promotion and disease prevention objectives*. DHHS Pub. No. (PHS)91-50212. Washington, DC: U.S. Department of Health and Human Services.

42. Dollinger, M., Rosenbaum, E. H., & Cable, G. (1991). *Everyone's guide to cancer therapy: How cancer is diagnosed, treated, and managed day to day*. Kansas City, MO: Andrews & McMeel (Somerville House).

43. Dollinger, Rosenbaum, & Cable, 1991.

44. Mitchell, M. S. (1991). Melanoma. In Dollinger, Rosenbaum, & Cable (Eds.), 428.

45. American Cancer Society (1990). *Cancer facts and figures*. Atlanta: American Cancer Society.

46. U.S. Public Health Service. (1987). *Testicular cancer: Research report*. Pub. No. (NIH)87-654. Washington, DC: U.S. Department of Health and Human Services.

47. Dollinger, M., & Rosenbaum, E. H. (1991). How cancer is diagnosed. In Dollinger, Rosenbaum, & Cable (Eds.), 11–20.

48. Cassileth, B. R. Questionable and unproven cancer therapies. (1991). In Dollinger, Rosenbaum, & Cable (Eds.), 91–96.

49. Cassileth, 1991.

50. Rosenbaum, E. H., Dollinger, M., & Newell, G. R. (1991). Risk assessment, cancer screening and prevention. In Dollinger, Rosenbaum, & Cable (Eds.), 186–92.

51. Finklestein, J. Z. Childhood cancers. (1991). In Dollinger, Rosenbaum, & Cable (Eds.), 285–93.

52. Slater-Freedberg, J. R., & Arndt, K. A. Skin. (1991). In Dollinger, Rosenbaum, & Cable (Eds.), 503–509.

53. U.S. Public Health Service, 1990.

54. Rosenbaum, Dollinger, & Newell, 1991.

55. U.S. Public Health Service, 1990.

56. Rosenbaum, Dollinger, & Newell, 1991.

57. Davis, W. (1990, December). High-touch medicine. *AH*, 46–48.

58. Cousins, N. (1976). Anatomy of an illness (as perceived by the patient). *NEJM, 295*, 1458–63.

59. Cousins, N. (1979). *Anatomy of an illness*. New York: Norton.

60. Cousins, N. (1983). *The healing heart: Antidotes to panic and helplessness*. New York: Norton.

61. O'Regan, B. (1989, Winter). Healing, remission, and miracle cures. *Whole Earth Review*, 126–35.

62. Spiegel, D., Bloom, J. R., Kraemer, H. C. et al. (1989). Effect of psychosocial treatment on survival of patients with metastatic breast cancer. *Lancet, 2*(8668), 888–91.

63. Levoy, G. (1990). Mind over medicine. *SFC, Sunday Punch*, 6; reprinted from *Longevity*.

64. Straus, H. (1989, May). The Lazarus file:

When the "spontaneous" cure comes from within. *AH*, 67–75.

65. O'Regan, 1989.

66. Weinstock, C. Quoted in: Levoy, 1990.

67. Papac, R. J. Quoted in: Hall, S. S. (1992, April). Cheating fate. *Health*, 38–46.

68. Papac, R. J. (1990). Spontaneous regression of cancer. *Connecticut Medicine, 54*, 179–82.

69. Glaser, R., & Kiecolt-Glaser, J. Cited in: Jaret, P. (1992, November/December). Mind over malady. *Health*, 87–94.

70. Kiecolt-Glaser, J. K, & Glaser, R. (1992). Psychoneuroimmunology: Can psychological interventions modulate immunity? *Journal of Consulting & Clinical Psychology, 60*, 569–75.

71. Davis, 1990.

72. O'Regan, 1989.

73. Siegel, B. (1986). *Love, medicine, and miracles*. New York: Harper & Row.

74. Siegel, B. Quoted in: Zuromski, P., & Zuromski, L. (1989, September/October). Medical visionary Bernie Siegel, M.D. [interview]. *Medical SelfCare*, 66–67.

75. O'Regan, B. Cited in: Straus, 1989.

76. Glick, D. (1992, July 13). New Age meets Hippocrates. *Newsweek*, 58.

77. Levy, S. Quoted in: Ludtke, M. (1990, March 12). Can the mind help cure disease? *Time*, 76–78.

78. Marantz, P. R. (1990). Blaming the victim: The negative consequence of preventive medicine. *AJPH, 80*, 1186–87.

79. Siegel, B. Quoted in: Straus, 1989, 75.

80. Simonton, S. Quoted in: Levoy, 1990.

UNIT 14: USING HEALTH RESOURCES

1. Moog, C. (1990). *"Are they selling her lips?": Advertising and identity*. New York: Morrow.

2. Klaidman, S. (1991). *Health in the headlines: The stories behind the stories*. New York: Oxford University Press.

3. Kahane, H. (1988). *Logic and contemporary rhetoric: The use of reason in everyday life* (5th ed.). Belmont, CA: Wadsworth.

4. Fishman, S. (1993, April). The powerful patient. *Health*, 74–78.

5. Ferguson, T. (1992, January–February). Patient, heal thyself: Health in the information age. *The Futurist*, 9–14.

6. Fiorello, J., & Siegel, B. Cited in: Ferguson, 1992.

7. Ferguson, 1992, 10.

8. U.S. Preventive Services Task Force. Cited in: Anonymous. (1991, May). Preventive care: From self-care to lab tests. *University of California, Berkeley, Wellness Letter*, 4–5.

9. Ferguson, 1992.

10. Editors of the University of California, Berkeley, *Wellness Letter*. (1991). *The wellness encyclopedia: The comprehensive family resource for safeguarding health and preventing illness*. Boston: Houghton Mifflin.

11. Angier, N. (1992, June 21). Bedside manners improve as more women enter medicine. *NYT*, sec. 4, 18.

12. Rosenthal, E. (1991, January 16). Don't call 'em 'Doctor.' *SFC*, B5; reprinted from *NYT*.

13. Hamilton, J. (1988, March). Shopping-mall medicine. *AH*, 106–13.

14. Council on Scientific Affairs. (1990, March 2). Home care in the 1990s. *JAMA, 263*, 1241–44.

15. Public Citizen Health Research Group. (1991). *9,479 questionable doctors disciplined by states or the federal government*. Washington, DC: Public Citizen Health Research Group (2000 P St. NW, Washington, DC 20036).

16. Maher, V. F. (1992). International migration and medical credentialling. *Medicine & Law, 11*, 275–79.

17. Goleman, D. (1991, November 26). Doctors find comfort is a potent medicine. *NYT*, B5, B8.

18. Nazario, S. L. (1992, March 17). Medical science seeks a cure for doctors suffering from boorish bedside manner. *WSJ*, B1, B10.

19. Nazario, 1992.

20. Nazario, 1992.

21. Belkin, L. (1992, June 4). In lessons on empathy, doctors become patients. *NYT*, A1, A13.

22. Anonymous. (1992, October 4). Wanted—doctors who are human. *SFC, Sunday Punch*, 2; reprinted from *NYT*.

23. Seligmann, J., Murr, A., Rosenberg, D., & Barrett, T. (1991, August 12). Making TLC a requirement. *Newsweek*, 56–57.

24. Winslow, R. (1989, October 5). Sometimes, talk is the best medicine. *WSJ*, B1.

25. American Medical Association. Cited in: Colburn, D. (1991, October 24). Are physicals worth it? *SFC*, B5.

26. American Society of Internal Medicine. Cited in: Editors of the University of California, Berkeley, *Wellness Letter*. (1991).

27. Anonymous. (1990). Complete blood count. *Medical Times, 118*, C26–C27.

28. Weil, A. (1990). *Natural health, natural medicine*. Boston: Houghton Mifflin.

29. Kolata, G. (1993, February 26). Studies say mammograms fail to help many women. *NYT*, A1, A10.

30. Willensky, D. (1992, March). Vital signs. *AH*, 100–103.

31. Brody, J. E. (1992, September 16). Ignoring the doctor's orders has become a costly and deadly epidemic. *NYT*, B6.

32. National Council on Patient Information and Education. Cited in: Brody, 1992.

33. Bronson, G. (1991, April). A consumer's guide to making your surgery as painless as possible. *AH*, 34–40.

34. Dowie, S. (1988, September/October). Your personal hospital survival kit. *Medical SelfCare*, 32–36.

35. Anonymous. (1991). *Physicians' desk reference* (44th ed.). Oradel, NJ: Medical Economics.

36. Anonymous. (1991). The top 200 Rx drugs of 1990. *American Druggist, 203*, 56–68.

37. Anonymous. (1990, May). Generic drugs: Still safe? *Consumer Reports*, 310–13.

38. Anonymous. (1991). Annual Rx review: No letup in Rx market expansion. *Drug Topics, 135*, 53–58.

39. Cramer, J. A., Mattson, R. H., Prevey, M. L. et al. (1989). How often is medication taken as prescribed? A novel assessment technique. *JAMA, 261*, 3273–77.

40. Anonymous. (1991). Are drugs approved by the FDA safe and risk free? *National Medical-Legal Journal, 2*, 8.

41. Hilts, P. J. (1990, May 27). Dangers of some new drugs go undetected, study says. *NYT*, 10.

42. Chastain, S. (1992, February–March). The accidental addict: Are you hooked on your prescriptions? *Modern Maturity*, 39.

43. Katzenstein, L. (1991, April). Rx to OTC: Who pays and who profits when prescription drugs go over the counter. *AH*, 49–53.

44. Edeson, E. (1991, November). What a relief: A guide to nonprescription pain medication. *AH*, 63–65.

45. Cowley, G., & Hager, M. (1990, March 12). Some counter intelligence. *Newsweek*, 82, 84.

46. Roine, R., Gentry, R. T., Hernandez-Munoz, R. et al. (1990). Aspirin increases blood-alcohol concentrations in humans after ingestion of ethanol. *JAMA, 264*, 2406–08.

47. Krieger, L. M. (1990, April 8). Beware what's over the counter. *SFE*, D-16, D-15.

48. Edeson, 1991.

49. Wootton, F. T., & Lee, W. M. (1990). Acetaminophen hepatotoxicity in the alcoholic. *Southern Medical Journal, 83*, 1047–49.

50. Foust, R. T., Reddy, K. R., Jeffers, L. J. et al. (1989). Nyquil-associated liver injury. *American Journal of Gastroenterology, 84*, 422–25.

51. Gengo, F. M. Cited in: Zoler, M. L. (1990). Antihistamines can bomb drivers. *Medical*

World News, *31*, 19.

52. National Consumers League. Cited in: Furtado, T. (1992, March). The over-the-counter culture. *Health*, 28–30.

53. Levy, L. Quoted in: Furtado, 1992, 30.

54. Taylor, M. G. (1990). *Insuring national health care: The Canadian experience*. Chapel Hill, NC: University of North Carolina Press.

55. Marmor, T. R., & Godfrey, J. (1992, July 23). Canada's medical system is a model. That's a fact. *NYT*, A17.

56. Farnsworth, C. H. (1992, February 17). Canadians defend care system against criticism. *NYT*, C8.

57. Garrison, J. (1990, October 10). Canada's system cuts costs for all, *SFE*, A-1, A-12.

58. Goad, G. P. (1991, December 3). Canada seems satisfied with a medical system that covers everyone. *WSJ*, A1, A10.

59. Canadian Medical Association. Cited in: Barnhill, W. (1992, November–December). Canadian health care: Would it work here? *Arthritis Today*, 35–44.

60. Roos, L. L., Fisher, E. S., Sharp, S. M. et al. (1990). Postsurgical mortality in Manitoba and New England. *JAMA*, *263*, 2453–58.

61. Schmitz, A. (1991, January/February). Health assurance. *In Health*, 39–47.

62. Farnsworth, 1992.

63. Morganthau, T., & Hagen, M. (1992, February 3). Cutting through the gobbledygook. *Newsweek*, 24–25.

64. Anonymous. (1992, July 27). Comparing health care. *Fortune*, 80.

65. Felsenthal, E. (1993, March 1). Doctors are spurring effort to remedy the nation's ailing malpractice system. *WSJ*, B1, B4.

66. Garland, S. B., & Freundlich, N. (1991, February 18). Insurers vs. doctors: Who knows best? *Business Week*, 64–65.

67. Garrison, J. (1990, October 9). Caught in a trap of technology. *SFE*,, A-1, A-10.

68. Fuchs, V. R., & Hahn, J. S. (1990). How does Canada do it? A comparison of expenditures for physicians' services in the United States and Canada. *NEJM*, *323*, 884–90.

69. Pear, R., & Eckholm, E. (1991, June 2). When healers are entrepreneurs: A debate over costs and ethics. *NYT*, 1, 17.

80. Anonymous, 1992. Comparing health care.

87. Veres, R. N., & Mason, J. (1991, October/November). To your health. *Investment Vision*, 61–63.

72. Anomymous. (1992, August). Are HMOs the answer? *Consumer Reports*, 519–31.

73. Mackowiak, P. A., Wasserman, S. S., & Levine, M. M. (1992). A critical appraisal of 98.6 degrees F, the upper limit of the normal body temperature, and other legacies of Carl Reinhold August Wunderlich. *JAMA*, *268*, 1578–80.

74. *Time*/CNN poll taken October 23, 1991, by Yankelovich Clancy Schuman. Cited in: Horowitz, J. M., & Lafferty, E. (1991, November 4). Why new age medicine is catching on. *Time*, 68–76.

75. Horowitz & Lafferty, 1991.

76. Begley, S. (1992, April). Alternative medicine: A cure for what ails us? *AH*, 39–40, 44, 46.

77. Fultz, O. (1992, April). Chiropractic: What can it do for you? *AH*, 41–43.

78. Shekelle, P. G., & Brook, R. H. (1991). A community-based study of the use of chiropractic services. *AJPH*, *81*, 439–42.

79. Brody, J. E. (1991, November 23). Acupressure eases morning sickness. *SFC*, C4; reprinted from *NYT*.

80. George, L. (1992, April). Acupuncture: Drug free pain relief. *AH*, 45.

81. Begley, 1992.

82. Horowitz & Lafferty, 1991.

83. Glick, D. (1992, July 13). New age meets Hippocrates. *Newsweek*, 58.

84. Newman, J. (1992, April). Homeopathy: Diluted or deluded? *AH*, 47.

85. Gorman, J. (1992, August 30). Take a little deadly nightshade and you'll feel better. *New York Times Magazine*, 23–25, 73.

86. Sears, C. (1991, October). Herbal confusion. *AH*, 78–82.

87. Nolen, W. A. (1974). *Healing: A doctor in search of a miracle*. New York: Random House.

88. Brenneman, R. J. (1990). *Deadly blessings: Faith healing on trial*. Buffalo, NY: Prometheus.

89. Randi, J. (1982). *Flim-flam! Psychics, ESP, unicorns, and other delusions*. Buffalo, NY: Prometheus.

90. Joyce, C. (1988, December 3). Cited in: Kaszuba, P. (1991, July/August). Psychics and suckers? *Utne Reader*, 27–30.

91. Barrett, S. (1991, March). Quack, quack: 30 ways to duck medicine's con artists. *AH*, 59–63.

92. Food and Drug Administration and Council of Better Business Bureaus. (1988). *Quackery targets teens*. HHS Pub. No. (FDA)88-1147. Rockville, MD: Department of Health and Human Services.

93. Masland, T., & Marshall, R. (1990, November 5). 'A really nasty business.' *Newsweek*, 36–43.

94. Federal Trade Commission. Cited in: Associated Press. (1992, May 25). How not to be fooled by diet programs. *SFC*, D4.

95. Adams, J. M. (1991, August 5). The clearest message may be: 'Buy this tape.' *Boston Globe*, 37, 40.

96. Bjork, R. A., & Druckman, D. (1991, November 5). The real message in human potential game. *SFC*, A19.

97. Barrett, 1991.

98. Wild, R. (1992, April). Maximize your brain power. *Men's Health*, 44–49.

99. Randi, J. (1992, April 13). Help stamp out absurd beliefs. *Time*, 80.

100. Ruchlis, H., & Oddo, S. (1990). *Clear thinking: A practical introduction*. Buffalo, NY: Prometheus, 109.

101. Kahane, H. (1988). *Logic and contemporary rhetoric: The use of reason in everyday life* (5th ed.) Belmont, CA: Wadsworth.

102. Rasool, J., Banks, C., & McCarthy, M.-J. (1993). *Critical thinking: Reading and writing in a diverse world*. Belmont, CA: Wadsworth, 132.

103. Rasool, Banks, & McCarthy, 1993, 132.

UNIT 15: AGING WELL AND COPING WITH DEATH

1. Gardner, J. W. (1991, June 16). Commencement address, Stanford University, Stanford, CA. Quoted in: Anonymous. (1991, June 17). Life is an endless unfolding Stanford graduates are told. *NYT*, 91.

2. Anonymous. (1991, April). You are what you were. *Johns Hopkins Medical Letter*, 3.

3. Field, D., & Millsap, R. E. (1991). Personality in advanced old age: continuity or change? *Journal of Gerontology*, *46*(6), P299–308.

4. Hagberg, B., Samuelsson, G., Lindberg, B., & Dehlin, O. (1991). Stability and change of personality in old age and its relation to survival. *Journal of Gerontology*, *46*(6), P285–91.

5. Field, D. (1991). Continuity and change in personality in old age—evidence from five longitudinal studies: Introduction to a special issue. *Journal of Gerontology*, *46*(6), P271–74.

6. Magnani, L. E. (1990). Hardiness, self-perceived health, and activity among independently functioning older adults. *Scholarly Inquiry for Nursing Practice*, *4*(3), 171–84.

7. Plouffe, L., & Gravelle, F. (1989). Age, sex, and personality correlates of self-actualization in elderly adults. *Psychological Reports*, *65*, 643–47.

8. Lafavore, M. (1990, October). Living long *and* well is a better revenge. *Men's Health*, 6.

9. Smith, P. (1991, January 13). The two great

ages. *SFC*, *This World*, 5–6.

10. Gallup, G. Jr., & Newport, F. (1991, January 7). Gallup Poll: Americans don't fret over death. *SFC*, B5.

11. Smith, 1991, 6.

12. Market Facts, Inc. Cited in: Anonymous. (1989, January–February). Age: All in your head. *PT*, 12.

13. Beck, M., Chideya, F., & Craffey, B. (1992, May 4). Attention, Willard Scott. *Newsweek*, 75.

14. Hocking-Vigie, P. (1992, May 17). 117-year-old woman's secret? Attitude. *LAT*, A6.

15. U.S. Census Bureau. Cited in: Beck et al., 1992.

16. Belden & Russonello survey, October 9–17, 1991, conducted for Alliance for Aging Research. Cited in: Associated Press. (1991, November 18). Two-thirds in U.S. survey want to be 100. *SFC*, A2.

17. Ignatius, A. (1990, March 9). Secrets of Bama: In a corner of China, they live to be 100. *WSJ*, A1, A14.

18. Olshansky, S. J., Carnes, B. A., & Cassel, C. (1990). In search of Methuselah: Estimating the upper limits to human longevity. *Science*, *250*, 634–40.

19. Otten, A. L. (1991, November 15). Charting future course of longevity gains. *WSJ*, B1.

20. Carey, J. R. Quoted in: Kolata, G. (1992, October 16). Fruit fly study challenges accepted longevity theory. *NYT*, A13.

21. Carey, J. R., Liedo, P., Orozco, D. et al. (1992). Slowing of mortality rates at older ages in large medfly cohorts. *Science*, *258*, 457–61.

22. Fries, J. Cited in: Waldholz, M. (1992, October 16). Fountain of youth may not be a fairy tale, study finds. *WSJ*, B1.

23. Fries, J. Cited in: Opatrny, D. J. (1991, November 24). Simple question: Why do we die? *SFE*, A-1, A-6.

24. Fries, J. F. (1992). Strategies for reduction of morbidity. *American Journal of Clinical Medicine*, *55*, 1257S–62S.

25. Fries, J. F., Williams, C. A., & Morfeld, D. (1992). Improvement in intergenerational health. *AJPH*, *82*, 109–12.

26. Fries, J. F. (1989). The compression of morbidity: Near or far? *Milbank Quarterly*, *67*(2), 208–32.

27. Kloeden, P. E., Rossler, R., & Rossler, O. E. (1990). Does a centralized clock for ageing exist? *Gerontology*, *36*, 314–22.

28. Carey, J. R., Liedo, P., Orozco, D. et al. (1992). Slowing of mortality rates at older ages in large medfly cohorts. *Science*, *258*, 457–61.

29. Curtsinger, J. W., Fukui, H. H., Townsend, D. R. et al. (1992). Demography of genotypes: Failure of the limited life-span paradigm in *Drosophila melanogaster. Science*, *258*, 461–63.

30. Ahlburg, D. A., & Vaupel, J. W. (1990). Alternative projections of the U.S. population. *Demography*, *27*, 639–52.

31. Vaupel, J., Gerontological Society of America meeting, San Francisco, October 1991. Quoted in: Opatrny, 1991, A-6.

32. Gaziano, J. M., Manson, J. E., Buring, J. E. et al. (1992). Dietary antioxidants and cardiovascular disease. *Annals of the New York Academy of Sciences*, *669*, 249–58.

33. Angier, N. (1990, April 17). Radical diet gives animals long lives. *SFC*, A1, A8.

34. Effros, R. B., Svoboda, K., & Walford, R. L. (1991). Influence of age and calorie restriction on macrophage IL-6 and TNF production. *Lymphokine & Cytokine Research*, *10*, 347–51.

35. Spindler, S. R., Grizzle, J. M., Walford, R. L. et al. (1991). Aging and restriction of dietary calories increases insulin receptor mRNA, and aging increases glucocorticoid receptor mRNA in the liver of female C3B10RF1 mice. *Journal of Gerontology*, *46*(6), B233–37.

36. Walford, R. L. (1990). The clinical promise of

diet restriction. *Geriatrics, 45,* 81–83, 86–87.

37. Walford, R. L., & Crew, M. (1989). How dietary restriction retards aging: An integrative hypothesis (editorial). *Growth, Development, & Aging, 53,* 139–40.

38. Walford, R. (1988). *The 120-year diet.* New York: Pocket.

39. Sobel, D. (1991, September). The 120-year man. *AH,* 18–21.

40. Roth, G. Cited in: Angier, 1990.

41. Roth, G. S., Ingram, D. K., & Cutler, R. G. (1991). Caloric restriction in non-human primates: A progress report. *Aging, 3,* 391–92.

42. Cutler, R. G., Davis, B. J., Ingram, D. K. et al. (1992). Plasma concentrations of glucose, insulin, and percent glycosylated hemoglobin are unaltered by food restriction in rhesus and squirrel monkeys. *Journal of Gerontology, 47*(1), B9–12.

43. Rudman, D., Fellder, A. G., Nagraj, H. S. et al. (1990). Effects of human growth hormone in men over 60 years. *NEJM, 323,* 1.

44. Stephens, R. (1990, September). Turning back the clock? *AARP Bulletin,* 10–12.

45. Anonymous. (1990, December). Human growth hormone: Fountain of youth? *Medical Aspects of Human Sexuality.*

46. Schneider, E. Quoted in: Opatrny, 1991, A-6.

47. Hall, H. (1988, December). Trying on old age. *PT,* 67.

48. Belkin, L. (1992, June 4). In lessons on empathy, doctors become patients. *NYT,* A1, A13.

49. Emerit, I. (1992). Free radicals and aging of the skin. *EXS, 62,* 328–41.

50. Anonymous. (1993, January–February). Baldness: The many stages of loss. *Men's Health,* 93.

51. Hilchey, T. (1992, November 25). Scientists pursue new ways to fight baldness. *NYT,* B6.

52. Brody, J. E. (1992, May 13). Perplexing syndrome of sudden baldness. *NYT,* C12.

53. Whitney, E. N., & Hamilton, E. M. N. (1987). *Understanding nutrition* (4th ed.). St. Paul: West.

54. Tanouye, E. (1992, July 1). Estrogen use cuts fracture rate for female osteoporosis sufferers. *WSJ,* B4.

55. Thomas, P. (1990, October). Osteoporosis might begin unnoticed in young women. *Medical World News,* 19–20.

56. Brody, J. (1992, October 14). Loss of weight is tied to the risk of osteoporosis. *NYT,* B7.

57. Dawson-Hughes, B., Dallal, G. E., Krall, E. A. et al. (1990). A controlled trial of the effect of calcium supplementation on bone density in postmenopausal women. *NEJM, 323,* 878–83.

58. Krall, E. A., Sahyoun, N., Tannenbaum, S. et al. (1989). Effect of vitamin D intake on seasonal variations in parathyroid hormone secretion in postmenopausal women. *NEJM, 321,* 1777–83.

59. Naessen, T., Persson, I., Adami, H. O. et al. (1990). Hormone replacement therapy and the risk for first hip fracture: A prospective, population-based cohort study. *AIM, 113,* 95–103.

60. Naessen, T., Persson, I., Ljunghall, S. et al. (1992). Women with climacteric symptoms: A target group for prevention of rapid bone loss and osteoporosis. *osteoporosis international, 2,* 225–31.

61. Riggs, B. L., Watts, N. B., Harris, S. T. et al. (1990). Intermittent cyclical etidronate treatment of postmenopausal osteoporosis. *NEJM, 323,* 73–79.

62. Love, R. R., Mazess, R. B., Barden, H. S. et al. (1992). Effects of tamoxifen on bone mineral density in postmenopausal women with breast cancer. *NEJM, 326,* 852–56.

63. Prince, R. L., Smith, M., Dick, I. M. et al. (1991). Prevention of postmenopausal osteoporosis: A comparative study of exercise, calcium supplementation, and hormone-replacement therapy. *NEJM, 325,* 1189–95.

64. Anonymous. (1990, November). Osteoarthritis. *Mayo Clinic Health Letter,* 6.

65. Ala-Kokko, L., Baldwin, C. T., Moskowitz, R. W. et al. (1990). Single base mutation in the type II procollagen gene (COL2A1) as a cause of primary osteoarthritis associated with a mild chondrodysplasia. *Proceedings of the National Academy of Sciences of the United States of America, 87,* 6565–68.

66. Turk, M. (1992, October). Warding off arthritis. *AH,* 7.

67. Kolata, G. (1991, April 16). The aging brain: The mind is resilient, it's the body that fails. *NYT,* B5, B8.

68. Terry, R. D. Quoted in: Chollar, S. (1988, December). Older brains don't fade away. *PT,* 22.

69. Toufexis, A., Blackman, A., Dolan, B. et al. (1991, October 28). When can memories be trusted? *Newsweek,* 86–88.

70. Associated Press. (1993, February 27). Forget something? You're not alone. *SFC,* C1.

71. Crook, T. H. Cited in: Trotter, B. (1991, April). Better memory through chemistry. *AH,* 12.

72. West, R. L., Crook, T. H., & Barron, K. L. (1992). Everyday memory performance across the life span: Effects of age and noncognitive individual differences. *Psychology & Aging, 7,* 72–82.

73. Crook, T. H., Larrabee, G. J., & Youngjohn, J. R. (1990). Diagnosis and assessment of age-associated memory impairment. *Clinical Neuropharmacology, 13,* Suppl. 3, S81–91.

74. Randal, J. (1990, November 16). It's true: Older people do forget more easily. *SFC,* B3, B5.

75. Salthouse, T. A., Legg, S., Palmon, R. et al. (1990). Memory factors in age-related differences in simple reasoning. *Psychology & Aging, 5*(1), 9–15.

76. Mitchell, D. Quoted in: Goleman, D. (1990, March 27). Not all memory fades with age, studies show. *SFC,* A2; reprinted from *NYT.*

77. National Institute on Aging. (1992). *Bound for good health: A collection of Age Pages.* Gaithersburg, MD: National Institute on Aging.

78. Alzheimer's Disease and Related Disorders Association. Cited in: Anonymous. (1992, December). Down with APP. *Living Well,* 21–22.

79. Kolata, G. (1991, February 28). Alzheimer's disease: Dangers and trials of denial. *NYT,* B15.

80. Wolf-Klein, G. P. (1990). Symptoms, diagnosis, and management of Alzheimer's disease. *Comprehensive Therapy, 16*(9), 25–29.

81. Associated Press. (1992, October 23). Genetic defect linked to Alzheimer's. *NYT,* A11.

82. Associated Press. (1992, December 22). Study backs theory on a cause of Alzheimer's. *NYT,* B9.

83. Kolata, 1991 (February 28).

84. Kantrowitz, B. (1989, December 18). Trapped inside her own world. *Newsweek,* 56–58.

85. Burden, D. (1989, August). Caring for the caregiver. *PT,* 22.

86. Anonymous. (1992, January 1). Avoiding 'caregiver burnout' in Alzheimer family groups. *NYT,* 13.

87. Konek, C. W. (1992). *Daddyboy: A memoir.* St. Paul: Graywolf.

88. Levine, D. (1991, December). Attacking Alzheimer's, 9–10.

89. Blakeslee, S. (1989, March). The return of the mind. *AH,* 94–96.

90. Lawren, B. (1992, December). Still creative after all these years. *Living Well,* 85–87.

91. Kolata, G. (1991, October 6). Mental gymnastics. *New York Times Magazine,* 15–17, 42.

92. Anonymous. (1990, June 1). Older women gain freedom by driving. *SFC,* A4; reprinted from *NYT.*

93. Fost, D. (1991, September). Who's too old to drive? *American Demographics,* 8–10.

94. National Institute on Aging. Cited in: Otten, A. L. (1992, June 1). Older drivers appear safer but more frail. *WSJ,* B1.

95. Opatrny, D. J. (1990, November 18). New tests planned for state's drivers. *SFE,* B-1, B-5.

96. Reinisch, J. M. (1991, May 7). Aging doesn't halt sexual functioning. *SFC,* D5.

97. Anonymous. (1991, September). Menopause and sexuality. *Medical Aspects of Human Sexuality,* 29–30.

98. Rauch, K. D. (1992, July 12). Sex for life. *SFC, This World,* 7.

99. Greeley, A. M. (1992). *Sex after sixty: A report.* Cited in: Woodward, K. L., & Springen, K. (1992, August 24). Better than a gold watch. *Newsweek,* p. 71.

100. Butler, R. N. Quoted in: Rovner, S. (1989, January 15). Older love. *SFC, This World,* 22; reprinted from *Washington Post.*

101. Weg, R. B. Cited in: Rovner, 1989.

102. Byer, C. O., & Shainberg, L. W. (1991). *Dimensions of human sexuality* (3rd ed.). Dubuque, IA: Wm. C. Brown.

103. Hamilton, J. A., Parry, B. L., & Blumenthal, S. J. (1988). The menstrual cycle in context, I: Affective syndromes associated with reproductive hormonal changes. *Journal of Clinical Psychiatry, 49,* 474–80.

104. Sutherland, F. N. (1990). Psychological aspects of menopause. *Maternal and Child Health, 15*(1), 13–14.

105. Matthews, K. A. (1992). Myths and realities of the menopause. *Psychosomatic Medicine, 54,* 1–9.

106. Kolata, G. (1991, September 17). Women face dilemma over estrogen therapy. *NYT,* B8.

107. Anonymous. (1991, September). The estrogen question: Is it a natural supplement or a dangerous drug? *Consumer Reports,* 587–91.

108. Ziegler, J. (1992, April). The dilemma of estrogen replacement. *AH,* 68–71.

109. Wright, K. (1992, December). Menopause: Change and choice. *Living Well,* 66–71.

110. Stampfer, M. J., Colditz, G. A., Willett, W. C. et al. (1991). Postmenopausal estrogen therapy and cardiovascular disease: Ten-year follow-up from the nurses' health study. *NEJM, 325,* 756–62.

111. Colditz, G. A., Stampfer, M. J., Willett, W. C. (1990). Prospective study of estrogen replacement therapy and risk of breast cancer in postmenopausal women. *JAMA, 264,* 2648–53.

112. Bewley, S., & Bewley, T. H. (1992). Drug dependence with oestrogen replacement therapy. *Lancet, 339,* 290–91.

113. Brody, J. E. (1992, May 20). For menopausal women, there are effective and painless alternatives to hormone replacement. *NYT,* B7.

114. Angier, N. (1992, May 20). Is there a male menopause? Jury is still out. *NYT,* A1, B7.

115. Miles, W. Cited in: Rauch, 1992.

116. Hamilton, E. (1992, November 5). Ailing oldsters can have sex. *Point Reyes Light* (Calif.), 6.

117. Barasch, D. (1992, December). Urinary incontinence. *Living Well,* 94.

118. Leary, W. E. (1992, March 24). U.S. issues guidelines on bladder problems. *NYT,* B6.

119. Goleman, D. (1991, May 16). A modern tradeoff: Longevity for health. *NYT,* B8.

120. Rubinstein, C., & Shaver, P. (1982). *In search of intimacy: A report on loneliness and what to do about it.* New York: Delacorte.

121. Corwin, N. Quoted in: Beck, M., Carroll, G., King, P. et al. (1992, December 7). The new middle age. *Newsweek,* 50–56.

122. Levinson, D. (1978). *The seasons of a man's life.* New York: Alfred A. Knopf.

123. Clausen, J. (1990, October 9). Study fails to find 'midlife crisis.' *SFE,* A2.

124. American Board of Family Practice. Cited in: McLeod, R. G. (1990, December 5). Midlife stress over parents, children. *SFC,* A2.

125. National Opinion Research Center General Social Survey. Cited in: Riche, M. F. (1991, January 4). Zestful outlook starts to get on in years. *WSJ,* B1.

126. New World Decisions, Inc. 1990 survey for American Board of Family Practice. Cited in:

Anonymous. (1990, August–September). Mapping out middle age...crisis or conquest? *Modern Maturity*, 88.

127. Goldstein, R. E. (1989, July). Taking the crisis out of mid-life. *San Francisco Focus*, 42–45, 94–102.

128. New World Decisions, Inc. survey, 1990.

129. Kalat, J. W. (1990). *Psychology* (2nd ed). Belmont, CA: Wadsworth.

130. Anonymous. Quoted in: Smith, P. (1991, September 15). Voices of experience. *SFC, This World*, 5–6.

131. Daniel Yankelovich Group survey, 1989, for American Association for Retired People. Cited in: Stephens, R. (1989, December). *AARP Bulletin*, 1, 4.

132. IFC study for Commonwealth Fund, 1991. Cited in: Teltsch, K. (1991, May 21). New study of older workers find they can become good investments. *NYT*, A10.

133. Bennet, J. (1992, January 21). Older job applicants find fewer opportunities. *NYT*, 21.

134. Lewis, R. (1991, December). Advantage: bosses. *AARP Bulletin*, 1, 12.

135. Older Women's League. Cited in: Lewin, T. (1991, May 9). *SFC*, B3; reprinted from *NYT*.

136. Older Women's League. Cited in: Cox News Service. (1990, May 10). Pension report says women lagging. *SFC*, A16.

137. Longino, C. F. Jr., & Crown, W. H. (1991, August). Older Americans: Rich or poor? *American Demographics*, 48–54.

138. Smith, L. (1992, January 13). The tyranny of America's old. *Fortune*, 68–72.

139. Longino & Crown, 1991.

140. Otten, A. I. (1990, December 24). Healthy aging hinges on income, education. *WSJ*, 9.

141. Kessler, R. C., Foster, C., Webster, P. S. et al. (1992). The relationship between age and depressive symptoms in two national surveys. *Psychology & Aging*, 7, 119–26.

142. Herzog, A. R., House, J. S., & Morgan, J. N. (1991). Relation of work and retirement to health and well-being in older age. *Psychology & Aging*, 6, 202–11.

143. House, J. S., Kessler, R. C., & Herzog, A. R. (1990). Age, socioeconomic status, and health. *Milbank Quarterly*, 63, 383–411.

144. Robinson, J. P. (1991, May). Quitting time. *American Demographics*, 34–36.

145. Kaplan, R. M. Cited in: Goleman, 1991.

146. Wingard, D. Cited in: Goleman, 1991.

147. Kaplan, R. M., Anderson, J. P., & Wingard, D. L. (1991). Gender differences in health-related quality of life. *Health Psychology*, 10, 86–93.

148. Stewart, R. B., Blashfield, R., Hale, W. E. et al. (1991). Correlates of Beck Depression Inventory scores in an ambulatory elderly population: Symptoms, diseases, laboratory values, and medications. *Journal of Family Practice*, 32, 497–502.

149. Friedhoff, A. Cited in: Medical Tribune News Service. (1991, November 7). Depressed elderly ignored. *SFC*, B5.

150. Rosenberg, M. Cited in: Rauch, K. D. (1992, July 12). Red flags of depression. *SFC, This World*, 10.

151. National Academy of Sciences. Cited in: Altman, L. K. (1990, November 6). More preventive care sought for older people. *NYT*, B8.

152. Elias, M. (1991, February 19). Reactions to medicine affect 20% of seniors. *USA Today*, 1A.

153. Kolata, G. (1992, February 2). Elderly become addicts to drug-induced sleep. *NYT*, sec. 4, 4.

154. Associated Press. (1989, December 15). Tranquilizers linked to hip fractures. *SFC*, A7.

155. Ray, W. A., Griffin, M. R., & Downey, W. (1989) Benzodiazepines of long and short elimination half-life and the risk of hip fracture. *JAMA*, 262, 3303–7.

156. Beresford, T. P., Blow, F. C., & Brower, K. J. (1990). Alcoholism in the elderly.

Comprehensive Therapy, 16(9), 38–43.

157. National Institute on Alcohol Abuse and Alcoholism. (1988, October). Alcohol and aging. *Alcohol Alert*, 1–3.

158. Anonymous. (1991, June). Mental illness clue to elder suicides. *AARP Bulletin*, 7.

159. Associated Press. (1991, April 8). Study on suicide by older people. *SFC*, 53.

160. Centers for Disease Control. Cited in: Associated Press. (1991, September 19). Suicide rate rises for the elderly. *NYT*, A14.

161. Freedman, M. (1992, May 16). Suicide rates high among the elderly. *SFC*, A8.

162. Oldham, J. Cited in: Anonymous. (1991, August). The middle of life: A good place to be. *University of California, Berkeley, Wellness Letter*, 4–5.

163. Kutner, L. (1991, May 23). Some adult children still look to their parents for much of their emotional and financial support. *NYT*, B5.

164. Associated Press. (1990, May 17). Elderly prefer to live alone. *SFC*, B4.

165. Sommers, T., & Fields, L. (1988). *Women take care: The consequences of caregiving in today's society*. Gainesville, FL: Triad.

166. Kutner, L. (1992, August 6). A growing number of people must care for children and dependent parents at the same time. *NYT*, B4.

167. Bennet, J. (1992, October 4). More and more, the elderly find themselves taking care of their parents. *NYT*, sec. 1, 21.

168. Sukosky, D. G. (1990/91). The paradox and perplexity of elder abuse. *Family Life Educator*, 9(2), 7–12.

169. Lewin, T. (1992, November 24). A.M.A. asking doctors to note abuse of elderly. *NYT*, A7.

170. Nordheimer, J. (1991, December 16). A new abuse of elderly: Theft by kin and friends. *NYT*, A1, A12.

171. Leonard, F. (1992/93, December–January). Home alone. *Modern Maturity*, 46–51, 77.

172. Mothner, I. (1991, March). Take care. *AH*, 64–68.

173. Stout, H. (1991, November 21). Godsend for many, home-care industry also has potential for fraud and abuse. *WSJ*, B1, B5.

174. O'Reilly, B. (1992, May 18). How to take care of aging parents. *Fortune*, 108–12.

175. Hennenberger, M. (1992, December 17). 'Home' vanishes from 'nursing home.' *NYT*, B8.

176. McCarthy, M. J. (1992, December 3). Older people will do anything to avoid life in nursing home. *WSJ*, A1, A6.

177. Cooper, M. (1992, November 12). Scientists study how some centenarians have managed to stay hale and hearty. *WSJ*, B1, B7.

178. Belden & Russonello survey, October 1991, for Alliance for Aging Research. Cited in: Associated Press, November 18, 1991.

179. Anonymous. (1989, January–February). Pickled brains. *PT*, 23.

180. House, J. R., Landis, K. R., & Umberson, D. (1988). Social relationships and health. *Science*, 241, 540–45.

181. Gerzon, M. Quoted in: Lipstein, O., Mauro, J., & Scanlon, M. (1992, October). Act II: Why it's not such a drag getting old. *PT*, 54–60, 94.

182. Eckel, H. Quoted in: Bill Moyers' "Healing and the mind," television documentary, February 24, 1993, Public Broadcasting System.

183. Dominguez, J., & Robin, V. (1992). *Your money or your life*. Bergenfield, NJ: Penguin.

184. Anonymous. Quoted in: Moyers, "Healing and the mind," 1993.

185. Leming, M. R., & Dickinson, G. E. (1990). *Understanding dying, death, and bereavement* (2nd ed.). Fort Worth, TX: Holt, Rinehart & Winston.

186. Cordes, H. (1991, September/October). Facing death. *Utne Reader*, 65.

187. Levine, S. (1982). *Who dies?* New York: Doubleday.

188. Chartrand, S. (1992, March 29). Baby miss-

ing part of brain challenges legal definition of death. *NYT*, sec. 1, 10.

189. Dowie, M. (1990, October). The biomort factor. *AH*, 18–19.

190. Dowie, 1990.

191. Dowie, 1990.

192. Dowie, 1990.

193. Chartrand, 1992.

194. Lewis, A. (1990, June 29). Conscience and the court. *NYT*, A11.

195. Greenhouse, L. (1990, June 27). Right to reject life. *NYT*, A13.

196. U.S. Supreme Court. Quoted in: Anonymous. (1990, June 26). Excerpts from court opinions on Missouri right-to-die case. *NYT*, A12.

197. Associated Press. (1990, December 15). Missouri judge says comatose woman can die. *SFC*, 1.

198. Malcolm, A. H. (1990, December 7). Right-to-die case nearing a finale. *NYT*, A14.

199. Lewin, T. (1990, December 27). Nancy Cruzan dies, outlived by debate over right to die. *NYT*, A1, A13.

200. Anonymous. (1990, December 27). Nancy Cruzan's accomplishment (editorial). *NYT*, A18.

201. Dowie, 1990.

202. *JAMA*. Reported in: Hilton, B. (1990, February 4). Making the toughest decisions. *SFE*, D-19.

203. Youngner, S. Quoted in: Dowie, 1990, 18.

204. Dowie, 1990.

205. Elber, L. (1990, May 27). Experimental drug saves woman. *SFC*, B-8.

206. Rosenthal, E. (1990, October 4). Rules on reviving the dying bring undue suffering, doctors contend. *NYT*, A1, B6.

207. Associated Press. (1991, July 6). Brain-damaged woman at center of lawsuit over life-support dies. *NYT*, 8.

208. Hilton, B. (1991, January 13). In the news: Right to die turned around. *SFE*, D-14.

209. Gladwell, M. (1990, September 19). Controversy over futile life-saving attempts. *SFC*, Briefing section, 9; reprinted from *Washington Post*.

210. Hilton, 1991.

211. Altman, L. K. (1991, October 23). Computing a hospital patient's chance of survival. *NYT*, B9.

212. Winslow, R. (1991, October 18). New system helps evaluate chance of dying. *WSJ*, B11.

213. Seligmann, J., & Sulavik, C. (1992, April 27). Software for hard issues. *Newsweek*, 55.

214. Brown, D. (1992, February 9). Medical computer with a godlike role. *SFC, Sunday Punch*, 4; reprinted from *NYT*.

215. Belkin, L. (1990, June 6). Doctor tells of first death using his suicide device. *NYT*, A1, A13.

216. Wilkerson, I. (1990, June 7). Physician fulfills a goal: Aiding a person in a suicide. *NYT*, A13.

217. Schmidt, W. E. (1990, December 15). Prosecutors drop criminal case against doctor in suicide case. *NYT*, 9.

218. Wilkerson, I. (1991, October 25). Rage and support for doctor's role in suicide. *NYT*, A1, A8.

219. Gibbs, N., & Gregory, S. S. (1991, November 4). Dr. Death strikes again. *Time*, 78.

220. Associated Press. (1992, July 22). Murder charges against Kevorkian are dismissed. *NYT*, A6.

221. Associated Press. (1992, November 24). 'Dr. Death' assists in his 6th suicide. *SFC*, A3.

222. American Hospital Association. Cited in: Malcolm, A. H. (1990, December 23). What medical science can't seem to learn: When to call it quits. *NYT*, sec. 4, 6.

223. Vorenberg, J. (1991, November 5). Going gently, with dignity. *NYT*, A15.

224. Altman, L. K. (1991, March 12). More physi-

cians broach forbidden subject of euthanasia. *NYT*, B6.

225. Quill, T.E. (1991). Death and dignity—a case of individualized decision making. *NEJM*, *324*, 691–94.

226. Altman, L. K. (1991, July 27). Jury declines to indict a doctor who said he aided in a suicide. *NYT*, 1, 7.

227. Simons, M. (1991, September 11). Dutch survey casts new light on patients who choose to die. *NYT*, B8.

228. Steinfels, P. (1991, November 2). Dutch study is euthanasia vote issue. *NYT*, 10.

229. Gallup Poll. (1991, January 8). Most adults support euthanasia. *SFC*, B5.

230. Princeton Survey Research Associates poll for Times Mirror Center for the People and the Press. Reported in: Anonymous. (1990, June 11). 'Right to die' supported for terminally ill. *SFC*, A9; reprinted from *Newsday*.

231. New York Times/CBS News Poll. (1990, June 26). Right to die: The public's view. *NYT*, A12.

232. Boston Globe and Harvard School of Public Health poll. Reported in: Associated Press. (1991, November 4). Euthanasia favored in poll. *NYT*, A9.

233. Conwell, Y., & Caine, E. D. (1991). Rational suicide and the right to die. *NEJM*, *325*, 1100–2.

234. Carton, R. W. (1990). The road to euthanasia (editorial). *JAMA*, *263*, 2221.

235. Sprung, C. L. (1990). Changing attitudes and practices in forgoing life-sustaining treatments. *JAMA*, *263*, 2211–15.

236. Singer, P. A., & Siegler, M. (1990). Euthanasia—a critique. *NEJM*, *322*, 1881–83.

237. Cassel, C. K., & Meier, D. E. (1990). Morals and moralism in the debate over euthanasia and assisted suicide. *NEJM*, *323*, 750–52.

238. Humphry, D. (1991). *Final exit: The practicalities of self-deliverance and assisted suicide for the dying*. Eugene, OR: The Hemlock Society.

239. American Hospital Association. Cited in: Malcolm, 1990, December 23.

240. Steinfels, P. (1991, October 28). At crossroads, U.S. ponders ethics of helping others die. *NYT*, A1, A15.

241. Associated Press. (1990, September 14). Dying have right to refuse food, Florida high court rules. *NYT*, A14.

242. McEnroe, C. (1990, July 1). The future of suicide on demand. *SFC, This World*, 24; reprinted from *Hartford Courant*.

243. Miles, R. E. (1990, June 19). Quick and painless death should be a right (letter). *NYT*, A14.

244. Angell, M. (1990, July 23). The right to die in dignity. *Newsweek*, 9.

245. Rowland, M. (1992, March 22). Planning for the end of life. *NYT*, sec. 3, 17.

246. Anonymous. (1990, March). Why you need a living will. *University of California, Berkeley, Wellness Letter*, 1–2.

247. Rosenthal, E. (1990, October 4). Rules on reviving the dying bring undue suffering, doctors contend. *NYT*, A1, B6.

248. Ames, K., Wilson, L., Sawhill, R. et al. (1991, August 26). Last rights. *Newsweek*, 40–41.

249. Decarlo, T. (1990, November 12). Looking for families willing to make a final gift of life. *SFC*, B3, B5.

250. Thomas, S. (1991). The gift of life. *Nursing Times*, *87*(37), 28–31.

251. Ring, K. (1980). *Life at death: A scientific investigation of near-death experience*. New York: Coward, McCann & Geohegan.

252. Perry, P. (1988, September). Brushes with death. *PT*, 14–17.

253. Ring, K. Quoted in: Peay, P. (1991, September/October). Back from the grave. *Utne Reader*, 72–73; reprinted from *Common Boundary*.

254. Moody, R. A. Jr. (1991). *Coming back*. New York: Bantam.

255. Krier, B. A. (1990, September 21). New reports from the great beyond. *SFC*, B3, B5; reprinted from *LAT*.

256. Owens, J., Stevenson, I., & Cook, E. Cited in: Farrell, J. (1991, May). Near-death trips may start when stress blows a brain circuit. *AH*, 14.

257. Gallup Poll. Cited in: Ferris, T. (1991, December 15). A cosmological event. *New York Times Magazine*, 44. 52–53.

258. Moody, R. A. Jr. (1975). *Life after life*. Cited in: Ferris, 1991.

259. Kubler-Ross, E. (1969). *On death and dying*. New York: Macmillan.

260. Kubler-Ross, 1969.

261. Hilton, B. (1991, January 27). All about lying at death's door. *SFE*, D-14.

262. Anonymous. Cited in: Hilton, 1991, January 27.

263. National Institute on Aging. (1981). *Aging and the circumstances of death*. Bethesda, MD: National Institute on Aging.

264. Somerville, J. (1991, January 7). The final days. *American Medical News*, p. 7.

265. Malcolm, A. H. (1991, July 5). Giving a dose of empathy to the dying. *NYT*, A12.

266. Egan, T. (1991, January 8). Creating a pleasant stop on the journey to death. *NYT*, A10.

267. Belkin, L. (1992, March 2). Choosing death at home: Dignity with its own toll. *NYT*, A1, B12.

268. Kutner, L. (1992, January 9). A parent's impending death can lead family members to reassess relationships with the parent. *NYT*, B3.

269. Veninga, R. Cited in: Kutner, 1992.

270. Frankel, M. R., & Canepa, L. (1988, September/October). Telling your kids you have cancer or any serious illness. *Medical SelfCare*, 37–41, 69–71.

271. Leming & Dickinson, 1990.

272. Leary, W. E. (1991, August 27). Not even death ends anti-pollution crusade. *NYT*, B8.

273. Horn, P. (1992, May 31). Death: The bottom line. *Reno Gazette-Journal*, 11A.

274. Carlson, L. (1991, September/October). Caring for our own dead. *Utne Reader*, 79–81; excerpted from *Woman of Power*.

275. Schwartz, N. (1992, September 3). Trend in gravestones is highly personal; it's 'cemetery art.' *WSJ*, A1, A4.

276. Rosenthal, E. (1992, December 6). Struggling to handle bereavement as AIDS rips relationships apart. *NYT*, sec. 1, 1, 21.

277. Chance, L. Cited in: Malcolm, A. H. (1991, October 11). *NYT*, B16.

278. Kalish, R. A. (1985). The social context of death and dying. In Binstock, R. H., & Shanas, E. (Eds.). *Handbook of aging and the social sciences*. New York: Van Nostrand Reinhold.

279. Kastenbaum, R. (1986). *Death, society, and the human experience*. Columbus, OH: Merrill.

280. Berger, K. S. (1988). *The developing person through the life span* (2nd ed.). New York: Worth.

281. Black, V. Quoted in: Greene, B. (1990, February 25). Some wounds never really heal. *SFC, This World*, 5–6.

282. Chance, S. (1992). *Stronger than death*. New York: W. W. Norton.

283. Higuera, E. Quoted in: Larsen, D. (1990, February 2). The 'orphaned' adult. *SFC*, B5; reprinted from *LAT*.

284. Scharlach, A. E. Cited in: Larsen, 1990.

285. Kutner, L. (1990, December 6). The death of a parent can profoundly alter the relationships of adult siblings. *NYT*, B7.

286. Cole, D. (1988, December). Grief's lessons: His and hers. *PT*, 60–61.

287. Bowling, A. (1987). Mortality after bereavement: A review of the literature on survival periods and factors affecting survival. *Social Science Medicine*, *24*(2), 117–24.

288. Smith, K. R. Cited in: Breecher, M. M. (1989, November). When death does us part: The difference between widows and widowers. *PT*, 14.

289. Townsend, L. (1992, March 16). Widowed men meet to share support. *SFC*, D4.

290. Nemy, E. (1992, June 28). Widows are choosing independent new lives rather than marriages. *NYT*, B1, B5.

291. Springer, I. (1992, July/August). Helping children grieve. *AH*, 86.

292. Meltz, B. F. (1991, March 1). How children respond to grief and loss. *Boston Globe*, 68.

293. Berger, 1988.

294. Joseph, N. (1991, January 7). Harder days at the office. *Newsweek*, 61.

295. Rosenthal, 1992.

296. Osterweis, M., Soloman, F., & Green, M. (Eds.). (1984). *Bereavement: Reactions, consequences, and care*. Washington, DC: National Academy Press.

297. Trunnell, E. P., Caserta, M. S., & White, G. L. (1992, July/August). Bereavement: Current issues in intervention and prevention. *Journal of Health Education*, *23*, 275–79.

298. Berger, 1988.

299. Goleman, D. (1991, March 25). People good at predicting own deaths. *SFC*, D3; reprinted from *NYT*.

300. Anonymous. (1992, September 10). Those who blame woes on aging die sooner. *SFC*; reprinted from *Washington Post*.

301. Associated Press. (1990, April 11). Some people just tell death to wait. *SFC*, A1.

302. Richardson, G. E., Neiger, B. L., Jensen, S. et al. (1990, November/December). The resiliency model. *Health Education*, 33–39.

303. Wels, S. (1986, Winter). The long road back: Coping with chronic illness. *Stanford Magazine*, 49–52.

304. LeMaistre, J. Quoted in: Wels, 1986.

305. Peck, M. S. (1978). *The road less traveled: A new psychology of love, traditional values and spiritual growth*. New York: Touchstone, p. 15.

306. Peck, M. S. Quoted in: Watts, J. (1993, June 13). Still searching for real community. *SFE*, p. D-2; reprinted from *London Observer*.

307. Kobasa, S. C. (1984, September). How much stress can you survive? *AH*, 64–77.

308. Kobasa, S.C., Maddi, S. R., & Khan, S. (1982). Hardiness and health: A prospective study. *Journal of Personality & Social Psychology*, *42*(1), 168–77.

309. Maddi, S. Cited in: Japenga, A. (1991, April). You're tougher than you think: The ability to bounce back. *Self*, 174–75, 187.

310. Flach, F. F. (1988). *Resilience: Discovering new strength at times of stress*. New York: Ballantine.

311. Flannery, R. (1990). *Becoming stress-resistant*. New York: Crossroads/Continuum.

312. Flannery, R. Cited in: Springer, I. (1991, March). The tough get going. *AH*, 12.

313. Werner, E. E., & Smith, R. S. (1982). *Vulnerable but invincible*. New York: McGraw-Hill.

314. Werner, E. E. Cited in: Japenga, 1991.

315. McKee, S. (1991, March). Just do it. *AH*, 12.

316. Haskall, A. (1992, November). Stop worrying. *Self*, 134–37.

317. Haskall, 1992, 137.

UNIT 16: ENVIRONMENTAL HEALTH

1. Ravo, N. (1991, October 6). Noise police crackdown takes boom out of Bronx. *NYT*, sec. 1, 20.

2. Browne, M. W. (1992, May 14). Noise experts agree: America is land of battered eardrums. *NYT*, B13.

3. Krieger, L. M. (1990, October 21). Hunh? I can't hear you. *SFE*, D-16.

4. Anonymous. (1990). Noise and hearing loss: National Institutes of Health Consensus Development Conference on Noise and Hearing Loss. *JAMA*, *263*, 3185.

5. Flodin, K. C. (1992, January/February). Now hear this. *AH*, 58–62.

6. U.S. Public Health Service. Cited in: Wing, E. (1992, February). Now hear this. *Self*, 116–17, 149.

7. Resen, S. V., & Hausman, C. (1985). *Coping with hearing loss: A guide for adults and their families*. New York: Dembner.

8. Barron, J. (1990, August 14). Above the clamor of New York City, more clamor. *NYT*, A16.

9. U.S. Public Health Service. (1990). *Healthy people 2000: National health promotion and disease prevention objectives*. DHHS Pub. No. (PHS)91-50212. Washington, DC: U.S. Government Printing Office.

10. Flodin, 1992.

11. Anonymous. (1991, October). Play it softly, Sam: Decibel overload. *Consumer Reports*, 660.

12. Monroe, L. R. (1990, December 13). Personal stereos called a threat to kids' hearing. *SFC*, A14; reprinted from *LAT*.

13. Flodin, 1992.

14. Monroe, 1990.

15. Peters, J. M., & London, S. J. Cited in: Petit, C. (1991, January 20). Electrical links to leukemia studied. *SFC*, A3.

16. Kirkpatrick, D. (1993, March 8). Do cellular phones cause cancer? *Fortune*, 82–89.

17. Kirkpatrick, 1993.

18. Elmer-DeWitt, P. (1993, February 8). Dialing "P" for panic. *Time*, 56.

19. Kirkpatrick, 1993.

20. Petit, C. (1991, June 11). Fear of man-made magnetism. *SFC*, A1, A4.

21. Kirkpatrick, D. (1990, December 31). Can power lines give you cancer? *Fortune*, 80–85.

22. Hacinli, C. (1992, January/February). A gauss in the house. *Garbage*, 40–43.

23. Kirkpatrick, 1990.

24. Kirkpatrick, 1993.

25. Gibson, R. (1992, March 9). Despite vocal critics, wary consumers, food makers move toward irradiation. *WSJ*, B1, B4.

26. Delaney, L. (1993, January/February). X-ray vision. *Men's Health*, 32–34.

27. Dollinger, M., Rosenbaum, E. H., & Cable, G. (1991). *Everyone's guide to cancer therapy*. Kansas City, MO: Somerville House.

28. Elias, M. (1989, March). The radon that came in from the cold. *AH*, 15.

29. Office of Health and Environmental Research. (1990). *Indoor radon and decay products: Concentration, causes, and control strategies*. Washington, DC: U.S. Department of Energy.

30. Office of Health and Environmental Research. (1991). *Radon research program—annual report, FY 1990*. Washington, DC: U.S. Department of Energy.

31. Leary, W. E. (1991, February 2). U.S. study finds reduced danger from radon seeping into homes. *NYT*, 9.

32. Brody, J. E. (1991, January 8). Some scientists say concern over radon is overblown by EPA. *NYT*, B7.

33. Broad, W. J., & Wald, M. L. (1992, December 1). Milestones of the nuclear era. *NYT*, B8.

34. Wald, M. L. (1991, June 24). Due up for license renewal: The future of nuclear power. *NYT*, A1, B1.

35. Anonymous. (1992, November 25). Cleanup resumes at 3 Mile Island. *SFC*, A8.

36. Hatch, M. C., Wallenstein, S., Beyea, J., Nieves, J. W., & Susser, M. (1991). Cancer rates after the Three Mile Island nuclear accident and proximity of residence to the plant. *AJPH*, *81*, 719–24.

37. Brooke, J. (1991, November 3). Chernobyl said to affect health of thousands in a Soviet region. *NYT*, sec. 1, 1, 6.

38. Kolata, G. (1992, September 3). A cancer legacy from Chernobyl. *NYT*, A4.

39. Medvedev, Z. A. (1990). *The legacy of Chernobyl*. New York: W. W. Norton.

40. Associated Press. (1991, April 26). Safety of U.S. A-plants questioned. *SFC*, A10.

41. Schneider, K. (1991, May 12). Is nuclear winter giving way to nuclear spring? *NYT*, sec. 4, 4.

42. Shabecoff, P. (1990, September 20). No added cancer risk is found near A-plants. *NYT*, A15.

43. Wald, 1991.

44. Wald, M. L. (1992, August 16). Nuclear power plants take early retirement. *NYT*, sec. 4, 7.

45. Rubin, J. (1992, September 15). U.S. 'atomic vets' push VA for compensation, information. *SFC*, A15.

46. Burns, R. (1990, July 14). U.S. knew in 1948 of A-plant's risks. *SFC*, A2.

47. Wing, S., Shy, C. M., Wood, J. L. (1991). Mortality among workers at Oak Ridge National Laboratory: Evidence of radiation effects in follow-up through 1984. *JAMA*, *265*, 1397–1402.

48. Atchison, S. D. (1990, October 15). 'These people were used as guinea pigs.' *Business Week*, 98.

49. Schneider, K. (1990, July 13). Report warns of impact of Hanford's radiation. *NYT*, A8.

50. Abramson, R. (1990, July 13). Thousands found exposed to Hanford plant radiation. *LAT*, A1, A32.

51. Schneider, K. (1992, November 25). Troubled nuclear factory is to be shut in Oklahoma. *NYT*, A7.

52. Wald, M. L. (1991, July 25). As U.S. struggles to restart Colorado bomb plant, critics question its need. *NYT*, A12.

53. Anonymous. (1991, March 22). Workers in jeopardy at A-plants. *SFC*, A15.

54. Associated Press. (1990, December 16). Agency tightens radiation exposure rules. *NYT*, 20.

55. Pfeiffer, M. B. (1992, September 5). The enemy below. *NYT*, 13.

56. Associated Press. (1992, November 4). Carpet fumes may be linked to health woes. *SFC*, D8.

57. Kreiss, K. (1990). The sick building syndrome: Where is the epidemiologic basis. *AJPH*, *80*, 1172–73.

58. Anonymous. (1991, July). Can a building really make you sick? *University of California, Berkeley, Wellness Letter*, 1–2.

59. Rice, F. (1990, July 2). Do you work in a sick building? *Fortune*, 86–87.

60. Shaughnessy, R. Quoted in: Griffin, K. (1993, February 14). When your office calls in sick. *SFC, This World*, 8–10; reprinted from *Health*.

61. Stevens, W. K. (1991, September 26). Study asserts intact asbestos poses little risk for most inside buildings. *NYT*, C19.

62. Stevens, W. K. (1991, August 7). Doctors reassess risk of asbestos. *NYT*, A15.

63. Associated Press. (1992, August 11). Asbestos settlements may reach $1 billion. *SFC*, A6.

64. Harris, T. (1993, December/January). The asbestos mess. *Garbage*, 44–49.

65. Norris, R. (1992, March). Safe houses. *AH*, 88–90.

66. Yulsman, T. (1991, April 28). Lead hazards at home. *New York Times Magazine, The Good Health Magazine*, 28, 46–51.

67. Needleman, H. L. (1991). Childhood lead poisoning: a disease for the history texts. *AJPH*, *81*, 685–87.

68. Rosewicz, B. (1991, May 8). EPA issues rules to reduce lead levels in drinking water of American homes. *WSJ*, B4.

69. Specter, M. (1992, October 21). E.P.A. tests find high lead levels. *NYT*, A15.

70. Anonymous. (1992, December 16). California lawsuit says faucets leach dangerous levels of lead. *NYT*, p. C18.

71. Brody, J. E. (1992, November 18). Lead is public enemy no. 1 for American children. *NYT*, p. B8.

72. McCoy, C. (1991, November 13). Ceramic-tableware lead levels spur California lawsuits; firms deny peril. *WSJ*, B7.

73. Reinhold, R. (1991, November 13). California moves to limit leaching of lead from tableware. *NYT*, A11.

74. Burros, M. (1992, February 26). With concerns being raised about lead in ceramics, you are what you eat on. *NYT*, B5.

75. Leary, W. E. (1991, September 11). F.D.A. seeks a limit on lead content in wine and a ban on foil capsules. *NYT*, B8.

76. Brody, J. E. (1992, October 29). Study documents lead-exposure damage in middle-class children. *NYT*, A14.

77. Pear, R. (1992, September 13). U.S. orders testing of poor children for lead poisoning. *NYT*, 1, 18.

78. Bellafante, G. (1990, March/April). Minimizing household hazardous waste. *Garbage*, 44–48.

79. *Consumer Reports*. Cited in: Anonymous. (1991, July). Fascinating facts. *University of California, Berkeley, Wellness Letter*, 1.

80. National Academy of Sciences. Cited in: Krattenmaker, T. (1990, October 14). Environmentally ill cry for medical recognition. *LAT*, B3.

81. Krattenmaker, 1990.

82. Poore, P. (1990, March/April). Clinical ecology: Medicine for the chemical-sensitive? *Garbage*, 30–35.

83. Anonymous. (1990, December 26). New flap over environmental illness. *SFC*, A10; reprinted from *NYT*.

84. Krattenmaker, 1990.

85. Poore, 1990, 30.

86. Hong, P. (1992, September 28). Do two pollutants make you sicker than one? *Business Week*, 77–78.

87. Louie, E. (1992, December 3). Building a home designed to keep a man healthy. *NYT*, B6.

88. Marinelli, J. (1990, March/April). Plants for healthier homes. *Garbage*, 36–43.

89. Marinelli, 1990.

90. Anonymous. (1991, October–November). Plants help cut indoor pollution. *Modern Maturity*, 12.

91. Sharp, D. (1992, December/January). What a dump! *In Health*, 56–60.

92. Bellafante, G. (1990, March/April). Minimizing household hazardous waste. *Garbage*, 44–48.

93. Tuller, D. (1993, March 8). Clear products sell healthy image. *SFC*, A1, A13.

94. Anonymous. (1990, October 8). U.S. is faulted for role in water quality. *NYT*, A7.

95. Associated Press. (1992, December 8). $500 billion may be needed to fix urban water systems. *SFC*, A4.

96. Bashin, B. J. (1992, August 23). Fear of faucets. *SFC, This World*, 7, 12–14; reprinted from *Eating Well*.

97. Miller, G. T. Jr. (1990). *Resource conservation and management*. Belmont, CA: Wadsworth.

98. Miller, 1990.

99. National Academy of Sciences. Cited in: Miller, 1990.

100. Gutfeld, R. (1992, October 21). Lead in water of many cities is found excessive. *WSJ*, B6.

101. Altman, L. K. (1992, July 1). Tiny cancer risk in chlorinated water. *NYT*, A12.

102. Sears, C. (1989, October). Fluoridation: Friends and foes. *AH*, 36–38.

103. Brody, J. E. (1991, March 21). Water fluoridation: A much-hailed measure still hampered by lingering doubts. *NYT*, B7.

104. Miller, 1990.

105. Bashin, 1992.

106. Bashin, 1992.

107. Simons, A. (1989, March/April). Diarrhea: On the runs. *Medical SelfCare*, 60–61.

108. Anonymous. (1991, November 23). Evidence piling up that smog is L.A. health hazard to all. *SFC*, A16; reprinted from *Los Angeles Daily News*.

109. Phalen, R. Quoted in: Siegel, L. (1990, March 25). Smog detective studies effects on humans. *LAT*, B5.

110. Secter, B., & Abramson, R. (1990, May 3). U.S. poised to clean up the air in Grand Canyon. *SFC*, A12; reprinted from *LAT*.

111. Anonymous. (1990, November 24). Smog is hurting trees in Yosemite. *SFC*, A6.

112. Ayres, B. D. Jr. (1991, May 2). Pollution shrouds Shenandoah Park. *NYT*, A10.

113. Stevens, W. K. (1990, July 17). If it's east of the Mississippi, it's blanketed in pollution's haze. *NYT*, B10.

114. Anonymous. (1991, January 26). Wood smoke called a health hazard. *SFC*, A17; reprinted from *LAT*.

115. Sonenshine, R. (1992, January 6). Wood-stove fad going up in smoke. *SFC*, A1.

116. Associated Press. (1991, June 3). A Lamborghini wins the pollution title. *SFC*, A14.

117. Associated Press. (1990, July 27). Council ranks states as world polluters. *SFC*, A12.

118. Reinhold, R. (1990, September 14). Citing medical evidence on smog, California lowers threshold for its health alerts. *NYT*, A10.

119. Anonymous, 1991. Evidence piling up that smog is L.A. health hazard to all.

120. Sherwin, R. Cited in: Boly, W. (1992, April). Smog City wants to make this perfectly clear. *Health*, 54–64.

121. Winslow, R. (1990, September 4). Air polluted by carbon monoxide poses risk to heart patients, study shows. *WSJ*, B4.

122. California Air Resources Board. Cited in: Dolan, M. (1992, July 22). 50% cut in smog in L.A. since '82. *SFC*, A13; reprinted from *LAT*.

123. Ivins, M. (1989, July/August). Too much stuff! Our accumulating crisis. *Utne Reader*, 77–79; reprinted from *Ms.*

124. Kotzsch, R. E. (1989, July/August). Just say no to junk. *Utne Reader*, 79; reprinted from *East West*.

125. Koch-Gonzalez, G. Quoted in: Ferriss, S. (1992, September 20). Urban garden tenders face filth in parks. *SFE*, B-5.

126. Schneider, K. (1991, October 25). Minorities join to fight toxic waste. *NYT*, A12.

127. Suro, R. (1993, January 11). Pollution-weary minorities try civil rights tack. *NYT*, A1, A12.

128. Environmental Protection Agency. Cited in: Suro, 1993.

129. Grimes, W. (1992, August 13). Finding truth in refuse at landfills; garbage as a window to the soul. *NYT*, A14.

130. Rathje, W., & Murphy, C. (1992). *Rubbish! The archaeology of garbage.* New York: HarperCollins.

131. Rathje & Murphy, 1992.

132. Rathje, W. L. (1991, May). Once and future landfills. *National Geographic*, 116–34.

133. Liddle, A. (1990, November 12). McDonald's pulls plastic packaging. *Nation's Restaurant News*, 1, 10.

134. Holusha, J. (1990, November 2). Packaging and public image: McDonald's fills a big order. *NYT*, A1, C5.

135. Rathje & Murphy, 1992.

136. Ratheje & Murphy, 1992.

137. Anonymous. (1991, August). Which are best for the environment? *Consumer Reports*, 555–56.

138. Specter, M. (1992, October 23). Among the earth baby set, disposable diapers are back. *NYT*, A1, A20.

139. Rathje, 1991.

140. Breen, B. (1990, September/October). Landfills are #1. *Garbage*, 42–47.

141. Schneider, K. (1992, January 6). Rules force towns to pick big new dumps or big costs. *NYT*, A1, A10.

142. Breen, 1990.

143. Barrett, P. M. (1992, March 23). High Court to enter waste-disposal war. *WSJ*, B1, B8.

144. Passell, P. (1992, February 26). The garbage problem: It may be politics, not nature. *NYT*, C1, C6.

145. Schneider, 1992.

146. Brown, P. (1992, July). Addressing public distrust. *Technology Review*, 68.

147. Passell, P. (1991, September 1). Experts question staggering costs of toxic cleanups. *NYT*, sec. 1, 1, 12.

148. Miller, 1990.

149. Passell, 1991.

150. Kay, J. (1990, September 23). Global dumping of U.S. toxics is big business. *SFE*, A-2.

151. Nash, N. C. (1991, December 16). Latin nations getting others' waste. *NYT*, A6.

152. Environmental Protection Agency. Cited in: Anonymous. (1992, April 10). U.S. says 45,000 sites may be nuclear hazards. *International Herald Tribune*, 3.

153. Grossman, D., & Shulman, S. (1993, December/January). Doing their low-level best. *Garbage*, 32–37.

154. Wald, M. L. (1992, September 20). As nuclear plants close, costs don't shut down. *NYT*, sec. 4, 18.

155. Wald, M. L. (1992, October 3). Nuclear plants held hostage to old fuel. *NYT*, 6.

156. Bauerlein, M. (1992, July/August). Plutonium is forever. *Utne Reader*, 34–37.

157. Breen, B. (1992, March/April). Dismantling nuclear power plants. *Garbage*, 40–47.

158. Wald, M. L. (1992, December 24). Nuclear hazard festers after alarm. *NYT*, A1, A10.

159. Schneider, K. (1992, February 26). Nuclear disarmament raises fear on storage of 'triggers.' *NYT*, A1, A8.

160. Broad, W. J. (1992, July 6). Nuclear accords bring new fears on arms disposal. *NYT*, A1, A4.

161. Grossman & Shulman, 1993.

162. Long, R. L. (1991, November 11). NIMBYism stalls action on nuclear waste sites. *SFC*, A21.

163. Lippman, T. W. (1992, December 19). Energy Dept. can't store nuclear fuel by deadline. *SFC*, A3; reprinted from *Washington Post*.

164. Wald, M. L. (1992, October 20). States' pressure over nuclear waste. *NYT*, C5.

165. Coates, J. (1992, July 12). Damage forces officials to rethink nuclear dump site. *SFE*, A-2; reprinted from *Chicago Tribune*.

166. Kenyon, Q. (1991, October 6). Nuclear waste starts rolling into Idaho. *Albuquerque Journal*, A3.

167. Schneider, K. (1991, October 10). U.S. delays opening of a waste site. *NYT*, A19.

168. Schneider, K. (1992, August 30). Wasting away. *New York Times Magazine*, 42–45, 56–58.

169. Bauerlein, 1992.

170. Skerrett, P. J. (1992, February/March). Nuclear burial at sea. *Technology Review*, 22–23.

171. Browne, M. C. (1991, October 29). Modern alchemists transmute nuclear waste. *NYT*, B5, B7.

172. Fialka, J. J. (1991, June 18). Salute the jimson! The noxious weed may save our planet. *WSJ*, A1, A7.

173. Anonymous. (1991, April 9). Bacterium may combat nuclear waste. *SFC*, A9; reprinted from *NYT*.

174. Piller, C. (1992). *The fail-safe society: Defiance and the end of American technological optimism.* New York: Basic.

175. World Health Organization. (1992, June 24). *Reproductive health: A key to a brighter future.* Cited in: Anonymous. (1992, June 25). Report on world sex adds up to millions. *SFC*, A1.

176. McLeod, R. G. (1992, March 2). Poll finds U.S. concern about world population. *SFC*, A3.

177. Ehrlich, P. R., & Ehrlich, A. H. (1990, April 11). People a lethal disease for earth. *SFC*, Briefing section, 8; reprinted from *Los Angles Times*.

178. Anonymous. (1991, May 14). New prediction on world's population. *SFC*, A7.

179. Ehrlich, P. Cited in: Reuters. (1992, June 19). Author still predicting a world 'population bomb.' *SFC*, A6.

180. Allen, F. E. (1991, September 13). Overpopulation takes center stage in 1990s. *WSJ*, B1.

181. Crossette, B. (1992, September 16). Population policy in Asia is faulted. *NYT*, A7.

182. U.S. Census Bureau. Cited in: Pear, R. (1992, December 4). New look at the U.S. in 2050: Bigger, older and less white. *NYT*, A1, A10.

183. United Nations. Cited in: Nash, N. C. (1992, October 11). Squalid slums grow as people flood Latin America's cities. *NYT*, sec. 1, 1, 10.

184. Lowe, M. D. (1992, July–August). Alternatives to shaping tomorrow's cities. *The Futurist*, 28–34.

185. Roberts, S. (1990, June 25). 'Mega-cities' join to fight problems. *NYT*, A13.

186. U.S. Census Bureau. Cited in: Vobejda, B. (1991, February 21). Half of population lives in urban areas. *Washington Post*, A1, A12.

187. Garreau, J. (1991). *Edge city: Life on the new frontier.* New York: Doubleday.

188. Gordon S. Black Corp. survey for Population Crisis Committee. Cited in: McLeod, R. G. (1992, March 2). Poll finds U.S. concern about world population. *SFC*, A3.

189. Fornos, W. (1991, February/March). Population politics. *Technology Review*, 45–51.

190. World Bank. Cited in: Fornos, 1991.

191. *IRED Forum* [a publication of the Geneva-based Innovations et Reseaux pour le Developpement], cited in: Anonymous. (1990, July/August). The global village. *Utne Reader*, 144; excerpted from *World Development Forum* (1990, April 15).

192. Sadik, N. (1991, March–April). World population continues to rise. *The Futurist*, 9–14.

193. United Nations Food and Agricultural Organization. Cited in: Associated Press. (1992, September 21). World producing enough food, U.N. study says. *SFC*, A10.

194. Sadik, 1991.

195. Anonymous. (1992, June 29). Notes and comment. *New Yorker*, 25–26.

196. Ehrlich, P. Cited in: Associated Press. (1990, April 6). Americans accused of ruining the planet. *SFC*, A11.

197. Durning, A. (1992). *How much is enough?* Washington, DC: The Worldwatch Institute.

198. Sadik, 1991.

199. United Nations. Cited in: Allen, 1991.

200. Jungerman, E. (1992, May 29). Confronting a threatened planet. *SFC*, A7.

201. Hofheinz, P. (1992, July 27). The new Soviet threat: Pollution. *Fortune*, 110–14.

202. Fesbach, M., & Friendly, A. Jr. (1992). *Ecocide in the U.S.S.R.: Health and nature under seige.* New York: Basic.

203. Bogert, C. (1992, November 2). Get out the geiger counters. *Newsweek*, 64–65.

204. Lewis, P. (1992, May 21). U.S. and six plan nuclear cleanup in Eastern Europe. *NYT*, A1, A7.

205. Kinzer, S. (1992, July 8). 7 leaders fail to agree on pact for A-plant safety. *NYT*, A6.

206. Intergovernmental Panel on Climate Change, 1990. Cited in: Jungerman, 1992.

207. Reuters. (1991, June 14). Expert says deforestation is suicidal. *SFC*, A16.

208. United Nations Food and Agriculture Organization. *Forest resources assessment, 1990 project.* Cited in: Jungerman, 1992.

209. Egan, T. (1990, April 20). Canada rain forest falling like Brazil's. *SFC*, A26; reprinted from *NYT*.

210. Durham, W. Cited in: Seawell, M. A. (1990, April–May). *Stanford Observer*, 5.

211. Larmer, B. (1991, August 12). The rain forest at risk. *Newsweek*, 42.

212. Shabecoff, P. (1990, June 8). Loss of tropical forests is found much worse than was thought. *NYT*, A1, A9.

213. Jungerman, 1992.

214. Kolata, G. (1991, May 13). Tree yields a cancer treatment, but ecological costs may be high. *NYT*, A1, A9.

215. Egan, T. (1991, May 31). Carving out a market for Oregon's yew tree. *NYT*, A8.

216. Sears, C. (1992, October). Jungle potions. *AH*, 70–75.

217. Barnum, A. (1992, December 22). Taking stock in the rain forest. *SFC*, C1

218. Anonymous. (1990, April 30). The rain forest goes commercial. *SFC*, C2; reprinted from *NYT*.

219. Starr, C., & Taggart, R. (1992). *Biology: The unity and diversity of life* (6th ed.). Belmont, CA: Wadsworth.

220. Shabecoff, P. (1990, June 24). Scientists report more deterioration in earth's ozone layer. *NYT*, sec. 1, 16.

221. Anonymous. (1992, September 30). Dramatic increase in ozone hole. *SFC*, A5.

222. Larmer, B. (1991, December 9). Life under the ozone hole. *Newsweek*, 43.

223. Kamm, T. (1993, January 12). Sheep and trees are acting strangely at 'end of the world.' *WSJ*, A1, A7.

224. Associated Press. (1992, November 26). New timetable for ban on ozone-depleting chemicals. *SFC*, A13.

225. Makhijani, A., Bickel, A., & Makhijani, A. (1990, May/June). Still working on the ozone hole. *Technology Review*, 53–56.

226. Revelle, R. Quoted in: Jungerman, 1992.

227. Boutros-Ghali, B. Cited in: Stevens, W. K. (1992, June 4). U.N. chief charts the defense of nature, saying arms spending should be diverted. *NYT*, A4.

228. Lentz Peace Research. Cited in: Farhat, L. (1990, October 23). Computer analysis tells a grim tale of war. *SFC*, A21.

229. Perlman, D. (1992, December 3). World still lives in nuclear fear. *SFC*, A1, A4.

230. Deutch, J. M. (1992, February/March). Nuclear weapons in the new world order. *Technology Review*, 68.

231. Rathjens, G. W., & Miller, M. M. (1991, August/September). *Technology Review*, 25–32.

232. Church, G. J. (1991, December 16). Who else will have the bomb? *Time*, 42–48.

233. Sivard, R. L. (1986). *World military and social expenditures, 1986*. Washington, DC: World Priorities, 26.

234. Farhat, 1990.

235. Pear, R. (1991, August 11). U.S. ranked no. 1 in weapons sales. *NYT*, 8.

236. Klare, M. T. (1990, May/June). Who's arming who? The arms trade in the 1990s. *Technology Review*, 42–50.

237. Meadows, D. H., Meadows, D. L., & Randers,

J. (1992). *Beyond the limits: Confronting global collapse, envisioning a sustainable future*. Post Mills, VT: Chelsea Green.

238. Paulsen, M. (1991, May/June). How to undermine overpopulation. *Garbage*, 49, 51.

239. Dominguez, J., & Robin, V. (1992). *Your money or your life*. Bergenfield, NJ: Penguin.

240. Nix, S. (1991, January 22). Living on less, enjoying it more. *SFC*, B3, B5.

241. Schlender, B. R. (1992, January 27). The values we will need. *Fortune*, 75.

242. Gitlin, T. Quoted in: Schlender, 1992, 76.

243. Luks, A. Cited in: Flippin, R. (1992, November). Good Luks: A champion of volunteerism insists helping is healthy. *AH*, 27–29.

244. House, J. Cited in: Growald, E. R., & Luks, A. (1988, March). Beyond self. *AH*, 51–53.

245. Luks, A. Quoted in: Flippin, 1992, 27–28.

246. Theiler, (1990, November/December). The power of one. *Common Cause Magazine*, 36–40.

247. Wade, J. (1992, November/December). Volunteering on vacation. *Arthritis Today*, 60–62.

248. Walls, D. (1993). *The activist's almanac: The concerned citizen's guide to the leading advocacy organizations in America*. New York: Simon & Schuster.

249. Robertson, I. (1987). *Sociology* (3rd ed.). New York: Worth.

250. Waldron, I. The role of genetic and biological factors in sex differences in mortality. In A. D. Lopez, & L. T. Ruzicka (Eds.), (1983). *Sex differences in mortality*. Canberra: Department of Demography, Australian National University.

251. Robertson, P., 1987, 325.

252. Fuller, K. S. (1991, November 23). Third World women caught in vicious cycle. *SFC*, A17.

253. United Nations International Fund for Agricultural Development. Cited in: Associated Press. (1991, July 29). Poverty among women up sharply around world. *SFC*, A8.

254. Sen, A. (1990, December 20). More than 100 million women are missing. *New York Review of Books*, 61–66.

255. Parales, C. A. (1987). Preface: Women, health, and poverty. *Women & Health*, 12(3/4), 1–20.

256. General Accounting Office. Cited in: Kolata, G. (1990, June 19). N.I.H. neglects women, study says. *NYT*, B11.

257. Watkins, T. (1990, October). Bypassed women. *AH*, 16.

258. Anomyous. (1991, July 26). Taking women's health to heart (editorial). *NYT*, A12.

259. National Opinion Research Center. Cited in: Lewin, T. (1992, January 8). Study points to increase in tolerance of ethnicity. *NYT*, A10.

260. National Center for Health Statistics. (1990). *Health, United States, 1989 and prevention profile*. DHHS Pub. No. (PHS)90-1232. Hyattsville, MD: U.S Department of Health and Human Services.

261. Department of Health and Human Services. Cited in: Stout, H. (1991, April 9). Life expectancy of black Americans fell in 1988 for fourth year in a row. *WSJ*, B4.

262. Cooper, R. Cited in: Duke, L. (1992, January 29). Analysis of death rates to look beyond race. *SFC*, A2; reprinted from *Washington Post*.

263. Rosenberg, H. Cited in Duke, 1992.

264. Rogers, R. Cited in: Krafft, S. (1991, December). Black death: The demographic difference. *American Demographics*, 12–13.

265. Rogers, 1991.

266. Reuters. (1991, April 17). Poverty blamed for blacks' high cancer rate. *NYT*, A12.

267. Thomas, S. B. (1992, January/February). Health status of the black community in the 21st century: A futuristic perspective for health education. *Journal of Health Education*, 7–13.

268. Editors, *AH*. (1990, November). Forgotten Americans. *AH*, 41–42.

269. Winslow, R. (1992, March 18). Study finds blacks get fewer bypasses. *WSJ*, B1. [Report of study by Arthur J. Hartz et al. of article in 3/18/92 JAMA article.]

270. Cohn, L. Cited in: Associated Press. (1992, March 18). Blacks on Medicare get fewer heart bypasses than whites. *NYT*, A14.

271. Gorman, C. (1991, September 16). Why do blacks die young? *Time*, 50–52.

272. *NEJM* (1990, January 18). Quoted in: Editors, *AH*, 1990.

273. Hilton, B. (1990, July 22). The No. 1 cause of poor health. *SFE*, D-15.

274. Frank, D. Quoted in: Anonymous. (1992, September 9). Study hints of hard choice for poor: Heat or food. *NYT*, C20.

275. Public Health Service. (1990). *Healthy people 2000*. DHHS Pub. No. (PHS)91-50212. Washington, DC: Department of Health and Human Services.

276. Public Health Service, 1990, 29.

277. Nasar, S. (1992, March 5). The 1980's: A very good time for the very rich. *NYT*, A1, C13.

278. Nasar, S. (1992, May 18). Those born wealthy or poor usually stay so, studies say. *NYT*, A1, C7.

279. Pear, R. (1992, September 4). Ranks of U.S. poor reach 35.7 million, the most since '64. *NYT*, A1, A10.

280. *United Nations human development report*.(1993). New York: Oxford University Press. Cited in: Lewis, P. (1993, May 23). New U.N. index measures wealth as quality of life. *NYT*, sec. 1, 1.

281. National Center for Health Statistics. Cited in: Otten, A. L. (1992, January 3). Poor health is linked to lack of education. *WSJ*, B1.

282. U.S. Census Bureau. (1993). *What's it worth? Educational background and economic status: Spring 1990*. Washington, DC: U.S. Census Bureau.

Index

Boldface page numbers indicate definitions.

Sources and Credits

F stands for Figure, **T** for Table, **SD** for Self Discovery, **P** for Page.

UNIT 1. F1.1 Centers for Disease Control. **F1.2** Adapted from Combs, B., Hales, D., & Williams, B. (1983). *Invitation to health* (2nd ed.). Menlo Park, CA: Benjamin/Cummings, 3. **F2.1** Vickery, D. M. (1990). *LifePlan*. Evergreen, CO: Health Decisions, 23. **F2.3** U.S. Public Health Service (1990). *Healthy people 2000*. Washington, DC: U.S. Government Printing Office, 16, 19. **F2.4** Brody, J. E. (1991, January 31). In pursuit of the best possible odds of preventing or minimizing the perils of major diseases. *New York Times*, B6. Copyright © 1991 by The New York Times Company. Reprinted by permission.

UNIT 2. F3.1 Lazarus, R. S. (1981, July). Little hassles can be hazardous to health. *Psychology Today*, 61. **F3.2** *(Top)* Kalat, J. W. (1990). *Introduction to psychology* (2nd ed.). Belmont, CA: Wadsworth, 78. Copyright © 1990, 1986 by Wadsworth, Inc. Reprinted by permission of Brooks/Cole, Pacific Grove, CA. *(Bottom)* Myers, D. G. (1989). *Psychology* (2nd ed.). New York: Worth, 26. **SD3.1** Copyright 1978 by the American Psychological Association. Adapted by permission. **F4.2** Starr, C., & Taggart, R. (1992). *Biology* (6th ed.). Belmont, CA: Wadsworth, 643. **F5.4** Kabat-Zinn, J. (1990). *Full catastrophe living*. New York: Delacorte.

UNIT 3. F6.1 Adapted from Menninger, K. (1963). *The vital balance*. New York: Viking; Combs, B., Hales, D., & Williams, B. (1980). *An invitation to health*. Menlo Park, CA: Benjamin/Cummings, 51; and Hales, D. (1992). *An Invitation to health* (5th ed). Redwood City, CA: Benjamin/Cummings, 70. **F6.6** Reprinted with permission from *Psychology Today Magazine*. Copyright © 1989 (Sussex Publishers, Inc.). **F8.1** Kalat, J. W. (1990). *Introduction to psychology* (2nd ed.). 509. (Adapted from Myers et al., 1984, *Arch. Gen. Psychiatry*, *41*, 949–58, and Robins et al., 1984, *Arch. Gen. Psychiatry*, *41*, 959–67. Copyright 1984 by the American Medical Association. **F8.2** Kalat, J. W. (1990). *Introduction to psychology* (2nd ed.). Belmont, CA: Wadsworth, 540. Copyright © 1986, 1990 by Wadsworth, Inc. Reprinted by permission of Brooks/Cole, Pacific Grove, CA. **F8.4** Phears and phobias. (1984, August/September). *Public Opinion Quarterly*, 32. Reprinted by permission of the University of Chicago Press. **F8.5** Nicol, S. E., & Gottesman, I. I. (1983). Clues to the genetics and neurobiology of schizophrenia. *American Scientist*, *71*, 398–404. **P. 3.46** Cult Awareness Network. Quoted in: Irving, C. (1990, March 4). Cults prey on university students. *San Francisco Examiner*, B-1.

UNIT 4. F10.1 Data on coffee, tea, tea products, and chocolate products: Institute of Food Technologists. (1987, June). *Evaluation of caffeine safety*. Data on soft drinks: National Soft Drink Association. **SD10.1** Reprinted by permission. **F11.2** *Smoking and health*. (1990). Rockville, MD: Health and Human Services. **F11.4** Adapted from Zaret, B. L. et al. (1992). *Yale University School of Medicine heart book*. New York: Hearst, p. 76. **F12.1** Adapted from Wechsler and McFadden for AAA Foundation for Traffic Safety, survey of 1669 college freshmen at 14 Massachusetts institutions. By permission. **F12.5** Starr, C., & Taggart, R. (1992). *Biology* (6th ed.). Belmont, CA: Wadsworth, 643. **F12.7** CDC. (1990). Alcohol-related mortality and years of potential life lost—United States, 1987. *MMWR*, *39*(11), 175. **F12.9** American Psychiatric Association (1987). *Diagnostic and statistical manual of mental disorders*, third edition—revised). Reprinted by permission. **F12.10** Kinney, J., & Leaton, G. (1987). *Loosening the grip* (3rd ed.). St. Louis: Times Mirror/Mosby. **F12.11** Kinney, J., & Leaton, G. (1987). *Loosening the grip: A handbook of alcohol information* (3rd ed.). St. Louis: Times Mirror/Mosby, pp. 153–8. **F12.12** Reprinted with permission © *American Demographics*, August, 1991. For subscription information, please call (800)828-1133. **P. 4.53** The Twelve Steps are reprinted with permission of Alcoholics Anonymous World Services, Inc. Permission to reprint this material does not mean that AA has reviewed or approved the contents of this publication, nor that AA agrees with the views expressed herein. AA is a program of recovery from alcoholism—use of the Twelve Steps in connection with programs and activities which are patterned after AA, but which address other problems, does not imply otherwise.

UNIT 5. F13.1 Pope, H. G., et al. (1990). Drug use and life style among college undergraduates in 1989: A comparison with 1969 and 1978. *American Journal of Psychiatry*, *147*, 999. Copyright 1971, the American Psychiatric Association. Reprinted by permission. **F13.4** Maisto, S. A., Galizio, M., & Connors, G. J. (1991). *Drug use and misuse*. Copyright © 1991 by Holt, Rinehart and Winston, Inc., reprinted by permission of the publisher. **SD14.2** Reprinted from *Shopaholics*, © 1988 by Janet Damon, published by Price Stern Sloan, Inc., Los Angeles, CA.

UNIT 6. F15.6 Reprinted by permission of Frances Moore Lappe and her agents, Raines & Raines, New York, NY. Copyright © 1971, 1975, 1982, 1991 by Frances Moore Lappe. *Diet for a small planet*. New York: Ballantine, 181. **F15.7** Adapted from Welsh, S. O., & Marston, R. M. (1982). Review of trends in food use in the United States, 1909 to 1980. *Journal of the American Dietetic Association*, *81*, 120. **F15.12** Starr, C., & Taggart, R. (1992). *Biology* (6th ed.). Belmont, CA: Wadsworth, 643. **F15.15** Adapted from *The label table*, California Dietetic Association, San Diego, CA. **F15.16** U.S. Department of Agriculture. **F16.1** Adapted from Britton, A. G. (1988, July/August). Thin is out, fit is in. *American Health*, 68–69. *American Health* © A. G. Britton. **SD16.1** From Rodin, J. (1992). *Body traps*. New York: William Morrow. **F16.2** Accentuating the negative, by Megan Jaegerman, October 21, 1991. Copyright © 1991 by The New York Times Company. Reprinted by permission. **F16.6** Excerpted from the *University of California at Berkeley Wellness Letter*, © Health Letter Associates, 1991. **SD16.5** *American Health* © 1986 by Susan Wooley, Ph.D., and O. Wayne Wooley, Ph.D.

UNIT 7. F17.1 Centers for Disease Control. (1990). Coronary heart disease attributable to sedentary lifestyle—selected states, 1988. *Journal of the American Medical Association*, *264*, 1392. **SD17.1** Reprinted by permission of *Prevention*. Copyright 1993 Rodale Press, Inc. All rights reserved. **SD17.2** Reprinted by permission of Warner Books/New York from *Fitness without exercise*. Copyright © 1990 by B.A. Stamford and P. Shimer. **F17.4** Graph from *Newsweek*, The Health Connection, May 13, 1991. Reprinted by permission. **F17.6** From "Staying Loose" by James M. Rippe, M.D., *Modern maturity*, June-July 1990, 73–74. Used with permission of the author. **F17.7** Stretching before—and after. *American Health* © 1990 by Marc Bloom. **F17.9** Adapted from Borg, G. (1973). Perceived exertion: A note on history and methods. *Medicine & Science in Sports*, *5*, 90. © by American College of Sports Medicine, 1973. **F17.12** (table). Adapted from DeWitt, J., & Roberts, T. (1991, September). Pumping up an adult fitness program. *Journal of Physical Education, Recreation, & Dance*, table 4, p. 70. **SD17.6** *American Health* © 1990 by J. Morrow. **F17.13** *(Top)* Data compiled from *The physiological basis of physical education and athletics* (3rd ed.) (p. 475) by E. L. Fox and D. K. Mathews, 1982, Philadelphia: Saunders College Publishing, and *Physiology of exercise: Responses and adaptations* (p. 281), 1978, D. R. Lamb, New York: Macmillan Publishing Co.. As shown in *Environment and human performance* by E. M. Haymes and C. L. Wells (p. 27), Champaign, IL: Human Kinetics Publishers. Copyright 1986 by Emily M. Haymes and Christine L. Wells. Adapted and reprinted by permission. *(Bottom)* Adapted from Sharkey, B. J., 1975, *Physiology and physical activity*, New York: Harper & Row Publishers, pp. 108–109. As found in *Environment and human performance* by E. M. Haymes and C. L. Wells (p. 27), Champaign, IL: Human Kinetics Publishers. Copyright 1986 by Emily M. Haymes and Christine L. Wells. Adapted and reprinted by permission. **T17.2** Adapted from Group Health Cooperative of Puget Sound. **SD18.1** © San Francisco Chronicle. Reprinted by permission. **F17.13** Weiten, W., Lloyd, M. A., & Lashley, R. L. (1991). *Psychology applied to modern life* (3rd ed.). Pacific Grove, CA: Brooks/Cole, 406. Copyright © 1991, 1986, 1983 by Wadsworth, Inc. Reprinted by permission of Brooks/Cole, Pacific Grove, CA.

UNIT 8. F19.3 After Sternberg, R. (1988). *The triangle of love*. New York: Basic Books. **F19.4** Census Bureau, National Center for Health Statistics. Adapted from Barringer, F. (1991, June 7). Changes in U.S. households: Single parents amid solitude. *New York Times*, A1, A13. **F20.4** Adapted from Kinsey, A., Pomeroy, W., & Martin, C. (1948). *Sexual behavior in the human male*. Philadelphia: W. B. Saunders, 638. **SD20.1** Adapted from the book *The Kinsey Institute new report on sex* by J. Reinisch & R. Beasley and reprinted with permission from St. Martin's Press, Inc., New York, NY.

UNIT 9. F21.1 Based on data from Katzenstein, L. (1991, January/February). When he has AIDS—and she doesn't know. *American Health*, 58–62. **F21.5** Based on data from: Centers for Disease Control. (1990). *Contraceptive options: Increasing your awareness.* Washington, DC: NAACOG. Hatcher, R. et al. (1990). *Contraceptive technology, 1990-1992.* New York: Irvington. Leads from the MMWR. (1988). Condoms for prevention of sexually transmitted diseases. *Journal of the American Medical Association, 259*, 1925–27. Harlap, S. et al. (1991). *Preventing pregnancy, protecting health: A new look at birth control choices in the United States.* New York: Alan Guttmacher. Anonymous. (1991, December). Deconstructing the condom. *Self*, 122–23. Consumers Union. (1989, March). Can you rely on condoms? *Consumer Reports*, 135–41. **F22.1** Adapted from Starr, C., & Taggart, R. (1992). *Biology* (6th ed.). Belmont, CA: Wadsworth, 768. **F22.2** Adapted from Kost, K., Forrest, J. D., & Harlap, S. (1991). Comparing the health risks and benefits of contraceptive choices. *Family Planning Perspectives, 23*, 54–61, table 1. **SD, p. 9.31** Adapted with permission from the *Journal of Health Education* (1992), *23*, 209–214. *Journal of Health Education* is a publication of the American Alliance for Health, Physical Education, Recreation and Dance, 1900 Association Dr., Reston, VA 22091. **SD, p. 9.34** Reproduced by permission of McGraw-Hill.

UNIT 10. F24.2 U.S. Census Bureau. **F24.3** Excter, T. (1991, August). The costs of growing up. *American Demographics*, 59. Reprinted with permission © *American Demographics* (August 1991). For subscription information, please call (800)828-1133. **F24.4** After Luke, B., & Keith, L. G. (1992). The contribution of singletons, twins and triplets to low birth weight, infant mortality and handicap in the United States. *Journal of Reproductive Medicine, 37*, 661–62. **F24.6** Adapted from Myers, D. G. (1989). *Psychology* (2nd ed.). New York: Worth Publishers, 59; and from Bevan, J. (1978). *The Simon & Schuster handbook of anatomy and physiology.* New York: Simon & Schuster, 17. **F24.7** Adapted from Bevan, J. (1978). *The Simon & Schuster handbook of anatomy and physiology.* New York: Simon & Schuster, 19. **F24.9** American College of Obstetrics and Gynecologists. Adapted from Anonymous. (1990, December). Older mothers: Chromosome defects. *American Health*, 11. **F25.2** Adapted from Starr, C., & Taggart, R. (1992). *Biology* (6th ed). Belmont, CA: Wadsworth, 768. **F25.4** Reproduced by permission from Jensen et al. (1979). *Biology.* Belmont, CA: Wadsworth, 237. **F25.7** Adapted from Zyla, G. (1990, November). Expectant moms expected to eat more. *American Health*, 89; and from Hegarty, V. (1988). *Decisions in nutrition.* St. Louis: Times Mirror/Mosby, 366. **F25.12** Adapted from Starr, C., & Taggart, R. (1992). *Biology* (6th ed). Belmont, CA: Wadsworth, 775. **P. 10.53** Reproduced by permission.

UNIT 11. F26.4 Adapted from Starr, C., & Taggart, R. (1992). *Biology* (6th ed.). Belmont, CA: Wadsworth, 677; Creager, J. C. (1983). *Human anatomy and physiology.* Belmont, CA: Wadsworth, 521; and Martini, F. (1989). *Fundamentals of anatomy and physiology.* Englewood Cliffs, NJ: Prentice Hall, 606. **F26.6** Centers for Disease Control and Prevention. **F26.8** *(Top left)* Centers for Disease Control and Prevention. *(Bottom and right)* Adapted from Anonymous. (1992, October 11). Anatomy of a disease: A primer on tuberculosis. *New York Times*, sec. 1, 20. **F27.1** Data from World Health Organization. Adapted from Gorman, C. (1992, August 3). Invincible AIDS. *Time*, 30–37. **F27.2** Data from World Health Organization Global Program on AIDS. Adapted from Krieger, L. M. (1992, July 19). Global attack on AIDS. *San Francisco Examiner*, A-1, A-10. **F27.3** Centers for Disease Control and Prevention.

UNIT 12. T29.1 Copyright © 1991 by The New York Times Company. Reprinted by permission. **T29.2** Copyright 1980, American Medical Association. **F29.1** From *The American Medical Association family medical guide* by the American Medical Association. Copyright © 1982 by the American Medical Association. Reprinted by permission of Random House, Inc. **F29.2** Adapted from data from American Automobile Association, in Blyskal, J. (1993, January/February). Crash course. *American Health*, 74–79. **F29.3** Adapted from San Jose State University Police Department. (1989). *Safety & security.* San Jose, CA: San Jose State University, 26–27. **F29.4, F29.7** From *The American Medical Association family medical guide* by the American Medical Association. Copyright © 1982 by the American Medical Association. Reprinted by permission of Random House, Inc. **F29.8** National Safety Council, cited in Milbank, D. (1991, March 29).

Companies turn to peer pressure to cut injuries as psychologists join the battle. *Wall Street Journal*, B1. Reprinted by permission of The Wall Street Journal, © 1991 Dow Jones & Company, Inc. All rights reserved worldwide. **F29.10** Fingerhut, L. A., & Kleinman, J. C. (1990). International and interstate comparisons of homicide among young males. *Journal of the American Medical Association, 263*, 3292–95. Copyright 1990, American Medical Association. **SD29.1** Copyright © 1992 by The New York Times Company. Reprinted by permission. **F29.12** National Victim Center. Adapted from Anonymous. (1992, May 4). Unsettling report on an epidemic of rape. *Time*, 15. **SD, p. 12.37** By permission of Donna K. Darden. This questionnaire was originally published in *Self*. **P. 12.39** Adapted from Scitovsky, T. (1980, October). Why do we seek more and more excitement? *Stanford Observer*, 13.

UNIT 13. F30.1 Adapted from Starr, C., & Taggart, R. (1992). *Biology* (6th ed.). Belmont, CA: Wadsworth, 664. Reprinted with permission of Wadsworth, Inc. **F30.2** Adapted from Curtis, H., & Barnes, N. S. (1989). *Biology* (5th ed.). New York: Worth, 755. **F30.3** *(Left)* Adapted from Fowler, I. (1983). *Human anatomy.* Belmont, CA: Wadsworth, 408. *(Right)* Starr, C., & Taggart, R. (1992). *Biology.* Belmont, CA: Wadsworth, 665–666; reprinted with permission of Wadsworth, Inc. and Joel Ito. **F30.5** Public Health Service (1990). *Healthy people 2000.* Washington, DC: U.S. Government Printing Office, 3. **F30.6** Right: Starr, C., & Taggart, R. (1992). *Biology.* Belmont, CA: Wadsworth, 671; reprinted with permission of Wadsworth, Inc. **F30.8** Starr, C., & Taggart, R. (1992). *Biology.* Belmont, CA: Wadsworth, 672; reprinted with permission of Wadsworth, Inc. **SD30.1** Adapted from Luckmann, J. (1990). *Your health!* Englewood Cliffs, NJ: Prentice Hall, 337–38; American Heart Association, 1985. **F30.9** National Health and Nutrition Examination Survey II, 1976–80. **F31.1** American Cancer Society. (1990). *Cancer facts and figures.* Atlanta: American Cancer Society. **F31.4** This excerpt first appeared in *Everyone's guide to cancer therapy: How cancer is diagnosed, treated, and managed day-to-day* by Malin Dollinger, M.D., Ernest H. Rosenbaum, M.D., and Greg Cable (adapted by The Canadian Medical Association, Richard Hasselback, M.D., editor) © 1992 Somerville House Books Limited and is published by the kind permission of Somerville House Books Limited. **F31.5** Adapted from Cohen, L. A. (1987). Diet and cancer. *Scientific American, 257*(5), 43. Copyright © 1987 by Scientific American, Inc. All rights reserved.

UNIT 14. F32.1 Health Strategy Group, New York, in Ferguson, T. (1992, January-February). Patient, heal thyself: Health in the information age. *The Futurist*, 9–14. Reproduced, with permission, from *The Futurist*, published by the World Future Society, 7910 Woodmont Ave., Suite 450, Bethesda, MD 20814. **T32.1** From *The wellness encyclopedia*, edited by the Editors of the University of California, Berkeley, Wellness Letter. Copyright © 1991 by Health Letter Associates. Reprinted by permission of Houghton Mifflin Co. All rights reserved.

UNIT 15. F34.4 Roper Organization. Adapted from Robertson, I. (1987). *Sociology* (3rd ed.). New York: Worth, 337. **SD35.1** Reprinted with permission from *Psychology Today* magazine. Copyright © 1970 (Sussex Publishers, Inc.). **F35.2** Reprinted by permission of Choice In Dying (formerly Concern for Dying/Society for the Right to Die), 200 Varick St., New York, NY 10014-4810; 212/366-5540. **SD35.2** Reprinted by permission of The Wall Street Journal, © 1990 Dow Jones & Company, Inc. All rights reserved worldwide. **F35.3** Taken from a "Dear Abby" column by Abigail Van Buren. © 1990. Distributed by Universal Press Syndicate. Reprinted by permission.

UNIT 16. SD36.1 Reprinted by permission of *Men's Health Magazine.* Copyright 1993 Rodale Press, Inc. All rights reserved. **F36.2** Patrick, D. (1993, March 8). Do cellular phones cause cancer? *Fortune*, 79–80. © 1993 Time Inc. All rights reserved. **SD36.2** Adapted with permission. **F36.3** Adapted from Luckmann, J. (1990). *Your health!* Englewood Cliffs, NJ: Prentice-Hall, 523. **F36.5** The Garbage Project, University of Arizona. Adapted from Rathje, W. L. (1991, May). Once and future landfills. *National Geographic*, 123. **F36.6** Environmental Protection Agency. **F37.1** United Nations, World Bank estimates.

Photo Credits

Credits are indicated by page numbers on which photos appear.